Hensley's Practical Approach to Cardiothoracic Anesthesia

Seventh Edition

Hensley's Practical Approach to Cardiothoracic Anesthesia

Seventh Edition

Editors

KARSTEN BARTELS, MD, PhD, MBA
Professor with Tenure
Robert Lieberman Endowed Chair in Anesthesiology
University of Nebraska Medical Center
Omaha, Nebraska

AMANDA A. FOX, MD, MPH
Professor, Vice Chair of Research
A.H. "Buddy" Giesecke, Jr, MD, Distinguished Professorship
Department of Anesthesiology and Pain Management
The University of Texas Southwestern Medical Center
Dallas, Texas

ANDREW D. SHAW, MB, FRCA, FFICM
Chair, Department of Intensive Care and Resuscitation
Cleveland Clinic Foundation
Cleveland, Ohio

KIMBERLY HOWARD-QUIJANO, MD, MS, FASE
Associate Professor, Chief of Cardiac Anesthesiology
Department of Anesthesiology and Perioperative Medicine
University of Pittsburgh School of Medicine
University of Pittsburgh Medical Center
Pittsburgh, Pennsylvania

ROBERT H. THIELE, MD, MBA
Professor, Departments of Anesthesiology and Biomedical Engineering
Division Chief, Critical Care Anesthesiology
University of Virginia School of Medicine
Charlottesville, Virginia

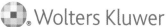 Wolters Kluwer

Philadelphia • Baltimore • New York • London
Buenos Aires • Hong Kong • Sydney • Tokyo

Acquisitions Editor: Keith Donnellan
Senior Development Editor: Ashley Fischer
Editorial Coordinator: Erin E. Hernandez
Editorial Assistant: Kristen Kardoley
Marketing Manager: Kristen Watrud
Production Project Manager: Frances Gunning
Manager, Graphic Arts & Design: Stephen Druding
Manufacturing Coordinator: Bernard Tomboc
Prepress Vendor: S4Carlisle Publishing Services

Seventh Edition

9 8 7 6 5 4 3 2 1

Printed in Mexico

Library of Congress Cataloging-in-Publication Data

Names: Bartels, Karsten, editor. | Shaw, Andrew D., editor. | Fox, Amanda, editor. | Thiel, Robert H., editor. | Howard-Quijano, Kimberly, editor.
Title: Hensley's practical approach to cardiothoracic anesthesia / editors, Karsten Bartels, Andrew D. Shaw, Amanda Fox, Robert H. Thiel, Kimberly Howard-Quijano.
Other titles: Practical approach to cardiothoracic anesthesia
Description: Seventh edition. | Philadelphia: Wolters Kluwer Health, [2025] | Includes bibliographical references and index.
Identifiers: LCCN 2023054677 (print) | LCCN 2023054678 (ebook) | ISBN 9781975209100 (paperback) | ISBN 9781975209117 (ebook)
Subjects: MESH: Anesthesia, Cardiac Procedures | Thoracic Surgical Procedures—methods
Classification: LCC RD87.3.H43 (print) | LCC RD87.3.H43 (ebook) | NLM WG 460 | DDC 617.9/67412—dc23/eng/20240130
LC record available at https://lccn.loc.gov/2023054677
LC ebook record available at https://lccn.loc.gov/2023054678

QUADM0524

Contributors

Darryl Abrams, MD
Associate Professor of Medicine
Department of Pulmonary and Critical Care Medicine
New York/Presbyterian Hospital
Columbia University Irving Medical Center
New York, New York

Rabia Amir, MD
Fellow
Department of Anesthesia, Critical Care and Pain
  Medicine
Beth Israel Deaconess Medical Center
Boston, Massachusetts

James M. Anton, MD
Associate Professor and Chair
Department of Anesthesiology
Texas Heart Institute
Baylor College of Medicine
St. Luke's Medical Center
Houston, Texas

Promise Ariyo, MD, MPH
Assistant Professor
Department of Anesthesia, Critical Care Medicine
The Johns Hopkins University School of Medicine
Baltimore, Maryland

Rebecca A. Aron, MD
Associate Professor, Program Director Cardiothoracic
  Anesthesiology
Department of Anesthesiology
University of Nebraska Medical Center
Omaha, Nebraska

Dalia Banks, MD, FASE
Clinical Professor
Department of Anesthesiology
UC San Diego School of Medicine
La Jolla, California

Atilio Barbeito, MD, MPH
Associate Professor
Chief, Division of Veterans Affairs
Department of Anesthesiology
Duke University School of Medicine
Durham, North Carolina

Karsten Bartels, MD, PHD, MBA
Professor of Anesthesiology
Department of Anesthesiology
University of Nebraska Medical Center
Omaha, Nebraska

Kiran Belani, MD, FASE, FACC
Assistant Professor, Director of Perioperative
  Echocardiography
Staff Cardiothoracic Anesthesiologist
Department of Anesthesiology
Inova Fairfax Hospital/Inova Heart and Vascular Institute,
  UVA Affiliate
Falls Church, Virginia

Juan C. Bianco, MD, MSc, PhD
Cardiovascular Anesthesiologist
Department of Anesthesiology
Hospital Italiano de Buenos Aires
Buenos Aires, Argentina

Daniel Brodie, MD
Professor of Medicine
Department of Medicine
Columbia University Vagelos College of Physicians
  and Surgeons
New York, New York

Jessica Brodt, MBBS
Clinical Associate Professor
Department of Anesthesiology, Perioperative and Pain Medicine
Stanford University School of Medicine
Stanford, California

Anna Budde, MD
Assistant Professor of Anesthesiology
Department of Anesthesiology
University of Minnesota Medical School
University of Minnesota Medical Center
Minneapolis, Minnesota

Michael T. Cain, MD
Fellow
Division of Cardiothoracic Surgery
Department of Surgery
University of Colorado School of Medicine
University of Colorado Anschutz Medical Center
Aurora, Colorado

Sreekanth Cheruku, MD, MPH, FASE
Assistant Professor
Department of Anesthesiology and Pain Management
The University of Texas Southwestern Medical Center
Dallas, Texas

Kenneth Cheung, BMedSci (Hons), MBBS, MMed
Fellow
Department of Anaesthesia and Perioperative Medicine
Westmead Hospital
Sydney, New South Wales, Australia

Christine Choi, MD
Assistant Clinical Professor
Department of Anesthesiology
UC San Diego School of Medicine
La Jolla, California

Joseph C. Cleveland, Jr., MD
Division Chief, Cardiothoracic Surgery
Department of Surgery
University of Colorado School of Medicine
University of Colorado Anschutz Medical Center
Aurora, Colorado

Joshua B. Cohen, MD
Assistant Professor
Department of Anesthesiology
Texas Heart Institute
Baylor College of Medicine
Houston, Texas

John R. Cooper, Jr., MD
Clinical Professor of Anesthesia
Department of Cardiovascular Anesthesia
Texas Heart Institute
Baylor College of Medicine
Houston, Texas

Etienne J. Couture, MD
Anesthesiologist and Intensivist
Department of Anesthesiology
Institut universitaire de cardiologie et de pneumologie de Quebec
Quebec City, Quebec, Canada

André Y. Denault, MD, PhD
Cardiac Anesthesiologist
Department of Anesthesiology
Montreal Heart Institute
Montreal, Quebec, Canada

Stefan Dieleman, MD, PhD
Assistant Professor of Anaesthesia
Department of Anaesthesia and Perioperative Medicine
Westmead Hospital
Western Sydney University
Sydney, New South Wales, Australia

Rohesh Joseph Fernando, MD, FASE, FASA
Assistant Professor of Anesthesiology
Medical Director, Cardiothoracic Anesthesia
Associate Section Head for Research
Department of Anesthesiology
Wake Forest School of Medicine
Winston-Salem, North Carolina

Janis Fliegenschmidt, BSc
Doctoral Student
Institute of Anesthesiology and Pain Therapy
Heat and Diabetes Center NRW
Bad Oeynhausen, Germany

Amanda A. Fox, MD, MPH
Professor, Vice Chair of Research
A.H. "Buddy" Giesecke, Jr, MD, Distinguished Professorship
Department of Anesthesiology and Pain Management
The University of Texas Southwestern Medical Center
Dallas, Texas

Steven M. Frank, MD
Professor
Department of Anesthesiology and Critical Care Medicine
The Johns Hopkins University School of Medicine
Baltimore, Maryland

Daniela Garcia, MD
Fellow
Department of Anesthesia, Critical Care and Pain Medicine
Beth Israel Deaconess Medical Center
Boston, Massachusetts

Thomas E. J. Gayeski, MD, PhD
Professor
Department of Anesthesiology and Perioperative Medicine
UAB Heersink School of Medicine
Birmingham, Alabama

Jeffrey B. Geske, MD
Professor of Medicine
Department of Cardiovascular Diseases
Mayo Clinic
Rochester, Minnesota

Mariya Geube, MD, FASE
Cardiothoracic Anesthesiologist and Intensivist
Department of Cardiothoracic Anesthesiology
Cleveland Clinic Foundation
Cleveland, Ohio

Thomas Graetz, MD
Chief of Cardiothoracic Anesthesiology
Department of Anesthesiology
Washington University School of Medicine in St. Louis
St. Louis, Missouri

Richard Greendyk, MD
Fellow
Division of Pulmonary, Allergy, and Critical Care
Columbia University Vagelos College of Physicians and Surgeons
New York, New York

Lars Grønlykke, MD, PhD
Anesthesiologist
Department of Cardiothoracic Anesthesiology
Copenhagen University Hospital, Rigshospitalet
Copenhagen, Denmark

John Hartnett, MD
Fellow
Department of Cardiovascular Anesthesia
Texas Heart Institute
Baylor College of Medicine
Houston, Texas

Jonathan Hastie, MD
Director of Cardiothoracic Intensive Care Unit
Department of Anesthesiology
Columbia University Medical Center
New York, New York

Nadia B. Hensley, MD
Assistant Professor
Department of Anesthesiology
The Johns Hopkins University School of Medicine
Baltimore, Maryland

Jordan R. H. Hoffman, MD
Cardiothoracic Surgeon
Department of Surgery
University of Colorado School of Medicine
University of Colorado Anschutz Medical Center
Aurora, Colorado

Kimberly Howard-Quijano, MD, MS, FASE
Associate Professor, Chief of Cardiac Anesthesiology
Department of Anesthesiology and Perioperative
    Medicine
University of Pittsburgh School of Medicine
University of Pittsburgh Medical Center
Pittsburgh, Pennsylvania

Alexander Huang, MD, FRCPC
Anesthesiologist
Department of Anesthesia and Pain Management
University Health Network—Toronto General Hospital
Toronto, Ontario, Canada

Steven Insler, DO
Anesthesiologist
Department of Intensive Care and Resuscitation
Cleveland Clinic Foundation
Cleveland, Ohio

Eric A. JohnBull, MD, MPH
Anesthesiologist
Department of Anesthesiology
Duke University School of Medicine
Durham, North Carolina

Ken Johnson, MD, MS, FASA
Vice Chair for Research
Department of Anesthesiology
University of Utah School of Medicine
Salt Lake City, Utah

Ashley Jones, MD
Fellow
Department of Anesthesiology
Baylor College of Medicine
Houston, Texas

Ravi V. Joshi, MD, FASE
Associate Professor, Program Director
Department of Cardiovascular and Thoracic
    Anesthesiology
The University of Texas Southwestern Medical Center
Dallas, Texas

Ali Khalifa, MD
Assistant Professor
Department of Cardiothoracic Anesthesiology
Baylor College of Medicine
Baylor St. Luke's Hospital
Houston, Texas

Colleen G. Koch, MD, MS, MBA
Dean
University of Florida College of Medicine
Gainesville, Florida

Megan P. Kostibas, MD
Assistant Professor
Department of Anesthesiology and Critical Care Medicine
The Johns Hopkins University School of Medicine
Baltimore, Maryland

Xiang Li, MBBS
Fellow
Department of Intensive Care and Resuscitation
Cleveland Clinic Foundation
Cleveland, Ohio

Daniel Lotz, MD
Assistant Professor
Divisions of Critical Care Medicine and Cardiac
    Anesthesia
University of Minnesota Medical School
Minneapolis, Minnesota

Feroze Mahmood, MD, FASE
Professor of Anesthesia
Harvard Medical School
Director, Cardiac Anesthesia
Beth Israel Deaconess Medical Center
Boston, Massachusetts

Bruno Maranhao, MD, PhD
Assistant Professor
Department of Anesthesiology
Washington University School of Medicine
    in St. Louis
St. Louis, Missouri

Jonathan B. Mark, MD
Professor of Anesthesiology
Department of Anesthesiology
Duke University School of Medicine
Veterans Affairs Healthcare System
Durham, North Carolina

Teuta Marsic, MD
Fellow
Anesthesiology Institute
Cleveland Clinic Foundation
Cleveland, Ohio

Christina Massoth, MD
Anesthesiologist
Department of Anesthesiology, Intensive Care and Pain
    Medicine
University Hospital Münster
Münster, Germany

John Steven McNeil, MD
Assistant Professor
Department of Anesthesiology
University of Virginia School of Medicine
Charlottesville, Virginia

J. Bradley Meers, MD
Associate Professor
Department of Anesthesiology and Perioperative
    Medicine
UAB Heersink School of Medicine
Birmingham, Alabama

Lachlan F. Miles, MBBS (Hons), PhD, FANZCA
Honorary Principal Fellow
Department of Critical Care
The University of Melbourne
Melbourne, Victoria, Australia

Ingrid Moreno-Duarte, MD
Assistant Professor of Anesthesiology
Divisions of Adult and Pediatric Cardiothoracic
    Anesthesiology
Department of Anesthesiology and Pain Management
Children's Medical Center Dallas
The University of Texas Southwestern Medical Center
Dallas, Texas

Alina Nicoara, MD
Attending Anesthesiologist
Department of Anesthesiology
Duke University School of Medicine
Durham, North Carolina

Nishank P. Nooli, MD
Assistant Professor
Department of Anesthesiology and Perioperative Medicine
UAB Heersink School of Medicine
Birmingham, Alabama

Michael O'Connor, DO, MPH, MA
Emeritus Staff Anesthesiologist
Department of Intensive Care and Resuscitation
Cleveland Clinic Foundation
Cleveland, Ohio

Robert O'Neal, MD
Cardiothoracic Anesthesiologist
Department of Anesthesiology
University of Utah Hospital
Salt Lake City, Utah

Alessia Pedoto, MD, FASA
Professor
Department of Anesthesiology and Critical Care
    Medicine
Memorial Sloan Kettering Cancer Center
New York, New York

Davinder S. Ramsingh, MD
Associate Professor
Department of Anesthesiology
Loma Linda University Medical Center
Loma Linda, California

Mark Robitaille, MD
Anesthesiologist
Department of Anesthesia, Critical Care and Pain
    Medicine
Harvard Medical School
Beth Israel Deaconess Medical Center
Boston, Massachusetts

James R. Rowbottom, MD
Vice Chair, Clinical Affairs Anesthesiology Institute
Department of Intensive Care and Resuscitation
Cleveland Clinic Foundation
Cleveland, Ohio

Furqaan Sadiq, MD
Fellow
Cleveland Clinic Foundation Fellow
Department of Anesthesiology
Washington University School of Medicine
    in St. Louis
St. Louis, Missouri

Julia Scarpa, MD, PhD
Chief Resident and Van Poznak Scholar
Department of Anesthesiology
New York Presbyterian Hospital—Weill Cornell
New York, New York

Hartzell V. Schaff, MD
Cardiovascular Surgeon
Department of Cardiovascular Surgery
Mayo Clinic
Rochester, Minnesota

Peter M. Schulman, MD
Professor
Department of Anesthesiology and Perioperative Medicine
Oregon Health & Science University
Portland, Oregon

Shahzad Shaefi, MD, MPH
Cardiac Anesthesiologist and Intensivist
Department of Anesthesia, Critical Care and Pain
  Medicine
Beth Israel Deaconess Medical Center
Boston, Massachusetts

Aidan Sharkey, MD
Instructor in Anesthesia
Department of Anesthesia, Critical Care and Pain
  Medicine
Harvard Medical School
Beth Israel Deaconess Medical Center
Boston, Massachusetts

Andrew D. Shaw, MB, FRCA, FFICM
Chair, Department of Intensive Care and Resuscitation
Cleveland Clinic Foundation
Cleveland, Ohio

Richard D. Sheu, MD, FASE
Assistant Professor, Director of Perioperative
  Echocardiography
Program Director, Adult Cardiothoracic Anesthesiology
  Fellowship
Department of Anesthesiology and Pain Medicine
University of Washington Medical Center
Seattle, Washington

Peter Slinger, MD, PRCPC
Professor
Department of Anesthesiology
University of Toronto
Toronto, Ontario, Canada

Warner Smith, MD
Associate Professor
Department of Anesthesiology
University of Utah School of Medicine
Salt Lake City, Utah

Eric C. Stecker, MD, MPH
Professor of Medicine, Electrophysiology
Knight Cardiovascular Institute
Oregon Health & Science University
Portland, Oregon

P. Andrew Stephens, MD, FACEP
Cardiothoracic and Surgical Intensivist
Department of Intensive Care and Resuscitation
Anesthesiology Institute
Cleveland Clinic Foundation
Cleveland, Ohio

Erik Strauss, MD
Anesthesiologist
Department of Anesthesiology
University of Maryland School of Medicine
Baltimore, Maryland

Erin A. Sullivan, MD, FASA
Professor of Anesthesiology and Perioperative Medicine
Department of Anesthesiology and Perioperative
  Medicine
University of Pittsburgh School of Medicine
University of Pittsburgh Medical Center
Pittsburgh, Pennsylvania

Elena Ashikhmina Swan, MD, PhD
Assistant Professor of Anesthesiology
Director, Congenital Cardiac Anesthesia
Department of Anesthesiology and Perioperative Medicine
Mayo Clinic
Rochester, Minnesota

Angela M. Taylor, MD, MS, MBA
Professor of Medicine
Department of Cardiology
University of Virginia School of Medicine
Charlottesville, Virginia

Robert H. Thiele, MD
Professor, Departments of Anesthesiology and Biomedical
  Engineering
Division Chief, Critical Care Anesthesiology
University of Virginia School of Medicine
Charlottesville, Virginia

Daniel A. Tolpin, MD
Associate Professor
Department of Anesthesiology
Texas Heart Institute
Baylor College of Medicine
Houston, Texas

Matthew M. Townsley, MD, FASE
Professor
Department of Anesthesiology and Perioperative Medicine
UAB Heersink School of Medicine
Birmingham, Alabama

Christopher A. Troianos, MD, FASE, FASA
Professor and Chair
Anesthesiology Institute
Cleveland Clinic Learner College of Medicine
Cleveland, Ohio

Ban Tsui, MD, MSc
Professor
Department of Anesthesiology, Perioperative and Pain
  Medicine
Stanford University School of Medicine
Stanford, California

Markus Velten, MD
Professor Section Chief, Cardiac Anesthesiology
Department of Anesthesiology and Intensive Care Medicine
Department of Anesthesiology and Pain Management
The University of Texas Southwestern Medical Center
Dallas, Texas

Vera von Dossow, MD
Institute of Anaesthesiology and Pain Therapy
Herz- und Diabeteszentrum NRW
Ruhr-University Bochum
Bochum, Germany

Benjamin Walker, MB, BCh, BAO
Anesthesiologist
Department of Anesthesiology
University of Utah School of Medicine
University of Utah Health Care
Salt Lake City, Utah

Michael H. Wall, MD, FCCM, FASA
JJ Buckley Professor and Chair
Department of Anesthesiology
University of Minnesota Medical School
Minneapolis, Minnesota

Tiffany Williams, MD, PhD
Assistant Professor-in-Residence
Department of Anesthesiology and Perioperative Medicine
David Geffen School of Medicine at UCLA
Los Angeles, California

Julie A. Wyrobek, MD
Assistant Professor of Anesthesiology and Perioperative
  Medicine
Department of Anesthesiology and Perioperative Medicine
University of Rochester School of Medicine and Dentistry
Rochester, New York

Jaclyn Yeung, DO
Fellow
Department of Anesthesiology
Washington University School of Medicine in St. Louis
St. Louis, Missouri

Alexander Zarbock, MD
Chair and Professor
Department of Anesthesiology, Intensive Care and Pain
  Medicine
University Hospital Münster
Münster, Germany

Preface

THE SEVENTH EDITION OF *Hensley's Practical Approach to Cardiothoracic Anesthesia* is aimed at preserving a trusted source of practical education for all those engaged in the practice of cardiothoracic anesthesia. In recognition of the foundational work put forth by the book's longtime past editors, Glenn Gravlee and the late Frederick Hensley, the editors of the seventh edition would like to express their gratitude for the opportunity to adapt the book's content to the constant evolution in the field.

To ensure diverse and up-to-date perspectives, Karsten Bartels and Andrew D. Shaw welcome three new editors to the editorial team: Amanda A. Fox, Kimberly Howard-Quijano, and Robert H. Thiele. The new editors are leaders in the field and bring additional expertise in perioperative organ injury, electrophysiology, monitoring, and clinical outcomes to the seventh edition. We are especially grateful to the returning and new chapter authors of this new edition. While they updated some of the existing content, more than half of the chapters in the seventh edition are completely new or rewritten. We also want to highlight the international perspective of the new edition, with authors from three continents describing cutting-edge approaches to cardiothoracic anesthesia.

With the ever-growing need to shepherd increasingly ill patients through high-fidelity cardiothoracic surgical procedures, we are hopeful that this book will provide practical and evidence-based information to learners and experienced clinicians alike.

Karsten Bartels, MD, PhD, MBA
Amanda A. Fox, MD, MPH
Andrew D. Shaw, MB, FRCA, FFICM
Kimberly Howard-Quijano, MD, MS, FASE
Robert H. Thiele, MD, MBA

Acknowledgments

EACH EDITION OF THIS BOOK HAS INVOLVED a broad team effort of authors, physician editors, development editors, copy editors, typesetters, and publishing and graphics experts. The editors thank the 91 authors representing 54 institutions for their timely and tireless efforts. On the publishing side, we thank Wolters Kluwer for their continued support of this book. Keith Donnellan gets warm thanks and appreciation for his dedication, experience, and wisdom. Special thanks go to Erin E. Hernandez and Ashley Fischer, whose expertise, persistence, and detail orientation during developmental editing proved indispensable.

Contents

Foundations and General Principles

1 Practical Anatomy of the Heart

Markus Velten

KEY POINTS

1. Two atria and two ventricles separated by atrioventricular (AV) leaflets are the main components.
2. While the right ventricle transports deoxygenated blood through the pulmonary valve into the lungs, the left ventricle perfuses the body through the aortic valve with oxygenated blood.
3. Cardiomyocytes are basic elements of the heart, providing the structure and function of this complex organ.
4. Blood perfuses the heart via the coronary arteries originating from the aorta and is drained by the coronary veins into the right atrium.

I. Introduction

The heart, as the fundamental organ of the cardiovascular system, perfuses the body with blood and is of central importance not just for the human body but also for every clinician in cardiac medicine. The basic anatomy consisting of the atria, ventricle, valves, and corresponding vessels represents a fixture in our daily practice since the first days of medical training. The heart is surrounded by the pericardium, a protective sac, and is supplied with blood by its own network of blood vessels, the coronary arteries and veins. Understanding the cardiac anatomy is crucial for diagnosing and treating various cardiac conditions. The present chapter will capitulate the basic anatomy of the cardiovascular system with a focus on anatomic correlations important for the management of patients with cardiac conditions during open heart surgeries in the operating room (OR), as well as interventional procedures in the interventional suite or hybrid OR, and during intensive care treatment.

II. Content

A. Embryologic Development of the Heart

Cardiac development is a complex interplay starting with molecular pathways and progenitor cells differentiating into myofibroblasts, vasculogenesis of blood islands leading to the so-called cardiogenic field initially constituted in a horseshoe form surrounded by myoblasts. Then primitive ventricles and outflow tracts develop. Through rotations, the primitive heart tube is formed from three layers, with the endothelial lining forming the endocardium, the myocardium resulting in the muscular wall, and the external surface resulting in the visceral pericardium in analogy to the adult heart.

Septa develop between 4 and 5 weeks of gestational age, contributing to the formation of atria and ventricles, AV canals, valves, and great vessels.

The fetal heart has two shunts. The foramen ovale moves blood from the right atrium of the heart to the left atrium, while the ductus arteriosus moves blood from the pulmonary artery to the aorta, both bypassing the pulmonary circulation. After birth, the lungs expand, and subsequently, both ductus arteriosus and foramen ovale closure occur due to pressure changes, resulting in pulmonary perfusion and transition from fetal to newborn blood circulation.

B. Structural Basics

In the regularly developed and not diseased organs, each side of the heart consists of an atrium and a ventricle. Atria collect blood from the great vessels when entering the heart, regulating the transfer into the ventricle. Ventricles eject blood from the heart into the great arteries. While the right ventricle (RV) perfuses deoxygenated blood at a low pressure into the pulmonary circulation, the left ventricle (LV) carries out the body perfusion with oxygenated blood.

Functional units of contraction are cardiomyocytes that are composed of a tubular structure containing myofibrils, which are rod-like units within the cell. The myofibrils consist of repeating sections of sarcomeres, representing the fundamental contractile units of the cardiomyocyte. Cardiomyocytes join together, forming an intricate system of muscle layers and in conjunction with fibroblast and endothelial cell chambers, valves, and nodes, which are only present in the heart. The heart's coronary arteries and veins, including the sinus venosus, comprise its own circulatory system. The heart independently produces electric impulses, leading to contraction and relaxation, resulting in the so-called cardiac cycle.[1]

C. Right Atrium

The right atrium consists of the lateral and dorsal part of the atrial sinus (sinus venarum cavarum), between the superior and inferior vena cava. Both veins drain deoxygenated blood from the body freely into the atrium without intervening valves. From the right atrium, the blood flows through the tricuspid valve (TV) into the RV. The ostium of the coronary sinus (coronary venous sinus) is located at the medial bottom of the right atrium, just above the septal leaflet of the TV. The ostium is closed by the Valvula sinus coronary (Valvula Thebesii). The coronary sinus is a confluence of several cardiac veins, located on the back surface (facies posterior) of the heart, running transverse to the heart axis in the sulcus between the left atrium and the LV, draining up to 75% of the venous blood of the heart muscle (Figure 1.1).

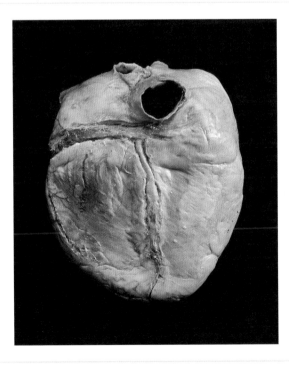

FIGURE 1.1   Cardiac view from posterior with coronary sinus.

D. Right Ventricle

The RV is asymmetrical, has a smaller muscle mass compared to the LV, and consists of the interventricular septum and the so-called free wall. Due to the cupped geometry, the RV appears smaller than the LV, even though both ventricles contain almost the same blood volume. Along with the right atrium and pulmonary artery, the RV is part of the "low-pressure system," passing blood into the pulmonary circulation.

E. Tricuspid Valve

The TV consists of a fibrous triangular or ovoid annulus, connecting the atrium and ventricle, the three leaflets, and papillary muscles, including the chordal attachments.[2,3] The anteroseptal leaflet is located upstream (apical) close to the RV outflow tract and aortic valve, while the posterolateral portion is displaced upward (atrial). The posteroseptal portion near the inflow of the coronary sinus is displaced downward (apical) to the anterolateral segment.[4] In healthy subjects, the TV annular area is 11 ± 2 cm^2 with a significant increase to 29.6 ± 5.5 cm^2 during systole.[5]

The three TV leaflets are highly variable, among the anterior being the longest with the largest area and greatest motion, while the septal is the shortest and least mobile, attached to the tricuspid annulus directly above the interventricular septum. The posterior leaflet may consist of multiple scallops but in 10% of individuals is not separated from the anterior leaflet.[6] Anatomic landmarks for each leaflet vary significantly depending on the size and shape of the annulus; however, the commissure between the septal and posterior leaflets (which are always clearly separated) is usually located near the entrance of the coronary sinus to the right atrium (RA).

CLINICAL PEARL

The ostium of the coronary sinus is an important structure for some electrophysiologic procedures. Furthermore, a persistent left superior vena cava is a prevalent cardiac malformation, draining blood through the coronary sinus into the RA that needs to be considered when difficulties occur draining the right-sided structure during cardiopulmonary bypass.

The TV consists of three highly variable papillary muscles, with the anterior and posterior distinct and a third being inconsistent. The anterior papillary muscle is the largest, with the moderator band joining and chordae supporting the anterior and posterior leaflets. The posterior frequently bi- or trifid papillary muscle lends chordal support to the posterior and septal leaflets. The septal papillary muscle is highly variable: absent in up to 20% of normal patients or small and multiple. Unlike the mitral valve, chordae may arise directly from the septum to the anterior and septal leaflets. Accessory chordae may attach to the RV-free wall and the moderator band (Figure 1.2).

F. Pulmonary Valve

The pulmonary valve (PV) constitutes from the ventricular muscle and, in contrast to the aortic valve that is in close connection to the left-sided AV valve, lacks fibrous continuity with the TV. Similar to the aortic valve, the PV consists of a tricuspid structure. However, its cusps are thinner due to the lower pressures.

CLINICAL PEARL

Thinner and less tissue may be one of the reasons for the limited durability of a Ross procedure (replacement of an aortic valve with the patient's own pulmonary valve).

Regurgitation is present in up to 75% of individuals without clinical pathology.[7] Mild to moderate pulmonary regurgitation (PR) is most frequently seen in patients with pulmonary arterial dilatation as a consequence of pulmonary hypertension (PH). Severe PR and pulmonary stenosis (PS) are commonly associated with congenital heart disease after previous

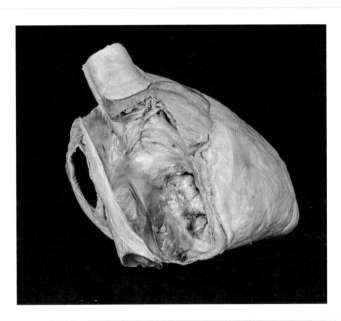

FIGURE 1.2   Overview of the right heart from the atrium to the tricuspid valve.

interventions, for example, valvotomy or valvuloplasty for PS or pulmonary atresia, and repaired tetralogy of Fallot, endocarditis, blunt chest trauma, carcinoid, myxomatous degeneration, rheumatic heart disease, and drug-induced causes (eg, pergolide).

G. Left Atrium

The two right and two left-sided pulmonary veins open into the roof of the left atrium, draining oxygenated blood from the lungs into the heart. The atrial septum (septum interatriale), which contains the fused foramen ovale, separates the left from the RA. The inner wall consists of delicate pectinate muscles (musculi pectinati). Anteriorly, the left atrium has a bulge, the left atrial appendage (auricula sinistra). An opening, the ostium atrioventriculare sinistrum, leads from the left atrium into the LV through the mitral valve, preventing the regurgitation of blood from the LV into the left atrium during systole.

H. Left Ventricle

The LV is the thickest and strongest chamber, located in the lower left portion of the heart and separated from the RV by the interventricular septum, responsible for pumping oxygenated blood to the rest of the body. Blood enters the LV from the RA through the oval-shaped mitral valve opening and exits the LV through the aorta.

The LV is supplied with blood by the left coronary artery, which branches off from the aorta and supplies oxygen and nutrients to the cardiac muscle. The anatomy of the LV can be visualized through various imaging techniques, such as echocardiography, cardiac MRI, or CT scans, which can provide detailed images of the heart and its structures.

CLINICAL PEARL

LV size and function provide valuable information about the overall cardiac condition such as hypertension, myocardial infarction, and heart failure. Enlargement of the LV, or left ventricular hypertrophy, can be an indicator of underlying cardiac disease and is associated with an increased risk of cardiovascular morbidity. LV ejection fraction is another important parameter that is used to assess the function of the heart. Understanding the clinical significance of the LV and its parameters can aid in the diagnosis and management of various cardiac conditions.

I. **Mitral Valve**

The complex anatomy of the mitral valve (MV), including its relation to proximate structures, most importantly the aortic valve, is of central importance for both interventional and surgical procedures. The MV consists of the annulus, the anterior and posterior leaflet, chordae tendineae, and the anterolateral and posteromedial papillary muscle. The MV is, unlike the TV, in proximate conjunction with the AV complex.[8] The MV has a characteristic D shaped anulus, with the anterior (aortic) leaflet being rounded, omitting into the intervalvular fibrosa, consisting of a third of the entire circumference. This connection needs to be considered for various cardiac pathologies, including the systolic anterior movement (SAM) phenomenon as well as reconstructions as for severe endocarditis, most notably a comprehensive reconstruction of the aortomitral passage, the so-called "commando" or "UFO" procedure.[9] Like the TV, the MV annulus is nonplanar, with an area change during the cardiac cycle. The posterior leaflet presents the other two-thirds of the circumference and tends to be narrower in radial extent, with the approximate areas of the two portions of the valve being equal. The coaptation line corresponds to an arch whose ends are called the anterolateral and posteromedial commissure. These do not extend to the annulus and although there may sometimes be clear cusps of the commissure, this region is more often less well defined. The posterior leaflet is characteristic, creating three unequal scallops, with the middle scallop being quite variable in size but typically larger than the medial and lateral scallops. The most lateral segment, at the anterolateral commissure, is designated P1, the middle, central segment P2, and the medial and posterior segment P3. No individual scallops can be identified on the anterior cusp, but corresponding areas in the systole connecting to the posterior leaflet are regarded accordingly (A1, A2, and A3). The anterolateral papillary muscle is associated with the lateral commissure and gives off chordae to the lateral halves of both, the anterior and posterior leaflet. The posteromedial papillary muscle is oriented below the medial commissure and gives off the corresponding chordae to the medial halves of both leaflets. Each tendon of the papillary muscles divides several times before inserting into the mitral leaflets. Primary chordae (first order) insert on the free edge of the leaflets, while secondary chordae insert on the body of the leaflet (second order), and tertiary chordae (third order) insert at the base of the posterior leaflet and at the annulus of the LV free wall, respectively; direct myocardial tendon attachments to the anterior leaflet are not usually seen.[10]

CLINICAL PEARL

It needs to be acknowledged that the anterolateral papillary muscle has a dual blood supply and is perfused with blood originating from the left ascending coronary and circumflex coronary artery, whereas the posteromedial papillary muscle regularly is perfused only from one coronary artery, most commonly the posterior descending coronary making it more vulnerable for reduced perfusion resulting in ischemia. Thus, the posteromedial papillary muscle is more vulnerable to rupture following a myocardial infarction (MI), inducing significant mortality.

J. **Aortic Valve**

The aortic valve (AV), composed of three crescent-shaped leaflets, is located near the center of the heart with a proximate connection to the MV. The leaflets are identified by the coronary arteries arising from the corresponding Valsalva sinuses (left coronary, right coronary, and noncoronary cusp). These three crescent-shaped protuberances form part of the Valsalva sinuses and fibrous interleaflet triangles. Each semilunar protuberance is curvedly attached to the aortic wall, with the basal attachment in the LV below the anatomical ventricular-aortic junction and the distal attachment at the sinotubular junction. Valsalva sinuses and sinotubular junction are integral parts of the valve mechanism, so any significant dilatation of these structures results in AV incompetence.[11]

In relation to the AV, the MV is located posteriorly and to the left, while the TV is located inferiorly and to the right, both in immediate proximity to the AV. In contrast, the PV is located anterior to the AV without any relation to the mitral or TV (Figure 1.3).

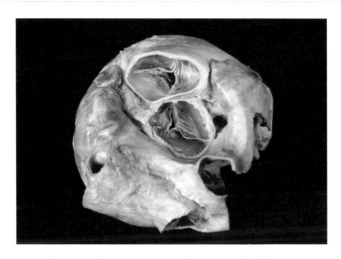

FIGURE 1.3   En face view and relation of the aortic and pulmonary valves.

III.   Summary

The heart, located in the chest cavity, is made up of four chambers separated by four valves that organize the blood through the body. Understanding the heart's complex anatomy is essential for diagnosing and treating various conditions. Echocardiography is frequently used to visualize different structures guiding surgeries as well as interventional procedures.

REFERENCES

1. U.S. National Institutes of Health, National Cancer Institute. *SEER Training Modules: Structure of the Heart*. NIH; 2023.
2. Shah PM, Raney AA. Tricuspid valve disease. *Curr Probl Cardiol*. 2008;33(2):47-84.
3. Martinez RM, O'Leary PW, Anderson RH. Anatomy and echocardiography of the normal and abnormal tricuspid valve. *Cardiol Young*. 2006;16(Suppl 3):4-11.
4. Rogers JH, Bolling SF. The tricuspid valve: current perspective and evolving management of tricuspid regurgitation. *Circulation*. 2009;119(20):2718-2725.
5. Fukuda S, Saracino G, Matsumura Y, et al. Three-dimensional geometry of the tricuspid annulus in healthy subjects and in patients with functional tricuspid regurgitation: a real-time, 3-dimensional echocardiographic study. *Circulation*. 2006;114(Suppl 1):I492-I498.
6. Henning RJ. Tricuspid valve regurgitation: current diagnosis and treatment. *Am J Cardiovasc Dis*. 2022;12(1):1-18.
7. Zoghbi WA, Adams D, Bonow RO, et al. Recommendations for noninvasive evaluation of native valvular regurgitation: a report from the American Society of Echocardiography developed in collaboration with the Society for Cardiovascular Magnetic Resonance. *J Am Soc Echocardiogr*. 2017;30(4):303-371.
8. Muresian H. The clinical anatomy of the mitral valve. *Clin Anat*. 2009;22(1):85-98.
9. Misfeld M, Davierwala PM, Borger MA, Bakhtiary F. The "UFO" procedure. *Ann Cardiothorac Surg*. 2019;8(6):691-698.
10. Carpentier AF, Lessana A, Relland JY, et al. The "physio-ring": an advanced concept in mitral valve annuloplasty. *Ann Thorac Surg*. 1995;60(5):1177-1185; discussion 1185-1186.
11. De Paulis R, Salica A. Surgical anatomy of the aortic valve and root-implications for valve repair. *Ann Cardiothorac Surg*. 2019;8(3):313-321.

2

Cardiovascular Physiology: A Primer

P. Andrew Stephens, Thomas E. J. Gayeski, Xiang Li, Teuta Marsic, and James R. Rowbottom

KEY POINTS

1. The heart has a fibrous skeleton that provides an insertion site at each valvular ring. This fibrous structure also connects cardiac myocytes so that "stretch" or preload results in coordinated lengthening of sarcomeres and not cardiac myocytes sliding past each other.

2. Understanding action potentials and how they differ between cardiac myocytes and cardiac pacemaker cells is key to understanding how and why anesthesia and cardiac medications affect the heart.

3. Contractility changes as a result of Ca^{2+} concentration change in the cytoplasm of the cardiac myocytes during systole.

4. Relaxation following contraction is an active process requiring adenosine triphosphate (ATP) consumption to pump Ca^{2+} into the sarcoplasmic reticulum as well as across the sarcolemma.

5. The endocardium receives blood flow only during diastole while the epicardium receives blood flow throughout most of the cardiac cycle. The endocardium is more susceptible to infarction.

6. The external stroke volume (SV) work the ventricle does is to raise the pressure of an SV from left or right ventricular end-diastolic pressure to mean arterial pressure (pulmonary or systemic, respectively).

7. Oxygen or ATP consumption occurs during release of actin-myosin bonds during the relaxation of this bond. The main determinants of myocardial oxygen consumption are heart rate (HR), contractility, and wall tension.

8. The primary role of the cardiovascular system is to provide sufficient cardiac output (CO) to meet the ever-changing metabolic demands of body tissues. Physiologic reserves are expansion factors allowing the cardiovascular system to respond to changes in blood pressure. The reserves include HR, contractility, systemic vascular resistance, and venous capacitance.

9. The two main mechanisms through which the body regulates arterial pressure include a fast, neuronally mediated baroreceptor reflex and a slower, hormonally regulated renin-angiotensin-aldosterone mechanism.
10. Understanding and integrating the physiologic reserves of the cardiovascular system to best provide care in the perioperative period allows individualized care that applies objective variables in adjunct to clinical assessment.

I. Introduction

As a physiologic primer for cardiac anesthesiology, this chapter requires compromise and choices, as entire textbooks are dedicated to this topic. The studies of cardiac anatomy, physiology, pathology, and genomics are decades to centuries old, continue to evolve, and have a vast literature. The focus of this chapter is on teaching key principles of cardiovascular physiology that are important to adult clinical management in the perioperative period. This chapter focuses on adult cardiac physiology, and, therefore, only briefly touches upon cardiovascular embryology and does not include concepts specific to pediatric cardiac physiology. A solid understanding of cardiovascular physiology is essential to delivering anesthetic care to both healthy patients and those with cardiovascular disease.

II. Embryologic Development of the Heart

A. The cardiovascular system begins to develop during week 3 of gestation as the primitive vascular system is formed from mesodermally derived endothelial tubes. At day 21, bilateral cardiogenic cords from paired endocardial heart tubes fuse into a single heart tube (primitive heart). This fusion initiates forward flow and begins the heart's transport function.

B. The primitive heart evolves into four chambers: Bulbus cordis, ventricle, primordial atrium, and sinus venosus, with the aortic arch coming from the truncus arteriosus. Initial contraction commences on days 21-22. These contractions result in unidirectional blood flow in week 4.

C. On day 23, the primitive tubular heart begins morphogenesis or cardiac folding. During this critical time, the primitive heart folds back onto itself giving a more adult appearance by day 24. It is important to note that the right ventricle and left ventricle form from different segments of the primitive tubular heart. The right ventricle is made up of the distal bulbus cordis, becoming the trabecular proximal arterial bulb, called the primitive right ventricle. The left ventricle arises from the primitive ventricle. This is an important difference, as in adults the right and left ventricles have different shapes, contractility patterns, and functions. It is wise to think of them, particularly in the ill patient.

D. From weeks 4-7, heart development enters a critical period, as it divides into the fetal circulation and the four chambers of the adult heart.

E. A fibrous skeleton composed of fibrin and elastin forms the framework of four rings encircling the four heart valves as well as intermyocyte connections.

F. **The Fibrous Skeleton**
1. Serves as an anchor for the insertion into the valve cusps
2. Resists overdistention of the annuli of the valves (resisting incompetence)
3. Provides a fixed insertion point for the muscular bundles of the ventricles
4. Minimizes intermyocyte sliding during ventricular filling and contraction

III. Organization of Myocytes

A. A cardiac myocyte measures approximately 25 µm in diameter and 100 µm in length. It appears to have a cross-striated pattern similar to skeletal muscle but with only one to two nuclei per cell. Around each myocyte is connective tissue rich in capillaries. Each cardiac capillary is approximately 1 mm in length, hence it serves about 80 cardiac myocytes along its length.

B. Each myocardial cell houses myofibrils, long chains of sarcomeres.

C. **Sarcomere**
1. Sarcomeres are composed of myosin, actin, troponin, and tropomyosin (Figure 2.1), and are responsible for the fundamental unit of tension development in the cell.
2. Actin molecules link to form a chain, and two chains intertwine to form a helix. Within each groove of this helix, tropomyosin sits with troponin bound to it intermittently along its length. This complex is known as a thin filament. The length of the thin filament is

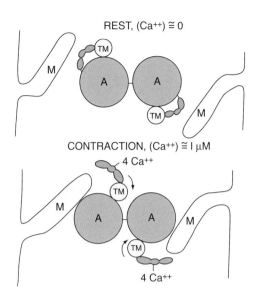

FIGURE 2.1   Schematic representation of actin-myosin dependence on Ca^{2+}-troponin binding for tension development to occur. A, actin; M, myosin; TM, tropomyosin; Ca^{++}, ionized calcium. (Derived from Honig C. *Modern Cardiovascular Physiology*. Little, Brown and Company; 1981.)

approximately 2 µm. In the absence of calcium, the actin sites of the thin filament are not available for binding to myosin.

3. About midway along the thin filament, the Z disc anchors the thin filaments in place in a regular pattern as schematized below. The Z disc is a strong meshwork of filaments that forms a band to anchor the interdigitated thin filaments.

4. Myosin molecules aggregate spontaneously, thereby forming thick filaments. These filaments are approximately 1.6 µm long. These thick filaments are held in place by M filaments and are interdigitated among the thin filaments. At the center of each thick filament is a zone that has no myosin "heads." Each myosin head contains an actin-binding site and ATPase.

5. Together, troponin, tropomyosin, and intramyocyte Ca^{2+} concentration regulate the percentage of possible actin and myosin interactions that participate in the shortening strength of the sarcomere.

6. As long as Ca^{2+} is bound to troponin, actin and myosin remain adjacent to each other. During exposure of unbound actin to myosin, they bind together to shorten a sarcomere. After this binding, uncoupling occurs because of the ATPase bound to myosin. This energy-dependent step, requiring oxygen consumption, occurs multiple times within each sarcomere during a cardiac cycle. As long as actin and myosin continue to bind and unbind, the actin-myosin complex continues to shorten the sarcomere as the ventricular chamber contracts in systole.

7. Depending on preload (preexisting "stretch" prior to contraction), the sarcomere length, or the distance between Z discs, has ideal physiologic ranges from 1.8 to 2.5 µm.

8. Intracellular calcium concentration establishes how many actin-myosin sites interact at any instant. The sarcomere length (Z-disc separation length) establishes the maximum number of actin and myosin heads that could potentially interact at any instant. Increasing the number of heads that do interact results in an increase in contractility (see section that follows).

D. As mentioned under embryology, collagen fibers link cardiac myocytes together. In a given layer, myocytes are approximately in parallel. These collagen fiber links connect adjacent, parallel myocytes and form a skeleton. This cross-banding can be seen under light microscopy and is noted as Z-lines. During the cardiac cycle, the overall sarcomere length varies from 2.5 µm during diastole to 1.8 µm during systole.

E. The sarcolemma (SL) is the name of the specialized myocardial cell membrane, further specializing at the end of each myocyte at the intercalated disk. The intercalated disk is made up of three components and serves three functions:

1. Fascia adherens is an anchoring site for actin.
2. Desmosomes prevent separation and anchor cells together during contraction.
3. Gap junctions are direct connections of the cytoplasm of neighboring cells allowing for rapid electrical activity of the action potential.[1]

F. T tubules (T) or the transverse tubular system (Figure 2.2) is another specialized feature of the cell membrane. These are deep, narrow invaginations of the cell membrane or SL. These invaginations increase the surface area of the cell membrane that come into contact with the extracellular interface, allowing for more rapid ion flow and therefore faster depolarization and repolarization, in a synchronized fashion.

G. The sarcoplasmic reticulum (SR) is the intracellular form of the T tubules. These intracellular tubules interface with the T tubules at a 90° angle, with a sac-like structure called the terminal cisternae or just cisterna (C). The cisterna house most of the intracellular calcium. These structures all run along the very visible Z-line.

H. Coupled with the Purkinje system's coordinated stimulation of myocytes, this skeleton (composed of the intercalated discs, T tubules, and SR) allows for rapid propagation of the action potential and for a summation of the simultaneous shortening of each myocyte into a concerted shortening of the ventricle.

I. 30%-35% of the myocardial cell volume is made up of mitochondria to support the tremendous energy requirements of cardiac cells, to allow for rapid and continuous phosphate reactions.[2]

J. This collagen structure also limits the cardiac myocyte from being overstretched, thereby minimizing the risk of destroying a cell or reducing actin-myosin exposure through overstretching.[3]

K. To add complexity, the longitudinal alignment of the cardiac myocytes differs in overlapping layers from epicardium to endocardium. Hence, shortening in each layer results in distortion between the layers.

L. Given that blood supply comes from the surface of the heart, this distortion results in partial occlusion of penetrating arteries supplying blood to the inner layers of the myocardium during systole.

M. Consequently, the endocardium is more vulnerable to ischemia than the epicardium. Blood flow to the endocardium occurs only during diastole, while that to the epicardium occurs during the majority of the cardiac cycle.

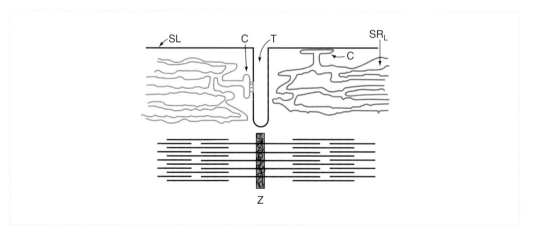

FIGURE 2.2   Relation of cardiac sarcoplasmic reticulum to surface membrane and myofibrils. The SRL and C overlie the myofilaments; they are shown separately for illustrative purposes. C, cisterna; SL, sarcolemma; SR$_L$, longitudinal sarcoplasmic reticulum; T, transverse tubule; Z, Z disc.

CLINICAL PEARL

Systolic contraction impairs coronary arterial blood flow penetrating from the epicardium to the endocardium, which potentially places the endocardium at risk for ischemia.

IV. Electrical Conduction

A. The action potential is a sequence of ion movements through specific channels, in the sarcolemma, that propagates cardiac activity through the heart's specialized cells:

1. Pacer cells of the sinoatrial (SA) node and atrioventricular (AV) node
2. Conduction tissues of the bundle of His and Purkinje fibers
3. Atrial and ventricular muscle cells

B. Reviewing in-depth the action potential is necessary for key topics discussed later in this book to include cardiac dysrhythmias, anesthetic effects, and antiarrhythmic medications.

C. As in most cells, the SL is made up of a phospholipid bilayer, which is impermeable to ions except through ion channels, active transport, and passive transport. The SL helps maintain ionic concentration gradients across the cell membrane (see Figure 2.3).

1. Passive movement of ions across the cell membrane depends on two variables: concentration gradient and transmembrane voltage potential. Ions always want to move down their gradient and are pulled toward their opposite charge. If we use sodium as our example ion, Na^+ will want to move from the extracellular concentration of 145 mM to the intracellular contraction of 15 mM. In order to establish a transmembrane voltage potential, the positively charged sodium ion is drawn intracellularly toward the negatively charged, −90 mV, intracellular space.

2. There is a predominance of potassium (K^+) and negatively charged proteins (anions, A^-) inside the cell and sodium (Na^+) and chloride (Cl^-) outside the cell (Figure 2.3).

3. At rest, the negative ions within the cell predominate, resulting in a negative transmembrane voltage. The resting voltage is referred to as the resting membrane potential, −90 mV.

4. The permeability of these ion channels is based on the voltage sensitivity of each ion channel. Voltage sensitivity is the ability of an ion channel to be turned on (opened) or turned off (closed), based on the voltage potential of the cell. The prime example of this in the cardiac cell is the fast-acting sodium channels that are closed, at the resting potential of −90 mV, but open at the threshold potential of −70 mV, flooding the intracellular space with the positively charged sodium ion.

5. Once the membrane has fully depolarized, these Na^+ channels will remain in the closed state until cell repolarization and a suitable membrane potential has been reached again below their threshold level, less than −70 mV, when they are returned to a resting state.

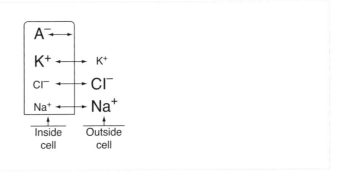

FIGURE 2.3   Major ionic content inside and outside a cell. A^- represents negatively charged proteins within the cell. Under normal conditions at rest, membrane potentials are negative, meaning that the voltage is more negative within the cell than outside of it.

6. At resting potential −90 mV, potassium ions can cross the membrane readily while sodium and chloride ions have a greater difficulty in doing so.
7. Membrane differences in ion channel concentrations and characteristics are cell-type specific.
8. Stimulation of a cell results in a change in membrane potential characteristic for that cell type because of a choreographed sequence of ion channels opening and closing. The plot of this sequence is referred to as an action potential.
9. The action potential of the sinoatrial node and atrioventricular node has a slightly different appearance. This is secondary to the fact that the resting potential of both the SA node and AV node is −70 mV. This difference, −70 mV in SA and AV nodes, versus −90 mV in the rest of the cardiac cells, keeps the fast-acting sodium channels in the SA and AV nodes, from playing a role in the action potential, and explains the difference in appearance of this action potential.
10. The remainder of the cardiac cells, other than the SA and AV nodes, has a more traditional appearing action potential:
    a. **Phase 0:** All processes that makes the membrane potential even slightly less negative will start Na$^+$ channels to begin to open, making the inside of the cell even less negatively charged. Once the threshold potential −70 mV is reached all fast-acting Na$^+$ channels, rapidly depolarizing the cell, give the near vertical upstroke. During this rapid depolarization, the cell membrane potential becomes positive and decreases K$^+$ permeability (Figure 2.4).
    b. **Phase 1:** With a positive membrane potential, all Na$^+$ channels are closed. Transiently activated channels transport K$^+$ out of the cell, returning the membrane potential to ≈0 mV, creating the sharp spike appearance.
    c. **Phase 2:** K$^+$ continues out of the cell and slow Ca^{2+} channels activate, transporting Ca^{2+} into the cell. The movements of K$^+$ out of the cell and Ca^{2+} into the cell are nearly balanced from an electrochemical standpoint giving a "plateau" appearance to the action potential. The influx of Ca^{2+} into the cell during this phase plays a major role in the release of the internal Ca^{2+} from the SR for myocyte contraction.
    d. **Phase 3:** Makes up the majority of the repolarization phase. Substantial outward movement, that exceeds the slow inward anion movement, quickly returns the cell to −90 mV. During this phase, Ca^{2+} is moved back into the sarcolemma by two mechanisms: a Na$^+$-Ca^{2+} exchanger and a Ca^{2+}-ATPase pump. At the cell membrane, there is Na$^+$-K$^+$-ATPase that actively corrects the Na$^+$/K$^+$ gradient, returning the cell to phase 4.

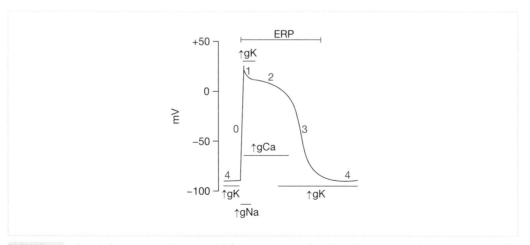

FIGURE 2.4   A typical myoctye action potential, for a non-pacemaker. Note the near vertical phase 0, owing to the "Fast" channels. g, conductance; ERP, effective refractory period. (Reprinted with permission from Klabunde RE, ed. Electrical activity of the heart. In: *Cardiovascular Physiology Concepts.* 3rd ed. Wolters Kluwer; 2022:36. Figure 3-5.)

e. **Phase 4:** The resting phase, which is maintained by passive K^+ movement in and out of the cell. This keeps the resting potential stable until the next action potential is generated, making the cell less negative enough to start opening the Na^+ channels and moving back into phase 0. During phase 4, K^+ movement is passive, moving out of the cell down the concentration gradient, making the intracellular space more negative, this in turn draws the K^+ back into the cell being attracted to the negative charge. All Na^+ and Ca^{2+} channels are closed in phase 4.

D. **Specialized Cells of the Conduction System**

1. Pacemaker cells, SA and AV nodes, have the property of automaticity because they are able to spontaneously depolarize, secondary to a less negative membrane potential and slow spontaneous depolarization during phase 4 (Figure 2.5). This slow spontaneous depolarization, of phase 4, takes place secondary to leakage of Na^+ into the cell. Because this takes place at approximately -40 mV, fast Na^+ channels are not involved, as they only repolarize close to -90 mV. Therefore, during phase 0 of the SA and AV nodes, depolarization is dependent on the slower Ca^{2+} channels, giving a less steep appearing action potential.

   a. The SA node is the "Native" pacemaker of the heart. It is located in the sulcus terminalis, situated at the junction of the superior vena cava (SVC) and right atrium posteriorly.

   b. The AV node, which is located anterior to the opening of the coronary sinus and above the tricuspid valve septal leaflet, has three different regions: upper junctional, middle node, and lower junctional. Only the upper and lower regions have automaticity at a rate of 40-60 beats per minute (bpm). The AV nodal myocardial fibers are small and conduct the action potential slower than the SA node.

   c. The bundle of His is made up of the lower fibers of the AV node coming together as they dive into the interventricular septum, giving rise to the right bundle branch (RBB) and left bundle branch (LBB), and finally the Purkinje fiber complex. The His-Purkinje fiber system has the fastest conduction in the heart.

2. Normal conduction starts in the SA node and spreads through the atrial region via specialized tracts in the atrial tissue, as well as propagation through all the atrial muscle cells. The atrial impulse usually takes about 0.04 seconds, in a healthy individual. Once the impulse reaches the AV node, there is a delay of ≈ 0.1 seconds, owing to the small AV nodal fibers. This delay allows for the passive and active filling of the ventricles, during diastole. Finalizing with the fastest conduction speeds through the His-Purkinje system taking only 0.03 seconds, it is conducted to the myocardial cells. Of note, the RBB is slightly shorter than the LBB, which allows for a spatially synchronized ventricular contraction pattern.

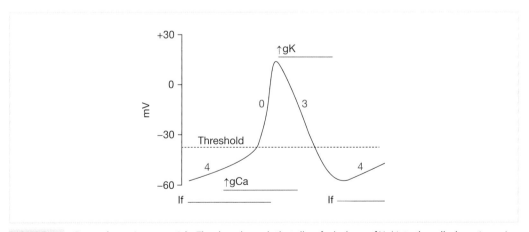

FIGURE 2.5   Pacemaker action potential—The slow channels that allow for leakage of Na^+ into the cell, phase 4, causing spontaneous depolarization of pacemaker cells, are called "funny" channels, If. (Reprinted with permission from Klabunde RE, ed. Electrical activity of the heart. In: *Cardiovascular Physiology Concepts*. 3rd ed. Wolters Kluwer; 2022:38. Figure 3-6.)

3. Conduction from myocyte to myocyte is through low-resistance gap junctions. These gap junctions have large amounts of ion channels, chemically coupling cardiac myocytes together. The conduction in the myocardial cells spreads from the endocardial layer outward to the epicardial layer and is completed in ≈0.03 seconds, secondary to this coupling.

4. The refractory period is the time period between depolarizing and when the cell has repolarized, -70 mV minimum, to allow another depolarization. The refractory period in the cardiac system is longer than that of other systems in the body. This is secondary to a longer action potential that gives more time for Ca^{2+} entry and binding to allow for maximal muscle contraction. This longer refractory period gives more time for both relaxation, chamber filling, and resetting of the Ca^{2+} system. The atrial refractory period is shorter than that of the ventricles and explains why the atrium has an underlying contraction rate of 270-300 bpm.

E. **Excitation-Contraction Coupling in the Heart**

1. The intricacies of ion channel opening due to a Purkinje action potential are beyond the scope of this chapter. However, these intricacies are important for anesthesiologists because patients take drugs that directly affect their characteristics.

2. Excitation-contraction coupling starts when a Purkinje cell action potential triggers Ca^{2+} ion channels to open resulting in the diffusion of Ca^{2+} ions (flux) across the sarcolemma principally within the T-tubule system (Figure 2.2).

3. The flux of Ca^{2+} across the sarcolemma is only about 1% of the Ca^{2+} needed for contraction. However, this Ca^{2+} serves as a trigger for SR Ca^{2+} ion channel opening and causes a graded release of Ca^{2+} to create the Ca^{2+} concentration needed for tension development. Graded release refers to the fact that the internal SR release of Ca^{2+} is dependent on the initial cytoplasmic Ca^{2+} concentration resulting from the external Ca^{2+} influx. This graded response is very different than the all-or-none response of skeletal muscle.

4. Three very important proteins within the SR are responsible for controlling calcium flux: the Ca^{2+} release channel, the sarcoendoplasmic reticulum calcium ATPase (SERCA-2), and the regulatory protein of SERCA-2 (phospholamban).

5. From relaxation to contraction, cytosolic Ca^{2+} concentration varies approximately 100-fold.

6. The myoplasmic (intracellular) Ca^{2+} concentration principally depends on the external Ca^{2+} concentration, the sympathetic tone (sarcolemma Ca^{2+} ion channel conductance), and the amount of Ca^{2+} stored in the SR.

7. Any increase in contractility via any drug results from increased myoplasmic Ca^{2+} concentration during systole! During systole, Ca^{2+} binds to troponin and results in a conformational change of tropomyosin. This change allows actin and myosin to interact, resulting in the shortening of a sarcomere (Figure 2.1) and oxygen consumption (see later).

CLINICAL PEARL

Intracellular calcium flux is critical to the initiation of myocardial sarcomere contraction, and many anesthetic drugs impair this flux.

8. Myoplasmic Ca^{2+}, and hence contractility, is affected by all inhalational agents and some intravenous anesthetic induction drugs.

9. Intracellular acidosis presents a common physiologic reason for decreased Ca^{2+}-troponin affinity. As compared to extracellular pH, intracellular pH is greatly buffered because of intracellular proteins. Intracellular pH is normally less than extracellular pH. When either intracellular or extracellular pH changes, transmembrane re-equilibration occurs. Because of the greater intracellular buffering capacity, the rate of intracellular pH change is delayed relative to extracellular pH changes.

10. Finally, for contraction to cease, Ca^{2+} must be unbound from troponin and removed from the myoplasm. Ca^{2+} is actively pumped into the SR as well as across the sarcolemma. Normally, approximately 99% of calcium is pumped back into the SR at a price of about 20% of total myocyte oxygen consumption.

V. Length-Tension Relationship

   A. Consider this thought experiment. There is an idealized, single cardiac myocyte that is 100 μm long with 40 sarcomeres in series. All distances between Z discs (sarcomere lengths) are equal for each of the 40 sarcomeres (100 μm = 40 × 2.5 μm) at rest. As the cardiac myocyte length changes, the length of each sarcomere changes proportionately. This single myocyte is suspended so that a strain gauge measures the tension that the myocyte generates at rest and during contraction.

   1. The idealized myocyte is stretched between two fixed points.
   2. The tension caused by the force of stretching the muscle at rest and created by the muscle during contraction is measured.
   3. The muscle is stretched at rest over a range of 72-100 μm. Consequently, the sarcomere lengths vary between 1.8 and 2.5 μm as this myocyte contracts.
   4. At each sarcomere length, two fixed myoplasmic Ca^{2+} concentrations are set within the cell: zero concentration (rest) and a known value (contraction).
   5. Myocyte tension is measured for both Ca^{2+} concentrations.
   6. Plotting resting tension as a function of length results in a resting length-(passive) tension plot.
   7. Recording peak tension as a function of myocyte length, a length-(active) tension curve can be plotted for the given Ca^{2+} concentration as depicted in Figure 2.6.

   B. Compliance

   1. In our idealized myocyte model, a measured amount of tension resulted when the sarcomere was stretched between 1.8 and 2.5 μm. In plotting this passive tension resulting from passive stretch of the sarcomeres, note that there is very little passive tension required to stretch the sarcomeres until the compliance of the cell membrane started to play a role.

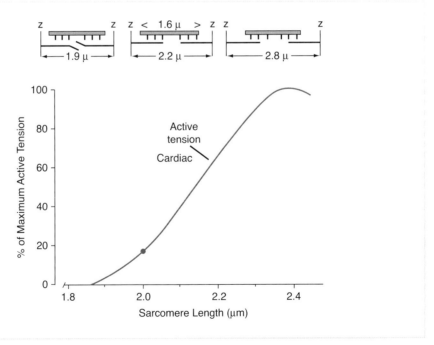

FIGURE 2.6 Top three schematic diagrams represent actin (thick filaments penetrating Z disc) and myosin (thin filaments forming sheaf between Z disc) filaments at three sarcomere lengths 1.9, 2.2, and 2.8 μm. Bottom graph represents a percent of maximum tension development versus sarcomere length for strips of cardiac muscle. Note that the fibrous cardiac skeleton inhibits sarcomere stretch from approaching a sarcomere length of 2.8 μm. (Derived from Honig C. *Modern Cardiovascular Physiology*. Little, Brown and Company; 1981.)

2. As the sarcomeres become stretched beyond 2.5 μm in intact cardiac muscle, the fibrous skeleton restricts further stretching. The fibrous skeleton resistance to stretch results in a rapid change in tension with very little change in length (very low compliance).

3. The slope of the line of this resting relationship between length and tension is the equivalent of ventricular compliance as will be discussed below.

C. Contractility

1. At a given Ca^{2+} concentration, a fraction of troponin molecules will bind Ca^{2+} molecules.

2. This Ca^{2+} binding to each troponin results in a conformational change in its corresponding tropomyosin that allows opposing actin and myosin head pairs, their exposure regulated by these tropomyosin molecules, to interact.

3. For this conformational change at the given Ca^{2+} concentration, the percentage of the actin and myocyte heads opposed to each other is determined.

4. If one repeats the above mental experiment with a different known Ca^{2+} concentration, a new contracting length-(active) tension curve is plotted.

5. For a range of Ca^{2+} concentrations in cardiac myocytes, a family of length-tension curves results.

6. For a given length, only through a change in myoplasmic Ca^{2+} concentration can active tension change.

7. In considering the family of curves in the context of ventricular contractility, the contractility is higher when for any given length, the developed tension is greater. In vivo, determining the contractility of the ventricle is complicated by the interactions of preload and afterload on any measurements.

D. Intracellular Ca^{2+} Concentration

1. The range of myoplasmic Ca^{2+} concentrations during contraction varies depending upon Ca^{2+} fluxes across the sarcolemma at the initiation of contraction and the Ca^{2+} released from the SR.

2. The transmembrane flux of Ca^{2+} across the sarcolemma is only about 1% of Ca^{2+} present during contraction. However, small changes in this transmembrane flux impressively alter the amount of Ca^{2+} released from the SR.

3. The SR response is graded. The more Ca^{2+} that crosses the sarcolemma, the more Ca^{2+} is released from the SR.

4. Examples of increasing sarcolemmal Ca^{2+} flux include increasing epinephrine levels and increasing external Ca^{2+} concentration (a $CaCl_2$ bolus).

5. Increased acute SR Ca^{2+} stores result from increased Ca^{2+} flux across the sarcolemma and increased heart rate (HR)—Treppe effect.

E. Oxygen Consumption

1. As described above, each interaction of actin and myosin results in a submicron shortening of the sarcomere.

2. Physiologic (15%) shortening requires multiple submicron shortenings.

3. For the sarcomere to shorten by 15%, many actin-myosin interactions take place.

4. Each submicron interaction requires adenosine triphosphate (ATP) for the release of the actin-myosin head. It is the relaxation of the actin-myosin interaction that requires energy and consumes oxygen.

5. Remember that the more actin-myosin cycles in a unit of time, the greater the oxygen consumption!

6. The three main determinants of myocardial oxygen consumption are as follows:
   a. **HR:** More beats at the same number of actin-myosin interactions
   b. **Contractility:** More interactions per beat
   c. **Wall tension:** More interaction for a given sarcomere length change

CLINICAL PEARL

The main determinants of myocardial oxygen consumption are HR, contractility, and wall tension.

VI. **Heart Chambers and External Work**

A. **The Chamber Wall**

1. Atrial and ventricular walls are formed, by individual myocytes which are joined together via collagen fibrin strands. This joining of myocytes, along a general overlapping orientation (not end to end), results in a sheet of muscle with myocytes oriented along a similar axis.

2. Several such layers form the chamber wall. These layers are oriented in different directions and are inserted on a fibrous cartilaginous skeleton at the base of the heart which includes the valvular annuli.

3. The nonalignment of the muscle layers allows for a twisting and pumping function with contraction.

4. The nonconductive fibrous skeleton isolates the atria from the ventricles allowing delayed conduction and atrioventricular synchrony. Because of the rapid electrical distribution of the signal through the conduction system, the layers of a chamber contract synchronously resulting in shortening of the muscle layers and a reduction in the volume of the chamber itself.

B. **Atria**

1. Composed of two thin muscle sheets

2. Atrial contraction contributes approximately 20% of the ventricular filling volume in a normal heart and may contribute even more when left ventricular end-diastolic pressure (LVEDP) is increased. In addition to the volume itself, the rate of ventricular volume addition resulting from atrial contraction may play a role in ventricular sarcomere lengthening.

C. **Ventricle**

1. Composed of three thick muscle sheets

2. For a given state of contractility (myoplasmic Ca^{2+} concentration), sarcomere length determines the wall tension the ventricle can achieve as discussed above. The aggregate shortening of the sarcomeres in the layers of cardiac myocytes results in wall tension that leads to the ejection of blood into the aorta and pulmonary artery (PA).

3. The active range of sarcomere length is only 1.8-2.5 μm (2.2 is the optimal length for maximal contraction) or ~15% of its length. Falling below 1.8 μm results from an empty ventricle while the collagen fiber network inhibits the stretching of sarcomeres much beyond 2.2 μm. This integration of structure and function is important in permitting response to increased demand and if there were no skeleton, overstretch would lead to reduced emptying that would lead to more overstretch and no cardiac output (CO).

4. Although the discussion below applies to both atria and ventricles, we will focus on the left ventricle below.

D. **Preload, Contractility, and Compliance**

1. **Preload**

   a. Preload is the volume of blood in the chamber at the end of diastole (end-diastolic volume—EDV), which will determine a specific sarcomere length and resultant muscle tension.

   b. Increasing EDV will increase muscle tension until it reaches its optimal length. Further stretching will decrease active tension since it will become "overstretched" where there are fewer cross-linked actin and myosin components.

   c. At rest, our EDV is less than maximal, which can be increased giving us cardiac reserve to meet increased demand.

   d. This length-tension relationship within the chamber is described by the Frank-Starling curve (described later).

   e. The best determinant of preload is EDV and not chamber pressure, as pressure does not always equate to volume.

2. Contractility is determined by myoplasmic Ca^{2+} concentration. This strength of contraction is primarily sympathetically mediated by increased calcium entry into the cell, increased SR Ca^{2+} concentrations, and increased clearance of calcium from the cell (faster relaxation). Faster relaxation with increased HR helps preserve diastolic time for enhanced coronary perfusion.

   a. Ventricular reserve is supported by increased stretch (to a point) and increased contractility.

3. Compliance, a variable that can be dynamic, relates to pressure and length.
   a. As discussed earlier, the preload (sarcomere length determined by EDV) determines how many actin-myosin heads interact for a given contractility at any instant.
   b. Measuring sarcomere length is essentially impossible clinically. As a surrogate for an indirect estimate of sarcomere length, clinicians measure a chamber pressure during chamber diastole. This pressure measurement is used as the equivalent of the myocyte resting tension measurement above and requires assumptions about compliance.
   c. More direct surrogate estimate of sarcomere length is chamber volume. Using echo-cardiography, measurement of volumes serves as a direct estimate of preload (EDV) and eliminates assumptions about chamber compliance that are necessary when using a pressure estimate.
   d. A plot of the relationship between resting chamber pressure and resting chamber volume results in a curve similar to the resting length-tension curve for the myocyte.
   e. The slope of this curve at any point (change in volume over the change in pressure at that point) is the compliance of the chamber at that point. The pressure-volume curve is nonlinear, and its slope varies depending on ventricular volume (Figures 2.7 and 2.8). Ventricles become much less compliant as sarcomere length surpasses 2.2 μm because of restriction by the collagen fiber skeleton.
   f. Nonischemic changes in compliance generally occur over long time periods. However, acute ischemia can change ventricular compliance very quickly. Thick ventricles, ventricles with scar formation, or ischemic ventricles have a lower compliance than normal ventricles. Less compliant ventricles require a higher pressure within them to contain equal volume as compared to a more compliant ventricle.
   g. While preload is most commonly considered in the left ventricle, it is important in all four chambers. Both congenital heart disease and cardiac tamponade can make that very apparent.

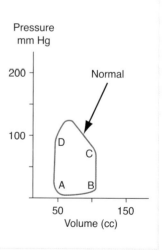

Ventricular Pressure–Volume Loops

Breakdown of a Pressure–Volume Loop
- P–V loop depicts IV volume and pressure relationship
- A = MV opening & LVESV
  B = MV closure & LVEDV/LVEDP
- C = AV opening & systemic aortic diastolic pressure
- D = AV closure & LVESV/LVESP & dicrotic notch in Ao pressure tracing
- AB → LV Filling
- BC → Isovolumetric contraction
- CD → LV ejection
- DA → Isovolumetric relaxation
- LV compliance is ΔP/ΔV during filling of LV (slope of AB)
- Stroke volume = EDV − ESV
- Ejection fraction = SV/EDV

FIGURE 2.7 Idealized pressure-volume loop. Area within the loop represents LVSW. Dividing SV (Point B minus Point A volumes) by BSA results in SVI. The area within this indexed loop is the LVSWI. AV, aortic valve; EDV, end-diastolic volume; ESV, end-systolic volume; IV, intraventricular; LV, left ventricle; LVEDP, left ventricular end-diastolic pressure; LVESV, left ventricular end-systolic volume; LVESP, left ventricular end-systolic pressure; LVSW, left ventricular stroke work; MV, mitral valve; P, pressure; P-V, pressure-volume; V, volume; SV, stroke volume.

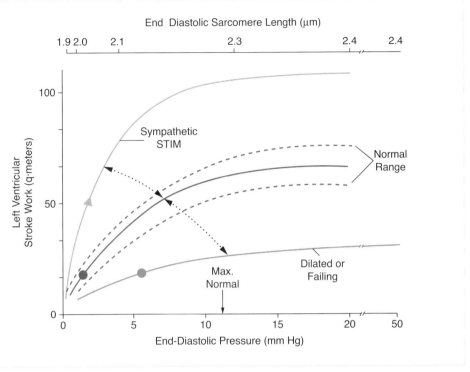

FIGURE 2.8 The Starling curve. Max., maximum; STIM, stimulation.

6

E. Ventricular Work

1. Afterload is the amount of pressure exerted by the heart in order to eject blood with each contraction. Afterload is mainly determined by arteriolar smooth muscle.
2. For a specific preload with a given contractility, the cardiac myocyte will shorten, develop tension, and eject blood from the ventricle when the pressure generated overcomes the afterload. The amount of blood ejected is the stroke volume (SV).
3. In ejecting this SV, the ventricle performs external work. This work comprises raising intraventricular pressure from end-diastolic pressure to peak systolic pressure. In the absence of valvular heart disease, the systolic left and right ventricular pressures closely match those in the aorta and PA, respectively.
4. Normal blood pressures (BPs) in the aorta and PA are not dependent on body size and vary little among normal subjects. By normalizing SV to stroke volume index (SVI) (SV divided by body surface area [BSA]), the variability of SVI among subjects becomes relatively small.
5. Hydrodynamically, the external work of a ventricle is the area within the pressure-volume loop seen in Figure 2.7. The definitions of various points and intervals are defined in the legend. This indexed work for the left ventricle (LVSWI) is derived by multiplying the SVI in milliliters times the difference in arterial mean pressure and ventricular pressure at the end of diastole (commonly estimated as atrial pressure or PA wedge pressure) times a constant (0.0136) to convert to clinical units:

$$\text{LVSWI} = \text{SVI} \times (\text{SBP mean} - \text{LVEDP}) \times 0.0136 \ (\text{g m/m}^2)$$

6. The normal resting values for SVI and LVSWI are approximately 50 mL/m^2 and 50 g m/m^2, hence they are relatively easy to remember.
7. **Myocardial efficiency:** Most of the energy expended by the myocytes goes to producing heat with the rest to myocardial work. Efficiency is work/total energy expenditure. In performing this work, the efficiency of the ventricle is 20%-25% at maximum and can be as low as 5% in severe heart failure. This can be an astonishingly inefficient process.

8. Heart failure (HF) is the inability of the heart to pump enough blood to meet the body's demands.
   a. Systolic heart failure, often termed heart failure with reduced ejection fraction (HFrEF), is characterized by ejection fraction (EF) <40%, decreased SV with increased EDV resulting in myocyte hypertrophy, and increased sympathetic stimulation causing increased renin and aldosterone levels with retention of Na and water.
   b. Diastolic HF often termed heart failure with preserved ejection fraction (HFpEF) is characterized by EF >40%, decreased myocardial elasticity, and high ventricular filling pressures. This is usually accompanied by concentric left ventricular hypertrophy further leading to decreased ventricular volumes and resultant backup of volume into the lungs and tissues.
   c. These changes have important implications for ventricular loading responses during the use of volatile anesthetics, IV anesthetics, and CPB.
   d. Treatment of HFrEF is based on angiotensin-converting enzyme (ACE) inhibitors (to decrease aldosterone and blood pressure), other vasodilators (to decrease preload and afterload), and diuretics (to decrease intravascular volume). β-Blockers have been shown to decrease morbidity and mortality in HF as well.
   e. Since external work is the product of pressure difference and SV, work does not distinguish between these two variables. Evidence suggests that the ventricles can do volume work somewhat more efficiently (requires less oxygen) than pressure work. The reasoning may relate to how many actin-myosin cycles are required to shorten a sarcomere to a given distance. The hypothesis is that it takes fewer actin-myosin cycles to shorten the same distance for volume work compared to pressure work. This principle may explain an underlying reason for the success of using vasodilators to treat HF as noted above.

F. **Starling Curve**
   1. For a given contractile state, varying the sarcomere length between 1.9 and 2.2 μm increases the amount of external work done. For a ventricle with normal compliance, a sarcomere length of 2.2 μm corresponds to one with an LVEDP of 10 mm Hg.
   2. By plotting the relationship of LVEDP with LVSWI, a Starling curve is generated.
   3. By changing the contractile state and replotting the same relationship, a new curve develops, resulting in a family of Starling curves idealized in Figure 2.8.

G. **Myocardial Oxygen Consumption and ATP Production**
   1. **Basal O_2 consumption:** 2 mL/100 g/min
   2. **Resting O_2 consumption:** 9 mL/100 g/min
   3. With activity, there is increased O_2 consumption with O_2 demand met by increasing coronary and capillary perfusion since venous O_2 is low (due to high myocyte O_2 extraction).
   4. O_2 consumption is determined by HR, contractility, and intramyocardial tension.
   5. ATP is the energy source utilized by the myocyte.
   6. Adequate production of ATP is dependent on mitochondrial function. Approximately 30% of cardiac cell volume is occupied by mitochondria. Given the substrate distribution and the ability to produce ATP within this volume, oxygen availability is the limiting factor for maintaining ATP availability. Mitochondria can maximally produce ATP when their cell Po_2 is 0.1 Torr.
   7. Phosphocreatine (PCr) is an intracellular buffer for the ATP concentration. The cell readily converts ATP into PCr and vice versa. PCr is an important energy reserve and also serves to transport ATP between mitochondria and myosin ATPase.
   8. Myosin ATPase activity is responsible for 75% of myocardial ATP consumption. The remaining 25% is consumed by Ca^{2+} transport into the SR and across the sarcolemma.
   9. The mitochondrion's role in determining the response to ischemia is important. Intracellular signaling pathways in response to hypoxia may direct the cell to necrosis or even apoptosis.
   10. Except for very unusual circumstances, substrate for ATP and phosphocreatine (PCr) production is readily available. Without external oxygen delivery, the intracellular oxygen content is capable of keeping the heart contracting for a very limited time. Carbohydrate and lipid stores can fuel the heart for almost an hour, albeit very inefficiently and unsustainably. Hence, capillary blood flow is crucial to maintain oxidative metabolism.

11. Myoglobin is an intracellular oxygen store. Its affinity for oxygen falls between those for hemoglobin and cytochrome aa3 (part of the respiratory chain). As noted, the maximum oxygen concentration required in mitochondria for maximal ATP production is just 0.1 Torr.

12. Myoglobin oxygen concentration is high enough to buffer interruptions in capillary flow only for seconds. Compared to high-energy phosphate buffers, this myoglobin buffer is small relative to ATP consumption rates.

13. Nevertheless, myoglobin's intermediate oxygen affinity enhances unloading of oxygen from the red cell into the myocyte and also serves to distribute oxygen within the cell.

14. Commonly atherosclerotic disease limits blood flow to regions of the heart, reducing oxygen delivery and cell oxygen tension. When this Po_2 falls below 0.1 Torr, ATP production decreases along with myocardial wall motion. Before ATP production is compromised, the entire oxygen difference from ambient air ($\sim$150 Torr) to 0.1 Torr has already happened!

H. **Oxygen Supply by Capillaries**

1. Capillaries are approximately 1 mm (1,000 µm) in length, regardless of the organ system in which they are located. In the heart, a cardiac myocyte is $\sim$100 µm in length, so each capillary supplies multiple cardiac myocytes. In contrast, a skeletal muscle fiber (cell) can be significantly longer (>20-100 mm). Since capillary length is the same (1 mm), each skeletal muscle capillary supplies a very small fraction of any given muscle cell.

2. There are multiple levels of arteriolar structure. The lower-order, or initial, arterioles are the primary determinants of systemic vascular resistance (SVR), and the higher-order, or distal, arterioles regulate regional blood flow distribution at the local level.

3. Capillary perfusion is organized so that several capillaries are supplied from a single higher-order arteriole.

4. This structure yields regions of perfusion on the scale of cubic millimeters for the regional blood flow unit. Hence, the smallest volumes for "small vessel infarcts" should be this order of magnitude. As the vessel occlusions become more proximal, the infarct size grows.

5. Because the length of cardiac myocytes is small relative to the capillary length, infarction due to small vessel disease only affects local zones. If the cardiac myocyte was significantly longer, like a skeletal myocyte, the consequences of a local infarct would affect the whole length and have a much larger impact.

VII. **Control Systems**

A. The space program put man in space. As importantly, it brought many technological advances. In the world of systems development, control systems were central. These systems allowed us to perform tasks in unexplored environments under unimagined conditions. In simplest concept, they permitted real-time sensing of system variables that resulted in the regulation of system output. In the jargon, **a feedback loop** is that portion of the system that takes a signal from within the system and returns that signal to a system input that in turn affects system output.

B. A feedback loop is referred to as a **negative feedback loop** if a deviation of the system output from the desired output, called set point, is **returned toward** that set point through the system response to that deviation. As considered below, perhaps the most studied biologic negative feedback loop is the cardiovascular reflexes.

C. In contrast, **positive feedback loops** increase the deviation from the normal level in response to deviation. Outside the physiology of the immune system, physiologic systems with positive feedback loops are generally pathologic. When a positive feedback loop occurs, the system frequently becomes unstable and usually leads to system failure. An example of this pathology is the response of the cardiovascular system to hypotension in the presence of coronary artery disease. Hypotension leads to a demand for an increase in HR, SVR, and contractility. If the resulting increase in oxygen consumption leads to ischemia, contractility will decrease, leading to further demands that eventually result in system failure.

VIII. **The Cardiovascular Control System**

A. The simple control system model can be used to develop a model of the cardiovascular system. This model is useful if it predicts the system response to system disturbances. Modified from Honig,[3(p249)] components in Figure 2.8 can be broken down into sensor, controller, and effector functions. The following discussion will summarize concepts for each function.

B. For the sensor functions, the two best-characterized sensors—the baroreceptors in the carotid sinus and the volume and HR sensors in the right atrium—will be outlined in detail.

C. The primary role of the cardiovascular system is to provide sufficient oxygen delivery to satisfy the ever-changing metabolic demands of body tissues, that is oxygen consumption. This ability is captured by the oxygen delivery (DO_2) equation:

Oxygen Delivery = (Cardiac Output [CO]) (Hemoglobin $\times$ 1.34 $\times$ Oxygen Saturation + 0.003 Partial Pressure of Dissolved Oxygen).

D. **Cardiac output** is the volume of blood pumped to body tissues per minute; it is equal to the product of HR and SV. The cardiac **index** is a normalized value for CO based on BSA, normally 2.5-3.5 L/min/m². The Fick equation can be used to calculate CO if the patient's O_2 consumption (Vo_2), arterial O_2 content (Cao_2), and mixed venous O_2 content (Cvo_2) are determined. The Fick equation is as follows:

$$CO = \frac{Vo_2}{C_a - C_v}$$

E. **Regulation** of a variable is defined as the variable remaining fixed despite changes in its determinants. In the cardiovascular system, mean arterial BP is the variable that remains fixed since BP changes only by perhaps $\pm 25\%$ from our being asleep to maximal exercising. BP is the product of CO and SVR. Unsurprisingly, our survival requires a wide range of CO and SVR. CO increase is offset by SVR decreasing and vice versa. The physiologic range for each is approximately 4- to 6-fold.

F. Both CO and SVR are under the control of the arterial baroreflex and autonomic nervous system. Since CO is the product of HR and SV, changes in either of these parameters also influence BP (Figure 2.9).

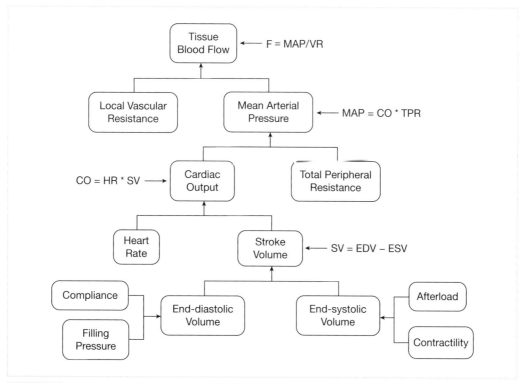

FIGURE 2.9 Determinants of oxygen delivery. CO, cardiac output; EDV, end-diastolic volume; ESV, end-systolic volume; F, flow; HR, heart rate; MAP, mean arterial pressure; SV, stroke volume; TPR, total peripheral resistance; VR, vascular resistance. (Derived from Rothe CF. Cardiodynamics. In: Selkurt EE, ed. *Physiology*. Little, Brown and Company; 1971:321.)

CLINICAL PEARL

Baroreceptors typically regulate BP within a range of ±25% even with 4- to 6-fold variations in CO and SVR.

G. The brain is the site of the controller. The medulla oblongata, specifically the medullary cardiovascular center, is the primary site of cardiovascular and baroreflex integration. In this region, the nucleus of the solitary tract (NTS) serves as the primary site for the first synapse of the baroreceptor afferents and is the key integrating site for all baroreceptor inputs including the cardiopulmonary baroreceptors.[4]

H. As outputs from the controller, the nervous system signals recruit and de-recruit the effectors in a predictable fashion through the sympathetic and parasympathetic nervous system and the release of norepinephrine (NOR) and acetylcholine (ACH).

I. The **effectors of the cardiovascular system—heart, venous system, and arterial system**—respond to changes in system demand. Globally, each effector has an expandable range known to physiologists as the **physiologic reserve**. The physiologic reserve of each effector will be discussed in detail in "Effectors and Physiologic Reserves for the Healthy Individual" section.

IX. **Arterial Baroreceptors**

A. The baroreceptors in the carotid sinus are the first described sensors of arterial blood pressure. Additional arterial baroreceptors have been discovered in the pulmonary and systemic arterial trees including the aortic arch.

B. **The baroreceptor reflex** is a negative feedback system that is responsible for the minute-to-minute maintenance of arterial blood pressure.

C. The carotid sinus and the aortic baroreceptors are innervated by the sinus nerve of Hering (a branch of the glossopharyngeal nerve) and the vagus nerve, respectively. In Figure 2.10, the single neural fiber signal from the sinus nerve of Hering correlates with a pulsatile "BP waveform."

D. The cardiovascular center in the medulla oblongata receives and integrates the sensory impulses from the baroreceptors. The responses are changes in CO and SVR via the autonomic nervous system (Figure 2.11).

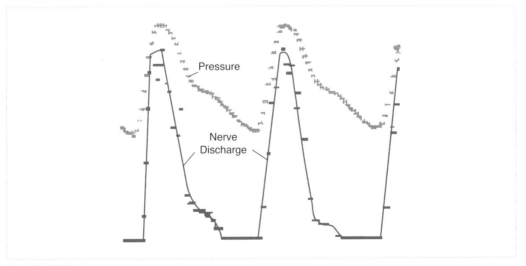

FIGURE 2.10 Note the relationship between the upslope of arterial pressure (dP/dt), the downslope (SVR), and the notch (SVR) and the action potential characteristics.

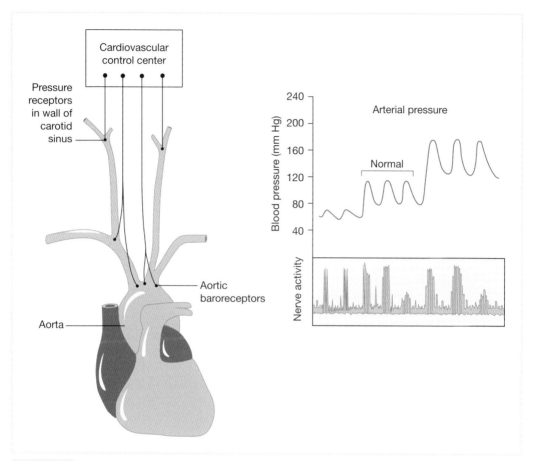

FIGURE 2.11   The major components of the baroreceptor reflexes. (Reprinted with permission from Campagna JA, Carter C. Clinical relevance of the Bezold-Jarisch reflex. *Anesthesiology.* 2003;98(5):1250-1260. © 2003 American Society of Anesthesiologists.)

E. A rise in arterial pressure reduces arterial baroreceptor afferent activity, resulting in further inhibition of the sympathetic and increased parasympathetic output. This results in decreased SVR and reductions in CO by decreasing HR and SV, which eventually normalizes arterial pressure. A decrease in arterial pressure has opposite effects.[5]

F. Patients with chronic hypertension often exhibit decreased baroreceptor reflex response and thus are more likely to experience intraoperative blood pressure lability.

G. Certain volatile anesthetics (such as halothane, sevoflurane, and desflurane) depress the baroreceptor reflex-mediated control of HR and blood pressure.

H. The aortic baroreceptor is located near or in the aortic arch. Infrequently, cardiac anesthesiologists can become acutely aware of its presence. When distorted, secondary to the placement of any aortic clamp, the resulting aortic baroreceptor signal results in an acute and dramatic increase in BP. The presumed mechanism is that the clamp distorts the aortic baroreceptor. This distortion results in a signal that BP has precipitously fallen. Even though the carotid baroreceptor has no such indication, hypertension ensues, thus representing imperfect system integration. Immediately releasing a partial-occlusion clamp (when possible) usually promptly returns the BP to a more normal level. When the release is not feasible, a short, rapid-acting intervention—pharmacologic vasodilation or reverse Trendelenburg positioning—is required.

I. Blood flow to the individual organs can be locally adjusted and/or centrally integrated. This organization allows for individual independent organ perfusion as long as aortic or PA pressure is maintained.

X. **Atrial Receptors**

A. All known pressure-sensitive sensors in the cardiovascular system are stretch receptors. The compliance of the receptor site impacts the receptor signal. Compliance pathology becomes central to understanding the disease of this aspect. In addition to the volume of a chamber, the rate of change of that volume is sensed and commensurate afferent signals are sent to the brain.

B. Within the right atrium, there are receptors at the junction of the superior and inferior venae cavae with the atrium (B fibers) and in the body of this atrium (A fibers), Figure 2.12. The corresponding impulses from the respective nerves are seen on the left. **A fibers**, seen in both atria, generate impulses during atrial contraction, indicating that they **detect** HR (Figure 2.12). **B fibers** are located only in the right atrium. B fibers are activated by atrial stretch and detect atrial volume filling. When combined with A fiber information, CO can be derived potentially.

C. Atrial stretch receptors respond to decreased atrial volume filling by causing the release of vasopressin from the posterior pituitary. Vasopressin has two effects that tend to increase blood pressure toward normal:

  1. It is a potent **vasoconstrictor** that increases SVR by activating **V1 receptors** on the arterioles.

  2. It increases **water reabsorption** by the renal distal tubule and collecting ducts by activating **V2 receptors.**

D. **Bainbridge Reflex**

  1. The Bainbridge reflex refers to an increase in HR in response to an increase in central blood volume.

  2. An increase in venous return serves to increase the pressure in the superior and inferior vena cava. This results in an increase in the pressure of the right atrium, which stimulates the B fibers. These atrial stretch receptors in turn signal the medullary control centers to increase the HR by increasing sympathetic activity to the sinoatrial node, thereby resulting in a decrease in the venous pressure of the great veins by drawing more blood out of the right atrium.

  3. Bainbridge reflex is involved in respiratory sinus arrhythmia. During inhalation, intrathoracic pressure decreases and leads to increased venous return. As a result, atrial stretch receptors sense the signal and via the Bainbridge reflex, increase the HR momentarily during inspiration.[6]

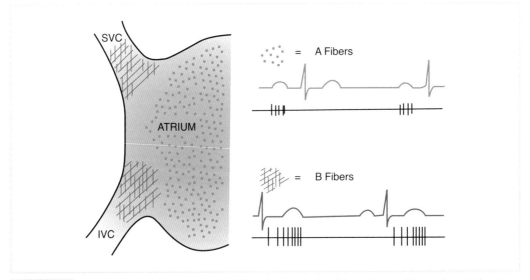

FIGURE 2.12 The A fibers (stretch receptors) are located in the body of the atrium and fire during atrial contraction and sense atrial contraction rate or HR. The B fibers (stretch receptors) are located at the intersection of the inferior vena cava (IVC) and superior vena cava (SVC). Their neural signals occur during ventricular systole when the atria are filling. Hence, they sense atrial volume. (Derived from Honig C. *Modern Cardiovascular Physiology*. Little, Brown and Company; 1981.)

XI. Chemoreceptors

- **A.** Peripheral chemoreceptors are located in the carotid body and aortic body. They are sensitive to blood O_2 content and blood pH.
- **B.** In conditions of hypoxia or acidosis, the carotid body elicits afferent impulses along the sinus nerve of Hering to the nucleus tractus solitarius. In response, the central respiratory center is stimulated and thus minute ventilation will be increased. In addition, the parasympathetic system is activated, and reduction in HR ensues.
- **C.** In the case of persistent hypoxia, the central nervous system is directly stimulated, resulting in sympathetic activation causing increased HR, CO, and vasoconstriction.
- **D. Benzold-Jerisch Reflex**
  - **1.** The Benzold-Jerisch reflex is a triad of bradycardia, vasodilation, and hypotension resulting from noxious stimulation of cardiac mechanical and chemosensitive receptors in the left ventricular wall.
  - **2.** Noxious stimuli may include myocardial ischemia and contraction of a poorly filled ventricle. Once stimulated, nonmyelinated vagal c-fibers signal the medulla, and result in the inhibition of sympathetic outflow and increased parasympathetic outflow (bradycardia, vasodilation, and hypotension).
  - **3.** This cardioprotective reflex has been implicated in the physiologic response to cardiovascular conditions such as myocardial ischemia, severe hypovolemia, and syncope.[7]

XII. Effectors and Physiologic Reserves for the Healthy Individual

- **A.** Each of the effectors contributes to maintaining BP through increasing CO, changing SVR, or shifting venous blood into or out of the thorax. In the face of everyday life, the variability for each effector can be referred to as a physiologic reserve.
- **B.** Knowing the range of reserve for each effector provides a perspective on how each can be utilized to support BP in the OR.
- **C.** Clinical situations in which physiologic reserves are reduced or, because of pharmacologic effects or clinical pathology, reduce options to support BP.
- **D. Heart Rate**
  - **1.** A normal resting HR range is 60-100 bpm. Maximum heart rate is age dependent and normally accepted as Maximum HR = 220 − age in years. For example, an attainable HR in a 25-year-old is 195 while it is 165 in a 55-year-old.
  - **2.** When using or allowing increases in HR, it must be kept in mind that increasing HR correlates with an increasing risk of ischemia specifically for patients under anesthesia.
- **E. Systemic Vascular Resistance**
  - **1.** The systemic and pulmonic distribution vessels are the aorta and PA, and their drainage vessels are the central vein system and pulmonary vein, respectively. Because of the large diameters of the normal aorta and PA, there is no physiologically important decrease in mean BP along either of their lengths.
  - **2.** These vessels (aorta to central vein; PA to pulmonary vein) have organ blood flow running between them. This configuration results in the organs being in parallel with the other organs in the systemic or pulmonic circulation.
  - **3.** Each organ experiences the same mean BP. Consequently, each organ autoregulates its individual blood flow by altering its own resistance. If BP is maintained, blood flows to organs are not dependent on other organ blood flows.
  - **4.** The total systemic and pulmonary vascular resistances are dependent on the organ resistances of each individual in that circulation. Because of the parallel structure of the organs, the resulting resistance change of an individual organ has less of an effect on the total resistance of the circulation.
  - **5.** In healthy individuals, organ blood flow requirements (regulated through organ resistance changes) are met without compromising BP. Metabolic requirements—substrate supply, oxygen supply, oxygen demand, and waste removal—are met through local adjustment of each organ's own blood flow.
  - **6.** The cardiovascular system maintains BP through its effectors via central nervous system (CNS) control responding to the impact of local organ resistance.

7. Based on the following equation:

$$SVR\ (dyne/s/cm^{-5}) = MAP\ (mm\ Hg) - CVP\ (mm\ Hg)/CO\ (L/min) \times 80$$

and assuming BP is regulated; when SVR is high then CO must be proportionally lower and vice versa. What is the observed range of SVR? For a severely dehydrated person or one with a very bad left ventricle, the cardiac index might be 33% of normal ($1.2\ LPM/M^2$). The corresponding SVR would be 3 times the normal value ($3,600\ dyne \cdot s/cm^5$). For a well-trained athlete who, during maximal exercise, would increase CO 7-fold, the SVR would be $\sim$15% of normal ($\sim$200 dyne$\cdot$s/cm^5).

F. **Contractility**
1. Contractility is the innate ability of a heart muscle to shorten for a given initial (resting) length and at a final contracted tension. It is not measured clinically because of the difficulty in direct measurement. Both afterload (arterial pressure) and preload (end-diastolic volume) effect its estimate.
2. Increasing contractility results in a reduced end-systolic volume (ESV) resulting in greater SVs and CO.
3. In healthy individuals, increasing contractility and wall tension can contribute to a modest increase of left ventricular ejection fraction (LVEF) from a value of 0.60-0.80. However, in patients with underlying heart disease, this modest change in EF may not be present requiring interventions to augment preload and afterload.

G. **Intravascular Volume: Venous Capacitance**
1. Total blood volume can be estimated from body weight. In the ideal 70-kg person, an estimate of blood volume is 70 mL/kg or about 5 L. This blood volume is considered euvolemia.
2. The distribution of that volume between intrathoracic and extrathoracic (or systemic) circulations is roughly 30% and 70%.
3. In each of these two compartments, approximately one-third of the blood is in the arteries and capillaries and two-thirds are in the venous system.
4. The pulmonary veins hold 1,100 mL, and the systemic veins hold 2,400 mL (totaling about two-thirds of the blood volume).
5. Relaxation of venous tone increases venous capacity for blood. If there is no change in blood volume, this decreases right atrial volume, which leads in turn to decreases in volume in the other cardiac chambers.
6. Since atrial pressure equals ventricular end-diastolic pressure (VEDP), returning those pressures to their original values requires an infusion of volume. When venous capacitance is at its largest, the amount of intravascular volume required to return these volumes to their original values is referred to as the venous capacitance reserve.
7. In addition to the blood volume defined as euvolemia, the intrathoracic and extrathoracic compartments can expand by 30%, or approximately 300 and 1,200 mL, respectively.
8. Thus, 1,500 mL of intravascular volume is a quantitative estimate of this venous capacitance reserve for this 70-kg person.
9. This reserve intravascular volume, when added to a euvolemic blood volume (5 L in a 70-kg subject), and the total intravascular volume would be 6.5 L.
10. While sustaining (ie, "defending") BP as the primary regulated variable, maintaining CO in the face of any reduction in total blood volume, for example, standing or hemorrhage, is another important task of the cardiovascular system. Through shifting blood into the thoracic circulation from the systemic veins, the sympathetic nervous system attempts to maintain pulmonary blood volume at the expense of systemic volume. In the setting of reduced circulating blood volume, protection of pulmonary blood volume coupled with increasing HR and contractility defends BP maintenance.
11. Recognize that anesthetics, both regional and general, alter the ability of the sympathetic nervous system to defend BP. In the presence of pathology, understanding how individual anesthetics interfere with each of the reserves may reduce the anesthetic risk through choosing the anesthetic approach that preserves the most physiologic reserves.
12. In pathologic states that chronically elevate right- or left-sided atrial pressures, venous dilation results in an increase in "euvolemic" blood volume.

13. Particularly in the systemic venous system, this increase in capacity can be large. While there is no experimental data, anecdotal observations of mitral valve patients going on cardiopulmonary bypass clearly demonstrate this fact. However, the extent to which increased volumes can be recruited to maintain intrathoracic volume in normal life, which is the key to maintaining preload, remains unknown. For any patient, a portion of that additional volume is available in circulatory emergencies (eg, hemorrhage), but the intravascular volume at the time of the emergency critically impacts this response.

14. Like hemorrhage, chronic diuresis leads to a contracted venous bed. Hence, caring for patients who are chronically or acutely hypovolemic secondary to diuresis must include understanding the state of their venous volume status (capacitance).

15. Of note, chronic diuretic administration leads to venoconstriction. However, an acute dose of furosemide will venodilate the patient with HF and actually lower intrathoracic blood volume by shifting blood into the dilated systemic veins.

H. **Lymphatic Circulation: A Final Reserve?**

1. The interstitial space lies between the capillaries and intracellular space. Clinically, this system is rarely discussed except as part of the so-called "third spacing," but physiologically, it plays a vital role. For our purposes, the lymphatic system protects organs from edema.

2. The characteristics of this space help prevent fluid accumulation in two ways—its low compliance and transport of fluid through the lymphatic conduits.[8]

3. The gel collagen matrix results in the interstitial space having a low compliance. Consequently, fluid entering the interstitial space raises interstitial pressure rapidly opposing further transudation of fluid across capillaries.

4. The lymphatics are tented open by a collagen matrix. Because of this tenting, lymphatics are not compressed when the interstitium is edematous. On the contrary, lymphatic diameter and drainage increase during edematous states.

5. This increased interstitial pressure also increases lymphatic drainage as the higher interstitial pressure increases the pressure gradient between interstitial space and right atrial pressure (the lymphatics drain into the systemic venous system).

6. Consequently, more fluid leaves the interstitium via lymphatic drainage when more fluid enters the lymphatics across the capillary.

7. Proteins pass across the capillary membrane although at markedly reduced rates compared to water and solutes. With normal capillary integrity, approximately 4% of intravascular proteins cross the capillary membrane each hour.

8. Interstitial fluid exchange between capillary blood and interstitial space is dynamic during the convective transport of blood down a capillary. Exchange occurs as fluid leaves the capillary at the arteriole end and returns at the venous end. The expansion factor for this exchange is approximately 8-fold. Hence, crystalloid administration equilibrates across the vascular and interstitial volumes rapidly (minutes). Colloid, if capillary integrity is intact, remains longer (hours).

9. Remember that the time constant for colloids remaining intravascular can be markedly reduced in the presence of the inflammatory response. The inflammatory response is part of every surgical procedure.

10. With severe hemorrhage accompanied by maximal sympathetic stimulation, interstitial and intracellular fluid may contribute up to 2.5 L of fluid to intravascular volume.[9] While this recruitment of intracellular and interstitial fluid compensates for intravascular depletion acutely, this depletion, particularly of intracellular volume, does so at the expense of cell function. This eventually induces cellular acidosis, which compromises cell function.

11. All three of these compartments—intracellular, interstitial, and intravascular—have a dynamic relationship with equilibrium being reached in minutes after volume administration, change in sympathetic tone, or administration of vasoactive drugs.

12. Physiologists define the interstitial space as a fluid space outside the intracellular and intravascular spaces that contains protein and solutes. Its structural composition causes it to be a markedly noncompliant space. This space equilibrates with the intracellular and intravascular spaces by dynamically exchanging fluid, electrolytes, and proteins with both. This results in a so-called "third space" volume that is very difficult to measure. The clinical impact of this third space appears minimal in the average surgical case. However, in

severe hemorrhage as described above in H.10, failure to account for its contribution to intravascular replenishment may lead to volume under resuscitation. Since the inflammatory response during surgery affects the integrity of all membranes, the normal equilibrium among intracellular, intravascular, and interstitial fluid spaces changes. Most often, the noncompliant nature of interstitial space likely minimizes its effects on fluid homeostasis.

13. Under normal conditions, minimal fluid accumulation occurs in space outside of organs, referred to here as potential space. However, when fluid leaks out into this potential space due to reduced oncotic pressure or capillary integrity, pathologic accumulations such as pleural effusions and/or ascites can ensue. If fluid is removed from these spaces during surgery, fluid from the adjacent organs will rapidly replace this extra-organ fluid and subsequently reduce intravascular volume and potentially induce hypotension.

14. In summary, for major hemorrhage, consideration of volume resuscitation requirements must include intracellular, interstitial, intravascular, and potential space compartments. Particularly when sympathetic tone is abruptly altered, the extent of circulatory collapse may be greater than anticipated as fluid within these compartments equilibrates at the new level of sympathetic tone.

I. **Brain: The Controller**

1. It is beyond the scope of this chapter, and to an extent of our knowledge, to detail the neural pathways, interactive signaling, and psychological influences on the cardiovascular system response. Accordingly, our brain as the controller is considered a black box. In this view, this controller is designed to maintain BP assuming that all the effectors are recruitable.

2. Making the controller a black box may be justifiable on another level. Although system integration can be characterized for a given patient at the moment, the medications clinicians utilize affects system integration through direct and indirect effects on effectors and perhaps on the controller and sensors as well. Other medications affect the ability of the CNS to stimulate responses through receptor or ganglion blockade. For anesthesiologists, in many situations, our clinical management must replace system integration. By understanding the pharmacology present and its effect on the cardiovascular system, clinical judgment dictates a plan to control BP regulation. This control responsibility must include temporizing and maintaining BP variability. Unable to rely on the cardiovascular system alone, the clinician physiologist manipulates the effector responses to maintain BP while remaining cognizant of the state (presence or absence) of physiologic reserves in the face of upcoming disturbances.

3. Understanding the impact of patient comorbidities anticipates the limitations in physiologic reserves and their availability for recruitment during stress. Through goal-directed therapy, recognition of necessary compromises for adjustment of the anesthetic approach can reduce the risk of morbidity and mortality.

4. One aspect of goal-directed therapy is fluid management. It is now understood that both hypovolemia and hypervolemia are associated with postoperative morbidity. Therefore, the previously thought notion of providing excessive fluid administration in the setting of hypotension is no longer recommended. Despite multiple methods of volume status assessment, including CVP, PA catheter, transesophageal echocardiography (TEE), arterial waveform analysis, and bioimpedance-based technologies, it is difficult to truly determine intravascular volume status in the perioperative course. It is up to the clinician to apply measured objective variables to the clinical situation so that short- and long-term outcome benefits are incorporated into volume management. This individualized guided fluid management has been shown to decrease mortality and surgical complications.[10]

XIII. **The Cardiovascular System Integration**

A. In normal healthy subjects, the cardiovascular system response to physiologic stress is predictable and reproducible. In its simplest form, if BP is altered, the integrated system response—sensors, controller, and effectors—senses the alteration and returns BP toward the original set point. This negative feedback permits us to lead our lives without considering the consequences or preparing for the disturbances to this system. As each effector is recruited to regulate BP, it can contribute less to compensating for an additional stress. It is easy to take the range and automaticity of this system response for granted.

B. The utilization of reserves depends on training levels, hydration status, and psychological state, among others. The compensatory limits of healthy humans are set through a complex physio-psycho state that ends with not being able to go on, that is, hitting the wall.

C. For patients, the response of effectors may be limited by pathology. The most common limiting factor is ischemic heart disease.

D. To maintain BP in the setting of hypotension, the cardiovascular system responses are predictable.

1. HR and contractility increase resulting in increased myocardial oxygen consumption. Wall tension may be increased or decreased. Since HR is a primary determinant of the onset of myocardial ischemia under anesthesia, its elevation is of particular concern.

2. Oxygen supply response is complex. Assuming no blood loss or alteration of oxygenation, increased HR leads to a reduction of diastolic time. Hence, endocardial perfusion time will be reduced. A decrease in diastolic systemic pressure may decrease the capillary perfusion pressure gradient (systemic diastolic pressure minus LVEDP) depending on the impact of hypotension on LVEDP.

3. **Intervention:** The anesthesiologist will most likely provide a small fluid bolus and administer phenylephrine in response to patient's hypotension. Preload and SVR will increase, allowing for a rise in SV. Normally, BP will rise, HR will fall, contractility will be reduced, diastolic time will lengthen, and perhaps coronary perfusion pressure will rise as well. Phenylephrine alone has a finite half-life and should only be used to mitigate hypotension quickly until the underlying cause is established.

4. **Response Time Required**

    a. Responding to hypotension is urgent and an everyday occurrence. Maintaining BP within 25% of the baseline is the goal. Defining hypotension can be difficult and in healthy patients considered a mean arterial pressure (MAP) of <65 mm Hg, for which end-organ perfusion may be compromised.

    b. However, in patients with significant disease burden, including but not limited to, hypertension, ischemic heart disease, valvular disease, and HF (systolic or diastolic), intraoperative hypotension measures need to be taken more vigorously, for which a MAP of 65 mm Hg alone may be inadequate.

    c. Ultimately, the goal is to maintain adequate perfusion to the cellular level.

    d. For the kidney, renal hypoperfusion secondary to hypovolemia, or low circulating volumes, can recover if identified and treated appropriately. This may progress to acute tubular necrosis and significant cellular injury. Injury has been linked to elevated mortality rates, longer hospital stays, and secondary detrimental clinical outcomes for patients.

    e. For a cardiac myocyte, the time constant falls somewhere between several minutes and several hours. The exact time constant is unclear for an individual myocyte, but normally it approaches an hour. After 4 hours, 50% of the myocytes will survive. Therefore, it is absolutely essential to be vigilant for ischemic changes.

    f. As an aside, cardiac anesthesiologists in the post-bypass period are confronted with BP management in the patient who frequently has a history of hypertension, renal insufficiency, peripheral vascular disease, and whose aorta has been recently cannulated (potentially increasing the risk of rupture with even modest hypertension). Systolic pressures are often kept under 100 mm Hg in this setting.

5. How long will it take at that pressure to cause damage? The answer is unclear, but such pressures are routinely maintained way beyond a few minutes.

6. As outlined above, phenylephrine administration elicits a potentially adverse physiologic impact if sustained. As the new controller of the sympathetic system, the anesthesia provider needs to consider why the hypotension occurred, if that reason is going to continue or get worse, how long the remaining physiologic reserves can maintain homeostasis in the face of further challenges, and finally the extent to which the ongoing management will negatively affect renal function.

7. These considerations are crucial in determining the likelihood of sustained—that is, through the course of the operation and the early postoperative period—hemodynamic stability of the patient.

8. Volume management is critical to this decision. Measures should be taken to assess volume status as "masking" hypovolemia with vasopressors can lead to long-term detrimental outcomes. Achieving the balance between the need for short-term intervention and long-term stability is the responsibility of the controller, that is, the anesthesia team's brain, during anesthesia.

CLINICAL PEARL

Masking hypovolemia with vasopressors can lead to detrimental outcomes, and objective variables should be used to provide goal-directed fluid therapy.

XIV. **Effect of Anesthesia Providers and Our Pharmacology on the Cardiovascular System**

A. **The Surgical Patient**
1. In the immediate preoperative period, perioperative hypertension is common, and its importance should be further investigated. Long-standing, uncontrolled hypertension has been shown to increase the risk of impaired myocardial function, stroke, and carotid atherosclerosis. Undergoing an anesthetic may increase short-term risks when hypertension is uncontrolled preoperatively.

2. Multiple factors contribute to perioperative hypertension including baseline sustained hypertension, anxiety, white-coat hypertension, and pain.

3. Obtaining a thorough history and physical is the first step to delineate the cause of perioperative hypertension. Is this patient on prescribed antihypertensives? Were they taken appropriately for the day of surgery? If not, providing the prescribed medication may be needed, especially in the setting of β-blockade.

4. White-coat hypertension, a probable symptom of anxiety, is well described in the literature without consensus about its prognostic significance. Some attribute this to the fight-or-flight response. It may contribute to cardiac-related complications and thus may be a predictor of increased cardiovascular risk alone.[11]

5. Assessing and treating pain should be prioritized. If hypertension does not improve despite initial efforts, a concern for sustained, poorly controlled hypertension is likely. Risks and benefits, as ill-defined as they are, should be considered prior to proceeding.

B. **The Anesthetic Choice**
1. For a healthy patient undergoing low-risk surgery, numerous retrospective studies suggest that in the presence of today's monitoring standards, anesthetic technique has little bearing on adverse patient outcomes.[12] Low surgical risk in the setting of normal physiologic reserves (HR, SVR, and venous volume) protects homeostasis to the extent that the margin for error is great. Provocative statement? Perhaps, but the American Society of Anesthesiologists' closed claims database supports this view.

2. For the high-risk patient with comorbidities, such as diabetes, vascular disease, ischemic, or valvular heart disease, consideration of their physiologic cardiac reserves becomes extremely important. The entire perioperative period subjects the patient to increased risk. Understanding the consequences of the patient's pathology on their physiologic reserves and the use of clinical management approaches to reduce the risk should influence the anesthetic choice through goal-directed therapy.[13]

3. In this chapter, physiologic reserves in the context of normal physiology were presented. The principles related to ventricular function, determinants of myocardial oxygen consumption, and physiologic reserves apply in the pathologic situation as well.

4. Of all the physiologic reserves discussed, one reserve is especially utilized in the intraoperative period and in the critically ill patient: venous capacitance. Volume management

is critical to constrict, replenish, or expand venous capacitance reserve. Resuscitation of hypovolemia is necessary for intravascular repletion to prevent organ hypoperfusion. However, multiple studies have elucidated that liberal fluid therapy and excessive fluid balance increase ICU complications and mortality. Therefore, incorporating goal-directed therapy is of paramount importance if we are to minimize overall risk for the patient with cardiovascular disease.

10   **C. Treating the Cause: Goal-Directed Therapy**

1. Despite a thorough understanding of physiology and pharmacology, there are times when clinical assessment is simply inadequate. Two very useful monitors in the setting of unresponsive hypotension (shock) under general anesthesia may be the PA catheter and the TEE examination.

2. The use of a PA catheter is one of the most debated issues. A national survey demonstrated that clinicians did not understand or know how to apply the physiologic principles underlying the interventions guided by PA catheter data.

3. Multiple trials have tried to assess the effectiveness of routine use of PA catheters in critically ill patients. The studies have concluded that the routine use of PA catheter-guided therapy is not recommended; however, these studies have their limitations in regard to the inadequate evaluation of the cardiac patient alone.[14]

4. Shock states can be attributed to intravascular volume depletion, significant vasodilation, decreased contractility, or mechanical obstruction. The use of the PA catheter may help identify the etiology with objective measures and identify the trajectory and need for escalation of care. Isseh et al,[14] eloquently reveal that PA catheters are significantly beneficial to cardiogenic shock patients and that the accurate interpretation of data actually may improve outcomes.

5. Certainly, the mere presence of a PA catheter could not improve outcome, in other words, "The yellow snake does no good when inserted."[15] Its use is reserved for high-risk patients and needs to be accompanied by a thorough understanding of its principles and technology, both in the OR and the intensive care unit.

CLINICAL PEARL

Many clinicians who use PA catheters lack adequate understanding of the physiologic information provided by these catheters.

6. TEE is the optimal tool for assessing ventricular volume status and regional wall motion abnormalities. An experienced echocardiographer can assess the volume status of the ventricle (intrathoracic blood volume) within a minute and almost as quickly can assess ventricular systolic function. These two data elements provide immediate help in the clinical management of unresponsive hypotension. Particularly in a setting where ventricular compliance can change rapidly (ischemia, acidosis, and sepsis), filling pressures from the PA catheter may or may not reflect volume status (actually more physiologically: sarcomere length or end-diastolic volume) of the ventricles. TEE is an essential tool precisely because it more accurately assesses cardiac preload under all conditions. As an example, TEE can assess the state of venous capacitance through observation of the impact of Trendelenburg and reverse Trendelenburg positions on diastolic volumes. With the increasing availability of three-dimensional echocardiography, real-time echocardiographic measurement of CO becomes more and more accessible. The availability of all physiologic reserves—HR, contractility, venous capacitance—can then be assessed. A drawback to TEE monitoring is its limited availability in the postoperative period (ie, once the patient has been awakened and extubated), hence transthoracic echocardiography (TTE) skills can contribute importantly to intravascular volume assessment both before and after surgery.

7. However, if the physiologic principles of preload, afterload, and contractility are not well understood, then their application to a circulatory problem such as hypotension will be unsound. There are two approaches to this problem: ignore it or develop goal-directed protocols. Learning the principles of goal-directed therapy can allow you to scientifically manage fluid therapy for most patients. The detailed application of goal-directed therapy is complex and varied, and it extends beyond the scope of this chapter. The studies of Walsh et al[16] and Hamilton et al[17] demonstrate the complexity of this topic.

REFERENCES

1. Wikipedia. *Intercalated disc.* https://en.wikipedia.org/wiki/Intercalated_disc#:~:text=Intercalated%20discs%20are%20complex %20structures,connect%20to%20the%20closest%20sarcomere
2. Lilly LS. *Pathophysiology of Heart Disease: An Introduction to Cardiovascular Medicine.* 7th ed. Wolters Kluwer; 2021.
3. Honig C. *Modern Cardiovascular Physiology.* Little, Brown and Company; 1981.
4. Wehrwein EA, Joyner MJ. Regulation of blood pressure by the arterial baroreflex and autonomic nervous system. *Handb Clin Neurol.* 2013;117:89-102.
5. Hemmings HC, Egan TD. *Pharmacology and Physiology for Anesthesia.* Elsevier Health Sciences; 2012.
6. Crystal GJ, Salem MR. The Bainbridge and the "reverse" Bainbridge reflexes: history, physiology, and clinical relevance. *Anesth Analg.* 2012;114:520-532.
7. Warltier DC, Campagna JA, Carter C. Clinical relevance of the Bezold-Jarisch reflex. *Anesthesiology.* 2003;98:1250-1260. doi:10.1097/00000542-200305000-00030
8. Mellander S, Johansson B. Control of resistance, exchange, and capacitance functions in the peripheral circulation. *Pharmacol Rev.* 1968;20:117-196.
9. Mellander S. Comparative studies on the adrenergic neuro-hormonal control of resistance and capacitance blood vessels in the cat. *Acta Physiol Scand Suppl.* 1960;50(176):1-86.
10. Kendrick JB, Kaye AD, Tong Y, et al. Goal-directed fluid therapy in the perioperative setting. *J Anaesthesiol Clin Pharmacol.* 2019;35(suppl 1):S29-S34.
11. Nuredini G, Saunders A, Rajkumar C, Okorie M. Current status of white coat hypertension: where are we? *Ther Adv Cardiovasc Dis.* 2020;14:1753944720931637.
12. Neumann MD, Fleisher LA. Risk of anesthesia. In: Miller RD, Eriksson LI, Fleisher LA, et al, eds. *Miller's Anesthesia.* 8th ed. Elsevier Saunders; 2015:1056-1084.
13. Gan TJ, Soppitt A, Maroof M, et al. Goal-directed intraoperative fluid administration reduces length of hospital stay after major surgery. *Anesthesiology.* 2002;97:820-826.
14. Isseh IN, Lee R, Khedraki R, Hoffman K. A critical review of hemodynamically guided therapy for cardiogenic shock: old habits die hard. *Curr Treat Options Cardiovasc Med.* 2021;23(5):29. doi:10.1007/s11936-021-00903-8
15. Iberti TJ, Fischer EP, Leibowitz AB, et al. A multicenter study of physicians' knowledge of the pulmonary artery catheter. Pulmonary Artery Catheter Study Group. *JAMA.* 1990;264(22):2928-2932.
16. Walsh SR, Tang TY, Farooq N, et al. Perioperative fluid restriction reduces complications after major gastrointestinal surgery. *Surgery.* 2008;143(4):466-468.
17. Hamilton MA, Mythen MG, Ackland GL. Less is not more: a lack of evidence for intraoperative fluid restriction improving outcome after major elective gastrointestinal surgery. *Anesth Analg.* 2006;102(3):970-971.

Pharmacology 3

Benjamin Walker, Robert O'Neal, Warner Smith, and Ken Johnson

KEY POINTS

1. Starting a vasoactive infusion can require up to 15 minutes to reach near steady state. In the fast tempo perioperative environment, this may be too long. Administering a small bolus before starting the infusion markedly reduces the time to reach near steady state.

2. The onset and duration of effect for intravenous administration of vasoactive drugs are not well described by half-life. Caution should be used when using half-life to characterize the pharmacologic behavior of fast-acting intravenous agents.

3. Characterizing cardiovascular function in terms of changes in preload, contractility, heart rate, systemic vascular resistance (SVR), and pulmonary vascular resistance (PVR) provides a useful construct when selecting the appropriate inotrope, vasoconstrictor, or vasodilator to treat hemodynamic instability.

4. Inotropes are often combined with vasopressor drugs to offset the side effects (eg, milrinone in combination with phenylephrine).

5. Antiarrhythmic drugs are classified based on their mechanism of action: sodium channel blockers (class I), β-adrenergic receptors (class II), potassium channel blockers (class III), and calcium channel blockers (class IV).

6. Inhaled pulmonary vasodilators are effective in treating perioperative pulmonary hypertension and increased PVR while minimizing unwanted systemic vasodilation.

7. Antifibrinolytics are an essential blood conservation strategy in cardiac surgery.

I. Introduction

Cardiac anesthesiologists are often called upon to care for patients with hemodynamic instability or intravascular coagulation issues. Potent medications play an important role in managing these problems. A working knowledge of pharmacologic principles, cardiovascular physiology, and blood coagulation function is useful when selecting medications and formulating their appropriate dose. Given the large repository of available pharmacology, cardiovascular, and coagulation literature, the aim of this chapter is to distill out clinically relevant information that can be efficiently adapted to patient care. To that end, the chapter presents a concise and structured summary of frequently used vasoactive and anticoagulation medications. It is organized into sections that cover inotropes, vasopressors, vasodilators, antiarrhythmic drugs, pulmonary vasodilators, anticoagulants, and antifibrinolytics. Each drug is described by its mechanism of action, dose, pharmacokinetics, clinical uses, advantages, and disadvantages. Where appropriate, cardiovascular drugs will be also characterized by their impact on preload, contractility, afterload, heart rate, and rhythm. Given that sources of hemodynamic instability vary, this is a useful construct to consider when identifying which agent is best to use.

II. Pharmacologic Principles

A. **Pharmacokinetics:** Describes the relationship between drug dose and plasma or effect site drug concentrations over time. Important descriptors of pharmacokinetics include distribution, metabolism, and elimination.[1]

1. **Distribution**
   a. Represents the volume within the body that a drug is diluted to achieve a measured blood concentration
   b. Characterizes how drug distributes between the vascular compartment and peripheral tissues and how drug binds to proteins within plasma and peripheral tissues

2. **Metabolism**
   a. Describes the biotransformation of drugs, so they are more efficiently eliminated
   b. Biotransformation includes chemical structure modification through hydrolysis, oxidation, reduction or conjugation, or attachment to another molecule, making it inert and water-soluble and rendering it more readily excretable.
   c. Most drug metabolism is done by liver cytochrome P450 enzymes and other enzymes such as monoamine oxidase (MAO) and catechol-*O*-methyltransferase (COMT) found in the liver, central nervous system, and other organs.

3. **Elimination**
   a. Describes removal of drug from the body
   b. Drug is excreted either unchanged or following biotransformation.
   c. Drugs are typically excreted by the kidneys into urine or by the liver into bile.
   d. Some drugs are also excreted by the lungs, tears, saliva, sweat, and breast milk.

4. **Pharmacokinetic models**
   a. Characterize how the body interacts with drugs.
   b. Use parameters to estimate how drug concentrations behave over time.
   c. Model parameters include volume of distribution, clearance, half-life, context-sensitive half-life, peak concentrations, time to peak concentrations, area under the concentration over time curve, among others.

    d. Through simulation, models are used to estimate how long a patient will be exposed to a drug following selected dosing regimens and illustrate clinically relevant concepts that influence approaches to dosing medications.

    e. **Sample simulation:** Plasma epinephrine concentrations that result from an infusion, or a bolus and an infusion of epinephrine (Figure 3.1) using published pharmacokinetic parameters[2]

    f. This simulation illustrates an infusion that was run for 60 minutes and then turned off:

      (1) Simply starting an infusion requires up to 15 minutes to reach a near steady state. In the fast tempo perioperative environment, this lag time may be too long.

      (2) Administering a small bolus before starting the infusion reduces the time to 5 minutes to reach near steady state.

      (3) The time it takes for plasma concentrations to drop once the infusion has ended is rapid. Plasma concentration drops by 50% within 2 minutes, suggesting that once the infusion is terminated, the drug effect will quickly dissipate.

B. Drug Delivery Time

   1. An important consideration when administering a vasoactive drug in an acute setting to treat hemodynamic instability is understanding the lag time between administration and achieving the desired effect.

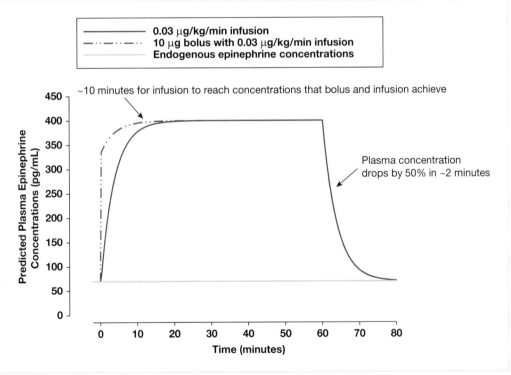

FIGURE 3.1 Simulation of predicted plasma epinephrine concentrations for a 1-hour continuous infusion at 0.03 μg/kg/min with and without a 10-μg bolus based on published epinephrine pharmacokinetic model parameters.[2] The left arrow highlights the difference in plasma concentrations that result from a bolus followed by infusion versus just an infusion. The time difference between the two dosing regimens to achieve the near-steady-state concentration of 400 pg/mL is 10 minutes. The right arrow highlights the 50% decrement time once the infusion is stopped. The gray line indicates the baseline endogenous epinephrine concentrations. These simulations assume instantaneous drug delivery and do not account for the time required for the drug to go from an infusion pump to the distal end of the catheter. Once an infusion pump is started, it can take an additional 3-6 minutes to achieve steady-state concentrations at the end of a catheter. Assumptions in this estimate include the epinephrine concentration of 16 μg/mL, a patient weight of 80 kg, the carrier infusion rate of between 10 and 30 mL/h, and the dead space volume of 0.6-0.8 mL in a multiport manifold and the 16-gauge lumen of a 16 cm 7 French triple-lumen catheter.

2. Elements that contribute to this lag time include the time required for a drug to
   a. Be delivered from the infusion pump to the bloodstream.
   b. Circulate through the cardiovascular system.
   c. Diffuse to the site of action and elicit an effect.
3. Investigators have studied the time required for a drug to go from an infusion pump to the distal end of vascular access using conventional infusion pumps, multiport manifolds, and central venous access catheters.
   a. Based on in vitro work with a multiport manifold connected to a triple-lumen catheter, Moss et al studied the time to reach a steady-state concentration of methylene blue dye administered at various carrier infusion and drug infusion rates.[3]
   b. Applying their methods to the epinephrine infusion presented in Figure 3.1, it takes approximately 3-6 minutes to achieve a steady-state concentration at the end of the triple-lumen catheter.
      (1) Circulation time, assuming a normal cardiac output (CO), is 45-60 seconds.
      (2) The time required for a drug to diffuse and elicit an effect depends on the location of the target tissue bed. This time period, known as *biophase*, is characterized by the lag between the peak concentration and peak effect.
      (3) The target tissue is the vascular endothelium for many vasoactive drugs, which have an almost negligible biophase lag time.
      (4) Other drugs that act in the central nervous system or in muscle tissue have longer biophase times (eg, digoxin can require 5-30 minutes to achieve effect following intravenous [IV] administration).

C. **Pharmacodynamics**
   1. Describe drug concentration-effect relationships.
   2. Models use parameters to estimate these relationships.
   3. Common pharmacodynamic parameters include the concentration associated with a 50% likelihood of effect and the slope of the concentration-effect relationship.

D. **Combined Pharmacokinetic and Pharmacodynamic Models**
   1. By combining pharmacokinetic and pharmacodynamic models, simulations can be used to estimate two parameters of interest: the onset and duration of effect.
   2. Figure 3.2 presents a simulation of predicted plasma epinephrine concentrations for a small bolus and 1-hour infusion, and the plasma concentrations associated with selected effects of epinephrine based on previously published data as presented in Table 3.1.[4]
      a. Although there is some overlap, each effect has a different epinephrine concentration range.
      b. A rise in heart rate occurs at low plasma concentrations, a rise in systolic blood pressure occurs at moderate concentrations, and a decrease in diastolic blood pressures and increase in blood glucose occur at higher plasma concentrations.
      c. Because plasma concentrations rise quickly with administration and rapidly fall with infusion termination, all these effects have an onset within seconds and dissipate within minutes of infusion termination.
      d. The duration of effect is the duration of the infusion.
   3. With IV administration, most vasoactive drugs achieve an onset of effect within minutes but may require more than 10 minutes to achieve their maximal concentrations and effects.
      a. Onset and duration of effect time estimates require high-quality clinically validated models.
      b. For most drugs presented in this chapter, however, combined pharmacokinetic-pharmacodynamic models and corresponding simulations are not yet available.
      c. Given this limitation, where available, estimates of onset and duration of action are presented based on published clinical observations rather than model predictions.

E. **Drug Variability**
   1. One of the vexing challenges faced when administering drugs is the marked variability in how they behave across patient populations.
   2. Following conventional dosing regimens, desired or undesired effects may be excessive, last too long, not long enough, etc.

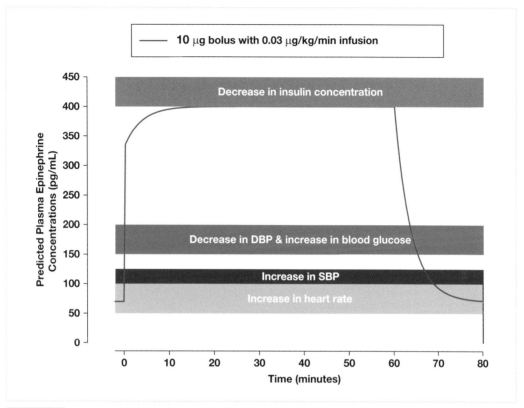

FIGURE 3.2 Simulations of predicted plasma epinephrine concentrations for a 1-hour continuous infusion at 0.03 µg/kg/min with a 10 µg bolus and predicted plasma concentration ranges for changes in heart rate (light gray), systolic blood pressure (SBP, purple), diastolic blood pressure and rise in plasma glucose (DBP, green), and reduction in insulin concentrations (dark yellow) based on published epinephrine pharmacokinetic model parameters and hemodynamic measurements and measured epinephrine, glucose, and insulin concentrations. (Derived from Clutter WE, Bier DM, Shah SD, Cryer PE. Epinephrine plasma metabolic clearance rates and physiologic thresholds for metabolic and hemodynamic actions in man. *J Clin Invest.* 1980;66(1):94-101.)

TABLE 3.1   Changes in Hemodynamic and Metabolic Measures in Response to Increasing Infusion Rates of Epinephrine and Their Corresponding Plasma Epinephrine Concentrations Observed in Human Volunteers

Epinephrine Infusion Rate (µg/kg/min)	Observed Mean Plasma Epinephrine Concentration	Heart Rate Change (bpm)	Systolic Blood Pressure Change (mm Hg)	Diastolic Blood Pressure Change (mm Hg)	Change in Plasma Glucose Concentration (mg/dL)	Change in Insulin Concentration (µU/L)
0.005	114	+9	+8	+1	+2	−1
0.01	219	+8	+6	−2	+12	+1
0.03	412	+13	+16	−10	+36	−2
0.06	715	+21	+22	−13	+68	−16

Data from Clutter WE, Bier DM, Shah SD, Cryer PE. Epinephrine plasma metabolic clearance rates and physiologic thresholds for metabolic and hemodynamic actions in man. *J Clin Invest.* 1980;66(1):94-101.

3. Sources of variability that are not readily apparent before drug administration include the following:
    a. Patient conditions such as intravascular volume status, cardiac function, metabolic derangements, plasma pH, temperature, circulating inflammatory substances, plasma protein concentrations, etc
    b. How a drug is taken up into circulating blood and then surrounding tissues (volume of distribution)
    c. Drug metabolism and elimination (clearance)
    d. Variability in drug sensitivity
    e. Drug-drug interactions

F. **Pharmacogenomics**
    1. Variability in proteins that code for enzymes responsible for metabolism, drug transport into and out of cells, membrane receptors and ion channels, and intracellular function can contribute to interindividual variability in drug responses.
    2. Many genes have been well studied, leading to the discovery of numerous gene variants some of which have been shown to alter drug behavior. There has been substantial discovery in this domain[5] showing promise in developing tools to refine dosing regimens and minimize the risk of drug-related adverse events.
        a. As an example, investigators have studied the use of introducing pharmacogenomics into perioperative care using a genomic prescribing system embedded into an electronic health record.[6]
        b. This included genotype data for selected genes known to influence nearly 50 medications frequently used during the perioperative period. These include genes for adrenergic receptors, nitric oxide synthase (NOS), cytochrome P450 enzymes, and G proteins, among others.
        c. A personalized list of medications and their associated pharmacogenomic information were graded according to risk of adverse conditions with a green, yellow, and red stop light advisory display.
        d. Although innovative, this type of practice advisory will require validation of its feasibility and clinical relevance.

III. **Inotropes**
    Positive inotropes increase myocardial contractility. Although pathways are different, inotropes all increase calcium availability in cardiac myocyte, increasing contractility (Table 3.2). Comparing the relative changes in preload, contractility, heart rate, systemic vascular resistance (SVR), and pulmonary vascular resistance (PVR) provides a useful construct when selecting the appropriate inotrope for each clinical situation (Figure 3.3).

TABLE 3.2 Inotropic Drugs and Their Adrenergic Receptor Activity

Drug	α_1-Activity	β_1-Activity	β_2-Activity	D_1-Activity
Epinephrine				
0.01-0.05 μg/kg/min	+	++	++	0
>0.05 μg/kg/min	+++	++	++	0
Norepinephrine	+++	++	0	0
Dobutamine	0	+++	+	0
Isoproterenol	0	+++	+++	0
Dopamine				
0.5-3 μg/kg/min	0	0	0	+
3-10 μg/kg/min	0	+	0	++
>10 μg/kg/min	+++	++	0	++
Ephedrine	+	+	+	0
Phenylephrine	+++	0	0	0

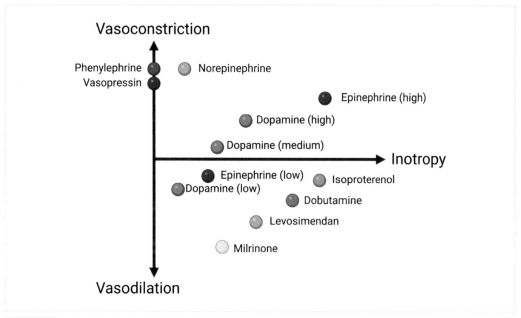

FIGURE 3.3   Summary of physiologic effects of inotropes and vasopressors. (Created with BioRender.com.)

A. **Epinephrine (Adrenaline)**[7]
1. **Action:** Potent adrenergic α_1-, β_1-, and β_2-agonist. β_1 (inotropic) effects predominate at low concentrations, α_1 (vasoconstrictor) effects predominate at high concentrations.

Preload	↑
Contractility	↑↑↑
Heart rate	↑↑
SVR	↑↑
PVR	↑

2. **Dose**

IV bolus	Hypotension: 5-10 µg Cardiac arrest: 1 mg
Infusion	0.02-0.3 µg/kg/min
Endotracheal tube	1 × IV bolus dose

3. **Pharmacokinetics**

Onset	1-3 min
Duration of action	2-5 min
Metabolism	COMT and MAO
Excretion	Urine unchanged

4. **Clinical uses**
   a. Separation from cardiopulmonary bypass (CPB) when CO is low
   b. **Anaphylaxis:** Reduces mucosal edema, bronchodilator, and stabilizes mast cells

    c. Cardiac arrest: Increases mean arterial pressure (MAP) to improve cerebral blood flow

    d. Local anesthetic toxicity: Low dose (1 µg/kg) to enhance myocardial contractility. High-dose administration is discouraged.

    e. Severe hypotension with bradycardia

    f. Acute right ventricular (RV) dysfunction

    g. Severe asthma

5. **Advantages**
   a. Short duration of action, predictable response, and easily titratable
   b. Tachycardia attenuated by vagal response
   c. No absolute contraindications against use

6. **Disadvantages (Figure 3.4)**
   a. Increases myocardial oxygen consumption, worsening ischemia
   b. Potent α_1-agonism at high doses can cause renal, mesenteric, and peripheral limb ischemia.
   c. Causes increase in serum concentrations of lactic acid and glucose
   d. Can precipitate hemodynamic instability in patients with dynamic outflow obstruction
   e. Administration with β-blocker can result in severe hypertension from unopposed α_1-agonism.

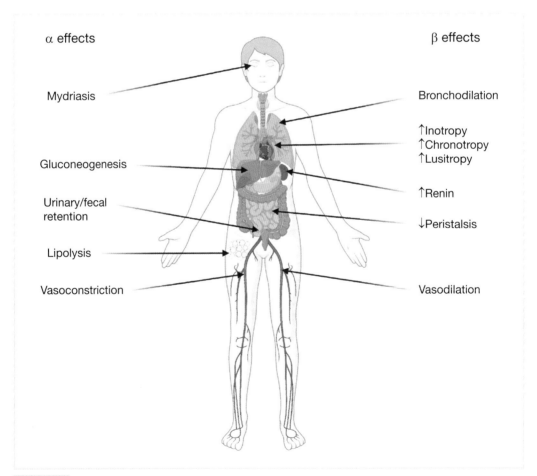

FIGURE 3.4 Physiologic effects of α- and β-stimulation. (Created with BioRender.com.)

CLINICAL PEARL

Epinephrine is widely used during separation from CPB. At lower doses it is effective at promoting contractility (eg, 0.03 μg/kg/min), and at higher doses, it is effective at treating low SVR (eg, 0.1 μg/kg/min).

    B. Norepinephrine (Levophed)[8]

      1. Action: Potent sympathomimetic with α_1-, α_2-, and β_1-agonism. Promotes arteriole vasoconstriction and cardiac inotropy. Has limited β_2-activity. Primary physiologic postganglionic sympathetic neurotransmitter

Preload	↑
Contractility	↑
Heart rate	↓↓
SVR	↑↑↑
PVR	↑↑

      2. Dose

IV bolus	5-10 μg
Infusion	0.02-0.5 μg/kg/min

      3. Pharmacokinetics

Onset	1-3 min
Duration of action	3-5 min
Metabolism	COMT and MAO
Excretion	Urine unchanged

      4. Clinical use

        a. Hypotension due to low SVR states. Effective in septic shock, vasoplegic syndrome, and patients taking angiotensin-converting enzyme inhibitors (ACEi) and angiotensin receptor blockers (ARBs)

        b. Temporary therapy for hypovolemia until blood volume is restored

      5. Advantages

        a. Short duration of action and easily titratable

        b. β_1-Agonism may be useful in states with low SVR and an increase in cardiac contractility is desired.[9]

        c. Redistributes blood flow to brain and heart from other vascular beds

        d. Elicits intense α_1-, α_2-agonism; may be effective as vasoconstrictor when phenylephrine lacks efficacy

      6. Disadvantages

        a. Reduced end-organ perfusion: Risk of renal, skin, hepatic, mesenteric, and extremity ischemia with high doses

        b. Increased afterload and contractility may precipitate myocardial ischemia.

        c. Increase in PVR

        d. May precipitate coronary vasospasm

        e. Higher rate of atrial fibrillation and severe postoperative outcomes when compared to vasopressin for post-pump vasoplegia[10]

CLINICAL PEARL

Although norepinephrine improves blood pressure, vasoconstriction reduces renal/mesenteric/peripheral perfusion and may cause ischemia to these organs.

C. Dobutamine (Dobutrex, Inotrex)[11]

1. **Action:** Synthetic selective catecholamine with primarily β_1-agonism

Preload	0
Contractility	↑↑
Heart rate	↑
SVR	↓
PVR	↓

2. **Dose**

IV bolus	No bolus dosing
Infusion	2-20 µg/kg/min

3. **Pharmacokinetics[12]**

Onset	1 min
Duration of action	3-5 min
Metabolism	COMT and MAO
Excretion	Urine unchanged

4. **Clinical uses**
   a. Used for noninvasive pharmacologic stress echocardiography
   b. Short-term management of cardiogenic shock, especially in patients with high SVR
   c. Patients requiring epinephrine perioperatively will often be transitioned to dobutamine postoperatively once the effect of vasodilatory anesthetics dissipates.

5. **Advantages**
   a. Short duration of action, predictable response, and easily titratable
   b. High β-agonism and minimal α-agonism result in reduced afterload and reduced cardiac filling pressures.
   c. Better than dopamine for improving cardiac index[13,14]
   d. Causes less tachycardia and hypotension than isoproterenol[15]

6. **Disadvantages**
   a. Increases myocardial oxygen consumption, worsening ischemia
   b. Pro-arrhythmogenic, can precipitate rapid ventricular response in patients with atrial fibrillation
   c. No survival benefit. May increase mortality in patients with severe heart failure[16]

CLINICAL PEARL

Dobutamine has limited perioperative use without the addition of vasopressors due to a synergistic interaction between its β_2-mediated vasodilation and general anesthetics leading to hypotension.

D. Isoproterenol (Isuprel)[17,18]

1. **Action:** Synthetic catecholamine with nonselective β-agonism

Preload	0
Contractility	↑↑
Heart rate	↑↑
SVR	↓↓
PVR	↓

2. **Dose**

IV bolus	No bolus dosing
Infusion	0.01-0.2 µg/kg/min

3. **Pharmacokinetics**[19]

Onset	1 min
Duration of action	3-4 min
Metabolism	COMT and MAO
Excretion	Urine unchanged

4. **Clinical uses**
   a. To treat refractory bradycardia (until temporary pacing established)
   b. Unmasks underlying arrhythmias in electrophysiology lab for mapping and ablation
   c. To provoke dynamic left ventricular outflow obstruction
5. **Advantages**
   a. Short duration of action, predictable response, and easily titratable
   b. Increases heart rate without being attenuated by vagal response
6. **Disadvantages**
   a. Significant increase in myocardial oxygen consumption that worsens ischemia[18]
   b. Pro-arrhythmogenic

CLINICAL PEARL

Side-effect profile, high cost, and lack of availability limit its intraoperative use.

E. **Dopamine (Intropin)**[20,21]
   1. **Action:** D_1-, α_1-, and β_1-agonist. At low doses, it is a D_1 receptor agonist causing renal, mesenteric, and coronary vasodilation. At medium doses, it adds β_1-receptor agonism and causes release of norepinephrine. At high doses, it adds α_1-receptor agonism.
   2. **Dose**

Dose	Low 0.5-2 µg/kg/min	Medium 2-10 µg/kg/min	High >10 µg/kg/min
Preload	0	0	0
Contractility	0	↑	↑↑
Heart rate	0	↑	↑↑
Afterload	↓	↓	↑↑
PVR	0	↓	↑

   a. Clinical effects at different doses vary significantly between patients and are difficult to predict.
   3. **Pharmacokinetics**

Onset	1 min
Duration of action	3-4 min
Metabolism	COMT and MAO
Excretion	Urine unchanged

   4. **Clinical uses:** Due to multiple disadvantages, rarely used clinically
   5. **Advantages:** Low dose selectively improves renal blood flow and natriuresis.

6. **Disadvantages**
   a. Higher mortality for treatment of shock compared to norepinephrine[22]
   b. Worse than dobutamine for the management of cardiogenic shock[14]
   c. No evidence that it reduces the risk of renal dysfunction[23]
   d. Pro-arrhythmic and increases myocardial oxygen demand
   e. Reduces ventilatory response to hypoxemia
   f. Extravasated IV will cause skin necrosis.

CLINICAL PEARL

Promotes renal blood flow and natriuresis; however, there is no proven outcome benefit. Rarely used intraoperatively due to side effects, variable clinical response, and better alternative agents.

F. **Ephedrine (Akovaz, Corphedra):** See "Vasopressors" section
G. **Milrinone (Primacor)**[24,25]
   1. **Action:** Synthetic inodilator that inhibits phosphodiesterase type III

Preload	0
Contractility	↑↑
Heart rate	0
SVR	↓
PVR	↓

   2. **Dose**

Loading dose	10-50 µg/kg over 10 min
Infusion	0.2-0.75 µg/kg/min
Inhaled dose	2-4 mg (in nebulizer)

   a. Dose should be reduced in low renal clearance.
   b. Loading dose can cause profound hypotension. Use caution in low SVR states; consider avoiding or administering a lower bolus dose.
   3. **Pharmacokinetics**

Onset	5-10 min
Duration of action	3-6 h
Metabolism	Renal
Excretion	Urine unchanged

   4. **Clinical uses**
   a. Cardiogenic shock, especially when weaning from bypass
   b. Right heart failure; it increases inotropy while decreasing PVR.
   c. Pulmonary hypertension
   5. **Advantages**
   a. Maintains potency in patients with chronic heart failure who have downregulated catecholamine receptors
   b. Increases success of weaning from bypass in high-risk patients[26]
   c. Improves flow in bypass grafts[27]
   d. Inhaled milrinone decreases PVR and increases inotropy without decreasing MAP.[28]
   6. **Disadvantages**
   a. Vasodilation may require pressors to maintain MAP.
   b. Vasopressin is preferred over norepinephrine for management of milrinone induced low SVR as it does not increase PVR.
   c. Pro-arrhythmogenic

4

CLINICAL PEARL

Milrinone is a slow-acting phosphodiesterase 3 (PDE3) inhibitor that acts as an inodilator and reduces PVR. It is particularly effective in right heart failure as it increases RV contractility and decreases afterload.

H. **Digoxin (Lanoxin)**[29]
   1. **Action:** Inhibits Na^+, K^+, ATPase in myocyte, increasing cytosolic Ca^{2+} to interact with myosin/actin

Preload	0
Contractility	↑↑
Heart rate	↓
Afterload	↓
PVR	0

   2. **Dose**

IV loading dose	0.5-1 mg over 10 min
Infusion	No infusion dosing

      a. Therapeutic serum digoxin level: 0.5-2.5 ng/mL
   3. **Pharmacokinetics**

Onset	5-30 min
Duration of action	3-6 h
Metabolism	None
Excretion	Urine unchanged

   4. **Clinical uses**
      a. Systolic heart failure, especially concomitant atrial fibrillation
      b. Control of supraventricular arrhythmias
   5. **Advantages**
      a. Increased inotropy without increase in myocardial oxygen demand (in congestive heart failure [CHF])
      b. Therapeutic benefit greater in patients with a dilated ventricle
      c. Slows ventricular response to atrial fibrillation
   6. **Disadvantages**
      a. Long-term use increases mortality in patients with systolic heart failure.[30]
      b. Narrow therapeutic index results in high incidence of side effects.
      c. Contraindicated in patients with an accessory electrical pathway
      d. Exogenous administration of calcium in digitalized patients can precipitate ventricular arrhythmias.
      e. **Digoxin toxicity:** Arrhythmias, yellow-green visual disturbance, gastrointestinal upset
      f. **Digoxin toxicity treatment:** Digitalis antibodies, correct hypokalemia, lidocaine, magnesium

I. **Levosimendan (Simdax)**[31]
   1. **Action:** Binds to cardiac troponin C, increasing sensitivity to calcium and increasing cardiac contractility

Preload	0
Contractility	↑↑
Heart rate	0
Afterload	↓
PVR	↓

2. **Dose**

IV bolus (loading dose)	6-12 µg/kg
Infusion	0.005-2 µg/kg/min

   a. Not approved for use in the United States. Oral version under review by the U.S. Food and Drug Administration
   b. Loading dose not recommended if low blood pressure
3. **Pharmacokinetics**

Onset	5 min
Duration of action	12 h
Metabolism	Hepatic
Excretion	Urine/feces

4. **Clinical uses**
   a. Acute heart failure
   b. Exacerbation of CHF
5. **Advantages**
   a. Increases inotropy via separate mechanism from β-agonists and PDEi
   b. Does not change intracellular Ca^{2+} levels and does not impair diastolic function
   c. Increases contractility without increasing myocardial oxygen demand
   d. Reduces afterload and improves coronary perfusion
   e. Effects are not diminished by β-blocker effect.
6. **Disadvantages**
   a. Not available in the United States
   b. Reduces afterload that can decrease myocardial perfusion pressure
   c. Active metabolites cause refractory tachycardia and hypotension.
J. **Glucagon (Glucagen)**[32]
   1. **Action:** Peptide hormone that binds to G-protein-coupled receptor, resulting in increased cyclic adenosine monophosphate (cAMP) and thus increased contractility (separate mechanism from β-receptor agonism)

Preload	0
Contractility	↑↑
Heart rate	↑↑
Afterload	0
PVR	0

   2. **Dose**

IV bolus	1-5 mg IV (slowly)
Infusion	25-75 µg/min

   3. **Pharmacokinetics**

Onset	Rapid: 3-5 min
Duration of action	20-30 min
Metabolism	Proteolysis in liver/kidney/plasma
Excretion	Unknown

   4. **Clinical uses**
      a. Severe hypoglycemia from insulin overdose
      b. Bradycardia from β-blocker overdose
      c. Sphincter of Oddi spasm

5. **Advantages:** Positive inotropic effect even in the presence of β-blockade
6. **Disadvantages**
    a. Can result in significant tachycardia
    b. High risk of severe nausea and vomiting

CLINICAL PEARL

Glucagon is used as a treatment for iatrogenic β-blocker overdose; it is a positive inotrope that maintains efficacy in the presence of overwhelming β-blockade.

IV. Vasopressors

Vasopressors are medications that induce vasoconstriction and elevate MAP. Vasopressors differ from inotropes, which increase cardiac contractility; however, many drugs have both vasopressor and inotropic effects (Table 3.3). Although the pathways by which these medications act are different, they share the common endpoint of increasing SVR. α-Adrenergic, angiotensin II, and vasopressin receptors mediate vasoconstriction (both arterial and venous).

A. **Phenylephrine (Neo-Synephrine)**[33]
    1. **Action:** Selective α_1-agonist. Primarily arteriole vasoconstriction (arteriole > venous). Transient increase in preload from hepatic and splanchnic vasoconstriction

Preload	↑
Contractility	0
Heart rate	↓↓
SVR	↑↑↑
PVR	↑↑↑

    2. **Dose**

IV bolus	50-100 µg
Infusion	0.1-2 µg/kg/min

    3. **Pharmacokinetics**

Onset	1-3 min
Duration of action	5-20 min
Metabolism	Redistribution and metabolism by MAO
Excretion	Urine 80% (2.6% unchanged)

    4. **Clinical use**
        a. Hypotension due to low SVR states
        b. Temporary therapy of hypovolemia until blood volume is restored

TABLE 3.3   Receptor Types and Vasoactive Effects

Receptor	Effect
Alpha 1 (α_1)	Vasoconstriction
Alpha 2 (α_2)	Norepinephrine reuptake Transient vasoconstriction
Beta 1 (β_1)	Inotropy, chronotropy, vasoconstriction (high doses)
Beta 2 (β_2)	Vasodilation
Vasopressin 1 (V_1)	Vasoconstriction
Angiotensin 1 (AT_1)	Vasoconstriction

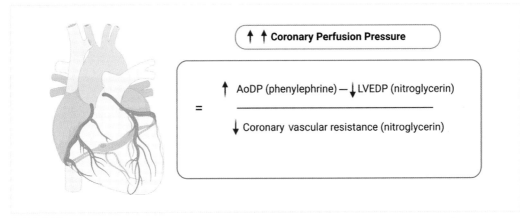

FIGURE 3.5 Schematic presenting a pharmacologic balloon pump to improve coronary perfusion pressure. Vasoactive drugs that make up the balloon pump include phenylephrine and nitroglycerin. Their opposing actions improved coronary perfusion pressure in similar fashion to a mechanical balloon pump. AoDP, aortic diastolic pressure; LVEDP, left ventricular end-diastolic pressure.

    c. Maintain or increase coronary perfusion pressure in patients with significant coronary artery disease (CAD) or aortic stenosis (Figure 3.5)
    d. Reduces dynamic left ventricular outflow tract (LVOT) obstruction during systolic anterior motion (SAM) of the mitral valve
    e. Component of the pharmacologic balloon pump when used with nitroglycerin
  5. Advantages
    a. Short duration of action, predictable response, and easily titratable
    b. Increases perfusion to brain, kidney, and heart in low SVR states
  6. Disadvantages
    a. Can cause significant reflex bradycardia. Caution in patients who are bradycardic at baseline
    b. May reduce stroke volume (SV) and CO secondary to increased afterload
    c. Increase in PVR. Vasopressin may be a better choice for systemic hypotension in pulmonary hypertension.[9]
    d. Significant microvascular vasoconstriction may cause decreased renal, mesenteric, and extremity perfusion. Caution with high doses, especially in patients who are profoundly hypovolemic

CLINICAL PEARL

Phenylephrine is an effective vasoconstrictor for the management of hypotension. It often reduces heart rate. Caution should be used in patients with low heart rates. Although it can improve blood pressure, it can reduce CO and increase PVR. This may lead to poor splanchnic and hepatic perfusion.

  B. Vasopressin (Vasostrict)[34]
    1. Action: Endogenous antidiuretic hormone (ADH) that activates smooth muscle V_1 receptors

Preload	0
Contractility	0
Heart rate	↓↓
SVR	↑↑↑
PVR	0

2. Dose

IV bolus	0.2-1 unit
Infusion	0.02-0.1 units/min

   a. One unit bolus is equivalent to 25 minutes of a 0.04 unit/min infusion.
3. Pharmacokinetics

Onset	Rapid
Duration of action	5-20 min
Metabolism	Hepatic and renal
Excretion	Urine (6% unchanged)

4. Clinical use
   a. Hypotension due to low SVR states. Effective in septic shock, vasoplegic syndrome, and patients taking ACEi/ARBs[35]
   b. Temporary therapy for hypovolemia until blood volume is restored
   c. Clinical uses are like phenylephrine.
5. Advantages
   a. Short duration of action and easily titratable
   b. Vasopressor of choice in the setting of pulmonary hypertension and systemic hypotension[36]
   c. Increases perfusion to brain, kidney, and heart in low SVR states
   d. Reduction in acute kidney injury (AKI) relative to norepinephrine[10]
   e. Lower rate of atrial fibrillation and severe postoperative outcomes when compared to norepinephrine for post-pump vasoplegia[10,36]
6. Disadvantages
   a. Very potent. Blood pressure response can be unpredictable to bolus doses.
   b. May reduce SV and CO secondary to increased afterload
   c. Reduces splanchnic blood flow and can contribute to gut ischemia, especially when combined with other agents
   d. No longer recommended during cardiac arrest as an alternative to epinephrine[37]
   e. Disadvantages are similar to phenylephrine.

CLINICAL PEARL

Vasopressin is most useful in the setting of post-pump vasoplegia, hypotension, and pulmonary hypertension.

   C. Norepinephrine (Noradrenaline, Levophed)[8]: See "Inotropes" section
   D. Ephedrine (Akovaz, Corphedra)[38]
      1. Action: Synthetic sympathomimetic alkaloid that acts directly on α-, and β-receptors and indirectly via release of norepinephrine. Rarely used in cardiac surgery[39]

Preload	0
Contractility	↑↑
Heart rate	↑↑
SVR	↑↑
PVR	↑↑

2. **Dose**

IV bolus	5-10 mg
Infusion	No infusion dosing
Intramuscular (IM) dose	50 mg

   a. Much longer duration of action (1 hour) with IM dosing
3. **Pharmacokinetics**

Onset	1-2 min
Duration of action	5-10 min
Metabolism	Hepatic
Excretion	Urine

4. **Clinical use**
   a. Hypotension due to low SVR states
   b. Temporary therapy for hypovolemia until blood volume is restored
5. **Advantages**
   a. In general, ephedrine is useful in the setting of low SVR and low heart rate.
   b. Useful in the setting of blood pressure management during the induction of regurgitant lesions (mitral regurgitation, aortic insufficiency). Will promote a "fast and forward" state
   c. β_1-Agonism will increase cardiac contractility.
6. **Disadvantages**
   a. **Caution:** Unpredictable response during the post-bypass period. Small doses of ephedrine may produce extreme increases in blood pressure.
   b. Rise in heart rate and contractility may be undesirable in significant CAD, precipitating a supply-demand mismatch.
   c. Efficacy is reduced when norepinephrine stores are depleted (eg, sepsis and methamphetamine abuse).
   d. Tachyphylaxis with repeated doses (rarely used as an infusion as noted earlier)
   e. Contraindicated in dynamic outflow obstruction

CLINICAL PEARL

Ephedrine is an indirect sympathomimetic with an unpredictable response. It is most useful in the setting of hypotension, low heart rate, and low myocardial contractility.

   E. **Angiotensin II (Giapreza)**
   1. **Action:** Naturally occurring vasopressor as part of the renin-angiotensin-aldosterone system (RAAS). Binds to AT_1 receptors. ACE is located within the pulmonary endothelium and converts angiotensin I to angiotensin II (Figure 3.6). During CPB, the lungs are also bypassed, reducing angiotensin I to angiotensin II.[40]

Preload	0
Contractility	0
Heart rate	0
SVR	↑↑↑
PVR	↑↑

   2. **Dose**

IV bolus	Not recommended
Infusion	1.25-80 ng/kg/min

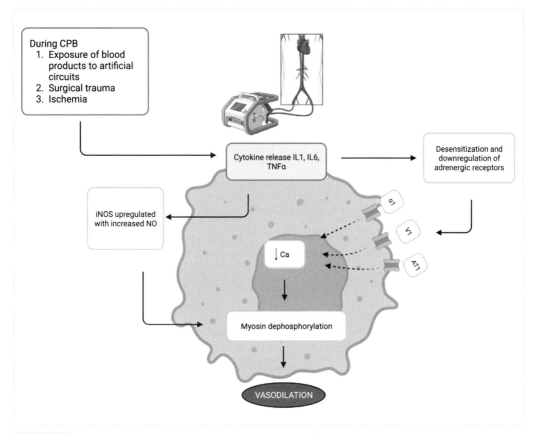

During CPB
1. Exposure of blood products to artificial circuits
2. Surgical trauma
3. Ischemia

Cytokine release IL1, IL6, TNFα

Desensitization and downregulation of adrenergic receptors

iNOS upregulated with increased NO

α1

V1

AT1

↓ Ca

Myosin dephosphorylation

VASODILATION

FIGURE 3.6 Schematic of the major pathway for the development of post–cardiopulmonary bypass (CPB) vasoplegia. Inflammatory cytokines lead to downregulation of the target receptors for vasoconstriction as well as upregulation of nitric oxide synthase (iNOS). IL, interleukin; NO, nitric oxide; TNF, tumor necrosis factor.

    a. Infusion through central access recommended
    b. Increase in increments of up to 15 ng/kg/min
  3. Pharmacokinetics

Onset	~5 min
Half-life	<1 min
Metabolism	Aminopeptidase A and ACE2
Excretion	Unknown

  4. Clinical use: Increased blood pressure in adults with septic or other distributive shock states
  5. Advantages
    a. Effective at rapid increases in blood pressure for catecholamine-resistant vasoplegia[41]
    b. Rapid blood pressure response with a significant vasopressor-sparing effect in cardiac surgery[42]
    c. Increasing evidence that angiotensin II is safe in cardiac surgery and mechanical circulatory support
  6. Disadvantages
    a. Expensive and not widely available
    b. Higher incidence of arterial and venous thrombotic and thromboembolic events[41]

CLINICAL PEARL

Angiotensin II acts independent of the catecholamine pathway and is useful in patients with post-pump vasoplegia who are catecholamine and vasopressin resistant. Catecholamine-resistant vasoplegia is defined as a cardiac index >2.2 L/min/m^2 despite adequate volume resuscitation with refractory hypotension (receipt of >0.2 µg/kg/min of norepinephrine-equivalent dose).[43]

F. Corticosteroids (Hydrocortisone)[44]

1. **Action:** Functional adrenal insufficiency resulting in a depleted adrenal axis can occur in critical illness. The two primary mechanisms of action include immune (anti-inflammatory) and cardiovascular modulation (improved vasopressor responsiveness).

2. **Dose**

IV bolus	100 mg
Infusion	Not recommended

   a. Continued in the intensive care unit 50 mg q6h if response detected[45]
   b. Maximum dose 200-300 mg/d for 7 days

3. **Pharmacokinetics**

Onset	~1 h
Duration of action	Complete excretion within 12 h
Metabolism	Hepatic (CYP3A4)
Excretion	Urine

4. **Clinical use:** Reduces the duration of shock[45,46]
5. **Advantages**
   a. Reduces shock duration
   b. Inexpensive and readily available
6. **Disadvantages**
   a. May cause hyperglycemia and associated increased risk of infection
   b. Maximal benefits may not be realized for more than 48 hours.

CLINICAL PEARL

Hydrocortisone offers mineralocorticoid and glucocorticoid activity in patients in shock who are presumed to have a functional adrenal insufficiency. As a non-catecholamine adjunct, it is most useful in patients who are catecholamine resistant.

G. Nitric Oxide Scavengers (Methylene Blue, Hydroxocobalamin [Cyanokit])[47,48]

1. **Action:** The listed non-vasopressor therapies are theorized to act either through the direct inhibition of NOS or scavenging of nitric oxide (NO).[35,49]

2. **Dose**

Methylene blue	2.5 mg/kg IV
Hydroxocobalamin	5 g IV over 15 min (can repeat)

3. **Pharmacokinetics**
   a. Methylene blue

Onset	~30 min
Half-life	24 h
Metabolism	Hepatic (UDP-glucuronosyltransferase enzymes)
Excretion	Urine primarily, biliary

b. Hydroxocobalamin

Onset	~1 min
Half-life	26-31 h
Metabolism	None
Excretion	Urine

4. **Clinical use (Figure 3.7)**
   a. Methylene blue used for the treatment of methemoglobinemia
   b. Hydroxocobalamin used for the treatment of cyanide toxicity
   c. Variable efficacy in vasoplegic shock
5. **Advantages:** May be vasopressor sparing if response detected
6. **Disadvantages**
   a. Use in cardiac surgery supported by low-level evidence
   b. There is significant heterogeneity in level of response.
   c. Methylene blue
      (1) Associated with serotonin syndrome
      (2) Elevations in PVR[50]
      (3) Hemolytic anemia in patients who are glucose-6-phosphate dehydrogenase deficient
   d. Hydroxocobalamin
      (1) Associated with oxalate nephropathy and renal failure
      (2) False blood-leak alarms on dialysis machines
      (3) Interference with laboratory values

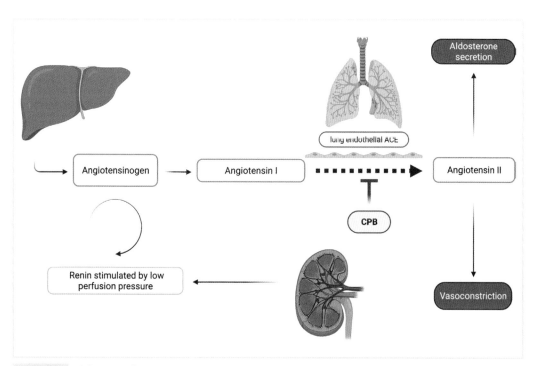

FIGURE 3.7   Schematic of angiotensin metabolism. Bypass of the pulmonary endothelium during CPB leads to a functional deficiency of angiotensin II and its downstream targets. ACE, angiotensin-converting enzyme; CPB, cardiopulmonary bypass.

CLINICAL PEARL

Methylene blue and hydroxocobalamin are NO scavengers with variable efficacy. They are most useful in the setting of profound catecholamine and vasopressin-resistant shock when other adjuncts have failed. Historically, vitamin C and thiamine have been used to manage vasoplegic shock. A recent large, randomized controlled trial (RCT) showed no benefit from use.[51,52]

V. **Vasodilators**

Vasodilators reduce vasomotor tone via various pathways, lower SVR, and lower blood pressure.

A. **Nitroglycerin (Glyceryl Trinitrate)[52]**

1. **Action:** Direct vasodilator, venous > arterial. Results in reduced left ventricular end-diastolic pressure (LVEDP) and pulmonary capillary wedge pressure (PCWP). Dilation of the coronary arteries also occurs.

Preload	↓↓↓
Contractility	0
Heart rate	↑↑
SVR	↓↓
PVR	↓↓↓

2. **Dose**

IV bolus	25-50 µg
Infusion	0.25-0.5 µg/kg/min

3. **Pharmacokinetics**

Onset	1 min
Duration of action	Serum half-life of 3 min
Metabolism	Hepatic to nitrite
Excretion	Urine

4. **Clinical use**
   a. Acute reduction in blood pressure prior to aortic cannulation
   b. Reduced LVEDP for optimization of coronary perfusion pressure (see Figure 3.5)
   c. Prevention of vasospasm when free arterial grafts are harvested

5. **Advantages**
   a. Rapid-acting, easily titratable, short-duration vasodilator
   b. Improved coronary perfusion pressure and reduced myocardial oxygen demand
   c. Minimal risk of coronary steal syndrome

6. **Disadvantages**
   a. Severe hypotension and shock with small doses in the setting of volume depletion, hypotension, or sildenafil use
   b. Tachyphylaxis with infusions
   c. Reflex tachycardia

CLINICAL PEARL

Nitroglycerin is a rapid-acting, potent vasodilator that primarily acts by venodilation and venous pooling.

B. **Nitroprusside (Nipride)[53]**

1. **Action:** Direct vasodilator through the production of NO, venous > arterial but less marked than NO. Coronary vasodilator

Preload	↓↓
Contractility	0
Heart rate	↑↑↑
SVR	↓↓↓
PVR	↓↓↓

2. **Dose**

IV bolus	Not recommended
Infusion	0.1-2 µg/kg/min

   a. Doses >2 µg/kg/min generate cyanide ion (CN^-) faster than the body can dispose of it.
   b. Doses >10 µg/kg/min should be limited to <10 minutes.

3. **Pharmacokinetics**

Onset	1 min
Duration of action	1-2 min
Metabolism	Intra-erythrocyte (see Figure 3.8)
Excretion	Urine

4. **Clinical use**
   a. Immediate reductions in blood pressure
   b. Treatment of acute heart failure (reduces LVEDP, PCWP, and SVR)

5. **Advantages:** Potent, rapid acting, and easily titratable

6. **Disadvantages**
   a. Dose-related production of CN^-, thiocyanate, and methemoglobinemia (Figure 3.8)
   b. Hepatic dysfunction predisposes to cyanide toxicity.
   c. Glomerular filtration rate (GFR) <30 mL/min/1.73 m^2 predisposes to thiocyanate toxicity.
   d. Rapid lowering of blood pressure may precipitate ischemia in other vascular territories.
   e. Rebound hypertension when stopped abruptly
   f. Significant risk of coronary steal syndrome

CLINICAL PEARL

Nitroprusside is a rapid-acting, easily titratable, and potent vasodilator. Use is limited by the production of cyanide, thiocyanate, and methemoglobin.

C. **Hydralazine (Apresoline)**[54,55]
   1. **Action:** Direct vasodilator, arterial more than venous. Reduces SVR

Preload	0
Contractility	0
Heart rate	↑↑↑
SVR	↓↓↓
PVR	↓↓↓

   2. **Dose**

IV push	2.5-5 mg every 15 min
Infusion	Not recommended

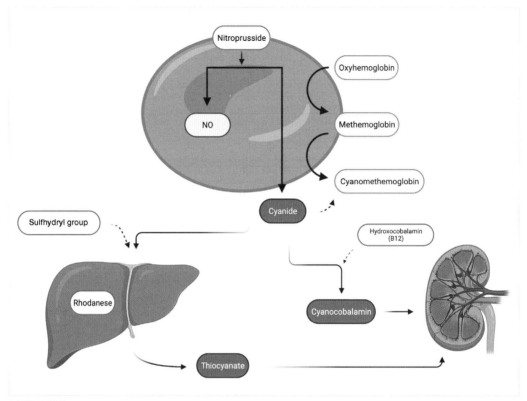

FIGURE 3.8 Schematic of the major pathways involved in the metabolism of sodium nitroprusside. Nitroprusside combines with oxyhemoglobin and is metabolized to five cyanide ions and cyanomethemoglobin. Cyanide converts to thiocyanate via rhodanese-mediated donation of a sulfur group to cyanocobalamin. Large quantities overwhelm this metabolic pathway, leading to an increase in cyanide, methemoglobin, and thiocyanate.

3. **Pharmacokinetics**

Onset	5-15 min
Duration of action	3-6 h
Metabolism	Hepatic (acetylation)
Excretion	Urine 52%-90%, feces 10%

4. **Clinical use:** Treatment of hypertension
5. **Advantages:** Selective vasodilation of arteries
6. **Disadvantages**
   a. Slow onset, long duration, and poorly titratable in the acute setting
   b. Reflex tachycardia can precipitate coronary ischemia.
   c. Significant risk of coronary steal syndrome

CLINICAL PEARL

Hydralazine has a slow onset and prolonged duration of action, which limits use in cardiac surgery.

D. **Nicardipine (Cardene)**[55]
   1. **Action:** Dihydropyridine calcium channel blocker. More selective to vascular smooth muscle than cardiac muscle. Minimal reduction in cardiac inotropy. Coronary vasodilator

Preload	0
Contractility	0
Heart rate	↑
SVR	↓↓↓
PVR	↓↓↓

2. **Dose**

IV bolus	100-200 µg
Infusion	2.5-15 mg/h

3. **Pharmacokinetics**

Onset	1 min
Duration of action	50% offset of action in 30 min
Metabolism	Hepatic (CYP2C8, 2D6, 3A4)
Excretion	Urine 49%-60%, feces 35%-43%

   a. Consider lower doses when hepatic or renal function is impaired.
4. **Clinical use**
   a. Treatment of perioperative hypertension
   b. Increases CO and forward flow. Useful in patients with CAD and heart failure with reduced ejection fraction
5. **Advantages**[56]
   a. Rapid acting and easily titratable
   b. No rebound hypertension when stopped
   c. Minimal electrophysiologic effects
   d. Can be reversed with IV calcium
   e. Coronary dilation improves perfusion in ischemic myocardium without coronary steal.
6. **Disadvantages:** Offset is slower than nitroprusside or nitroglycerin.

CLINICAL PEARL

Useful for the management of acute perioperative hypertension.

E. **Clevidipine (Cleviprex)**[57]
   1. **Action:** Dihydropyridine calcium channel blocker. Effects are similar to Nicardipine with faster onset and shorter duration of action.

Preload	0
Contractility	0
Heart rate	↑
SVR	↓↓↓
PVR	↓↓↓

   2. **Dose**

IV bolus	250-500 µg
Infusion	1-32 mg/h

   a. Starting dose at 1-2 mg/h
   b. Dose can be doubled at short intervals initially.
   c. Desired response in most patients occurs at 4-6 mg/h.
   d. There is limited evidence of effectiveness at doses >32 mg/h.

3.   **Pharmacokinetics**

Onset	1 min
Duration of action	5-15 min
Metabolism	Plasma and tissue esterases
Excretion	Urine 63%-74%, feces 7%-22%

4.   **Clinical use:** Treatment of perioperative hypertension
5.   **Advantages**
   a.   The most rapid acting and titratable antihypertensive available
   b.   Elimination is independent of hepatic and renal metabolism.
   c.   Minimal electrophysiologic effects
6.   **Disadvantages**
   a.   Prepared in a lipid emulsion. Restrictions may be necessary with disorders of lipid metabolism.
   b.   Contraindicated in pathologic hyperlipidemia and allergies to soy or egg products
   c.   High risk of drug error with resemblance to Propofol

CLINICAL PEARL

Clevidipine is an ultra-rapid-acting, potent, easily titratable dihydropyridine calcium channel blocker. Useful for the management of acute perioperative hypertension.

VI.   **Antiarrhythmic Drugs**
   Antiarrhythmic drugs (Table 3.4) are commonly classified by the Singh and Vaughan Williams classification, which divides them into four groups based on the receptors they act on. This chapter focuses on drugs frequently encountered in the perioperative setting.
   A.   **Class I Antiarrhythmics: Sodium Channel Blockers (Figure 3.9)**
      Sodium channel blockers block cardiac Na^+ channels, preventing myocardial depolarization (phase 0) and reducing myocyte excitability.
      1.   **Procainamide (Pronestyl)**[58]
         a.   **Action:** Blocks cardiac Na^+ channels, stabilizing membrane and prolonging myocardial repolarization
         b.   **Dose**

IV bolus (every 5 min)	100 mg (max dose 15 mg/kg)
Infusion	0-6 mg/min

         (1)   **Renal dosing:** Loading 12 mg/kg, infusion 1.4 mg/kg/h
         (2) N-acetylprocainamide levels should be monitored in long duration of therapy. Maintain <12 μg/mL

TABLE 3.4   Overview of Antiarrhythmic Medications

Class	Mechanism	Examples
1a	Na^+ channel blocker (intermediate binding kinetics)	Procainamide, Quinidine
1b	Na^+ channel blocker (fast-binding kinetics)	Lidocaine, Phenytoin
1c	Na^+ channel blocker (slow-binding kinetics)	Flecainide, Propafenone
2	β-Blockers	Labetalol, Metoprolol
3	K^+ channel blockers	Amiodarone, Sotalol
4	Ca^{2+} channel blockers	Verapamil, Diltiazem

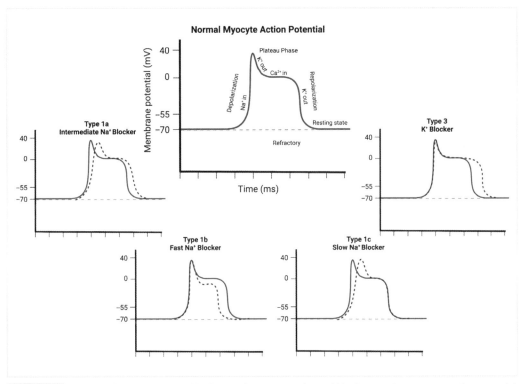

FIGURE 3.9 Effects of sodium channel blockers and potassium channel blockers on the myocyte action potential. Type 1a delays the entire action potential, prolonging the QRS and QT interval. Type 1b reduces the action potential length reducing the QT interval. Class 1c maintains the normal action potential length, but significantly increases the QRS interval. Class 3 will prolong repolarization. (Created with BioRender.com.)

   c. Pharmacokinetics

Onset	Rapid: 1-2 min
Duration of action	Long: 4-6 h
Metabolism	Hepatic and renal
Excretion	Urine (65% unchanged)

   d. Clinical uses
      (1) Conversion and maintenance of acute atrial fibrillation to sinus rhythm
      (2) Wolff-Parkinson-White syndrome: Converts accessory pathway supraventricular tachycardia (SVT)
      (3) Treatment of life-threatening ventricular arrhythmias
   e. Advantages: Effective for emergency ventricular arrhythmias when lidocaine fails
   f. Disadvantages
      (1) Renal impairment causes buildup of toxic metabolite *N*-acetylprocainamide.
      (2) Causes Q-T prolongation resulting in torsades de pointes
      (3) Long durations of treatment can result in lupus-like symptoms.
      (4) Hypotension with rapid administration

CLINICAL PEARL

Procainamide is a type 1a Na^+ channel blocker used in Wolff-Parkinson-White and unstable ventricular arrhythmias.

2. **Lidocaine (Xylocaine)**[59]
   a. **Action:** Blocks cardiac Na^+ channels, stabilizing membrane and shortening myocardial repolarization
   b. **Dose**

IV bolus	1-1.5 mg/kg
Infusion	20-50 µg/kg/min

       (1) Lidocaine levels should be monitored in infusions >24 hours, therapeutic range is 1.5-5 µg/mL.
       (2) In patients with hepatic dysfunction, reduce dose by 50%.
   c. **Pharmacokinetics**

Onset	Rapid: 1-2 min
Duration of action	Medium: 30-60 min
Metabolism	Hepatic
Excretion	Urine (10% unchanged)

   d. **Clinical uses**
       (1) Treatment of life-threatening ventricular arrhythmias
   e. **Advantages**
       (1) Fast acting and easily accessible
       (2) Single bolus is low risk.
       (3) Effects are exaggerated at high and diminished at lower heart rates.
   f. **Disadvantages**
       (1) Toxicity can be unrecognized under general anesthetic.
       (2) Less effective in patients with hypokalemia
       (3) May increase mortality in arrhythmias precipitated by ischemia[60]
       (4) Caution in patients in atrioventricular (AV) nodal block as it will slow or stop ventricular excitation

CLINICAL PEARL

Lidocaine is a type 1b Na^+ channel blocker effective for membrane stabilization in ventricular arrhythmias. It is a safe, rapidly available, and inexpensive medication.

B. **Class II Antiarrhythmics: β-Blockers**
   β-Blockers prevent tachyarrhythmias through the competitive antagonism of β-adrenergic pathways. They are particularly effective perioperatively as many arrhythmias during this period are precipitated by adrenergic stimulation. β-Blocking drugs are categorized by their selectivity to the β-receptors.

α- and β-blockers	Nonselective (β1 + β2)	Cardioselective (β1)
Carvedilol	Nadolol	Atenolol
Labetalol	Propranolol	Bisoprolol
	Timolol	Esmolol
	Sotalol	Metoprolol

1. **Common advantages**
   a. Reduce myocardial oxygen consumption by decreasing contractility and heart rate
   b. Increase the duration of diastole increasing myocardial oxygen supply
   c. Reduce left ventricular ejection velocity (useful in aortic dissection/aneurysm)
   d. Reduce dynamic left ventricular outflow obstruction (useful in hypertrophic obstructive cardiomyopathy and SAM of the mitral valve)
   e. Long-term use post–myocardial infarction reduces remodeling and improves survival.

2. **Common disadvantages**
    a. Can precipitate or worsen degree of heart block and bradycardia
    b. Acute withdrawal increases sensitivity to catecholamines, resulting in hyperdynamic function and potential myocardial infarction.
    c. Initiation can acutely worsen systolic dysfunction in patients with reduced ejection fraction.
    d. Increase in all-cause mortality when course started perioperatively for noncardiac surgery[61]
    e. Can exacerbate Raynaud disease and intermittent claudication in peripheral vascular disease
    f. Will mask symptoms of hypoglycemia (flushing, tachycardia, sweating)
3. **Labetalol (Trandate)[62]**
    a. **Action:** α- and β-blocker (α:β ratio IV—1:7, oral—1:3)

Preload	0
Contractility	↓
Heart rate	↓
Afterload	↓
PVR	↓

    b. **Dose**

IV bolus	10-20 mg
Infusion	0.5-10 mg/min

    c. **Pharmacokinetics**

Onset	1-2 min
Duration of action	3-6 h
Metabolism	Hepatic
Excretion	Urine (5% unchanged)

    d. **Clinical uses:** Treatment of acute hypertension
    e. **Advantages**
        (1) Produces vasodilation without reflex tachycardia
        (2) Predictable response
        (3) Proven safe in pregnancy
    f. **Disadvantages**
        (1) Can precipitate bronchospasm in reactive airways
        (2) Long duration of action
        (3) Postural hypotension

CLINICAL PEARL

Labetalol is a long-acting α- and β-blocker that is effective at treating hypertension. It is avoided in perioperative cardiac cases due to long duration of action.

4. **Propranolol (Inderal)[63]**
    a. **Action:** Potent nonselective ($\beta_1 + \beta_2$) β-blocker
    b. **Dose**

IV bolus	0.5-1 mg
Infusion	1-3 mg/h

c. **Pharmacokinetics**

Onset	1-2 min
Duration of action	4-6 h
Metabolism	Hepatic
Excretion	Urine (<1% unchanged)

d. **Clinical uses**
   (1) Treatment of heart failure
   (2) CAD
   (3) Rate control of atrial fibrillation
   (4) Thyrotoxicosis
   (5) Performance anxiety
e. **Advantages**
   (1) Reduces inotropy without reduction in afterload
   (2) Anxiolytic properties
   (3) Has electrical membrane–stabilizing properties independent of β-blockade
f. **Disadvantages**
   (1) Can precipitate bronchospasm in reactive airway disease
   (2) Increases blood glucose, caution in people with diabetes
   (3) β_2-Blockade can increase SVR.
   (4) Heparinization increases the free fraction of propranolol that was previously protein bound by up to 50%. Reversed with protamine

CLINICAL PEARL

Propranolol is a potent nonselective β-blocker with additional anxiolytic properties. It is typically avoided in cardiac operating room due to long duration of action and undesirable side effects.

5. **Metoprolol (Lopressor)**[64]
   a. **Action:** Cardioselective β_1-blocker
   b. **Dose**

IV bolus	1-5 mg
Infusion	20-50 µg/kg/min

   c. **Pharmacokinetics**

Onset	1-2 min
Duration of action	4-6 h
Metabolism	Hepatic
Excretion	Urine (<5% unchanged)

   d. **Clinical uses**
      (1) Treatment of heart failure
      (2) CAD
      (3) Rate control of atrial fibrillation
      (4) Control of SVT that are adrenergically mediated
   e. **Advantages:** Minimal effects on bronchoconstriction
   f. **Disadvantages**
      (1) Long duration of action
      (2) Slow hydroxylators will have prolonged duration of action.
      (3) Caution in patients with elevated levels of catecholamines (pheochromocytoma, cocaine, methamphetamine) as selective β-blockade will precipitate a hypertensive crisis through unopposed α-stimulation.

Metoprolol is a long-acting cardioselective β_1-blocker with minimal adverse effects.

6. **Esmolol (Brevibloc)**[65]
   a. **Action:** Cardioselective β_1-blocker
   b. **Dose**

IV bolus	10-50 mg
Infusion	20-250 µg/kg/min

   c. **Pharmacokinetics**

Onset	1-2 min
Duration of action	10-20 min
Metabolism	Red blood cell esterases
Excretion	Urine (<1% unchanged)

   d. **Clinical uses**
      (1) Treatment of heart failure
      (2) CAD
      (3) Rate control of atrial fibrillation
      (4) Treatment of acute tachycardia
      (5) Sympathectomy for induction
   e. **Advantages**
      (1) Well tolerated with minimal adverse effects
      (2) Short duration of action, predictable response, and easily titratable
      (3) Minimal increase in airway resistance
      (4) No known metabolic interactions
      (5) The esterase responsible for metabolism is not affected by cholinesterase inhibitors.
   f. **Disadvantages:** Prolonged infusions result in substantial fluid administration.

Esmolol is a very-short-acting cardioselective β_1-blocker with minimal adverse effects.

C. **Class III Antiarrhythmics: Potassium Channel Blockers**
   Blockade of K^+ channels reduces repolarizing potassium currents, which increases the refractory period where additional impulses do not result in electrical stimuli. Many have other mechanisms of action that contribute to their electrophysiologic effects.
   1. **Amiodarone (Pacerone, Cordarone, Nexterone) (Figure 3.10)**[66]
      a. **Action:** K^+ channel blocker with Na^+, β, and Ca^{2+} blocking action
      b. **Dose**

IV bolus (load over 15 min)	150-300 mg
Infusion	0.5-1 mg/min

      c. **Pharmacokinetics**

Onset	1-2 min
Duration of action	Days-months
Metabolism	Hepatic
Excretion	Bile

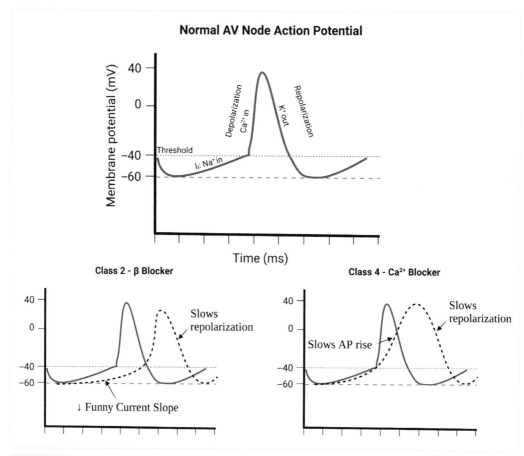

FIGURE 3.10 Effects of β-blocker and Ca^{2+} blockers on the sinoatrial and atrioventricular nodal action potential. β-Blockade will slow the rise of the funny current and slow repolarization resulting in a slower heart rate. Ca^{2+} blockade slows the rise of the action potential and slows repolarization slowing heart rate. (Created with BioRender.com.)

    d. **Clinical uses**
       (1) Treatment of refractory ventricular tachycardia (VT) and ventricular fibrillation (VF)
       (2) Supraventricular arrhythmia rate and rhythm control
    e. **Advantages**
       (1) Selectively increased effect in ischemic tissue
       (2) Effective in arrhythmias refractory to other antiarrhythmic therapy
       (3) Reduces rate of atrial fibrillation and VT or VF post–cardiac surgery; however, American College of Cardiology guidelines still recommend β-blockers as first line.[67]
    f. **Disadvantages**
       (1) Numerous side effects with chronic therapy (pulmonary fibrosis, thyroid derangements)
       (2) Acutely can precipitate or worsen heart block and bradycardia
       (3) Negative inotropic and vasodilatory effects potentiated by volatile anesthetics[68]
       (4) Peak therapeutic effects may take up to 6 weeks of therapy.
       (5) Rapid injection of loading dose will cause hypotension.
       (6) QTc is not prolonged with acute administration but becomes prolonged with chronic use.

CLINICAL PEARL

Amiodarone is an extremely long duration K^+ channel blocker that also blocks numerous other receptors. It is effective for supraventricular and ventricular arrhythmia management.

    D. **Class IV: Calcium Channel Blockers**

Blockade of Ca^{2+} channels in tissues where depolarization is Ca^{2+} dependent (sinoatrial node and AV node) results in prolonged discharge and recovery rate.

        1. **Diltiazem (Cardizem) and Verapamil (Calin, Isoptin)**[69,70]

            a. **Action:** Benzothiazepine calcium channel blocker (non-dihydropyridine)

            b. **Dose**

	Diltiazem	Verapamil
IV bolus	0.25-0.3 mg/kg	0.075-0.15 mg/kg
Infusion	10-20 mg/h	5-15 mg/h

            c. **Pharmacokinetics**

	Diltiazem	Verapamil
Onset	1-2 min	1-2 min
Duration of action	6-12 h	6-12 h
Metabolism	Hepatic and renal	Hepatic
Excretion	Bile/urine (<2% unchanged)	Urine (<4% unchanged)

            d. **Clinical uses**

                (1) Conversion of supraventricular arrhythmias

                (2) Rate control of atrial fibrillation and flutter with rapid ventricular rate

            e. **Advantages**

                (1) Less likely to precipitate heart failure in patients with reduced ejection fraction than β-blockers

                (2) Option for patients who can't tolerate side effects of β-blockers

            f. **Disadvantages**

                (1) Negative inotropy exaggerated by volatile anesthetics[71]

                (2) Little effect if tachycardia is due to an accessory pathway

                (3) Potentiates neuromuscular blockade

                (4) Increases digoxin levels approximately 50%, can precipitate toxicity

                (5) Not effective for ventricular arrhythmias, can cause hypotension

CLINICAL PEARL

Diltiazem and verapamil are long-acting non-dihydropyridine Ca^{2+} blockers effective for the management of supraventricular arrhythmias.

    E. **Class V Antiarrhythmics: Other**

        1. **Adenosine (Adenocard)**[72]

            a. **Action:** Binds to adenosine receptors in AV nodal tissue slowing conduction time by increasing K^+ efflux and decreasing Ca^{2+} influx

            b. **Dose**

IV bolus	6 mg → 12 mg → 18 mg
Infusion	150-300 μg/kg/min

      (1) Caffeine and methylxanthines block adenosine receptor requiring larger doses for clinical effect.

      (2) Dipyridamole and carbamazepine potentiate adenosine; consider 3 mg starting dose

  c. Pharmacokinetics

Onset	15-30 s
Duration of action	30-60 s
Metabolism	Cellular adenosine deaminase
Excretion	Not excreted

  d. Clinical uses

      (1) Treatment of SVT originating at the AV node

      (2) Transient slowing of ventricular rate to identify arrhythmia

      (3) Transient asystole for management of acute hemorrhage

      (4) Used in cardiac stress tests to cause coronary vasodilation inducing coronary steal and subsequent ischemia

  e. Advantages

      (1) Extremely short duration of action

      (2) Minimal toxic effects

  f. Disadvantages

      (1) Can precipitate bronchospasm in reactive airways

      (2) Effects are short lived if arrhythmia does not originate from AV node.

CLINICAL PEARL

Adenosine slows conduction through AV node converting patients with arrhythmias originating from the AV node.

  2. Magnesium

    a. Action: Required for proper functioning of Na^+/K^+ ATPase, which maintains K^+ cellular gradient. Deficiency mimics electrical abnormalities of hypokalemia.

    b. Dose

IV bolus	2-4 g
Infusion	0-2 g/h

    c. Pharmacokinetics

Onset	1-2 min
Duration of action	30-60 min
Metabolism	None
Excretion	Urine

    d. Clinical uses

      (1) Hypomagnesemia

      (2) Ventricular arrhythmias

      (3) Digoxin-induced arrhythmias

      (4) Torsades de pointes (prolonged QT)

      (5) Postoperative atrial fibrillation

    e. Advantages: Safe to administer empirically with wide therapeutic index

    f. Disadvantages

      (1) Causes hypotension and reduced inotropy with rapid administration

      (2) Potentiates neuromuscular blockade

CLINICAL PEARL

Magnesium is an essential electrolyte for cardiac electrical activity that is commonly depleted in patients who are critically ill and those on diuretics. Arrhythmias precipitated by hypomagnesemia are typically refractory to treatment with other antiarrhythmics and electrical cardioversion.

   3. **Digoxin:** See Section III.H.
VII. Pulmonary Vasodilators
   Pulmonary arterial hypertension and increased PVR are present in many patients presenting for cardiac surgery. If untreated, this can cause or exacerbate RV failure and decrease CO. Treatment with IV medications is limited by reductions in SVR, leading to systemic hypotension (Table 3.5). There are a number of newer oral medications used to treat pulmonary hypertension, but they have limited use perioperatively. Therefore, inhaled pulmonary vasodilators have become the primary perioperative treatment for pulmonary hypertension and increased PVR.
A. Inhaled Nitric Oxide
   1. **Action:** Binds and activates guanylate cyclase in vascular smooth muscle increasing cyclic guanosine monophosphate (cGMP) that activates protein kinase, leading to smooth muscle relaxation and vasodilation (Figure 3.11)[73]
   2. **Dose:** Continuous inhaled delivery: 20 ppm; 1 to 80 ppm is the possible range. Most delivery systems can deliver up to 80 ppm, but there is little additional hemodynamic benefit above 20 ppm.[74]
   3. **Pharmacokinetics**[74]

Onset	1 min
Duration of action	<30 s
Metabolism	Inactivation by hemoglobin → various metabolites
Excretion	Urine

   4. **Clinical use**
      a. Treatment of pulmonary arterial hypertension
      b. Treatment of right heart failure during cardiac surgery
      c. Treatment of hypoxic respiratory failure including acute respiratory distress syndrome (ARDS)
      d. Diagnostic testing for vasoreactivity during right heart catheterization
   5. **Advantages**
      a. Rapid onset and short duration of action
      b. Minimal to no systemic vasodilation
      c. Inhaled NO can also improve ventilatory/perfusion (*V/Q*) matching by selectively vasodilating ventilated portions of the lung.

TABLE 3.5 Three Pathways to Treat Pulmonary Hypertension

Pathway	Effect
Nitric oxide	Increase cyclic guanosine monophosphate (cGMP) in smooth muscle → vasodilation and antiproliferation of smooth muscle
Prostacyclin	Increases cyclic adenosine monophosphate (cAMP) in smooth muscle → vasodilation and antiproliferation of smooth muscle
Endothelin	Endothelin 1 binds smooth muscle endothelin A and B receptors causing vasoconstriction. Antagonist causes vasodilation.

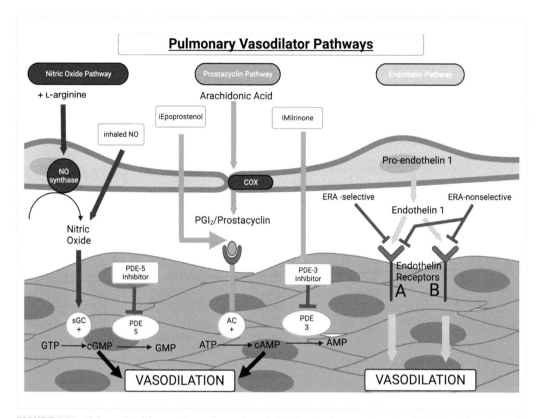

FIGURE 3.11   Schematic of three major pathways targeted to treat pulmonary hypertension. The nitric oxide pathway and the prostacyclin pathways are the primary targets for acute intraoperative management due to their inhaled delivery. The endothelin receptor antagonists (ERA) are used for long-term management and only available in oral formulations.

6. **Disadvantages**
   a. High cost and proprietary equipment required
   b. Rebound pulmonary hypertension with abrupt discontinuation
   c. Methemoglobinemia formation
   d. Nitrogen dioxide (NO_2) production can lead to pulmonary edema.
   e. Increased left-sided filling pressures can lead to pulmonary edema in patients with isolated postcapillary pulmonary hypertension.

CLINICAL PEARL

Inhaled NO is a potent pulmonary vasodilator with minimal systemic effects. Its use is limited by cost and proprietary equipment.

   B. **Inhaled Epoprostenol/Prostacyclin/Prostaglandin I_2 (Flolan, Veletri)**[75]
      1. **Action:** Activates prostacyclin receptors, increasing cAMP (Figure 3.11)
         a. In endothelial smooth muscle, this causes vasodilation.
         b. In platelets, this inhibits aggregation and adhesion.
      2. **Dose**

Bolus	Not recommended
Continuous nebulization	50 ng/kg/min

3. **Pharmacokinetics**

Onset	1 min
Duration of action	1 min
Metabolism	Spontaneous and enzymatic degradation
Excretion	Urine excretion of metabolites

4. **Clinical use**
   a. Treatment of pulmonary arterial hypertension
   b. Treatment of right heart failure during cardiac surgery
   c. Treatment of hypoxic respiratory failure including adult respiratory distress syndrome
   d. Diagnostic testing for vasoreactivity during right heart catheterization
5. **Advantages**
   a. Rapid onset and short duration of action
   b. No activity outside pulmonary circulation
   c. Efficacy at least equal to inhaled NO but more cost-effective[73]
   d. No toxic metabolites
6. **Disadvantages**
   a. Rebound pulmonary hypertension with abrupt discontinuation
   b. Requires expiratory high-efficiency particulate air (HEPA) filter that can clog and needs to be replaced every 2 hours

CLINICAL PEARL

Inhaled epoprostenol is an effective pulmonary vasodilator with minimal systemic effects that is more cost-effective than inhaled NO.

C. **Inhaled Milrinone**
   1. **Action:** PDE3 inhibitor decreases the breakdown of cAMP in the pulmonary smooth muscle leading to pulmonary vasodilation (Figure 3.11).
   2. **Dose:** Intermittent nebulization 2-4 mg
   3. **Pharmacokinetics**[76]

Onset	10 min
Duration of action	30 min
Metabolism	Glucuronidation
Excretion	Urine (83% unchanged)

4. **Clinical use**
   a. Treatment of pulmonary arterial hypertension
   b. Treatment of right heart failure during cardiac surgery
5. **Advantages**
   a. Does not require reconstitution or dilution
   b. Additive pulmonary vasodilation when administered with epoprostenol[77]
   c. Minimal reduction in SVR compared to IV milrinone[28]
6. **Disadvantages**
   a. Requires expiratory HEPA filter that can clog and needs to be replaced every 2 hours
   b. Accumulation in severe renal dysfunction

CLINICAL PEARL

Milrinone, a PDE3 inhibitor, when nebulized is a potent pulmonary vasodilator with minimal reduction in SVR. Its effects are additive to inhaled epoprostenol.

VIII. Anticoagulants

    A. **Heparin—Unfractionated Heparin (UFH)** is a heavily sulfated glycosaminoglycan polymer that is negatively charged. Commercial preparations include a wide range of molecular weights from 3,000 to 40,000 Da (15,000 Da average).

        1. **Action:** Binds antithrombin III (AT III), potentiating its activity 1,000-fold to inhibit thrombin and Xa most importantly, but also IXa, XIa, and XIIa

        2. **Dose:** IV bolus: 300-400 U/kg for CPB

            a. Heterogeneous response requires clot inhibition testing before initiation of CPB.[78]

            b. Heparin dose-response monitoring may be used to determine heparin dose (Figure 3.12) but has not been shown to be superior to weight-based dosing.

            c. Activated clotting time (ACT) is the most common assay of heparin anticoagulation with a goal of 480 seconds. ACT precision worsened in hemodilution, hypothermia, and thrombocytopenia.

            d. Whole blood concentrations of heparin can be monitored with a target of 3-4 units/mL.[79]

            e. CPB priming solution should contain 5,000-10,000 units of heparin.

        3. **Pharmacokinetics**

Onset	1 min
Duration of action	4-6 h
Metabolism	Reticuloendothelial system and hepatic uptake
Excretion	Minimal excretion in urine

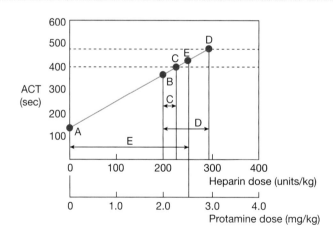

FIGURE 3.12 Graph of a heparin (and protamine) dosing algorithm. In the graph, the control activated clotting time (ACT) is shown as point A, and the ACT resulting from an initial heparin bolus of 200 units/kg is show as point B. The line connecting A and B then is extrapolated and a desired ACT is selected. Point C represents the intersection between this line and a target ACT of 400 seconds, theoretically requiring an additional heparin dose represented by the difference between points C and B on the horizontal axis (arrow C). Similarly, to achieve an ACT of 480 seconds (higher horizontal dotted line intersecting the ACT vs heparin dose line at point D), one would administer the additional heparin dose represented by arrow D. To estimate heparin concentration and calculate protamine dose at the time of heparin neutralization, the most recently measured ACT value is plotted on the dose-response line (point E in the example). The whole blood heparin concentration present theoretically is represented by the difference between point E and point A on the horizontal axis (arrow E). The protamine dose required to neutralize the remaining heparin then may be calculated. Protamine 1 mg/kg is administered for every 100 units/kg of heparin present. (Modified from Bull BS, Huse WM, Brauer FS, Korpman RA. Heparin therapy during extracorporeal circulation. II. The use of a dose-response curve to individualize heparin and protamine dosage. *J Thorac Cardiovasc Surg.* 1975;69(5):685-689; Gravlee GP. Anticoagulation for cardiopulmonary bypass. In: Gravlee GP, Davis RF, Kurusz M, Utley JR, eds. *Cardiopulmonary Bypass: Principles and Practice.* 2nd ed. Lippincott Williams & Wilkins; 2000:435-472.)

4. **Clinical use**
   a. Anticoagulation for CPB
   b. Anticoagulation for off-pump coronary interventions
   c. Anticoagulation for extracorporeal membrane oxygenation (ECMO) circuits
   d. Anticoagulation for bridging mechanical heart valves
   e. Anticoagulation for acute coronary syndrome
5. **Advantages**
   a. Rapid onset and reversibility
   b. Real-time clinical effect monitoring
   c. Well tolerated with rare anaphylaxis
6. **Disadvantages**
   a. Heparin boluses can decrease SVR.
   b. Heparin resistance
      (1) AT III deficiency is the most commonly cited cause but it is frequently multifactorial.
      (2) **Risk factors:** AT III <60%, preoperative heparin administration, platelet >300,000/mm^3, age >65 years
      (3) Treatment
         (a) Additional heparin up to 600 U/kg
         (b) AT III concentrates 500-1,000 U[80]
            (i) AT III preferred over fresh frozen plasma (FFP) to avoid risks of transfusion[81]
         (c) Transient *decrease* in platelets with heparin administration
   c. **Heparin rebound:** Delayed appearance of heparin effect after protamine reversal
      (1) Increased risk when higher doses of heparin are required
      (2) Possibly from redistribution of sequestered heparin
      (3) Can be treated with additional protamine
   d. **Heparin-induced thrombocytopenia (HIT) type I:** Transient decrease in platelets with heparin administration
      (1) Nonimmunologic in origin
   e. **HIT type II:** Immune-mediated thrombocytopenia and thrombosis[82]
      (1) Immunoglobulin G (IgG) antibodies to the heparin-platelet factor 4 (PF4) complex
      (2) Antibodies 5-10 days after continuous exposure
      (3) 20% have thrombosis, mortality as high as 40%
      (4) Antibodies undetectable within 100 days of discontinuation
      (5) Testing
         (a) Enzyme-linked immunosorbent assay (ELISA) for heparin-PF4 antibodies is sensitive but not specific.
         (a) Heparin-induced serotonin release assay is a functional test and is the gold standard.

CLINICAL PEARL

Heparin is the preferred anticoagulant for cardiac surgery due to its rapid onset, predictable response, and most importantly reversibility. Heparin's use can rarely be complicated by HIT, which is life-threatening and requires an alternative anticoagulant.

B. **Protamine:** Strongly positively charged nitrogenous alkaline derived from salmon sperm is used for the reversal of heparin anticoagulation.
   1. **Action:** Cation that strongly bonds to the anion heparin to create a stable complex without anticoagulant activity
   2. **Dose:** Slow bolus infusion over 10 minutes, 0.6-1.3 mg per 100 units heparin
      a. Should be based on heparin remaining in circulation
      b. Dose can be as follows:
         (1) Empiric 0.6-1.3 mg/100 units heparin

      (2) Based on heparin dose-response curve (Figure 3.12)

      (3) Calculated by automated protamine titration curve

    c. Dilute to 60 mL and deliver over 10 minutes with an infusion pump to minimize adverse effects.

3. Pharmacokinetics

Onset	5 min
Duration of action	2 h
Metabolism	Unknown
Excretion	Unknown

4. Clinical use

    a. Reversal of heparin after CPB

    b. Treatment of heparin overdose or bleeding in patient who are heparinized

    c. Reversal of low-molecular-weight heparin (less effective)

5. Advantages

    a. Effective and rapid elimination of heparin effect

    b. Real-time clinical effect monitoring

6. Disadvantages

    a. Type I protamine reaction: Decreased SVR

      (1) Proposed mechanisms include histamine displacement from mast cells and endothelial NO.

      (2) Reduced risk with slow administration

    b. Type II protamine reaction: Anaphylaxis or anaphylactoid reactions

      (1) **IIA:** True anaphylaxis

        (a) Risks factors include prior protamine exposure, protamine containing insulin, fin fish allergy, and vasectomy.

      (2) **IIB:** Nonimmunologic anaphylactoid reaction

      (3) **IIC:** Delayed noncardiogenic pulmonary edema

    c. Type III protamine reaction: Catastrophic pulmonary hypertension, RV failure, and cardiovascular collapse

      (1) Large heparin-protamine complexes entering the pulmonary circulation lead thromboxane release and pulmonary vasoconstriction.

      (2) Treatment involves supportive care, heparin administration, and frequently reinitiation of CPB.

      (3) Slow administration likely decreases risk by reducing size and rate of protamine heparin complexes entering the pulmonary circulation.

    d. Protamine causes platelet activation and consumption.

CLINICAL PEARL

Protamine is a large cation that binds and reverses the anticoagulant effects of heparin. Type III protamine reactions cause life-threatening pulmonary hypertension. The risk of a type III reaction is reduced by slow administration.

  C. Bivalirudin (Angiomax) is a synthetic, direct thrombin inhibitor that can be used as an alternative to heparin anticoagulation.

    1. Action: Inhibits thrombin by reversibly binding the catalytic site and fibrinogen binding site[83]

    2. Dose[78]

IV bolus	1.0 mg/kg, 50 mg in pump prime
Infusion	2.5 mg/kg/h

    a. Clinical effect should be monitored using ACT with a goal ACT of 2.5 times the baseline ACT.

    b. Infusion rate should be reduced in patients with severe renal dysfunction or patients on hemodialysis.

3. **Pharmacokinetics**[83,84]

Onset	1 min
Duration of action	1-2 h
Metabolism	80% proteolytic cleavage in plasma
Excretion	20% urine

    a. Duration is prolonged in the setting of renal dysfunction or hypothermia.

    b. Elimination can be enhanced with ultrafiltration, hemodialysis, and hyperthermia.

4. **Clinical use**

    a. Anticoagulant for percutaneous coronary intervention (PCI) with or without HIT

    b. Anticoagulation for cardiac surgery for patients with or without HIT

5. **Advantages**

    a. Fast onset and short duration of action allow for return of normal coagulation shortly after CPB.

    b. Safe to use in patients with HIT

    c. Real-time clinical effect monitoring

    d. Can be partially eliminated through dialysis to shorten duration of action

    e. Multiple RCTs and prospective clinical trials have demonstrated safety as alternative to heparin.

6. **Disadvantages**

    a. There is no reversal agent.

    b. Duration of action is profoundly extended in renal failure.

    c. Stasis in grafts or lines allows thrombin cleavage of bivalirudin and thrombus formation. Modifications to perfusion techniques and surgical techniques are required.

CLINICAL PEARL

Bivalirudin is a direct thrombin inhibitor that can be used as an alternative to heparin for cardiac surgery and is safe in HIT. It is not reversible but has a short duration of action in patients with normal renal function and can be removed by ultrafiltration.

D. Argatroban: Argatroban is a synthetic, direct thrombin inhibitor that is used in the treatment of HIT and as an alternative to heparin anticoagulation.

1. **Action:** Inhibits thrombin by reversibly binding the active site of thrombin[83]

2. **Dose**

IV bolus	0.1 mg/kg
Infusion	2.5-15 µg/kg/min

    a. ACT goal of 500-600 seconds[85]

    b. Activated partial thromboplastin time (aPTT) goal of 70-80 seconds[86]

3. **Pharmacokinetics**

Onset	30 min (delayed peak 2 h)
Duration of action	Variable, >1 h
Metabolism	Hepatic
Excretion	Feces 65%, urine 22%

4. **Clinical use**
   a. Treatment of HIT
   b. Anticoagulant for PCI in patients with or at risk of HIT
   c. Anticoagulation for cardiac surgery in patients with HIT
5. **Advantages**
   a. Renal and temperature-independent elimination
   b. Safe in patients with HIT
   c. Reasonable correlation with real-time clinical effect monitoring
6. **Disadvantages**
   a. Slow onset and delayed peak make dosing complicated and often result in overdosing.[85]
   b. No reversal agent
   c. Duration prolonged in hepatic dysfunction
   d. Limited clinical data on dosing regimens and monitoring for CPB
   e. Can cause thrombosis as well as excessive bleeding

CLINICAL PEARL

Argatroban is a direct thrombin inhibitor that can be used as an alternative to heparin to cardiac surgery and is safe in HIT. Argatroban pharmacokinetics are less favorable for cardiac surgery than bivalirudin.

IX. Antifibrinolytics

Antifibrinolytics are utilized to inhibit fibrinolysis during cardiac surgery, thereby limiting blood loss and transfusion requirements. They are considered an essential part of a comprehensive blood conservation strategy in cardiac surgery. The Society of Thoracic Surgeons and Society of Cardiac Anesthesiologists guidelines show level IA evidence that "Use of synthetic antifibrinolytic agents such as Epsilon Aminocaproic Acid (EACA) or Tranexamic Acid (TXA) reduces blood loss and blood transfusion during cardiac procedures and is indicated for blood conservation."[87]

A. **EACA (Amicar):** Epsilon-aminocaproic acid (EACA) is a synthetic lysine analogue that is used as an antifibrinolytic for blood conservation in cardiac surgery.
   1. **Action:** Competitively blocks the conversion of plasminogen to plasmin as well as blocking lysine binding site on fibrinogen, resulting in the inhibition of fibrinolysis (Figure 3.13)
   2. **Dose**

IV bolus	5-10 g
Infusion	1-2 g/h

   3. **Pharmacokinetics**

Onset	~60 min
Duration of action	Several hours
Metabolism	Minimal hepatic
Excretion	Urine (65% unchanged)

   4. **Clinical use**
      a. Enhancement of coagulation in active bleeding
      b. Enhancement of coagulation for blood conservation in cardiac and other surgeries
   5. **Advantages**
      a. Extensive clinical data demonstrating its efficacy
      b. Well tolerated with rare side effects
   6. **Disadvantages**
      a. Degree of bleeding reduction is typically modest.
      b. Most studies do not demonstrate a mortality benefit.

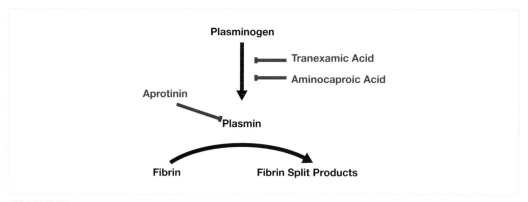

FIGURE 3.13 Diagram of site of action of the antifibrinolytics contrasting the lysine analogues (tranexamic acid and aminocaproic acid) and the serine protease inhibitor (aprotinin).

    B. **TXA (Cyklokapron, Lysteda)** is a synthetic lysine analogue that is used as an antifibrinolytic for blood conservation in cardiac surgery.

        1. **Action:** Competitively blocks the conversion of plasminogen to plasmin as well as blocking lysine binding site on fibrinogen, resulting in the inhibition of fibrinolysis (Figure 3.13)

        2. **Dose**

IV bolus	10-20 mg/kg
Infusion	1-2 mg/kg/h

            a. Recent modeling meta-analysis determined a 10 mg/kg bolus followed by 1 mg/kg/h for 12 hours or one 20 mg/kg was the optimal dose.[88]

        3. **Pharmacokinetics**[89]

Onset	1 min
Duration of action	3 h
Metabolism	None
Excretion	Urine (95% unchanged)

        4. **Clinical use**

            a. Enhancement of coagulation in active bleeding

            b. Enhancement of coagulation for blood conservation in cardiac and other surgeries, trauma, postpartum bleeding

            c. Hereditary angioedema prophylaxis

        5. **Advantages**

            a. Extensive clinical data demonstrating its efficacy in many clinical scenarios

            b. Well tolerated with rare side effects

        6. **Disadvantages**

            a. Increased risk of seizures in many studies, appears dose dependent, and is rare with lower dose regimen[88]

            b. Degree of bleeding reduction is typically modest.

            c. Most studies do not demonstrate a mortality benefit.

CLINICAL PEARL

EACA and tranexamic acid (TXA) are antifibrinolytics with a demonstrated reduction in blood loss and transfusion in cardiac surgery. Both have similar mechanisms of action. TXA has a 6- to 10-fold increased affinity in binding plasminogen compared with EACA, but TXA has a dose-dependent risk of seizure.

C. **Aprotinin**[90] is a serine protease inhibitor that was used until 2008 in the United States for blood conservation in cardiac surgery. It was removed from the U.S. market due to concerns of increased mortality that was demonstrated in several trials, culminating with the Blood Conservation Using Antifibrinolytics in a Randomized Trial (BART) in 2008.[91] These trials have been questioned since 2008 and aprotinin was reintroduced in Europe and Canada for coronary artery bypass graft (CABG) surgery, but not in the United States.

1. **Action:** A serine protease inhibitor that inhibits free plasmin limiting pathologic fibrinolysis (Figure 3.13). It has minimal effect on bound plasmin.

2. **Dose**

IV bolus	2 million KIU
Infusion	500,000 KIU/h

   a. Dose is in kallikrein inhibitor units (KIU).
   b. 2 million KIU in pump prime as well

3. **Pharmacokinetics**[90]

Onset	1 min
Duration of action	4-5 h
Metabolism	Renal lysosomal enzymes
Excretion	Urine

4. **Clinical use**
   a. Not currently approved or used in the United States
   b. Limited use in Europe and Canada for blood conservation in high-risk CABG surgery

5. **Advantages:** Some studies show superior blood conservation compared to TXA and EACA.

6. **Disadvantages**[90]
   a. Controversial increase in mortality and renal injury
   b. Risk of anaphylaxis, especially with repeat exposure within 6 months
   c. Prolongs celite ACTs necessitating the use of kaolin ACTs

CLINICAL PEARL

Aprotinin is an antifibrinolytic with proven blood conservation in cardiac surgery that was pulled from the U.S. market in 2008 for concerns over increased mortality and renal injury. These concerns have been challenged and it is currently approved for high-risk CABG surgery in Europe and Canada.

ACKNOWLEDGMENTS

The authors acknowledge the contributions of coauthors in previous editions: Drs. Nirvik Pal and John F. Butterworth.

REFERENCES

1. Grogan S, Preuss CV. Pharmacokinetics. In: StatPearls [Internet]. *Treasure Island* (FL): StatPearls Publishing; 2023. PMID: 32491676.
2. Abboud I, Lerolle N, Urien S, et al. Pharmacokinetics of epinephrine in patients with septic shock: modelization and interaction with endogenous neurohormonal status. *Crit Care*. 2009;13(4):R120.
3. Moss DR, Bartels K, Peterfreund GL, Lovich MA, Sims NM, Peterfreund RA. An in vitro analysis of central venous drug delivery by continuous infusion: the effect of manifold design and port selection. *Anesth Analg*. 2009;109(5):1524-1529.
4. Clutter WE, Bier DM, Shah SD, Cryer PE. Epinephrine plasma metabolic clearance rates and physiologic thresholds for metabolic and hemodynamic actions in man. *J Clin Invest*. 1980;66(1):94-101.
5. Davis BH, Limdi NA. Translational pharmacogenomics: discovery, evidence synthesis and delivery of race-conscious medicine. *Clin Pharmacol Ther*. 2021;110(4):909-925.
6. Truong TM, Apfelbaum JL, Danahey K, et al. Pilot findings of pharmacogenomics in perioperative care: initial results from the first phase of the ImPreSS trial. *Anesth Analg*. 2022;135(5):929-940.
7. Epinephrine. Package insert. JHP Pharmaceuticals, LLC; 2012.
8. Norepinephrine. Package insert. Hospira Inc; 2020.
9. Jentzer JC, Coons JC, Link CB, Schmidhofer M. Pharmacotherapy update on the use of vasopressors and inotropes in the intensive care unit. *J Cardiovasc Pharmacol Ther*. 2015;20(3):249-260.

10. Hajjar LA, Vincent JL, Barbosa Gomes Galas FR, et al. Vasopressin versus norepinephrine in patients with vasoplegic shock after cardiac surgery. *Anesthesiology*. 2017;126(1):85-93.

11. Dobutamine. Package insert. Hospira Inc; 2016.

12. Daly AL, Linares OA, Smith MJ, Starling MR, Supiano MA. Dobutamine pharmacokinetics during dobutamine stress echo-cardiography. *Am J Cardiol*. 1997;79(10):1381-1386.

13. Salomon NW, Plachetka JR, Copeland JG. Comparison of dopamine and dobutamine following coronary artery bypass grafting. *Ann Thorac Surg*. 1982;33(1):48-54.

14. Stoner JD, Bolen JL, Harrison DC. Comparison of dobutamine and dopamine in treatment of severe heart failure. *Br Heart J*. 1977;39(5):536-539.

15. Kersting F, Follath F, Moulds R, et al. A comparison of cardiovascular effects of dobutamine and isoprenaline after open heart surgery. *Heart*. 1976;38(6):622-626.

16. Tacon CL, McCaffrey J, Delaney A. Dobutamine for patients with severe heart failure: a systematic review and meta-analysis of randomised controlled trials. *Intensive Care Med*. 2012;38(3):359-367.

17. Isoproterenol. Package insert. Hospira Inc; 2013.

18. Krasnow N, Rolett EL, Yurchak PM, Hood WB, Gorlin R. Isoproterenol and cardiovascular performance. *Am J Med*. 1964;37(4):514-525.

19. Conway WD, Minatoya H, Lands AM, et al. Absorption and elimination profile of isoproterenol. *J Pharm Sci*. 1968;57(7):1135-1141.

20. Dopamine. Package insert. Hospira Inc; 2014.

21. Goldberg L, Rajfer S. Dopamine receptors: applications in clinical cardiology. *Circulation*. 1985;72(2):245-248.

22. De Backer D, Biston P, Devriendt J, et al. Comparison of dopamine and norepinephrine in the treatment of shock. *N Engl J Med*. 2010;362(9):779-789.

23. Kellum JA, Decker JM. Use of dopamine in acute renal failure: a meta-analysis. *Crit Care Med*. 2001;29(8):1526-1531.

24. Milrinone. Package insert. Sanofi-Synthelabo Inc; 2003.

25. Hilleman DE, Forbes WP. Role of milrinone in the management of congestive heart failure. *Ann Pharmacother*. 1989;23(5):357-362.

26. Lobato EB, Florete O, Bingham HL. A single dose of milrinone facilitates separation from cardiopulmonary bypass in patients with pre-existing left ventricular dysfunction. *Br J Anaesth*. 1998;81(5):782-784.

27. Arbeus M, Axelsson B, Friberg Ö, Magnuson A, Bodin L, Hultman J. Milrinone increases flow in coronary artery bypass grafts after cardiopulmonary bypass: a prospective, randomized, double-blind, placebo-controlled study. *J Cardiothorac Vasc Anesth*. 2009;23(1):48-53.

28. Patel J, Patel K, Garg P, Patel S. Inhaled versus intravenous milrinone in mitral stenosis with pulmonary hypertension. *Asian Cardiovasc Thorac Ann*. 2021;29(3):170-178.

29. Digoxin. Package insert. Concordia Pharmaceuticals Inc; 2016.

30. Heidenreich PA, Bozkurt B, Aguilar D, et al. 2022 AHA/ACC/HFSA guideline for the management of heart failure: a report of the American College of Cardiology/American Heart Association Joint Committee on Clinical Practice Guidelines. *Circulation*. 2022;145(18):e895-e1032.

31. Landoni G, Lomivorotov VV, Alvaro G, et al. Levosimendan for hemodynamic support after cardiac surgery. *N Engl J Med*. 2017;376(21):2021-2031.

32. Glucagon. Package insert. Eli Lilly and Company; 2021.

33. Phenylephrine. Package insert. West-Ward Pharmaceuticals; 2012.

34. Vasopressin. Package insert. American Regent, Inc; 2015.

35. Busse LW, Barker N, Petersen C. Vasoplegic syndrome following cardiothoracic surgery-review of pathophysiology and update of treatment options. *Crit Care*. 2020;24(1):36.

36. Guarracino F, Habicher M, Treskatsch S, et al. Vasopressor therapy in cardiac surgery—an experts' consensus statement. *J Cardiothorac Vasc Anesth*. 2021;35(4):1018-1029.

37. Neumar RW, Shuster M, Callaway CW, et al. Part 1: Executive Summary: 2015 American Heart Association guidelines update for cardiopulmonary resuscitation and emergency cardiovascular care. *Circulation*. 2015;132(18 suppl 2):S315-S367.

38. Ephedrine. Package insert. Éclat Pharmaceuticals; 2022.

39. Limberger RP, Jacques ALB, Schmitt GC, Arbo MD. Pharmacological effects of ephedrine. In: Ramawat KG, Mérillon J-M, eds. *Natural Products*. Springer; 2013:1217-1237.

40. Chow JH, Wittwer ED, Wieruszewski PM, Khanna AK. Evaluating the evidence for angiotensin II for the treatment of vasoplegia in critically ill cardiothoracic surgery patients. *J Thorac Cardiovasc Surg*. 2022;163(4):1407-1414.

41. Khanna A, English SW, Wang XS, et al. Angiotensin II for the treatment of vasodilatory shock. *N Engl J Med*. 2017;377(5):419-430.

42. Klijian A, Khanna AK, Reddy VS, et al. Treatment with angiotensin II is associated with rapid blood pressure response and vasopressor sparing in patients with vasoplegia after cardiac surgery: a post-hoc analysis of Angiotensin II for the Treatment of High-Output Shock (ATHOS-3) study. *J Cardiothorac Vasc Anesth*. 2021;35(1):51-58.

43. Barnes TJ, Hockstein MA, Jabaley CS. Vasoplegia after cardiopulmonary bypass: a narrative review of pathophysiology and emerging targeted therapies. *SAGE Open Med*. 2020;8:2050312120935466.

44. Hydrocortisone (systemic): drug information. *UpToDate*. Pharmacia & Upjohn; 2023.

45. Venkatesh B, Finfer S, Cohen J, et al. Adjunctive glucocorticoid therapy in patients with septic shock. *N Engl J Med*. 2018;378(9):797-808.

46. Annane D, Renault A, Brun-Buisson C, et al. Hydrocortisone plus fludrocortisone for adults with septic shock. *N Engl J Med*. 2018;378(9):809-818.

47. Hydroxocobalamin. Package insert. Merck Santé; 2018.

48. Methylene Blue. Package insert. American Regent; 2016.

49. Shapeton AD, Mahmood F, Ortoleva JP. Hydroxocobalamin for the treatment of vasoplegia: a review of current literature and considerations for use. *J Cardiothorac Vasc Anesth*. 2019;33(4):894-901.

50. Park BK, Shim TS, Lim CM, et al. The effects of methylene blue on hemodynamic parameters and cytokine levels in refractory septic shock. *Korean J Intern Med*. 2005;20(2):123-128.
51. Fujii T, Luethi N, Young PJ, et al. Effect of vitamin C, hydrocortisone, and thiamine vs hydrocortisone alone on time alive and free of vasopressor support among patients with septic shock: the VITAMINS randomized clinical trial. *JAMA*. 2020;323(5):423-431.
52. Divakaran S, Loscalzo J. The role of nitroglycerin and other nitrogen oxides in cardiovascular therapeutics. *J Am Coll Cardiol*. 2017;70(19):2393-2410.
53. Friederich JA, Butterworth JF IV. Sodium nitroprusside: twenty years and counting. *Anesth Analg*. 1995;81(1):152-162.
54. Hydralazine. Package insert. Ciba-Geigy Corporation; 2015.
55. Nicardipine. Package insert. Baxter Healthcare Corporation; 2010.
56. Tobias JD. Nicardipine: applications in anesthesia practice. *J Clin Anesth*. 1995;7(6):525-533.
57. Clevidipine. Package insert. The Medicines Company; 2011.
58. Procainamide. Package insert. Hospira Inc; 2021.
59. Lidocaine. Package insert. APP Pharmaceuticals, LLC; 2010.
60. Hine LK, Laird N, Hewitt P, Chalmers TC. Meta-analytic evidence against prophylactic use of lidocaine in acute myocardial infarction. *Arch Intern Med*. 1989;149(12):2694-2698.
61. Bouri S, Shun-Shin MJ, Cole GD, Mayet J, Francis DP. Meta-analysis of secure randomised controlled trials of β-blockade to prevent perioperative death in non-cardiac surgery. *Heart*. 2014;100(6):456-464.
62. Labetalol. Package insert. Hikma Pharmaceuticals USA Inc; 2020.
63. Propranolol. Package insert. Wyeth Pharmaceuticals, Inc; 2010.
64. Metoprolol. Package insert. AstraZeneca AB; 2006.
65. Esmolol. Package insert. Baxter Healthcare Corporation; 2012.
66. Amiodarone. Package insert. Wyeth Pharmaceuticals; 2018.
67. Bagshaw SM, Galbraith PD, Mitchell LB, Sauve R, Exner DV, Ghali WA. Prophylactic amiodarone for prevention of atrial fibrillation after cardiac surgery: a meta-analysis. *Ann Thorac Surg*. 2006;82(5):1927-1937.
68. Feinberg B, LaMantia K, Levy W. Amiodarone and general anesthesia: a retrospective analysis. *Anesth Analg*. 1986;65:S49.
69. Diltiazem. Package insert. Valeant Pharmaceuticals North America LLC; 2014.
70. Verapamil. Package insert. G.D. Searle, LLC; 2017.
71. Kapur P, Bloor B, Flacke W, Olewine S. Comparison of cardiovascular responses to verapamil during enflurane, isoflurane, or halothane anesthesia in the dog. *Anesthesiology*. 1984;61(2):156-160.
72. Adenosine. Package insert. Hospira Inc; 2014.
73. Cheng JW, Tonelli AR, Pettersson G, Krasuski RA. Pharmacologic management of perioperative pulmonary hypertension. *J Cardiovasc Pharmacol*. 2014;63(4):375-384.
74. Ichinose F, Roberts JD, Zapol WM. Inhaled nitric oxide: a selective pulmonary vasodilator: current uses and therapeutic potential. *Circulation*. 2004;109(25):3106-3111.
75. FLOLAN. Package insert. GlaxoSmithKline; 2008.
76. Sablotzki A, Starzmann W, Scheubel R, Grond S, Czeslick EG. Selective pulmonary vasodilation with inhaled aerosolized milrinone in heart transplant candidates. *Can J Anesth*. 2005;52(10):1076-1083.
77. Thunberg C, Morozowich S, Ramakrishna H. Inhaled therapy for the management of perioperative pulmonary hypertension. *Ann Card Anaesth*. 2015;18(3):394-402.
78. Shore-Lesserson L, Baker RA, Ferraris VA, et al. The Society of Thoracic Surgeons, The Society of Cardiovascular Anesthesiologists, and The American Society of ExtraCorporeal Technology: clinical practice guidelines—anticoagulation during cardiopulmonary bypass. *Ann Thorac Surg*. 2018;105(2):650-662.
79. Despotis GJ, Joist JH, Hogue CW Jr, et al. More effective suppression of hemostatic system activation in patients undergoing cardiac surgery by heparin dosing based on heparin blood concentrations rather than ACT. *Thromb Haemost*. 1996;76(6):902-908. PMID: 8972609.
80. Lemmer JH, Despotis GJ. Antithrombin III concentrate to treat heparin resistance in patients undergoing cardiac surgery. *J Thorac Cardiovasc Surg*. 2002;123(2):213-217.
81. Beattie GW, Jeffrey RR. Is there evidence that fresh frozen plasma is superior to antithrombin administration to treat heparin resistance in cardiac surgery? *Interact Cardiovasc Thorac Surg*. 2014;18(1):117-120.
82. Pishko AM, Cuker A. Heparin-induced thrombocytopenia and cardiovascular surgery. *Hematology*. 2021;2021(1):536-544. https://ashpublications.org/hematology/article/2021/1/536/483002/Heparin-induced-thrombocytopenia-and
83. Koster A, Faraoni D, Levy JH. Argatroban and bivalirudin for perioperative anticoagulation in cardiac surgery. *Anesthesiology*. 2018;128(2):390-400.
84. Food and Drug Administration label for bivalirudin. https://www.accessdata.fda.gov/drugsatfda_docs/label/2016/020873s036lbl.pdf.
85. Agarwal S, Ullom B, Al-Baghdadi Y, Okumura M. Challenges encountered with argatroban anticoagulation during cardiopulmonary bypass. *J Anaesthesiol Clin Pharmacol*. 2012;28(1):106-110.
86. Hillebrand J, Sindermann J, Schmidt C, Mesters R, Martens S, Scherer M. Implantation of left ventricular assist devices under extracorporeal life support in patients with heparin-induced thrombocytopenia. *J Artif Organs*. 2015;18(4):291-299.
87. Tibi P, McClure RS, Huang J, et al. STS/SCA/AmSECT/SABM update to the clinical practice guidelines on patient blood management. *Ann Thorac Surg*. 2021;112(3):981-1004.
88. Zufferey PJ, Lanoiselée J, Graouch B, Vieille B, Delavenne X, Ollier E. Exposure-response relationship of tranexamic acid in cardiac surgery: a model-based meta-analysis. *Anesthesiology*. 2021;34(2):165-178.
89. Chauncey JM, Wieters JS. Tranexamic acid. In: *StatPearls*. StatPearls Publishing; 2022.
90. Aggarwal NK, Subramanian A. Antifibrinolytics and cardiac surgery: the past, the present, and the future. *Ann Card Anaesth*. 2020;23(2):193-199.
91. Fergusson DA, Hébert PC, Mazer CD, et al. A comparison of aprotinin and lysine analogues in high-risk cardiac surgery. *N Engl J Med*. 2008;358(22):2319-2331.

Equipment and Technology

4

Cardiac Ultrasound

Rohesh Joseph Fernando, Davinder S. Ramsingh, and Alina Nicoara

KEY POINTS

1. Transesophageal echocardiography (TEE) uses piezoelectric crystals to generate ultrasound waves that are processed to produce an image. Several modes, such as color flow Doppler and three-dimensional imaging, allow for displaying additional information beyond the standard two-dimensional imaging.

2. Pulsed-wave Doppler is useful for measuring velocities at a specific location but is subject to aliasing. Continuous-wave Doppler is useful for measuring high velocities since aliasing does not occur but is subject to range ambiguity.

3. Understanding knobology is important to optimize imaging.

4. The comprehensive TEE examination includes 28 views obtained from either the esophagus or the stomach. This allows for evaluation of structure and/or function of the ventricles, atria, valves, thoracic aorta, and pericardium.

5. Point-of-care ultrasonography (POCUS) has demonstrated utility for hemodynamic monitoring and assessment of cardiopulmonary function.

6. Although pulmonary POCUS image acquisition is straightforward, the ideal image acquisition windows for cardiac POCUS have more variability and often require multiple ultrasound planes to visualize the entire anatomy.

7. Lung ultrasound is noninvasive and allows for immediate bedside diagnosis of lung pathology such as pulmonary edema, pleural effusion, and pneumothorax.

I. Introduction

Transesophageal echocardiography (TEE) is an invaluable tool in the armamentarium of cardiac anesthesiologists. In addition to cardiac surgical procedures, TEE is utilized in areas outside the operating room such as the intensive care unit as well as the cardiac catheterization lab where interventional procedures are performed.[1] Proficiency in perioperative TEE is therefore paramount. This chapter focuses on the basic tenets of ultrasound and the approach for comprehensive TEE evaluation. In addition, given the expanding role of the cardiac anesthesiologist, focused cardiac and lung ultrasound will be discussed (see ⊙ **Video 4.1** for summary of chapter).

II. Basic Principles of Ultrasound

A. Physics[2]

1. Electricity applied to a piezoelectric crystal causes vibration that produces ultrasound. Returning ultrasound waves similarly cause vibration of the crystal, which can then be used to create a scan line. The process of sending and receiving an ultrasound is a cycle.

2. A two-dimensional (2D) image, known as a frame, is created from up to 100 scan lines per sector by excitation of multiple crystals in a sequential manner. The creation of multiple frames per second (frame rate) allows for live imaging with cardiac motion.

3. The ultrasound systems spend less than 1% of the cycle transmitting ultrasound waves and a very large percentage of time (99%) receiving them. When continuous-wave Doppler is used, a pair of piezoelectric crystals is employed, one transmits 100% of the time and one listens for the reflected waveform 100% of the time.

4. The sound wave weakens or attenuates as it travels through the tissues. The processes that contribute to attenuation are reflection, scattering, and absorption. Reflection decreases the portion of the sound wave that continues to transmit in a forward direction. The percentage of sound waves reflected backward versus transmitted forward depends on the impedance between media separated by a boundary and the angle of incidence of the sound wave at the boundary. Normal incidence of the sound wave to the surface boundary leads to optimal transmission.

5. The Doppler effect can be used to calculate the velocity (v) of moving objects using the Doppler equation. As an object moves, there is a change in the transmitted frequency reflected off the object. The difference between the frequency of the reflected sound wave (F_r) and the transmitted frequency (F_t) can be used together with other parameters such as the speed of sound (c) in tissue (1,540 m/s) and the cosine of the angle (θ) between the Doppler beam and moving object to calculate the velocity of the moving object using the Doppler equation, $v = \dfrac{(F_r - F_t)c}{(\cos \theta)2F_t}$.

6. **Nyquist limit:** The limit above which ultrasound velocities cannot be accurately measured due to inadequate sampling frequency when using pulsed wave Doppler. Mathematically defined as pulse repetition frequency divided by 2. The higher the sampling rate, the higher the velocity of blood flow that can be accurately measured.

   a. Aliasing can sometimes be corrected by changing the baseline and always be corrected by using continuous-wave Doppler.

CLINICAL PEARL

When using the Doppler effect, calculating velocities of objects moving at 90° to the ultrasound beam is not possible, and nonparallel angles lead to underestimation.

B. Probe Selection

1. The current age of TEE started in 1982 with the use of phased array probes. Multiplane imaging was subsequently developed with the ability to rotate the transducer angle up to 180°.[1] Currently, matrix-array transducers offer the ability to obtain three-dimensional (3D) images of the heart by using ~3,000 piezoelectric elements in the 5-8 MHz range.[3]

C. **Ultrasound Modes**
   1. **M-mode[4]**
      a. Displays returning echoes in one dimension (*y*-axis) over time (*x*-axis) with *very* high temporal resolution. This is not routinely recommended for measurements but can be helpful for specific situations such as tricuspid annular plane systolic excursion (TAPSE), assessing aortic valve leaflet motion, or detecting systolic anterior motion (SAM) of the mitral valve (MV).
   2. **Two-dimensional[1]**
      a. This is the standard mode used for TEE imaging.
   3. **Three-dimensional[1,3]**
      a. A 3-D TEE probe allows for multiplane imaging (simultaneous display of orthogonal 2D images) or the creation of a three-dimensional dataset.
      b. A dataset can be single or multi-beat. Single-beat allows for live imaging. Multi-beat acquisition, in which gating based on the electrocardiogram allows for individual sub-volumes (slices) of a desired volume to be independently acquired and stitched together into a final dataset, offers high temporal (30 Hz or higher for multi-beat, full-volume acquisition) and spatial resolution. Arrhythmias or movement, such as respiratory motion, can lead to image compilation problems (stitch artifact).
      c. A narrow-angle volume (narrow sector) is a 30° × 60° dataset. A wide-angle volume (wide sector) offers the ability to include more structures at the expense of temporal resolution. A zoom mode allows for a focused, wide-sector option that should be kept as small as possible to maximize temporal resolution.
      d. Color flow Doppler (CFD) can be used with 3D, but this mode decreases temporal resolution (a multi-beat, full-volume acquisition may be in the range of 15-25 Hz).

CLINICAL PEARL

A good-quality 3D dataset requires a good-quality 2D image.

   4. **Pulsed-wave Doppler[4]**
      a. Spectral Doppler mode is used to display the velocity of blood flow (*y*-axis) at a specific location (sample volume) over time (*x*-axis). Blood flow away from the TEE probe is displayed below the baseline, whereas flow toward the probe is displayed above the baseline. When velocities exceed the Nyquist limit (see section II.A.6), aliasing occurs, resulting in partial or "overlapping" (discontinuous) waveforms.
   5. **Continuous-Wave Doppler[4]**
      a. Spectral Doppler mode that employs two crystals, continuously sending and receiving signals along the line of the Doppler beam. It is used to measure high velocities over time since aliasing does not occur as with pulsed-wave Doppler (PWD). However, the location where the velocities originate is unknown, a limitation known as range ambiguity.
   6. **Color flow Doppler[4]**
      a. Uses PWD to determine the speed and direction of blood flow and conveys this information by superimposing color on a 2D image.
   7. **Tissue Doppler imaging[4]**
      a. Imaging that can be combined with CFD and PWD to assess high-amplitude and low velocities originating from the myocardium.
      b. Typically used to assess myocardial velocities and at the MV and tricuspid valve (TV) annuli.

III. **Appropriate Use of Transesophageal Echocardiography**
   A. **Indications for Intraoperative Transesophageal Echocardiography[1,5]**
      1. Intraoperative TEE is indicated for all open-heart and thoracic aortic surgery. When TEE would significantly impact patient care, additional uses that may be appropriate include coronary artery bypass graft surgery, noncardiac surgery with notable cardiac comorbidities, interventional cardiac procedures, major vascular surgery, and in the intensive care unit when the information is not obtainable by transthoracic ultrasound.

TABLE 4.1   Contraindications for TEE Probe Placement

Absolute Contraindications	Relative Contraindications
Perforated viscus	History of radiation to neck and mediastinum
Esophageal stricture	History of gastrointestinal surgery
Esophageal tumor	Recent upper gastrointestinal bleed
Esophageal perforation/laceration	Barrett esophagus
Esophageal diverticulum	History of dysphagia
Active upper gastrointestinal bleed	Restriction of neck mobility (severe cervical arthritis, atlantoaxial disease)
	Esophageal varices
	Coagulopathy, thrombocytopenia
	Active esophagitis
	Active peptic ulcer disease

Reprinted from Hahn RT, Abraham T, Adams MS, et al. Guidelines for performing a comprehensive transesophageal echocardiographic examination: recommendations from the American Society of Echocardiography and the Society of Cardiovascular Anesthesiologists. *J Am Soc Echocardiogr.* 2013;26(9):921-964. © 2013 Elsevier. With permission.

   B. Contraindications for Transesophageal Echocardiography[1]
   1. The risks and benefits should be weighed before insertion of the TEE probe. Absolute and relative contraindications are listed in Table 4.1.
   C. Complications[1]
   1. Intraoperative TEE has a cumulative complication rate of 0.2%. Significant morbidity occurs in up to 1.2%. Possible complications include major bleeding (up to 0.8%), esophageal perforation (up to 0.3%), severely painful sore throat (0.1%), unintentional displacement of the endotracheal tube (0.03%), and dental injury (0.03%).

CLINICAL PEARL

The presence of contraindications should always be assessed prior to TEE probe placement. This may be challenging with emergencies but is nevertheless important.

   IV. Probe Insertion, Manipulation, and Machine Knobology[1]
   A. TEE Probe Insertion
   1. Probe insertion is performed at the head of the bed. A small degree of anteflexion can be useful, and jaw thrust with head flexion facilitates probe placement. Direct laryngoscopy may be required for difficult cases. A bite block should be used after probe placement.[1]

CLINICAL PEARL

A bite block is important to protect the TEE probe. It is typically easier to place the bite block *after* probe insertion.

   B. TEE Probe Manipulation
   1. Several movements/adjustments are possible with a TEE probe (**Figure 4.1**). These include advancement/withdrawal, rotation of the probe to the patient's right/left, anteflexion/retroflexion (large wheel), and right/left flexion (small wheel). Extreme flexion should be avoided to reduce the risk of injury, especially with probe advancement/withdrawal. The omniplane angle can be electronically adjusted to rotate forward to 180° or backward to 0°. Views can be obtained in the upper esophagus (UE), mid-esophagus (ME), and stomach (transgastric [TG]). Structures can be viewed in long axis (LAX) and short axis (SAX).[1]
   C. Transesophageal Echocardiography Machine Knobology[4]
   1. **Sector width:** The narrowest width to include the structure of interest should be used.
   2. **Depth:** The lowest depth needed for the structure of interest should be used.

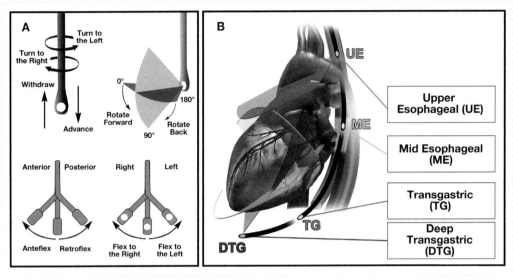

FIGURE 4.1   (A) Various TEE probe manipulations are possible and are named according to their action; **(B)** the different probe positions and their relationship to the heart are shown. (Reprinted from Hahn RT, Abraham T, Adams MS, et al. Guidelines for performing a comprehensive transesophageal echocardiographic examination: recommendations from the American Society of Echocardiography and the Society of Cardiovascular Anesthesiologists. *J Am Soc Echocardiogr.* 2013;26(9):921-964. © 2013 Elsevier. With permission.)

3. **Focus:** The narrowest area of the beam where lateral resolution is improved. The focus should be set at the same depth as the structure of interest.
4. **Gain:** Amplification of received ultrasound signals prior to display. Increasing gain shows as increased brightness.
5. **Time-gain compensation:** Allows for adjusting gain based on depth
6. **Color gain:** Should be increased until random color speckles are seen outside the area being evaluated and then decreased until the speckles are no longer seen. This may need to be adjusted more than once. Blood flow may be masked by color gain that is too low.
7. **Color map:** Typically, flow toward the probe is red and flow away from the probe is blue. The Nyquist limit is generally 50-70 cm/s. Turbulent flow is typically bright with several colors seen.

CLINICAL PEARL

Take the time to adjust knobology to ensure the image is optimized.

V. **Intraoperative Transesophageal Echocardiography Examination**
  A. **Comprehensive Exam**
    1. The Society of Cardiovascular Anesthesiologists and the American Society of Echocardiography (ASE) have proposed a standard comprehensive examination (Figure 4.2). Additional views may be necessary, and angles and probe movements required for each view may be patient-specific.[1]
  B. **Left Ventricle**
    1. **Transesophageal echocardiography views:** ME 4-chamber (▶ **Video 4.2**), ME 2-chamber (▶ **Video 4.3**), and TG SAX (▶ **Video 4.4**) views may be particularly helpful.[1]
    2. **Left ventricle systolic function**[6]
      a. Fractional shortening is a method based on the percentage decrease in left ventricle (LV) chamber diameter between systole and diastole. Regional wall motion abnormalities may render this less accurate.

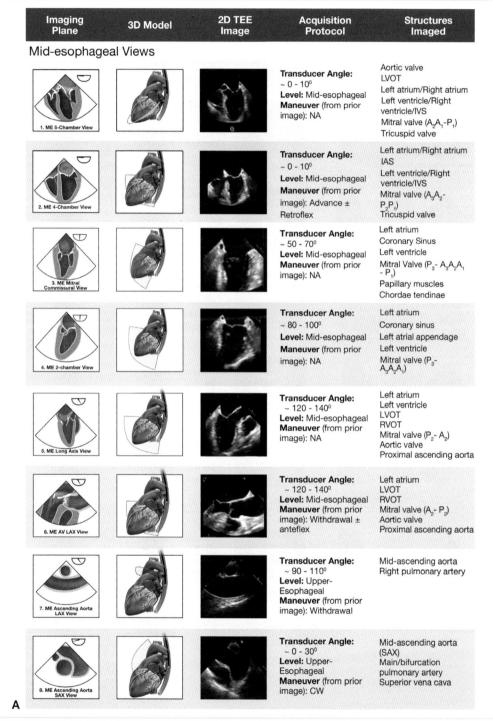

Imaging Plane	3D Model	2D TEE Image	Acquisition Protocol	Structures Imaged
Mid-esophageal Views				
1. ME 5-Chamber View			**Transducer Angle:** ~ 0 - 10° **Level:** Mid-esophageal **Maneuver** (from prior image): NA	Aortic valve LVOT Left atrium/Right atrium Left ventricle/Right ventricle/IVS Mitral valve (A_2A_1-P_1) Tricuspid valve
2. ME 4-Chamber View			**Transducer Angle:** ~ 0 - 10° **Level:** Mid-esophageal **Maneuver** (from prior image): Advance ± Retroflex	Left atrium/Right atrium IAS Left ventricle/Right ventricle/IVS Mitral valve (A_3A_2-P_2P_1) Tricuspid valve
3. ME Mitral Commissural View			**Transducer Angle:** ~ 50 - 70° **Level:** Mid-esophageal **Maneuver** (from prior image): NA	Left atrium Coronary Sinus Left ventricle Mitral Valve (P_3- $A_3A_2A_1$ - P_1) Papillary muscles Chordae tendinae
4. ME 2-chamber View			**Transducer Angle:** ~ 80 - 100° **Level:** Mid-esophageal **Maneuver** (from prior image): NA	Left atrium Coronary sinus Left atrial appendage Left ventricle Mitral valve (P_3- $A_3A_2A_1$)
5. ME Long Axis View			**Transducer Angle:** ~ 120 - 140° **Level:** Mid-esophageal **Maneuver** (from prior image): NA	Left atrium Left ventricle LVOT RVOT Mitral valve (P_2- A_2) Aortic valve Proximal ascending aorta
6. ME AV LAX View			**Transducer Angle:** ~ 120 - 140° **Level:** Mid-esophageal **Maneuver** (from prior image): Withdrawal ± anteflex	Left atrium LVOT RVOT Mitral valve (A_2- P_2) Aortic valve Proximal ascending aorta
7. ME Ascending Aorta LAX View			**Transducer Angle:** ~ 90 - 110° **Level:** Upper-Esophageal **Maneuver** (from prior image): Withdrawal	Mid-ascending aorta Right pulmonary artery
8. ME Ascending Aorta SAX View			**Transducer Angle:** ~ 0 - 30° **Level:** Upper-Esophageal **Maneuver** (from prior image): CW	Mid-ascending aorta (SAX) Main/bifurcation pulmonary artery Superior vena cava

A

FIGURE 4.2 Comprehensive transesophageal echocardiographic examination with 28 views as suggested by the Society of Cardiovascular Anesthesiologists and the American Society of Echocardiography. The mid-esophageal (ME) views (**A, B**), transgastric (TG) views (**C**), and aortic views (**D**) are depicted. AV, aortic valve; CW, clockwise; CCW, counter-clockwise; IAS, interatrial septum; IVS, interventricular septum; LAX, long axis; LVOT, left ventricular outflow tract; MV, mitral valve; NA, not applicable; RV, right ventricle; RVOT, right ventricular outflow tract; SAX, short axis; TV, tricuspid valve. (Reprinted from Hahn RT, Abraham T, Adams MS, et al. Guidelines for performing a comprehensive transesophageal echocardiographic examination: recommendations from the American Society of Echocardiography and the Society of Cardiovascular Anesthesiologists. *J Am Soc Echocardiogr.* 2013;26(9):921-964. © 2013 Elsevier. With permission.)

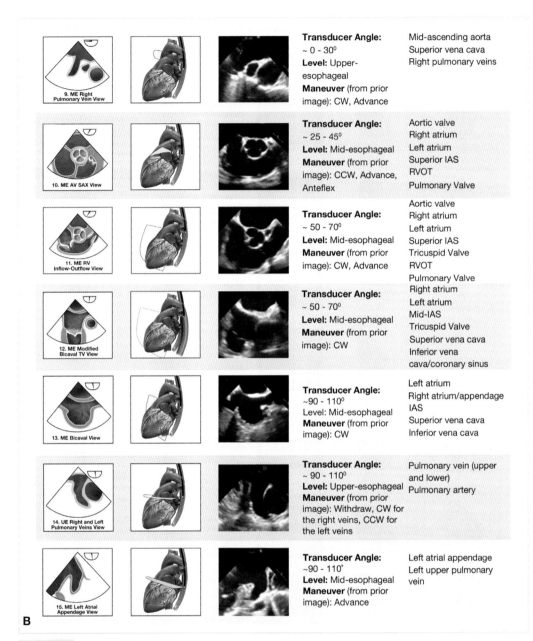

			Transducer Angle: ~ 0 - 30° **Level:** Upper-esophageal **Maneuver** (from prior image): CW, Advance	Mid-ascending aorta Superior vena cava Right pulmonary veins
			Transducer Angle: ~ 25 - 45° **Level:** Mid-esophageal **Maneuver** (from prior image): CCW, Advance, Anteflex	Aortic valve Right atrium Left atrium Superior IAS RVOT Pulmonary Valve
			Transducer Angle: ~ 50 - 70° **Level:** Mid-esophageal **Maneuver** (from prior image): CW, Advance	Aortic valve Right atrium Left atrium Superior IAS Tricuspid Valve RVOT Pulmonary Valve
			Transducer Angle: ~ 50 - 70° **Level:** Mid-esophageal **Maneuver** (from prior image): CW	Right atrium Left atrium Mid-IAS Tricuspid Valve Superior vena cava Inferior vena cava/coronary sinus
			Transducer Angle: ~90 - 110° Level: Mid-esophageal **Maneuver** (from prior image): CW	Left atrium Right atrium/appendage IAS Superior vena cava Inferior vena cava
			Transducer Angle: ~ 90 - 110° **Level:** Upper-esophageal **Maneuver** (from prior image): Withdraw, CW for the right veins, CCW for the left veins	Pulmonary vein (upper and lower) Pulmonary artery
			Transducer Angle: ~90 - 110° **Level:** Mid-esophageal **Maneuver** (from prior image): Advance	Left atrial appendage Left upper pulmonary vein

9. ME Right Pulmonary Vein View

10. ME AV SAX View

11. ME RV Inflow-Outflow View

12. ME Modified Bicaval TV View

13. ME Bicaval View

14. UE Right and Left Pulmonary Veins View

15. ME Left Atrial Appendage View

B

FIGURE 4.2   (continued)

Transgastric Views

16. TG Basal SAX View

Transducer Angle: ~ 0 - 20°
Level: Transgastric
Maneuver (from prior image): Advance ± Anteflex

Left ventricle (base)
Right ventricle (base)
Mitral valve (SAX)
Tricuspid valve (short-axis)

17. TG Mid Papillary SAX View

Transducer Angle: ~ 0 - 20°
Level: Transgastric
Maneuver (from prior image): Advance ± Anteflex

Left ventricle (mid)
Papillary muscles
Right ventricle (mid)

18. TG Apical SAX View

Transducer Angle: ~ 0 - 20°
Level: Transgastric
Maneuver (from prior image): Advance ± Anteflex

Left ventricle (apex)
Right ventricle (apex)

19. TG RV Basal View

Transducer Angle: ~ 0 - 20°
Level: Transgastric
Maneuver (from prior image): Anteflex

Left ventricle (mid)
Right ventricle (mid)
Right ventricular outflow tract
Tricuspid Valve (SAX)
Pulmonary Valve

20. TG RV Inflow-Outflow View

Transducer Angle: ~ 0 - 20°
Level: Transgastric
Maneuver (from prior image): Right-flex

Right atrium
Right ventricle
Right ventricular outflow tract
Pulmonary valve
Tricuspid Valve

21. Deep TG 5-chamber View

Transducer Angle: ~ 0 - 20°
Level: Transgastric
Maneuver (from prior image): Left-flex, Advance, Anteflex

Left ventricle
Left ventricular outflow tract
Right ventricle
Aortic valve
Aortic root
Mitral Valve

22. TG 2-Chamber View

Transducer Angle: ~ 90 - 110°
Level: Transgastric
Maneuver (from prior image): Neutral flexion, Withdraw

Left ventricle
Left atrium/appendage
Mitral valve

23. TG RV Inflow View

Transducer Angle: ~ 90 - 110°
Level: Transgastric
Maneuver (from prior image): CW

Right ventricle
Right atrium
Tricuspid valve

24. TG LAX View

Transducer Angle: ~ 120 - 140°
Level: Transgastric
Maneuver (from prior image): CCW

Left ventricle
Left ventricular outflow tract
Right ventricle
Aortic valve
Aortic root
Mitral valve

C

FIGURE 4.2 *(continued)*

Aortic Views

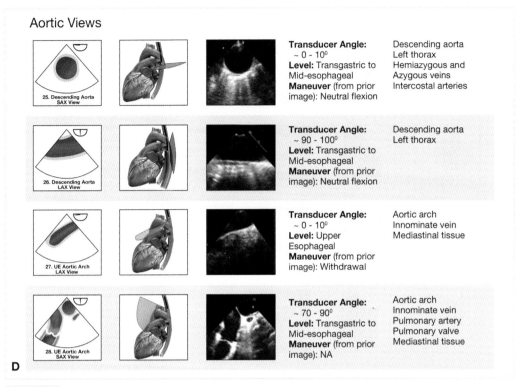

| | | | Transducer Angle: ~ 0 - 10⁰ **Level:** Transgastric to Mid-esophageal **Maneuver** (from prior image): Neutral flexion | Descending aorta Left thorax Hemiazygous and Azygous veins Intercostal arteries |

25. Descending Aorta SAX View

Transducer Angle: ~ 0 - 10⁰
Level: Transgastric to Mid-esophageal
Maneuver (from prior image): Neutral flexion

Descending aorta
Left thorax
Hemiazygous and
Azygous veins
Intercostal arteries

26. Descending Aorta LAX View

Transducer Angle: ~ 90 - 100⁰
Level: Transgastric to Mid-esophageal
Maneuver (from prior image): Neutral flexion

Descending aorta
Left thorax

27. UE Aortic Arch LAX View

Transducer Angle: ~ 0 - 10⁰
Level: Upper Esophageal
Maneuver (from prior image): Withdrawal

Aortic arch
Innominate vein
Mediastinal tissue

28. UE Aortic Arch SAX View

Transducer Angle: ~ 70 - 90⁰
Level: Transgastric to Mid-esophageal
Maneuver (from prior image): NA

Aortic arch
Innominate vein
Pulmonary artery
Pulmonary valve
Mediastinal tissue

D

FIGURE 4.2 *(continued)*

(1) Fractional shortening (%) measured at the endocardium is classified as normal (male: 25-43, female: 27-45), mildly decreased (male: 20-24, female 22-26), moderately decreased (male: 15-19, female 17-21), or severely decreased (male: ≤14, female ≤16).[7]

b. **Left ventricle ejection fraction (LVEF):** The recommended 2D method is modified Simpson's rule (biplane technique that divides the LV into disks and adds them up); 3D EF is accurate and reproducible and should be used whenever possible.

c. EF (%) can be classified as normal (male: 52-72, female: 54-74), mildly decreased (male: 41-51, female: 41-53), moderately decreased (male and female: 30-40), or severely decreased (male and female: <30).

d. A 17-segment model exists (Figure 4.3), and regional wall motion can be scored based on myocardial wall thickening: 1 = normal/hyperkinetic, 2 = hypokinetic (less than normal but noticeable thickening), 3 = akinetic (no significant thickening), 4 = dyskinetic (thinning during systole rather than thickening—also known as aneurysmal).

CLINICAL PEARL

A new regional wall motion abnormality should raise concern for adequate perfusion from the corresponding coronary artery that supplies the territory.

3. **Left ventricle diastolic function**[8]

a. Mitral annular e' velocities (obtained by tissue Doppler imaging (TDI) at lateral and septal mitral annulus), transmitral E and A velocities (Figure 4.4), peak tricuspid regurgitation (TR) velocity, pulmonary vein S/D velocities, and left atrium (LA) volume should be measured. Notably, these criteria may be affected by age and hemodynamics. Diagnosis of

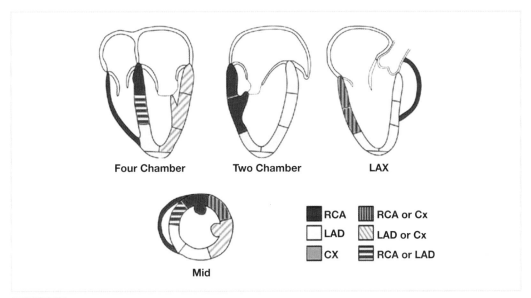

Four Chamber   Two Chamber   LAX

Mid

■ RCA	▥ RCA or Cx
□ LAD	▨ LAD or Cx
▨ CX	▤ RCA or LAD

FIGURE 4.3   Depiction of the different segments of the left ventricle and their respective coronary artery supply. Cx, circumflex; LAD, left anterior descending; LAX, long axis; RCA, right coronary artery. (Reprinted from Reeves ST, Finley AC, Skubas NJ, et al. Basic perioperative transesophageal echocardiography examination: a consensus statement of the American Society of Echocardiography and the Society of Cardiovascular Anesthesiologists. *J Am Soc Echocardiogr.* 2013;26(5):443-456. © 2013 Elsevier. With permission.)

diastolic dysfunction can be assessed and graded (Figure 4.5). Grade II is also known as pseudonormalization, named because the *E/A* ratio resembles that of normal.[8] The LA volume will be difficult to obtain by TEE given incomplete visualization of the LA.[6]

4. **Size**[6]
   a. LV size (cm) in end-diastole can be classified as normal (male: 4.2-5.8, female: 3.8-5.2), mildly abnormal (men: 5.9-6.3, female: 5.3-5.6), moderately abnormal (male: 6.4-6.8, female: 5.7-6.1), and severely abnormal (male: >6.8, female: >6.1).
   b. The TG SAX view can be helpful to assess preload at the extremes. Hypovolemia may be suggested by low LV end-diastolic diameter/area.[9]

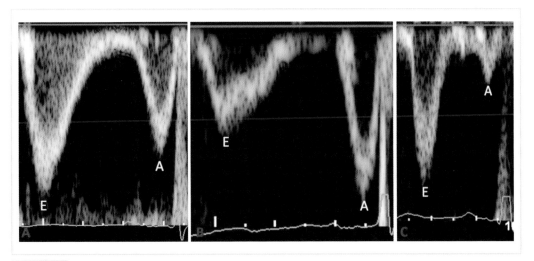

FIGURE 4.4   Transmitral spectral Doppler profile demonstrating the E and A waves, obtained by placing the PWD sample gate between the MV leaflet tips. **(A)** Normal (also pseudonormal [grade II diastolic dysfunction]), **(B)** impaired relaxation (grade I diastolic dysfunction) with E/A ≤0.8, and **(C)** restrictive pattern (grade III diastolic dysfunction) with E/A >2 are shown.

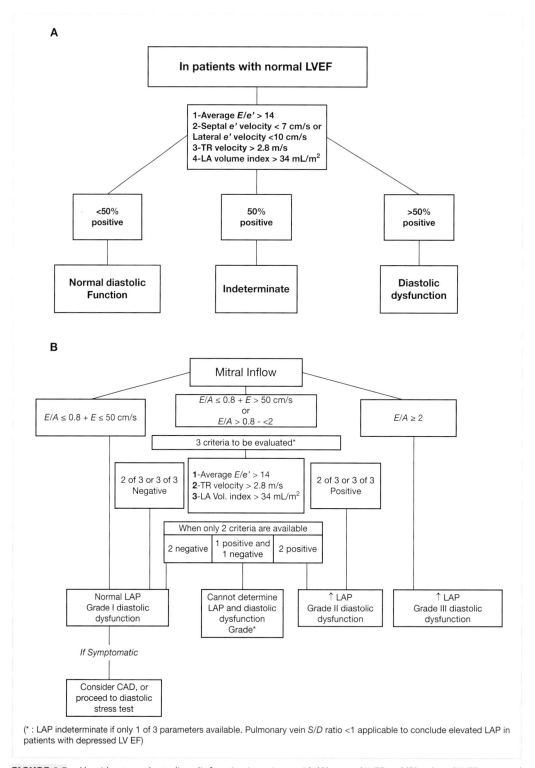

FIGURE 4.5   Algorithm to evaluate diastolic function in patients with **(A)** normal LVEF and **(B)** reduced LVEF or normal LVEF with myocardial disease. CAD, coronary artery disease; LAP, left atrial pressure; LVEF, left ventricle ejection fraction; Vol, volume. (Reprinted from Nagueh SF, Smiseth OA, Appleton CP, et al. Recommendations for the evaluation of left ventricular diastolic function by echocardiography: an update from the American Society of Echocardiography and the European Association of Cardiovascular Imaging. *J Am Soc Echocardiogr.* 2016;29(4):277-314. © 2016 American Society of Echocardiography. With permission.)

5. **Wall thickness[6]**
   a. Septal and posterior wall thickness (cm) can be classified as normal (male: 0.6-1.0, female: 0.6-0.9), mildly abnormal (male: 1.1-1.3, female: 1.0-1.2), moderately abnormal (male: 1.4-1.6, female: 1.3-1.5), and severely abnormal (male: >1.6, female: >1.5).
   b. Hypertrophic cardiomyopathy (HCM) is diagnosed by wall thickness ≥1.5 cm without cause (≥1.3 cm if genetic predisposition or family history of HCM). Obstruction is suggested by turbulence in the LV outflow tract (LVOT) with CFD and a mid-late peaking dagger-shaped waveform with continuous-wave Doppler (CWD) in the LVOT.[10]

C. **Right Ventricle[6]**
   1. **Transesophageal echocardiography views:** ME four-chamber, ME right ventricle (RV) inflow-outflow (⊙ **Video 4.5**), and TG SAX views may be particularly helpful.[1]
   2. Dilation is indicated by basal diameter >41 mm or a mid-diameter >35 mm. Normal wall thickness is 1-5 mm in end-diastole.
   3. **Right ventricle systolic function**
      a. Parameters used for assessment include TAPSE (<17 mm abnormal), fractional area change as measured in ME 4-chamber view (<35% abnormal), s' velocity obtained by TDI at the lateral tricuspid annulus (<9.5 cm/s abnormal), and RV myocardial performance index (RIMP) (PWD value >0.43 or TDI >0.54 abnormal).

      (1) $$RIMP = \frac{\text{Isovolemic Contraction Time + Isovolemic Relaxation Time}}{\text{RV Ejection Time}}$$

      (a) May be inaccurate when right atrium (RA) pressure is increased.
      (2) Despite preserved RV EF, TAPSE and s' values may decrease after opening the pericardium and/or cardiopulmonary bypass.[11]

D. **Interventricular Septum[1,10,12,13]**
   1. **Transesophageal echocardiography views:** The interventricular septum (IVS) can be seen in multiple ME views, but the ME four-chamber, ME LAX (⊙ **Video 4.6**), and TG SAX views may be particularly helpful.[1]
   2. The IVS separates the RV and LV.
   3. A ventricular septal defect may be congenital or iatrogenic (after septal myectomy) and typically results in left → right systolic flow.

CLINICAL PEARL

Flattening of the IVS during systole suggests RV pressure overload, whereas during diastole suggests RV volume overload.[13]

E. **Right Atrium**
   1. **Transesophageal echocardiography views:** The RA can be seen in many ME views, but the ME four-chamber and ME bicaval (⊙ **Video 4.7**) views may be particularly helpful.[1]
   2. The ME four-chamber view is likely the best for measuring the RA size.[6]
   3. A eustachian valve, a fetal remnant designed to point blood toward the fossa ovalis, can be seen at the inferior vena cava (IVC)/RA junction in the ME bicaval view. A net-like structure of fibers is more consistent with a Chiari network, which can be associated with an aneurysmal interatrial septum (IAS) and/or patent foramen ovale (PFO).[1]
   4. The crista terminalis, seen in the ME bicaval view at the opening of the superior vena cava (SVC) in the RA, is a ridge that separates the smooth part of the RA from the right atrial appendage.[1]
   5. The opening of the coronary sinus can be found in the vicinity of the IVC and the septal leaflet of the TV. A Thebesian valve may be present near the ostium. The coronary sinus can be visualized in LAX by advancing the probe slightly from an ME four-chamber view or using an ME bicaval view with slight advancement and rightward rotation of the probe.[1]

F. **Interatrial Septum**
1. **Transesophageal echocardiography views:** The IAS can be seen in multiple ME views, but the ME four-chamber and ME bicaval views may be particularly helpful.[1]
2. The IAS separates the left and right atria. An atrial septal defect (ASD) creates a shunt and may risk paradoxical embolism; ASD types include primum, secundum, sinus venosus, and coronary sinus.[14]
3. **Aneurysmal interatrial septum:** A fixed protrusion or hypermobility of the fossa ovalis area with combined or one-sided movement toward the right or left atria from midline of ≥15 mm; it is frequently associated with a PFO.[14]

CLINICAL PEARL

A PFO can be diagnosed by injection of agitated saline with >3 bubbles seen in the LA within three beats after bubbles are visualized in the RA. Visualization of bubbles after 3-8 beats may suggest intrapulmonary shunt. CFD can also be used to diagnose a PFO but cannot exclude it.[1]

G. **Left Atrium**
1. **Transesophageal echocardiography views:** The LA can be seen in all ME views, but the ME four-chamber, ME two-chamber, and ME bicaval views may be particularly helpful. The LA is typically the closest chamber to the TEE probe in the ME views.[1]
2. Size is measured at the end of ventricular systole, but TEE is not recommended for this since the LA cannot be seen in its entirety by TEE.[6]
3. The left atrial appendage (LAA) is a common area for thrombus with atrial fibrillation. The LAA can be imaged at 0°, 45°, 90°, and 135°.[15]
4. **Pulmonary veins**
   a. PWD sample gate is placed 1-2 cm into the pulmonary vein.[1]
   b. Normal pattern is triphasic and includes antegrade systolic (S) and diastolic (D) waves, and a retrograde atrial (A) wave.[16]

H. **Aortic Valve**
1. **Transesophageal echocardiography views:** The aortic valve (AV) can be evaluated in the ME SAX (Video 4.8) and LAX, and deep TG five-chamber (TG-5ch) (LAX) view (Video 4.9).[1]
2. **Anatomy:** The AV has three cusps: left, right, and noncoronary cusps.[1]
3. **Aortic stenosis**[17]
   a. **Etiology:** Most commonly calcific tricuspid, calcific bicuspid, and rheumatic
   b. Level 1 recommendations (for all patients) for diagnosing aortic stenosis are mean gradient, peak velocity, or calculated aortic valve area (AVA) by continuity equation.
      (1) The mean gradient and peak velocity are obtained from a deep TG-5ch using CWD across the AV.
      (2) Calculating the AVA requires measurement of the LVOT diameter (D_{LVOT}) in the ME LAX view to calculate the LVOT area (A_{LVOT}), the LVOT velocity time integrals (VTI) (VTI_{LVOT}) using PWD in the deep TG-5ch, the AV VTI (VTI_{AV} using CWD in deep TG-5ch).
         (a) $A_{LVOT} = \pi(D_{LVOT}/2)^2$
         (b) $AVA = \dfrac{A_{LVOT} \times VTI_{LVOT}}{VTI_{AV}}$
   c. Planimetry (tracing out area on 2D/3D) and dimensionless index (DI), similar to velocity ratio, are level 2 criteria.
      (1) $DI = \dfrac{VTI_{LVOT}}{VTI_{AV}}$

    d. LV dysfunction and low-flow, low-gradient AS

        (1) Severe AS (AVA <1.0 cm^2) can exist despite not meeting traditional velocity/gradient criteria due to the inability to generate adequate flow across the stenotic aortic valve (eg, as a result of LV dysfunction).

        (2) If the LV dysfunction is caused by increased afterload from AS, then this may represent true severe AS. If the LVEF is reduced due to another reason (myocardial infarction), then this may be pseudosevere AS. An increase in AVA >1.0 cm^2 after administration of dobutamine suggests against true severe AS.

  4. Aortic regurgitation[13]

    a. Etiology: Type 1 refers to normal leaflet motion, but aortic regurgitation (AR) occurs due to (1a) dilation of the sinotubular junction (STJ) and ascending aorta, (1b) dilation of sinuses of Valsalva (SoV) and STJ, (1c) dilation of aortic annulus, or (1d) cusp perforation/tear. Type II is excessive motion (prolapse), and type III refers to restriction.

    b. Qualitative measures

        (1) Pressure half-time (ms) obtained by CWD (mild >500, moderate 200-500, severe <200) or holo-diastolic flow reversal in the descending aorta

    c. Semi-quantitative

        (1) Vena contracta (mm) (mild <3, moderate 3-6, severe >6) or ratio of jet width/LVOT width (%) for central jet (mild <25, moderate 25-64, severe ≥65). Vena contracta is the narrowest portion of the jet that is either at the orifice of regurgitation or immediately after.

    d. Quantitative

        (1) Regurgitant volume (mL/beat) (mild <30, moderate 30-59, severe ≥60) or effective regurgitant orifice area (EROA) (cm^2) (mild <0.10, moderate 0.10-0.29, severe ≥0.30)

I. Mitral Valve

  1. Transesophageal echocardiography views: The MV can be evaluated in multiple views, including ME four-chamber, ME mitral commissural (⊙ **Video 4.10**), ME LAX, and TG SAX.[1]

  2. Anatomy: The MV has two leaflets (anterior and posterior). The posterior leaflet has three scallops from lateral to medial (P$_1$, P$_2$, and P$_3$). The anterior leaflet does not have scallops, but corresponding segments are referenced (A$_1$, A$_2$, and A$_3$).[1]

  3. Mitral stenosis

    a. Etiology: Despite low incidence in affluent countries, rheumatic disease is a significant cause of MS throughout the world, with a greater prevalence in women. Classic findings are diastolic doming and commissural fusion. Older patients in affluent countries may develop nonrheumatic calcific MS where calcification develops on the mitral annulus and progresses toward the leaflet bases.[18]

    b. Planimetry and pressure half-time (PHT) are typically the most important measurements for assessing severity. Planimetry refers to tracing of the orifice and while a basal TG SAX can be used, 3D TEE allows for accurate assessment. PHT is the time (ms) necessary for the peak mitral gradient to decrease by half. Pulmonary artery systolic pressure (PASP) can also be useful in grading severity.[18-20]

        (1) Mitral valve area (MVA) by PHT: $\text{MVA} = \dfrac{220}{\text{PHT}}$.

    c. Calculating MVA by continuity equation and proximal isovelocity surface area (PISA) is reserved for when routine measurements are discordant.[20]

        (1) The continuity equation assumes that the volume of blood going through the MV is the same as the volume of blood ejected through the LVOT (conservation of mass). The VTI and area of the LVOT (A_{LVOT}) must be determined.[19]

$$\textbf{(a)} \quad \text{MVA} = A_{\text{LVOT}} \times \left(\frac{\text{VTI}_{\text{LVOT}}}{\text{VTI}_{\text{MV}}} \right)$$

        (b) The continuity equation should not be used if there is significant mitral regurgitation (MR) or AR.[19] It may be more useful in calcific MS when planimetry is challenging due to acoustic shadowing.[18]

(2) **PISA:** A method that assumes hemispheric-shaped flow convergence in the LA as blood crosses the stenotic MV (Figure 4.6). The PISA radius (r) of the hemisphere created where aliasing occurs is measured. The aliasing velocity (Velocity$_{aliasing}$), the Nyquist limit for the direction of stenotic flow, the peak diastolic velocity (Vmax$_{MV}$) through the MV as measured by CWD, and the angle of the MV leaflets (α) on the atrial side must also be determined. MVA can then be calculated by:

(a) $MVA = 2\pi r^2 \left(\dfrac{\text{Velocity}_{aliasing}}{\text{Vmax}_{MV}} \right) \left(\dfrac{\alpha}{180} \right)$

 d. The ASE classifies MS as mild (MVA >2.5 cm^2, PHT <100 ms, mean gradient <5 mm Hg, PASP <30 mm Hg), moderate (MVA 1.6-2.5 cm^2, PHT 100-149 ms, mean gradient 5-9 mm Hg, PASP 30-49 mm Hg), or severe (MVA ≤1.5 cm^2, PHT ≥150 ms, mean gradient ≥10 mm Hg, PASP ≥50 mm Hg). Gradients assume a heart rate of 60-80 beats per minute. ASE guidelines emphasize that MS should not be graded solely based on one criterion.[19] The American College of Cardiology and American Heart Association do not focus on the mean gradients due to their variability with heart rate and flow.[18]

4. **Mitral regurgitation**[13]
   a. **Etiology:** MR is classified as primary (abnormal leaflets) or secondary (abnormal MV coaptation due to LV or LA remodeling). Leaflet motion is classified based on Carpentier system where type 1 is normal motion (leaflet perforation, annular dilation), type II is excess motion (prolapse [leaflet moves into LA >2 mm above annular plane during systole] or flail [leaflet tip is moving freely in LA, typically with ruptured chord]), and type III is restriction due to thickening (IIIa) such as with rheumatic disease, or restriction due to LV dilation (type IIIb) (Figure 4.7).

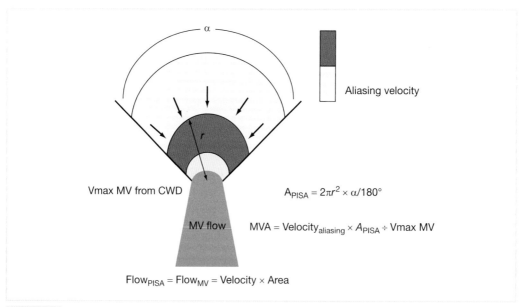

FIGURE 4.6 Diagram of the PISA method to measure MV area in mitral stenosis. The thick lines represent the MV with a central stenotic orifice. As the blood flow converges on the orifice, the velocity increases and causes aliasing of the CFD signal, changing the color from blue to red creating the PISA (small arrows) on the atrial side of the valve. The aliasing velocity (Velocity$_{aliasing}$) is taken from the CFD scale. A_{PISA} is calculated by measuring its radius (r, large arrow) and using the formula for the surface area of a hemisphere and is modified based on the ratio of the angle formed by the leaflets (α) and 180°: $A_{PISA} = 2\pi r^2 \times \alpha/180°$. The peak velocity of the transmitral inflow (Vmax$_{MV}$) is measured by using CWD aimed through the stenotic orifice. Flow$_{PISA}$ = Velocity$_{aliasing}$ $\times$ A_{PISA} and Flow$_{MV}$ = Vmax$_{MV}$ $\cdot$ MVA. By the continuity principle, Flow$_{MV}$ = Flow$_{PISA}$, so MVA = (Velocity$_{aliasing}$ $\times$ A_{PISA})/Vmax$_{MV}$. CFD, Color flow Doppler; MV, mitral valve; PISA, proximal isovelocity surface area.

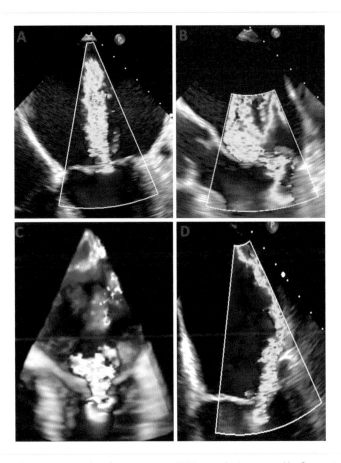

FIGURE 4.7   MR based on Carpentier classification system. **(A)** Type 1 depicts normal leaflet motion. **(B)** Type II depicts excessive leaflet motion (posterior leaflet in this example). **(C)** Type IIIA is leaflet restriction during systole and diastole. **(D)** Type IIIB shows leaflet restriction during systole (posterior leaflet in this example). MR, mitral regurgitation.

b. Methods for assessment
   (1) Vena contracta: Flow convergence must be seen well for accuracy.
   (2) PISA: It is less accurate for eccentric jets. The baseline on CFD is shifted toward the direction of MR such that the Nyquist limit is 30-40 cm/s to produce a hemispheric shape in the area of flow convergence. The Nyquist limit in the direction of the MR jet is the aliasing velocity ($Velocity_{aliasing}$). The PISA radius (r) is then measured in cm from the vena contracta to the area where flow convergence aliases (Figure 4.8). CWD can be used to measure the peak velocity ($Vmax_{MR}$) and VTI of the MR jet (VTI_{MR}), and then the EROA and the regurgitant volume (Rvol) can be calculated.
      (a) $Flow_{MR} = 2\pi r^2 \times Velocity_{aliasing}$
      (b) $EROA = \dfrac{Flow_{MR}}{VMax_{MR}}$
      (c) $Rvol = EROA * VTI_{MR}$
c. Qualitative assessment
   (1) A dense MR jet or triangular jet on CWD, an eccentric wall-hugging jet (Coanda effect), a flail leaflet, and ruptured papillary muscle are associated with severe MR.
d. Semi-quantitative assessment
   (1) Vena contracta (mm) (mild <3, ≥ 3 moderate <7, severe ≥ 7)
   (2) Pulmonary S-wave reversal suggests severe MR but absence does not exclude it.

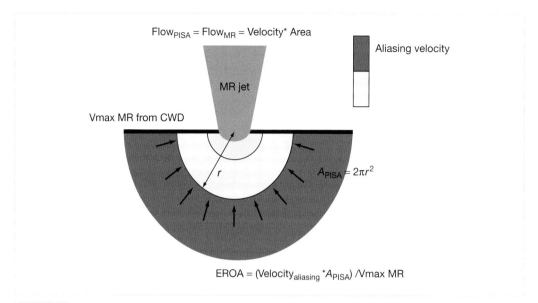

Flow$_{PISA}$ = Flow$_{MR}$ = Velocity* Area

Aliasing velocity

MR jet

Vmax MR from CWD

r

$A_{PISA} = 2\pi r^2$

EROA = (Velocity$_{aliasing}$ *A_{PISA}) /Vmax MR

FIGURE 4.8 Diagram of the PISA method to measure EROA in central MR. The horizontal line represents the MV with a central regurgitant orifice. As the blood flow converges on the orifice, the velocity increases and causes aliasing of the CFD signal, changing the color from red to blue creating the PISA hemisphere (small arrows) on the ventricular side of the valve. The aliasing velocity (Velocity$_{aliasing}$) is taken from the CFD scale. A_{PISA} is calculated by measuring its radius (r, large arrow) and using the formula for the surface area of a hemisphere: $A_{PISA} = 2\pi r^2$. The peak velocity of the MR (Vmax$_{MR}$) is measured by using CWD aimed through the orifice. Flow$_{PISA}$ = Velocity$_{aliasing}$ × A_{PISA} and Flow$_{MR}$ = Vmax$_{MR}$ × EROA. By the continuity principle, Flow$_{MR}$ = Flow$_{PISA}$, so EROA = (Velocity$_{aliasing}$ × A_{PISA})/Vmax$_{MR}$. CFD, Color flow Doppler; EROA, effective regurgitant orifice area; MR, mitral regurgitation; PISA, proximal isovelocity surface area.

   e. Quantitative assessment
      (1) Rvol (mL/beat) (mild <30, moderate 30-59, severe ≥60) or EROA (cm^2) (mild <0.20, moderate 0.20-0.39, severe ≥0.40)
J. **Tricuspid Valve**
   1. **Transesophageal echocardiography views:** ME four-chamber, ME RV inflow-outflow, and ME-modified TV bicaval (⊙ **Video 4.11**) views may be particularly helpful.[1]
   2. **Anatomy:** The TV has three leaflets (anterior, posterior, and septal).[13]
   3. **Tricuspid stenosis**[20]
      a. Lowest incidence of valve stenosis. Causes include rheumatic (diastolic doming), carcinoid (frozen leaflets), endocarditis, tumor, and adhesions from a pacemaker lead.
      b. Hemodynamically significant stenosis is suggested by mean gradient ≥5 mm Hg, inflow VTI >60 cm, PHT ≥190 ms, valve area by continuity equation ≤1 cm^2. A moderate or severely dilated RA and/or IVC may be seen.
   4. **Tricuspid regurgitation**[13]
      a. Leaflet motion is evaluated using Carpentier classification as with the MV. TR is typically a secondary problem such as annular dilation but could also be iatrogenic (pacemaker lead) or congenital (Ebstein anomaly). Trace or mild TR can be normal.
      b. The peak velocity of the TR jet (TR$_{Vmax}$), measured by CWD, can be used to estimate right ventricular systolic pressure (RVSP) based on the modified Bernoulli equation if the central venous pressure (CVP) is known.[9]
      (1) RVSP = 4(TR$_{Vmax}$)^2 + CVP
      (2) In the absence of RV outflow obstruction, the RVSP will be the same as the PASP.
      c. Qualitative assessment
      (1) A dense TR jet or triangular jet on CWD and a flail leaflet are associated with severe TR.

   d. Semi-quantitative assessment
      (1) Vena contracta (mm) (mild <3, ≥3 moderate <7, severe ≥7)
      (2) Hepatic S-wave reversal may suggest severe TR but is affected by numerous factors.
   e. Quantitative assessment
      (1) Rvol (mL/beat) (mild <30, moderate 30-44, severe ≥45) or EROA (cm²) (mild <0.20, moderate 0.20-0.39, severe ≥0.40)

K. Pulmonic Valve
   1. **Transesophageal echocardiography views:** ME RV inflow-outflow and the UE aortic arch SAX (**▶ Video 4.12**) views may be particularly helpful. The pulmonic valve (PV) may be difficult to visualize, given the anterior location.[1]
   2. **Anatomy:** The PV has three cusps: left, right, and anterior.[1]
   3. **Pulmonic stenosis**[20]
      a. Pulmonic stenosis (PS) is usually congenital and may be part of a collection of malformations such as tetralogy of Fallot or double outlet RV.
      b. Severity can be assessed by peak velocity (m/s) (mild <3, moderate 3-4, severe >4) and peak gradient (mm Hg) (mild <36, moderate 36-64, severe >64).
   4. **Pulmonic regurgitation**
      a. Trace-mild pulmonic regurgitation (PR) can be normal. Quantification of PR is not well defined.[13]

L. Aorta
   1. **Transesophageal echocardiography views:** The aortic arch can be visualized using the UE Aortic Arch SAX and LAX (**▶ Video 4.13**). The ascending aorta can be evaluated using ME LAX, ME AV LAX, ME ascending aorta SAX (**▶ Video 4.14**), and LAX (**▶ Video 4.15**). The distal ascending aorta and proximal aortic arch are often not visualized due to interference from the trachea. The descending aorta is seen using the descending aorta SAX (**▶ Video 4.16**) and LAX (**▶ Video 4.17**).[1]
   2. Aortic evaluation includes the aortic root, ascending aorta, aortic arch, and descending aorta.[21]
      a. Size should be measured using leading-edge to leading-edge method at end-diastole. Normal size may vary depending on body surface area, age, and sex (larger in males).
   3. The aorta should be evaluated for atheroma.[21]
      a. Grade 1 (normal): Intimal thickness <2 mm; grade II (mild): intimal thickness 2-3 mm; grade III (moderate): atheroma 3-5 mm; grade IV (severe): atheroma >5 mm; grade V (complex): any atheroma that is ulcerated or mobile.
   4. Examine for evidence of acute aortic syndrome, including ascending aortic aneurysm rupture, dissection, intramural hematoma, or penetrating ulcer (Figure 4.9).[21]
      a. Aortic dissection
         (1) The dissection flap separates true and false lumen and is often mobile. It must be distinguished from artifacts.
            (a) True lumen often expands during systole.

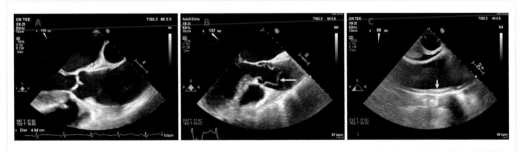

FIGURE 4.9 **(A)** Ascending aortic aneurysm, and acute aortic syndromes such as **(B)** type A dissection, and **(C)** intramural hematoma, are shown.

        (b) False lumen often expands during diastole. Velocities are often slower in false lumen when visualized with CFD, and blood flow may be retrograde. It may contain spontaneous echo contrast or thrombus. It is usually larger than the true lumen in the descending aorta.

CLINICAL PEARL

An aortic dissection may be associated with ventricular dysfunction if the coronary ostia are affected, AR due to dilation or prolapse of the AV, or a pericardial effusion.

---

    b. Intramural hematoma
        (1) Aortic wall appears thickened (often >5 mm) with no evidence of a dissection flap. The wall may look like a crescent that wraps around the aorta or may be circular. The thickening of the wall pushes in intima inward along with displacement of atheroma toward the center of the aortic lumen. The aortic lumen still appears round.
    c. Aortic penetrating ulcer
        (1) An ulceration of an atheroma that extends into the media and often associated with significant burden of atheroma
    d. Thoracic aortic aneurysm
        (1) Occurs when an area of the artery is permanently dilated to a diameter ≥50% normal.
    e. Aortic coarctation
        (1) Uncommon congenital anomaly that typically results in narrowing distal to the left subclavian artery
        (2) CFD may reveal flow acceleration during systole, and a gradient may also exist during diastole. A gradient may be difficult to obtain using TEE due to blood flow being perpendicular to the Doppler beam.

M. Pericardium
    1. Transesophageal echocardiography views: It can be seen in multiple views, but the ME four-chamber and TG SAX may be particularly helpful.[1]
    2. A transudative pericardial effusion is seen as an anechoic space between the visceral and parietal pericardium. The width of the effusion should be measured at end-diastole and classified based on Table 4.2.[22]
    3. A transudative effusion should be differentiated from epicardial fat, which is typically more hyperechoic and moves with cardiac motion.[22]
    4. A pericardial effusion may be loculated or circumferential, transudative or exudative (possibly with strands), or contain thrombus.[22]
    5. Cardiac tamponade is suggested by reduced left ventricular size, right heart chamber collapse, dilated IVC, and variation in transvalvular velocity with respiration.[22]
        a. RA collapse for >1/3 of the cardiac cycle is both very sensitive and specific for cardiac tamponade. Right ventricular diastolic collapse can occur. A ventricular septal bounce may be seen although this is not a specific sign.

TABLE 4.2   Classification of a Pericardial Effusion Based on Size

Effusion Measurement	Classification
Only visualized in systole	Trivial
<10 mm	Small
10-20 mm	Moderate
20-25 mm	Large
>25 mm	Very large

Data from Klein AL, Abbara S, Agler DA, et al. American Society of Echocardiography clinical recommendations for multimodality cardiovascular imaging of patients with pericardial disease: endorsed by the Society for Cardiovascular Magnetic Resonance and Society of Cardiovascular Computed Tomography. *J Am Soc Echocardiogr.* 2013;26(9):965-1012.e15.

    b. The variation in peak E-wave velocity (v) can be calculated as $[(v_{expiration} - v_{inspiration})/ v_{expiration}]$. Significant variation is >30% for the MV and >60% for the TV (value will be negative for TV). Notably, respiratory variation of transvalvular velocities (a) will be reduced with positive pressure ventilation, (b) may be seen in other conditions such as chronic obstructive pulmonary disease, and (c) should not be the sole criteria to diagnose tamponade.

  6. Constrictive pericarditis[22]

    a. Pericardial thickening and calcification are seen: Other signs include a dilated IVC, premature end of diastolic filling, and a ventricular septal bounce.

    b. Variation in transvalvular velocity with respiration can be seen and is calculated similarly as with cardiac tamponade; however, the cutoff for significant variation is >25% for the MV and >40% for the TV.

    c. TDI of the mitral annulus is normal. However, annulus reversus can be seen whereby the septal e' velocity > lateral e' velocity.

  7. Restrictive cardiomyopathy[22]

    a. Reduced septal e' with TDI

CLINICAL PEARL

Pericardial thickening suggests constrictive pericarditis rather than restrictive cardiomyopathy.

VI. POCUS

  A. Definition of POCUS

    1. POCUS can be defined as ultrasonography brought to the patient and performed by the provider in real time. This section highlights areas of POCUS that are relevant to cardiac anesthesia.[23]

  B. Evaluation of Cardiac Function

    1. A complete transthoracic echocardiography examination involves five probe placement windows for cardiac imaging. The three common windows utilized for POCUS cardiovascular assessment are the parasternal, apical, and subcostal windows (Figure 4.10).

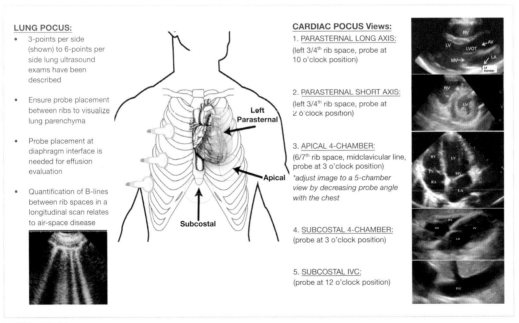

LUNG POCUS:
- 3-points per side (shown) to 6-points per side lung ultrasound exams have been described
- Ensure probe placement between ribs to visualize lung parenchyma
- Probe placement at diaphragm interface is needed for effusion evaluation
- Quantification of B-lines between rib spaces in a longitudinal scan relates to air-space disease

CARDIAC POCUS Views:
1. PARASTERNAL LONG AXIS: (left 3/4th rib space, probe at 10 o'clock position)

2. PARASTERNAL SHORT AXIS: (left 3/4th rib space, probe at 2 o'clock position)

3. APICAL 4-CHAMBER: (6/7th rib space, midclavicular line, probe at 3 o'clock position) *adjust image to a 5-chamber view by decreasing probe angle with the chest*

4. SUBCOSTAL 4-CHAMBER: (probe at 3 o'clock position)

5. SUBCOSTAL IVC: (probe at 12 o'clock position)

FIGURE 4.10 Image acquisition and interpretation for lung (left) and cardiac (right) point-of-care ultrasound. The Subcostal IVC view is shown with the on-screen orientation indicator on the left side of the screen, whereas the other cardiac views are shown with the on-screen orientation indicator on the right side of the screen. AV, aortic valve; IVC, inferior vena cava; LA, left atrium; LV, left ventricle; LVOT, left ventricular outflow tract; MV, mitral valve; RA, right atrium; RV, right ventricle; TV, tricuspid valve.

2. For imaging windows involving the thorax (apical, parasternal), the ultrasound probe is placed between ribs and requires a low-frequency probe with a small footprint (phased array probe). The subcostal window can be insonated via any low-frequency probe (curved linear, phased array).

3. Left ventricular cardiac function is commonly assessed via the parasternal SAX and LAX views that allow for the calculation of fractional shortening and fractional area change.

4. Gross valvular assessment, RV function, and diastolic function are often evaluated via the apical four-chamber view as it provides optimal insonation angles for Doppler ultrasound.

5. The subcostal window assesses pericardial fluid, right ventricular function, and right atrial pressure (RAP) via two views (Figure 4.10).

CLINICAL PEARL

It is important to recognize differences in insonation between TEE (probe posterior to the heart) and surface cardiac POCUS (probe anterior to the heart) to facilitate accurate image interpretation.

C. **Hemodynamic Monitoring**

1. **Assessment of filling pressures**

    a. The diameter of the IVC and its percentage collapsibility from respiration has been shown to correlate to RAPs in spontaneously breathing as well as mechanically ventilated patients.[24]

    b. Common reference diameter values are <1.5 cm = RAP <5 mm Hg; >1.5 cm to <2 cm with >50% respiratory collapsibility = RAP 5-10 mm Hg; >1.5 to <2 cm with <50% respiratory collapsibility = RAP 10-15 mm Hg; and >2 cm with no respiratory collapsibility = RAP >15 mm Hg.

    c. Another modality involves the direct measurement of the left ventricular end-diastolic area from a parasternal SAX view, with a referenced value of an area <8 cm^2 associated with a reduced filling state.[24]

2. **Assessment of fluid responsiveness**

    a. Dynamic flow parameters are used to identify whether a patient is on the steep portion of the Frank-Starling curve (fluid responsive). This requires obtaining particular measurements through several cardiac cycles to monitor the effects of controlled pressure changes in the thorax from mechanical ventilation. This cyclic change stresses the filling condition of the heart to the degree that is directly related to intravascular volume of the patient.

    b. Specific dynamic ultrasound measurements for fluid responsiveness in mechanically ventilated patients include assessment of the IVC diameter at end expiration (D_{min}) and at end inspiration (D_{max}) to determine the distensibility index (dIVC), which is $[D_{max} - D_{min}]/D_{min}$. A threshold dIVC of 18% has been demonstrated to differentiate responders and nonresponders with 90% sensitivity and 90% specificity.[24]

    c. More intricate methods include using Doppler ultrasonography to measure the area under the flow curve (VTI) for structures that transmit the pulsatile systemic blood flow. For example, from the apical views, assessment of the respiratory variation during positive pressure mechanical ventilation of the VTI across the LVOT has been shown to indicate fluid responsiveness.[24]

        (1) The percentage of variation threshold indicating "fluid responsive" has been reported between 15% and 20%.[24]

    d. The same concepts mentioned earlier are the basis for similar measurements performed across the brachial and other peripheral arteries.

D. **Assessment of Pulmonary Disorders**

1. The fundamental principle for lung ultrasound is that fluid is present in more dependent areas while gases rise to the top. Therefore, the patient's position will be important at the time of examination, that is, supine or upright.

2. The position of the ultrasound probe placement is similar to that of the stethoscope and can be anterior/superior or posterior/inferior for the diagnosis of dependent versus nondependent pathologies (Figure 4.10).

3. A longitudinal ultrasound plane is often used as the ribs provide landmarks. A low-frequency probe is ideal for visualizing both the lung pleura and parenchyma, while a high-frequency probe will only allow pleural evaluation.

4. Lung ultrasound provides noninvasive, immediate bedside diagnosis and has proven to be superior to chest x-ray (CXR) for various pulmonary disorders, including pneumothorax, pleural effusion, and parenchymal air-space disease.[23]

5. For pneumothorax assessment, ultrasound is used to visualize pleural lung sliding, which is the movement of the visceral pleura across the parietal pleura during respiration.[24] Importantly, anterior lung fields are adequate for detecting pneumothoraces >25% of the lung field.

6. For pleural effusion assessment, the probe should be placed in the dependent area of the lung. The fluid is bound inferiorly by the diaphragm and around the pleura. Ultrasound is more sensitive and specific than auscultation and CXR for pleural effusion detection.[23] A referenced equation to estimate effusion volume with the patient supine, with 15° trunk elevation, and placement of transducer perpendicular to the dorsolateral chest wall with measurements taken at end expiration is as follows: pleural effusion volume (mL) = (measured distance [mm]) $\times$ 20.[25]

7. POCUS is used to assess for parenchymal air-space disease via the detection/quantification of ultrasound lung comets, also known as B-lines (Figure 4.10), which are ultrasound artifacts of fluid-thickened interlobular septa. In a longitudinal plane, $\geq$3 B-lines between two ribs suggest pathologic interstitial edema.[26] The number of B-lines correlates with extracellular lung water and pulmonary wedge pressures.[26] The presence of B-lines in the setting of acute dyspnea correlates with NT-proBNP and the Framingham criteria as a means to distinguish cardiogenic and noncardiogenic dyspnea.[27]

8. **Lung ultrasound-guided chest tubes:** In addition to diagnostic applications, lung ultrasound can be employed to guide the placement of chest tubes. Lung ultrasound not only leads to an improvement in the diagnosis but also allows for the detection of the best puncture site and facilitates quantification of the pleural effusion.[28] Some practitioners use ultrasound to facilitate the procedure "live," continuously monitoring the needle or catheter placement in relation to the pleural space and lung tissue. Other clinicians use ultrasound to mark the point of entry for chest tube placement before initiating the procedure. Both approaches enhance the safety and effectiveness of the procedure by ensuring proper positioning and reducing the risk of complications.[28] Additionally, it is recommended to perform a bilateral complete lung ultrasound examination at the end of the procedure to exclude potential complications such as pneumothorax and to confirm the position of the chest tube.[28]

VII. Summary

TEE allows for a comprehensive evaluation of the structure and function of the heart. Understanding the physics and knobology facilitates optimizing imaging, and being cognizant of the indications, contraindications, and complications of TEE allows for safe and appropriate use. The TEE skillset places the cardiac anesthesiologist in a favorable vantage point to perform cardiac and lung POCUS, which can be useful for evaluation in the preoperative and postoperative arena.

REFERENCES

1. Hahn RT, Abraham T, Adams MS, et al. Guidelines for performing a comprehensive transesophageal echocardiographic examination: recommendations from the American Society of Echocardiography and the Society of Cardiovascular Anesthesiologists. *J Am Soc Echocardiogr*. 2013;26:921-964.
2. Rengasamy S, Subramaniam B. Basic physics of transesophageal echocardiography. *Int Anesthesiol Clin*. 2008;46:11-29.
3. Lang RM, Badano LP, Tsang W, et al. EAE/ASE recommendations for image acquisition and display using three-dimensional echocardiography. *J Am Soc Echocardiogr*. 2012;25:3-46.
4. Mitchell C, Rahko PS, Blauwet LA, et al. Guidelines for performing a comprehensive transthoracic echocardiographic examination in adults: recommendations from the American Society of Echocardiography. *J Am Soc Echocardiogr*. 2019;32:1-64.

5. American Society of Anesthesiologists and Society of Cardiovascular Anesthesiologists Task Force on Transesophageal Echo-cardiography. Practice guidelines for perioperative transesophageal echocardiography. An updated report by the American Society of Anesthesiologists and the Society of Cardiovascular Anesthesiologists Task Force on Transesophageal Echocardiography. *Anesthesiology*. 2010;112:1084-1096.
6. Lang RM, Badano LP, Mor-Avi V, et al. Recommendations for cardiac chamber quantification by echocardiography in adults: an update from the American Society of Echocardiography and the European Association of Cardiovascular Imaging. *J Am Soc Echocardiogr*. 2015;28:1.e14-39.e14.
7. Lang RM, Bierig M, Devereux RB, et al. Recommendations for chamber quantification: a report from the American Society of Echocardiography's Guidelines and Standards Committee and the Chamber Quantification Writing Group, developed in conjunction with the European Association of Echocardiography, a branch of the European Society of Cardiology. *J Am Soc Echocardiogr*. 2005;18:1440-1463.
8. Nagueh SF, Smiseth OA, Appleton CP, et al. Recommendations for the evaluation of left ventricular diastolic function by echo-cardiography: an update from the American Society of Echocardiography and the European Association of Cardiovascular Imaging. *J Am Soc Echocardiogr*. 2016;29:277-314.
9. Reeves ST, Finley AC, Skubas NJ, et al. Basic perioperative transesophageal echocardiography examination: a consensus state-ment of the American Society of Echocardiography and the Society of Cardiovascular Anesthesiologists. *J Am Soc Echocardiogr*. 2013;26:443-456.
10. Nagueh SF, Phelan D, Abraham T, et al. Recommendations for multimodality cardiovascular imaging of patients with hyper-trophic cardiomyopathy: an update from the American Society of Echocardiography, in Collaboration with the American So-ciety of Nuclear Cardiology, the Society for Cardiovascular Magnetic Resonance, and the Society of Cardiovascular Computed Tomography. *J Am Soc Echocardiogr*. 2022;35:533-569.
11. Donauer M, Schneider J, Jander N, et al. Perioperative changes of right ventricular function in cardiac surgical patients assessed by myocardial deformation analysis and 3-dimensional echocardiography. *J Cardiothorac Vasc Anesth*. 2020;34:708-718.
12. Nicoara A, Skubas N, Ad N, et al. Guidelines for the use of transesophageal echocardiography to assist with surgical decision-making in the operating room: a surgery-based approach: from the American Society of Echocardiography in Col-laboration with the Society of Cardiovascular Anesthesiologists and the Society of Thoracic Surgeons. *J Am Soc Echocardiogr*. 2020;33:692-734.
13. Zoghbi WA, Adams D, Bonow RO, et al. Recommendations for noninvasive evaluation of native valvular regurgitation: a report from the American Society of Echocardiography Developed in Collaboration with the Society for Cardiovascular Mag-netic Resonance. *J Am Soc Echocardiogr*. 2017;30:303-371.
14. Saric M, Armour AC, Arnaout MS, et al. Guidelines for the use of echocardiography in the evaluation of a cardiac source of embolism. *J Am Soc Echocardiogr*. 2016;29:1-42.
15. Vainrib AF, Harb SC, Jaber W, et al. Left atrial appendage occlusion/exclusion: procedural image guidance with transesopha-geal echocardiography. *J Am Soc Echocardiogr*. 2018;31:454-474.
16. Puchalski MD, Lui GK, Miller-Hance WC, et al. Guidelines for performing a comprehensive transesophageal echocardio-graphic: examination in children and all patients with congenital heart disease: recommendations from the American Society of Echocardiography. *J Am Soc Echocardiogr*. 2019;32:173-215.
17. Baumgartner H, Hung J, Bermejo J, et al. Recommendations on the echocardiographic assessment of aortic valve stenosis: a focused update from the European Association of Cardiovascular Imaging and the American Society of Echocardiography. *J Am Soc Echocardiogr*. 2017;30:372-392.
18. Otto CM, Nishimura RA, Bonow RO, et al. 2020 ACC/AHA guideline for the management of patients with valvular heart disease: a report of the American College of Cardiology/American Heart Association Joint Committee on Clinical Practice Guidelines. *Circulation*. 2021;143:e72-e227.
19. Pandian NG, Kim JK, Arias-Godinez JA, et al. Recommendations for the use of echocardiography in the evaluation of rheu-matic heart disease: a report from the American Society of Echocardiography. *J Am Soc Echocardiogr*. 2023;36:3-28.
20. Baumgartner H, Hung J, Bermejo J, et al. Echocardiographic assessment of valve stenosis: EAE/ASE recommendations for clinical practice. *J Am Soc Echocardiogr*. 2009;22:1-23; quiz 101-102.
21. Goldstein SA, Evangelista A, Abbara S, et al. Multimodality imaging of diseases of the thoracic aorta in adults: from the American Society of Echocardiography and the European Association of Cardiovascular Imaging: endorsed by the Society of Cardiovascular Computed Tomography and Society for Cardiovascular Magnetic Resonance. *J Am Soc Echocardiogr*. 2015;28:119-182.
22. Klein AL, Abbara S, Agler DA, et al. American Society of Echocardiography clinical recommendations for multimodality car-diovascular imaging of patients with pericardial disease: endorsed by the Society for Cardiovascular Magnetic Resonance and Society of Cardiovascular Computed Tomography. *J Am Soc Echocardiogr*. 2013;26:965-1012.e15.
23. Ramsingh D, Bronshteyn YS, Haskins S, et al. Perioperative point-of-care ultrasound: from concept to application. *Anesthesiol-ogy*. 2020;132:908-916.
24. Ramsingh D, Singh S, Ross M, Williams W, Cannesson M. Review of point of care (POC) ultrasound for the 21st century perioperative physician. *Curr Anesthesiol Rep*. 2015;5:452-464.
25. Balik M, Plasil P, Waldauf P, et al. Ultrasound estimation of volume of pleural fluid in mechanically ventilated patients. *Intensive Care Med*. 2006;32:318.
26. Lichtenstein D, Meziere G, Biderman P, et al. The comet-tail artifact. An ultrasound sign of alveolar-interstitial syndrome. *Am J Respir Crit Care Med*. 1997;156:1640-1646.
27. Gargani L, Frassi F, Soldati G, et al. Ultrasound lung comets for the differential diagnosis of acute cardiogenic dyspnoea: a comparison with natriuretic peptides. *Eur J Heart Fail*. 2008;10:70-77.
28. Vetrugno L, Guadagnin GM, Orso D, et al. An easier and safe affair, pleural drainage with ultrasound in critical patient: a technical note. *Crit Ultrasound J*. 2018;10:18.

5

Perianesthetic Monitoring

Eric A. JohnBull, Atilio Barbeito, and Jonathan B. Mark

KEY POINTS

1. For cardiac anesthesia, a five-lead electrocardiogram (ECG) monitor should be used. Ischemic ST-segment changes should be verified using a diagnostic bandpass filter mode (0.05-150 Hz band pass filter), which is less likely to miss ST changes than the monitoring mode (0.5-40 Hz band pass filter).

2. The dynamic response of the arterial blood pressure monitoring system can be assessed using a "fast flush" test and inspecting the oscillations in the pressure waveform. An underdamped system will show multiple pressure oscillations, and an overdamped system will not oscillate. Underdamped systems artifactually overestimate systolic blood pressure ("systolic pressure overshoot"), and conversely, overdamped systems will underestimate peak systolic pressure. A critically damped system will demonstrate one or two pressure oscillations and measure systolic pressure most accurately.

3. Air within the pressure monitoring tubing or transducer is a common cause of monitoring errors.

4. Direct arterial pressure monitoring initiated *prior to induction of anesthesia* is recommended for high-risk patients undergoing cardiac procedures and should be considered for other patients undergoing cardiac, major thoracic, or vascular operations.

5. The radial artery pressure may be significantly lower than the aortic pressure at the completion of cardiopulmonary bypass (CPB) and for a variable period thereafter.

6. The central venous pressure (CVP) waveform components (*a*, *c*, and *v* waves) are best identified in reference to the ECG waveform components.

7. Current evidence supports the use of pulmonary artery catheter (PAC) monitoring for patients at very high risk and undergoing complex cardiac surgery.

8. The PAC should be withdrawn a few centimeters when initiating CPB to decrease the risk of pulmonary artery injury. The pulmonary artery pressure waveform should be continually monitored to identify unintentional catheter wedging or tip occlusion when the balloon is not inflated.

9. Svo_2 provides a global assessment of whether oxygen delivery (Do_2) is meeting oxygen consumption (Vo_2) requirements. Normal Svo_2 is 75% and most commonly decreases when oxygen delivery is reduced.

10. Systolic pressure variation (SPV), pulse pressure variation (PPV), and stroke volume variation (SVV) depend on the interaction between intrathoracic pressure, lung volume, and arterial blood pressure. These measures may help identify when a patient is volume responsive, are inaccurate when the chest is open during surgery, and are dependent on tidal volumes.

11. Temperature monitoring should be performed at multiple sites including the nasopharynx (or tympanic membrane), bladder (a more core measurement), and pulmonary artery blood temperature (when PAC monitoring is utilized).

12. In patients undergoing cardiac surgery with ascending aortic atheroma identified by epiaortic scanning, modification of the surgical technique and neuroprotective strategies may reduce the incidence of neurologic complications.

I. Introduction

Patients presenting for cardiac surgery require extensive monitoring due to the frequent occurrence of acute hemodynamic changes related to the patient's underlying medical problems and the surgical procedure, including cardiopulmonary bypass (CPB). Although the evidence base for monitoring practices is generally limited, certain practices have been widely studied and are core recommendations from practice guidelines. For example, central venous catheterization of the internal jugular vein, which is routinely performed for most cardiac surgical procedures, should be guided using real-time ultrasound monitoring to reduce mechanical complications.[1] In contrast, the use of pulmonary artery catheter (PAC) monitoring (including continuous cardiac output (CO) and mixed venous hemoglobin saturation [SvO_2] monitoring) remains controversial and is not recommended for routine cardiac surgical procedures, but is often utilized for complex procedures in patients with severe cardiovascular derangement (eg, cardiogenic shock).[2,3]

Transesophageal echocardiography (TEE) has become a routine monitor during cardiac surgical procedures and has supplanted PAC monitoring for patients at lower risk, given its minimally invasive nature and the wealth of information provided. This monitoring modality, as well as point-of-care coagulation testing, is discussed elsewhere (Chapters 4 and 28, respectively). Other aspects of patient monitoring unique to cardiac surgical procedures (eg, temperature, renal, and neurologic function monitoring) are also briefly discussed.

II. Cardiovascular Monitors

A. Electrocardiogram

The electrocardiogram (ECG) serves as the primary monitor of heart rate and allows detection of dysrhythmias, myocardial ischemia, and cardiac electrical silence during cardioplegic arrest. Typically, two leads (II, V_5) are displayed continually, although with a five-electrode system all limb and modified limb leads can be displayed along with a single precordial lead.

1. **Indications**[4]
   a. Monitor heart rate
   b. Diagnose dysrhythmias
   c. Diagnose myocardial ischemia
   d. Detect proper functioning of cardiac pacemakers
   e. Diagnose electrolyte disturbances
   f. Monitor effect of cardioplegia to achieve asystole

2. **Techniques**
   a. **The five-electrode system:** ECG monitoring systems for cardiac surgery utilize five leads with standard American Heart Association (AHA) color coding: right arm (white), left arm (black), right leg (green), left leg (red), and precordial lead (brown). Of note, this color scheme is not an international standard. Typically, the four limb leads are placed behind the shoulders and above the hips, although the right leg (green) lead may be placed anywhere on the body because it is a ground electrode, and its location will not alter the display of any of the selected standard leads. The single precordial lead should be placed in the V_5 position directly lateral to V_4 in the fifth intercostal space

in the anterior axillary line. When the surgical procedure involves a left thoracic incision, the precordial lead must be located in another position. The precordial V_5 lead is the most sensitive lead for the detection of myocardial ischemia[5] and will often display subendocardial (demand-mediated) ST-segment depression when the limb leads are unchanged. Although other precordial leads such as V_4 may be slightly more sensitive than V_5 for detecting ST-segment changes,[6] maintaining a sterile surgical field for median sternotomy generally precludes this lead position.

b. **Epicardial electrodes:** Cardiac surgeons routinely place ventricular and/or atrial epicardial pacing wires at the conclusion of CPB prior to sternal closure. In addition to atrioventricular (AV) pacing, these pacing wires can be utilized to record atrial and/or ventricular epicardial ECGs (Figure 5.1).

c. **Computer-assisted ST-segment analysis:** Computerized ST-segment analysis identifies the ST segment 60 or 80 ms after the J point (border between QRS complex and ST segment) and compares it with the isoelectric point measured during the PR interval. One millimeter of ST-segment deviation is equivalent to a 0.1 mV difference. The changes in ST-segment level over time in each lead can be displayed as ST-segment trends.

d. **ECG artifacts:** The most common cause of ECG artifacts in the operating room is the electrosurgical unit (ESU), and current filtering techniques cannot fully eliminate this interference. Depending on the ECG filter being used (see later), 60 Hz interference is common and easily recognized. Unique to the cardiac operating room, the CPB machine may introduce an ECG artifact owing to a piezoelectric effect or static electricity generated during pump operation.[7]

e. **ECG pacing mode:** Most bedside ECG monitors now include a pacing mode selection, which when activated, employs an algorithm to detect and highlight pacing spikes that may not be apparent, particularly when the monitor bandpass filter mode is utilized (see later). The resulting ECG display shows regular markers, often in a different color than the ECG tracing, which indicate and highlight the presence of a pacemaker stimulus output. While particularly helpful in the operating room and intensive care unit, this modality may both under- and overdetect pacemaker stimuli.

f. **ECG filters:** Because the surface ECG signal is subject to artifacts (noise) both in the low-frequency and high-frequency ranges, ECG monitors use bandpass filters to narrow

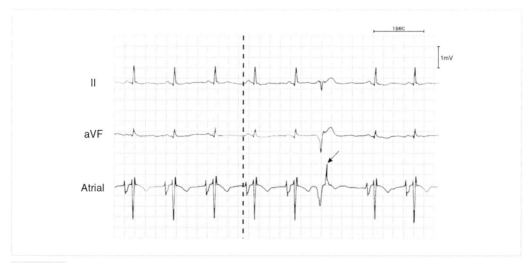

FIGURE 5.1 Simultaneous recording of surface ECG leads II and aVF and an atrial epicardial lead (atrial) recorded from a pacing wire attached to the surface of the right atrium. Onset of atrial electrical activity is denoted by the *P* wave in the surface leads and marked by the dashed vertical line. Note that the amplitude of the atrial electrical signal is greatest in the atrial lead recording. In addition, the sixth beat is a ventricular premature beat, and the resulting retrograde atrial depolarization is clearly evident in the atrial lead (arrow) but not seen as easily in standard surface ECG leads II or aVF.

the signal bandwidth and reduce artifacts. Low-frequency artifact is typically caused by respiration or patient movement that causes the ECG tracing to wander above and below the baseline. *Low-frequency filters* (also called *high-pass filters*) will eliminate this artifact and are typically set to attenuate signals at frequencies below 0.5 Hz. However, at the same time, such filters may distort the ECG waveform, particularly the ST segment, typically exaggerating the magnitude of ST-segment depression.

High-frequency ECG artifacts are typically caused by muscle fasciculations, tremors, and most importantly, the ever-present 60-cycle (Hz) electromagnetic interference caused by other electrical equipment. These artifacts can be eliminated with *high-frequency filters* (also termed *low-pass filters*) but simultaneously may also distort the ECG signal in undesirable ways. For example, pacemaker spikes, which are high frequency and low amplitude, are often eliminated by high-frequency filters, thereby making pacemaker function difficult to determine.

In general, the ECG *diagnostic filter mode* has a bandpass of 0.05-150 Hz and is the standard filter applied to 12-lead ECG recordings. This filter should always be selected for the most undistorted and accurate display of the ST segment and identification of pacing spikes. The *monitor filter mode* typically has a bandpass of 0.5-40 Hz, which helps attenuate low-frequency (respiratory drift) and high-frequency (60 Hz) artifacts but commonly distorts ST-segment deviations (Figure 5.2).

3. **Myocardial ischemia detection via ECG monitoring:** During cardiac surgery, early and accurate detection of myocardial ischemia is an important role for ECG monitoring.[8] Most commonly, *demand-mediated* or *subendocardial ischemia* is identified by ST-segment depression. In contrast, *supply-mediated* or *transmural ischemia* causes ST-segment elevation (Figure 5.3). The former is much more common and as emphasized earlier, the anterolateral precordial leads (V_5 or V_4) are the single most sensitive leads for observing these changes. Note that ST-segment depressions are *nonlocalizing;* they appear first and often only in an anterior precordial lead regardless of the coronary territory responsible for the ischemic event. In contrast, intraoperative ST-segment elevation, which is rarely seen outside the cardiac operating rooms, *localizes* the myocardial region at risk. For example,

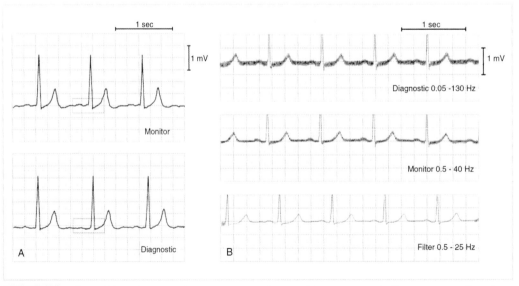

FIGURE 5.2   Effects of filter selection on the ST segment. Application of the monitor mode filter **(A, top panel)** produces artifactual J-point depression and upsloping ST-segment depression (box). These abnormalities are not seen when the diagnostic mode filter **(A, bottom panel)** is used to record the ECG. Filter selection also effects ECG electrical interference originating from the wall power source **(B panels)**. Compared to the diagnostic mode filter (bandpass 0.05-130 Hz), the narrower bandpass of the monitor mode (0.5-40 Hz) reduces this high-frequency artifact, and the filter mode (0.5-25 Hz) that incorporates an additional notch filter at 60 Hz eliminates this electrical artifact entirely.

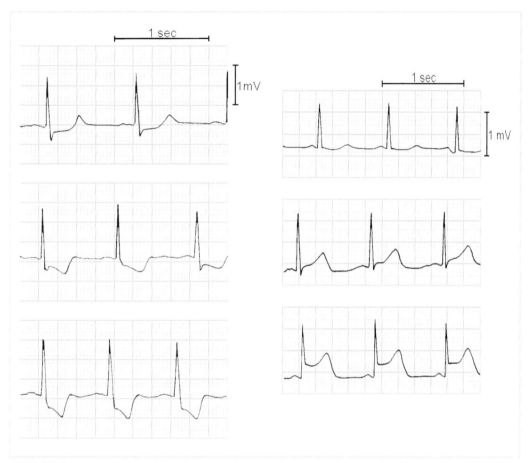

FIGURE 5.3 Myocardial ischemia. Shown are ECG tracings depicting subendocardial ischemia (**left**) and transmural ischemia (**right**). ST-segment depression results from subendocardial ischemia. This patient had left main coronary disease and the ST depression worsened as heart rate increased (63 → 75 → 86 beats/min). Transmural ischemia (full thickness) produces ST-segment elevation and frequently results from proximal coronary artery occlusion. This patient underwent a redo coronary artery bypass grafting and had acute thrombosis of a saphenous vein graft. (From Mark JB. *Atlas of Cardiovascular Monitoring*. Churchill Livingstone; 1998. Figures 11.1 and 11.2. Reprinted with permission of Jonathan B. Mark, MD.)

acute thrombosis or air embolism of the right coronary artery would cause ST-segment elevation in the inferior leads (II, III, aVF).

B. **Blood Pressure**

While standard oscillometric intermittent blood pressure (BP) monitoring[9] used routinely during all surgical procedures should be applied as a backup method during cardiac surgery, continuous direct arterial pressure measurement is always required for these procedures. Oscillometry will not function during periods of nonpulsatile flow, as occurs during CPB or in patients with left ventricular assist devices (LVADs). In cases in which arterial catheters are not available or not functioning, oscillometry may be used as an alternative, with the caveat that they can be quite inaccurate in this population.[10]

1. **Continuous noninvasive blood pressure monitors:** A number of newer technologies have been used for deriving continual displays of an arterial pressure waveform.[11-13] The majority of these devices use the *volume clamp technique*, in which measurements are obtained via one or more finger cuffs with integrated photoplethysmography sensors. BP is measured by dynamic inflation of the finger cuff so that a constant volume is measured in the finger via the sensor. An arterial waveform can then be reconstructed based on the pressure in the cuff.

2. **Direct invasive arterial pressure monitoring:** Direct arterial BP monitoring is invaluable during cardiac procedures for detecting rapid and severe changes in blood pressure and providing vascular access for frequent blood sampling for blood testing. The procedure should be performed with a suitable sterile prep, field, and gloves. In general, direct arterial pressure measurements are considered the "gold standard" or reference values that guide therapy. To meet this standard, certain technical aspects[14] of the monitoring system must be addressed.

   a. **Technical aspects for direct pressure monitoring:** Pressure waves in the cardiovascular system can be characterized as complex periodic sine waves. These complex waves are a summation of a series of simple sine waves of differing amplitudes and frequencies, which represent the natural harmonics of a fundamental frequency. The first harmonic, or fundamental frequency, is equal to the heart rate (Figure 5.4A,B), and the first 10 harmonics of the fundamental frequency will contribute significantly to the waveform.

   b. Frequency response (or amplitude ratio) is the ratio of the measured amplitude versus the input amplitude of a signal at a specific frequency. The frequency response should be constant over the desired range of input frequencies—that is, the signal should not be distorted (amplified or attenuated). The ideal amplitude ratio is close to 1. The signal frequency range of an intravascular pressure wave response is determined by the heart rate. For example, if a patient's heart rate is 120 beats/min, the fundamental frequency is 2 Hz. Because the first 10 harmonics contribute to the arterial waveform, frequencies up to 20 Hz will contribute to the morphology of an arterial waveform at this heart rate.

   c. Natural frequency (or resonant frequency), a property of all matter, refers to the frequency at which a monitoring system resonates and amplifies the signal. The natural frequency (f_n) of a monitoring system is directly proportional to the catheter lumen diameter (D) and inversely proportional to the square root of three parameters: the tubing connection length (L), the system compliance ($\Delta V/\Delta P$), and the density of fluid contained in the system (δ). To increase f_n and thereby reduce distortion, it is imperative that a pressure-sensing system be composed of short, low-compliance (stiff) tubing, and filled with a low-density fluid (such as normal saline). Ideally, the f_n of the measuring system should be at least 10 times the fundamental frequency to reproduce the first 10 harmonics of the pressure wave without distortion.[13] In clinical practice, the f_n of most measuring systems is between 10 and 20 Hz. If the input frequency is close to the system's f_n (which is usually the case in clinical situations), the system's response will be amplified (Figure 5.4C). Therefore, these systems require the correct amount of *damping* to minimize distortion.

   d. The *damping coefficient* reflects the rate of dissipation of the energy of a pressure wave. Figure 5.4D shows the relationship among frequency response, f_n, and damping coefficient.

      Typical clinical monitoring systems have a low f_n and are slightly *underdamped*. The problem is compounded when the heart rate is fast, which increases the demands of the system by increasing the input frequency and in turn, requires a higher f_n to avoid resonance within the system. As a result, most clinical monitoring systems artifactually increase the systolic BP and decrease the diastolic BP. In contrast, an *overdamped* system, which is most often the result of air within the monitoring tubing, will not oscillate at all but will settle to baseline slowly, thus underestimating systolic and overestimating diastolic pressures. A critically damped system will settle to baseline after only one or two oscillations and will reproduce the arterial pressure waveform accurately. An optimally or *critically* damped system will exhibit a constant (or *flat*) frequency response in the range of frequencies up to the f_n of the system (Figure 5.4D). If a given system does not meet this criterion, components should be checked, especially for air, or the system replaced. Even an optimally damped system will begin to distort the waveform at higher heart rates because the 10th harmonic exceeds the system's f_n (Figure 5.5).

      Both the f_n and the damping coefficient of a system can be estimated using an adaptation of the square wave method known as the *"pop" test* or *"fast flush" test*. The f_n

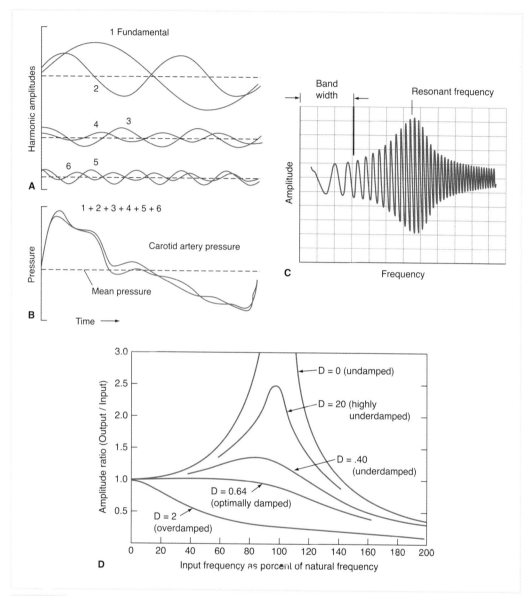

FIGURE 5.4 **(A)** Generation of the harmonic waveforms from the fundamental frequency (heart rate) by Fourier analysis. **(B)** The first six harmonics are shown. The addition of the six harmonics reproduces an actual BP wave. The first six harmonics are superimposed, showing a likeness to, but not a faithful reproduction of, the original wave. The first 10 harmonics of a pressure wave must be sensed by a catheter-transducer system, if that system is to provide an accurate reproduction of the wave. **(C)** Pressure recording from a pressure generator simulator, which emits a sine wave at increasing frequencies (horizontal axis). The frequency response (ratio of signal amplitude$_{OUT}$ to signal amplitude$_{IN}$) is plotted on the vertical axis for a typical catheter-transducer system. The useful bandwidth (range of frequency producing a "flat" response) and the amplification of the signal in the frequency range near the natural frequency of the system are shown. (**A-C:** Reprinted with permission from Welch JP, D'Ambra MN. Hemodynamic monitoring. In: Kofke WA, Levy JH, eds. *Postoperative Critical Care Procedures of the Massachusetts General Hospital*. Little, Brown and Company; 1986:146. **D:** Reprinted with permission from Grossman W. *Cardiac Catheterization and Angiography*. 3rd ed. Lea & Febiger; 1986:22.) **(D)** Amplitude ratio (or frequency response) on the vertical axis is plotted as a function of the input frequency as a percentage of the natural frequency (rather than as absolute values). In the undamped or underdamped system, the signal output is amplified in the region of the natural frequency of the transducer system; in the overdamped system, a reduction in amplitude ratio for most input frequencies is seen. This plot exhibits several important points: (i) If a catheter-transducer system has a high natural frequency, less damping will be required to produce a flat response in the clinically relevant range of input frequencies (10-30 Hz). (ii) For systems with a natural frequency in the clinically relevant range (usual case), a level of "critical" (optimal) damping exists that will maintain a flat frequency response. *D*, damping coefficient. (From Grossman W. *Cardiac Catheterization*. 3rd ed. Lea & Febiger; 1985:122, with permission.)

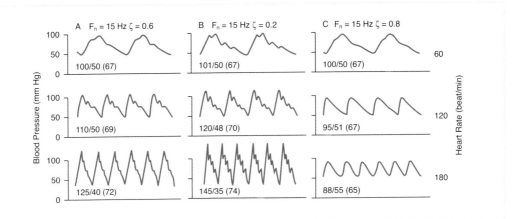

FIGURE 5.5 Comparison of three catheter-transducer systems with the same natural frequency (15 Hz) under different conditions of heart rate. Pressures are displayed as systolic-diastolic (mean). The reference BP for all panels is 100/50. **(A)** A critically damped system ($\zeta = 0.6$) provides an accurate reproduction until higher heart rates (>150) are reached. **(B)** An underdamped system ($\zeta = 0.2$) shows distortion at lower rates, leading to overestimation of systolic and underestimation of diastolic pressures. **(C)** An overdamped system ($\zeta = 0.8$) demonstrates an underestimation of systolic pressure and an overestimation of diastolic pressure. Also, note that diastolic and mean pressures are affected less by the inadequate monitoring systems. f_n, natural frequency; ζ, damping coefficient.

is calculated by measuring the time period of one oscillation as the system settles to baseline after a high-pressure flush. The damping coefficient is calculated by measuring the amplitude ratio of two successive peaks and using a graphical solution (Figure 5.6).[13]

After a rapid pressure change (performed by flushing the pressure line), an underdamped system will continue to oscillate for a prolonged time. In terms of blood pressure monitoring, this translates to an overestimation of systolic BP (*systolic pressure overshoot*) and an underestimation of diastolic BP. An overdamped system will not oscillate at all but will settle to baseline slowly, thus underestimating systolic and overestimating diastolic pressures. A critically damped system will settle to baseline after only one or two oscillations and will reproduce systolic pressures accurately. Notably, most pressure monitoring systems in clinical practice have a low f_n and are underdamped, resulting in the common observation of systolic pressure overshoot.[15]

e. **Pressure transducers:** Pressure transducers have a diaphragm, which acts to link the input pressure wave to an electrical output. When the diaphragm of a transducer is distorted by a change in pressure, voltages are altered across the variable resistor of a Wheatstone bridge contained in the transducer. This in turn produces a change in current, which is electronically converted and displayed as a pressure waveform. Prior to the onset of monitoring, the transducer is *zeroed* by exposing it to ambient atmospheric pressure and performing the zeroing function on the bedside monitor. The next step is to adjust the transducer level to the appropriate *reference level* on the patient, which is typically the fourth intercostal space at the midaxillary line in a supine patient.[16] Note that this level corresponds to the mid-left atrium, and some authors have suggested that a more appropriate reference level for the transducer would be ~5 cm posterior to the sternum to best approximate the level of the right atrium (RA).[17,18] The most important thing to recognize is that when invasive pressure monitoring is being utilized, the transducer location (*reference level*) influences the resulting pressure values recorded in direct proportion to the hydrostatic pressure difference at various heights. For example, during the course of a cardiac surgical procedure, the operating room table is often repositioned. If the "height" of the pressure transducer is not adjusted accordingly to the appropriate level, the resulting measurement will be in error. A 10 cm water (or saline) column is the equivalent of 7.4 mm Hg, a small relative error in BP measurement but a significant error in measuring other central vascular pressures.

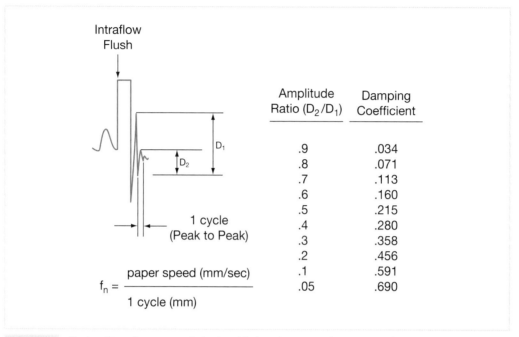

FIGURE 5.6 The "pop" test allows one to derive f_n and ζ of a catheter-transducer system. The test should be done with the catheter in situ, as all components contribute to the harmonics of the system. The test involves a rapid flush (with the high-pressure flush system used commonly), followed by a sudden release. This produces a rapid decrease in the flush bag pressure and, owing to the inertia of the system, an overshoot of the baseline. The subsequent oscillations about the baseline are used to calculate f_n and ζ. For example, the arterial pulse at the far left of the figure is followed by a fast flush and sudden release. The resulting oscillations have a definite period, or cycle, measured in millimeters. The natural frequency f_n is the paper speed divided by this period, expressed in cycles per second, or Hz. If the period were 2 mm and the paper speed 25 mm/s, $f_n = 12.5$ Hz. For determining f_n, a faster paper speed will give better reliability. The ratio of the amplitude of one induced resonant wave to the next, D_2/D_1, is used to calculate damping coefficients (**right column**). A damping coefficient of 0.2-0.4 describes an underdamped system, 0.4-0.6 an optimally damped system, and 0.6-0.8 an overdamped system. (Reprinted from Bedford RF. Invasive blood pressure monitoring. In: Blitt CD, ed. *Monitoring in Anesthesia and Critical Care Medicine*. Churchill Livingstone; 1985:59. © 1985 Elsevier. With permission.)

  f. Sources of error in intravascular pressure measurement

   (1) **Inadequate dynamic response:** Monitoring systems with low f_n will only record an accurate BP waveform if the damping is within a narrow range. As noted earlier, most pressure monitoring systems in clinical practice have a low f_n and are underdamped, resulting in the common observation of systolic pressure overshoot. In contrast, air bubbles or blood clots within the monitoring tubing are the most common cause of an overdamped system. Intentional introduction of a small air bubble into the monitoring system to increase the damping of an underdamped system may paradoxically worsen the systolic pressure overshoot because the air bubble will simultaneously lower the f_n. This should be avoided.

   (2) **Catheter whip:** Catheter "whip" is a phenomenon in which the motion of the catheter tip itself produces a noticeable pressure swing. This artifact usually is not observed with peripheral arterial catheters but is more common with PACs that traverse the right heart chambers and valves.

   (3) **Resonance in peripheral vessels:** The arterial pressure waveform changes morphology as it travels from the aorta peripherally. *Peripheral pulse amplification* is a normal physiologic phenomenon related to the propagation of the arterial waveform through the vascular tree with wave reflection from branch points and resonance within the vascular system. As a consequence, a normal radial artery waveform will always have a slightly wider pulse pressure (with higher systolic and lower diastolic pressure) than the pressure within the aortic root[14,19] (Figure 5.7).

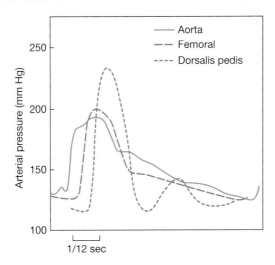

FIGURE 5.7 Change of pulse pressure waveform morphology in different arteries. Arterial waveforms do not have a single morphology. The central aortic waveform is more rounded and has a definite dicrotic notch. The dorsalis pedis and, to a lesser extent, the femoral artery show a delay in pulse transmission, sharper initial upstrokes (and thus higher systolic pressure), and slurring (femoral) and loss (dorsalis) of the dicrotic notch. The dicrotic notch is better maintained in the upper-extremity pressure wave (see Figure 5.8). The small second "hump" in the dorsalis wave probably is due to a reflected wave from the arterial-arteriolar impedance mismatching. (Reprinted with permission from Welch JP, D'Ambra MN. Hemodynamic monitoring. In: Kofke WA, Levy JH, eds. *Postoperative Critical Care Procedures of the Massachusetts General Hospital*. Little, Brown and Company; 1986:144.)

    (4) **Changes in electrical properties of the transducer:** Electrical balance, or electrical zero, refers to the adjustment of the Wheatstone bridge within the transducer so that zero current flows to the detector at zero pressure. The zero value should be periodically confirmed during a surgical procedure because the zero point may drift, for instance, if the room temperature changes. The pressure waveform morphology may not change with the baseline drift of a transducer.

    (5) **Transducer position errors:** As noted earlier, the location of the pressure transducer is a critical factor in accurate intravascular pressure measurement. Consequently, any adjustment in patient position that alters the reference level of the transducer will introduce an error directly equal to the hydrostatic (vertical) pressure difference. In the operating room and intensive care unit, adjustments in bed and patient position require simultaneous repositioning of the transducer, so that it remains at the same reference level.

3. **Arterial catheterization:** Direct arterial BP monitoring by arterial catheterization is universally required during cardiac surgery. Placement of an art line *prior to induction* is imperative for a safe, smooth anesthetic induction in patients at high risk for hemodynamic instability. Complications are uncommon but widely recognized, including localized bleeding, vascular thrombosis, infection, and peripheral ischemia.

    a. **Radial artery:** The radial artery is the most utilized site, although some institutions prefer brachial artery pressure monitoring, owing to the common observation that at the end of CPB, the radial artery pressure may transiently underestimate central aortic pressure.[20] Prior to arterial cannulation, the BP should be measured noninvasively in both arms to assure that there is not a significant pressure difference. Either radial artery may be used, most typically in the nondominant hand unless there are surgical plans for radial artery harvest. Although commonly used and recommended, the *modified Allen test* is not useful for predicting ischemic complications following radial artery catheterization.[21,22] Although radial artery cannulation is still often guided by arterial palpation alone, increasingly cannulation with ultrasound guidance is chosen.[23] This technique is invaluable for use when there is nonpulsatile blood flow, such as that occurs in patients on venoarterial extracorporeal membrane oxygenation (ECMO) or those with LVAD support.

b. **Ulnar artery:** The ulnar artery is less commonly chosen than the radial and may even be used when there is failed cannulation of the ipsilateral radial artery. Although clinicians may avoid this owing to concerns for ischemic complications, there is limited evidence that this practice is unsafe.

c. **Femoral artery:** A femoral arterial line may be chosen when upper extremity arterial catheterization cannot be used. On occasion, a femoral arterial catheter may be placed by the surgeon at the end of bypass if the radial artery pressure line is not working or is displaying values significantly lower than the pressure in the ascending aorta. The latter can be directly measured from the aortic cannula when the patient has been weaned from bypass. Of note, unlike peripheral arterial catheterization, vascular injury during femoral artery access may be occult and result in life-threatening retroperitoneal hemorrhage.

d. **Brachial artery:** The brachial artery is an easily accessible artery located medially in the antecubital fossa. Although there is a theoretical concern that the absence of collateral flow at the level of the antecubital fossa presents an increased risk for ischemic complications, this has not been born out in clinical experience.[20] When brachial arterial monitoring is utilized, a longer catheter should be employed to assure that the catheter remains intravascular in an awake moving postoperative patient.

e. **Axillary artery:** The axillary artery may be cannulated for arterial pressure monitoring.[24] Since this is a more central monitoring site, the problem of underestimating aortic pressure at the end of bypass (noted earlier) with radial pressure monitoring is obviated. However, flushing of this line must be meticulous to avoid cerebral embolization. In addition, hemothorax is a known complication.

f. **Dorsalis pedis, posterior tibialis, and superficial temporal arteries:** These sites are utilized in pediatric patients but uncommonly in adult patients. When necessary, consider cannulating with a 22-gauge intravenous catheter to minimize complications.

4. **Arterial pressure waveforms**
   a. **Normal waveforms:** A typical radial artery pressure waveform is shown in Figure 5.8. In addition to the heart rate recorded from the ECG, the arterial pressure waveform provides the true pulse rate, which may not be identical to the heart rate. This difference is noted as a pulse deficit and may be observed during frequent atrial or ventricular ectopic beats and tachydysrhythmias (owing to reduced cardiac filling), and in the most extreme case, during pulseless electrical activity (PEA). Even when there is no real difference between perfusing beats and the heart rate, the arterial pressure waveform alone can be useful in circumstances where the ECG-derived heart rate is obscured by electrocautery, such as during chest opening and closing.

   b. One critical and common situation during cardiac surgery, *intra-aortic balloon counterpulsation timing*, requires proper interpretation of the arterial pressure waveform (Figure 5.9).

   c. In mechanically ventilated patients, the arterial pressure waveform can be used to identify *respiratory-circulatory interactions* such as systolic pressure variation (SPV), pulse pressure variation (PPV),[25] or derived stroke volume variation (SVV). The use of these metrics to guide fluid therapy is discussed further in Section II.E.3 and II.E.4.

   d. **Abnormal arterial pressure waveforms:** While rarely diagnostic in the absence of other supportive data, abnormalities in the arterial pressure waveform often reveal underlying cardiovascular pathophysiology (Figure 5.10).

C. **Central Venous Pressure Monitoring**
   1. **Indications for central venous cannulation**
      Placement of a central venous catheter (CVC) is indicated in most cardiac surgical procedures to provide a large-bore conduit for rapid fluid administration and delivery of vasoactive drugs into the central circulation. In addition to these therapeutic indications, a CVC is used to measure central venous pressure (CVP) and allow the insertion of a PAC. Other

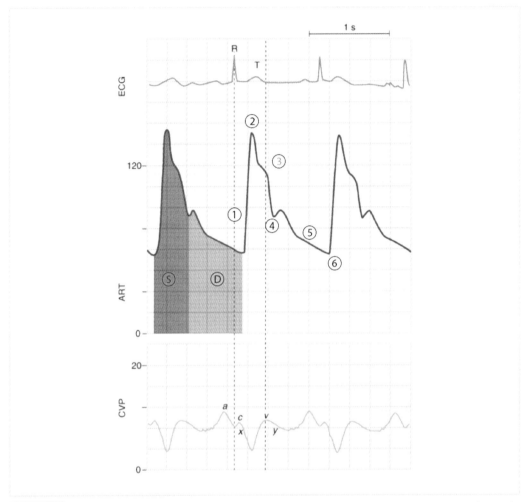

FIGURE 5.8 Normal arterial waveform morphology. Components of the normal arterial waveform include (1) the systolic upstroke, (2) systolic peak pressure, (3) systolic decline, (4) the dicrotic notch, (5) diastolic runoff, and (6) end-diastolic pressure. The area underneath the curve (shaded area on the left) divided by the beat period equals the mean arterial pressure (MAP). CVP, central venous pressure; ECG, electrocardiogram; D, diastole; S, systole. (Modified from Mark JB. *Atlas of Cardiovascular Monitoring.* Churchill Livingstone; 1998. Figures 8.1 and 8.2. Reprinted with permission of Jonathan B. Mark, MD.)

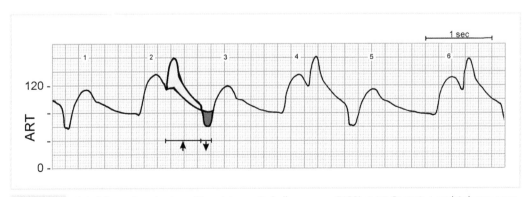

FIGURE 5.9 Arterial waveform tracing with an intra-aortic balloon pump (IABP) at 1:2. Beats 2, 4, and 6 show a properly timed inflation of the balloon at the dicrotic notch, resulting in increased diastolic arterial pressure. Deflation of the balloon just prior to the systolic upstroke results in a drop in arterial pressure at the onset of systole and a reduced peak in the following beat. (From Mark JB. *Atlas of Cardiovascular Monitoring.* Churchill Livingstone; 1998. Figure 20.1. Reprinted with permission of Jonathan B. Mark, MD.)

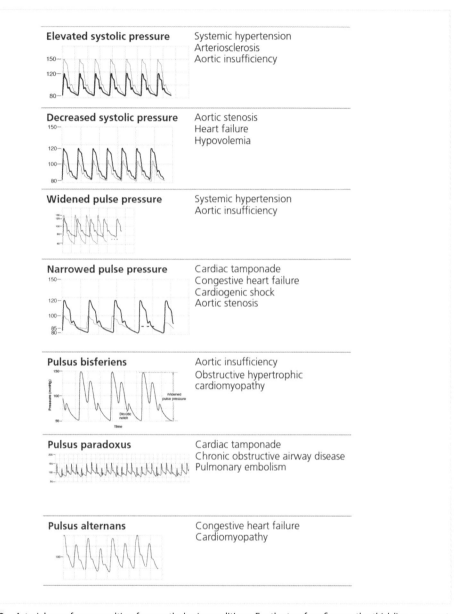

FIGURE 5.10 Arterial waveforms resulting from pathologic conditions. For the top four figures, the *thick line* represents a normal arterial waveform. (From *Quick Guide to Cardiopulmonary Care*. 3rd ed. Edwards Critical Care Education; 2015. Used with permission from Edwards Critical Care Education.)

less common indications for CVC placement in cardiac surgery include the need for hemodialysis and the placement of transvenous pacing or percutaneous cardioplegia delivery cannulae. The decision to perform central venous cannulation before or following the induction of anesthesia is typically guided by institutional practice and physician preferences.

2. **Cannulation of a central vein**

   a. **Catheter selection:** Introducer sheaths with one or two integrated ports are preferred over multilumen CVCs in cardiac surgery. These devices allow insertion of a catheter through the hemostasis valve for continuous CVP monitoring or fluid and drug infusion, or insertion of a PAC if needed. Because most CVCs are significantly longer than the typical peripheral IV cannula and flow is inversely proportional to catheter length (Poiseuille law), not all CVCs provide adequate flow rates for very rapid fluid or blood product administration, as is sometimes needed during cardiac surgery.[26]

For example, the maximal flow rate through the proximal or central lumens of a typical 16 cm triple-lumen CVC is only one third of the flow rate achievable through the side port of an 8.5F introducer sheath.[27]

b. **Site selection:** The internal jugular (IJ), subclavian (SV), and femoral vein (FV) are the most common sites for catheter access to the central circulation.

 (1) **Internal jugular:** Due to their superficial location in the neck, the IJ veins are readily compressible, allowing for easier control of bleeding in the patient with co-agulopathy. The IJ site is also the preferred cannulation site in patients with severe pulmonary disease in whom a pneumothorax could be life-threatening. The *right* IJ vein is most commonly used by the cardiac anesthesiologist because it provides a straight pathway to the RA. This is especially relevant during the insertion of a PAC or temporary pacing wire. Additionally, most anesthesiologists are right-handed, making the right IJ vein ergonomically easier to access. When positioning the patient for IJ venous cannulation, excessive rotation of the head should be avoided as this may cause the carotid to lie immediately posterior to the jugular vein, increasing the chances of unintentional arterial puncture. Relative contra-indications for IJ CVC placement include significant ipsilateral carotid disease, recent cannulation of the same vein, contralateral diaphragmatic dysfunction, and thyromegaly or prior neck surgery or radiation. Note that when left IJ vein cannulation is being performed, the thoracic duct lies in close proximity. Furthermore, left IJ vein catheterization carries a higher risk of injuring the left brachiocephalic vein or superior vena cava owing to the more acute angle between the left IJ and innominate veins.

 (2) **Subclavian:** The subclavian approach is common during cardiopulmonary and trauma resuscitation. The main advantage to SV cannulation is its relative ease of access with concomitant cervical spine stabilization and the stability of the cathe-ter during long-term cannulation. Subclavian vein cannulation carries the highest rate of pneumothorax. If SV cannulation is unsuccessful on one side, a chest x-ray should be obtained to rule out pneumothorax before attempting contralateral SV cannulation. One problem of SV catheters unique to cardiac surgery is the poten-tial for catheter kinking and compression during sternal retraction. In addition, using a right SV approach, insertion of a PAC into the RA is more difficult be-cause of the acute angle that the catheter must negotiate. When PAC monitoring is planned, the left subclavian approach is preferred.

 (3) **Axillary:** The axillary vein is the lateral extension of the subclavian vein but does not lie underneath the clavicle. This makes the axillary vein visible under ultrasound.

 (4) **Femoral:** The femoral approach is less commonly used in cardiac surgery for sev-eral reasons. Early postoperative ambulation is restricted by FV catheters. In ad-dition, venous drainage for CPB may require FV cannulation. Finally, FV catheters may carry a higher risk of infection and thrombosis.

 (5) **External jugular:** The external jugular vein courses superficially across the ster-nocleidomastoid muscle to join the subclavian vein close to the junction of the IJ and subclavian SV veins. Its course is more tortuous, and the presence of valves makes CVC placement more difficult. The placement of rigid catheters (eg, intro-ducer sheaths) via the external jugular vein increases the risk of vessel trauma and is not recommended. Pliable central catheters and short catheters may be used when no other intravenous access is available.

c. **Cannulation process:** Certain basic principles should be adhered to when cannulat-ing a central vein for cardiac surgery. Among these, the routine use of standardized equipment, involvement of an assistant, meticulous hand washing, and maximal barrier precautions all contribute to minimizing complications. The use of the Trendelenburg position is recommended to maximize the size of the venous target and reduce the risk of venous air embolism. A modified Seldinger technique (catheter-over needle, then wire-through-catheter) is a common cannulation method. It is important to verify venous cannulation using at least two different methods such as pressure manometry plus ultrasound confirmation that the wire resides in the vein before advancing the larger catheter.

   d. Ultrasound guidance: A preinsertion ultrasound scan is recommended to confirm the location, size, and patency of the target vein prior to central vein cannulation (Figure 5.11). A patent vein should be compressible using minimal pressure. Real-time ultrasound guidance is now the standard of care for right IJ cannulation and is recommended for cannulation of the subclavian and femoral veins.[28]

   e. Complications of CVC placement: Complications may be mechanical, thromboembolic, or infectious. The most severe complications of CVC insertion are usually preventable. When using longer catheters, it is important to verify catheter location using TEE or radiographic imaging to ensure the tip is located outside the RA, as mechanical irritation of the RA or superior vena cava (SVC)-RA junction may lead to thrombus formation, endocarditis, SVC syndrome, and in rare cases cardiac tamponade.[29,30] Catheters inserted in the left IJ vein are especially predisposed to malpositioning, as the tip of the catheter may abut the lateral wall of the SVC as the catheter enters more horizontally from the left innominate vein. The final positioning of the CVC should be confirmed by a chest x-ray demonstrating that its tip lies parallel to the wall of the SVC.

3. **Central venous pressure interpretation**

   Cannulation of the central veins allows monitoring of CVP during cardiac surgery. Important information is derived from both the mean CVP value as well as interpretation of the CVP waveform morphology.[31] Consistent and proper transducer height is critical, as analysis of transducer placement has revealed very high interoperator variability.[32]

   a. Mean CVP value: Normal mean CVP is 2-5 mm Hg in awake, healthy individuals and slightly higher in mechanically ventilated patients. Mean CVP reflects mean RA pressure and is affected by circulating blood volume, venous tone, juxtacardiac pressures, and right ventricle (RV) function. The interaction of these physiologic variables is complex, and therefore a single CVP value cannot be used as a direct predictor of volume status.[33]

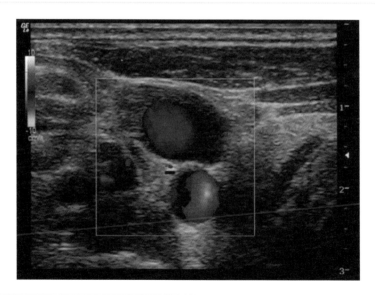

FIGURE 5.11 Ultrasound image of the internal jugular vein and carotid artery. Note that color flow visualizes blood flowing away from the transducer as blue, while blood flowing toward the transducer is red. So, with the probe angled caudally, blood flow in the internal jugular vein returning to the heart is blue, while the blood traveling up from the aortic arch into the carotid artery is red. (Reprinted with permission from Perrino AC Jr, Popescu WM, Jadbabaie F, Skubas NJ. Echocardiography. In: Barash PG, Cahalan MK, Cullen BF, et al, eds. *Clinical Anesthesia*. 8th ed. Wolters Kluwer; 2018:731-766. Figure 27.44.)

b. **CVP, circulating blood volume, and venous tone:** Venous return, defined as the flow of blood from the peripheral circulation into the RA, equals CO and is determined by the pressure gradient between the mean circulatory filling pressure (which cannot be measured clinically but is estimated to be 8-10 mm Hg) and CVP. This means that small changes in CVP (the downstream pressure) can greatly affect venous return and CO.[33] Also, factors that affect the tone of the various venous capacitance vessel beds (such as sympathetic tone and local vasomotor reflexes) are activated in response to reductions in venous return. These compensatory mechanisms maintain a stable CVP at various levels of intravascular volume and cardiac function, emphasizing the difficulty in interpreting a single CVP value as an indicator of blood volume.[34,35]

c. **Juxtacardiac pressure:** CVP is referenced to atmospheric pressure, but the RA is contained within the pericardium and thorax, and changes in pressure surrounding the RA influence the pressure measurements within the atrium. This means that the same measured CVP, referenced to atmospheric pressure, can be associated with markedly different transmural pressures and chamber volumes, depending on whether juxtacardiac pressure is high or low.[30]

d. **RV function:** CVP reflects RV filling pressure and is dependent on RV inotropic state and compliance. An RV that is operating on the flat portion of its pressure-volume curve may exhibit large changes in filling volume with only minimal changes in filling pressure (CVP), whereas the same increase in filling volume will result in large changes in CVP in an RV that is less compliant and operating on the steep portion of the pressure-volume curve. It is therefore important to always interpret the mean CVP value in the context of RV function.[33]

4. **Central venous pressure waveform morphology:** The normal CVP waveform consists of three pressure peaks, termed *a*, *c*, and *v* waves, and two pressure descents, termed *x* and *y* descents. The CVP waveform components represent mechanical events that are altered by changes in heart function and arrhythmias (Tables 5.1 and 5.2). Correct identification of the CVP waveform components is facilitated by examining the accompanying ECG waveform, which allows easy identification of the systolic and diastolic portions of the cardiac cycle. Note that when present, the typically small CVP *c* wave *always* follows the ECG *R* wave because it results from tricuspid valve closure and isovolumic right ventricular contraction (Figure 5.8, bottom).

a. **Abnormal waves:** A common abnormality in the CVP trace is loss of the *a* wave in patients with atrial fibrillation. In the presence of AV dissociation, which may be observed in patients with ventricular pacing or junctional rhythm, RA contraction against a closed tricuspid valve produces a large "cannon *a* wave" (Figure 5.12). Tall, abnormal *v* waves may be seen with tricuspid valve regurgitation when holosystolic retrograde flow through the incompetent valve increases RA pressure during systole (Figure 5.13, top).

TABLE 5.1   Components of the Central Venous Pressure (CVP) Waveform

Waveform Component	Cardiac Event
a wave	RA contraction following ECG *P* wave at end-diastole
x descent	RA relaxation
c wave	Isovolumic ventricular contraction in early systole
x′ descent	Systolic descent of tricuspid annulus toward RV apex
v wave	Mid to late systolic RA filling
y descent	Early diastolic collapse in RA pressure resulting in RV filling

The normal CVP waveform components are produced by distinct mechanical events. Factors that influence these events produce alterations in the CVP waveform. Note that the *c* wave *always* follows the ECG *R* wave and marks the separation of the *x* descent into the *x* and *x′* components. Aligning the ECG with the CVP assists identification of waveform components and abnormalities.
ECG, electrocardiogram; RA, right atrium; RV, right ventricle.

TABLE 5.2 Differential Diagnosis of RA-RV Hemodynamic Abnormalities

Abnormal Waveform Chart

Right Atrial Waveforms

Decreased mean pressure	Hypovolemia
	Transducer zero reference level too high
Increased mean pressure	Hypervolemia
	Right ventricular (RV) failure
	Tricuspid stenosis or regurgitation
	Pulmonic stenosis or regurgitation
	Pulmonary hypertension
Tall *a* wave	Tricuspid stenosis
	Decreased RV compliance
	RV failure
	Pulmonic stenosis
	Pulmonary hypertension
Absent *a* wave	Atrial fibrillation
	Atrial flutter
	Junctional rhythm
Cannon *a* wave	Junctional rhythm
	Atrioventricular dissociation
Tall *v* wave (or *cv* wave)	Tricuspid regurgitation
Tall *a* and *v* waves	Cardiac tamponade
	Pericardial constriction
	Hypervolemia
	RV failure

RV Waveforms

Elevated systolic pressure	Pulmonary hypertension
	Pulmonic stenosis
Decreased systolic pressure	Hypovolemia
Increased diastolic pressure	Hypervolemia
	Cardiac tamponade
	Pericardial constriction
Decreased diastolic pressure	Hypovolemia

Modified from *Quick Guide to Cardiopulmonary Care*. 3rd ed. Edwards Critical Care Education; 2015. Used with permission from Edwards Critical Care Education.

D. **Pulmonary Artery Catheter**

The PAC allows continuous and simultaneous monitoring of important hemodynamic variables that are essential in many pre-, intra-, and post-cardiac surgical scenarios. For example, in the setting of RV dysfunction, the PAC will allow the clinician to differentiate increased RV afterload (high pulmonary artery pressure [PAP]) from primary RV failure (low PAP and high CVP). Similarly, simultaneous measurement of filling pressures and CO aids diagnosis of the different types of shock: cardiogenic shock will manifest as low CO and high left- and right-sided filling pressures (pulmonary artery wedge pressure [PAWP] and CVP, respectively); hypovolemic shock will present as low CO and low filling pressures; and vasoplegic shock as high CO and low systemic vascular resistance.

1. **Indications for pulmonary artery catheterization:** PACs are useful in high-risk patients such as those with pulmonary hypertension, RV dysfunction, or complex valvular pathology because these catheters provide continuous hemodynamic information that is not available through alternative means such as echocardiography.[36,37] However, patients undergoing routine cardiac surgery with preserved left ventricle (LV) and RV function can generally be managed with CVP and TEE monitoring alone. Despite a reduction in overall

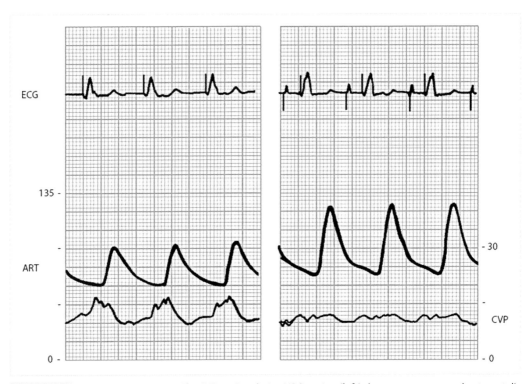

FIGURE 5.12 VOO versus AV pacing. The CVP tracing during VOO pacing (**left**) shows cannon waves due to systolic contraction of the right atrium (RA) from retrograde conduction. AV pacing (**right**) shows a normal CVP tracing and a substantial improvement in arterial blood pressure, as demonstrated by the arterial waveform. (From Mark JB. *Atlas of Cardiovascular Monitoring*. Churchill Livingstone; 1998. Figure 14.16. Reprinted with permission of Jonathan B. Mark, MD.)

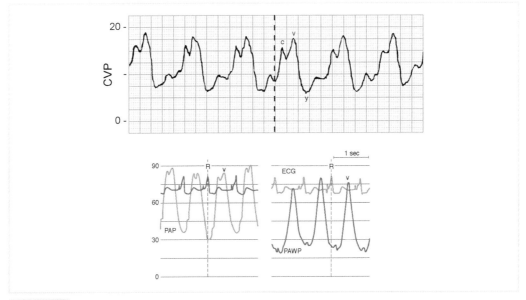

FIGURE 5.13 (**Top**) CVP tracing showing a large *v* wave and steep *y* descent due to tricuspid regurgitation. The regurgitant flow during systole obscures the *x* descent, causing a fusion of *c* and *v* waves. RV end-diastolic pressure is best estimated from the tracing prior to the *v* wave, at the time of the *R* wave on the ECG. (**Bottom**) *V* waves secondary to severe mitral regurgitation. The tall systolic *v* wave in the pulmonary artery wedge pressure (PAWP) trace also distorts the PA tracing, thereby giving it a bifid appearance. LVEDP is best estimated by measuring PAWP at the time of the ECG *R* wave before the onset of the regurgitant *v* wave. CVP, central venous pressure; ECG, electrocardiogram; PAP, pulmonary artery pressure. (From Mark JB. *Atlas of Cardiovascular Monitoring*. Churchill Livingstone; 1998. Figures 17.1 and 17.11. Reprinted with permission of Jonathan B. Mark, MD.)

use over the past two decades, PAC use in cardiac surgery has increased recently, probably related to the increased utilization of mechanical support devices.[38] In fact, PAC is recommended by scientific societies for the management of cardiogenic shock.[39,40]

2. **Contraindications to pulmonary artery catheter placement**
   a. Tricuspid or pulmonary valve stenosis, endocarditis, or mechanical prosthetic tricuspid or pulmonic valves
   b. Presence of a right-sided mass (tumor/thrombosis) that could embolize if dislodged
   c. Left bundle branch block (LBBB) is a relative contraindication owing to the risk of PAC-induced right bundle branch block (RBBB)[41] and resulting complete heart block (CHB). When PAC monitoring is required in patients with preexisting LBBB, external pacing should be immediately available. In addition, insertion of the PAC can be delayed until the chest is open so that CPB may be rapidly initiated should refractory CHB occur.

3. **Common catheter features:** A large variety of PACs are currently available for clinical use. The standard PAC is 7F, 110 cm in length, with markings every 10 cm to aid insertion and positioning. These catheters have the following features:
   a. A distal port for monitoring pressures during insertion and for continuous monitoring of PAP once the catheter is in place
   b. A proximal port, 26 cm from the catheter tip, used for CVP monitoring
   c. A venous infusion port (VIP), 30 cm from the tip, used for central drug and fluid infusion
   d. A thermistor near the catheter tip for measurement of blood temperature. This thermistor allows the calculation of CO via the intermittent bolus thermodilution method when cold or room temperature saline is injected into the RA.
   e. A lumen for inflation of the distal tip balloon with air

CLINICAL PEARL

A common error is to forget that the VIP and CVP ports will remain outside of the patient and lie within the protective insertion sheath if the PAC has not yet been floated fully into the PA. Medications administered via these ports will not be delivered into the patient's circulation under this circumstance.

4. **Additional catheter features:** A variety of PAC models are currently available for clinical use. Some of the additional features included in these catheters are as follows:
   a. **Continuous CO (CCO) measurement:** These PACs use low-power thermal filaments located in the RA/RV segment of the catheter that impart small temperature changes to RV blood. The thermistor at the catheter tip allows for semicontinuous (every 60-180 seconds) CO determinations. A "stat" option allows for faster (every 60 seconds) display of CO readings.[42]
   b. **Mixed venous oxygen saturation (Svo$_2$):** Several PAC models also incorporate fiberoptic bundles that allow continuous hemoglobin oxygen saturation of the pulmonary artery blood (Svo$_2$) using two or three wavelength reflectance oximetry.
   c. **Pacing:** PACs with pacing capabilities have a separate lumen terminating 19 cm from the catheter tip. When the catheter tip lies in the PA in a patient with a normal-sized heart, this more proximal port will be positioned in the RV. A separate sterile, prepackaged pacing wire can be inserted through this port until it makes contact with the RV endocardium, allowing for RV pacing. Pacing PACs are seldom used in cardiac surgery as epicardial pacing wires are routinely placed by the surgeon intraoperatively.
   d. **Ejection fraction PACs:** PACs with faster thermistor response times can be used to determine RV ejection fraction in addition to CO. Using proprietary algorithms that combine fast-response thermodilution with pulse contour analysis of the PA waveform, these catheters display RV stroke volume, end-diastolic volume, and end-systolic volume with each beat. Monitoring these parameters can be helpful in patients with RV dysfunction.

5. **Insertion technique:** An introducer sheath is inserted into a central vein as described in "Central Venous Pressure Interpretation" section. Recommendations related to PAC insertion technique include the following:

   a. **Patient monitoring:** The patient should be fully monitored during the PAC insertion procedure. ECG monitoring is especially important as dysrhythmias are the most common complication of PAC insertion. Pulse oximetry gives an audible tone reflecting oxygenation and pulse rate and may alert the physician to desaturation, an abnormal heart rate, or irregular rhythm.

   b. **Preferred approach:** The right IJ approach offers the most direct route to the RA and thus results in the highest rate of successful PA catheterization. The left subclavian vein is the second best option.

   c. **Catheter advancement**

      (1) With help from a trained assistant, the catheter is inserted through the hemostatic valve of the introducer sheath to a depth of ~20 cm (RA position). A typical CVP waveform is seen at this point (Figure 5.14).

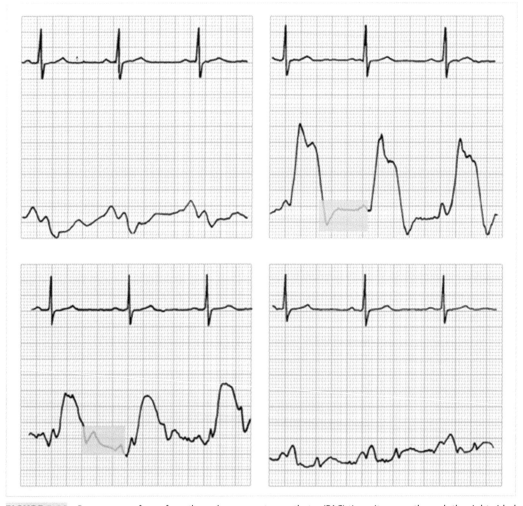

FIGURE 5.14 Pressure waveforms from the pulmonary artery catheter (PAC) tip as it passes through the right-sided heart chambers and into the pulmonary vasculature. The upper left panel shows the central venous pressure (CVP) or right atrial pressure waveform, the right upper panel shows the right ventricular (RV) pressure waveform, the left lower panel shows the pulmonary artery (PA) pressure waveform, and the right lower panel shows the pulmonary artery wedge pressure (PAWP) waveform. Note that both CVP and PAWP waveforms exhibit *a*, *c*, and *v* waves (See Figure 5.8). The shaded boxes in the RV and PA waveforms demonstrate the upward slope during diastolic filling in the RV versus the downward-sloping diastolic runoff in the PA. This diastolic pressure feature helps distinguish RV from PA waveforms when inserting a PAC. (From Mark JB. *Atlas of Cardiovascular Monitoring*. Churchill Livingstone; 1998. Figure 3.1. Reprinted with permission of Jonathan B. Mark, MD.)

(2) The balloon is then inflated fully with air (1.5 mL) and the catheter advanced slowly while observing the transduced waveform. The tricuspid valve is typically crossed at ~30-35 cm, at which point an RV waveform is observed, with clear systolic and diastolic pressures.

(3) The catheter is advanced further until the pulmonic valve is crossed (~40-45 cm), at which point a step-up in diastolic pressure will occur and a PAP waveform observed.

(4) The catheter is then advanced slowly until the pulsatile PA waveform disappears and the PAWP waveform is displayed. The PAWP waveform is a *delayed and dampened* reflection of downstream left atrial pressure, with a similar morphology to CVP (Figure 5.14).

(5) The PAWP is recorded and the balloon is deflated.

CLINICAL PEARL

(1) It is sometimes difficult to ascertain the location of the PAC as it is advanced from RV to PA, especially when focusing entirely on the systolic and diastolic numeric values displayed on the bedside monitor rather than on the pressure waveform. Inspection of the waveform will allow differentiation between an *up-sloping* diastolic wave that represents RV filling versus a *down-sloping* wave representing PA diastolic runoff. PAC position in the PA can also be confirmed using TEE.[43] (2) Always be sure to completely flush all air bubbles from the PA catheter. Failure to do so will lead to a dampened, difficult-to-interpret waveform.

    d. Safety: The following may increase the safety of PAC insertion and use:

      (1) Always check the balloon for proper inflation and symmetry before insertion. The balloon should always be inflated fully with air (1.5 mL) and should extend just beyond the catheter tip lumen.

      (2) Verify that the displayed pressure waveform corresponds to the pressure recorded from the tip of the catheter (rather than from a more proximal lumen) before proceeding with catheter insertion.

      (3) Use closed-loop communication between the proceduralist and the assistant (call-outs and check-backs) during insertion and balloon inflation/deflation.

      (4) Following catheter insertion into the RA, if the expected pressure waveforms do not appear at typical insertion depths (eg, 30-35 cm for RV, 40-45 cm for PA, and 45-50 cm for PAWP when accessed from the RIJ), deflate the balloon, withdraw the catheter into the RA, and restart the procedure.

      (5) Once the catheter is wedged, deflate the balloon and withdraw the catheter ~2 cm. Slight catheter withdrawal should also precede the institution of CPB because, with hypothermia, the catheter will stiffen making pulmonary artery injury more common.

      (6) Always observe the PA waveform in real time during balloon inflation to measure PAWP. A display of the PAWP waveform with only partial balloon inflation indicates distal migration of the catheter. In this situation, full balloon inflation may injure the pulmonary artery.

      (7) Recognize and correct "overwedging." This occurs when the catheter migrates distally and eccentric balloon inflation forces the catheter tip against the vessel wall, resulting in a gradually rising, nonpulsatile pressure waveform.

  6. Complications

    a. Vascular access: See in "Central Venous Pressure Interpretation" section

    b. PAC placement/manipulation

      (1) Cardiac arrhythmias: The reported incidence ranges from 12.5% to 70%.[15] PVCs are the most common arrhythmia. Fortunately, most arrhythmias are transient or resolve with either catheter withdrawal or with the advancement of the catheter tip from RV into PA. There appears to be a higher incidence of arrhythmias during catheter insertion when the patient is positioned in the Trendelenburg position versus the right-tilt position.[39]

(2) **Injury to cardiac structures:** Catheter knotting and entanglement of cardiac structures, although rare, can occur. Damage to intracardiac structures such as valves, chordae, and even RV perforation has been reported. The presence of inferior vena cava (IVC) filters, other indwelling catheters, and pacemakers can increase the risk of such complications. The incidence of knotting is estimated at 0.03%, and this complication can be decreased with careful attention to depth of insertion and waveform morphology.[44] To reduce the risk of knotting, a catheter should be withdrawn if the RV waveform is still present 20 cm after its initial appearance or when the absolute depth of 60 cm is reached without a PAP tracing.

(3) **PA rupture:** This is a rare complication with a very high mortality rate.[45] Risk factors include pulmonary hypertension, age >60, hyperinflation of the balloon, improper (distal) catheter positioning, and coagulopathy.[41] During CPB, distal migration of the catheter tip may occur, and it is recommended that the PAC be withdrawn ~2 cm prior to initiating bypass (see earlier).

c. **Thrombosis:** Although thrombus formation on PACs has been noted at 24 hours, the incidence of thrombogenicity substantially increases after 72 hours.

d. **Pulmonary infarction:** It can occur as a complication of continuous distal wedging from catheter migration or embolization of a previously formed thrombus.

e. **Infection:** The incidence of bacteremia and bloodstream infection related to PAC monitoring is low. However, the PAC can contribute to endothelial damage of the tricuspid and pulmonary valves leading to endocarditis.

f. **Errors in equipment and data acquisition:** Examples include inappropriate pressure transducer level and over/underdamping of the catheter-tubing-transducer system.

g. **Misinterpretation or misapplication of data:** Misinterpretation can occur when not considering ventilation modes, ventricular compliance changes, or intrinsic cardiac or pulmonary pathology.

h. **Other:** Balloon rupture, heparin-induced thrombocytopenia (HIT) secondary to heparin-coated catheters, anaphylaxis from latex (balloon) allergy, and hepatic venous placement have all been reported as uncommon PAC-related complications.

7. **Parameters measured**

a. **Central venous pressure:** A proximal port of the PAC is located in the RA and allows measurement of the CVP.

b. **RV pressure:** RV pacing-capable PACs allow continuous monitoring of RV pressure waveforms and have been used for monitoring RV function during cardiac surgery.[46] Elevated RV end-diastolic pressure has been associated with difficult separation from CPB[47] (Table 5.2).

c. **Pulmonary artery pressure:** The distal lumen of the PAC will record systolic, diastolic, and mean PAP. Normal mean PAP is <20 mm Hg.[48] PAP is determined by the resistance of the pulmonary vasculature (PVR), its compliance (not typically measured but defined as stroke volume divided by PA pulse pressure), RV function, and left atrial (LA) pressure.

d. **Pulmonary artery wedge pressure:** PAWP is an indirect estimate of LA pressure. With the balloon inflated and "wedged" in a branch of the PA, a continuous fluid column connects the distal PAC port and the LA. The end-diastolic PAWP approximates left ventricular end-diastolic pressure (LVEDP). Like all central vascular pressure measurements, recording PAWP at end expiration will obviate the confounding effects of intrathoracic pressure changes that occur during the respiratory cycle (Table 5.3).

e. **Cardiac output:** A thermistor located at the tip of the PAC allows measurement of RV output by the thermodilution technique. In the absence of intracardiac shunts, this measurement equals LV output. It is important to note that CO represents a measure of blood flow and not cardiac contractility. In addition to contractility, CO is dependent on ventricular preload and afterload. CO is used to calculate oxygen delivery (Table 5.4).

f. **Blood temperature:** The thermistor can provide a constant measurement of blood temperature, which is an accurate reflection of core temperature.

TABLE 5.3 Differential Diagnosis of Pulmonary Artery Pressure and Pulmonary Artery Wedge Pressure (PAWP) Hemodynamic Abnormalities

Pulmonary Artery Pressure Waveforms

Increased systolic pressure	Pulmonary disease
	Increased blood flow, left to right shunt
	Increased pulmonary vascular resistance (PVR)
Increased diastolic pressure	Left heart failure
	Intravascular volume overload
	Mitral stenosis or regurgitation
Decreased systolic and diastolic pressure	Hypovolemia
	Pulmonic stenosis
	Tricuspid stenosis

Pulmonary Artery Wedge Pressure Waveform

Decreased (mean) pressure	Hypovolemia
	Transducer zero reference level too high
Increased (mean) pressure	Fluid overload states
	Left ventricular (LV) failure
	Mitral stenosis or regurgitation
	Aortic stenosis or regurgitation
	Myocardial infarction
Tall PAWP *a* wave	Mitral stenosis
Absent PAWP *a* wave	Atrial fibrillation
	Atrial flutter
	Junctional rhythm
Tall PAWP *v* wave (or *cv* wave)	Mitral regurgitation
	Ventricular septal defect
Tall PAWP *a* and *v* waves	Cardiac tamponade
	Pericardial constriction
	Hypervolemia
	LV failure

Modified from *Quick Guide to Cardiopulmonary Care*. 3rd ed. Edwards Critical Care Education; 2015. Used with permission from Edwards Critical Care Education.

TABLE 5.4 Oxygen Delivery Variables and Normal Values

Oxygen Parameters—Adult

Parameter	Equation	Normal Range
Arterial oxygen content (Cao_2)	$(0.0138 \times Hgb \times Sao_2) + 0.0031 \times Pao_2$	16-22 mL/dL
Venous oxygen content (Cvo_2)	$(0.0138 \times Hgb \times Svo_2) + 0.0031 \times Pvo_2$	15 mL/dL
A-V oxygen content difference ($C[a-v]o_2$)	$Cao_2 - Cvo_2$	4-6 mL/dL
Oxygen delivery (Do_2)	$Cao_2 \times CO \times 10$	950-1,150 mL/min
Oxygen delivery index (Do_2I)	$Cao_2 \times CI \times 10$	500-600 mL/min/m^2
Oxygen consumption (Vo_2)	$C(a-v)o_2 \times CO \times 10$	200-250 mL/min
Oxygen consumption index (Vo_2I)	$C(a-v)o_2 \times CI \times 10$	120-160 mL/min/m^2
Oxygen extraction ratio (O_2ER)	$(Cao_2 - Cvo_2)/Cao_2 \times 100$	22%-30%
Oxygen extraction index (O_2EI)	$(Sao_2 - Svo_2)/Sao_2 \times 100$	20%-25%

Modified from *Quick Guide to Cardiopulmonary Care*. 3rd ed. Edwards Critical Care Education; 2015. Used with permission from Edwards Critical Care Education.

g. **Mixed venous oxygen saturation (Svo₂):** Oximetric PACs measure real-time PA blood hemoglobin saturation. This value is inversely proportional to CO, and during periods of stable oxygen consumption and arterial hemoglobin saturation, provides additional indication of the direction and magnitude of changes in CO. Figure 5.15 presents a treatment algorithm utilizing SvO_2 to guide management. Decreased oxygen delivery or increased oxygen utilization results in a decreased SvO_2. Four mechanisms can result in a significant decrease in SvO_2.
   (1) Decreased CO
   (2) Decreased hemoglobin concentration
   (3) Decreased hemoglobin saturation (SaO_2)
   (4) Increased O_2 consumption

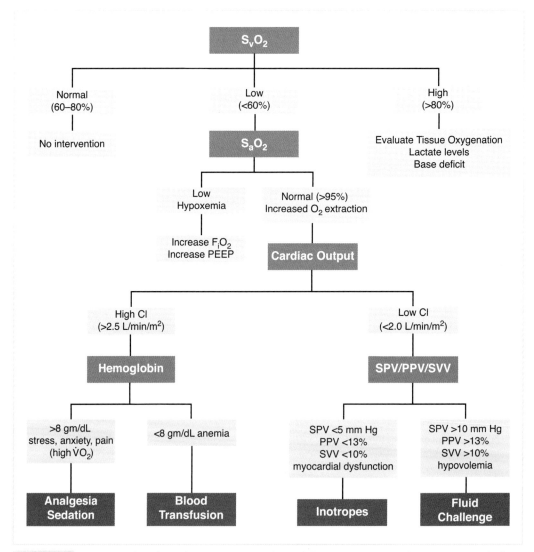

FIGURE 5.15   Treatment algorithm utilizing SvO_2, SaO_2, CO, hemoglobin concentration, and a measurement of volume status. CO, cardiac output; PEEP, positive end-expiratory pressure; PPV, pulse pressure variation; SvO_2, mixed venous oxygen saturation; SaO_2, arterial oxygen saturation; SPV, systolic pressure variation; SVV, stroke volume variation. (Adapted from *Quick Guide to Cardiopulmonary Care*. 3rd ed. Edwards Critical Care Education; 2015. Used with permission from Edwards Critical Care Education.)

These mechanisms can be understood by reviewing the oxygen consumption equation:

$$\text{VO}_2 = \text{CO} \times \text{Hgb} \times 13.8 \times (\text{SaO}_2 - \text{SvO}_2)$$

where VO_2 is oxygen consumption, CO is cardiac output in L/min, Hgb is the hemoglobin in g/dL, 13.8 is the amount of oxygen that can combine hemoglobin (1 g of Hgb can bind 1.38 mL of O_2, this factor is multiplied by 10 to convert dL to L as Hgb is measured in g/dL), SaO_2 is arterial saturation, and SvO_2 is mixed venous saturation.

8. **Other derived hemodynamic parameters:** Advanced indices of ventricular performance and cardiovascular status can be derived using parameters measured by the PAC (Table 5.5).

   a. **Systemic vascular resistance:** Represents the total resistance offered to the LV by the systemic vasculature. It is mostly determined by the diameter of the vessels but is also affected by blood viscosity.

   b. **Pulmonary vascular resistance:** Represents the resistance offered to the RV by the pulmonary vasculature and is calculated as the ratio of the transpulmonary gradient (mPAP-PAWP) over CO.

   c. Transpulmonary gradient (TPG) and diastolic pulmonary vascular pressure gradient (DPG). TPG—the difference between mean PAP and mean PAWP (normal $\leq$12 mm Hg) and DPG (diastolic PAP $-$ PAWP, normal $<$7 mm Hg) have been used as additional

TABLE 5.5 Hemodynamic Variables and Normal Values

Normal Hemodynamic Parameters—Adult

Parameter	Equation	Normal Range
Arterial blood pressure (BP)	Systolic (SBP)	100-140 mm Hg
	Diastolic (DBP)	60-90 mm Hg
Mean arterial pressure (MAP)	SBP + (2 × DPB)/3	70-105 mm Hg
Right atrial pressure (RAP)		2-6 mm Hg
Right ventricular pressure (RVP)	Systolic (RVSP)	15-30 mm Hg
	Diastolic (RVDP)	0-8 mm Hg
Pulmonary artery pressure (PAP)	Systolic (PASP)	15-30 mm Hg
	Diastolic (PADP)	8-15 mm Hg
Mean pulmonary artery pressure (MPAP)	PASP + (2 × PADP)/3	9-18 mm Hg
Pulmonary artery occlusion pressure (PAOP)		6-12 mm Hg
Left atrial pressure (LAP)		4-12 mm Hg
Cardiac output (CO)	HR × SV/1,000	4.0-8.0 L/min
Cardiac index (CI)	CO/BSA	2.5-4.0 L/min/m²
Stroke volume (SV)	CO/HR × 1,000	60-100 mL/beat
Stroke volume index (SVI)	CI/HR × 1,000	33-47 mL/m²/beat
Stroke volume variation (SVV)	$SV_{max} - SV_{min}/SV_{mean} \times 100$	<10%-15%
Systemic vascular resistance (SVR)	80 × (MAP − RAP)/CO	800-1,200 dynes·s/cm⁵
Systemic vascular resistance index (SVRI)	80 × (MAP − RAP)/CI	1,970-2,390 dynes·s/cm⁵·m²
Pulmonary vascular resistance (PVR)	80 × (MPAP − PAOP)/CO	<250 dynes· s/cm⁵
Pulmonary vascular resistance index (PVRI)	80 × (MPAP − PAOP)/CI	255-285 dynes·s/cm⁵·m²
Left ventricular stroke work index (LVSWI)	SVI × (MAP − PAOP) × 0.0136	50-62 g/m²/beat
Right ventricular stroke work index (RVSWI)	SVI × (MPAP − CVP) × 0.0136	5-10 g/m²/beat
Coronary artery perfusion pressure	Diastolic BP − PAOP	60-80 mm Hg
Right ventricular end-diastolic volume (RVEDV)	SV/EF	100-160 mL
Right ventricular end-diastolic volume index (RVEDVI)	RVEDV/BSA	60-100 mL/m²
Right ventricular end-systolic volume (RVESV)	EDV − SV	50-100 mL
Right ventricular ejection fraction (RVEF)	SV/EDV × 100	40%-60%

Modified from *Quick Guide to Cardiopulmonary Care*. 3rd ed. Edwards Critical Care Education; 2015. Used with permission from Edwards Critical Care Education.

hemodynamic criteria for the differential diagnosis of isolated pre-capillary (iPc-PH) versus combined pre- and post-capillary (cPc-PH) pulmonary hypertension. The most recent criteria include the use of PVR alone (cPc-PH is identified by a PVR ≥3 Wood units).[49,50]

d. **Pulmonary artery pulsatility index:** Defined as PA pulse pressure divided by CVP, pulmonary artery pulsatility index (PAPi) has been proposed as a predictor of long-term RV failure in several patient populations but may not be as useful in predicting acute adverse events.[51,52] A computationally more simplistic variable calculated as mPAP-CVP has been proposed. Compared to the PAPi, this alternative hemodynamic variable is more resistant to errors in transducer leveling and over or underdampened signals, which may lead to under or overestimation of PA pulse pressure, respectively. Furthermore, 1-year mortality was predicted by the mPAP-CVP gradient but not by the PAPi in a cardiac surgical patient cohort.[53]

e. Other indices that characterize ventriculoarterial coupling using hemodynamic data have been described. For example, the systemic congestive index combines systemic pulse pressure and CVP and may represent ventriculoarterial coupling.[54]

9. **Considerations when interpreting PAC data**

a. **Effects of ventilation:** The effects of ventilation on CVP and PAP readings can be significant in the low-pressure system of the right-sided circulation because intrathoracic juxtacardiac (airway or transpleural) pressure is transmitted to the pulmonary vasculature. The negative intrapleural pressure generated during spontaneous breathing, particularly in a patient experiencing dyspnea, will decrease the monitored intravascular pressures, occasionally resulting in negative (subatmospheric) PA diastolic, PAWP, and CVP pressures. In contrast, positive airway pressures are transmitted to the vasculature during mechanical ventilation, leading to elevations in monitored vascular pressures. Mean airway pressure is the parameter that correlates most closely with the changes in PAP and CVP measurements. The established convention is to evaluate all central vascular pressures at *end expiration* to obviate the effects of the respiratory cycle. The digital monitor numerical readout may not appropriately identify the pressure values at this phase in the respiratory cycle. Thus, inspection of the pressure waveforms is required for correct interpretation.

b. **Location of the catheter tip:** PA pressure measurements depend on where the tip of the catheter resides in the pulmonary vascular tree. In areas of the lung that are well ventilated but poorly perfused (West zone I), the PAC readings may be altered substantially by the changes in airway pressure. Likewise, even when the tip is in a good location in the middle or lower lung fields, high positive end-expiratory pressure (>10 mm Hg) may affect PAP values.

E. **Cardiac Output**

1. **Methods**

a. **Thermodilution with cold injectate:** This method is commonly utilized because of its ease of use and ability to repeat measurements over time. The indicator is an aliquot of saline (typically 10 mL, which is at a lower temperature than the temperature of blood) injected into the RA. The change in temperature produced by injection of this indicator is measured in the PA by a thermistor and is integrated over time to generate a value for RV output, which is equal to systemic CO if no intracardiac shunts are present (Figure 5.16). This method requires no withdrawal of blood and no arterial line, uses an inexpensive indicator, and is not greatly affected by recirculation.

CLINICAL PEARL

Thermodilution CO underestimates the CO with right-side valvular lesions but remains accurate with mitral and aortic valve lesions.

---

b. **Continuous thermodilution:** A thermal filament in the PAC heats blood ~15-25 cm before its tip, thus generating a PA temperature change that is measured via a distal thermistor. The input and output signals are correlated to generate CO values.

c. **RV ejection fraction:** Improved preload estimates might be obtained with this type of PAC.[55]

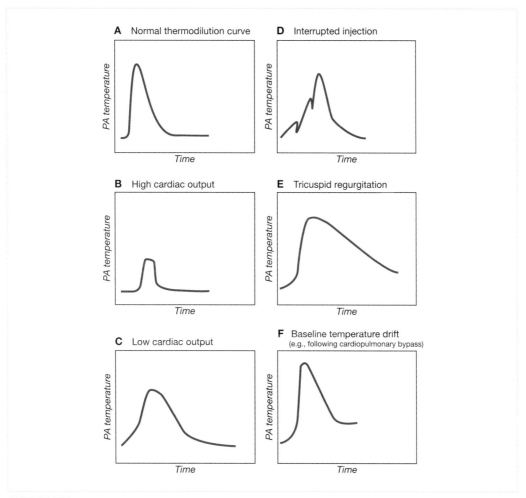

FIGURE 5.16 Thermodilution curves recorded from a PAC thermistor. Cardiac output (CO) is inversely related to the area under the curve. The curves on the left **(A-C)** demonstrated normal, high, and low CO, respectively. Curve **(D)** demonstrates an error in thermodilution technique. Curve **(E)** demonstrates a thermodilution curve in a patient with TR, where recirculation of the injected fluid results in distortion of the descending limb of the curve, causing an increase in the area under the curve and an underestimation of the CO. Curve **(F)** is representative of a patient who was recently liberated from cardiopulmonary bypass (CPB). Blood from cooled parts of the body will decrease the overall temperature of the overall circulation, leading to a drift in baseline, which will cause an overestimation of CO. PA, pulmonary artery; TR, tricuspid regurgitation. (Used with permission of McGraw Hill LLC from Bar-Yosef S, Schroeder RA, Mark JB. Hemodynamic monitoring. In: Longnecker DE, Brown DL, Newman MF, Zapol WM, eds. *Anesthesiology*. 2nd ed. McGraw-Hill Medical; 2012:420. Figure 30.14; permission conveyed through Copyright Clearance Center, Inc.)

2. **Assumptions and errors with thermodilution:** Specific errors in CO determination are mentioned later:
   a. **Volume of injectate:** Because the output computer will base its calculations on a specific volume, an injectate volume less than that for which the computer is set will cause a falsely high value of CO, and vice versa.
   b. **Temperature of injectate:** If the injectate temperature parameter is incorrect, errors can occur. For example, an increase of 1 °C will cause a 3% overestimation of CO. The controversy over iced versus room temperature injectate centers around the concept that a larger difference between the injectate temperature and blood temperature should increase the accuracy of the CO determination. Studies have not supported this hypothesis, and the extra inconvenience of keeping syringes on ice, together with the increased risk of infection (nonsterile water surrounding the Luer tip), makes the iced saline method a less attractive alternative.

c. **Shunts:** Intracardiac shunts will cause erroneous values for thermodilution CO values. This technique should not be used if a communication exists between the pulmonary and systemic circulations. A shunt should always be suspected when thermodilution CO values do not fit the clinical findings.

d. **Timing with the respiratory cycle:** As much as a 10% difference in CO will result, depending on when injection occurs during the respiratory cycle. These changes are most likely due to actual changes in pulmonary blood flow during respiration.

e. **Catheter position:** The tip of the pulmonary catheter must be in the PA and must not be "wedged"; otherwise, nonsensical curves are obtained.

f. **Accuracy:** Studies have shown variable and sometimes poor correlation of thermodilution with the gold-standard direct Fick method.[56]

3. **Minimally invasive CO monitoring:** The desire to assess cardiac function and adequate tissue perfusion in patients who are critically ill is traditionally accomplished using the PAC. The controversy about its invasive nature and potential harm has led to the development of less invasive CO monitoring devices.[57,58]

a. **Pulse contour analysis:** Monitors based on the assumption that SV can be tracked continuously by analysis of the arterial waveform. These monitors require an optimal arterial waveform, thus arrhythmias, IABPs, LVADs, and even properties of the arterial line monitoring systems (such as over/underdamping) can alter accuracy of the CO measurement. Four common pulse contour analysis devices are compared in Table 5.6.

b. **Doppler:** CO can be measured using the change in frequency of an ultrasonic beam as it measures blood flow velocity. To achieve accurate measurements, at least three conditions must be met: (1) The cross-sectional area of the vessel must be known; (2) the ultrasound beam must be directed parallel to the flow of blood; and (3) the beam direction cannot move to any great degree between measurements. This is discussed in greater detail in Chapter 4.

TABLE 5.6 Pulse Contour Analysis Devices

	FloTrac System	PiCCO*plus* System	LiDCO*plus* System	Argos CO Monitor
Requires external calibration	No	Yes	Yes	No
Requires central line	No	Yes	No	No
Type of calibration	—	Transpulmonary thermodilution via CVL	Pulmonary lithium indicator	—
Special arterial catheter	No	Yes, thermistor-tipped catheter	No	No
Preferred arterial site	Any site	Femoral	Any site	Any site
Alternative sites	—	Radial/brachial (require longer catheter)	—	—
Main advantages	Minimally invasive Operator independent Easy to use	Broad range of hemodynamic parameters More robust during hemodynamic instability (with frequent recalibration)	Minimally invasive Easy to use More robust during hemodynamic Instability (with frequent recalibration)	Multi-beat analysis avoids confounding effects of wave reflection No proprietary consumable per patient
Main disadvantages	Reliability in vasoplegic patients low in older versions Less robust during hemodynamic instability	More invasive Requires recalibration	Disturbing factors (lithium use, neuromuscular blocking agents) Requires recalibration	

TABLE 5.6   Pulse Contour Analysis Devices *(continued)*

	FloTrac System	PiCCO*plus* System	LiDCO*plus* System	Argos CO Monitor
Method	Concept that the area under the curve of the systolic arterial waveform is proportional to SV Standard deviation of pulse pressure is correlated with "normal" SV based on a database of patient demographics (age, sex, weight, height). Impedance is also derived from this demographic data	Concept that the area under the curve of the systolic arterial waveform is proportional to SV. Calibration is used to determine the individual aortic impedance. Recalibration recommended every 8 h in stable patients; increased frequency of recalibration (up to every 1 h) is needed in patients with hemodynamic instability (significant changes of vascular resistance)	Concept of conservation of mass (power). Suggests that after calibration and correction for compliance, the relationship between net power and net flow is linear. Calibration was used to determine resistance of vasculature; recalibration is recommended q8h. Lithium calibration is negatively affected by: 1. Changes in electrolytes 2. Changes in hematocrit 3. High peak doses of muscle relaxant 4. Patient on lithium 5. Patients <40 kg	Concept that the area under the curve of the systolic arterial waveform is proportional to SV
Additional assessments provided	SVV	Global end-diastolic volume; extravascular lung volume; SVV	SVV	

Goal-directed assessment of fluid-responsive hypovolemia can be automatically measured by several commercially available devices. Comparison of these devices is depicted.
CVL, central venous line; PPV, pulse pressure variation; SPV, systolic pressure variation; SV, stroke volume; SVV, stroke volume variation.

   c. **TEE:** In addition to the Doppler-based measurements of CO, TEE can utilize the Simpson method of disks or 3D volumes to estimate CO without the use of Doppler. End-diastolic and end-systolic dimensions measured by echocardiography are converted to volumes, allowing SV and CO to be determined.

  4. **Measurements of volume responsiveness:** Fluid management is an integral part of anesthetic care. Fluid administration is regularly administered intraoperatively to improve CO. Due to the complex physiology associated with both cardiac surgery and general anesthesia, the determination of volume responsiveness can be complex. Studies have shown that static pressure measurements that have historically been used to assess for volume responsiveness, specifically, CVP and pulmonary capillary occlusion pressure (PAOP), are unreliable.[33] Dynamic parameters (Table 5.7) such as SPV, PPV, and SVV have shown very promising correlations with volume responsiveness.[59] However, because all of these parameters rely on cardiopulmonary interaction, it has been noted that their utility during open

TABLE 5.7   Measurements of Fluid Responsiveness

Parameter	Normal	Fluid Responsive
SPV (mm Hg)	5 mm Hg	>10 mm Hg
PPV (%)	<13%	>13%
SVV (%)	<10%	>10%-15%

Comparison of SPV/PPV/SVV. Goal-directed assessment of fluid responsiveness in patients with hypovolemia.
PPV, pulse pressure variation; SPV, systolic pressure variation; SVV, stroke volume variation.

heart surgery may be limited. SVV/PPV have been shown to have a good correlation with preload surrogates before sternotomy and after sternal closure, but poor correlation while the chest is open.[60] Additionally, the shift toward lung-protective smaller tidal volumes has been found to nullify the usefulness of these measures. This has been addressed by the more recently developed tidal volume challenge.

10

CLINICAL PEARL

Generally, SPV, PPV, and SVV require a regular heart rhythm to be accurate.

    a. **Systolic pressure variation:** Increased intrathoracic pressure generated during a positive pressure breath leads to decreased LV stroke volume, and subsequently a drop in systolic blood pressure (sBP). The drop in the systolic pressure from baseline to after delivery of a fixed tidal volume the delta down (ΔDown) has been shown to correlate with volume status. The advantage of this parameter is that only a standard arterial line is required (Figure 5.17A).

    b. **Pulse pressure variation:** A similar concept to SPV, PPV compares changes in pulse pressure, that is, the difference between systolic and diastolic pressures throughout the respiratory cycle in a mechanically ventilated patient. It has been demonstrated that PPV is a more accurate surrogate of SV, most likely because SPV is influenced by both aortic transmural pressure (from the LV stroke volume) and extramural pressure from

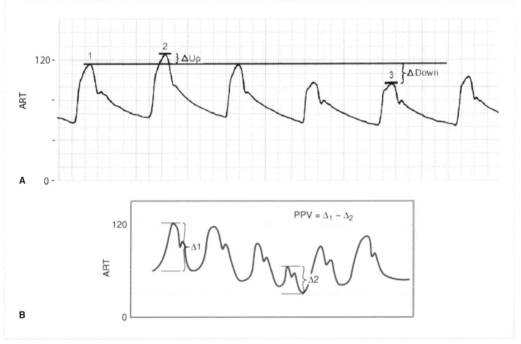

FIGURE 5.17 **(A)** Arterial waveform tracing demonstrating systolic pressure variation (SPV). The first cycle is recorded during apnea, giving a baseline from which ΔUp and ΔDown are measured. In this case, ΔUp is ~7 mm Hg, while ΔDown is 5 mm Hg, giving an SPV of 22 mm Hg, indicating that this patient would likely respond to a fluid challenge. (Reprinted with permission from Pittman JA, Ping JS, Mark JB. Arterial and central venous pressure monitoring. *Int Anesthesiol Clin*. 2004;42(1):13-30.) **(B)** An illustration of pulse pressure variation (PPV). In this case, the maximal pulse pressure, Δ1, is ~60 mm Hg, and the minimal, Δ2, is 35 mm Hg, giving a pulse pressure difference of Δ1 − Δ2 = 25 mm Hg. The pulse pressure difference divided by the mean of the two values (47.5 mm Hg) gives a pulse pressure variation of 53%, which is >12%, indicating that this patient would also likely respond to a fluid challenge. (Used with permission of McGraw Hill LLC from Bar-Yosef S, Schroeder RA, Mark JB. Hemodynamic monitoring. In: Longnecker DE, Brown DL, Newman MF, Zapol WM, eds. *Anesthesiology*. 2nd ed. McGraw-Hill Medical; 2012:425. Figure 30.18; permission conveyed through Copyright Clearance Center, Inc.)

changes in pleural pressure, whereas PPV eliminates the effects of pleural pressure as systolic and diastolic pressures would be affected equally. While this parameter can also be measured by a standard arterial line, many of the minimally invasive CO measurement devices that rely on pulse contour analysis will automatically calculate this number (Figure 5.17B).

   c. **Stroke volume variation:** Real-time measurement of variations in SV has been made possible using the same arterial waveform analysis used for minimally invasive continuous CO monitoring (see earlier). These devices determine SV using an algorithm based on the contour of the arterial pressure tracing. SVV is also measured, using the formula $SVV = (SV_{max} - SV_{min})/SV_{mean}$. SVV has been shown to very accurately predict volume responsiveness in critical care patients.[61]

   d. **Tidal volume challenge:** PPV and SVV are unreliable during lung-protective low tidal volume ventilation. The change in these dynamic indicators can be measured after a standardized, temporary increase in tidal volume to 8 mL/kg predicted body weight. A significant change in the indicators has good predictive value for fluid responsiveness.[62,63]

F. Echocardiography

  1. **TEE:** TEE is discussed extensively in Chapter 4.

III. Temperature

Cardiac anesthesia is unique in that therapeutic hypothermia is utilized frequently and aggressively in many cases. Distribution of thermal energy can be manipulated, via CPB, more rapidly and extensively than in other anesthetic cases. As an extreme example, circulatory arrest procedures[64] typically involve cooling to <28 °C. Temperature monitoring pertaining specifically to cardiac anesthesia will be discussed later. General principles of perianesthetic temperature monitoring are reviewed elsewhere.[65]

A. Indications: Cardiopulmonary Bypass CPB and Hypothermia

  1. **"Warm" or normothermic CPB:** 36-37 °C

  2. **"Mild" hypothermic or tepid CPB:** 32-34 °C

  3. **"Moderate" hypothermic CPB:** 28-32 °C

  4. **"Deep" hypothermic circulatory arrest (DHCA):** <28 °C. This unique therapeutic technique is discussed in Chapter 23.

    Cardiac surgery utilizes the capabilities of the CPB circuit to cool or warm patients. Despite most literature comparing normothermic CPB with hypothermic CPB showing no benefit,[66,67] mild hyperthermia is widely utilized for brain and other organ protection.[68] However, hypothermia leading to coagulation abnormalities and bleeding remain major concerns. Below 32 °C, the myocardium is irritable and susceptible to arrhythmias, especially ventricular tachycardia and fibrillation. By communicating with the perfusionists, the anesthesiologist should be aware of the rate of temperature change during rewarming and gradients between CPB inflow and outflow temperatures. Most importantly during the rewarming period, the CPB arterial outflow temperature should not exceed 37 °C.[69] Even mild hyperthermia is associated with postoperative cognitive dysfunction,[70] and enzyme denaturation and cell damage occur with temperatures ≥41 °C.

B. Sites of Measurement

Temperature may be measured at numerous sites, which can be grouped into the brain, core, or shell. Brain and core temperature should both be continually monitored.

  1. **Brain temperature**

   a. **Nasopharyngeal temperature:** Nasopharyngeal temperature provides an accurate reflection of brain temperature during CPB. The probe should be inserted into the nasopharynx to a depth equivalent to the distance from the naris to the tip of the earlobe and not over inserted to avoid unintentional measurement of esophageal temperature.[69]

   b. **Tympanic membrane temperature:** Temperature at this site reflects brain temperature and may provide an alternative to nasopharyngeal temperature.

   c. **CPB arterial line temperature:** This is the temperature of the heat exchanger (ie, the lowest temperature during active cooling and the highest temperature during active rewarming). During either of these phases, a gradient always exists between the arterial line temperature and temperature measured at sites in the patient.

2. **Core temperature:** The core temperature, which represents the temperature of the vital organs, is perhaps a misnomer because, during the rapid cooling and warming phases on CPB, temperature gradients will exist between the vessel-rich group and less highly perfused portions of the body.

   a. **Pulmonary artery blood temperature:** In patients with PAC monitoring, the thermistor near the catheter tip will record this temperature. This is the best estimate of core temperature when pulmonary blood flow is present (ie, before and after CPB).

   b. **Bladder temperature:** This modality has been used to measure core temperature, although it may be inaccurate in instances when urine production is decreased.

   c. **Esophageal temperature:** Because the esophagus is a mediastinal structure, it will be greatly affected by the temperature of the blood returning from the extracorporeal pump and the iced saline slush used for topical cooling of the myocardium. Consequently, this monitoring site should not be used for cases involving CPB.

   d. **Rectal temperature:** This monitoring site is occasionally used if bladder temperature cannot be obtained. However, if the tip of the probe rests in stool, a significant lag will exist with changing temperatures.

   e. **CPB venous line temperature:** This is the temperature of the venous blood draining from the patient into the CPB circuit and probably best reflects core temperature during CPB when no active warming or cooling is occurring.

3. **Shell temperature:** The shell compartment represents the majority of the body (muscle, fat, bone), which receives a smaller proportion of blood flow, thus acting as an energy sink that can significantly affect temperature fluxes. Shell temperature lags behind core temperature during CPB cooling and rewarming. At the point of bypass separation, the core temperature will be significantly higher than the shell temperature. Subsequently, as heat redistributes from the core to the shell, the patient's core temperature will decrease. In general, some active heating methods, like those used in the general operating rooms, will be employed to prevent post-bypass hypothermia.

   a. **Skin temperature:** Skin temperature is rarely utilized in cardiac surgery.

IV. Renal Function

A. **Indications for Monitoring**

1. **Increased incidence of acute kidney injury (AKI) after CPB:** AKI occurs in 5%-31% of cases and is strongly associated with postoperative mortality.[71] AKI is multifactorial and related to preoperative renal function and the presence of coexisting disease.

2. **Use of diuretics in CPB prime:** Mannitol may be used in the priming volume for CPB to promote diuresis and reduce the obligatory volume load of bypass. It may also maintain urine output in the setting of CPB-related hemolysis and thereby reduce the risk of renal tubular cell damage. However, studies have not demonstrated a reduction in AKI with the use of mannitol.[72,73]

B. **Urinary Catheter**

This is the single most important monitor of renal function during surgical cases involving CPB. In addition, a thermistor in the catheter is used to monitor bladder temperature.

C. **Electrolytes**

Serum electrolytes, especially potassium, calcium, and magnesium, should be checked throughout the procedure including at the start of the case, prior to separation from CPB, and following weaning from CPB.

V. Neurologic Function

A. **General Considerations**

Neurocognitive dysfunction is common following cardiac surgery and is multifactorial in origin. Patients undergoing cardiac surgery frequently have increased baseline susceptibility to neurocognitive insults from atherosclerosis, diabetes mellitus, and genetic predisposition. Factors contributing to the stroke or cognitive impairment include perioperative hemodynamic instability leading to cerebral hypoperfusion and central nervous system (CNS) emboli, including air, atheromatous material, and thrombus.[74] Some cardiac centers employ newer neurologic monitoring techniques in an attempt to reduce these adverse events.[75-78]

B. **Indications for Monitoring Neurologic Function**
   1. Monitor depth of anesthesia and prevent unintentional awareness
   2. Avoidance of burst suppression during CPB and associated POCD
   3. Diagnose cerebral embolism
   4. Diagnose aortic cannula malposition leading to brain malperfusion
   5. Diagnose globally inadequate arterial flow on CPB
   6. Confirm adequate brain cooling
   7. Ensure suppression of brain activity prior to and during deep hypothermic circulatory arrest
   8. Ensure adequate spinal cord perfusion during thoracic aortic surgery, particularly thoracoabdominal aneurysm repair

C. **Physiologic and Metabolic Monitoring**
   1. **Cerebral perfusion pressure:** Maintaining adequate cerebral perfusion is the primary intervention for any neuroprotective strategy. Cerebral blood flow (CBF) is autoregulated across a wide range of mean arterial pressure (MAP). Traditionally this range in MAP was considered to be 50-150 mm Hg, but there is considerable interpatient variability, and the average lower limit of CBF autoregulation more likely occurs at a MAP closer to 70 mm Hg in awake normal adults.[79] Of note, however, a randomized controlled trial targeting a higher MAP during bypass (70-80 mm Hg) compared to a lower MAP (40-50 mm Hg) did not reduce the incidence of cerebral injury.[80] Consequently, the primary approach to neurologic monitoring during cardiac surgery involves ensuring adequate MAP and maintaining normal targeted blood flows while on CPB.
   2. **Blood glucose monitoring:** Hyperglycemia markedly worsens neurologic outcomes when present during ischemia/reperfusion[81] and is associated with mortality in patients undergoing cardiac surgery.[82] An insulin infusion should be titrated to a target blood glucose of ≤180 mg/dL.[83] It is important to note that the effects of insulin are diminished with hypothermia and increased catecholamine states. β-Adrenergic stimulation from the stress response to CPB increases blood glucose. Since insulin causes potassium shifting, potassium levels should also be monitored during blood glucose treatment.
   3. **Clinical observation:** Observation of the face for evenly distributed blanching and reperfusion when starting CPB is a crude method to identify gross malposition of the aortic cannula, particularly in patients with aortic dissection.

D. **Monitors of Central Nervous System Electrical Activity**
   1. **Electroencephalogram** (EEG; see Chapter 23): In general, hypothermia or cerebral ischemia causes EEG changes, including increased latency and decreased signal amplitude. EEG monitoring may be employed to establish a neurophysiologic end point for the cerebral effects of cooling (electrocortical silence) in patients undergoing procedures involving the ascending aorta or aortic arch that require the use of deep hypothermic circulatory arrest (DHCA), as well as to detect cerebral hypoperfusion and monitor anesthetic depth.[84] EEG monitoring generally requires specialized expertise.
   2. **Processed EEG:** To increase its intraoperative utility, the EEG data are processed by fast Fourier analysis into a single power versus time spectral array that is more easily interpreted. Examples of power spectrum analysis include *compressed spectral array, density spectral array*, and the more widely familiar *bispectral index (BIS)*. The BIS monitor analyzes the phase relationships between different frequency components over time. The result is reduced via a proprietary method to a single number scaled between 0 (electrical silence) and 100 (alert wakefulness). Most commonly used as an indicator of anesthetic depth, the BIS monitor may also be used to identify electrocortical silence during cases requiring DHCA, as indicated by an isoelectric EEG and a BIS value near 0. Evidence supporting BIS data as a monitor of neurologic function in patients at risk for hypoxic or ischemic brain injury continues to accumulate.[85] Abnormally low BIS scores and prolonged low BIS scores may be associated with poor neurologic outcomes.[86]
   3. **Evoked potentials:** In general, monitoring of evoked potentials is used in selected surgical cases involving the descending aortic to ensure adequate spinal cord perfusion. It requires

specialized expertise and a dedicated technician working in the operating room. Evoked potentials in aortic surgery are discussed in greater detail in Chapter 23.

    a. **Somatosensory evoked potentials (SSEPs):** SSEPs monitor the integrity of the posterior-lateral spinal cord. A stimulus is applied to a peripheral nerve, and the resultant brainstem and brain activity is monitored.

    b. **Motor evoked potentials (MEPs):** MEPs monitor the anterior spinal cord, which is at greatest risk during surgery of the descending aorta.

    c. **Visual evoked response and brainstem audio evoked responses:** These techniques do not have routine clinical application in cardiac surgical procedures.

E. Near-Infrared Spectroscopy Cerebral Oximetry

Near-infrared spectroscopy (NIRS) is a noninvasive method to monitor regional cerebral oxygen saturation. Red and near-infrared light is transmitted from the surface of the scalp and penetrates the scalp, skull, cerebrospinal fluid, and brain. The light is reflected by tissue but differentially absorbed by hemoglobin-containing moieties. It is imperative that baseline cerebral oximetry measurements are acquired to allow intraoperative interpretation of the data because changes from baseline are more important than absolute values.[87] A reduction of 20% from baseline values is often considered the threshold for interventions to restore the values toward baseline.[88] Although this monitoring technique is often employed, there is limited evidence that the use of cerebral oximetry and treatment of low values leads to reduced neurologic complications, mortality, or other postoperative complications.[89]

F. Monitors of Central Nervous System Embolic Events

    1. **Transcranial Doppler ultrasonography (TCD):** TCD is a sensitive method to detect emboli in the cerebral circulation. Incorporation into clinical practice has been hindered by difficulty obtaining a reliable and stable signal, thus limiting its use primarily as a research tool. Of note, embolic showers are particularly associated with aortic cross-clamp application and removal.

    2. **Epiaortic scanning:** The importance of aortic atheromas, especially in the ascending aorta and/or aortic arch, in association with poor neurologic outcomes, has long been recognized. Aortic atheromas with a mobile component may present the greatest risk. The introduction and use of TEE to detect aortic atheroma was a significant improvement over surgical palpation. However, TEE had significant limitations particularly in the detection of disease near the typical aortic cannulation site in the distal ascending aorta owing to acoustic shadowing from intervening airway structures. As an alternative, epiaortic scanning is a highly sensitive and specific monitoring modality to detect atheroma in the thoracic aorta including regions where TEE evaluation is not possible.[90] Studies have shown that the use of epiaortic ultrasound can dramatically reduce the risk for embolic stroke.[91]

REFERENCES

1. Apfelbaum JL, Rupp SM, Tung A, et al. Practice guidelines for central venous access 2020: an updated report by the American Society of Anesthesiologists Task Force on Central Venous Access. *Anesthesiology.* 2020;132(1):8-43.
2. Practice guidelines for pulmonary artery catheterization: an updated report by the American Society of Anesthesiologists Task Force on Pulmonary Artery Catheterization. *Anesthesiology.* 2003;99:988-1014.
3. Arias-Ortiz J, Vincent J-L. The pulmonary artery catheter. *Curr Opin Crit Care.* 2023;29(3):231-235.
4. Sandau KE, Funk M, Auerbach A, et al. American Heart Association Council on Cardiovascular and Stroke Nursing; Council on Clinical Cardiology; and Council on Cardiovascular Disease in the Young. Update to practice standards for electrocardiographic monitoring in hospital settings: a scientific statement from the American Heart Association. *Circulation.* 2017;136(19):e273-e344.
5. London MJ, Hollenberg M, Wong MG, et al. Intraoperative myocardial ischemia: localization by continuous 12-lead electrocardiography. *Anesthesiology.* 1988;69(2):232-241.
6. Landesberg G, Mosseri M, Wolf Y, Vesselov Y, Weissman C. Perioperative myocardial ischemia and infarction: identification by continuous 12-lead electrocardiogram with online ST-segment monitoring. *Anesthesiology.* 2002;96(2):264-270.
7. Khambatta HJ, Stone JG, Wald A, Mongero LB. Electrocardiographic artifacts during cardiopulmonary bypass. *Anesth Analg.* 1990;71(1):88-91.
8. Mark JB. Multimodal detection of perioperative myocardial ischemia. *Tex Heart Inst J.* 2005;32(4):461-466.
9. Bartels K, Esper SA, Thiele RH. Blood pressure monitoring for the anesthesiologist: a practical review. *Anesth Analg.* 2016;122(6):1866-1879.
10. Wax DB, Lin HM, Leibowitz AB. Invasive and concomitant noninvasive intraoperative blood pressure monitoring: observed differences in measurements and associated therapeutic interventions. *Anesthesiology.* 2011;115(5):973-978.

11. Saugel B, Cecconi M, Hajjar LA. Noninvasive cardiac output monitoring in cardiothoracic surgery patients: available methods and future directions. *J Cardiothorac Vasc Anesth.* 2019;33(6):1742-1752.
12. Saugel B, Hoppe P, Nicklas JY, et al. Continuous noninvasive pulse wave analysis using finger cuff technologies for arterial blood pressure and cardiac output monitoring in perioperative and intensive care medicine: a systematic review and meta-analysis. *Br J Anaesth.* 2020;125(1):25-37.
13. Truijen J, van Lieshout JJ, Wesselink WA, Westerhof BE. Noninvasive continuous hemodynamic monitoring. *J Clin Monit Comp.* 2012;26(4):267-278.
14. Gardner RM. Direct blood pressure measurement—dynamic response requirements. *Anesthesiology.* 1981;54(3):227-236.
15. Mark JB., Chapter 9: Technical requirements for direct blood pressure measurement. In: *Atlas of Cardiovascular Monitoring.* Churchill Livingstone; 1998:99-126.
16. Ortega R, Connor C, Kotova F, Deng W, Lacerra C. Use of pressure transducers. *N Engl J Med.* 2017;376(14):e26.
17. Courtois M, Fattal PG, Kovacs SJ, Tiefenbrunn AJ, Ludbrook PA. Anatomically and physiologically based reference level for measurement of intracardiac pressures. *Circulation.* 1995;92(7):1994-2000.
18. Kovacs G, Avian A, Olschewski A, Olschewski H. Zero reference level for right heart catheterisation. *Eur Respir J.* 2013;42(6):1586-1594.
19. Ackland GL, Brudney CS, Cecconi M, et al. Perioperative Quality Initiative consensus statement on the physiology of arterial blood pressure control in perioperative medicine. *Br J Anaesth.* 2019;122(5):542-551.
20. Bazaral MG, Welch M, Golding LA, Badhwar K. Comparison of brachial and radial arterial pressure monitoring in patients undergoing coronary bypass surgery. *Anesthesiology.* 1990;73(1):38-45.
21. Brzezinski M, Luisetti T, London MJ. Radial artery cannulation: a comprehensive review of recent anatomic and physiologic investigations. *Anesth Analg.* 2009;109(6):1763-1781.
22. Bertrand OF, Carey PC, Gilchrist IC. Allen or no Allen: that is the question! *J Am Coll Cardiol.* 2014;63(18):1842-1844.
23. Ailon J, Mourad O, Chien V, Saun T, Dev SP. Videos in clinical medicine. Ultrasound-guided insertion of a radial arterial catheter. *N Engl J Med.* 2014;371(15):e21.
24. Htet N, Vaughn J, Adigopula S, Hennessey E, Mihm F. Needle-guided ultrasound technique for axillary artery catheter placement in critically ill patients: a case series and technique description. *J Crit Care.* 2017;41:194-197.
25. Cannesson M, Manach YL, Hofer CK, et al. Assessing the diagnostic accuracy of pulse pressure variations for the prediction of fluid responsiveness: a "gray zone" approach. *Anesthesiology.* 2011;115(2):231-241.
26. Proctor RD, Beckett D, Oakes JL. Over the limit: use of peripheral venous cannulae above the manufacturer's recommended flow rates. *Clin Radiol.* 2011;66(5):456-458.
27. Traylor S, Bastani A, Butris-Daut N, et al. Are three ports better than one? An evaluation of flow rates using all ports of a triple lumen central venous catheter in volume resuscitation. *Am J Emerg Med.* 2018;36(5):739-740.
28. Practice guidelines for central venous access 2020: an updated report by the American Society of Anesthesiologists Task Force on Central Venous Access. *Anesthesiology.* 2020;132(1):8-43.
29. Gilon D, Schechter D, Rein AJ, et al. Right atrial thrombi are related to indwelling central venous catheter position: insights into time course and possible mechanism of formation. *Am Heart J.* 1998;135(3):457-462.
30. Barbeito A, Bar-Yosef S, Lowe JE, Atkins BZ, Mark JB. Unusual cause of superior vena cava syndrome diagnosed with transesophageal echocardiography. *Can J Anaesth.* 2008;55(11):774-778.
31. Barbeito A, Mark JB. Arterial and central venous pressure monitoring. *Anesthesiol Clin.* 2006;24(4):717-735.
32. Figg KK, Nemergut EC. Error in central venous pressure measurement. *Anesth Analg.* 2009;108(4):1209-1211.
33. Gelman S. Venous function and central venous pressure: a physiologic story. *Anesthesiology.* 2008;108(4):735-748.
34. Magder S. Central venous pressure: a useful but not so simple measurement. *Crit Care Med.* 2006;34(8):2224-2227.
35. Marik PE, Cavallazzi R. Does the central venous pressure predict fluid responsiveness? An updated meta-analysis and a plea for some common sense. *Crit Care Med.* 2013;41(7):1774-1781.
36. Milam AJ, Ghoddoussi F, Lucaj J, et al. Comparing the mutual interchangeability of ECOM, FloTrac/Vigileo, 3D-TEE, and ITD-PAC cardiac output measuring systems in coronary artery bypass grafting. *J Cardiothorac Vasc Anesth.* 2021,35(2):514-529.
37. Rong LQ, Kaushal M, Mauer E, et al. Two- or 3-dimensional echocardiography-derived cardiac output cannot replace the pulmonary artery catheter in cardiac surgery. *J Cardiothorac Vasc Anesth.* 2020;34(10):2691-2697.
38. Brovman EY, Gabriel RA, Dutton RP, Urman RD. Pulmonary artery catheter use during cardiac surgery in the United States, 2010 to 2014. *J Cardiothorac Vasc Anesth.* 2016;30(3):579-584.
39. Baran DA, Grines CL, Bailey S, et al. SCAI clinical expert consensus statement on the classification of cardiogenic shock: this document was endorsed by the American College of Cardiology (ACC), the American Heart Association (AHA), the Society of Critical Care Medicine (SCCM), and the Society of Thoracic Surgeons (STS) in April 2019. *Catheter Cardiovasc Interv.* 2019;94(1):29-37.
40. Saxena A, Garan AR, Kapur NK, et al. Value of hemodynamic monitoring in patients with cardiogenic shock undergoing mechanical circulatory support. *Circulation.* 2020;141(14):1184-1197.
41. Evans DC, Doraiswamy VA, Prosciak MP, et al. Complications associated with pulmonary artery catheters: a comprehensive clinical review. *Scand J Surg.* 2009;98(4):199-208.
42. Swanz Ganz Pulmonary Artery Catheters. Published 2023. Accessed April 14, 2023. https://www.edwards.com/healthcare-professionals/products-services/hemodynamic-monitoring/swan-ganz-catheters
43. Baer J, Wyatt MM, Kreisler KR. Utilizing transesophageal echocardiography for placement of pulmonary artery catheters. *Echocardiography.* 2018;35(4):467-473.
44. Bossert T, Gummert JF, Bittner HB, et al. Swan-Ganz catheter-induced severe complications in cardiac surgery: right ventricular perforation, knotting, and rupture of a pulmonary artery. *J Card Surg.* 2006;21(3):292-295.
45. Bussieres JS. Iatrogenic pulmonary artery rupture. *Curr Opin Anaesthesiol.* 2007;20(1):48-52.
46. Denault A, Canevet M, Couture EJ. Pro: we should use a pulmonary artery catheter with right ventricular pressure waveforms in cardiac surgical patients. *J Cardiothorac Vasc Anesth.* 2023;37(4):659-662.

47. Couture EJ, Gronlykke L, Denault AY. New developments in the understanding of right ventricular function in acute care. *Curr Opin Crit Care.* 2022;28(3):331-339.

48. Simonneau G, Montani D, Celermajer DS, et al. Haemodynamic definitions and updated clinical classification of pulmonary hypertension. *Eur Respir J.* 2019;53(1):1801913.

49. Sugimoto K, Yoshihisa A, Nakazato K, et al. Significance of pulmonary vascular resistance and diastolic pressure gradient on the new definition of combined post-capillary pulmonary hypertension. *Int Heart J.* 2020;61(2):301-307.

50. Naeije R, Vachiery JL, Yerly P, Vanderpool R. The transpulmonary pressure gradient for the diagnosis of pulmonary vascular disease. *Eur Respir J.* 2013;41(1):217-223.

51. Martin-Suarez S, Gliozzi G, Cavalli GG, et al. Is pulmonary artery pulsatility index (PAPi) a predictor of outcome after pulmonary endarterectomy? *J Clin Med.* 2022;11(15):4353.

52. Kochav SM, Flores RJ, Truby LK, Topkara VK. Prognostic impact of pulmonary artery pulsatility index (PAPi) in patients with advanced heart failure: insights from the ESCAPE trial. *J Card Fail.* 2018;24(7):453-459.

53. Knio ZO, Thiele RH, Wright WZ, Mazimba S, Naik BI, Hulse MC. A novel hemodynamic index of post-operative right heart dysfunction predicts mortality in cardiac surgical patients. *Semin Cardiothorac Vasc Anesth.* 2022;26(3):200-208.

54. Knio ZO, Morales FL, Shah KP, et al. A systemic congestive index (systemic pulse pressure to central venous pressure ratio) predicts adverse outcomes in patients undergoing valvular heart surgery. *J Card Surg.* 2022;37(10):3259-3266.

55. Cheatham ML, Nelson LD, Chang MC, et al. Right ventricular end-diastolic volume index as a predictor of preload status in patients on positive end-expiratory pressure. *Crit Care Med.* 1998;26(11):1801-1806.

56. Narang N, Thibodeau JT, Parker WF, et al. Comparison of accuracy of estimation of cardiac output by thermodilution versus the fick method using measured oxygen uptake. *Am J Cardiol.* 2022;176:58-65.

57. Funk DJ, Moretti EW, Gan TJ. Minimally invasive cardiac output monitoring in the perioperative setting. *Anesth Analg.* 2009;108(3):887-897.

58. Lee AJ, Cohn JH, Ranasinghe JS. Cardiac output assessed by invasive and minimally invasive techniques. *Anesthesiol Res Pract.* 2011;2011:475151.

59. Preisman S, Kogan S, Berkenstadt H, Perel A. Predicting fluid responsiveness in patients undergoing cardiac surgery: functional haemodynamic parameters including the Respiratory Systolic Variation Test and static preload indicators. *Br J Anaesth.* 2005;95(6):746-755.

60. Rex S, Schälte G, Schroth S, et al. Limitations of arterial pulse pressure variation and left ventricular stroke volume variation in estimating cardiac pre-load during open heart surgery. *Acta Anaesthesiol Scand.* 2007;51(9):1258-1267.

61. Reuter DA, Felbinger, TW, Schmidt, C, et al. Stroke volume variations for assessment of cardiac responsiveness to volume loading in mechanically ventilated patients after cardiac surgery. *Intensive Care Med.* 2002;28(4):392-398.

62. Myatra SN, Prabu NR, Divatia JV, Monnet X, Kulkarni AP, Teboul JL. The changes in pulse pressure variation or stroke volume variation after a "tidal volume challenge" reliably predict fluid responsiveness during low tidal volume ventilation. *Crit Care Med.* 2017;45(3):415-421.

63. Messina A, Montagnini C, Cammarota G, et al. Tidal volume challenge to predict fluid responsiveness in the operating room: an observational study. *Eur J Anaesthesiol.* 2019;36(8):583-591.

64. Reed H, Berg KB, Janelle GM, et al. Aortic surgery and deep-hypothermic arrest: anesthetic update. *Semin Cardiothorac Vasc Anesth.* 2014;18(2):137-145.

65. Insler SR, Sessler DI. Perioperative thermoregulation and temperature monitoring. *Anesthesiol Clin.* 2006;24(4):823-837.

66. Rees K, Beranek-Stanley M, Burke M, Ebrahim S. Hypothermia to reduce neurological damage following coronary artery bypass surgery. *Cochrane Database Syst Rev.* 2001;2001(1):CD002138.

67. Boodhwani M, Rubens F, Wozny D, Rodriguez R, Nathan HJ. Effects of sustained mild hypothermia on neurocognitive function after coronary artery bypass surgery: a randomized, double-blind study. *J Thorac Cardiovasc Surg.* 2007;134(6):1443-1450.

68. Belway D, Tee R, Nathan HJ, Rubens FD, Boodhwani M. Temperature management and monitoring practices during adult cardiac surgery under cardiopulmonary bypass: results of a Canadian national survey. *Perfusion.* 2011;26(5):395-400.

69. Engelman R, Baker RA, Likosky DS, et al. The Society of Thoracic Surgeons, The Society of Cardiovascular Anesthesiologists, and The American Society of ExtraCorporeal Technology: clinical practice guidelines for cardiopulmonary bypass—temperature management during cardiopulmonary bypass. *J Cardiothorac Vasc Anesth.* 2015;29(4):1104-1113.

70. Grocott HP, Mackensen GB, Grigore AM, et al. Postoperative hyperthermia is associated with cognitive dysfunction after coronary artery bypass graft surgery. *Stroke.* 2002;33(2):537-541.

71. Chertow GM, Lazarus JM, Christiansen CL, et al. Preoperative renal risk stratification. *Circulation.* 1997;95(4):878-884.

72. Ljunggren M, Sköld A, Dardashti A, Hyllén S. The use of mannitol in cardiopulmonary bypass prime solution—prospective randomized double-blind clinical trial. *Acta Anaesthesiol Scand.* 2019;63(10):1298-1305.

73. Brown JR, Baker RA, Shore-Lesserson L, et al. The Society of Thoracic Surgeons/Society of Cardiovascular Anesthesiologists/American Society for Extracorporeal Technology Clinical practice guidelines for the prevention of adult cardiac surgery-associated acute kidney injury. *Anesth Analg.* 2023;136(1):176-184.

74. Breuer AC, Furlan AJ, Hanson MR, et al. Central nervous system complications of coronary artery bypass graft surgery: prospective analysis of 421 patients. *Stroke.* 1983;14(5):682-687.

75. Newman MF, Wolman R, Kanchuger M, et al. Multicenter preoperative stroke risk index for patients undergoing coronary artery bypass graft surgery. Multicenter Study of Perioperative Ischemia (McSPI) Research Group. *Circulation.* 1996;94(Suppl. 9):II74-II80.

76. Bhatia A, Gupta AK. Neuromonitoring in the intensive care unit I. Intracranial pressure and cerebral blood flow monitoring. *Intensive Care Med.* 2007;33(7):1263-1271.

77. Bhatia A, Gupta AK. Neuromonitoring in the intensive care unit II. Cerebral oxygenation monitoring and microdialysis. *Intensive Care Med.* 2007;33(8):1322-1328.

78. Grocott HP, Davie S, Fedorow C. Monitoring of brain function in anesthesia and intensive care. *Curr Opin Anesthesiol.* 2010;23(6):759-764.

79. Drummond JC. Blood pressure and the brain: how low can you go? *Anesth Analg.* 2019;128(4):759-771.
80. Vedel AG, Holmgaard F, Rasmussen LS, et al. High-target versus low-target blood pressure management during cardiopulmonary bypass to prevent cerebral injury in cardiac surgery patients: a randomized controlled trial. *Circulation.* 2018;137(17):1770-1780.
81. Lindsberg PJ, Roine RO. Hyperglycemia in acute stroke. *Stroke.* 2004;35(2):363-364.
82. D'Alessandro C, Leprince P, Golmard JL, et al. Strict glycemic control reduces EuroSCORE expected mortality in diabetic patients undergoing myocardial revascularization. *J Thorac Cardiovasc Surg.* 2007;134(1):29-37.
83. Lazar HL, McDonnell M, Chipkin SR, et al. The Society of Thoracic Surgeons practice guideline series: blood glucose management during adult cardiac surgery. *Ann Thorac Surg.* 2009;87(2):663-669.
84. Gregory SH, Yalamuri SM, Bishawi M, Swaminathan M. The perioperative management of ascending aortic dissection. *Anesth Analg.* 2018;127(6):1302-1313.
85. Myles PS, Daly D, Silvers A, et al. Prediction of neurological outcome using bispectral index monitoring in patients with severe ischemic-hypoxic brain injury undergoing emergency surgery. *Anesthesiology.* 2009;110(5):1106-1115.
86. Pedemonte JC, Plummer GS, Chamadia S, et al. Electroencephalogram burst-suppression during cardiopulmonary bypass in elderly patients mediates postoperative delirium. *Anesthesiology.* 2020;133(2):280-292.
87. Hogue CW, Levine A, Hudson A, Lewis C. Clinical applications of near-infrared spectroscopy monitoring in cardiovascular surgery. *Anesthesiology.* 2021;134(5):784-791.
88. Subramanian B, Nyman C, Fritock M, et al. A multicenter pilot study assessing regional cerebral oxygen desaturation frequency during cardiopulmonary bypass and responsiveness to an intervention algorithm. *Anesth Analg.* 2016;122(6):1786-1793.
89. Thiele RH, Shaw AD, Bartels K, et al. American society for enhanced recovery and perioperative quality initiative joint consensus statement on the role of neuromonitoring in perioperative outcomes: cerebral near-infrared spectroscopy. *Anesth Analg.* 2020;131(5):1444-1455.
90. Glas KE, Swaminathan M, Reeves ST, et al. Guidelines for the performance of a comprehensive intraoperative epiaortic ultrasonographic examination: recommendations of the American Society of Echocardiography and the Society of Cardiovascular Anesthesiologists; endorsed by the Society of Thoracic Surgeons. *J Am Soc Echocardiogr.* 2007;20(11):1227-1235.
91. Biancari F, Santini F, Tauriainen T, et al. Epiaortic ultrasound to prevent stroke in coronary artery bypass grafting. *Ann Thorac Surg.* 2020;109(1):294-301.

Pacemakers and Implantable Cardioverter Defibrillators: Indications, Function, Perioperative Evaluation and Management

Rebecca A. Aron, Eric C. Stecker, and Peter M. Schulman

KEY POINTS

1. In addition to delivering antitachycardia therapy, all modern transvenous implantable cardioverter-defibrillators (ICDs) and cardiac resynchronization therapy defibrillators (CRT-Ds) are capable of also functioning as pacemakers.

2. A patient should be considered pacing dependent if the cessation of pacing results in an absent intrinsic heart rhythm, or functionally dependent if the cessation of pacing results in an inadequate intrinsic heart rhythm (eg, hemodynamic instability).

3. When a recent cardiac implantable electronic device (CIED) interrogation report is not available, and it is not possible to have the CIED interrogated, pacing dependence should be assumed if every complex is paced on an electrocardiogram (ECG). An exception is for patients with a CRT device, because the goal of CRT programming is to achieve 100% biventricular pacing.

4. The revised North American Society of Pacing and Electrophysiology and British Pacing and Electrophysiology Group ("NBG") Code describes the antibradycardia pacing capabilities of any CIED.

5. Right ventricular (RV) pacing causes electrical and mechanical dyssynchrony, which often increases heart failure and worsens systolic function. Algorithms that minimize RV pacing can create confusion and mimic device malfunction ("pseudomalfunction") by intermittently allowing a significantly prolonged atrioventricular (AV) delay or a dropped QRS.

6. Subcutaneous ICDs (S-ICDs) are entirely extracardiac. They are implanted for patients who meet the criteria for an ICD but have poor vascular access or are at high risk of infection, provided pacing or CRT is not needed or anticipated. Because S-ICDs do not have transvenous leads, they cannot pace. They are readily distinguished from all other ICDs by chest x-ray.

7. Intraoperative electromagnetic interference (EMI) can cause CIED malfunction. The most common source of intraoperative EMI is monopolar electrosurgery ("the bovie"). Serious sequelae include (1) pacing inhibition (the CIED fails to pace when it should) with resultant bradycardia or asystole in the patient who is pacing dependent, and (2) inappropriate antitachycardia therapy in the patient with an ICD.

8. For transvenous pacemakers (but not for ICDs), most generators will respond to magnet placement by pacing asynchronously at a manufacturer-specific rate that identifies battery performance. Leadless pacemakers respond differently than transvenous pacemakers to magnet placement. Some leadless pacemakers (Medtronic Micra) have no magnet response. Others (Abbott Aveir) will respond by VOO pacing at 100 bpm for five cycles before continuing to pace in the VOO mode at a rate reflecting the remaining battery life (assuming the magnet response is programmed on).

9. Placing a magnet over an ICD usually suspends antitachycardia therapy. Magnet placement never changes the pacing mode of an ICD. Patients with ICD requiring asynchronous pacing always require device reprogramming.

10. If a CIED was reprogrammed before a surgical procedure, its original settings should be restored postoperatively. In some instances, new settings may be indicated. If the antitachycardia therapy of an ICD was programmed off, the patient should remain in a monitored environment (eg, operating room, postanesthesia care unit, or intensive care unit) until this therapy is reactivated.

I. Overview/Prevalence

Cardiac implantable electronic devices (CIEDs) are used to treat a myriad of conditions, including cardiac conduction system abnormalities (eg, sinus node dysfunction, atrioventricular [AV] block), life-threatening arrhythmias, and heart failure. In the United States, upward of 3 million people have a conventional CIED, which includes transvenous pacemakers (PMs), implantable cardioverter-defibrillators (ICDs), and cardiac resynchronization therapy (CRT) devices.[1] Over the last decade, technologic advancements have brought leadless PMs and a subcutaneous ICD (S-ICD) to market, which have further increased the utility and prevalence of these devices. Since patients with CIEDs often undergo surgical procedures and the presence of a CIED might increase perioperative risk, anesthesiologists must understand how these devices function, the indications for their use, and how to manage them during the perioperative period.[2]

II. Cardiac Implantable Electronic Devices Types and Function

A. Basic Components of Transvenous Cardiac Implantable Electronic Devices

Transvenous CIEDs contain a pulse generator that is usually implanted in the infraclavicular region of the chest and houses the battery and electronic equipment. The pulse generator connects to one to three intracardiac leads that are typically placed in the right atrium (RA), right ventricle (RV), and/or coronary sinus (CS) (in lieu of in the left ventricle [LV]). All leads contain electrodes that contact the myocardium and are capable of sensing and pacing in their respective chambers. The RV lead of a transvenous ICD includes one, or less commonly two, shock coil capable of delivering high-voltage defibrillation (ie, antitachycardia) therapy. The presence of a shock coil can be used to distinguish an ICD from a PM on a chest x-ray (CXR) (Figure 6.1). In addition to delivering antitachycardia therapy, all modern transvenous ICDs and cardiac resynchronization therapy defibrillators (CRT-Ds) have antibradycardia pacing capability (ie, also fully functioning as a transvenous PM). Most CRT devices contain a CS lead that is used to pace the LV (Figure 6.1). The number of leads placed largely depends on the indications for implantation (see indications). One important distinction between transvenous CIEDs and much-less-common S-ICDs is that all transvenous CIEDs pace, while S-ICDs do not pace. S-ICDs have a distinctive appearance on CXR that allows them to be distinguished from transvenous CIEDs (Figure 6.2).

CLINICAL PEARL

The presence of a shock coil can be used to distinguish an ICD from a PM on a CXR.

B. Pacing/Implantable Pacemakers

1. **Normal cardiac conduction:** Normal cardiac conduction begins in the sinus node, propagates through the atrium, and results in atrial depolarization and contraction (ie, a p-wave on the electrocardiogram [ECG]). Next, electrical waves spread across the AV node, through the bundle of His to the left and right bundle branches and Purkinje fibers to

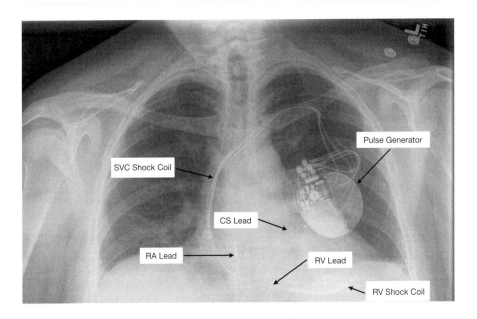

FIGURE 6.1 CXR showing a biventricular ICD. Note shock coils and CS lead. CS, coronary sinus; CXR, chest x-ray; ICD, implantable cardioverter-defibrillator; RA, right atrium; RV, right ventricle; SVC, superior vena cava.

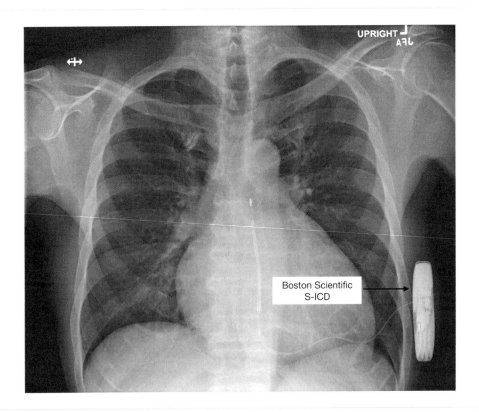

FIGURE 6.2 CXR showing Boston Scientific S-ICD. CXR, chest x-ray; S-ICD, subcutaneous implantable cardioverter-defibrillator.

depolarize the ventricles, resulting in the QRS complex on the ECG.[3] The normal QRS on the ECG has a narrow morphology with a duration of 60-100 msec.

2. **Electrophysiology of pacing:** Understanding how pacing impacts the ECG is essential, as the misinterpretation of paced rhythms might lead to adverse events.[4] Capture occurs when a CIED emits a pacing stimulus with sufficient electrical energy to force the myocardium to depolarize (contract). When the ventricles are depolarized by pacing, QRS widening occurs because of delayed ventricular activation that results from electrical activation outside of the normal conduction system. Thus, conventional RV pacing creates a left bundle branch block (LBBB) pattern because the depolarization begins in the RV before spreading through the septum to activate the LV.[4] This activation sequence produces a tall and broad R wave in leads 1, V5, and V6, and a deep QS in lead V1. LV pacing (typically via a CS lead) often creates a right bundle branch block (RBBB) pattern or intraventricular conduction delay (IVCD) pattern ending with an R wave in V1, because the LV is activated before the RV. Biventricular pacing often creates a narrower and somewhat normal-appearing QRS. However, the QRS can be wide and resemble a RBBB, LBBB, or nonspecific IVCD depending on the location of the leads and ventricular offset programming.

3. **Indications for permanent pacing:** A comprehensive list of indications for permanent pacing is beyond the scope of this chapter; however, permanent pacing is often needed to treat irreversible and symptomatic sinus node dysfunction or high-grade or symptomatic AV block. Although a heart rate of <40 bpm or pauses of >4 seconds often create symptoms, there is no numerical heart rate or pause length cutoff defining when a permanent PM is absolutely indicated. Another common class I indication is symptomatic chronotropic incompetence (ie, impaired heart rate response to exercise). A complete list of indications for permanent pacing is found in the 2018 American College of Cardiology (ACC)/American Heart Association (AHA)/Heart Rhythm Society (HRS) Guideline on the Evaluation and Management of Patients with Bradycardia and Cardiac Conduction Delay.[5]

4. **Pacing dependency:** Pacing-dependent patients require special attention during the perioperative period because they are at high risk for injury or death in the event of pacing system malfunction. A patient should be considered completely pacing dependent if the cessation of pacing results in an absent intrinsic heart rhythm or "functionally dependent" if the cessation of pacing results in an inadequate intrinsic heart rhythm (eg, hemodynamic instability). Testing for pacing dependency is generally performed during each in-person CIED follow-up visit. This assessment is made by temporarily programming the patient's CIED to a non-tracking mode (ie, VVI, DDI) at the lowest programmable pacing rate (ie, 30-40 bpm). If prior to a surgical procedure, a recent interrogation report is not available, and it is not possible to interrogate the CIED, it is sometimes possible to determine whether the patient is pacing dependent by reviewing their history or examining their ECG. Pacing dependency should be assumed if there is a history of AV node ablation. The patient might also be pacing dependent if their CIED was implanted for a symptomatic bradyarrhythmia or syncope. On the ECG, pacing dependence should be assumed if every complex is paced, except for patients with a CRT device, because CRT programming aims to achieve 100% biventricular pacing regardless of underlying rhythm/conduction.

CLINICAL PEARL

Pacing dependence should generally be assumed if every ventricular complex is paced, unless CIED interrogation proves otherwise. An exception is patients with a CRT device, because the goal of CRT programming is to achieve 100% biventricular pacing regardless of underlying rhythm.

5. **"Demand" versus "asynchronous" pacing:** All modern transvenous CIEDs provide "demand" pacing, meaning a pacing stimulus is only provided in the absence of an intrinsic event. "Asynchronous pacing" means that a CIED paces without regard for the patient's underlying rhythm. Examples of asynchronous pacing modes include DOO and VOO. More in-depth explanations of the most frequently used pacing modes are provided in the sections that follow.

CLINICAL PEARL

Asynchronous pacing means the CIED paces without regard for the patient's underlying rhythm.

6. **Modes of operation**

a. **NBG code:** The Generic Pacemaker Code (The North American Society of Pacing and Electrophysiology and British Pacing and Electrophysiology Group or "NBG code") describes the antibradycardia function of a CIED (see Table 6.1).[6]

b. **Common modes:** The most common single-chamber and dual-chamber pacing modes are VVI and DDD, respectively.

c. **VVI:** In the VVI mode, pacing and sensing only occur in the ventricle. Ventricular pacing occurs at the programmed lower rate limit; the "I" in the third position indicates that pacing is inhibited by a sensed ventricular event. Permanent atrial fibrillation is a common reason for selecting the VVI mode.

d. **DDD:** In the DDD mode, sensing and pacing occur in both the RA and RV. The "D" in the third position indicates that pacing in the atrium is inhibited by a sensed atrial event, pacing in the ventricle is inhibited by a sensed ventricular event, and an atrial event will "trigger" an ensuing ventricular pace when necessary (to maintain AV synchrony). In the absence of rate modulation or other esoteric advanced programmable features, atrial pacing in the DDD mode occurs at the programmed lower rate limit. Studies have shown better short- and long-term hemodynamics with AV synchronous pacing.[7] For patients with a significant ventricular pacing burden, DDD is preferable to VVI because of its ability to maintain AV synchrony and decrease the risk of "pacemaker syndrome" (ie, fatigue, dyspnea, hypotension related to decreased cardiac output from loss of AV synchrony).

e. **Other modes:** Other pacing modes that can preserve AV synchrony include AAI (which requires intact AV nodal function) and VDD (which can be used to maintain AV synchrony, but requires intact sinus node function since this mode does not provide atrial pacing).

7. **Minimizing right ventricular pacing:** Historically, the RV has been the most common site to deliver pacing. However, pacing from the RV creates ventricular electrical and mechanical dyssynchrony that may lead to heart failure, decreased systolic function, and increased hospitalizations.[8] Strategies and proprietary algorithms exist to minimize the detrimental effects of unnecessary RV pacing. Patients requiring little to no pacing (ie, a patient with an ICD for the treatment of ventricular tachyarrhythmias) often receive a single-chamber device programmed to the VVI mode with a lower rate limit of 40 bpm.

In addition, hybrid pacing modes incorporating AAI have been developed that provide atrial pacing with ventricular backup (ie, if native AV conduction is lost, the device automatically switches from AAI to DDD). In the hospital environment, algorithms that minimize ventricular pacing can create confusion and mimic device malfunction ("pseudo-malfunction") by intermittently allowing a significantly prolonged AV delay or a dropped QRS.[9] If ventricular pacing cannot be avoided, or programming modes to minimize it are not desirable, biventricular pacing (with a lead in a CS branch) or left bundle area pacing (with a lead deep into the interventricular septum, from the RV) can be utilized.

TABLE 6.1   NBG Generic Pacemaker Code

Chamber Paced	Chamber Sensed	Response	Rate Modulation	Multisite Pacing
A = Atrium	A = Atrium	I = Inhibited	O = None	A = Atrium
V = Ventricle	V = Ventricle	T = Triggered	R = Rate modulation	V = Ventricle
D = Dual/both	D = Dual/both	D = Both/dual		D = Dual/both
O = None	O = None	O = None		O = None

CLINICAL PEARL

While frequently necessary, RV pacing can result in dyssynchrony and increase the risk of heart failure.

8. **Rate modulation:** For the patient with chronotropic incompetence, all currently implanted transvenous CIEDs can detect increased physiologic demand (eg, exercise) and increase the pacing rate in response. Various mechanical and/or electronic sensors are utilized for this purpose. Knowledge of sensor type and settings can prevent inappropriate treatment and patient injury when iatrogenic sensor stimulation from skin prep or electrical interference might increase the paced heart rate inappropriately during the perioperative period.[10]

C. **Leadless Pacemakers:** Leadless PMs are implanted percutaneously via the femoral vein. The battery, generator, and electrodes of these devices are all contained in a unit about 10% the size of a conventional transvenous system. Two leadless pacing systems (Medtronic Micra and Abbott Aveir, CXRs shown in Figures 6.3 and 6.4) are now Food and Drug Administration (FDA) approved, and another (Boston Scientific EMPOWER) may be forthcoming. The Medtronic VR and Abbott Aveir systems are only capable of pacing and sensing in the RV. They are principally placed for patients with intact sinus node function with only rare episodes of AV block or sinus arrest, or permanent atrial fibrillation.[11,12] A newer version of the Micra (Micra AV) is now also capable of operating in the VDD mode; despite being implanted in the RV, it can provide dual-chamber sensing to maintain AV synchrony.[13] Leadless PMs additionally provide rate-modulated pacing for patients with chronotropic incompetence.

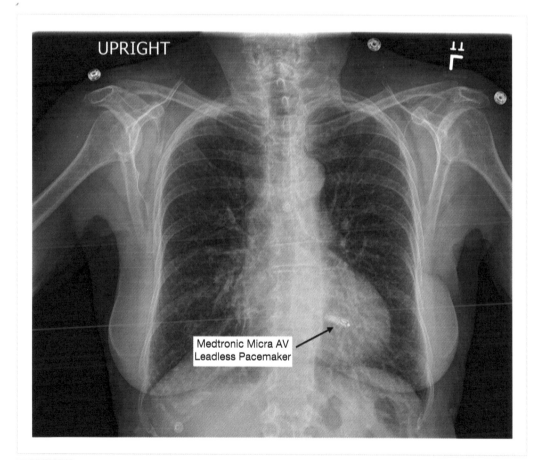

Medtronic Micra AV
Leadless Pacemaker

FIGURE 6.3 CXR showing Medtronic Micra AV Leadless Pacemaker implanted in the right ventricle. CXR, chest x-ray.

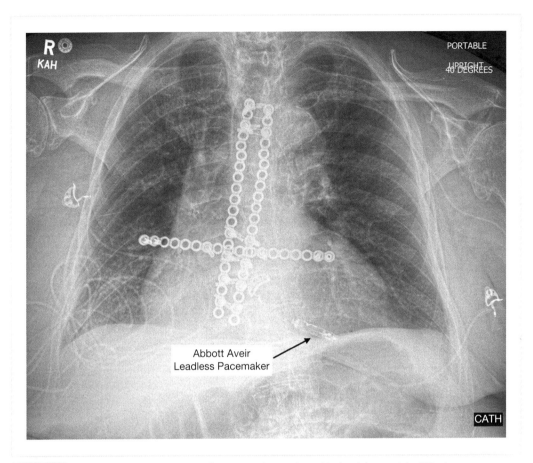

Abbott Aveir
Leadless Pacemaker

FIGURE 6.4 CXR showing Abbott Aveir Leadless Pacemaker implanted in the right ventricle. CXR, chest x-ray.

CLINICAL PEARL

Leadless PMs are most often placed for patients with intact sinus node function and rare episodes of AV block or sinus arrest, or permanent atrial fibrillation.

    D. Temporary Cardiac Pacing: Temporary pacing is indicated for both prophylactic and emergent reasons, and is utilized when a severe bradyarrhythmia is expected to be transient, or as a bridge to permanent PM placement. Common modalities include the following:

        1. Transcutaneous: This modality is the most readily available and rapidly employable in emergent situations until temporary transvenous pacing can be instituted. However, it has variable efficacy and is often not well tolerated in the awake patient because thresholds of 20-120 mA are usually required.[14]

        2. Transvenous: This modality is the most reliable and well-tolerated method of temporary cardiac pacing. With leads placed in both the RA and RV, AV synchrony is maintained, which may improve cardiac output. Disadvantages include the need for an experienced practitioner, insertion time, potential complications of catheter placement and manipulation, and need for x-ray or fluoroscopy. Rapid insertion of a balloon-tipped flow-directed RV pacing lead can be done at the bedside (without fluoroscopy) to treat high-grade AV block. Once the RV is entered, gently advance the catheter until capture is maintained (optimally <1 mA).[15] Then the generator output should be programmed to 2-3 times threshold as a safety margin.

3. **Epicardial:** Temporary epicardial pacing wires are often placed near the end of a cardiac operation to treat bradyarrhythmias and/or regulate the heart rate. Some surgeons routinely place both atrial and ventricular wires, while others frequently opt to place ventricular wires only (due to a higher risk of bleeding from the thinner atrial tissue) unless atrial wires are essential (ie, orthotopic heart transplant or low cardiac output due to sinus bradycardia).[16] Of note, many dual-chamber external pacing generators permit dual-chamber programming (ie, DDD) without an atrial lead (or with a nonfunctional atrial lead). Inappropriately programming a PM in this manner can result in the R-on-T phenomenon and cardiac arrest.[17]

CLINICAL PEARL

The DDD mode without an atrial lead (or with a nonfunctional atrial lead) can result in R-on-T pacing and cardiac arrest.

While epicardial pacing is usually extremely reliable in the immediate postoperative period, the amount of energy required to capture the myocardium decreases with time, and after multiple days they almost always eventually become nonfunctional. Consequently, these leads should be assessed daily to ensure they are still functioning appropriately by checking pacing sensing thresholds.[16]

E. **Pacing and Sensing Thresholds**
1. **Pacing threshold:** This threshold is the minimum amount of energy needed to reliably and consistently capture the myocardium (ie, produce a paced beat). To check this threshold the pacing rate is increased so that it is faster than the patient's underlying rate. The pacing output is programmed to a high enough value so that consistent capture is achieved. Then, the pacing output is reduced in a stepwise fashion until capture is lost (a pacing artifact does not produce a paced beat). The output is then programmed to provide an adequate margin of safety (typically 2-3 times the threshold).[16]
2. **Sensing threshold:** This threshold is the minimum intracardiac signal amplitude (mV) that is sensed by the PM. To check this threshold the pacing rate is decreased so that it is slower than the patient's underlying rate. (An intrinsic rhythm is required.) Starting at the lowest sensitivity (ie, highest value), the sensitivity is then increased in a stepwise fashion until sensing resumes. This threshold is the smallest intrinsic signal reliably recognized by the device. The sensitivity is then typically programmed to half of this value.

F. **Implantable Cardioverter-Defibrillators**
1. **Indications:** ICDs reduce mortality from malignant ventricular arrhythmias. Initially, ICDs were only implanted for the secondary prevention of sudden cardiac death after ventricular fibrillation (VF) arrest or sustained ventricular tachycardia (VT). Subsequent studies evaluating prophylactic placement in patients without a history of tachyarrhythmias have significantly increased the number of patients for whom ICD therapy is indicated. A comprehensive list of indications is provided by the AHA/ACC/HRS.[8] However, in general, the indications are as follows[8]:
   a. **Secondary prevention of sudden cardiac death:** Class I indications include (1) patients with ischemic heart disease who survive sudden cardiac arrest from VT/VF, (2) hemodynamically unstable or stable VT, (3) ischemic heart disease with unexplained syncope and inducible sustained monomorphic VT during an electrophysiologic study.
   b. **Primary prevention of sudden cardiac death:** Class I indications include patients with ischemic heart disease and who (1) have an LV ejection fraction (LVEF) ≤35% at least 40 days post–myocardial infarction and 90 days post-revascularization with New York Heart Association (NYHA) class II/III despite goal-directed medical therapy.
   c. Additional indications for primary prevention and regardless of LVEF include high-risk patients with hypertrophic cardiomyopathy, long QT or Brugada syndrome (RBBB, ST-segment elevation in leads V1-V3) with syncope, arrhythmogenic RV dysplasia, and infiltrative cardiomyopathy (sarcoidosis, amyloidosis).

2. **Antitachycardia therapy:** ICDs continuously measure the patient's intrinsic ventricular heart rate (R-R interval) and categorize it as normal, too fast, or too slow. An "antitachycardia event" begins when a fast ventricular rate (short R-R interval) is detected. If so programmed, the ICD can employ algorithmic discriminators (see later) to determine whether the tachyarrhythmia is malignant (VT/VF) or nonmalignant (ie, supraventricular tachycardia [SVT], atrial fibrillation with rapid ventricular response). For malignant rhythms, transvenous ICDs are programmed to deliver antitachycardia pacing (ATP) or shock(s), depending on the rhythm's presentation and programmed response. ATP is often employed first since it is painless, results in less battery consumption, and is approximately 85% efficacious at terminating hemodynamically stable VT. However, the use of ATP can delay the time to first shock, because each ATP cycle requires 8-15 seconds. ATP can also accelerate stable VT into unstable VT or VF. ICD shocks terminate VF in >98% of episodes. Despite improvements in detection of ventricular tachyarrhythmias, >10% of delivered shocks are still inappropriate.[18] To prevent an inappropriate shock, most ICDs are programmed to reconfirm VT or VF after charging.

3. **Ventricular tachycardia/supraventricular tachycardia discriminators:** Modern ICDs use a variety of methods to discriminate VT from SVT. Common examples include (1) heart rate and duration, (2) suddenness of rhythm onset, (3) interval (rate) stability, (4) AV relationship, and (5) electrogram morphology.

G. **Subcutaneous Implantable Cardioverter-Defibrillators**

S-ICDs are less invasive than transvenous ICDs; they consist of a pulse generator implanted in the left chest, and an electrode that is connected to the generator and tunneled subcutaneously to the sternum for sensing malignant ventricular rhythms and administer shocks (see Figure 6.3). Because these devices are entirely extracardiac, the potential for both immediate and long-term complications is substantially reduced. However, the drawback of an S-ICD is limited functionality. The high-voltage output of these devices is fixed at 80 J. Moreover, they do not provide antibradycardia pacing (aside from brief postshock pacing), ATP, or biventricular pacing (ie, CRT). Finally, S-ICDs are more prone to T-wave oversensing, which can cause double-counting of QRSs, causing the device to detect arrhythmia that is twice the rate of the actual rhythm.

Class I indications for an S-ICD include patients who meet the criteria for an ICD, but have inadequate vascular access, or are at high risk of infection and do not need pacing or CRT.[19]

CLINICAL PEARL

Subcutaneous ICDs have very limited pacing functionality and only provide temporary, external pacing for a short period after defibrillation.

H. **Cardiac Resynchronization Therapy**

1. **Indications:** In certain patients, CRT (also called biventricular pacing) improves functional status and heart failure symptoms, and has also been shown to reduce mortality in some studies. The restoration of electrical synchrony that occurs with CRT results in reverse remodeling of the LV and improved systolic function.[20] For patients with symptomatic heart failure despite optimal medical therapy, class I recommendations include LVEF ≤35%, QRS duration >150 msec with LBBB morphology, sinus rhythm, and NYHA class II, III, or ambulatory class IV symptoms.[21] As most patients with CRT also meet primary prevention criteria for ICD implantation, a CRT-D rather than a CRT-P (CRT with PM only) is much more frequently selected. Unfortunately, up to 30% of patients meeting standard criteria for CRT and who receive one do not show improvement with this therapy (CRT nonresponders).

2. **Left bundle pacing:** "Cardiac physiologic pacing" (currently left bundle pacing, formerly His bundle pacing) provides a new and alternative approach to RV apical and biventricular pacing. It can produce a more physiologic pattern of ventricular activation that may prevent or mitigate cardiomyopathy and heart failure from LV dyssynchrony.

III. **Cardiac Implantable Electronic Device Malfunction and Perioperative Considerations**
Although modern CIEDs are extremely reliable and outright failure is rare, malfunction does sometimes occur, and the presence of a CIED might be a risk factor for increased perioperative morbidity. Causes of CIED malfunction include the following:

A. **Battery Depletion:** Battery depletion can result in pacing system failure, or failure to deliver high-voltage therapy for an ICD. In addition, at detection of the elective replacement battery voltage, some CIEDs automatically change from dual-chamber to single-chamber pacing to further limit battery current drain. Low battery voltage also puts some CIEDs at increased risk for electromagnetic interference (EMI)-induced reset. Unexpected battery depletion was formerly extremely rare and remains uncommon, but challenges with new battery chemistry designs have resulted in many patients being monitored for potential accelerated battery depletion (based on manufacturer advisories).

B. **Lead Dislodgment:** Lead dislodgment is rare after the first 6 weeks of implant. However, lead tip fibrosis resulting in sensing or pacing threshold issues, and lead fracture or insulation failure, remain important longer-term issues.

C. **Electromagnetic Interference:** EMI is the most significant in-hospital/intraoperative concern (typically due to monopolar electrosurgical instruments—that is, the "bovie") and can cause temporary (and more rarely permanent) malfunction or "pseudomalfunction" (ie, proper function that is misinterpreted as malfunction). Numerous reports demonstrate that even pseudomalfunction can result in CIED damage and/or patient harm, and that these events occur with some regularity in patients undergoing surgical procedures.[10]

The risk of EMI is greatest when monopolar electrosurgery is used near the CIED (ie, above the umbilicus),[22] and it can cause significant bradycardia or asystole in the patient who is pacing dependent[23-25] and inappropriate antitachycardia therapy (ATP or shocks) in patients with an ICD.[1,24]

CLINICAL PEARL

Intraoperative EMI can cause significant bradycardia or asystole in the patient who is pacing dependent, and inappropriate antitachycardia therapy (ATP or shocks) in patients with an ICD.

IV. **Perioperative Assessment and Management**

A. **Preoperative Assessment**

1. **Cardiac implantable electronic device–related information:** Determine the CIED type, manufacturer, current settings, indication for placement, date the device was last interrogated, and that it was functioning properly at that time.

2. **Proper cardiac implantable electronic device function:** The American Society of Anesthesiologists (ASA) Practice Advisory recommends CIED interrogation 3-6 months prior to a scheduled procedure, while the HRS recommends interrogation within 12 months for a PM, 6 months for an ICD, and 3-6 months for CRT devices.[23,24] Prior to any scheduled procedure, a de novo interrogation should be performed if a recent interrogation report is not available, or if there is any concern about proper CIED function.

3. **Underlying rate and rhythm:** The patient's underlying rate and rhythm should be ascertained since EMI-induced pacing inhibition can cause severe bradycardia or asystole in patients who are completely or functionally pacing dependent (see "Pacing Dependency" section for more information).

4. **Coexisting disease:** Patients with a CIED often have coexisting disease. In particular, patients with an ICD or CRT device often have concomitant problems such as cardiomyopathy and/or heart failure, and might necessitate a more extensive workup and optimization prior to an elective surgical procedure.

5. **Additional information:** While specific laboratory or radiographic imaging is not needed simply because of the presence of a CIED, and radiography is insensitive for most lead-related problems, a CXR can be useful to help determine the CIED type and manufacturer if this

information is not known or not readily available. A CXR can also be used to document the location of transvenous leads (especially if invasive line placement or intracardiac or thoracic surgery is planned), since lead dislodgment (CS leads are highest risk) can occur.

6. **Surgical emergencies:** If records are not available and it is not possible to interrogate the CIED, as earlier a CXR may be used to identify the CIED type and manufacturer, since most CIEDs have a manufacturer-specific radiopaque alphanumeric code inscribed on the generator (Figure 6.5). Pertinent information can also be obtained from the patient's CIED identification card or by calling the manufacturer. There is also a smart phone application that uses CXRs to identify CIED manufacturers. In addition, a method to identify the generator manufacturer from the magnet response, assuming completely normal behavior (ie, the device has not undergone elective replacement or a safety reset), has been described.[26]

B. **Intraoperative Management**

1. **Monitoring:** In patients with a CIED, mechanical systoles must be evaluated by plethysmography or arterial waveform, since the misinterpretation of paced heart rhythms can occur with adverse consequences.[4] To demonstrate pacing pulses, most ECG monitors must be temporarily reconfigured to reduce high-frequency filtering.

2. **Electromagnetic interference:** EMI is the most important intraoperative consideration, and failure to mitigate its effects might lead to patient injury, increased mortality, and CIED damage.[27] Monopolar electrosurgery is the most frequent cause; the coagulation (high-voltage) mode creates more EMI than the nonblended cutting (low-voltage) mode.[1] The risk of EMI increases substantially when monopolar electrosurgery is used in close proximity to the CIED; it is considered significant when monopolar electrosurgery is used above the level of the umbilicus, and low when used below the level of the umbilicus.[22] Whenever monopolar electrosurgery is used, the risk of EMI should be mitigated by strategically positioning the dispersive electrode (ie, "bovie pad") to divert the current return path away from the CIED.[22] Other potential but less common sources of intraoperative EMI include radiofrequency scanners used to locate retained surgical instruments, radiofrequency ablation machines, electroconvulsive therapy, and lithotripsy.[1]

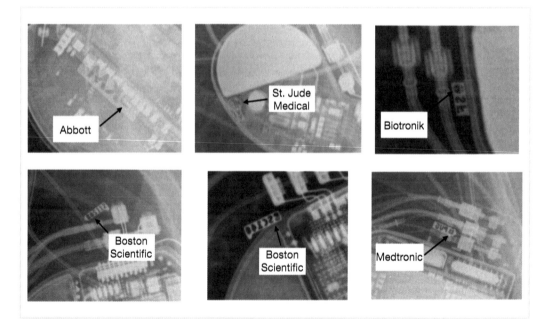

FIGURE 6.5 Cropped and magnified CXRs showing commonly encountered radiopaque logos from various CIED manufacturers. CIED, cardiac implantable electronic device; CXR, chest x-ray.

3. **Underbody dispersive electrode:** These electrodes are placed directly on the operating table rather than on a patient's skin, and are being used with increasing frequency. Since mounting evidence suggests the risk of EMI might be increased with underbody electrode use, consideration should be given to using an optimally positioned conventional dispersive electrode (see earlier) rather than an underbody electrode for patients with CIEDs undergoing surgical procedures until more conclusive evidence is available.[28]

4. **Cardiac implantable electronic device reprogramming:** In any patient with CIED, EMI can cause pacing inhibition and bradycardia or asystole in the patient who is pacing dependent, unwanted rapid pacing from inappropriate tracking or interference with rate-responsive algorithms, and more rarely pulse generator damage or electrical reset. In the patient with an ICD, EMI can cause inappropriate antitachycardia therapy (ie, ATP and shocks).[27] Therefore, if EMI is likely to occur (eg, monopolar electrosurgery will be used above the level of the umbilicus), the antitachycardia therapy function of an ICD should be suspended. In addition, the CIED of a patient who is pacing dependent should be reprogrammed to an asynchronous pacing mode. When reprogramming a CIED to an asynchronous pacing mode, it is important to select a pacing rate (ie, the lower rate limit) that is faster than the patient's underlying rate to prevent the R-on-T phenomenon, which can occur when there is competition between paced and intrinsic beats. For the patient who is pacing dependent, consideration should also be given to increasing the pacing output, because physiologic and metabolic derangements that occur during a major surgical procedure can increase the pacing threshold. Prior to a major surgical procedure, it might also be necessary to augment the cardiac output by increasing the patient's paced heart rate (ie, lower rate limit). Other changes to consider include programming rate responsiveness and pacing features which can mimic pacing system malfunction to off (ie, hysteresis, sleep rate, AV search), since inappropriately fast or slow pacing rates can create confusion and lead to patient injury. While reprogramming or magnet use (when appropriate—discussed in the following section) can be used to mitigate many EMI-related issues, neither of these interventions will protect a CIED from EMI-induced internal damage or electrical reset.

5. **Emergency equipment:** Backup equipment for external pacing and defibrillation should be readily available whenever a patient with a CIED undergoes a surgical procedure, and transcutaneous pacing/defibrillator pads should be placed on the patient whenever the antitachycardia therapy of an ICD has been suspended.

6. **Magnet use:** Magnet application is often recommended as an alternative to reprogramming because it is easy, quick, and does not require the services of specially trained personnel. However, magnet behavior remains non-standardized across manufacturers, and magnet application does not always produce the anticipated or desired effect.[29] Magnet placement will most often suspend the antitachycardia function of an ICD and cause a PM to pace asynchronously. Note that magnet placement will never alter the pacing mode of an ICD. Therefore, patients with ICD who require asynchronous pacing (eg, PM dependent) will always require device reprogramming.

While magnet application will usually produce these aforementioned effects, there are reasons why some CIEDs might not respond in these ways. Some CIEDs have a programmable magnet mode and might be programmed to respond differently or have no response to magnet placement. Some PMs (eg, Medtronic "Micra" leadless PM) have no magnet sensor. Although high-rate (85-100 bpm) asynchronous pacing occurs with magnet placement in the vast majority of PMs, by default, some PMs (eg, Biotronik) respond by asynchronous pacing for only 10 beats before reverting to the base pacing mode and rate. In patients who are obese or have a deep generator implant (ie, S-ICD), magnet application might fail to elicit the magnet response, and two stacked magnets might be needed. Magnet application might also fail to elicit the magnet response if the magnet is incorrectly positioned over the generator, and for some manufacturers the correct magnet position is actually off-center. There are additional reasons why magnet use might be problematic. When patients are in the prone or lateral position it is often difficult to maintain the magnet in a stable position. Magnet placement might not be feasible when the pulse generator is close to the operative site. Some ICDs do not emit a tone with magnet placement, meaning there is no way to confirm that the antitachycardia therapy has actually been suspended. Because of these caveats and concerns the ASA Practice Advisory cautions against the indiscriminate use of a magnet over an ICD, and reprogramming rather than magnet placement is generally the most reliable option.

C. **Postoperative Management:** If a CIED was reprogrammed prior to a surgical procedure, its original settings should be restored postoperatively. In some instances, new settings may be indicated. If the antitachycardia therapy of an ICD was programmed off, the patient should remain in a monitored environment (eg, operating room, postanesthesia care unit, or intensive care unit) until this therapy is reactivated. Postoperative CIED interrogation is also often indicated if (1) an urgent or emergent surgical procedure was performed without an appropriate preoperative CIED evaluation, (2) intraoperative antitachycardia therapy (appropriate or inappropriate) was delivered, (3) exposure to EMI near the pulse generator occurred, (4) the procedure could have caused CIED damage (eg, median sternotomy, thoracotomy), (5) there was significant intraoperative hemodynamic instability, and (6) there is any question of CIED malfunction. Although the antitachycardia function of some older ICDs can be permanently disabled by magnet application, these ICDs are unlikely to be encountered. Thus, a CIED does not have to be interrogated simply because a magnet was applied.

V. Summary

It is important for anesthesiologists to recognize the presence of a CIED, the type of CIED, its indication, and how these devices function to optimally manage them during the perioperative period.

REFERENCES

1. Schulman PM. Perioperative management of patients with a pacemaker or implantable cardioverter-defibrillator. In: Nussmeier N, ed. *UpToDate*. UpToDate Inc. Accessed January 9, 2023. https://www.uptodate.com/contents/perioperative-management-of-patients-with-a-pacemaker-or-implantable-cardioverter-defibrillator
2. Schulman PM, Rozner MA. The perioperative management of implantable pacemakers and cardioverter-defibrillators. *Adv Anesth*. 2016;34(1):117-141.
3. Mulpuru SK, Madhavan M, McLeod CJ, et al. Cardiac pacemakers: function, troubleshooting, and management: part 1 of a 2-part series. *J Am Coll Cardiol*. 2017;69(2):189-210.
4. Luan-Erfe BM, Sweitzer B, Soghikian MO, et al. Misinterpreting paced heart rhythms: a case report. *A A Pract*. 2020;14(14):e01363.
5. Kusumoto FM, Schoenfeld MH, Barrett C, et al. 2018 ACC/AHA/HRS guideline on the evaluation and management of patients with bradycardia and cardiac conduction delay: a report of the American College of Cardiology/American Heart Association Task Force on Clinical Practice Guidelines and the Heart Rhythm Society. *Heart Rhythm*. 2019;16(9):e128-e226.
6. Bernstein AD, Daubert JC, Fletcher RD, et al. The revised NASPE/BPEG generic code for antibradycardia, adaptive-rate, and multisite pacing. North American Society of Pacing and Electrophysiology/British Pacing and Electrophysiology Group. *Pacing Clin Electrophysiol*. 2002;25(2):260-264.
7. Kruse I, Arnman K, Conradson TB, et al. A comparison of the acute and long-term hemodynamic effects of ventricular inhibited and atrial synchronous ventricular inhibited pacing. *Circulation*. 1982;65(5):846-855.
8. Sweeney MO, Hellkamp AS, Ellenbogen KA, et al. Adverse effect of ventricular pacing on heart failure and atrial fibrillation among patients with normal baseline QRS duration in a clinical trial of pacemaker therapy for sinus node dysfunction. *Circulation*. 2003;107(23):2932-2937.
9. Abi-Saleh B, ElBaba M, Khoury M, et al. A confused pacemaker. *Card Electrophysiol Clin*. 2016;8(1):181-183.
10. Lau W, Corcoran SJ, Mond HG. Pacemaker tachycardia in a minute ventilation rate-adaptive pacemaker induced by electrocardiographic monitoring. *Pacing Clin Electrophysiol*. 2006;29(4):438-440.

11. Mickus GJ, Soliman GI, Reed RR, et al. Perioperative management of a leadless pacemaker: the paucity of evidence-based guidelines. *J Cardiothorac Vasc Anesth*. 2016;30(6):1594-1598.
12. Kotsakou M, Kioumis I, Lazaridis G, et al. Pacemaker insertion. *Ann Transl Med*. 2015;3(3):42.
13. Medtronic. Micra *physician portfolio brochure*. 2022. https://asiapac.medtronic.com/content/dam/medtronic-com/01_crhf/brady/pdfs/micra-physician-portfolio-brochure.pdf
14. Madsen JK, Meibom J, Videbak R, et al. Transcutaneous pacing: experience with the Zoll noninvasive temporary pacemaker. *Am Heart J*. 1988;116(1 pt 1):7-10.
15. Timperley J, Leeson P, Mitchell AR, et al, eds. Temporary cardiac pacing. In: *Pacemakers and ICDs*. Oxford University Press; 2007:155-176.
16. Cronin B, Dalia A, Goh R, et al. Temporary epicardial pacing after cardiac surgery. *J Cardiothorac Vasc Anesth*. 2022;36(12):4427-4439.
17. Schulman PM, Stecker EC, Rozner MA. R-on-T and cardiac arrest from dual-chamber pacing without an atrial lead. *Heart Rhythm*. 2012;9(6):970-973.
18. Reade MC. Temporary epicardial pacing after cardiac surgery: a practical review. Part 2: selection of epicardial pacing modes and troubleshooting. *Anaesthesia*. 2007;62(4):364-373.
19. Al-Khatib SM, Stevenson WG, Ackerman MJ, et al. 2017 AHA/ACC/HRS guideline for management of patients with ventricular arrhythmias and the prevention of sudden cardiac death: a report of the American College of Cardiology/American Heart Association Task Force on Clinical Practice Guidelines and the Heart Rhythm Society. *J Am Coll Cardiol*. 2018;72(14):e91-e220.
20. Keene D, Whinnett ZI. Advances in cardiac resynchronisation therapy: review of indications and delivery options. *Heart*. 2022;108(11):889-897.
21. Epstein AE, DiMarco JP, Ellenbogen KA, et al. 2012 ACCF/AHA/HRS focused update incorporated into the ACCF/AHA/HRS 2008 guidelines for device-based therapy of cardiac rhythm abnormalities: a report of the American College of Cardiology Foundation/American Heart Association Task Force on Practice Guidelines and the Heart Rhythm Society. *J Am Coll Cardiol*. 2013;61(3):e6-e75.
22. Schulman PM, Treggiari MM, Yanez ND, et al. Electromagnetic interference with protocolized electrosurgery dispersive electrode positioning in patients with implantable cardioverter defibrillators. *Anesthesiology*. 2019;130(4):530-540.
23. Practice advisory for the perioperative management of patients with cardiac implantable electronic devices: pacemakers and implantable cardioverter-defibrillators: an updated report by the American Society of Anesthesiologists task force on perioperative management of patients with cardiac implantable electronic devices. *Anesthesiology*. 2011;114(2):247-261.
24. Practice advisory for the perioperative management of patients with cardiac implantable electronic devices: pacemakers and implantable cardioverter–defibrillators 2020: an updated report by the American Society of Anesthesiologists task force on perioperative management of patients with cardiac implantable electronic devices. *Anesthesiology*. 2020;132(2):225-252.
25. Schulman PM, Stecker EC. How should we prepare the patient with a pacemaker/implantable cardioverter-defibrillator? In: *Evidence-Based Practice of Anesthesiology*. 4th ed. Elsevier; 2023:75-84.
26. Weinreich M, Chudow JJ, Weinreich B, et al. Development of an artificially intelligent mobile phone application to identify cardiac devices on chest radiography. *JACC Clin Electrophysiol*. 2019;5(9):1094-1095.
27. Rozner MA, Kahl EA, Schulman PM. Inappropriate implantable cardioverter-defibrillator therapy during surgery: an important and preventable complication. *J Cardiothorac Vasc Anesth*. 2017;31(3):1037-1041.
28. Tully BW, Gerstein NS, Schulman PM. Electromagnetic interference with an underbody dispersive electrode in a patient with an implantable cardioverter-defibrillator undergoing noncardiac surgery: a case report. *A A Pract*. 2020;14(11):e01285.
29. Schulman PM, Rozner MA. Use caution when applying magnets to pacemakers or defibrillators for surgery. *Anesth Analg*. 2013;117(2):422-427.

7

Cardiopulmonary Bypass

Janis Fliegenschmidt and Vera von Dossow

KEY POINTS

1. Initiating cardiopulmonary bypass (CPB) for cardiac surgery requires close communication and coordination between surgeon, perfusionist, and anesthesiologist.
2. Management of CPB should be governed by local standards and protocols that all medical professionals involved should be intimately familiar with.
3. Employment of Team Resource Management (TRM) principles for effective communication and team leadership contribute to procedural and patient safety.

I. Introduction: Patient Safety in the Cardiac Operating Room

The cardiac surgical operating room is a complex environment in which highly trained specialists interact with each other using sophisticated equipment to care for high-risk patients with severe cardiac disease and significant comorbidities. Thousands of patients' lives have been saved or significantly improved with the advent of modern cardiac surgery. Indeed, both mortality and morbidity for coronary artery bypass surgery have decreased during the past decade.[1] Nonetheless, the highly skilled and dedicated personnel in cardiac operating rooms are human and will make mistakes. Although the evolution of advanced technologies and enhanced coordination of care have led to significant improvements in cardiac surgery outcomes, there is little evidence that much progress has been achieved in reducing or preventing human errors. The tools to measure potential risks and interventions to improve patient safety are still in the early stages of development and testing. Preventable errors are often not related to failure of technical skill, training, or knowledge but represent cognitive, system, or teamwork failure. In a review of hazards in cardiac surgery, Martinez and colleagues[2] identified machines and technology to cause patient harm in four ways:

1. Misuse (poor training or negligence)
2. Inherent risks of using the device
3. Poor maintenance and upkeep
4. Poor machine design

Much of modern equipment is designed with the focus on mechanical efficiency and biocompatibility, with little emphasis on how design can impact human error. For example, studies found problems with placement, legibility, and format of warning displays; components were poorly integrated into the machine; and the space design and placement of the components was not ideal. Alarms were found to be too quiet or too loud or to have inappropriate tonality.

II. General Aspects of Cardiopulmonary Bypass

The first successful human cardiac surgery using cardiopulmonary bypass (CPB) was performed by John Gibbon in 1952 for repair of an atrioseptal defect. CPB provides optimal conditions for the surgeon and ensures a relatively bloodless surgical field. It incorporates an extracorporeal circuit to provide physiologic support in which venous blood is drained to a reservoir, oxygenated, and sent back to the body using a pump. The normal physiologic functions of the heart and lungs, especially circulation of blood and gas exchange, are temporarily taken over by the CPB machine. In most cases, the heart is also separated from the circulation (via aortic cross-clamping), and cardioplegia solution is administered to allow the cardiac surgeon to operate on a nonbeating heart, while other end organs remain adequately oxygenated and perfused.

1

The responsibility for safe CPB is shared by surgeons, anesthesiologists, and perfusionists alike, to manage cardiac surgery with the lowest possible risk to the patient. Despite technologic advances in circuit design over the past several decades, CPB imposes physiologic aberrations that may cause perioperative organ injury. This chapter focuses on the equipment needed for CPB, anesthesia preparations for initiation of CPB, maintenance of anesthesia during CPB, and the process of weaning from CPB. Complications that may be encountered in the post-bypass period are discussed separately.

A. Principle of the Cardiopulmonary Bypass Circuit

Central venous drainage into the CPB's reservoir enables the provision of a bloodless surgical field for cardiac surgery. The arterial pump functions as an extracorporeal circulation by withdrawing blood from the reservoir and propelling it through a heat exchanger, an oxygenator for gas exchange, and then through an arterial line filter. Finally, the blood is returned to the patient via an arterial cannula positioned in the ascending aorta. Additional CPB circuit components include pumps to suction blood from the surgical field, to deliver cardioplegia solution to produce cardiac electromechanical silence, and to decompress heart chambers via a vent and remove fluid (ultrafiltration).

CPB temporarily substitutes vital organ functions by providing circulation and organ perfusion (heart), oxygenation and removal of carbon dioxide (lung), and, to a lesser extent, hemofiltration (kidney). While providing these critical functions, however, CPB is also associated with an inflammatory response, sometimes culminating in a systemic inflammatory reaction syndrome (SIRS). This is due in large part to the contact of blood with the nonendothelial surfaces of the CPB circuit: Platelet activation and induction of the coagulation cascade result in decreased levels of circulating coagulation factors. In addition, endothelial cells and leukocytes are activated, releasing inflammatory mediators and causing capillary leakage and tissue edema. Furthermore, priming solutions for the CPB circuit (in adults, 1-2 L of crystalloid solution or colloid solution, depending on local protocols) result in hemodilution, temporary anemia, and dilution coagulopathy.

B. Equipment and Physiology

The CPB circuit includes pumps, cannulas, tubing, reservoir, oxygenator, heat exchanger, and an arterial line filter (Figure 7.1). The majority of modern CPB machines have systems for monitoring pressures, temperature, oxygen saturation, hemoglobin, blood gases, electrolytes,

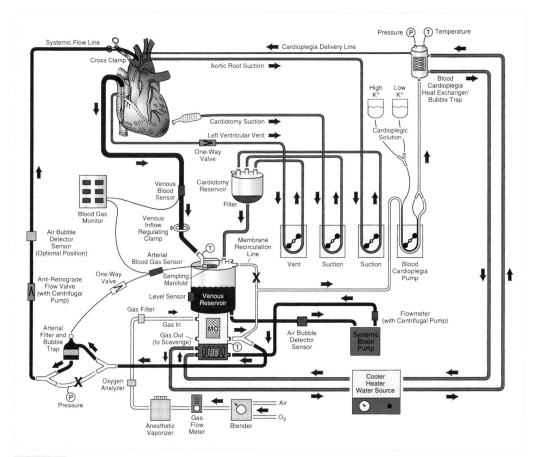

FIGURE 7.1 Detailed schematic diagram of arrangement of a typical cardiopulmonary bypass (CPB) circuit using a membrane oxygenator (MO) with integral hardshell venous reservoir and heat exchanger (HE) (lower center) and external *cardiotomy reservoir*. Venous cannulation is by a *cavoatrial* cannula and *arterial cannulation* is in the ascending aorta. Some circuits do not incorporate an MO *recirculation line*; in these cases, the cardioplegia blood source is a separate outlet connector built in to the oxygenator near the arterial outlet. The systemic blood pump may be either a roller or centrifugal type. The *cardioplegia delivery system* (right) is a one-pass combination blood/crystalloid type. The *heater-cooler water source* may be operated to supply water separately to both the oxygenator heat exchanger and cardioplegia delivery system. The *air bubble detector sensor* may be placed on the line between the venous reservoir and systemic pump, between the pump and MO inlet, or between the oxygenator outlet and arterial filter (neither shown) or on the line after the arterial filter (optional position on drawing). *One-way valves* prevent retrograde flow (some circuits with a centrifugal pump also incorporate a one-way valve after the pump and within the systemic flow line). Other safety devices include an *oxygen analyzer* placed between the *anesthetic vaporizer* (if used) and the oxygenator gas inlet and a *venous reservoir-level sensor* attached to the housing of the hardshell venous reservoir (on the left). *Arrows,* directions of flow; *X,* placement of tubing clamps; *P* and *T,* pressure and temperature sensors, respectively. Hemoconcentrator (described in text) not shown. (Reprinted with permission from Hessel EA II, Shann KG. Blood pumps, circuitry and cannulation techniques in cardiopulmonary bypass. In: Gravlee GP, Davis RF, Hammon J, Kussman B, eds. *Cardiopulmonary Bypass and Mechanical Support: Principles and Practice.* 4th ed. Wolters Kluwer; 2016:21. Figure 2.2.)

as well as safety features such as bubble detectors, oxygen sensors, and a low reservoir-level detection alarm.

1. **Pumps in the cardiopulmonary bypass circuit**

The two most commonly used types of pumps are roller pumps and centrifugal pumps (Table 7.1). Most heart-lung machines use roller pumps for aspirating wound blood, venting the cardiac chambers, and for cardioplegia. Roller pumps include two rollers positioned on a rotating arm, compressing a length of tubing twice per full revolution to produce forward flow. This might be associated with hemolysis during longer procedures. In contrast,

TABLE 7.1 Comparison Between Roller and Centrifugal Pump

Roller Pump	Centrifugal Pump
Afterload dependent	Afterload independent
No need for flowmeter	Need for flowmeter
Short-term use	Long-term use
Greater risk of air embolism	Lesser risk of air embolism
Higher blood trauma	Less blood trauma
No backflow occurs	Retrograde flow possible if pump stops
Lower priming volume	More priming volume

Modified with permission from Sarkar M, Prabhu V. Basics of cardiopulmonary bypass. *Indian J Anaesth*. 2017;61(9):760-767. © 2017 Indian Journal of Anaesthesia.

centrifugal pumps consist of impellers and stacked cones. Rotation rapidly causes a negative pressure at one side of the pump and positive pressure at the other, thereby generating forward flow along the pressure gradient. Hemodynamic alterations such as increases in afterload with systemic vascular resistance increments will result in a drop in cardiac output (CO) unless the flow through the pump is increased. There is significant evidence to support the claim that centrifugal pumps may improve platelet preservation, renal function, and neurologic outcomes in longer cases.[3]

CLINICAL PEARL

The use of centrifugal pumps should be considered for expected longer CPB times (Class IIa, EACTS[4]).

2. Cannulas

The arterial cannula is usually inserted into the distal ascending aorta. Before cannulation, the systolic arterial blood pressure is lowered below 100 mm Hg to reduce the risk of aortic dissection (0.06%-0.23% incidence). The femoral artery is the primary choice in case of emergency surgery such as cardiac arrest, aortic dissection, or severe bleeding. The axillary subclavian artery is increasingly used for cannulation, mostly in case of aortic dissection. Epiaortic scanning (EAS) is the preferred method of screening the cannulation site for at-risk plaques, as avoiding their mobilization may improve neurologic outcomes, especially in older patients. Systemic anticoagulation should be administered prior to aortic cannulation to avoid thrombus build-up on the aortic cannula.

Venous cannulation can be achieved with different types of cannulas: a "single-stage" cannula with a distal opening, a "two-stage," single-lumen cannula with a wide proximal portion with drainage slits as well as a distal opening, and bicaval cannulation. The latter uses two cannulas that are inserted into the superior and inferior vena cava (IVC) each, connected by a Y-piece. An alternative site for cannulation is via the femoral vein in minimally invasive or redo surgeries, where a long cannula is inserted up to the right atrium. Transesophageal echocardiography (TEE) is used to assess the correct position (bicaval view). A vent may be required to drain the left ventricle (LV) from blood entering through the bronchial and thebesian veins.

Cardiac anesthesiologists should be aware that 0.3%-0.5% of the general population and about 3%-10% of patients with congenital heart disease have a persistent left superior vena cava (LSVC). This remnant of fetal development drains blood from the junction of the left internal jugular and left subclavian veins into the coronary sinus. A dilated coronary sinus (≥~11 mm) seen on echocardiography may be a clue to an existing LSVC. In the presence of an LSVC, placing cannulas in the right superior vena cava (SVC) and IVC will not divert all systemic venous drainage away from the right atrium. One solution is for the surgeon to temporarily occlude ("snare") the LSVC, which may result in cerebral venous hypertension. In these cases, the surgeon may place a third venous cannula in the LSVC either retrograde via the coronary sinus or directly into the LSVC through a purse-string suture.

CLINICAL PEARL

It is recommended that the perfusionist and the surgeon agree preoperatively on the type and size of the venous and arterial cannulae in order to achieve and maintain optimal and safe venous return and an appropriate arterial flow (Class I recommendation, EACTS[4]).

3. **Oxygenators**

Membrane oxygenators consist of hollow microporous polypropylene fibers (100-200 μm internal diameter). Blood flows outside the fibers while gases pass inside the fibers, thus separating the blood and gas phases providing blood gas control and lowering the risk of air embolism. Newer designs have an integrated filter to collect emboli, thus making additional arterial filters unnecessary. A heat exchanger integrated proximal to the oxygenator further helps reduce the release of gaseous emboli due to alterations in the temperature of saturated blood.

4. **Tubing**

Tubes are generally made of polyvinyl chloride (PVC), due to PVC's durability and acceptable hemolysis rate. There is evidence that heparin-bonded circuits reduce inflammation and platelet activation, resulting in a reduction in bleeding and reduced transfusion requirements.[5]

5. **Reservoir**

The venous reservoir collects the blood drained from the patient and a cardiotomy reservoir collects shed mediastinal blood and blood from the venting lines. There is no conclusive evidence between open and closed reservoirs regarding biocompatibility.[6] Open reservoirs are more commonly used and allow passive removal of entrained venous air, along with the option of applying a vacuum to assist drainage. They integrate a separate cardiotomy and defoaming circuit to process suctioned blood. A safe level of blood in the reservoir is necessary to avoid air entry into the arterial circuit. Closed reservoirs have only limited volume capacity but offer a smaller area of blood contact with artificial surfaces. This might be associated with less inflammatory response and reduces postoperative transfusion rates.[7] A separate circuit for processing suctioned blood is required.

6. **Cardioplegia**

Cross-clamping of the aorta is necessary for intracardiac repair. The cardioplegia cannula is inserted proximally, while the aortic cannula is inserted distally to the cross-clamp positioned on the ascending aorta. The antegrade cardioplegia technique is achieved by administering the cardioplegia solution into the aortic root via a separate pump into the ascending aorta between the aortic valve and aortic clamp. The time between the placement of the cross-clamp and the administration of cardioplegia is kept to a minimum to prevent warm ischemia. In certain cases, such as in severe aortic regurgitation, antegrade cardioplegia solution is infused via ostial cannulas directly into the coronary arteries. Alternatively, cardioplegia solution can be administered in retrograde fashion into the coronary sinus. To maximize cardioprotective effects, retrograde cardioplegia is often administered in conjunction with antegrade cardioplegia. TEE can guide the placement of the balloon-tipped retrograde cannula into the coronary sinus. It has to be taken into consideration that retrograde cardioplegia alone might result in inadequate protection of the right ventricle.

Cardioplegia is a solution that causes electromechanical arrest of the heart. Arresting the heart improves myocardial protection via reduction of myocardial oxygen consumption. Cardioplegia solution can be crystalloid (cold) or blood based (warm or cold 8 °C-12 °C). It can be administered intermittently and/or continuously. Most myocardial protection techniques involve cold cardioplegia, and ice may be placed around the heart to provide further protection. Potassium-based solutions are commonly used. Blood cardioplegia is a combination of oxygenated blood and crystalloid in a ratio ranging from 1:1 to 8:1. Substances such as bicarbonate, mannitol, adenosine, glucose, and glutamate may be added.

7. **Other circuit components**
   a. The gas line and blender deliver fresh gas to the oxygenator in a controlled mixture.
   b. The set FIO_2 determines PaO_2, while total flow determines $PaCO_2$ during CPB.
   c. An arterial line filter is integrated distal to the pump and removes particles.

CLINICAL PEARL

It is recommended to use pressure monitoring on the arterial line and cardioplegia delivery systems (Class I recommendation, EACTS[4]) and a bubble detector in all inflow lines (Class I recommendation, EACTS[4]).

III. Type of Circuits

The traditional setup of CPB was uniformly focused on safety and versatility. Perfusionists tried to improve CPB setup by improving biocompatibility and reducing hemodilution. This minimalistic approach, the so-called minimally invasive extracorporeal circulation (MIECC),[8] incorporates small priming volumes, tip-to-tip coating of the CPB tubing, a closed CPB system, and the use of a centrifugal pump. Furthermore, no cardiotomy suction is used. However, there is still debate about the hypothetical outcome improvements with MIECC.[9]

IV. Priming Volume and Autologous Priming

De-airing of the CPB circuit is achieved through the use of priming solutions, usually consisting of a mixture of crystalloids and colloids. CPB prime also contains heparin (eg, 5,000-10,000 units), and an antifibrinolytic agent may also be added (eg, tranexamic acid [TA], 1 g). The volume of the prime depends on the circuit components and is typically about 1,400-2,000 mL for adults. Hence, the use of priming solutions is associated with hemodilution, which can adversely affect coagulation and subsequent blood loss.

Depending on the pre-bypass hematocrit and the priming volume, the addition of external blood may be required to maintain a target hematocrit on bypass (21%-24% in adults and 28%-30% in children). The following equations are used:

$$\text{Total circulating volume (TCV)} = \text{Patient's blood volume} + \text{priming volume}$$

$$\text{Target hematocrit (Hct) on CPB} = \text{Patient's blood volume (PBV)} \times \text{Hct/TCV}$$

$$\text{Blood required on prime} = (\text{Target Hct} \times \text{TCV}) - (\text{Pt. Hct} \times \text{PBV})/\text{Hct of donor blood}$$

Autologous priming has emerged as an alternative strategy to reduce priming volume, with a reservoir allowing blood flow in a retrograde or anterograde manner to displace fluid in the CPB circuit. The use of autologous priming is associated with a reduction in both the number of patients requiring perioperative transfusions and the number of units transfused.[10] However, based on currently available evidence, it is still unclear which priming strategy is superior.

Furthermore, despite its common use in priming solutions, there is no clear evidence for beneficial effects of mannitol. Synthetic colloids, however, such as hydroxyethyl starches have been associated with higher rates of kidney injury and should no longer be used.

CLINICAL PEARL

Retrograde and antegrade autologous priming strategies are recommended as a part of patient blood management strategy and to reduce transfusions (Class I recommendation, EACTS[4]). The use of low-molecular-weight starches in priming solutions to reduce transfusions is not recommended (CLASS III recommendation, EACTS[4]).

V. Pump Flow Management

The cardiac index of a 70-kg adult with normal metabolism at 37 °C is 2.2-2.4 $L/m^2/min$. For each 1 °C decrease in temperature, the required CO is reduced by 7%, and the pump flow can be reduced by an equivalent factor. Knowing the body surface area (BSA) of the patient, the required pump flow is as follows:

$$Pump\ flow\ rate = BSA \times Cardiac\ index$$

The target blood flow during CPB is determined by BSA and temperature. Depending on the temperature (normo- to mild hypothermia), the pump flow rate is set between 2.2 and 2.8 $L/min/m^2$. However, especially for patients who are obese, BSA might be not the ideal parameter to determine optimal pump flow. Pump flow should guarantee sufficient oxygen delivery (DO_2) to all organs (oxygen consumption, VO_2):

$$DO_2: Pump\ flow \times Oxygen\ content\ /HB\ (g/dL) + Sao_2$$

Lower pump flows are associated with a greater risk of acute kidney injury (AKI).[10] To date, it is not possible to give simple, one-size-fits-all recommendations on optimal pump flow rate. Signs of inadequate perfusion include:

1. Lower SVo_2
2. Lower DO_2
3. Lower cerebral oximetry values
4. Higher lactate levels
5. Higher O_2 extraction rate

Studies trialing a goal $SVo_2 > 75\%$ and goal-directed perfusion showed an association with a reduced incidence of AKI.[11]

CLINICAL PEARL

Pump flow rate should be determined before initiation of CPB based on BSA and the planned temperature (Class I recommendation, EACTS[4]).

A. Pulsatile Versus Continuous Flow

The majority of CPB use continuous flow (roller or centrifugal pumps). Pulsatile pumps are specially designed, and there are only a few clinical studies to judge efficacy. However, two meta-analyses of randomized controlled trials (RCTs) found better renal outcomes and lower lactate levels postoperatively.[12]

VI. Protocols and Standards

Surgical procedures requiring CPB follow a predictable sequence of events that includes priming and testing of the CPB circuit, anticoagulation, vascular cannulation, initiation and maintenance of CPB, and finally weaning and termination of CPB. Cardiac arrest with myocardial protection followed by myocardial reperfusion is employed when a stationary heart and bloodless field are desired.

A. Preparations for Cardiopulmonary Bypass

The perfusionist assembles the CPB circuit before commencement of surgery, so that CPB can be instituted rapidly if necessary. The circuit components are decided by institutional preference and should comply with the guidelines of professional organizations.

CLINICAL PEARL

It is recommended to have backups for vital systems of the heart-lung machine available at all times (Class I recommendation, EACTS[4]). Institutions should have a maintenance plan for CPB equipment (Class I recommendation, EACTS[4]).

It is recommended to use an institution-approved pre-CPB checklist during the setup of the CPB machine and prior to CPB initiation.

Continuous standard monitoring during CPB includes:

1. Pre- and post-oxygenator arterial line pressure
2. Temperature
3. SV_2 and Hct levels
4. Arterial blood gas analysis at regular intervals

CLINICAL PEARL

It is obligatory to objectively and adequately record all adverse events related to CPB and properly analyze them (Class I recommendation, EACTS[4]).

B. Initiation of Cardiopulmonary Bypass

Although institutional protocols for heparin dosage and the required activated clotting time (ACT) value for CPB vary to some degree, heparin 300-500 U/kg IV is administered before arterial cannulation with a target ACT of more than 480 seconds, measured 3 minutes after heparinization. Systolic pressure during aortic cannulation should be 90-100 mm Hg to reduce the risk of aortic dissection. The aortic cannulation is done first to provide volume resuscitation in case of hypotension associated with venous cannulation. Once the aortic cannula is connected to the tubing, line pressure is checked to rule out dissection. After venous cannulation, venous clamp is gradually released to establish full CPB and then ventilation is discontinued.

The anesthesiologist's pre-CPB checklist should be part of local CPB protocols. An example checklist is presented in Table 7.2.

CLINICAL PEARL

During central cannulation for CPB, the sequence of cannula placement is first aortic and then venous cannula. Should the patient suffer a cardiac arrest after aortic cannula placement, for example, from persistent ventricular fibrillation, CPB may be initiated without a venous cannula in place by using a scalpel to quickly open the right atrial appendage. Pump suckers are placed into the chest return the central venous blood to the CPB circuit, thereby rapidly establishing "pump-sucker" bypass. Then, a definitive cannula configuration can be established.

TABLE 7.2 Pre-Bypass Checklist

Anticoagulation	ACT > 480 s
Anesthesia	Continuous delivery ensured
Infusions	Review drug infusions and cease fluid infusions.
Monitoring	Withdraw PA catheter into the main PA (if used).
	Return TEE probe to neutral position.
	Check correct "zero" of pressure transducers.
	Ensure optimally placed core temperature measurement.
	Record pre-CPB EEG and cerebral oximetry measurements (if used).
	Empty/record urinary catheter drainage bag.
Hemodilution	Discuss safe Hct limits and transfusion triggers.
Blood pressure management	Discuss patient's individualized target mean arterial pressure (MAP) limits (according to cerebral vascular diseases, Doppler diagnostics etc).
Adherence to protocol	Remind all team members of diversions from the standard procedure if planned.

ACT, activated clotting time; CPB, cardiopulmonary bypass; EEG, electroencephalography; PA, pulmonary artery; TEE, transesophageal echocardiography.
The Checklist as Well as the Management of Its Items Should be Standardized in Local Protocols

C. **Blood Pressure Management on Cardiopulmonary Bypass**

To maintain adequate organ perfusion, in particular to the brain and the kidneys, it is critical to maintain adequate mean arterial blood pressure during CPB. There is growing evidence that low blood pressure is associated with a higher risk of postoperative cognitive dysfunction and AKI.[10,13] In addition, it is important to prevent vasoplegic syndrome as this is associated with pro- and anti-inflammatory response resulting in hyperinflammatory syndrome and excessive vasopressor need. Reasons for vasoplegic syndrome include, but are not limited to, preoperative angiotensin-converting enzyme inhibitors, angiotensin receptor blockers, calcium channel blockers, active endocarditis, and sepsis.

In contrast, hypertension might be due to an inadequate level of anesthesia (electroencephalography (EEG) monitoring during CPB should be strongly considered), vasoconstriction due to hypothermia, and/or release of catecholamines.[10] Commonly targeted mean arterial pressures (MAP) range between 60 and 80 mm Hg. It is important to discuss patient's individual safe MAP limits (with regard to cerebrovascular diseases, carotid Doppler diagnostics, etc) with the perfusionist, cardiac surgeon, and anesthesiologist. Untreated chronic hypertension may shift the lower inflection point of cerebrovascular autoregulation upward, resulting in a higher MAP being required for the maintenance of safe and organ-protective CPB.[14]

1. **Central venous pressure**

With appropriate venous drainage, the central venous pressure (CVP) should be low (0-5 mm Hg) during CPB. A persistently high CVP may indicate poor venous drainage, which may require adjustment of the venous cannula(e) by the surgeon. A rising CVP on CPB should prompt investigation. Venous drainage can also be improved slightly by increasing the hydrostatic gradient between the heart and the venous reservoir.

2. **Urine output**

Urine output should be quantified as a sign of adequate renal perfusion and to assist in appropriate fluid management. Very high urine flow rates (eg, >300 mL/h) may be seen during hemodilution (due to low plasma oncotic pressure). Oliguria (usually defined as <1 mL/kg/h) should prompt an investigation because it may indicate inadequate renal perfusion. The most important renal protective strategy is to ensure adequate renal perfusion during CPB by optimizing MAP, fluid loading, optimizing pump flow rates, paying close attention to the renal perfusion pressure, and avoiding intravascular hemolysis and hemoglobinuria.

D. **Aortic Cannulation**

In most cases, the arterial cannulation site will be the distal ascending aorta. The perfusionist then checks that the pressure trace through the arterial cannula matches the systemic blood pressure trace (MAP and pulsatility). This ensures that the arterial cannula has been placed within the aortic lumen. A short interval of pump flow is initiated to estimate if the pressure gradient, "bump," across the cannula is appropriate for the given cannula size and circuit setup. Depending on the type of aortic cannula, it may also be possible to check the correct position of the tip using TEE. Following successful aortic cannulation, central venous cannulation is performed. If a two-stage venous cannula is selected, the surgeon inserts the venous cannula into the right atrium and guides the distal stage of the cannula into the IVC.

Femoral or axillary arterial cannulation may be used if access to the distal ascending aorta is limited or in the case of minimal-invasive cardiac surgery. The axillary approach avoids retrograde flow in the often atherosclerotic thoracic and abdominal aorta. The venous cannula can also be inserted peripherally through a femoral vein, if necessary, but must be advanced to the right atrium for adequate drainage. In these cases, TEE is required to confirm correct positioning in the superior vena cava.

E. **Venting of the Left Ventricle**

During cross-clamping, vents are typically placed in the aortic root to ensure that the left heart does not distend. For open-chamber procedures, vents are also placed in the left atrium or LV to remove both blood and air. Inadequate venting may result in elevation of intracavitary pressures that increase the transmural pressure gradient across the LV wall. Especially in patients with coronary artery disease, potential subendocardial ischemia may result. The coronary perfusion pressure during cardioplegia is also reduced.

CLINICAL PEARL

TEE examination during CPB should be routinely performed to check for the presence of a distended LV that requires venting.

F. **Anticoagulation**

Unfractioned heparin serves as an anticoagulant during cardiac surgery with the use of CPB.[4] Heparin binds to antithrombin and inactivates thrombin and Factor Xa up to 1,000-fold. ACT is a point-of-care test used to assess the adequacy of heparinization. ACT is a whole-blood anticoagulation test for the intrinsic coagulation system. ACT values are influenced by temperature, hemodilution, platelet count, and by surgical factors. Normal ACT ranges from 80 to 120 seconds. Heparin for CPB is dosed based on patient's weight, with doses commonly ranging from 300 to 500 IU/kg. ACT must be monitored every 30-40 minutes during bypass as clotting of the CPB circuit is life-threatening. Target ACT levels are commonly >480 seconds during CPB. After weaning from CPB, protamine is used to neutralize heparin. The protamine-heparin complex leads to dissociation of heparin from antithrombin, restoring its procoagulant properties. The dosage of protamine is based on the initial dose of heparin. Inadequate protamine dosing may result in severe postoperative bleeding and might influence hemostasis. Protamine itself can cause severe hypotension, pulmonary hypertension, and severe anaphylactic reactions with subsequent cardiovascular collapse (<1%).[4] Individually, both heparin and protamine prolong ACT.

1. **Patient-individualized heparin and protamine management**

Other methods to titrate patient-individualized anticoagulation include the Hepcon-based heparin and protamine management using the Hepcon Haemostasis Management System (Medtronic), which provides more comprehensive hemostasis information like anti-Xa measurements or blood heparin measurements in addition to ACT. Although the rationale for utilizing patient-specific coagulation data for heparin dosing is convincing, clinical studies have provided conflicting results of the efficacy of such a strategy.

In some cases, patients fail to achieve target ACT levels even with additional doses of heparin due to an altered heparin response. Causes for the so-called heparin resistance despite high doses of heparin (800-1,000 U/kg) include advanced age, recent heparin exposure, nitroglycerin infusion, thrombocytosis, and antithrombin III deficiency (congenital/acquired).[15,16] Treatment consists of the administration of antithrombin III concentrates (1,000 units) or fresh frozen plasma (2-4 units).

Further exposure to heparin is a concern in patients with heparin-induced thrombocytopenia (HIT) requiring CPB. An alternative anticoagulant is bivalirudin. Bivalirudin has the advantage of a short half-life of 24 minutes due to metabolism by bivalirudin-bound thrombin. There is no specific reversal agent available for bivalirudin. The therapeutic level of bivalirudin is measured by using the ecarin clotting time or even ACT levels. The target ACT is 2.5 to baseline values during CPB. Clearance of bivalirudin is mainly driven by proteolytic cleavage, and 20% is cleared by the kidney. Even if the use of bivalirudin was associated with similar chest tube output, care must be taken to prevent stasis in the circuit, as bivalirudin will be consumed in static blood if not continuously circulated. Thus, the routine use of bivalirudin should be restricted to experienced teams of perfusionists, surgeons, and anesthesiologists.

CLINICAL PEARL

For patients recently treated with heparin infusions, checking plasma antithrombin III levels prior to cardiac surgery may identify the need for pre-CPB antithrombin III supplementation.

2. Antifibrinolytics

CPB causes qualitative and quantitative platelet dysfunction. The concentration of pro-coagulants decreases due to hemodilution. Inflammatory, coagulation, complement, and fibrinolytic pathways are activated. Thromboelastography can help define the cause of bleeding diathesis. Bleeding is greater with prolonged bypass time, redo surgery, and pre-operative use of anticoagulants. Studies have shown decreased blood loss and transfusion requirement in cardiac surgery patients with prophylactic anti-fibrinolytics.[17,18] Effective fibrinolysis inhibition requires a loading dose of 10-30 mg/kg of TA. Additional continuous delivery can be considered for long cases with high bleeding risk. Epsilon-aminocaproic acid can be considered as an alternative if needed. High doses of TA may increase the risk of seizures (~5%-7%), especially in patients with reduced renal function.[19]

G. Temperature Management

Core temperature monitoring sites include the rectum, urinary bladder, esophagus, and pulmonary artery. Nasopharyngeal temperature gives an estimate of cerebral temperature. Hypothermia is frequently used during CPB for its presumed organ protective effects. Blood viscosity increases with hypothermia and allows maintenance of a higher perfusion pressure despite hemodilution. However, hypothermia reversibly inhibits the clotting factors and platelet function. Currently, data are inconclusive regarding the superiority of hypothermic versus normothermic CPB. Hypothermia during CPB reduces metabolic rate and oxygen requirements and provides organ protection against ischemia. However, hypothermia may promote coagulation abnormalities and may increase the risk of microbubble formation during rewarming. Hypothermia shifts the Hb oxygen saturation curve to the left, reducing peripheral oxygen delivery, but this is countered by the reduced oxygen requirements. The rewarming phase may prolong CPB duration and may also risk overheating, particularly in the brain. Cerebral hyperthermia during CPB should be avoided as it is associated with a higher risk of cerebral injury.

Lack of response of the nasopharyngeal or tympanic temperature during the cooling phase may indicate inadequate brain cooling and should prompt investigation of the cause (eg, ineffective heat exchanger, inadequate cerebral perfusion). The position and function of the temperature monitor should also be checked to exclude artifactual causes.

For certain surgical procedures in which circulatory arrest is required (eg, repairs of the aortic arch), deep hypothermic circulatory arrest (DHCA) is used as part of a strategy to prevent cerebral injury. The typical target temperature prior to circulatory arrest is about 15 °C-17 °C, although if antegrade cerebral perfusion is planned, 22 °C-24°C may suffice. Deep neuromuscular blockade prior to DHCA is advisable to prevent shivering. Cerebral oximetry monitoring should be employed.

H. Ventilation, Acid-Base, Electrolyte, and Glucose Management

Ventilation, acid-base, and electrolyte management are of utmost importance during CPB. Arterial blood gases (ABGs) at regular intervals and following changes in management are imperative. Table 7.3 provides guidance for reacting to ABG results.

1. Alpha-stat and pH-stat

In cases of mild and moderate hypothermic CPB and especially for DHCA, acid-base management is of critical importance. There are two alternative strategies, the alpha-stat and pH-Stat approaches. During cooling, CO_2 becomes more soluble in the blood (partial pressure decreases), causing alkalosis. The "alpha" in alpha-stat, refers to the alpha-imidazole ring of histidine, which is an important intracellular buffer. The constancy of the charge state of this ring is important in the regulation of pH-dependent cellular processes. In α-stat, pH is not corrected, and $Paco_2$ is allowed to fall with hypothermia. Blood gases measured at 37 °C are uncorrected. Employing α-stat reduces microembolization by maintaining cerebral autoregulation. The disadvantage of α-stat management is inhomogeneous cerebral cooling. With the pH-stat method, pH and $Paco_2$ are maintained to be constant during hypothermia. CO_2 is added to the oxygenator causing increased cerebral blood flow and cooling. However, prolonged pH-stat management can lead to severe acidosis; therefore, a change to conventional α-stat during the rewarming phase is required.

TABLE 7.3   Acid-Base and Electrolyte Management

Arterial P_{O_2}	Typically maintained at 150-300 mm Hg Hypoxemia may indicate inadequate oxygenator gas flow, inadequate oxygen fraction, or a defective oxygenator.
Arterial P_{CO_2}	Typically maintained at ~40 mm Hg Controlled mainly by sweep gas flow through the oxygenator
Metabolic acidosis	Occurs with inadequate tissue perfusion Severe metabolic acidosis may be cautiously corrected with sodium bicarbonate, in the context of ventricular dysfunction. Unexplained acidosis occurring with signs of increased metabolism should prompt consideration of MH.
Hyperkalemia	Can occur with infusion of cardioplegia solution, usually mild or transient Severe hyperkalemia in patients with renal dysfunction or high doses of cardioplegia can be treated by promoting elimination (eg, loop diuretics) or ultrafiltration. A normal ionized calcium level should be ensured.
Hypokalemia	Might resolve after cardioplegia infusions If replacement is indicated, slow replacement during CPB is safer than quick replacement after weaning.
Sodium	Should be maintained in the normal range where possible Rapid corrections must be avoided due to the risk of acute change in ICP and neurologic sequelae.
Ionized calcium	Should be maintained within normal range
Hyperglycemia	Blood glucose should be maintained <180 mg/dL, by infusion of insulin if necessary. Hyperglycemia may exacerbate neuronal injury and promote risk of infection.
Hypoglycemia	Must be avoided during CPB due to the risk of serious neurologic injury within a short period of time Patients receiving insulin or hypoglycemic agents should be checked more frequently to avoid adverse events.

CPB, cardiopulmonary bypass; ICP, intracranial pressure; MH, malignant hyperthermia.

In adults with mild and moderate hypothermia, an α-stat approach is beneficial regarding the neurologic outcome.[20]

2. **Ultrafiltration**

A hemofiltration device (also referred to as an ultrafilter) consists of a semipermeable membrane that separates blood flowing on one side (under pressure) and air (sometimes under vacuum) on the other side. Water and small molecules (sodium, potassium, and water-soluble non-protein-bound anesthetic agents) can pass through it and be removed from the blood, but protein and cellular blood components do not. Hemoconcentrators are used to eliminate excess crystalloid and potassium and to raise hematocrit. They may also remove inflammatory mediators and hence reduce the systemic inflammatory response syndrome. The device is usually placed distal to the arterial pump with drainage into the venous limb or reservoir. It can also be placed in the venous limb of the circuit, which requires a separate pump. Five hundred to 2,000 mL or more of fluid may be removed during a typical adult cardiac surgery case.

Conventional ultrafiltration uses a hemofilter inserted into the bypass circuit. Modified ultrafiltration is used after completion of the surgical repair before protamine administration, with blood removed from the arterial line and returned to the venous line after passing through the hemofilter.

VII. Initiation of Cardiopulmonary Bypass: Establishing "Full Flow"

An initial CPB checklist is presented in Table 7.4. Once the cannulas are in place and all other checks and observations are satisfactory, the surgeon indicates that CPB should commence. The perfusionist gradually increases the flow of oxygenated blood through the arterial cannula into the systemic circulation. At the same time, the venous clamp is gradually released, allowing an increasing proportion of systemic venous blood to drain into the CPB reservoir. Care is taken to match the arterial flow to the venous drainage. Typically, the arterial inflow is increased over about 30-60 seconds to provide a "normal" CO, based on a cardiac index of about $2.2\text{-}2.4$ L/min/m^2. This is known as "full flow." At this stage, the LV should have ceased to eject, and the CVP should be close to zero.

A. Adequacy of Perfusion

Oxygen delivery (DO$_2$) is the central concept in establishing adequate perfusion (DO$_2$ = CaO$_2$ [blood oxygen content] × effective perfusion flow rate). The margin of error is often reduced due to hemodilution, but oxygen utilization may also be decreased by hypothermia. Inadequate DO$_2$ will cause a reduction in the mixed venous O$_2$ saturation due to increased oxygen extraction. However, below a critical point, tissue hypoxia and lactic acidosis will also begin to occur. DO$_2$ can be improved by raising hematocrit (by transfusion or hemoconcentration) or by increasing pump flow rates. Oxygen demand is reduced by hypothermia and muscle relaxation. Calculation of oxygen consumption may assist in ensuring that adequate oxygen is being delivered.

VIII. Anesthesia Management for Cardiopulmonary Bypass Cases

A. Preoperative Assessment

An adequate preoperative assessment of the patient allows the anesthesiologist to plan the procedure and anticipate possible complications. This early risk stratification and strategy (ERSAS) planning includes the evaluation of significant comorbidities such as arterial hypertension, heart failure, pulmonary hypertension, chronic renal dysfunction, diabetes mellitus, anemia, as well as cognitive and physical function (frailty assessment).

CLINICAL PEARL

It is highly recommended that a preoperative assessment should be a vital part of an institution-wide planning and clinical pathway for patients (Class I recommendation, EACTS[4]).

TABLE 7.4   Initial Cardiopulmonary Bypass Checklist

Cannula position	Arterial line: Pressure and pulsatility should match the patient's blood pressure. Face: Color and temperature should be symmetrical without plethora or edema. Eyes: Pupil sizes should be symmetrical with no conjunctival edema. Recheck with TEE if necessary.
Oxygenation	Arteriovenous color differences should be visible in pump lines. Confirm with inline Pao$_2$ or Sao$_2$. Check satisfactory SVo$_2$.
Hemodynamics	MAP 50-80 mm Hg. (as before) CVP <5 mm Hg PA pressure <15 mm Hg (if used)
Heart	Should be empty, with atria and ventricles decompressed
Perfusion flow	Should increase to "full flow" (PI 2.2-2.4 L/min/m^2) over 30-60 s in the absence of cardiac ejection as heart empties
Ventilation	Cease ventilation when full flow is achieved.
Monitoring	ECG, MAP, CVP, core temperature, urine output, ABG, depth of anesthesia monitoring, ACT, NIRS (if used)

ABG, arterial blood gas; ACT, activated clotting time; CVP, central venous pressure; ECG, electrocardiogram; MAP, mean arterial pressure; NIRS, near-infrared spectroscopy; PA, pulmonary artery; PI, perfusion index; TEE, transesophageal echocardiography.

B. **Pharmacologic Treatment During Cardiopulmonary Bypass**

CPB alters pharmacokinetic and pharmacodynamic effects of anesthetic drugs. At the onset of CPB, the circulating blood volume is increased by the addition of the priming solution in the extracorporeal circuit. Since intravenous anesthetics and opioids are hemodilution dependent, their concentration decreases with priming and during CPB. Furthermore, hemodilution causes a decrease of blood concentrations of proteins such as albumin, resulting in drug concentration reduction.

Hypothermia reduces the rate of drug metabolism and elimination, as does a reduction in blood flow to the liver and kidneys. Bypassing the lungs reduces pulmonary metabolism and sequestration of certain drugs and hormones. Reduced blood supply to vessel-poor tissues such as muscle and fat may result in sequestration of drugs given pre-CPB. The response to drugs may also be altered by hypothermia and hemodynamic alterations associated with CPB. The combined effect of these pharmacologic changes may be difficult to predict, so the principle of titrating drugs to achieve a certain endpoint is particularly important during CPB. Age-related alterations of pharmacokinetics and pharmacodynamics regarding dose reductions must be taken into consideration. Depth of anesthesia should be monitored in all patients with EEG and possibly auditory evoked responses to ensure adequate depth of anesthesia. Too deep anesthesia with burst suppression is associated with an increased risk of cognitive dysfunction and postoperative delirium, which is, in turn, associated with higher 1-year mortality. Providing too light anesthesia during CPB, however, might cause awareness and posttraumatic stress disorder.

Volatile anesthetics are temperature dependent and hemodilution dependent: Although hypothermia increases the blood/gas partition coefficient, hemodilution decreases it.[21] This means that in the case of rewarming, which is known to be faster than hematocrit increase, there is a lower blood/gas partition coefficient with faster washing and, therefore, a subsequent increase in depth of anesthesia. However, as modern CPB techniques use lower priming volumes and normothermia, these effects will often be negligible.

CLINICAL PEARL

Systemic hypothermia requires lower levels of volatile anesthetics, while higher levels are necessary during rewarming.

Volatile anesthetics commonly cross through the microporous polypropylene hollow fiber membrane oxygenator. Therefore, the concentration of volatile anesthetics in the exhaust oxygenator line should be continuously monitored.[4] During CPB, volatile anesthetics such as sevoflurane and isoflurane may cause vasodilation with severe hypotension and vasoplegia syndrome, especially during prolonged CPB.

A large international multicenter study from 2019 included 5,400 patients with coronary artery bypass graft (CABG) surgery and did not demonstrate superiority regarding 1-year mortality compared to intravenous anesthesia regimens (2,8% vs 3.0%; $P = .71$).[22] In addition, there is increasing evidence that volatile anesthetics may be associated with an increased risk of postoperative delirium.[23]

1. **Glycemic control**

Cardiac surgery and the use of CPB are associated with increased inflammatory response, stress response, and hyperglycemia. There is a high rate of patients with diabetes mellitus undergoing cardiac surgery. Current guidelines suggest treatment with insulin for intraoperative serum glucose values exceeding 180 mg/dL.[24] To prevent dangerous hypoglycemia, clinicians should be cautious about checking serum glucose at least hourly while treating with insulin.

IX. **Weaning From Cardiopulmonary Bypass**

Weaning is the process where extracorporeal support is gradually withdrawn as the heart takes over the circulation. Several steps are required for successful completion of weaning.

The use of hypothermia requires a period of rewarming. Caution must be taken to avoid too fast rewarming as hyperthermia is associated with cerebral injury. Nasopharyngeal temperature should not exceed 37 °C. The temperature gradient between the heater and venous blood should not exceed 10 °C. Use of vasodilators (nitroglycerine) can help with homogenous rewarming and with increasing venous capacitance during transfusion of circuit blood. Supplemental doses of anesthetics may be administered; acid-base balance, electrolytes, Pao_2, $Paco_2$, glucose levels, and hematocrit levels are kept within normal limits. Serum potassium of 4.5-5 mmol/L is targeted to prevent arrhythmias.

After open-heart procedures, de-airing maneuvers must be performed. TEE is useful to assess the adequacy of de-airing. Air embolism, frequently involving the *right coronary artery* due to its anterior location, can cause arrhythmias, ST elevation, and acute myocardial dysfunction. It is treated by increasing the perfusion pressure and maintaining pulsatile perfusion by partially clamping the venous line.

Heart rate, rhythm, and contractility are assessed. Epicardial pacing is used for managing persistent atrioventricular blockage. Removal of the aortic cross-clamp can be associated with ventricular fibrillation, especially in conditions causing left ventricular hypertrophy, like severe aortic stenosis. Defibrillation is achieved using internal paddles with a biphasic energy of 10-30 J. Antiarrhythmics such as amiodarone, lidocaine, and magnesium are possible options for the treatment of persistent dysrhythmias.

Anesthesiologists should prepare for the weaning of the bypass (Table 7.5). Mechanical ventilation is started, and the perfusionist gradually occludes venous return and fills the heart while incrementally reducing pump flows.

Difficulties in weaning manifested by systemic hypotension may be due to hypovolemia, low cardiac output syndrome (LCOS) with ventricular dysfunction, or low systemic vascular resistance (SVR). Hypovolemia is treated by giving controlled boluses of blood from the CPB circuit. Low SVR is treated with vasopressors such as phenylephrine, norepinephrine, or vasopressin. The need for inotropes should be evaluated by visually assessing contractility and with TEE. Prior left ventricular dysfunction, severe pulmonary hypertension, inadequate myocardial protection, and prolonged cross-clamp time are factors to consider in determining the post-bypass use of inotropes. A variety of inotropes are available, such as milrinone, dobutamine, epinephrine, and levosimendan. All can be used in the setting of ventricular dysfunction with increased afterload. Inhaled milrinone and inhaled nitric oxide may be used to reduce right ventricular afterload with minimal systemic hypotension. If, despite all measures, the patient fails to wean from CPB, mechanical support devices like an intra-aortic balloon pump, a ventricular assist device, or ECMO should be considered. The need for extensive inotropic support is an independent predictor of increased mortality.[25]

A. **Separation From Cardiopulmonary Bypass**

Once the patient is separated from CPB, heparin (100 units) is reversed with protamine (1 mg) in a ratio of 1:1-1:3. Protamine should be administered over 10-15 minutes. Protamine administration is associated with various negative reactions:

1. Type I (hypotension, due to fast infusion)
2. Type II (anaphylaxis)
3. Type III (pulmonary hypertensive crisis)

Depending on the severity of these different reactions, protamine should be stopped immediately. Adequate measures depend on the presentation and may include fluids, vasoconstrictors/inotropes, and/or return to bypass.

TABLE 7.5 Preparations for Weaning From CPB

Pacing preparations	Cardiac pacing equipment is checked and attached.
Electrolyte management	Electrolyte and acid-base disturbances are identified and corrected.
Hemodilution	Adequate Hb is ensured, and transfusion requirements are checked.
Pharmacologic circulatory support	Inotropic or vasopressor drug infusions are prepared and attached as needed.

Once protamine administration is complete, an ACT is checked to confirm normalization. In case of circuit blood transfusion, an additional bolus of protamine should be given. Caution is advised in case of high doses of protamine, as this can cause anticoagulation as well.

X. Prevention and Management of Adverse Events Associated With Cardiopulmonary Bypass

The safe conduct of perfusion requires vigilance on the parts of the perfusionist, anesthesiologist, and cardiac surgeon to ensure that perfusion-related problems are prevented where possible and diagnosed early and managed rapidly, if they occur.

A. The Human Factor: Standards, Checklists, and Communication

Team Resource Management (TRM) principles should be applied from the beginning of all cases. Although generally safe, placing patients on CPB is always a high-risk situation in which errors can lead to catastrophic consequences. Acknowledging human factors as a significant source of errors is the first step in managing them safely.

All persons involved in the operation should have a shared mental model of the procedure, with precise knowledge of their own responsibilities and a good understanding of the common goal in each step of the operation. Standard operating procedures (SOPs), including checklists and the communication of their completeness, should be established to this end.

Just as with the technical side of the operation, everyone involved needs to know the patient and their medical history. A structured patient handover according to the Situation-Background-Assessment-Recommendation (SBAR) mnemonic can achieve this goal for the interventional team and improve postoperative handover to ensure excellent care after the operation.

To harness the collective capabilities of all personnel involved, everyone should feel comfortable raising concerns and observations whenever they feel the need to do so. An atmosphere of collegiality and team spirit helps to achieve this goal, while rigid hierarchical structures tend to impede it. Team leaders can actively seek their team's input by employing "10-for-10" prompts: a 10-second recapitulation of the plan for the next 10 minutes, while also asking the team members to validate the plan.

Table 7.6 lists common adverse events.

B. Management of Unusual or Rare Conditions Affecting Bypass

1. Sickle cell trait and disease[26,27]

The congenital presence of abnormal HbS as the trait (heterozygote, Hb-AS) but especially as the disease (homozygote, Hb-SS) allows red blood cells (RBCs) to undergo sickle transformation and occlude the microvasculature or lyse. RBC sickling may be induced by exposure to hypoxemia, vascular stasis, hyperosmolarity, or acidosis. Hypoxia, acidosis, and conditions leading to vascular stasis (eg, hypovolemia, dehydration) should be avoided or minimized in all patients with sickle cell trait or disease. CPB should be avoided, especially with hypothermia and cold cardioplegia. Preoperative transfusion to an Hb level >10 g/dL will improve oxygen carriage and reduce the percentage of HbS. For deep hypothermia, exchange transfusion may be required. Expert preoperative hematologic consultation is advised before CPB for patients with sickle cell disease.

2. Cold agglutinin disease[26,28]

Autoantibodies against RBCs in patients with cold agglutinin disease are activated by cold exposure below a critical temperature. Below this temperature, hemagglutination will occur, resulting in vascular occlusion with organ ischemia or infarction. The organ at greatest risk of damage is the myocardium because RBCs are exposed to extreme hypothermia (4 °C-8 °C) during the preparation of blood cardioplegia solution. If cold agglutinins are suspected preoperatively, careful assessment by a hematologist is warranted, including characterizing the type of antibody, its titer, and its critical temperature. CPB should be avoided, but if it is required, systemic temperatures should be maintained above the critical temperature. Systemic temperatures of 28 °C or higher are generally safe in asymptomatic patients. Cardioplegia management includes avoidance of cold blood cardioplegia. If a reduction of the patient's core temperature below their critical temperature for hemagglutinin formation is unavoidable, preoperative plasmapheresis may be required.

TABLE 7.6 Common Adverse Events Under CPB

Malposition of the arterial cannula	If the cannula is situated in the arterial wall, there is a risk of aortic dissection upon starting CPB. Carotid or innominate artery hyperperfusion can occur if the cannula sits too close to their orifices. Consequences: Cerebral edema, arterial wall rupture. Symptoms: Facial flushing, anisocoria, conjunctival edema
Reversed cannulation	Can be avoided by ensuring an arterial pressure trace in the outflow cannula before the commencement of CPB Management requires cessation of CPB and execution of the massive gas embolism protocol (see Table 7.5).
Obstruction to venous return	Reduced venous drainage leads to higher CVP in turn reducing perfusion pressure while also emptying the venous reservoir, putting the patient at risk for gas embolism. The cause must be determined immediately since perfusion can only be kept up in the absence of effective drainage by transfusion of large volumes into the reservoir. Obstruction may be caused by air lock, the presence of large bubbles in the drainage tubing. Mechanical manipulation by the surgeon can also cause obstruction to venous return.
High pressure in the arterial line	May occur due to kinking of the line, increasing the risk of disconnection
Pump failure	May be caused by electrical or mechanical failure, tubing rupture or disconnection, or by automatic shutoff by a low reservoir or bubble detector. If the problem cannot immediately be resolved, deep hypothermia and open cardiac massage may be necessary.
Oxygenator failure	Oxygenator failure may be due to a manufacturing defect or mechanical obstruction from clot or debris, among other causes. A protocol for rapid replacement should be in place (eg PRONTO procedure, Groom et al[8]).
Clotted oxygenator or circuit	The main cause is inadequate anticoagulation, which may result from inadequate dose, heparin resistance, or the inadvertent administration of protamine during CPB. Management involves cessation of CPB and replacement of the oxygenator and tubing if necessary. Reheparinization using a different lot of heparin if possible, and satisfactory anticoagulation must be confirmed before reinstituting CPB. Deep hypothermia and open cardiac massage may be necessary to bridge replacement efforts.

CPB, cardiopulmonary bypass; CVP, central venous pressure; PRONTO, parallel replacement of the oxygenator that is not transferring oxygen.

3. Hereditary angioedema[29]

A deficiency of an endogenous inhibitor of the C1 esterase complement protein leads to exaggerated complement pathway activation, resulting in edema of the airway, face, gastrointestinal tract, and extremities. CPB *can cause fatal complement activation* in patients with hereditary angioedema; peak activation follows protamine administration. In the past, management of acute episodes has been mainly supportive. A purified human C1 esterase inhibitor replacement protein (C1-INHRP) concentrate (Cinryze, ViroPharma) is now available for prophylaxis and treatment, and another purified C1-INH concentrate (Berinert, CSL Behring) is available for treatment. Other drugs have been introduced recently to block bradykinin B2 receptors or inhibitor plasma kallikrein and reduce the severity of reactions.

REFERENCES

1. Wahr JA, Prager RL, Abernathy JH III, et al. Patient safety in the cardiac operating room: human factors and teamwork: a scientific statement from the American Heart Association. *Circulation*. 2013;128:1139-1169.
2. Martinez EA, Thompson DA, Errett NA, et al. High stakes and high risk: a focused qualitative review of hazards during cardiac surgery. *Anesth Analg*. 2011;112:1061-1074.
3. Saczkowski R, Maklin M, Mesana T, Boodhwani M, Ruel M. Centrifugal pump and roller pump in adult cardiac surgery: a meta-analysis of randomized controlled trials. *Artif Organs*. 2012;36:668-676.
4. Wahba A, Milojevic M, Boer C, et al. 2019 EACTS/EACTA/EBCP guidelines on cardiopulmonary bypass in adult cardiac surgery. *Eur J Cardiothorac Surg*. 2020;57:210-251. doi:10.1093/ejcts/ezz267
5. Ranucci M, Mazzucco A, Pessotto R, et al. Heparin-coated circuits for high-risk patients: a multicenter, prospective, randomized trial. *Ann Thorac Surg*. 1999;67:994-1000.
6. Koster A, Böttcher W, Merkel F, Hetzer R, Kuppe H. The more closed the bypass system the better: a pilot study on the effects of reduction of cardiotomy suction and passive venting on hemostatic activation during on-pump coronary artery bypass grafting. *Perfusion*. 2005;20:285-288.
7. Groom RC, Forest RJ, Cormack JE, Niimi KS, Morton J. Parallel replacement of the oxygenator that is not transferring oxygen: the PRONTO procedure. *Perfusion*. 2002;17(6):447-450.
8. Anastasiadis K, Murkin J, Antonitsis P, et al. Use of minimal invasive extracorporeal circulation in cardiac surgery: principles, definitions and potential benefits. A position paper from the Minimal invasive Extra-Corporeal Technologies international Society (MiECTiS). *Interact Cardiovasc Thorac Surg*. 2016;22:647-662.
9. Kanji HD, Schulze CJ, Hervas-Malo M, et al. Difference between pre-operative and cardiopulmonary bypass mean arterial pressure is independently associated with early cardiac surgery-associated acute kidney injury. *J Cardiothorac Surg*. 2010;5:1-9.
10. Sun P, Ji B, Sun Y, et al. Effects of retrograde autologous priming on blood transfusion and clinical outcomes in adults: a meta-analysis. *Perfusion*. 2013;28:238-243.
11. Ranucci M, Johnson I, Willcox T, et al. Goal-directed perfusion to reduce acute kidney injury: a randomized trial. *J Thorac Cardiovasc Surg*. 2018;156:1918-1927.
12. Sievert A, Sistino J. A meta-analysis of renal benefits to pulsatile perfusion in cardiac surgery. *J Extra Corpor Technol*. 2012;44:10.
13. Siepe M, Pfeiffer T, Gieringer A, et al. Increased systemic perfusion pressure during cardiopulmonary bypass is associated with less early postoperative cognitive dysfunction and delirium. *Eur J Cardiothorac Surg*. 2011;40:200-207.
14. Brown CH, Neufeld KJ, Tian J, et al. Effect of targeting mean arterial pressure during cardiopulmonary bypass by monitoring cerebral autoregulation on postsurgical delirium among older patients: a nested randomized clinical trial. *JAMA Surg*. 2019;154:819-826. doi:10.1001/jamasurg.2019.1163
15. Boer C, Meesters MI, Veerhoek D, Vonk ABA. Anticoagulant and side-effects of protamine in cardiac surgery: a narrative review. *Br J Anaesth*. 2018;120:914-927.
16. Finley A, Greenberg C. Heparin sensitivity and resistance: management during cardiopulmonary bypass. *Anesth Analg*. 2013;116:1210-1222.
17. Shi J, Zhou C, Pan W, et al. Effect of high-vs low-dose tranexamic acid infusion on need for red blood cell transfusion and adverse events in patients undergoing cardiac surgery: the OPTIMAL randomized clinical trial. *JAMA*. 2022;328:336-347. doi:10.1001/jama.2022.10725
18. Koster A, Hulde N, Zittermann A. High-vs low-dose tranexamic acid infusion and need for red blood cell transfusion and adverse events in cardiac surgery. *JAMA*. 2023;329:97.
19. Hulde N, Zittermann A, Deutsch M-A, von Dossow V, Gummert JE, Koster A. Moderate dose of tranexamic acid and complications after valvular heart surgery. *Thorac Cardiovasc Surg*. 2023;71(3):181-188.
20. Patel RL, Turtle MR, Chambers DJ, James DN, Newman S, Venn GE. Alpha-stat acid-base regulation during CPB improves neuropsychologic outcome in patients undergoing coronary artery bypass grafting. *J Thorac Cardiovasc Surg*. 1996;111:1267-1279.
21. Zhou J-X, Liu J. Dynamic changes in blood solubility of desflurane, isoflurane, and halothane during cardiac surgery. *J Cardiothorac Vasc Anesth*. 2001;15:555-559.
22. Landoni G, Lomivorotov VV, Nigro NC, et al. Volatile anesthetics versus total intravenous anesthesia for cardiac surgery. *N Engl J Med*. 2019;380:1214-1225.
23. Saller T, Hubig L, Seibold H, et al. Association between post-operative delirium and use of volatile anesthetics in the elderly: a real-world big data approach. *J Clin Anesth*. 2022;83:110957.
24. Lazar HL, McDonnell M, Chipkin SR, et al. The Society of Thoracic Surgeons practice guideline series: blood glucose management during adult cardiac surgery. *Ann Thorac Surg*. 2009;87:663-669. doi:10.1016/j.athoracsur.2008.11.011
25. Hyun J, Kim AR, Lee SE, et al. Vasoactive-inotropic score as a determinant of timely initiation of venoarterial extracorporeal membrane oxygenation in patients with cardiogenic shock. *Circ J*. 2022;86:687-694. doi:10.1253/circj.CJ-21-0614
26. Kurusz M, Mills NL, Davis RF. *Unusual Problems in Cardiopulmonary Bypass*. Lippincott Williams & Wilkins; 2015.
27. Firth PG, Head CA, Warltier DC. Sickle cell disease and anesthesia. *Anesthesiology*. 2004;101:766-785.
28. Atkinson VP, Soeding P, Horne G, Tatoulis J. Cold agglutinins in cardiac surgery: management of myocardial protection and cardiopulmonary bypass. *Ann Thorac Surg*. 2008;85:310-311.
29. Levy JH, Freiberger DJ, Roback J. Hereditary angioedema: current and emerging treatment options. *Anesth Analg*. 2010;110:1271-1280.

Extracorporeal Membrane Oxygenation for Pulmonary or Cardiac Support

Richard Greendyk, Jonathan Hastie, Daniel Brodie, and Darryl Abrams

KEY POINTS

1. Venovenous extracorporeal membrane oxygenation (ECMO) provides for gas exchange without cardiac support, whereas venoarterial ECMO provides support for both impaired gas exchange and impaired cardiac function.
2. Because carbon dioxide can be removed efficiently at low blood flow rates, extracorporeal carbon dioxide removal (ECCO$_2$R) has the potential to alter the paradigm of the management of respiratory failure through the use of minimization and avoidance of mechanical ventilation.
3. In femoral-femoral venoarterial ECMO, delivery of oxygenated blood to the aortic arch and great vessels may be compromised when native gas exchange is impaired and there is residual native cardiac output. Hybrid, upper-body, or central cannulation strategies may mitigate this problem.
4. Temporary venoarterial ECMO is used in patients in cardiac failure as part of several potential strategies, or bridges; the end points of these bridges may include recovery, heart transplantation, long-term mechanical circulatory support, or, when outcomes are uncertain, a decision. However, ECMO for respiratory failure can only be used as a bridge to recovery or transplantation, because no other bridge or destination device is currently in existence.
5. Extracorporeal cardiopulmonary resuscitation (ECPR) has the potential to significantly improve neurologically intact survival from cardiac arrest. However, appropriate patient selection is essential in optimizing outcomes and avoiding the widespread application of this resource-intensive strategy.

THE USE OF EXTRACORPOREAL MEMBRANE OXYGENATION (ECMO) for severe respiratory and cardiac failure has grown rapidly over the last several years in the context of both technologic advances in extracorporeal circuitry and a growing body of literature demonstrating favorable outcomes. As cannulation techniques and management strategies evolve, ECMO has the potential to transform the approach to severe cardiopulmonary failure. This chapter addresses the rationale for ECMO use, its potential indications and contraindications, including its use in the context of respiratory pandemics, management approaches to the circuit and patient, and common complications. Lastly, because ECMO is a resource-intensive technology that profoundly affects the ability to support critically ill patients, economic impact and ethically challenging situations are discussed.

I. History of Extracorporeal Membrane Oxygenation

    A. ECMO was first devised as an extension of cardiopulmonary bypass, with the idea that respiratory and cardiac function could be supported through extracorporeal circuitry beyond the operating room setting.

    B. The first successful application of ECMO for acute, severe respiratory failure was in 1971.

    C. Although such success held great promise for the future development of the field and expanding use in severe respiratory failure, initial prospective randomized trials failed to demonstrate a survival benefit from extracorporeal support compared to conventional management. Much of the failure of ECMO was attributed to high complication rates, particularly bleeding and thrombosis. These complications fundamentally relate to the circuitry components available at the time and limited practitioner experience with the technology.

    D. Over the last 20 years, substantial advances in extracorporeal technology include the following components:

        1. Novel cannula designs that optimize drainage and reinfusion of blood

        2. Biocompatible circuits that decrease the risk of thrombus formation and reduce the requirement for anticoagulation

        3. Oxygenators that improve efficiency through the use of semipermeable membranes to selectively allow for diffusion of gas

        4. Centrifugal pumps that reduce trauma to blood components and decrease the risk of damage to the circuit

    E. The combination of improved technology, with a more favorable risk profile, and concurrent advances in the overall critical care management of patients with severe cardiopulmonary failure has led to a growing body of literature that suggests improving survival in patients supported with ECMO.

II. Extracorporeal Membrane Oxygenation Physiology

    A. ECMO provides gas exchange support during severe respiratory failure by directly oxygenating and removing carbon dioxide from blood.[1]

    B. Deoxygenated blood is drained from a central vein and pumped through a gas exchange device called a membrane lung. The blood passes along one side of a semipermeable membrane, while gas, referred to as sweep gas, passes along the other side. The gas is typically a mixture of oxygen and air, the proportions of which (ie, the fraction of delivered oxygen, FDO_2) are controlled by a blender.

    C. The membrane allows for diffusion of oxygen down a gradient from high concentration in the sweep gas to low concentration in the blood compartment. Carbon dioxide also diffuses from high to low concentration (from the blood compartment to the gas compartment).

    D. Well-oxygenated blood leaving the membrane lung is then reinfused back to the patient. The carbon dioxide removed by the membrane lung is vented to the environment.

    E. When blood is drained from a vein and reinfused into a vein, the configuration is called venovenous ECMO. This configuration provides only gas exchange and relies upon the native cardiac function to circulate the reinfused, oxygenated blood.

CLINICAL PEARL

Venovenous ECMO provides gas exchange support, whereas venoarterial ECMO provides both gas exchange and hemodynamic support.

F. Venoarterial ECMO describes the configuration in which blood is drained from a vein and reinfused into an artery. This provides both gas exchange and hemodynamic support by reinfusing blood under pressure directly into the systemic arterial circulation.

CLINICAL PEARL

In cases of acute right ventricular failure due to severe hypoxemia or hypercapnia, venovenous ECMO may be sufficient to improve right heart function without the need for venoarterial support.

G. Extracorporeal oxygen delivery is proportional to extracorporeal blood flow; large cannulae are often required to achieve adequate flow rates. Extracorporeal carbon dioxide removal (EC-CO$_2$R) is predominantly determined by the sweep gas flow rate and can be achieved at much lower blood flow rates. This allows for the use of smaller cannulae, which may be associated with fewer complications.

CLINICAL PEARL

The main determinant of oxygenation through the ECMO circuit is blood flow rate. The main determinant of carbon dioxide removal through the ECMO circuit, during full-flow ECMO, is the sweep gas flow rate.

III. **Cannulation Strategies**
   A. **Venovenous**
      ECMO traditionally involves the insertion of two separate cannulae, one for drainage and one for reinfusion. Venous drainage commonly occurs from the inferior vena cava (IVC), which is accessed through a femoral vein, while reinfused blood is delivered to the superior vena cava (SVC) through an internal jugular vein (Figure 8.1).
      1. A two-site venovenous configuration has the advantage of ease of bedside insertion without the need for advanced imaging techniques (although ultrasound guidance is recommended). However, the orientation of the drainage and reinfusion cannulae may result in drainage of reinfused, well-oxygenated blood back into the circuit without first having passed through the systemic circulation. This phenomenon, known as recirculation, limits the efficiency of the circuit's gas exchange.
      2. An alternative single-site configuration may minimize recirculation through the use of a bicaval, dual-lumen cannula.
         a. This cannula is inserted into an internal jugular vein with its tip in the IVC. It is positioned so that SVC and IVC drainage ports drain blood into one lumen. After passing through the membrane lung, reinfused blood passes through a second lumen whose port is directed toward the tricuspid valve (Figure 8.2).
         b. Recirculation is minimized both by separating drainage and reinfusion ports and directing the reinfusion jet toward the tricuspid valve.
         c. By avoiding the cannulation of a femoral vein, this configuration may minimize infectious risks and allow for increased mobility, although mobilization is still feasible with femoral cannulation.
         d. In order to ensure correct placement and orientation, this cannula should ideally be placed with guidance from both transesophageal echocardiography and fluoroscopy.

CLINICAL PEARL

Two-site venovenous ECMO is the most common configuration when ECMO is used for respiratory failure; its downsides include femoral cannulation and tendency for recirculation. Single-site cannulation with a dual-lumen cannula avoids femoral cannulation and minimizes recirculation; however, such an approach requires advanced imaging techniques to ensure satisfactory placement.

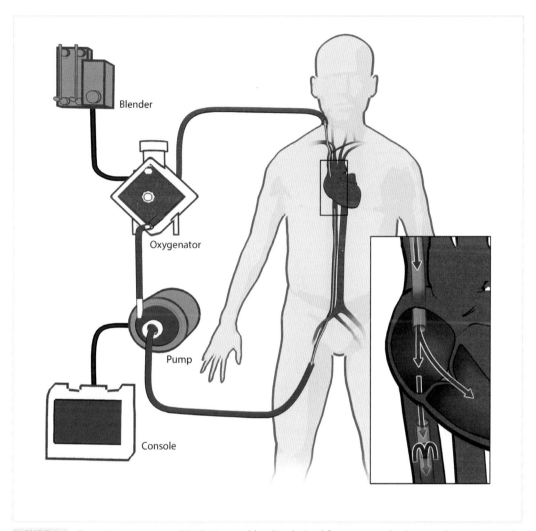

FIGURE 8.1 Two-site venovenous ECMO. Venous blood is drained from a central vein via a drainage cannula, pumped through an oxygenator, and returned to a central vein through a separate reinfusion cannula. Inset: Some reinfused blood may be taken back up by the drainage cannula (purple arrow) without passing through the systemic circulation, which is referred to as recirculation. ECMO, extracorporeal membrane oxygenation. (From Abrams D, Brodie D. Extracorporeal circulatory approaches to treat acute respiratory distress syndrome. *Clin Chest Med.* 2014;35(4):765-779. Reprinted with permission of Department of Surgery, Columbia University Irving Medical Center.)

B. Venoarterial

ECMO is most commonly performed with peripheral insertion of cannulae into the femoral vein and artery. This approach, much like two-site venovenous ECMO, can be performed rapidly at the bedside, which is particularly useful for supporting hemodynamically unstable patients. Such an approach is usually adequate to provide sufficient circulatory support to maintain adequate end-organ perfusion.

1. **Hybrid configurations:** Femoral venoarterial ECMO creates retrograde flow of reinfused blood in the aorta. In patients receiving venoarterial ECMO for cardiac failure who have concomitant severe respiratory failure, residual native cardiac function may pump deoxygenated blood into the ascending aorta. These competing blood flows can create dual circulations, potentially leading to the delivery of poorly oxygenated blood to the

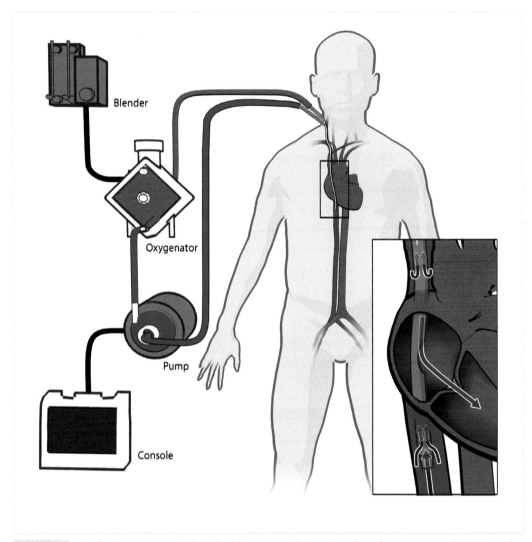

FIGURE 8.2 Single-site venovenous ECMO. Dual-lumen cannula insertion allows for venovenous ECMO through a single venous access point and may minimize recirculation when properly positioned. ECMO, extracorporeal membrane oxygenation. (From Abrams D, Brodie D. Extracorporeal circulatory approaches to treat acute respiratory distress syndrome. *Clin Chest Med.* 2014;35(4):765-779. Reprinted with permission of Department of Surgery, Columbia University Irving Medical Center.)

upper body (including the coronary and cerebral circulations) and well-oxygenated blood to the lower body, referred to as differential oxygenation (Figure 8.3). One remedy to this problem involves the addition of a second reinfusion limb into the internal jugular vein, which will improve the oxygenation of blood passing through the native cardiac circulation and into the upper body. This configuration is referred to as venoarterial venous ECMO (Figure 8.4).

2. In circumstances in which sufficient circulatory support cannot be provided by the cannulation of peripheral vessels, central cannulation may be necessary, with the use of shorter, larger bore cannulae. This configuration, which is analogous to typical cardiopulmonary bypass cannulation for open heart surgery, varies based on the patient's needs and may include, for example, right atrial drainage with either aortic or pulmonary venous reinfusion.

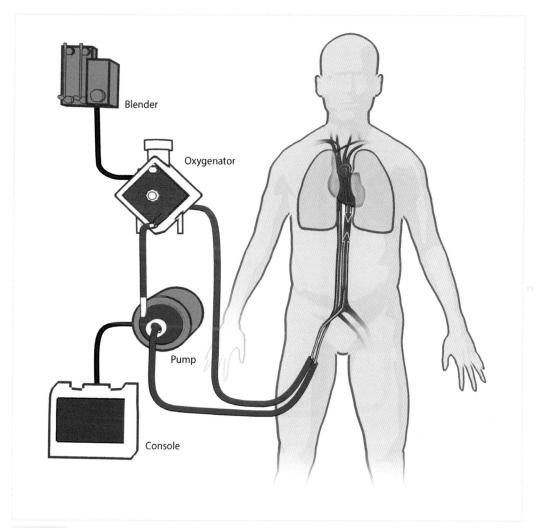

FIGURE 8.3 Femoral venoarterial ECMO in the setting of impaired gas exchange. Reinfused oxygenated blood flows retrograde up the aorta (red arrow) and may meet resistance from antegrade flow from the native cardiac output (purple arrow), which, in the context of impaired native gas exchange, may lead to poor upper body oxygenation. ECMO, extracorporeal membrane oxygenation. (From Abrams D, Brodie D. Extracorporeal circulatory approaches to treat acute respiratory distress syndrome. *Clin Chest Med.* 2014;35(4):765-779. Reprinted with permission of Department of Surgery, Columbia University Irving Medical Center.)

3. **Left ventricular venting:** The retrograde flow of reinfused blood in the aorta in femoral venoarterial ECMO may result in several adverse physiologic consequences related to an increase in left ventricular afterload. Increased left ventricular afterload increases wall stress, which both increases myocardial oxygen demand and decreases coronary arterial perfusion. Increased left ventricular afterload also leads to an increase in the end-diastolic volume, which may lead to acute pulmonary edema, along with stasis and risk of intracardiac thrombus formation, particularly when the aortic valve is not opening. Left ventricular venting—performed either percutaneously or surgically—mitigates each of these effects by decompressing the ventricle. Left ventricular venting (drainage) into the ECMO circuit also reduces the likelihood of upper-body hypoxemia in patients with impaired lung function.

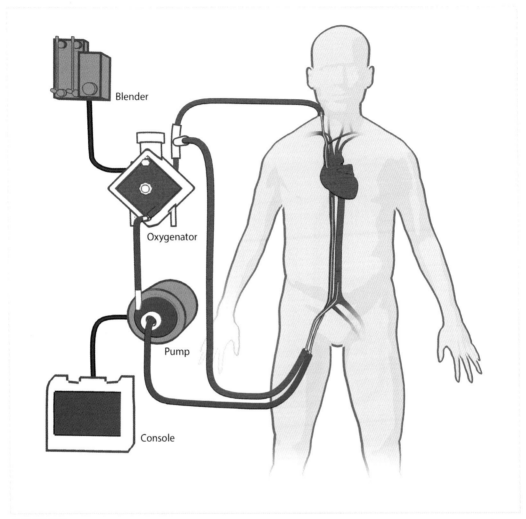

FIGURE 8.4   Venoarterial venous ECMO. Inadequate upper body oxygenation due to a combination of femoral veno-arterial ECMO and impaired native gas exchange may be partially overcome by the addition of a second reinfusion limb into an internal jugular vein. ECMO, extracorporeal membrane oxygenation. (From Abrams D, Brodie D. Extracorporeal circulatory approaches to treat acute respiratory distress syndrome. *Clin Chest Med*. 2014;35(4):765-779. Reprinted with permission of Department of Surgery, Columbia University Irving Medical Center.)

CLINICAL PEARL

The most common approach for venoarterial ECMO utilizes femoral venous drainage and femoral arterial reinfusion. However, this configuration may be associated with upper-body hypoxemia in the setting of impaired native gas exchange and residual native left ventricular function.

IV. **Indications for Extracorporeal Membrane Oxygenation in Respiratory Failure**
   A. **Bridge to Recovery**
      1. **Severe acute respiratory distress syndrome:** The most common indication for venovenous ECMO is severe acute respiratory distress syndrome (ARDS), defined by the acute onset of severe hypoxemia with bilateral infiltrates on chest imaging that cannot be fully explained by elevated left atrial pressure.

a. A volume- and pressure-limited ventilation strategy is standard of care in ARDS, with a proven mortality benefit over conventional higher volumes and plateau airway pressures.[2] Other strategies that confer a mortality benefit in ARDS include prone positioning and possibly the early use of neuromuscular blockade or high levels of positive end-expiratory pressure (PEEP).

b. The largest prospective randomized controlled trial of ECMO in severe, refractory ARDS was the *Extracorporeal Membrane Oxygenation for Severe Acute Respiratory Distress Syndrome* (EOLIA) trial, which demonstrated a nonstatistically significant difference in 60-day mortality by intention-to-treat analysis in patients with severe ARDS who received ECMO combined with an ultra-lung-protective ventilation strategy compared to patients who received optimal conventional management (35% in the ECMO arm vs 46% in the control arm; relative risk [RR] 0.76; 95% CI 0.55-1.04; $P = .09$). Of note, the trial was terminated early after enrollment of 249 patients based on prespecified stopping criteria. Furthermore, 28% of patients in the control arm crossed over to ECMO for indications including refractory hypoxemia, right heart failure, or other clinical worsening, thus biasing results to the null.

c. A follow-up Bayesian analysis of the data from the EOLIA trial demonstrated high probability of mortality benefit from ECMO in severe ARDS, with the magnitude of benefit varying by the priors applied.[3] A subsequent systematic review and meta-analysis as well as a separate individual patient data meta-analysis using data from the EOLIA trial and a prior randomized controlled trial evaluating the efficacy of ECMO for severe ARDS demonstrated a mortality benefit from ECMO at 60 days (RR 0.73; 95% CI 0.58-0.92; $P = .008$)[4] and 90 days (RR 0.75; 95% CI 0.6-0.94; $P = .013$).[5] A network meta-analysis—assessing the impact of multiple interventions—likewise demonstrated a 28-day mortality benefit from ECMO when combined with a lung-protective ventilation strategy.[6] In sum, the data suggest a clinically significant benefit from ECMO compared to conventional management in patients with severe ARDS when performed at experienced ECMO centers and used in concert with a ventilation strategy incorporating volumes and airway pressures below the current standard of care.

d. Recommended thresholds to initiate ECMO in ARDS, as defined by the EOLIA trial, as are follows[7]:

   (1) Partial pressure of arterial oxygen to fraction of inspired oxygen (Pao_2:Fio_2) <50 mm Hg for >3 hours or Pao_2:Fio_2 <80 mm Hg for >6 hours, despite an Fio_2 ≥0.8 and PEEP ≥10 cm H_2O

   (2) pH <7.25 and partial pressure of arterial carbon dioxide ($Paco_2$) ≥60 mm Hg for >6 hours with respiratory rate increased to 35 breaths per minute and mechanical ventilation settings adjusted to keep plateau airway pressure ≤32 cm H_2O

2. **COVID-19-related ARDS**

   a. Whereas initial observational studies demonstrated similar survival rates for patients receiving ECMO for COVID-19-related severe ARDS as for patients receiving ECMO for severe ARDS due to other prepandemic etiologies, there has been a trend toward worsening mortality in ECMO-supported patients with COVID-19 later in the pandemic, calling into question the benefit and appropriateness of ECMO in this population, particularly in the context of enormous strain on health care resource.[8,9]

   b. Despite these observed trends, a registry-based comparative effectiveness study of 7,345 patients with COVID-19-related ARDS found a significant reduction in mortality when a strategy of ECMO was applied to patients with a Pao_2:Fio_2 <80 mm Hg, compared to conventional mechanical ventilation alone.[10]

   c. Further investigation is needed to more clearly elucidate the role of ECMO in patients with COVID-19-related ARDS, especially in light of the economic and ethical implications of ECMO in the context of a worldwide pandemic.

3. **Primary graft dysfunction after lung transplantation:** Clinically similar to ARDS, though etiologically thought to be a consequence of ischemia-reperfusion injury, primary graft dysfunction (PGD) manifests as acute hypoxemic respiratory failure and

radiographic infiltrates in the allograft within 72 hours of lung transplantation. ECMO should be considered early in PGD to support severe gas exchange impairment and minimize harm from aggressive ventilator settings. In select patients, particularly those with pretransplantation pulmonary hypertension or right ventricular dysfunction, venoarterial ECMO may be considered intraoperatively as a means of accomplishing two goals: providing intraoperative hemodynamic support and controlling reperfusion to the allograft to minimize the risk of PGD. In some patients with severe pulmonary hypertension, venoarterial ECMO may be instituted preoperatively for respiratory failure associated with hemodynamic instability.[11]

4. **Acute hypercapnic respiratory failure:** $ECCO_2R$ may be used in the management of acute hypercapnic respiratory failure while minimizing or eliminating the need for invasive mechanical ventilation. Because carbon dioxide removal is more efficient than oxygenation, adequate carbon dioxide removal may be achieved at lower blood flow rates with smaller cannulae than what is required for hypoxemic respiratory failure, potentially mitigating some of the risks associated with ECMO.

   a. Potential benefits of this strategy include the following:
      (1) Minimization of dynamic hyperinflation and auto-PEEP
      (2) Minimization of ventilator-induced lung injury (VILI)
      (3) Avoidance of ventilator-associated pneumonia
      (4) Improved delivery of aerosolized medications
      (5) Facilitation of early mobilization through better control of dyspnea and work of breathing

   b. The feasibility of such a strategy has been demonstrated in small studies of subjects with acute exacerbations of chronic obstructive pulmonary disease. Prospective randomized studies demonstrating clinically meaningful benefits from $ECCO_2R$ versus conventional management are needed before this approach can be recommended for clinical use.

   c. A similar approach may be considered in severe cases of status asthmaticus in which patients have marked ventilatory impairment, often as a consequence of positive pressure ventilation and dynamic hyperinflation. Case series of patients with status asthmaticus receiving $ECCO_2R$ have demonstrated the viability of this strategy.

B. **Bridge to Transplant**

1. ECMO support for end-stage respiratory failure as a bridging therapy to lung transplantation has traditionally been associated with poor posttransplant outcomes, mostly due to poor patient selection and device-associated complications. However, there have recently been improvements in posttransplant outcomes for patients supported with ECMO pretransplant.[11] These improvements are at least in part attributable to the following:

   a. Careful patient selection and earlier initiation, thereby avoiding patients too moribund to successfully undergo lung transplantation

   b. Increased experience at high-volume centers with an associated reduction in complications

   c. Strategies that optimize physical conditioning and minimize intensive care unit (ICU) complications. These strategies include avoidance of sedation, endotracheal extubation, and early mobilization.

2. Because there is no destination device for respiratory failure equivalent to the left ventricular assist device (LVAD) in advanced cardiac failure, patients with end-stage respiratory failure should be selected for ECMO support only when they are candidates for lung transplantation.

CLINICAL PEARL

Indications for venovenous ECMO include bridge to recovery for severe ARDS and bridge to lung transplantation for end-stage respiratory failure. The use of $ECCO_2R$ for acute hypercapnic respiratory failure is a promising area of ongoing research.

V. Indications for Extracorporeal Membrane Oxygenation in Cardiac Failure

A. Bridge to Recovery

1. **Cardiogenic shock:** Several mechanical circulatory support systems can restore organ perfusion in the setting of cardiogenic shock. Venoarterial ECMO has two notable advantages of being able to be initiated at the bedside and providing gas exchange. The success of ECMO support as a bridge to recovery largely depends on the etiology, with cardiac failure due to acute sepsis-induced cardiomyopathy, fulminant myocarditis, refractory ventricular arrhythmias, myocardial infarction, and post–cardiac transplant allograft failure having the most favorable outcomes. The data for ECMO in cardiogenic shock are largely limited to case series, small cohort studies, and retrospective propensity analyses.[12] Pre-ECMO prognostication scores have been proposed to help maximize patient outcomes by identifying those most likely to benefit from ECMO support.

   a. Postcardiotomy cardiogenic shock is a complication of cardiac surgery that is associated with significant mortality. Postcardiotomy shock may be secondary to ischemia from coronary artery disease, poor preservation of the myocardium while the aorta is cross-clamped, or changes in valve function after separating from cardiopulmonary bypass. ECMO may be considered as temporary postoperative support when a patient cannot be weaned from cardiopulmonary bypass in the operating room.

   b. Primary graft failure (PGF), a complication of heart transplantation that is associated with a high rate of mortality, may be supported with venoarterial ECMO. Patients with PGF who are supported on ECMO and who survive beyond the early posttransplant period have comparable long-term survival to transplant recipients who never developed PGF.

   c. Evidence suggests that venoarterial ECMO may offer a significant mortality benefit for sepsis-induced cardiomyopathy. A multicenter cohort study with propensity score–weighted analysis demonstrated that patients receiving ECMO for sepsis-induced cardiomyopathy had significantly higher survival than those who did not receive ECMO (51% vs 14%; adjusted RR for mortality 0.57; 95% CI 0.35-0.93; $P = .0029$).[13]

   d. A randomized controlled trial of immediate venoarterial ECMO versus conventional management (with allowance for ECMO later in their course) in patients with severe or rapidly deteriorating cardiogenic shock—the majority of whom had cardiogenic shock related to myocardial infarction or acute decompensated heart failure—failed to show a statistically significant difference in the primary 30-day composite outcome of death, resuscitated circulatory arrest, or use of other mechanical circulatory support (hazard ratio [HR] 0.72; 95% CI 0.46-1.12; $P = .21$).[14]

2. **Extracorporeal cardiopulmonary resuscitation:** ECPR (the use of ECMO in refractory cardiac arrest) is a rapidly expanding indication for venoarterial ECMO with evolving data.

   a. A phase 2, single-center, open-label, randomized controlled trial of early ECPR (at hospital arrival) versus standard advanced cardiac life support (ACLS) for out-of-hospital cardiac arrest (OHCA) and refractory ventricular fibrillation demonstrated improved survival to hospital discharge and 6-month survival in patients receiving early ECPR versus those receiving standard ACLS.[15] Of note, the trial was terminated early—after enrollment of 30 patients—based on prespecified superiority criteria.

   b. A larger single-center randomized controlled trial of 256 patients with refractory OHCA of presumed cardiac origin did not find a significant improvement in survival with neurologically favorable outcome at 180 days in patients who received early ECPR versus those who received standard ACLS. However, this trial was possibly underpowered to detect a clinically relevant difference. Additionally, in a secondary analysis of patients who did not achieve prehospital return of spontaneous circulation, ECPR was associated with a significantly lower risk of death at 180 days compared to prolonged conventional ACLS alone (23.9% vs 1.2%).[16]

   Similarly, a multicenter, randomized controlled trial of 160 patient with OHCA of presumed cardiac origin did not find a significant difference in survival with a neurologically favorable outcome at 30 days in patients who received early ECPR versus those who received standard ACLS. However, early randomization led to a considerable number of patients in both arms of the study who had return of spontaneous circulation prior to hospital arrival, possibly biasing the results towards the null.[17]

c. Propensity analyses and meta-analysis have suggested a benefit of ECPR in select patients with in-hospital cardiac arrest.[18]

d. In sum, there is a growing body of evidence suggesting that the use of ECPR in carefully selected patients may lead to favorable outcomes.

3. **Pulmonary vascular disease**

a. Decompensated pulmonary hypertension with right ventricular failure, a condition associated with high mortality, is emerging as a potential target for ECMO support.[19] Traditionally, a venoarterial configuration is needed to decompress the right ventricle and bypass the high resistance of the pulmonary vasculature. However, such an approach may be inadequate to oxygenate the upper body when femoral vessels are used for venoarterial ECMO. Alternative strategies include the following approaches:

(1) Upper-body venoarterial ECMO with right internal jugular venous drainage and subclavian or innominate arterial reinfusion via an end-to-side graft

(2) Single-site, dual-lumen cannulation (with bicaval drainage) via the internal jugular vein with reinfusion directed across a preexisting atrial septal defect or intentionally created septostomy

(3) Pumpless arteriovenous ECMO between the main pulmonary artery and the left atrium

(4) Right atrial to left atrial ECMO: This configuration provides right ventricular support and gas exchange, but uses the native left ventricle for systemic circulation. Like venoarterial ECMO, it is associated with increased risk of stroke.

b. Pulmonary embolism, when associated with severe right ventricular dysfunction with or without hemodynamic collapse, may be appropriate for venoarterial ECMO support. Nonrandomized studies have demonstrated favorable survival rates when this strategy has been employed with concomitant consideration of systemic thrombolysis, catheter-directed therapies, or surgical embolectomy.

B. **Bridge to Left Ventricular Assist Device or Transplantation**

1. ECMO has been reported as a viable bridging strategy for both LVAD and heart transplantation. LVAD themselves are used as either a longer-term bridge to transplantation or as destination therapy for patients who are not eligible for transplantation. Because venoarterial ECMO is associated with significant morbidity, the duration of support is typically limited to 1 to 2 weeks. During this time, assessment of neurologic function and organ system recovery are significant factors in determining the timing of LVAD insertion. Pre-ECMO patient characteristics that have been associated with poor outcomes for ECMO as bridge to VAD or transplant include age >50 years, CPR prior to ECMO initiation, and high pre-ECMO severity of illness scores.[12]

2. In cases where it is unclear whether cardiac function will recover (eg, postacute myocardial infarction complicated by cardiogenic shock), ECMO may be considered as a bridge to decision. Serial assessments of myocardial function allow determination of whether a patient will recover or be eligible for VAD insertion or transplantation. Loss of end-organ function, such as kidney failure or neurologic injury, may preclude eligibility for transplantation or VAD insertion in many centers.

CLINICAL PEARL

Indications for venoarterial ECMO include bridge to recovery for potentially reversible cardiogenic shock or cardiac arrest and bridge to VAD or heart transplantation for irreversible cardiac failure. An emerging strategy is the use of venoarterial ECMO in patients with decompensated pulmonary hypertension as a bridge to either transplant or recovery.

VI. **Extracorporeal Membrane Oxygenation Management**

A. **Invasive Mechanical Ventilation Practices**

1. VILI is believed to be the main determinant of poor outcomes in ARDS, explaining why a volume- and pressure-limited ventilation strategy has such a significant impact on survival.

2. Several studies have demonstrated that tidal volumes and plateau pressures below the current standard of care could further reduce VILI. However, reductions in tidal volumes, airway pressures, and respiratory rates with conventional invasive mechanical ventilation alone are often limited by intolerable levels of respiratory acidosis that come with marked reductions in minute ventilation.

3. $ECCO_2R$ can facilitate even lower tidal volumes and airway pressures by managing the concomitant hypercapnia and acidemia, to the point where, in select cases, mechanical ventilation may be discontinued, and patients could be endotracheally extubated while on ECMO.

4. In cases of severe ARDS in which ECMO is initiated for refractory gas exchange abnormalities or excess plateau airway pressures, a strategy of very low tidal volumes, airway pressures, and respiratory rates, while maintaining a moderate amount of PEEP to minimize alveolar collapse, is recommended based on the results of the EOLIA trial. Occasionally, in select patients, mechanical ventilation can be discontinued altogether.

5. An ultra-lung-protective ventilation strategy may ultimately prove beneficial in less severe forms of ARDS, where oxygenation is better preserved and an approach targeting CO_2 removal alone with lower blood flows and smaller cannulae (ie, $ECCO_2R$) is sufficient.

   a. A phase 2 prospective, multicenter trial demonstrated the feasibility of $ECCO_2R$ to facilitate ultra-lung-protective ventilation, defined as tidal volumes <4 mL/kg predicted body weight and plateau airway pressure ≤25 cm H_2O, in patients with moderate ARDS.[20]

   b. A subsequent randomized, open-label, pragmatic clinical trial found no mortality difference in patients with acute hypoxemic respiratory failure treated with $ECCO_2R$ to facilitate ultraprotective ventilation (goal tidal volume <3 mL/kg) versus conventional low tidal volume ventilation. Factors that may have contributed to the negative result include early termination of the trial and subsequent lack of power to detect a difference, time-limited use of $ECCO_2R$ in the intervention arm, patient population not restricted to ARDS nor those most likely to benefit from the strategy, high rates of adverse events in the intervention arm, and inability to achieve the target tidal volume of <3 mL/kg in many patients in the intervention arm.[21]

   c. Further investigation is necessary to determine whether there is, in fact, a clinical benefit that outweighs the potential risks of extracorporeal support for this potential indication.

CLINICAL PEARL

The use of extracorporeal support for respiratory failure in mechanically ventilated patients may reduce VILI by permitting the use of tidal volumes and plateau airway pressures below the current standard of care.

B. **Anticoagulation and Transfusion Strategies**

1. Continuous systemic anticoagulation is generally needed to maintain ECMO circuit patency and minimize thrombotic risk to the patient. The degree of anticoagulation must be balanced with the risk of hemorrhagic complications. There are no universally accepted anticoagulation standards for ECMO, nor is there a consensus on how anticoagulation should be monitored, with activated clotting time, activated partial thromboplastin time (aPTT), and thromboelastography, among others, having been reported.

2. For venovenous ECMO, strategies that employ lower levels of anticoagulation, restrictive transfusion thresholds, and reinfusion of circuit blood at the time of decannulation have been associated with favorable outcomes with minimal transfusion requirements.[22] Furthermore, a multicenter, prospective cohort study of patients receiving venovenous ECMO found that a hemoglobin concentration of <7 g/dL was associated with higher risk of death in the ICU compared with other higher hemoglobin concentrations and that red blood cell transfusion was associated with lower risk of death only when transfused for a hemoglobin concentration of <7 g/dL.[23]

3. Prolonged heparin infusions may reduce available antithrombin III and thereby impair the efficacy of heparin. Antithrombin III is available in recombinant form and may be considered to restore the efficacy of heparin in the context of low antithrombin III levels.

4. If heparin cannot be used, for example, in the setting of heparin-induced thrombocytopenia (HIT), alternative anticoagulants include argatroban and bivalirudin.

CLINICAL PEARL

Low levels of systemic anticoagulation appear to be effective at maintaining ECMO circuit patency while minimizing the risk of significant bleeding.

C. **Early Mobilization**
1. Early mobilization of critically ill patients supported with ECMO has been demonstrated as safe and feasible, even in the presence of femoral venous and arterial cannulae.[24]
2. Extubation and cessation of mechanical ventilation during ECMO support, when feasible, may aid in early mobilization.
3. Physical rehabilitation, including early mobilization, is of critical importance in the bridge-to-transplant population in order to maintain transplant candidacy. Whether there is a benefit in the bridge-to-recovery population comparable to that seen in other critically ill patients has yet to be determined and is an area of active research.

D. **Weaning ECMO**
1. **Venovenous:** Patients should be evaluated for their readiness to wean from ECMO support after the underlying cause of respiratory failure is treated and the patient's native gas exchange and respiratory system mechanics improve. There are several approaches to weaning venovenous ECMO. An approach of incremental reductions in sweep gas flow rate (with or without concomitant decreases in F_{DO_2}) while monitoring the ability to maintain adequate gas exchange with native lung function is most commonly employed. A trial with sweep gas flow turned off for a prespecified period of time (eg, 30 minutes) with acceptable gas exchange, no excess work of breathing, and acceptable ventilator settings (if applicable) should be performed in most patients prior to consideration of decannulation and may be used as the sole determinant of weaning readiness.

2. **Venoarterial:** Weaning from venoarterial ECMO differs significantly from venovenous ECMO. Because venoarterial ECMO provides hemodynamic support, weaning can be performed with incremental reductions in extracorporeal blood flow with serial assessments of vasopressor and inotrope requirements, cardiac function, and end-organ perfusion. Ideally, vasopressors will be able to be minimized or discontinued entirely prior to decannulation from venoarterial ECMO, while it is more common to maintain some pharmacologic inotropic support. During weaning trials, a minimum extracorporeal blood flow rate of 2 L/min should be maintained through the circuit to avoid circuit thrombosis. Sweep gas F_{DO_2} is typically not weaned—and sweep gas should never be turned off entirely—in order to avoid the creation of a right-to-left shunt. If a patient appears ready for decannulation from a hemodynamic perspective but continues to require extracorporeal gas exchange support, conversion from venoarterial to venovenous ECMO (with its lower risk of systemic embolization) should be considered.

CLINICAL PEARL

When determining readiness for decannulation from venovenous ECMO, sweep gas flow should be discontinued to assess adequacy of native gas exchange. When weaning venoarterial ECMO, extracorporeal blood flow is typically reduced to assess hemodynamic readiness for decannulation. In venoarterial ECMO, sweep gas flow should always be maintained; discontinuation of sweep gas flow would lead to hypoxemia from a right-to-left shunt.

VII. **Extracorporeal Membrane Oxygenation Transport**

   A. Patients with severe, refractory respiratory or cardiac failure who would otherwise benefit from ECMO support may be at facilities without ECMO capabilities and yet be too unstable to transport to an ECMO-capable center. Under such circumstances, mobile ECMO transport teams may improve these patients' outcomes by performing ECMO cannulation at the origin hospital and transporting them to specialized centers capable of providing ongoing ECMO management.

   B. ECMO transport has been demonstrated to be safe and feasible. This highlights the potential role of regionalization of ECMO in order to maximize outcomes by referring patients to high-volume centers with greater experience and expertise.[25]

VIII. **Complications**

   A. Potential complications are inherent with any invasive intervention, especially among patients with severe underlying critical illness, and must be weighed against the potential benefit of the intervention. Complication rates for ECMO vary greatly based on center experience, management strategies, devices used, and patient characteristics.

      1. Commonly encountered hematologic complications include hemorrhage and thrombotic/thromboembolic events, the severities of which are heavily influenced by center-specific anticoagulation practices and patient-specific factors. Less common hematologic complications include hemolysis, thrombocytopenia, disseminated intravascular coagulation, acquired von Willebrand disease, and HIT.

         a. The diagnosis of HIT during ECMO should be made based on appropriate clinical criteria (eg, 4T score). If HIT is suspected, a heparin antibody test should be performed as an initial screening test, followed by a serotonin release assay if the heparin antibody test is positive. Alternate anticoagulants (eg, direct thrombin inhibitors) may be used for anticoagulation while awaiting the results of serologic testing.

      2. Infectious complication rates vary substantially by center and by the manner in which ECMO-related infections are defined. Standardized infection control practices should be used for ECMO insertion, maintenance, and removal.

      3. Other complications, such as limb ischemia, limb engorgement, and vascular perforation, may be a consequence of certain ECMO cannulation approaches and techniques, and will be influenced by the experience of the provider performing the procedure and the use of radiographic guidance. Prompt Doppler examination in the ICU will guide interventions.

IX. **Economic Considerations**

   A. The implementation across a health system of any novel technology, particularly for commonly encountered diseases, has to take into consideration the resources it may require, including financial resources that will vary greatly by region. There are limited data on the economic impact of ECMO use in ARDS, and even less for ECMO for cardiac failure. The CESAR trial, conducted within the United Kingdom's National Health Service, estimated that referral for consideration of ECMO led to a gain of 0.03 quality-adjusted life-years (QALYs) at 6-month follow-up, with the predicted cost per QALY of ECMO to be £19,252 (95% CI £7,622-59,200).

   B. Any future prospective randomized studies assessing the role of ECMO in cardiopulmonary failure would benefit from characterizing the economic impact in addition to the clinical outcomes, so that hospitals and health care systems can best decide how to allocate the resources appropriately.

C. The role of ECMO in the context of a global pandemic, such as that experienced with COVID-19, remains an area of active debate. When available medical resources are insufficient to meet the health care demands, there is a need for more judicious use of resource-intensive interventions such as ECMO, taking into consideration who is likely to derive the greatest benefit and at what cost—both in terms of resource utilization and the potential impact on the care of other patients.[26]

X. Ethical Considerations

With the advent of technology that is able to entirely support the respiratory or cardiac system, and to do so for prolonged periods of time, the creation of ethically challenging situations is inevitable.[27]

A. The ability of ECPR to improve survival beyond conventional CPR opens up the potential for ECPR to be used indiscriminately among patients suffering cardiac arrest, a practice that has the capacity to prolong suffering for many patients without changing the ultimate outcome. Whenever possible, evidence-based criteria ought to be used to identify patients most likely to benefit from ECPR.

B. The lack of destination device therapy in end-stage respiratory failure creates its own unique dilemma. Patients supported with ECMO as bridge to transplant who are no longer deemed transplant candidates and yet are dependent on ECMO for respiratory function have no viable long-term solution, often referred to as a "bridge to nowhere." Whether to continue supporting these patients and for how long, particularly those patients who are sentient, is a fraught situation that often requires ethics and palliative care consultations and extensive discussions with the patient and family. Potential bridge-to-transplant candidates ought to be carefully selected so as to avoid the "bridge to nowhere" scenario whenever possible.

C. Because venoarterial ECMO may adequately support end-organ perfusion in the absence of native cardiac function, the relevance of CPR, and thus a "Do Not Resuscitate" (DNR) order, may be murky. This highlights the need to understand not only the procedures to be performed but also the overall goals of care. Even in the absence of a physiologic benefit of CPR, a DNR order may still help convey the goals of care for the patient, particularly if it is deemed that meaningful recovery cannot be achieved. At that point, the conversation should focus on limiting or withdrawing life-sustaining treatments.

REFERENCES

1. Brodie D, Slutsky AS, Combes A. Extracorporeal life support for adults with respiratory failure and related indications: a review. *JAMA*. 2019;322(6):557-568.
2. The Acute Respiratory Distress Syndrome Network; Brower RG, Matthay MA, et al. Ventilation with lower tidal volumes as compared with traditional tidal volumes for acute lung injury and the acute respiratory distress syndrome. *N Engl J Med*. 2000;342(18):1301-1308.
3. Goligher EC, Tomlinson G, Hajage D, et al. Extracorporeal membrane oxygenation for severe acute respiratory distress syndrome and posterior probability of mortality benefit in a post hoc Bayesian analysis of a randomized clinical trial. *JAMA*. 2018;320(21):2251-2259.
4. Munshi L, Walkey A, Goligher E, et al. Venovenous extracorporeal membrane oxygenation for acute respiratory distress syndrome: a systematic review and meta-analysis. *Lancet Respir Med*. 2019;7(2):163-172.
5. Combes A, Peek GJ, Hajage D, et al. ECMO for severe ARDS: systematic review and individual patient data meta-analysis. *Intensive Care Med*. 2020;46(11):2048-2057.
6. Aoyama H, Uchida K, Aoyama K, et al. Assessment of therapeutic interventions and lung protective ventilation in patients with moderate to severe acute respiratory distress syndrome: a systematic review and network meta-analysis. *JAMA Netw Open*. 2019;2(7):e198116.
7. Combes A, Hajage D, Capellier G, et al. Extracorporeal membrane oxygenation for severe acute respiratory distress syndrome. *N Engl J Med*. 2018;378(21):1965-1975.
8. Barbaro RP, MacLaren G, Boonstra PS, et al. Extracorporeal membrane oxygenation support in COVID-19: an international cohort study of the Extracorporeal Life Support Organization registry. *Lancet*. 2020;396(10257):1071-1078.
9. Barbaro RP, MacLaren G, Boonstra PS, et al. Extracorporeal membrane oxygenation for COVID-19: evolving outcomes from the international Extracorporeal Life Support Organization registry. *Lancet*. 2021;398(10307):1230-1238.
10. Urner M, Barnett AG, Bassi GL, et al. Venovenous extracorporeal membrane oxygenation in patients with acute covid-19 associated respiratory failure: comparative effectiveness study. *BMJ*. 2022;377:e068723.
11. Abrams D, Brodie D, Arcasoy SM. Extracorporeal life support in lung transplantation. *Clin Chest Med*. 2017;38(4):655-666.
12. Combes A, Price S, Slutsky AS, et al. Temporary circulatory support for cardiogenic shock. *Lancet*. 2020;396(10245):199-212.
13. Brechot N, Hajage D, Kimmoun A, et al. Venoarterial extracorporeal membrane oxygenation to rescue sepsis-induced cardiogenic shock: a retrospective, multicentre, international cohort study. *Lancet*. 2020;396(10250):545-552.

14. Ostadal P, Rokyta R, Karasek J, et al. Extracorporeal membrane oxygenation in the therapy of cardiogenic shock: results of the ECMO-CS randomized clinical trial. *Circulation.* 2023;147(6):454-464.

15. Yannopoulos D, Bartos J, Raveendran G, et al. Advanced reperfusion strategies for patients with out-of-hospital cardiac arrest and refractory ventricular fibrillation (ARREST): a phase 2, single centre, open-label, randomised controlled trial. *Lancet.* 2020;396(10265):1807-1816.

16. Belohlavek J, Smalcova J, Rob D, et al. Effect of intra-arrest transport, extracorporeal cardiopulmonary resuscitation, and immediate invasive assessment and treatment on functional neurologic outcome in refractory out-of-hospital cardiac arrest: a randomized clinical trial. *JAMA.* 2022;327(8):737-747.

17. Suverein MM, Delnoij TSR, Lorusso R, et al. Early Extracorporeal CPR for Refractory Out-of-Hospital Cardiac Arrest. *N Engl J Med.* 2023;388(4):299-309.

18. Low CJW, Ramanathan K, Ling RR, et al. Extracorporeal cardiopulmonary resuscitation versus conventional cardiopulmonary resuscitation in adults with cardiac arrest: a comparative meta-analysis and trial sequential analysis. *Lancet Respir Med.* 2023;11(10):883-893.

19. Abrams DC, Brodie D, Rosenzweig EB, et al. Upper-body extracorporeal membrane oxygenation as a strategy in decompensated pulmonary arterial hypertension. *Pulm Circ.* 2013;3(2):432-435.

20. Combes A, Fanelli V, Pham T, et al. Feasibility and safety of extracorporeal CO_2 removal to enhance protective ventilation in acute respiratory distress syndrome: the SUPERNOVA study. *Intensive Care Med.* 2019;45(5):592-600.

21. McNamee JJ, Gillies MA, Barrett NA, et al. Effect of lower tidal volume ventilation facilitated by extracorporeal carbon dioxide removal vs standard care ventilation on 90-day mortality in patients with acute hypoxemic respiratory failure: the REST randomized clinical trial. *JAMA.* 2021;326(11):1013-1023.

22. Agerstrand CL, Burkart KM, Abrams DC, Bacchetta MD, Brodie D. Blood conservation in extracorporeal membrane oxygenation for acute respiratory distress syndrome. *Ann Thorac Surg.* 2015;99(2):590-595.

23. Martucci G, Schmidt M, Agerstrand C, et al. Transfusion practice in patients receiving VV ECMO (PROTECMO): a prospective, multicentre, observational study. *Lancet Respir Med.* 2023;11(3):245-255.

24. Abrams D, Madahar P, Eckhardt CM, et al. Early mobilization during extracorporeal membrane oxygenation for cardiopulmonary failure in adults: factors associated with intensity of treatment. *Ann Am Thorac Soc.* 2022;19(1):90-98.

25. Combes A, Brodie D, Bartlett R, et al. Position paper for the organization of extracorporeal membrane oxygenation programs for acute respiratory failure in adult patients. *Am J Respir Crit Care Med.* 2014;190(5):488-496.

26. Brodie D, Abrams D, MacLaren G, et al. Extracorporeal membrane oxygenation during respiratory pandemics: past, present, and future. *Am J Respir Crit Care Med.* 2022;205(12):1382-1390.

27. Abrams DC, Prager K, Blinderman CD, et al. Ethical dilemmas encountered with the use of extracorporeal membrane oxygenation in adults. *Chest.* 2014;145(4):876-882.

9

Devices for Cardiac Support and Replacement

Michael T. Cain, Joseph C. Cleveland, Jr., and Jordan R. H. Hoffman

KEY POINTS

1. In New York Heart Association class IV heart failure (minimal activity–induced symptoms), VADs provide better survival and quality of life than medical therapy.
2. Mechanical circulatory support devices (MCSDs) most often are ventricular assist devices (VADs), which are indicated for bridging to myocardial recovery, cardiac transplantation, or as a permanent assist device (destination therapy).
3. Historically, the principal growth area for VADs has been destination therapy; however, a greater proportion of development has recently focused on temporary bridging devices. The predominant device used for destination therapy is the Abbott HeartMate 3, which has largely replaced the use of the HeartMate II and HeartWare HVAD.
4. Short-term bridging VADs include the CentriMag, Tandem Heart, Protek Duo, and Impella pumps, all of which are continuous-flow pumps that implant and operate in separate and distinct ways.
5. Separation from cardiopulmonary bypass (CPB) after left ventricular assist device placement may be complicated by right ventricular (RV) failure, which may require various combinations of pulmonary

arterial vasodilators (eg, milrinone, nitric oxide), inotropes (eg, dobutamine, epinephrine), and systemic arterial vasoconstrictors (eg, vasopressin), or use of right ventricular assist device (RVAD).

6. Common early postoperative problems include bleeding and RV dysfunction. Late postoperative problems include device thrombosis, stroke, and infection.

7. Continuous-flow VAD patients presenting for noncardiac surgery pose a variety of clinical problems, which include obtaining accurate measurements of blood pressure (BP) and pulse oximetry, maintaining VAD blood flow, as well as challenges with hemostasis.

8. Intra-aortic balloon pumps (IABPs) are most often used to provide temporary left ventricle (LV) support. IABPs augment diastolic blood flow to increase coronary artery blood flow and reduce LV afterload.

9. IABP inflation and deflation must be synchronized to the cardiac cycle, which can be done using either electrocardiography (ECG) or an intra-arterial waveform.

I. Introduction

The use of mechanical circulatory support devices (MCSDs), most commonly left ventricular assist devices (LVADs), has grown significantly in recent years. As the population ages and the incidence of heart failure rises, the supply of donor hearts for transplantation remains insufficient. Therefore, a larger percentage of patients are undergoing LVAD surgery as a bridge to heart transplantation. In addition, a significant number of patients who are not eligible for transplantation are undergoing LVAD implantation as permanent, or destination, therapy. The development of newer, short-term MCSDs has led to increased growth of patients being supported for interventional cardiology and cardiac surgery procedures, as well as for bridging strategies for myocardial recovery after infarction or myocarditis.

CLINICAL PEARL

Relatively small intracardiac shunts can enlarge when the left-sided filling pressures are reduced after LVAD implantation.

CLINICAL PEARL

Right ventricular (RV) function will typically deteriorate after LVAD implantation and will often require significant inotropic or temporary mechanical support.

Devices are getting smaller, easier to implant, and more durable. This chapter will discuss the current state of mechanical circulatory support, including available devices and therapies.

II. History

Dr Michael DeBakey performed the first successful clinical implant of a ventricular assist device (VAD) for postcardiotomy cardiac failure in 1966,[1] followed by the first "bridge" to transplantation by Dr Denton Cooley in 1978.[2] The total artificial heart (TAH) was first used on Dr Barney Clarke, a retired dentist, by Dr William DeVries and Dr Lyle Joyce in 1982 at the University of Utah[3] using a Jarvik-7 TAH designed by Dr Robert Jarvik. Dr Clarke lived for 112 days but unfortunately died from sepsis and embolic events. Slow, steady advancements in pump design and understanding founded on this early work ultimately resulted in the first device to receive Food and Drug Administration (FDA) approval in the United States: the Abiomed BVS 5000 (Abiomed) in November, 1992. Multiple implantable and eventually dischargeable devices were subsequently developed and approved. In 2001, the landmark REMATCH (Randomized Evaluation of Mechanical Assistance for the Treatment of Congestive Heart Failure) trial led to the approval of the Thoratec VE for destination therapy, ushering in a new era for durable mechanical support.[4]

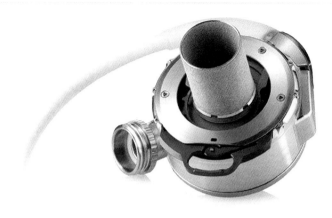

FIGURE 9.1 HeartMate 3 magnetically levitated centrifugal LVAD. (HeartMate 3 is trademark of Abbott or its related companies. Reproduced with permission of Abbott, © 2023. All rights reserved.)

The modern era has been defined by the development of smaller and safer devices. The HeartMate 3 (HM 3) (Figure 9.1) has been approved for bridge to transplantation and destination therapy after completion of the MOMENTUM 3 clinical trial and is currently the only approved durable LVAD after the FDA recall of the HeartWare HVAD (Medtronic) in June of 2021 due to increased adverse neurologic events and mortality associated with this device, as well as device malfunction.

Concurrent with the development of long-term, implantable LVADs, a number of short-term devices have been brought to market and are seeing increasing use. These devices are deployed by a variety of techniques and approaches but focus on providing short-term support as a bridge to recovery or destination therapy in acute ventricular failure.

III. Indications

2

There are three commonly described indications for the use of MCSDs: bridge to myocardial recovery, bridge to cardiac transplantation, and destination therapy.

A. Bridge to Recovery

The use of an MCSD as a recovery system has focused on short-term use. *Traditionally, this has been thought of as support for days to weeks.* Clinical indications for this use include cardiogenic shock in the following settings:

1. Postcardiotomy
2. Acute myocardial infarction
3. Viral cardiomyopathies
4. **Primary graft failure after cardiac transplantation**

The postcardiotomy use of these pumps has declined likely derived from improved perfusion and preservation techniques. Several devices are now employed as short-term bridge-to-recovery devices: the Abiomed Impella CP, 5.5, and RP (for right heart dysfunction); the CentriMag system and the TandemHeart systems; and the Protek Duo and Spectrum dual lumen cannula systems. These short-term devices are especially useful in catastrophic, sudden presentations of cardiogenic shock (eg, prolonged cardiac arrest during high-risk percutaneous coronary interventions) situations in which the likelihood of intact neurologic recovery remains unknown. These devices allow time to determine whether an irreversible neurologic injury, or other irreversible end-organ damage, would determine the patient's ultimate outcome.

B. Bridge to Transplantation

Mechanical support devices traditionally have been instituted in individuals who were listed for cardiac transplantation but failing conventional or inotropic therapy. *The MCSD can be employed to support the patient and improve the physiologic condition until they are suitable for transplantation.*

Currently, the most commonly used VAD in the United States is the Abbott HM 3, after the recall of the Medtronic HeartWare HVAD. The HM 3 is the immediate successor to the HM II and bolsters a fully magnetically levitated centrifugal-flow design. This reduces shear forces and heat generation, making this device more hemocompatible than previous devices. These design advantages have been studied in the MOMENTUM 3 clinical trials, which concluded that this device was superior to axial flow devices with respect to event-free survival, disabling stroke, need for pump replacement, and pump malfunction.[5,6] Historically, evaluation for LVAD candidacy has carried the requirement that individuals have been evaluated for heart transplantation as well; however, in a December 1, 2020 updated policy, the Center for Medicare and Medicaid Services (CMS) made significant changes to requirements for reimbursement for durable LVADs by removing the prior therapeutic intent-to-treat criteria of bridge to transplant (BTT) and destination therapy (DT) for LVAD. These changes, in effect, eliminate the need, on a reimbursement level, for a transplant evaluation prior to LVAD implantation, essentially uncoupling heart transplant and LVAD centers.

C. Destination Therapy

As experience with long-term use of MCSD led to successful outpatient use of this therapy, the concept of using MCSD as another option for patients with end-stage heart failure who were not transplant candidates emerged.

A landmark REMATCH study concluded that *patients with end-stage heart failure who received a Thoratec Heartmate VE LVAD experienced improved survival and quality of life when compared to optimal medical therapy*. The use of MCSD as permanent support for end-stage heart failure is now an accepted and viable therapy that is also supported by the Center for Medicare Services (CMS). The HM II received FDA approval for DT in 2009. The HeartWare HVAD subsequently was approved for use as DT following the HeartWare ENDURANCE clinical trial[7]; however, issues surrounding pump malfunction have resulted in the recall of this device. The MOMENTUM 3 clinical trials of the HM 3 have resulted in approval of this device for DT and BTT.

IV. Classification and Attachment Sites of Ventricular Assist Devices

VADs can be used as an isolated LVAD, an isolated right ventricular assist device (RVAD), or as a biventricular assist device (BIVAD). These devices can be surgically implanted or inserted percutaneously. TAHs differ from VADs in that a TAH is inserted by resecting both ventricles and anastomosing the sewing cuffs of the TAH to the mitral and tricuspid annuli (Figure 9.2).

A. Left Ventricular Assist Device

For left-sided circulatory support, the inflow for all of the approved devices resides in the LV, with the exception of TandemHeart, which has a cannula in the left atrium. *The LV apex is the preferred site of LVAD attachment for long-term devices.* The Impella platform is placed across the aortic valve, with the inflow in the LV. *The LVAD outflow graft is routinely anastomosed to the aorta*, usually the ascending aorta. The Impella outflow is immediately distal to the aortic valve, and the TandemHeart outflow is in the femoral artery for retrograde flow into the aorta.

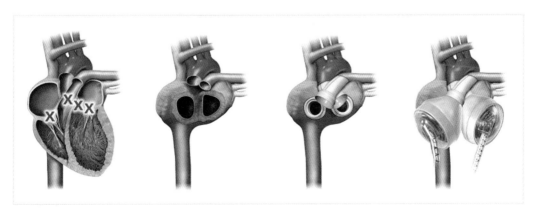

FIGURE 9.2 TAH implant requires resection of both ventricles. (Courtesy of syncardia.com.)

4

B. Right Ventricular Assist Device

For right-sided support, either *right atrial or right ventricular (RV) cannulation can be used successfully*. Substantial thrombus formation in the RV does not appear to result from right atrial cannulation even in long-term support, although this experience is limited. Right atrial cannulation is therefore the most common approach. *The RVAD outflow graft is anastomosed to the pulmonary artery (PA)*. VADs can be implanted without the support of cardiopulmonary bypass (CPB), but CPB is generally used to maintain patient stability.[7] Percutaneous RVAD support generates similar drainage and outflow by using a curved dual lumen cannula which drains blood from the right atrium endovascularly and ejects it out the cannula tip positioned distal to the pulmonic valve.

C. Biventricular Assist Device

A BIVAD consists of the simultaneous use of RVAD and LVAD with connections as noted earlier for the individual assist devices. A combination of short- and long-term devices can be used in a BIVAD configuration if required.

D. Total Artificial Heart

Placement of a TAH requires excision of the native ventricle. The SynCardia TAH requires the removal of the ventricles, preserving the tricuspid and mitral annulus for securing the device. Valves are located in both the inlet (atrioventricular) and the outlet (aortic or pulmonary) positions. Separate graft conduits connect the two pumping chambers to the aorta and main PA.

V. Mechanical Assistance Systems

5

A variety of mechanical support systems are used to treat patients with end-stage heart failure. While early-generation pumps were pulsatile, all currently available devices (with the exception of the SynCardia TAH) are continuous-flow devices. The current technologies include axial flow (Impella) and centrifugal designs (HM 3, TandemHeart).

A. Pulsatile

Pulsatile pumps are generally volume displacement pumps that work like the native heart. These are often called first-generation pumps. The pumping chamber fills for a set duration of time, and this volume of blood is ejected into the aorta. Pulsatile pumps all have inflow and outflow valves mimicking the native mitral and aortic valves. The SynCardia TAH is pneumatically driven to generate a pulsatile flow similar to the native heart. The device rate and percent systole (ejection time) are set to achieve normal values for cardiac output.

B. Continuous Flow

Axial flow devices with bearings are considered "second-generation" devices, whereas centrifugal pumps are considered "third-generation" devices.

1. **Short-term support:** Several continuous-flow pumps are currently being utilized in the United States as short-term support devices: CentriMag (Thoratec Corp.), the TandemHeart (TandemLife, Inc.), the Protek Duo (Livanova), the Spectrum RVAD (Spectrum Medical), and Impella (Abiomed).

2. **The CentriMag pump:** Is most commonly utilized with an open chest implantation with left atrial or LV inflow cannulation for the LVAD, and ascending aortic cannulation for outflow. The right atrium or RV can be cannulated for inflow and the PA as outflow for an RVAD.

3. **The TandemHeart pump:** Is unique as a percutaneous LVAD. The inflow is placed via the right common femoral vein, across the intra-atrial septum into the left atrium. The outflow is in the descending thoracic aorta via a cannula placed in the femoral artery. Given the more challenging transeptal nature of this device, the use of the TandemHeart has waned as other devices have come to market.

4. **The Impella system:** Comes in a variety of sizes and can be placed percutaneously or via cutdown through a graft, depending on the goals of treatment and device size. When placed percutaneously, it is placed via the common femoral artery, retrograde across the aortic valve into the LV. Inflow is through the LV and outflow is into the ascending aorta—the VAD is placed across the aortic valve. A larger Impella 5.5 is placed surgically through a cutdown and vascular graft in the femoral or axillary arteries and can provide up to 5.5 L/min of flow (Figure 9.3A and B).

5. **Long-term support:** Although previously the two most commonly used continuous-flow LVADs had been the HM II LVAD and the HeartWare ventricular assist device (HVAD),

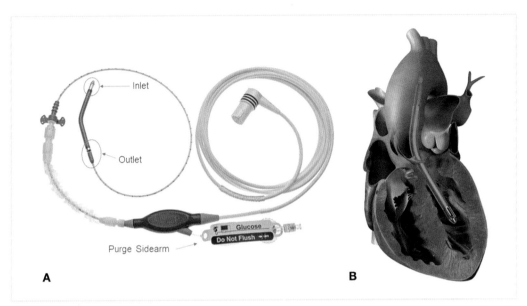

FIGURE 9.3 **(A)** Impella 5.5 catheter-based left ventricular assist device (LVAD). **(B)** Transaortic placement of Impella system with inflow port in left ventricle and outflow port in the proximal ascending aorta. **(A:** Reprinted with permission from ABIOMED, Inc. **B:** Reprinted with permission from Ramzy D, Soltesz E, Anderson M. New surgical circulatory support system outcomes. ASAIO J. 2020;66(7):746-752.)

recent results of the Abbot HM 3 clinical trials and withdrawal of the HVAD have restricted durable LVAD options. Currently, the HM 3 is the only FDA-approved LVAD, approved for DT and bridge to transplantation.

6. **Advantages and disadvantages:** *Continuous-flow devices offer the advantage of being much smaller than their pulsatile counterparts, as no "blood chamber" is needed.* Their smaller size often leads to easier implantation with less intraoperative dissection. This can reduce blood loss, shorten operative times, reduce infection rates, and provide the potential for more rapid patient recovery. Furthermore, smaller device size has allowed for sternal-sparing thoracotomy-based approaches to implantation, which may allow for reduced RV dysfunction following implantation. This sternal-sparing technique can facilitate a less challenging reoperation for heart transplantation for bridge-to-transplant candidates. The data generated from the outcomes with the utilization of continuous-flow devices as a bridge-to-transplant indication show excellent 1-year survival of 86.6%. The 2-year survival for the cohort that received the HM 3 was 79%, with event-free survival reaching 74.7% across this time frame. These outcomes were notably improved compared with axial flow devices, which showed an event-free survival of 60.6% across 2 years, and are a clinical representation of the technological advancement in the field.[7-10]

7. **Continuous-flow devices pose inherent challenges:** These devices do not have valves and need to flow at a minimum rate to prevent stasis and thrombus formation. In addition, as patients are managed with long-term devices, certain complications that are device related have emerged. The HM II LVAD, HVAD, and HM 3 universally cleave the von Willebrand factor (vWF). Nearly all patients with an HM II LVAD acquire a deficiency in vWF and are prone to mucosal bleeding events—particularly in the gastrointestinal tract.[11] The recently available HM 3 is a magnetically levitated centrifugal pump, and recent studies have demonstrated a decrease in the rate of pump thrombus while providing full circulatory support.[12] *Many patients have minimal arterial pulsatility when on full support.* This is not generally problematic when arterial pressure is monitored with an indwelling arterial catheter but may become so when the patient leaves the intensive care unit (ICU) or leaves the hospital for home or an extended care facility. In most cases, an automated blood pressure (BP) cuff is inaccurate, and manual Doppler monitoring of BP is required.

VI. **Intraoperative Considerations**
  A. **Anesthetic Considerations**
    1. **Monitoring:** Standard American Society of Anesthesiologists monitors (electrocardiography [ECG], pulse oximetry, temperature) are used with the exception of a noninvasive BP cuff. As noted earlier, an arterial catheter is essential. *Monitoring cerebral oxygenation using near-infrared spectroscopy (NIRS) technology is recommended, especially since the absence of pulsatile blood flow will render conventional pulse oximetry unreliable.* PA catheters can be very helpful for the assessment of RV function and pulmonary vascular resistance (PVR), but they may be mechanically infeasible after initiation of therapy with RVAD, BIVAD, or TAH. *Intraoperative transesophageal echocardiography is essential* for the assessment of aortic valve competency, patent foramen ovale (PFO), LV thrombus, adequacy of VAD inflow and outflow, cardiac preload assessment, and RV function (for isolated LVADs).

CLINICAL PEARL

Intraoperative transesophageal echocardiography should focus on aortic valve competence, intracardiac shunts, LV thrombus, positioning of LVAD inflow cannula, cardiac preload, and RV function.

    2. **Cardiac rhythm management device:** Many of these patients will have an implanted cardiac rhythm management device (automatic implantable cardioverter-defibrillator and/or pacemaker) that requires a management plan prior to proceeding with induction of anesthesia. The antiarrhythmic functions will need to be turned off, so they are not triggered by electrocautery during surgery. As soon as such deactivation occurs, patients require continuous ECG monitoring and external cardioversion capability needs to be immediately available. Management of the pacemaker function is dependent on the patient's underlying rhythm, the device's current settings, and its pacing activity. Please see Chapter 6 for these considerations. Once the procedure is completed, it is critical to reinstate antiarrhythmic functions and interrogate the device.

CLINICAL PEARL

Dysrhythmias can be particularly detrimental in the setting of depressed ventricular function. External defibrillator pads should be placed on the patient prior to induction of anesthesia.

    3. **Vascular access:** *Large-bore vascular access is required* because blood loss and coagulopathy can be substantial. This can be achieved with one large-bore (16 gauge or larger) peripheral intravenous catheter and a large-lumen (eg, 9Fr) central-access introducer or with its equivalent via central venous access (eg, a PA catheter introducer with additional double-lumen large-bore integral ports).
    4. **Anesthetic techniques:** Anesthetic drugs should be titrated carefully, accounting for slower circulation time and a lower volume of distribution for drugs in patients with heart failure. Hypoxia and hypercarbia can further impair myocardial function and increase PVR. Hence, periods of apnea should be avoided and ventilation continued even when performing a rapid sequence induction.

      Preexisting inotropic and vasoactive drugs should be continued. Patients often present with high levels of intrinsic sympathetic tone to the operating room and induction of anesthesia frequently is followed by marked hypotension. In addition to careful titration of anesthetic drugs, starting a low-dose vasoactive infusion, such as norepinephrine, prior to induction may preempt such effects.

      Secondary organ dysfunction should be considered in the choice of anesthetic drugs; for example, cisatracurium would be appropriate as a muscle relaxant in a patient with impaired liver function. Nitrous oxide probably should be avoided because of its potential to increase PVR and the high risk of intravascular air.

B. **Surgical Techniques**
   1. **Cannulation techniques**
      a. **VADs:** VAD implantation is most commonly performed using CPB without myocardial arrest. Atrial cannulation is the most common approach to gain inflow for short-term support when using either a right- or left-sided VAD system to allow for better hemostasis due to the low-pressure system. Cannulation of the LV apex for inflow minimizes blood stasis in the ventricle and provides the best decompression of the heart, which may aid in myocardial recovery. However, decannulation and repair of this high-pressure chamber can be difficult and often require placement back onto CPB. LV apex cannulation is highly recommended when a prosthetic mitral valve is present to maintain blood flow through the valve and prevent thrombus formation. *The LV apex is the sole acceptable inflow cannulation site for most long-term LVADs.*
      b. **TAH:** For implantation of a TAH, excision of the native ventricles must be performed while preserving the atria. After initiation of CPB with bicaval cannulation, the surgeon attaches sewing cuffs that will connect the atria to the TAH pumping chambers, after which the surgeon sews grafts to both the aorta and the main PA. The TAH is then attached to the atrial cuffs after a leak test, followed by the arterial grafts.

C. **Initiation of Support for Left Ventricular Assist Device**
   1. **Initial considerations:** Following implantation, ventilation is reestablished and the heart is gradually filled. The assist device is started at a slow rate until adequate preload and afterload are established. *If the ventricle(s) are not decompressed with the initiation of support, inflow obstruction (into the VAD) must be considered.* Transesophageal echocardiography (TEE) should be utilized to identify interventricular septal position. Displacement toward the LV may compromise right heart function by impairing the septal component of RV contraction. Treatment is reduction of LVAD speed and increased medical therapy for RV function, such as inotropes and inhaled pulmonary vasodilators. *Right-sided function may be further compromised by increased* PVR caused by thromboxane A2 and transfusion-induced cytokine activation as a result of CPB.[13]
   2. **Role of transesophageal echocardiography:** Use of TEE to separate from CPB is essential. TEE is used to assess the presence of ventricular air and inflow chamber decompression. *If the chamber is full, or has poor device flow, there is a technical issue that needs to be identified and corrected.* If the LV is empty and there is poor flow through the VAD, then there is either inadequate RV preload or right heart failure. The apical interventricular septum can occasionally deflect leftward and obstruct inflow into the LVAD, causing a phenomenon known as a suction event. TEE is also used to identify aortic insufficiency and the presence of intracardiac shunts, either of which may arise at the time of VAD support.
   3. **Aortic insufficiency:** *Aortic valve insufficiency (AI) can be challenging, and TEE is essential to identify its presence or absence and severity.* With the implementation of LVAD support, the left ventricular end diastolic pressure (LVEDP) will become very low and the mean arterial pressure (MAP) will increase, so the aortic transvalvular gradient (MAP-LVEDP) will be much greater. Mild preoperative AI, therefore, can become severe AI with LVAD support. This will result in high LVAD flow rates which are deceptive because much of the flow is "circular" from LV to LVAD to the ascending aorta and back via the incompetent aortic valve to the LV. AI should be treated aggressively; however, the ideal approach is still controversial (valve replacement vs permanent valve closure).[14-18]

CLINICAL PEARL

Aortic insufficiency in a patient being supported with a continuous-flow LVAD will typically be underestimated due to the continuous nature of the regurgitant jet.

4. **Intracardiac shunts:** *Quiescent intracardiac shunts may become clinically apparent and significant as a result of changes in chamber pressures when VAD support is initiated.* A PFO is present in up to 20% of the population but is clinically quiescent in the vast majority of patients. Upon unloading the LV and left atrium with LVAD support, right atrial pressure will become higher than left atrial pressure causing even a small PFO to produce a large right to left. These shunts should be closed when identified.

5. **Pharmacologic support:** *Inotropic agents (eg, dobutamine, milrinone, epinephrine) are important to support the right heart when only left-sided support is used. Inhaled nitric oxide or epoprostenol may be invaluable in the early management of these patients because of its capacity to vasodilate the pulmonary vasculature without the systemic hypotensive effects seen with other PA vasodilators.* Vasopressin offers an advantage over α-adrenergic agonists because it possesses minimal vasoconstrictive effects on the pulmonary arterial vasculature.

D. **Initiation of Support for Biventricular Assist Device**

1. **Initial considerations:** When initiating biventricular support, *the left system should be actuated first* to prevent LV overdistention and resultant pulmonary edema. The PA catheter should not be withdrawn as it will be difficult to reinsert it, although thermodilution cardiac outputs are not calculable when an RVAD is functioning. All available temporary RVADs have accurate flow measurement tools that can replace the need for Swan-Ganz cardiac output monitoring.

2. **Flow rates:** The RVAD and LVAD flow rates should be balanced at a 3:4 ratio. RVAD flow that exceeds LVAD flow early after initiating BIVAD support is worrisome. This can occur with two common scenarios:

   a. One or both left-sided cannulae are malpositioned to impede inflow to or from the device. If the obstruction is not corrected, the lungs can become flooded with the increased blood flow from the RVAD.

   b. The LV is beginning to recover and is ejecting some blood over and above the LVAD flow. This can be identified by the appearance of an arterial pressure waveform corresponding to the QRS complex of the ECG (see "**Weaning From Ventricular Assist Device Support**" section).

E. **Initiation of Support for Right Ventricular Assist Device**

1. **Initial considerations:** CPB is weaned as RVAD support is increased. All currently available devices can overcome elevated PVR; however, significantly elevated PA pressures may lead to pulmonary edema.

2. **Pharmacologic support:** In many instances, some inotropic support of the LV will be necessary to handle the increased RV output.

VII. **Postoperative Management and Complications**

7

A. **Right-Sided Circulatory Failure**

Right-sided circulatory management is the key to perioperative care for patients with LVAD. Attention to right heart management and PVR is critical. Strategies include chronotropy, inotropy, and pulmonary vasodilators to increase flow through the pulmonary vascular bed. For additional considerations, see "Initiation of Support for Left Ventricular Assist Device" section.

B. **Hemorrhage**

Postoperative hemorrhage is common in this patient population. Hepatic and renal dysfunction lead to imbalances in platelet function and the coagulation cascade, which are exacerbated by CPB. Use of a thromboelastogram (TEG) and thromboelastometry to help target the deficiency in the clotting process is gaining popularity.

C. **Thromboembolism**

Thromboembolism is associated with all current assist systems. The unique design characteristics of each system as well as the patient's underlying pathology establish the overall risk. Anticoagulation with heparin is required for short-term devices, and warfarin and aspirin are required with all long-term assist devices.

D. **Infection**

Device-related infection is the most common cause of morbidity in the chronically supported patient. Driveline and device "pocket" infections occur in up to 40% of these patients. The vast majority of these infections may be managed with chronic antibiotic therapy until transplantation. Device exchange for infection has not been demonstrated to be universally effective due to the necessary replacement of the new pump into an infected field.

E. **Device Malfunction**

Catastrophic device malfunctions occur infrequently but can be life threatening. These include mechanical device failure, device separation or fracture, graft or valve rupture, and console failure. Minor device malfunctions occur more frequently and are usually addressed at the bedside. These include driveline damage and controller malfunctions. All of these malfunctions are becoming increasingly rare as yearly device modifications and software upgrades are introduced.

VIII. **Weaning From Ventricular Assist Device Support**

A minority of patients will experience myocardial recovery sufficient for device explantation.[19] For patients in whom the heart recovers, the heart will be able to eject, and the arterial waveform will begin to display pulses corresponding to the QRS complex.[20] When the device flows are weaned downward and cardiac preload conditions move toward normal, these ejections will become more prominent. *If the device can be weaned to 1 L/min flow and the patient can maintain adequate perfusion with reasonable inotropic support, explantation can be considered.* Final weaning from the device is accomplished in the operating room with TEE as surgical cutdown on the access site is often needed for device explantation.

IX. **Management of the Patient With Ventricular Assist Device for Noncardiac Surgery**

These patients can be very ill if surgery is contemplated early after MCSD implantation. However, patients will often recover physiologically over the ensuing weeks and months. Patients who are stable on support may safely undergo noncardiac surgical procedures.[21,22] The optimal approach involves asking some basic questions:

A. What chamber(s) are being assisted (LVAD, RVAD, BIVAD, or TAH)?

B. What type of pump is being used? All continuous-flow pumps are preload dependent and afterload sensitive. Percutaneous and peripherally inserted pumps are also positional and patient movement may impact device functionality.

C. Is technical support personnel available to help manage and troubleshoot the pump? This is critical for transport as well as intraoperative management.

D. *How does one determine flow through the pump?* This can be quantitative or qualitative, depending upon the pump, but knowledge of pump flow clearly assists in determining systemic vascular resistance and PVR, which in turn guide anesthetic drug selection, pharmacologic support, and volume management.

E. Will TEE be helpful? If major volume shifts are anticipated, the use of TEE can be very helpful in assessing preload, valvular function, and intracardiac shunts.

F. What is the patient's clotting status? For most pumps, anticoagulation and antiplatelet medications are required. Reversal of warfarin and conversion to intravenous heparin may be indicated. In general, be prepared for transfusion of red blood cells and other components.

G. What is the patient's intravenous access? Central venous access is desirable in most situations, but large-bore peripheral access is acceptable for minor surgical procedures.

H. What pharmacologic support is the patient receiving? This will vary from no support to multiple inotropes, antiarrhythmics, vasoconstrictors, and pulmonary vasodilators. If nitric oxide is in use, this will require planning for transport and operating room use.

I. Will electrocautery affect the assist device? For most devices, this will not be a problem, but excessive electrocautery can intermittently interfere with the function of coexisting pacemakers or defibrillators.

    J. If defibrillation or electrical cardioversion is needed, how will it be most safely applied?

    K. If the patient does not have pulsatile blood flow, consider the use of NIRS technology to monitor cerebral oxygenation as conventional pulse oximetry relies on pulsatile blood flow.

X. Intra-aortic Balloon Pump Circulatory Assistance

A. Indications for Placement

Thought by some to be reserved for placement after one or more failed attempts at separation from CPB, the number of intra-aortic balloon pumps (IABPs) placed in the cardiac catheterization laboratory far exceeds the number placed intraoperatively. Interventional cardiologists often place IABPs when high-grade lesions of proximal coronary vessels supplying large regions of myocardium are diagnosed, when myocardial ischemia persists, or when myocardial infarction (MI) occurs after an intervention such as coronary stent placement. Retrospective outcome studies for preoperative versus intraoperative placement of IABP for coronary artery bypass graft (CABG) patients suggest that preoperative IABP placement improves outcome and shortens hospital stay, especially for patients with low ejection fractions or those undergoing urgent or emergent CABG[23]; however, RCTs including the SHOCK II trial have demonstrated no improvement in 30-day mortality in patients with cardiogenic shock complicating acute MI who receive an IABP.[24] As a result, there is ongoing robust debate about the utility of the IABP. Moderately severe LV failure despite reasonable inotropic support that is thought to derive from an injury that will resolve (or greatly improve) within 24-48 hours (eg, LV stunning) constitutes the most common intraoperative indication. Unfortunately, the definitions of "LV failure," "maximal inotropic support," and "ongoing regional myocardial ischemia" vary widely among surgeons and anesthesiologists, confounding its use.

B. Contraindications to Placement

    1. Aortic insufficiency: Use of the IABP is relatively contraindicated in patients with AI. As the IABP inflates in the descending aorta during diastole to promote retrograde flow into the ascending aorta, this potentially increases aortic valvular regurgitation, further distending the LV at the expense of coronary perfusion.

    2. Sepsis: As with any prosthetic intravascular device, bacteremic infections are difficult to treat if the prosthetic surfaces become seeded with bacteria.

    3. Severe peripheral vascular disease: Placement of an IABP may be technically difficult in patients with atherosclerosis or other vascular pathologies. Such patients are more prone to arterial thrombosis and iatrogenic dissection during the use of an IABP. Patients with abdominal aortic aneurysms are at increased risk for aortic rupture, although balloons have been successfully passed and used in such patients. For patients with severe aortoiliac or femoral arterial disease, placement may be performed through a small vascular graft sewn to the subclavian artery.

C. Functional Design

The IABP consists of an inflatable balloon at the end of a catheter that is typically advanced into the descending thoracic aorta percutaneously from the femoral artery (Figure 9.4). The balloon inflates during diastole, displacing blood from the thoracic aorta and increasing aortic diastolic pressure. Balloon inflation improves coronary perfusion pressure, increasing coronary blood flow. During early systole, rapid balloon deflation reduces LV afterload and wall tension. IABP can improve myocardial energy balance at most by 15%. The IABP drive console consists of a pressurized gas reservoir that is connected to the balloon supply line through an electronically controlled solenoid valve. The gas used to inflate the balloon is either CO_2 or helium. The advantage of CO_2 is its high blood solubility, which reduces the consequences of balloon rupture with potential gas embolization. The advantage of helium is its low density, which thereby decreases the Reynolds number and allows the same flow through a smaller device, decreasing the potential for injury to the artery.

D. Intra-aortic Balloon Pump Placement

Insertion of the IABP is usually accomplished either percutaneously or by surgical cutdown into the femoral artery using the Seldinger technique for placement of a large-diameter introducer. Accurate placement of the Seldinger wire is often confirmed intraoperatively using TEE following which the balloon is passed through the introducer.

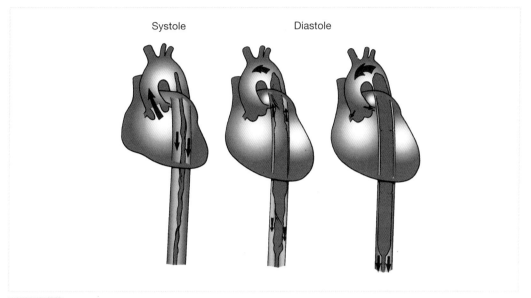

Systole   Diastole

FIGURE 9.4   Placement of the IABP in the aorta. The IABP is shown in the descending aorta, with the tip at the distal aortic arch. During systole, the balloon is deflated to enhance ventricular ejection. During diastole the balloon inflates, forcing blood from the proximal aorta into the coronary and peripheral vessels.

The balloon is positioned so that its tip is at the junction of the descending aorta and the aortic arch, just distal to the origin of the subclavian artery (Figure 9.5). This positioning minimizes the risk of subclavian or renal artery injury or occlusion. Radiographically, the tip should lie at the level of the carina on a chest x-ray.

When the IABP is placed intraoperatively, transesophageal echocardiography or fluoroscopy can confirm the proper tip location before initiation of balloon assistance.

CLINICAL PEARL

Intraoperative placement of an IABP will typically require TEE guidance for positioning: the tip of the catheter should be approximately 2 cm from the subclavian artery.

E. **Intra-aortic Balloon Pump Control**

Several parameters are important during the setup and operation of an IABP.

1. **Synchronization of the intra-aortic balloon pump:** Synchronization of the IABP with the cardiac rhythm is accomplished by using either the electrocardiographic QRS complex or the arterial pressure waveform. If there is a natural pulse pressure >40 mm Hg, use of the arterial waveform for synchronization is often preferred in the operating room because the electrical artifact produced by electrocautery inhibits ECG-triggered IABP control units. Most current consoles can differentiate pacer spikes from a QRS complex, allowing proper timing of IABP inflation even when atrial or atrioventricular pacing is in use, but pacer interference should be considered in the differential diagnosis of faulty IABP timing.

2. **Timing of balloon inflation and deflation:** When setting the timing of IABP inflation (Figure 9.5), it is important to time the onset of the pressure rise caused by balloon inflation with the dicrotic notch of the arterial waveform, which signifies aortic valve closure and the start of diastole. If inflation begins sooner, the IABP will impede ventricular ejection. If it begins later, the effectiveness of the balloon in augmenting coronary perfusion and reducing afterload will be limited. Deflation should be timed so that the arterial

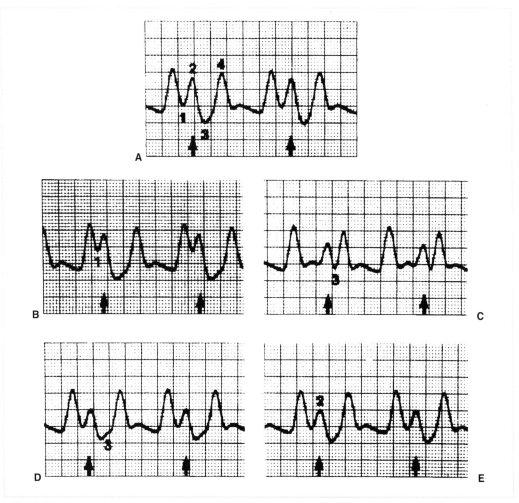

FIGURE 9.5 Manipulation of the timing of inflation and deflation of IABP. Tracings illustrate 1:2 support for the sake of clarity. **(A)** Normal tracing. Augmentation commences after the dicrotic notch (1), augments diastolic pressure (2), and reaches its nadir just before the next contraction (3). Peak systolic pressure in the next (nonaugmented) beat is decreased (4). **(B)** Early inflation. Augmentation commences before aortic valve closure (1), thereby increasing afterload and possibly inducing aortic regurgitation. **(C)** Late inflation. Diastolic augmentation is inadequate, and end-diastolic pressure is not different from that in the unassisted cycle (3). **(D)** Early deflation. Diastolic augmentation and afterload reduction are impaired. **(E)** Inadequate filling time. Timing is satisfactory, but diastolic augmentation is impaired. (Reprinted with permission from Sladen RN. Management of the adult cardiac patient in the intensive care unit. In: Ream AK, Fogdall RP, eds. *Acute Cardiovascular Management in Anesthesia and Intensive Care.* J.B. Lippincott Company; 1982:509.)

pressure just reaches its minimum level at the onset of the next ventricular pulse. If it deflates too soon, the aorta will not be maximally evacuated before ventricular contraction. If the balloon deflates too late, it will impede LV ejection. Most modern balloon devices use an intra-aortic arterial waveform obtained from the tip of the balloon catheter. If this mechanism should fail and synchronization should be monitored from another site, subtle differences in optimal timing may occur (eg, balloon inflation and deflation as judged by a femoral arterial waveform are delayed in comparison to an intra-aortic or radial arterial waveform).

3. **Ratio of native ventricle pulsations to intra-aortic balloon pump pulsation:** Pumping is frequently initiated at a ratio of 1:2 (one IABP beat for every two cardiac beats), so the natural ventricular beats and augmented beats can be compared to determine IABP timing and efficacy. If needed, the ratio can be increased to 1:1 to obtain maximal benefit.

4. **Stroke volume of the balloon:** The volume of gas used to inflate the balloon is determined by the balloon used and the patient's size. Typically, balloon volume is set to 50%-60% of the patient's ideal stroke volume.[25]

5. **Balloon filling:** The time required for the balloon to fill and empty is determined by the density of the gas used, gas pressure, the length and diameter of the gas line, and balloon volume. At high heart rates, the time required for balloon filling may limit balloon stroke volume.

F. **Intra-aortic Balloon Pump Weaning**

Weaning the patient from IABP circulatory assistance should be considered when inotropic support has been reduced substantially, allowing "room" to increase inotropic support as IABP support is reduced. Weaning is done primarily by gradually (over 6-12 hours) decreasing the ratio of augmented to native heartbeats (from 1:1 to 1:2 to 1:4 or less) and/or decreasing balloon inflation volume while monitoring hemodynamics. The balloon is never turned off while it remains in the aorta except when the patient is anticoagulated, as during CPB, due to the risk of thrombus formation. An IABP can be turned to a slow rate of 1:4 during a short weaning trial prior to removal, but this should not last longer than 30 minutes before being removed or returned to a rate of 1:2 or greater. As ventricular performance improves, the amplitude of the native pressure tracing will increase relative to the IABP augmented pressure tracing. Once the IABP is removed, it is important to closely examine the distal ipsilateral leg because partial or total femoral arterial occlusion may occur.

G. **Management of Anticoagulation During Intra-aortic Balloon Pump Assistance**

In the immediate post-CPB period, anticoagulants are not required for the first 6-12 hours or until drainage from the chest tubes is acceptable (<100-150 mL/h). Heparin can prevent IABP-related thrombosis and is used by some; however, evidence suggests that a no-heparin IABP protocol provides acceptable low rates of thrombus formation with fewer bleeding complications than when anticoagulation is used. The surgeon should weigh the risks of thrombus formation with prolonged heparin-free IABP use against the risk of excessive bleeding when using anticoagulation.[23]

H. **Complications**

The incidence of IABP complications has decreased significantly from its early use but significant morbidities persist. The most frequent complications are vascular complications, with a reported incidence of 6%-33%.[25] These complications include limb ischemia, compartment syndrome, mesenteric infarction, aortic perforation, and aortic dissection. Neurologic complications include paresthesia, ischemic neuritis, neuralgia, footdrop, and rarely paraplegia.[26] Balloon rupture with gas embolus can occur presumably as a result of severe aortic atherosclerotic calcifications. When this occurs, blood is usually seen in the gas driveline and the arterial pressure deflection caused by the IABP is lost. Air embolism from the pressure monitoring line to the brain is a larger risk from the IABP than from a radial artery catheter because the monitoring port is located at the tip of the balloon catheter, adjacent to the carotid arteries.

I. **Limitations**

The ability of the IABP to augment cardiac output and unload the LV is limited because the IABP does not directly affect LV function. With severe LV failure, an IABP will not provide sufficient flow to sustain the circulation. When the LV cannot eject blood into the aorta, the IABP will simply cause pulsations in the arterial waveform without increasing blood flow. In this situation, a VAD must be considered. Irregular heart rhythms persist as a limitation to IABP efficacy as the optimal timing of inflation and deflation cannot be achieved with large variations in the R-R interval.

REFERENCES

1. Ross JN Jr, Akers WW, O'Bannon W, et al. Problems encountered during the development and implantation of the Baylor-Rice orthotopic cardiac prosthesis. *Trans Am Soc Artif Intern Organs*. 1972;18:168-175, 179.

2. Norman JC, Brook MI, Cooley DA, et al. Total support of the circulation of a patient with post-cardiotomy stone-heart syndrome by a partial artificial heart (ALVAD) for 5 days followed by heart and kidney transplantation. *Lancet*. 1978;1(8074):1125-1127.

3. Joyce LD, DeVries WC, Hastings WL, et al. Response of the human body to the first permanent implant of the Jarvik-7 total artificial heart. *Trans Am Soc Artif Intern Organs*. 1983;29:81-87.

4. Rose E, Gelijns A, Moskowitz AJ, et al. Long-term use of a left ventricular assist device for end-stage heart failure. *N Engl J Med*. 2001;345(20):1435-1443.

5. Mehra MR, Uriel N, Naka Y, et al. A fully magnetically levitated left ventricular assist device—final report. *N Engl J Med*. 2019;380:1618-1627.

6. Bourque K, Cotter C, Dague C, et al. Design rationale and preclinical evaluation of the HeartMate 3 left ventricular assist system for hemocompatibility. *ASAIO J*. 2016;62:375-383.

7. Rogers JG, Pagani FD, Tatooles AJ, et al. Intrapericardial left ventricular assist device for advanced heart failure. *N Engl J Med*. 2017;376(5):451-460.

8. Mehra MR, Naka Y, Uriel N, et al. A fully magnetically levitated circulatory pump for advanced heart failure. *N Engl J Med*. 2017;376(5):440-450.

9. John R, Kamdar F, Eckman P, et al. Lessons learned from experience with over 100 consecutive HeartMate II left ventricular assist devices. *Ann Thorac Surg*. 2011;92(5):1593-1599; discussion 1599-1600.

10. Schmitto JD, Zimpfer D, Fiane AE, et al. Long-term support of patients receiving a left ventricular assist device for advanced heart failure: a follow-up analysis of the registry to evaluate the HeartWare left ventricular assist system. *Eur J Cardiothorac Surg*. 2016;50(5):834-838.

11. Crow S, Chen D, Milano C, et al. Acquired von Willebrand syndrome in continuous-flow ventricular assist device recipients. *Ann Thorac Surg*. 2010;90(4):1263-1269; discussion 1269.

12. John R, Naka Y, Smedira NG, et al. Continuous flow left ventricular assist device outcomes in commercial use compared with the prior clinical trial. *Ann Thorac Surg*. 2011;92(4):1406-1413.

13. Shenkar R, Coulson WF, Abraham E. Hemorrhage and resuscitation induce alterations in cytokine expression and the development of acute lung injury. *Am J Respir Cell Mol Biol*. 1994;10(3):290-297.

14. Atkins B, Hashmi ZA, Ganapathi AM, et al. Surgical correction of aortic valve insufficiency after left ventricular assist device implantation. *J Thorac Cardiovasc Surg*. 2013;146(5):1247-1252.

15. Bryant AS, Holman WL, Nanda NC, et al. Native aortic valve insufficiency in patients with left ventricular assist devices. *Ann Thorac Surg*. 2006;81(2):e6-e8.

16. Rajagopal K, Daneshmand MA, Patel CB, et al. Natural history and clinical effect of aortic valve regurgitation after left ventricular assist device implantation. *J Thorac Cardiovasc Surg*. 2013;145(5):1373-1379.

17. Savage EB, d'Amato TA, Magovern JA. Aortic valve patch closure: an alternative to replacement with HeartMate LVAS insertion. *Eur J Cardiothorac Surg*. 1999;16(3):359-361.

18. Pal JD, McCabe JM, Dardas T, et al. Transcatheter aortic valve repair for management of aortic insufficiency in patients supported with left ventricular assist devices. *J Card Surg*. 2016;31(10):654-657.

19. Helman DN, Maybaum SW, Morales DL, et al. Recurrent remodeling after ventricular assistance: is long-term myocardial recovery attainable? *Ann Thorac Surg*. 2000;70(4):1255-1258.

20. Birks EJ, Tansley PD, Hardy J, et al. Left ventricular assist device and drug therapy for the reversal of heart failure. *N Engl J Med*. 2006;355(18):1873-1884.

21. Garatti A, Bruschi G, Colombo T, et al. Noncardiac surgical procedures in patient supported with long-term implantable left ventricular assist device. *Am J Surg*. 2009;197(6):710-714.

22. Goldstein DJ, Mullis SL, Delphin ES, et al. Noncardiac surgery in long-term implantable left ventricular assist-device recipients. *Ann Surg*. 1995;222(2):203-207.

23. Kogan A, Preisman S, Sternik L, et al. Heparin-free management of intra-aortic balloon pump after cardiac surgery. *J Card Surg*. 2012;27(4):434-437.

24. Thiele H, Zeymer U, Neumann F, et al. Intraaortic balloon support for myocardial infarction with cardiogenic shock. *N Engl J Med*. 2012;367:1287-1296.

25. Webb CA, Weyker PD, Flynn BC. Management of intra-aortic balloon pumps. *Semin Cardiothorac Vasc Anesth*. 2015;19(2):106-121.

26. Hurlé A, Llamas P, Meseguer J, et al. Paraplegia complicating intraaortic balloon pumping. *Ann Thorac Surg*. 1997;63(4):1217-1218.

Cardiac Anesthesia

10

Preparation for Cardiac Surgery

Mark Robitaille, Daniela Garcia, and Shahzad Shaefi

KEY POINTS

1. Individual risk assessment is an important first step in preparing a patient for cardiac surgery.
2. The primary objectives of the preanesthetic evaluation are to evaluate cardiac and overall health risks, identify and optimize comorbidities, and anticipate any factors that may lead to complications during the intraoperative and postoperative periods.
3. Enhanced Recovery After Surgery (ERAS) is a perioperative multimodal care improvement initiative. Compared to conventional management, ERAS protocols have been associated with a reduction in perioperative complications and length of hospital stay. The first expert consensus on Enhanced Recovery After Cardiac Surgery (ERACS) provides preoperative recommendations for cardiac surgical patients.
4. While frailty is more common in the geriatric population, it can affect patients of all ages. Physiologic age predicts outcomes better after cardiac surgery than chronologic age.
5. Preoperative rehabilitation, commonly referred to as prehabilitation, aims to optimize current conditions and reduce postoperative morbidity. It involves tailored interventions targeting various systems based on individual patient needs to enhance functional and nutritional capacity and reduce postoperative morbidity.

I. Introduction

Preparation for cardiac surgery necessitates a comprehensive assessment of patient risk, including identifying preexisting comorbidities, a thorough understanding of perioperative medication management, and recognizing frailty and the potential benefits of prehabilitation. This chapter aims to provide insights into the overall risk assessment and prognostication, preanesthetic evaluation, and interventions that can optimize patients for cardiac surgery.

II. Risk Assessment

1

The initial step in preparing a patient for cardiac surgery involves assessing individual risk. Two widely employed risk models worldwide are the Society of Thoracic Surgeons (STS) Score and the European System for Cardiac Operative Risk Evaluation (EuroSCORE). These models are designed to enhance the predictive accuracy of risk based on patient characteristics.

A. **Society of Thoracic Surgeons Score**

The STS Adult Cardiac Risk Models were initially developed to incorporate risk adjustment into the outcomes analysis among individual providers. These risk models have been periodically re-calibrated to align with changes in surgical practices and patient risk profiles, thus ensuring their relevance to current healthcare features. Focused initially on mortality following coronary artery bypass grafting (CABG), these risk models have expanded to predict both morbidity and mortality in procedures such as CABG, aortic valve repair/replacement (AVR), mitral valve repair/replacement (MVR), and combined procedures. While the initial goal was to provide risk-adjusted outcomes for STS feedback reports and public reporting, these risk models now contribute to performance improvement initiatives and assist in patient counseling and shared decision-making.[1] The STS Score includes eight outcomes for each risk model, as presented in Table 10.1.[1,2] The online STS calculator can be accessed at https://riskcalc.sts.org/stswebriskcalc/calculate.

B. **European System for Cardiac Operative Risk Evaluation II**

The EuroSCORE was developed based on the European International database of cardiac surgical patients. This model was designed to predict mortality after cardiac surgery and has been widely used for risk assessment and analysis of cardiac surgical quality. In 2012, EuroSCORE II was published to ensure its ongoing accuracy. EuroSCORE II evaluates mortality, defined as

TABLE 10.1 STS Score Outcomes[a]

Outcome	Definition
Operative mortality	1. Occurring during the hospitalization in which the surgery was performed (even after 30 d). Or 2. All deaths occurring after discharge but before postoperative day 30
Stroke	Global neurologic dysfunction lasting >24 h and caused by a hemorrhage or infarction in the brain, spinal cord, or retinal vasculature
Renal failure	Risk, Injury, Failure, Loss of Kidney function, and End-stage kidney disease (RIFLE) classification: *Failure:* ↑ SCr × 3 or ↓ GFR >75% or if baseline SCr ≥353.6 µmol/L (≥4 mg/dL) ↑ SCr >44.2 µmol/L (>0.5 mg/dL) **or** UO <0.3 mL/kg/h × 24 h or anuria × 12 h *Loss of kidney function:* Complete loss of kidney function >4 wk *End-stage kidney disease:* Complete loss of kidney function >3 mo Or New requirement for dialysis
Prolonged ventilation	>24 h or reintubation
Reoperation	For bleeding, tamponade, or any cardiac reason
Major morbidity or mortality composite	Composite of outcomes above occurring
Prolonged PLOS	>14 d, alive or deceased
Short PLOS	<6 d, with the patient alive at discharge

GFR, glomerular filtration rate; PLOS, postoperative length of stay; SCr, serum creatinine; STS, Society of Thoracic Surgeons; UO, urine output.

[a]The STS Score is a validated risk model that provides risk-adjusted outcomes. It is commonly used to aid in patient counseling and shared decision-making. It estimates the risk of the outcomes defined by criteria in column 2.

Derived from Shahian DM, Jacobs JP, Badhwar V, et al. The Society of Thoracic Surgeons 2018 adult cardiac surgery risk models: part 1—background, design considerations, and model development. *Ann Thorac Surg.* 2018;105(5):1411-1418; Lopes JA, Jorge S. The RIFLE and AKIN classifications for acute kidney injury: a critical and comprehensive review. *Clin Kidney J.* 2013;6(1):8-14.

death during hospitalization when the operation took place. The risk factors associated with EuroSCORE II are listed in Table 10.2.[3]

The outcomes estimated by the STS and EuroSCORE II models were selected based on clinical and historical factors, resource considerations, and performance assessment. These scores derive from the presence or absence of specific risk factors, aiding shared decision-making, but not standalone management guidance. Preoperative optimization for cardiac surgery depends on individual comorbidities and characteristics, extending beyond STS Score and EuroSCORE factors. Guidelines offer illness severity-based recommendations but lack specific STS Score and EuroSCORE thresholds for management. Adjusted risk score models can identify at-risk patients but are not standard for optimizing cardiac surgery patients.

TABLE 10.2 EuroSCORE II Risk Factors[a]

Risk Factor	Description
NYHA class	I: No (dyspnea) symptoms on moderate exertion II: Symptoms on moderate exertion III: Symptoms on light exertion IV: Symptoms at rest
CCS class 4	Inability to perform any activity without angina or angina at rest
Extracardiac arteriopathy	One or more of the following: Claudication Carotid occlusion or >50% stenosis Amputation for arterial disease Previous or planned intervention on the abdominal aorta, carotids, or limb arteries
Poor mobility	Severe impairment secondary to musculoskeletal or neurologic dysfunction
Previous cardiac surgery	Major cardiac surgery requiring opening of the pericardium
Renal dysfunction	Assessed by the creatinine clearance (CC) using the Cockcroft-Gault formula CC 51-84 CC <50 On dialysis
Active endocarditis	Patient still under antibiotic treatment for endocarditis at the time of surgery
Critical preoperative state	Ventricular arrhythmias or sudden cardiac death Chest compressions Preoperative ventilation Preoperative inotropes or MCS Acute renal failure
LV function or LVEF	Good: LVEF ≥51% Moderate: LVEF 31%-50% Poor: LVEF 21%-30% Very poor: LVEF ≤20%
Urgency of procedure	Elective Urgent Emergency Salvage
Recent MI	Within 90 d before surgery
Type of procedure	Baseline is isolated CABG: Isolated non-CABG major procedure Two major procedures Three major procedures

CABG, coronary artery bypass grafting; CCS, Canadian Cardiovascular Society; IABP, intra-aortic balloon pump; LV, left ventricular; LVEF, left ventricular ejection fraction; MCS, mechanical circulatory support; MI, myocardial infarction; NYHA, New York Heart Association; VAD, ventricular assist device.

[a]The EuroSCORE II is another risk adjustment model used to calculate the risk of mortality during hospitalization when cardiac surgery took place. It considers the preoperative characteristics defined by criteria provided in column 2.

Adapted from Nashef SA, Roques F, Sharples LD, et al. EuroSCORE II. *Eur J Cardiothorac Surg*. 2012;41(4):734-745. Reproduced by permission of Oxford University Press.

III. Preanesthetic Evaluation

The primary objectives of the preanesthetic evaluation are to evaluate cardiac and overall health risks, identify and optimize comorbidities, and anticipate any factors that may lead to complications during the intraoperative and postoperative periods. In elective surgery cases, if comorbidities can be optimized before the procedure, it is essential to carefully consider the risks and benefits associated with postponing the surgery. During the preoperative period, the evaluation should encompass an assessment of patient-related factors and surgical risk factors, as summarized in Table 10.3.[4,5]

A. Assessment of Preoperative Medical Conditions

1. Stroke

Cardiac surgical patients who experience intraoperative and postoperative strokes have worse short- and long-term outcomes. These patients exhibit higher in-hospital mortality rates, 5- to 10-fold greater than patients without perioperative stroke, and are also at an increased risk of cognitive decline and disability.[6] Conversely, some cardiac surgical patients may have a history of previous strokes. This section aims to discuss the optimization of these patients before cardiac surgery and the prevention of recurrent strokes after cardiac surgery.

A history of stroke is a risk factor for recurrent stroke events and major adverse cardiovascular events (MACEs). Recurrent strokes are associated with higher functional disability, mortality, and financial burden than incident strokes. The risk of recurrent stroke and MACE is time dependent, with the highest risk occurring within the first month of the episode. The risk remains significantly increased within 3 months and gradually declines between 3-6, 6-12, and beyond 12 months.[7] After 9 months, the risk plateaus, indicating

TABLE 10.3   Patient-Related and Surgical Risk Factors[a]

Patient-related risk factors				Surgical risk factors
Cardiovascular conditions	Noncardiac comorbidities	Common comorbidities	Nonmodifiable risk factors	
Myocardial ischemia	Renal insufficiency	Hypertension	Female gender	Emergent surgery[b]
Ventricular dysfunction	Anemia	COPD	Older age	Urgent surgery[c]
Carotid artery disease	Tobacco use	Diabetes mellitus		Complexity of the procedure
Peripheral vascular disease	Respiratory disease	Hypothyroidism/ hyperthyroidism		Combined procedures
Cerebrovascular disease	Anemia	OSA		Prior cardiac surgery
Proximal aorta atherosclerosis/ calcification	RBC disorders			Cross-clamp time
Pulmonary hypertension	Hemostasis disorders			Institutional procedural volume/ experience

COPD, chronic obstructive pulmonary disease; OSA, obstructive sleep apnea; RBC, red blood cell.

[a]Preoperative comorbidities are associated with increased morbidity and mortality. These can be classified as patient-related risk factors or procedural risk factors. Risk factors presented by patients can be further divided into cardiovascular and noncardiovascular comorbidities. The most common comorbidities and nonmodifiable characteristics are included.

[b]Emergent surgery: life-threatening conditions in need of cardiac surgery immediately.[10]

[c]Urgent surgery: decompensated heart disease in need of surgery 72 h post admission.[10]

Derived from Andreasen C, Jørgensen ME, Gislason GH, et al. Association of timing of aortic valve replacement surgery after stroke with risk of recurrent stroke and mortality. *JAMA Cardiol*. 2018;3(6):506-513; Gaudino M, Benesch C, Bakaeen F, et al. Considerations for reduction of risk of perioperative stroke in adult patients undergoing cardiac and thoracic aortic operations: a scientific statement from the American Heart Association. *Circulation*. 2020;142(14):e193-e209.

that nonurgent elective surgeries should be delayed in patients with a history of stroke within the previous 9 months.[6-8] In cases where surgery must be performed urgently within 9 months of the stroke, appropriate arterial pressure control is crucial. Hypotension should be avoided, and blood pressure should be maintained as close to the patient's baseline as possible. Maintaining mean arterial pressure (MAP) >80 mm Hg and achieving a blood glucose target between 140 and 180 mg/dL while preventing hypoglycemia are reasonable in these situations.[7,8] For management recommendations regarding antiplatelet agents before cardiac surgery, refer to "Management of Preoperative Medications" section.

2. **Carotid artery stenosis**

Carotid artery stenosis (CAS) is a known risk factor for intraoperative stroke as it predisposes to cerebral hypoperfusion and atherosclerotic emboli. Intraoperative stroke is associated with operative and late mortality rates of 28% and 11%, respectively.[9] Approximately one-third of patients undergoing CABG have CAS (≥50% stenosis), and around 10% of patients with ischemic heart disease have significant CAS (>70% stenosis).[10] Screening for significant carotid artery disease is crucial in the prevention of stroke in cardiac surgical patients. Carotid duplex ultrasound, computed tomography angiography, and magnetic resonance angiography are recommended in patients who are ≥65 years of age, have a history of previous stroke, transient ischemic attack (TIA), or have an STS-predicted stroke risk >5%.[11] Preoperative imaging findings associated with an increased risk of perioperative stroke include:

   a. Men with symptomatic carotid stenosis of 50%-99%.
   b. Women with symptomatic carotid stenosis of 70%-99%.
   c. Unilateral asymptomatic carotid stenosis of 70%-99% and contralateral carotid occlusion.
   d. Bilateral severe carotid disease (80%-99%).

Patients with symptomatic stenosis of 50%-99% or those with severe bilateral disease should undergo carotid revascularization. However, individuals with unilateral asymptomatic carotid stenosis of 50%-99% do not require revascularization as they have a lower risk of perioperative stroke.[11] A staged rather than a combined approach is preferred unless there is an urgent indication for cardiac surgery in a patient with high-grade symptomatic carotid stenosis. Methods for revascularization include carotid endarterectomy (CEA) and carotid artery stenting. In cases where immediate CABG is indicated, and carotid revascularization is required, open CEA is preferred to carotid artery stenting.[9]

3. **Smoking and chronic obstructive pulmonary disease**

Smoking is a significant risk factor for respiratory, cardiovascular, and wound healing complications following cardiac surgery. Preoperative smoking cessation is effective in reducing postoperative morbidity and increasing abstinence rates.[12]

Smoking cessation interventions should be initiated as early as possible, as longer periods of preoperative abstinence are associated with better outcomes. Implementing cessation interventions at least 4 weeks before surgery has shown improved abstinence rates and decreased postoperative complications. Smoking cessation 3-4 weeks before surgery has been associated with fewer wound healing complications. High-intensity interventions have demonstrated the best outcomes, but even informal advice provided by physicians and trained nurses can promote cessation. Healthcare providers should engage in counseling focused on perioperative risks and identify barriers to abstinence as early as possible. Strategies such as motivational interviewing, education on the higher risk of surgical complications, and evidence of improved outcomes with smoking cessation can be implemented by any physician. Smoking cessation guidelines recommend utilizing the "5 A's" approach: Ask, Advise, Assess, Assist, and Arrange. Referral to smoking cessation and behavioral counseling programs can further improve adherence.[12]

Chronic obstructive pulmonary disease (COPD) is a significant risk factor for postoperative pulmonary complications (PPCs) following cardiac surgery, including prolonged intubation, reintubation, pneumonia, increased hospital length of stay, and mortality.[13,14]

Patients with known COPD should undergo assessment using tools and diagnostic evaluations, such as oximetry, pulmonary function tests, exercise tolerance testing, and assessment of the number of COPD exacerbations in the past year. High-risk patients may benefit from preoperative interventions, such as antibiotics, bronchodilators, intensive inspiratory muscle training, and incentive spirometry.[13] Adherence to guideline recommendations for COPD treatment with long-acting β-agonists, muscarinic agonists, and inhaled corticosteroids may decrease the incidence of PPCs.[14]

4. **Chronic kidney disease**

Cardiac surgery-associated acute kidney injury (CSA-AKI) is the second most common cause of AKI in the intensive care population. CSA-AKI is a clinically significant complication, with 1%-5% of patients requiring renal replacement therapy.[15] Cardiac surgery exposes patients to various factors contributing to kidney injury, including hemolysis, nephrotoxins, oxidative stress, inflammation, and reperfusion injury.[15] Diagnosing chronic kidney disease (CKD) before cardiac surgery (estimated glomerular filtration rate [eGFR] <60 mL/min/1.73 m^2), based on a serum creatinine measurement within 3 months of surgery, is crucial and should not be overlooked.[15]

Preoperative management of patients with CKD before cardiac surgery focuses on addressing modifiable risk factors. Optimal volume status should be achieved, and hypotension should be avoided. Minimizing exposure to nephrotoxic agents, such as iodinated radiocontrast agents and nonsteroidal anti-inflammatory drugs (NSAIDs), is essential to prevent further renal dysfunction. The use of angiotensin-converting enzyme (ACE) inhibitors and angiotensin receptor blockers (ARBs) should also be minimized, as they can cause volume depletion and efferent arteriolar vasodilation, leading to a decrease in eGFR. In addition, optimizing anemia due to severe CKD may decrease the risk of transfusion requirements associated with a high risk of CSA-AKI.[16] Some centers have preoperative transfusion management clinics, and erythropoietin (EPO) and iron are administered before surgery.

5. **Anemia**

Preoperative anemia, defined as hemoglobin levels <13 g/dL in men and 12 g/dL in women, affects 20%-50% of cardiac surgical patients and is an important contributor to adverse outcomes in this population.[17-19] It not only drives the need for perioperative red blood cell (RBC) transfusions and associated risks but also significantly elevates the likelihood of complications following cardiac surgery, including in-hospital mortality, stroke, AKI, myocardial infarction, infection, and reduced survival rates.[17-19] Blood management programs are available to address preoperative anemia, aiming to reduce intraoperative RBC transfusion requirements and improve outcomes. Early assessment of hemoglobin levels, ideally initiated 4-6 weeks before elective surgery, is crucial for timely detection and intervention. Diagnostics encompass complete blood counts, ferritin levels, transferrin concentration and saturation, and soluble transferrin receptor levels, aiding in anemia classification and management, particularly given that iron deficiency is a common underlying cause.[18] Notably, cardiac surgery patients frequently present with anemia of chronic disease coupled with EPO deficiency. Irrespective of etiology, correcting the underlying cause of anemia is paramount. Oral iron therapy suffices for iron deficiency anemia; however, intravenous (IV) iron supplementation may be preferred for rapid preoperative correction.[18] Clinical guidelines recommend initiating iron supplementation in patients with mild-to-severe anemia and introducing erythropoiesis-stimulating agents (ESAs) for those with anemia of chronic disease and absolute or relative EPO deficiency. The optimal duration of short-term (1-3 days) versus long-term (2-4 weeks) ESA interventions remains unclear. Therefore, assessing the requirement and duration of ESA interventions, along with the decision between oral or IV iron, requires a case-by-case evaluation considering surgical urgency and the accompanying risks and benefits of the therapies.[18] Optimizing hemoglobin levels before cardiac surgery is pivotal in reducing transfusion requirements, associated risks, and hospital readmissions, ultimately improving patient outcomes.[17-19]

6. **Hyperglycemia**

Hyperglycemia is associated with higher mortality rates, wound infections, AKI, and longer hospital length of stay in the context of cardiac surgery. Perioperative stress-induced hyperglycemia, defined as blood glucose levels >140 mg/dL, in patients without diabetes is linked to a 4-fold increase in complications and a 2-fold increase in death compared to patients without stress-induced hyperglycemia.[20] Patients with diabetes also experience worsening hyperglycemia during and after cardiac surgery due to the release of counter-regulatory hormones during stress. Severe hyperglycemia induces various detrimental effects, including osmotic diuresis, electrolyte abnormalities, impaired collagen synthesis and wound healing, reduced leukocyte function, upregulation of inflammatory cytokines, increased vascular permeability, impaired endothelial vasodilation, and increased platelet activation with reduced fibrinolytic activity. Therefore, risk stratification of all patients should include blood glucose and hemoglobin A1c (HbA1c) testing.[20]

Exogenous insulin administration is necessary to restore euglycemia and reduce postoperative morbidity and mortality. In cases of planned elective surgery, patients with poor glycemic control should undergo close glucose monitoring and receive education on dietary modifications and lifestyle changes before the scheduled surgery date. Blood glucose control should be initiated before surgery, and prolonged fasting should be avoided.[20] If a patient awaiting surgery is found to have a blood glucose level >180 mg/dL, continuous insulin infusion should be initiated to maintain glucose levels <150 mg/dL. Oral hypoglycemic agents should be discontinued at least 24 hours in advance to surgery, and insulin-dependent patients with diabetes should not receive short-acting insulin types after fasting the evening before surgery. Intermediate- or long-acting insulins should be reduced on the day of surgery to minimize the risk of hypoglycemia.[21,22]

7. **Blood disorders**

This section addresses RBC and hemostatic disorders that may present challenges in the context of cardiac surgery. RBC disorders with physiologic consequences that need to be identified include cold agglutinin disease and sickle cell disease. Relevant hemostatic disorders include von Willebrand disease (vWD) and heparin-induced thrombocytopenia (HIT).

Cold agglutinin disease is an autoimmune hemolytic anemia characterized by the presence of cold reactive immunoglobulin M (IgM) autoantibodies that bind to RBC antigens at temperatures of 0-4 °C, leading to erythrocyte agglutination and thrombotic complications. Some pathogenic cold agglutinins can cause RBC agglutination at higher temperatures (28-30 °C).[23] Early detection of patients with pathogenic cold agglutinins is crucial to reduce the risk. This involves thoroughly reviewing medical history for signs of hemolysis, acrocyanosis, and previous anemia studies. Symptomatic or potentially symptomatic cases should be referred to a hematologist for further testing to characterize the specific antibody present. Surgery without hypothermia should be planned for at-risk patients, and measures such as immunosuppression, plasmapheresis, or perfusion protocols with limited hypothermia may be considered. In addition, preoperative preparation of antigen-crossmatched compatible RBC units should be arranged, and vigilant monitoring for agglutination during surgery is essential, with prompt rewarming if agglutination occurs.[23,24]

Sickle cell disease is an autosomal recessive disorder that causes affected RBCs to lose their ability to pass through small capillaries, leading to thrombotic events. Cardiac surgical patients with sickle cell disease are at an increased risk of thrombotic and infectious complications. While there is no consensus on the preoperative management of patients with sickle cell disease, preoperative exchange transfusions have been used to reduce the proportion of hemoglobin S in whole blood. Warm cardioplegia and systemic normothermia (35-36 °C) may also minimize vaso-occlusive crises.[25]

vWD is characterized by defects in the von Willebrand factor (vWF), which impair clotting factor VIII (FVIII) and platelet adhesion and aggregation, leading to coagulopathy. This condition can be exacerbated by cardiac surgery and cardiopulmonary bypass (CPB). Patients with a history of prolonged bleeding should undergo laboratory tests to assess bleeding time and ristocetin cofactor activity for vWD diagnosis. Vasopressin (DDAVP) is the first-line agent for patients with vWD, as it induces the release of endothelial vWF. In cases where vasopressin is ineffective, manufactured vWF/FVIII concentrates can be used as an alternative, and their availability should be planned in advance.[26]

HIT is a prothrombotic disorder caused by platelet-activating antibodies specific to platelet factor 4 (PF4) and heparin. The incidence of HIT in cardiac surgical patients ranges from 1% to 2%.[27] Patients with a history of HIT should consult a hematologist and avoid heparin products before surgery. Diagnosis of acute, subacute, or remote HIT is based on platelet count, immunoassay for antibodies to PF4/heparin complexes, and serotonin release assay results. Surgery should be delayed when feasible in acute or subacute HIT. If surgery cannot be delayed, alternative anticoagulants such as bivalirudin may be used. Another strategy involves heparin administration in conjunction with preoperative or intraoperative plasma exchange or the use of a potent antiplatelet agent. Platelet transfusions should be avoided as they can exacerbate the underlying disease process and potentially lead to additional thrombotic complications.[27,28]

8. **Malnutrition**

Approximately 10%-50% of cardiac surgical patients are malnourished, depending on the assessment tool used. This increases morbidity and mortality, decreases quality of life, and increases hospital costs and the need for rehabilitation.[29,30] Assessing malnutrition in the preoperative setting is important for optimizing and mitigating perioperative complications. Over 40 diagnostic tools have been described, but few apply to cardiac surgery patients. The Nutritional Risk Screening 2002 (NRS-2002), the Malnutrition Universal Screening Tool (MUST), the Mini-Nutritional Assessment (MNA), the Short Nutritional Assessment Questionnaire (SNAQ), and the Nutrition Risk Screening Tool are commonly used.[31,32] The North American Surgical Nutrition Summit Consensus advises implementing perioperative nutritional care, including diet counseling, immunonutrition, and screening tools.[33] The European Society for Clinical Nutrition and Metabolism (ESPEN) recommends using the Nutrition Risk Screening Tool. In addition to identifying malnourished patients, this tool identifies patients at high nutrition risk who may present malnutrition in the highly catabolic postoperative period. It assesses the presence of low body mass index (BMI), recent weight loss of 5% or more in the previous 1-3 months, decrease in food intake, age 70 years and older, and severity of underlying disease. A score of ≥5 is considered a high nutrition risk. The ESPEN guidelines recommend 7-14 days of nutritional support for severely malnourished patients.[30] A consensus statement from an International Multidisciplinary Expert Group on Nutrition in Cardiac Surgery recommends nutritional support at least 2-7 days before surgery.[32]

B. **Optimization of Patients With Active COVID-19**

Patients with active COVID-19 infection and a history of cardiovascular disease face an increased mortality risk, which can range between 7% and 40%, and prolonged hospital stay.[5] These patients are more prone to myocardial injury and have an increased likelihood of experiencing arrhythmias and death. Furthermore, patients with an ongoing COVID-19 infection who undergo surgery encounter an elevated overall mortality rate of approximately 20%. Based on current data, the mortality rate for patients with active COVID-19 infection ranges between 16% and 44%.[5] It is crucial to stratify patients with active COVID-19 infection according to the urgency of surgical intervention.[34] Continuous assessment of patients with COVID-19 who require cardiac surgery should be conducted regularly in a multidisciplinary approach involving a cardiologist, a cardiac surgeon, an anesthesiologist, and an intensivist to ensure comprehensive care.[5]

C. **Indications for Intra-aortic Balloon Pump and Impella Insertion**

Intra-aortic balloon pumps (IABPs) and Impella devices are short-term mechanical circulatory assist devices used to provide hemodynamic support to failing left and/or right ventricles in patients with conditions such as cardiogenic shock, acute decompensated heart failure, cardiopulmonary arrest, and before high-risk invasive coronary artery procedures. Prompt initiation of support, especially in acute myocardial infarction–associated cardiogenic shock cases, before interventions has been shown to improve survival. The goals of these devices include maintaining end-organ and coronary perfusion, reducing myocardial wall stress and oxygen consumption, supporting cardiogenic shock, reducing pulmonary vascular congestion, and facilitating cardiac recovery. Among these devices, IABP is the most commonly used, while the use of Impella for cardiogenic shock is increasing. Although there is no standardized consensus on which cardiac surgical patients may benefit from these devices, high-risk patients should be evaluated and considered for mechanical circulatory support.[35]

D. Risk Factors for Developing Mediastinitis and Wound Infections

Mediastinitis and deep sternal wound infections (DSWIs) refer to infections occurring in the structures within the mediastinum, including the heart, great vessels, trachea, mainstem bronchi, esophagus, and vagus or phrenic nerves. Most cases of mediastinitis arise as a postoperative complication following median sternotomy and are considered life-threatening. DSWI occurs in approximately 0.4%-4% of cardiac surgical procedures, with reported in-hospital mortality rates ranging from 10% to 20%.[36,37] Several risk factors contribute to the development of DSWI, including previous sternotomy, advanced age, obesity, diabetes mellitus, COPD, peripheral vascular disease, renal failure requiring hemodialysis, tobacco use, low cardiac output states, history of endocarditis, preoperative colonization with *Staphylococcus aureus*, immunosuppression, mechanical support device utilization before or after cardiac surgery, and prolonged preoperative hospitalization. Obesity, in particular, is strongly associated with developing postoperative mediastinitis, with a 2.2- to 6.5-fold increased risk in patients with a BMI >30 kg/m^2.[38]

S. aureus accounts for up to 60% of DSWI cases; therefore, preoperative nasal screening and treatment for methicillin-susceptible *S. aureus* (MSSA) or methicillin-resistant *S. aureus* (MRSA) colonization are recommended in addition to routine administration of prophylactic IV antibiotics.[36-38] In cases where there is known or presumed staphylococcal colonization, an institution with a high incidence of MRSA, in-hospital length of stay exceeding 3 days, transfer from an inpatient facility, or procedures involving patients with prosthetic valves or vascular graft insertions, the addition of one or two doses of a glycopeptide, such as vancomycin, alongside a β-lactam antibiotic is advised.[37]

The World Health Organization (WHO) recommends the routine use of intranasal mupirocin with or without chlorhexidine body wash in patients with *S. aureus* colonization undergoing cardiac surgery. However, intranasal iodine may prove to be more effective.[39] Iodine rapidly penetrates Gram-positive and Gram-negative microorganisms, oxidizing essential cellular components such as fatty acids, nucleotides, and proteins. In vitro studies have confirmed that povidone-iodine (PVP-I) 10% solutions exhibit greater antimicrobial effects against MSSA and MRSA than chlorhexidine, even in chlorhexidine- and mupirocin-resistant strains. Ultimately, a combination of several preventive measures, including screening, isolation, surface disinfection, decolonization, and good hygiene practices, can significantly reduce the incidence of postoperative infectious complications.[39]

IV. Management of Preoperative Medications

A. Angiotensin-Converting Enzyme Inhibitors and Angiotensin Receptor Blockers

Chronic use of ACE inhibitors or ARBs is common in cardiac surgical patients due to their cardioprotective and vascular effects in conditions such as hypertension, heart failure, CKD, and diabetes. However, administration of these medications in the preoperative period has been associated with intraoperative and postoperative vasoplegia, postoperative kidney injury, increased use of inotropes and vasopressors in the postoperative period, prolonged ventilation, and longer intensive care unit (ICU) stays. Patients taking long-acting ACE inhibitors and ARBs with uncontrolled hypertension in the preoperative period may be switched to short-acting ACE inhibitors. Specific medications, such as enalapril, lisinopril, ramipril, losartan, and valsartan, should be discontinued 24 hours before cardiac surgery, while captopril should be discontinued 12 hours before surgery.[40]

B. Antiplatelet Therapy

Dual-antiplatelet therapy with aspirin and P2Y12 antagonists is commonly prescribed to cardiac surgical patients, particularly those with coronary artery disease. Aspirin should be continued throughout the perioperative period in patients already on the medication. The decision to start or continue aspirin preoperatively should consider increased bleeding risks. P2Y12 inhibitors should be discontinued before cardiac surgery due to the elevated risk of major bleeding complications. Table 10.4 provides guidance on when to discontinue these antiplatelet agents preoperatively.[41] In urgent cases where there is insufficient time to discontinue P2Y12 inhibitors, the administration of antifibrinolytics, desmopressin, or recombinant FVIIa is recommended to improve platelet function and reduce perioperative bleeding. There are

TABLE 10.4 Preoperative Management of Antiplatelets and Anticoagulants[a]

Antithrombotic/ Anticoagulant	D−8	D−7	D−6	D−5	D−4	D−3	D−2	D−1	Day of Surgery 0
VKA bridging									
Warfarin	✓	✓	✓						
LMWH							✓	✓[b]	
DOACs									
Apixaban	✓	✓	✓	✓	✓	✓			
Rivaroxaban	✓	✓	✓	✓	✓	✓			
Edoxaban	✓	✓	✓	✓	✓	✓			
Dabigatran CrCl ≥50 mL/min	✓	✓	✓	✓	✓	✓			
Dabigatran CrCl <50 mL/min	✓	✓	✓						
Antiplatelet agents									
Aspirin	✓	✓	✓	✓	✓	✓	✓	✓	✓ (Day of Surgery 0)
Ticagrelor	✓	✓	✓	✓	✓				
Clopidogrel	✓	✓	✓						
Prasugrel	✓								

CrCl, creatinine clearance; DOACs, direct oral anticoagulants; LMWH, low molecular weight heparin; VKA, vitamin K antagonist
[a]Cardiac surgery has an increased risk of bleeding complications. Patients receiving anticoagulants and antithrombotic agents must suspend their use before surgery while minimizing the risk of thrombotic events. Vitamin K antagonists, direct oral anticoagulant, and antiplatelet agents are also presented. Box with ✓ indicates on which preoperative days it is safe to administer each agent and how far ahead of surgery they should be suspended.
[b]Bridging with full-dose LMWH: enoxaparin 1 mg/kg twice daily or 1.5 mg/kg daily, or dalteparin 100 UI/kg twice daily or 200 IU/kg daily. The last dose is given the morning before surgery (d −1) at half the daily dose.
Derived from Brown JK, Singh K, Dumitru R, Chan E, Kim MP. The benefits of enhanced recovery after surgery programs and their application in cardiothoracic surgery. *Methodist Debakey Cardiovasc J*. 2018;14(2):77-88. doi:10.14797/mdcj-14-2-77.

methods for assessing platelet activity, especially via viscoelastic testing, but data are limiting regarding the timing of surgery, treatment options, and patient outcomes based on the results of this testing.[41]

C. Anticoagulation Bridging

Managing anticoagulation in patients undergoing cardiac surgery poses challenges, as it requires balancing the risks of thrombotic and bleeding complications.[41] Risk stratification based on the indication for anticoagulation is outlined in Table 10.5.

In cases of urgent or emergent cardiac surgery, anticoagulation reversal is warranted. If surgery is planned within the next 1-2 days, warfarin should be stopped, and 2.5-5 mg of oral or IV vitamin K should be administered. Ideally, the international normalized ratio (INR) should be ≤1.5 before surgery. Prothrombin complex concentrates are used to reverse the effects of warfarin for immediate reversal.[42] Dabigatran can be reversed with idarucizumab, while direct FXa inhibitors can be reversed with andexanet alfa or prothrombin complex concentrates.[41]

V. Management of Cardiac Implantable Electronic Devices

Pacemakers and implantable cardioverter-defibrillators (ICDs) play a crucial role in managing patients with abnormalities in the heart conduction system, protecting against sudden cardiac death in various arrhythmias. Therefore, it is essential to meticulously evaluate patients during the preoperative assessment to determine the presence and proper functioning of cardiac implantable electronic devices (CIEDs). Once the device has been identified, it is necessary to ascertain the indications for implantation and configure appropriate device settings. Evaluating the proper functioning of the CIED can be achieved through a comprehensive assessment of the device or, at the very least, by verifying that pacing impulses generate a paced rhythm.[43]

TABLE 10.5 Thromboembolic Risk Assessment[a]

Indication for Anticoagulation	Level of Thromboembolic Risk		
	Low Risk	Moderate Risk	High Risk
Venous thromboembolism (VTE)	VTE >12 mo ago	VTE 3-12 mo ago	Protein C & S deficiency
	Recurrent VTE	Heterozygous factor V Leiden mutation	Homozygous factor V Leiden mutation
	Active cancer	Prothrombin mutations	Antiphospholipid syndrome
			Antithrombin deficiency
Atrial fibrillation (AF)	CHA2DS2-VASc score 0-2	CHA2DS2-VASc score 3-4	CHA2DS2-VASc score >5
			Stroke/TIA in previous 3 mo
			Rheumatic valvular disease
Mechanical heart valve	Bileaflet aortic valve without risk factors	Bileaflet aortic valve prothesis with ≥1 risk factors[b]	Mechanical mitral valve
			Stroke/TIA in previous 3 mo
			Caged-ball/tilting disk aortic mechanical valves

TIA, transient ischemic attack

[a]Upon assessing thromboembolic vs bleeding risks, the indication for requiring anticoagulation is central to stratify thromboembolic risk. This table includes criteria to classify these indications into low, moderate, and high risk of developing thromboembolic events.

[b]Age ≥75, AF, congestive heart failure (CHF), hypertension, diabetes, stroke/transient ischemic attack.

Derived from Brown JK, Singh K, Dumitru R, Chan E, Kim MP. The benefits of enhanced recovery after surgery programs and their application in cardiothoracic surgery. *Methodist Debakey Cardiovasc J.* 2018;14(2):77-88. doi:10.14797/mdcj-14-2-77.

Upon completing a thorough evaluation of the CIED, a well-planned strategy should be devised to ensure the appropriate preservation of device function during surgery. This includes several considerations:

1. Reprogramming the pacemaker function to an asynchronous mode is recommended for patients who are pacemaker dependent.[43]
2. For patients who are not pacemaker dependent, programming the device to VVI mode during short bursts of electrocautery is advisable.[43]
3. In the preoperative area, it is important to disable antitachycardia therapies provided by the CIED. This step prevents unintended activation of the device due to external stimuli.[43]
4. An analysis of the possible consequences of anesthetic methods on the patient and the CIED should be conducted. Considering the effects of anesthetics and ensuring they do not interfere with the CIED's functioning are of paramount importance to ensure patient safety.[43]
5. Adequate arrangements should be made to ensure properly functioning temporary pacing and defibrillation devices are available. These backup measures are essential if any issues arise with the patient's CIED during surgery, allowing immediate intervention and support if necessary.[43]

VI. Enhanced Recovery After Surgery and Enhanced Recovery After Cardiac Surgery

Enhanced Recovery After Surgery (ERAS) is a perioperative multimodal care improvement initiative to improve patient outcomes. Compared to conventional management, ERAS protocols have been associated with a reduction in perioperative complications and length of hospital stay. The first expert consensus on Enhanced Recovery After Cardiac Surgery (ERACS) provides preoperative recommendations for cardiac surgical patients[44]:

1. Screening for diabetes and achieving adequate glycemic control with a target HbA1c level of <7%.[44]
2. Assessment of preoperative albumin levels, as hypoalbuminemia indicates increased preoperative risk and has shown a correlation with mortality, longer length of stay, AKI, infection, and prolonged ventilation.[44]

3. Initiation of preoperative oral nutritional supplementation in malnourished patients with serum albumin levels <3 g/dL, starting 7-10 days before surgery.[44]

4. Encouraging nonalcoholic clear liquid consumption 2-4 hours before anesthesia. Cardiac surgical patients are typically instructed to ingest nothing by mouth (NPO) after midnight for surgery the following day or fast for at least 6-8 hours from their last solid meal. However, clear liquids can be safely consumed without increasing the risks of aspiration.[44]

5. Carbohydrate loading with a 12-ounce clear beverage or a 24-g complex carbohydrate drink 2 hours before surgery to reduce insulin resistance, improve postoperative glucose control, and enhance gut function.[44]

6. Provision of education and counseling to reduce perioperative anxiety, fear, and discomfort, utilizing emerging software applications for improved compliance.[44]

7. Screening for smoking and hazardous alcohol use and promoting abstinence.[44]

8. Implementation of prehabilitation strategies (discussed in the subsequent section).[44]

A. Frailty and Prehabilitation

Frailty is a state of reduced multiorgan reserve and increased vulnerability characterized by self-reported fatigue, reduced muscle mass, and low activity levels. Frail patients have a higher risk of postoperative complications, longer hospital stays, and increased mortality compared to those with higher functional reserve. While frailty is more common in the geriatric population, it can affect patients of all ages. Physiologic age predicts outcomes better after cardiac surgery than chronologic age.[45,46] Evaluating the degree of frailty can help identify discrepancies between chronologic and physiologic age and between modifiable morbidity predictors for optimized preoperative care. The major barriers to routine assessment are the lack of standardization between frailty instruments and the multidisciplinary process required for the Comprehensive Geriatric Assessment (CGA), which requires multiple geriatric visits.[47]

Two main physiologic models of frailty, the deficit accumulation model and the phenotype model, provide insight into the assessment and management of frailty. The deficit accumulation model considers the cumulative effect of coexisting social, medical, and functional deficits. The phenotype model examines age-related body composition states, weakness, exhaustion, and slowness. Both model principles should be considered.[47] Table 10.6 includes frailty assessment methods that are more feasible to carry out during the preoperative period than the CGA.[46,47]

Preoperative rehabilitation, commonly referred to as *prehabilitation*, aims to optimize current conditions and reduce postoperative morbidity. It involves tailored interventions targeting various systems based on individual patient needs to enhance functional and nutritional capacity to reduce postoperative morbidity.[45]

Improving preoperative aerobic capacity has been associated with decreased mortality, reduced postoperative morbidity, and shorter hospital stays.[45] While some patients may be unable or unwilling to engage in preoperative exercise, education and psychological support can promote the benefits of increased cardiorespiratory fitness and the safety of physical activity. Interventions of at least 2 weeks duration, customized to patient preferences and exercise tolerance, have shown significant reductions in ICU and in-hospital length of stay. This includes a combination of cycle ergometers, treadmills, body weight, and resistance training based on predicted maximum workloads or achieving 50%-85% of individual maximal oxygen uptake capacity over a period of approximately 6 weeks.[45]

Preoperative inspiratory muscle training has demonstrated efficacy in reducing PPCs. Deep breathing exercises, forced expiration exercises, and incentive spirometry have shown improvements in muscular strength and sputum clearance, particularly in patients with chronic respiratory conditions. A combination of these exercises performed for approximately 20 minutes daily over 8 weeks has been associated with a reduction in the need for reintubation, pneumonia, and pleural effusions during the postoperative period. Further research is needed to provide definitive conclusions on the benefit of respiratory prehabilitation strategies in reducing PPCs.[45]

B. Nonsteroidal Anti-inflammatory Drugs

NSAIDs are generally avoided in cardiac surgery due to evidence of adverse cardiovascular events associated with nonselective and COX-2–specific inhibitors. Although NSAIDs were

TABLE 10.6 Tools for Preoperative Frailty Assessment[a]

Frailty Assessment Tools	Aim	What Does It Evaluate?	Interpretation
Gait speed	Determines the interplay of vision, proprioception, and aerobic capacity	Measures the time it takes an individual to walk 5 m	Gait speed >5 s for 4 m (<0.85 m/s) is associated with increased frailty <5 m in 6 s is an independent predictor of major postoperative morbidity and mortality
Hand grip strength (HGS)	Determines musculoskeletal function	Measures isometric hand strength using a hydraulic dynamometer	<25% of the total weight is associated with lower survival
Chair rise	Determines leg strength and endurance Increases likelihood of detecting impaired mobility	Measures how many times a patient can stand to a full upright position from a sitting position, with their arms crossed and placed in the opposite shoulder, in 30 s	Low chair rise scores (compared to a validated cohort for specified age ranges) predicts delayed functional recovery
Frailty scale	Assessment of: 1. Illnesses 2. Fatigue 3. Weight loss 4. Resistance 5. Aerobic capacity	5-question verbal assessment that yields an age, gender, and comorbidity adjusted score	0: Robust 1-2: Prefrail 3-5: Frail Shows significant association between frailty and postoperative complications, hospital length of stay
Comprehensive assessment of frailty (CAF) score	Predictor of 30-d and 1-y mortality	Factors assessed: • BMI • Laboratory tests including albumin and creatinine • FEV1 • Exhaustion phenotype via a questionnaire evaluating weekly energy used in physical activities. • Hand grip strength • Gait speed • Physical performance test[b]	1-10 points: Not frail 11-25 points: Moderately frail 26-35 points: Severely frail
Nutrition	Assessment of nutritional status	The ESPEN defines severe malnutrition when one is present: • Weight loss >10%-15% within 6 mo • BMI <18 kg/m^2 • Severely malnourished • Serum albumin <30 g/L (with no evidence of hepatic or renal dysfunction)	Perioperative nutrition plays an important role in modulating the surgical stress response

BMI, body mass index; ESPEN, European Society for Clinical Nutrition and Metabolism; FEV1, forced expiratory volume in 1 s.

[a]Assessing frailty is key to target modifiable risk factors of poor outcomes. Several frailty assessment tools that are feasible to carry out by any physician are given. Each tool and its interpretation are described.

[b]The physical performance test includes assessment of standing balance, chair rise, picking up a pen from the floor, putting on a removing a jacket, and turning 360°.

Derived from Van Schoonevelt T, Rupp M. Mediastinitis. In: Bennett JE, Dolin R, Blaser MJ, eds. *Mandell, Douglas and Bennett's Principles and Practice of Infectious Diseases.* 8th ed. Elsevier; 2015:1080-1090; Lepelletier D, Maillard JY, Pozzetto B, Simon A. Povidone iodine: properties, mechanisms of action, and role in infection control and Staphylococcus aureus decolonization. *Antimicrob Agents Chemother.* 2020;64(9):e00682-20.

previously used for perioperative analgesia in cardiac surgery, two randomized controlled trials (RCTs) investigating the use of valdecoxib and parecoxib reported adverse outcomes in cardiac surgical patients. As a result, the U.S. Food and Drug Administration (FDA) issued a "black box" warning for all NSAIDs immediately after CABG.[13] In addition, NSAIDs increase the risk of CSA-AKI, and in patients taking aspirin, NSAIDs can attenuate the antiaggregation properties of aspirin, thereby increasing the risk of bleeding. Therefore, administration of NSAIDs should be minimized in this patient population, and acetaminophen can be considered an alternative analgesic.[13,48]

C. Acetaminophen

Acetaminophen is commonly used as an adjuvant analgesic in cardiac surgery. It possesses central analgesic properties, reduces inflammation, and decreases opioid consumption. A recent RCT demonstrated that patients receiving acetaminophen had a lower incidence of postoperative delirium, lower opioid dose requirements, and a shorter ICU length of stay compared to those receiving placebo. Therefore, using IV acetaminophen as an adjuvant analgesic is reasonable, as it has shown promising results without an increase in adverse events.[48]

D. Gabapentinoids

Early studies favoring the routine use of gabapentinoids focused on their analgesic effects but overlooked their side effects. The use of perioperative gabapentinoids is associated with an increased risk of visual disturbances, ataxia, balance disorders, dizziness, somnolence, sedation, and cognitive impairment due to their binding to the $\alpha2\delta$ subunit of voltage-gated calcium channels in the cerebellum and hippocampus. Pregabalin has been associated with approximately a 3-fold greater risk of serious adverse events, and the use of gabapentinoids on the day of surgery increases the odds of PPCs and ICU admissions without reducing opioid requirements or length of stay. The potential analgesic benefits of gabapentinoids appear to be outweighed by their adverse side effects, and it is recommended to reconsider their inclusion in ERACS protocols.[49]

VII. Summary

Preparing a patient for cardiac surgery involves assessing their individual risks using validated risk models, optimizing baseline characteristics and functional status, and implementing strategies, such as hemodynamic optimization, optimal medical therapy for COPD, careful management of CKD, and weight loss and glycemic control for patients with diabetes. A multidisciplinary approach incorporating ERACS and prehabilitation is crucial for improving outcomes. ERACS protocols focus on evidence-based enhancements in perioperative care, while prehabilitation involves interventions to optimize the patient's physical capacity before surgery. By integrating these comprehensive strategies, healthcare providers can enhance surgical outcomes and patient well-being.

REFERENCES

1. Shahian DM, Jacobs JP, Badhwar V, et al. The Society of Thoracic Surgeons 2018 Adult Cardiac Surgery Risk Models: part 1—background, design considerations, and model development. *Ann Thorac Surg.* 2018;105(5):1411-1418.
2. Lopes JA, Jorge S. The RIFLE and AKIN classifications for acute kidney injury: a critical and comprehensive review. *Clin Kidney J.* 2013;6:8-14.
3. Nashef SAM, Roques F, Sharples LD, et al. Euroscore II. *Eur J Cardiothorac Surg.* 2012;41(4):734-745.
4. Barbeito, A. (2022). Preoperative evaluation for anesthesia for cardiac surgery. *UpToDate.* Retrieved October 13, 2022, from https://www.uptodate.com/contents/preoperative-evaluation-for-anesthesia-for-cardiac-surgery?search=preoperative%20evaluation%20for%20anesthesia%20for%20cardiac%20surgery&source=search_result&selectedTitle=1~150&usage_type=default&display_rank=1
5. Mihalj M, Mosbahi S, Schmidli J, et al. Providing safe perioperative care in cardiac surgery during the COVID-19 pandemic. *Best Practice & Research Clinical Anaesthesiology.* 2021;35(3): 321–332. doi:10.1016/j.bpa.2021.01.002.
6. Kleindorfer DO, Towfighi A, Chaturvedi S, et al. 2021 Guideline for the prevention of stroke in patients with stroke and transient ischemic attack; a guideline from the American Heart Association/American Stroke Association. *Stroke.* 2021;52(7):e364-e467.
7. Minhas JS, Rook W, Panerai RB, et al. Pathophysiological and clinical considerations in the perioperative care of patients with a previous ischaemic stroke: a multidisciplinary narrative review. *Br J Anaesth.* 2020;124:183-196.
8. Andreasen C, Jørgensen ME, Gislason GH, et al. Association of timing of aortic valve replacement surgery after stroke with risk of recurrent stroke and mortality. *JAMA Cardiol.* 2018;3(6):506-513.
9. Gaudino M, Benesch C, Bakaeen F, et al. Considerations for reduction of risk of perioperative stroke in adult patients undergoing cardiac and thoracic aortic operations: a scientific statement from the American Heart Association. *Circulation.* 2020;142:e193-e209.

10. Adhikary D, Ranjan R, Mandal S, Hawlader MDH, Mitra DK, Adhikary AB. Prevalence of carotid artery stenosis in ischaemic heart disease patients in Bangladesh. *SAGE Open Med*. 2019;7:205031211983083.

11. Lazar H, Wilson CA, Messé Steven R. Coronary artery bypass grafting in patients with cerebrovascular disease. *UpToDate*. Retrieved February 7, 2023, from https://www.uptodate.com/contents/coronary-artery-bypass-grafting-in-patients-with-cerebrovascular-disease?search=coronary%20artery%20bypass%20grafting%20in%20patients%20with%20cerebrovascular%20disease&source=search_result&selectedTitle=1~150&usage_type=default&display_rank=1

12. Wong J, An D, Urman RD, et al. Society for perioperative assessment and quality improvement (SPAQI) consensus statement on perioperative smoking cessation. *Anesth Analg*. 2020;131(3):955-968.

13. Hillis LD, Smith PK, Bittl JA, et al. 2011 ACCF/AHA guideline for coronary artery bypass graft surgery: executive summary: a report of the American College of Cardiology Foundation/American Heart Association Task Force on Practice Guidelines. *Circulation*. 2011;124(23):2610-2642.

14. Numata T, Nakayama K, Fujii S, et al. Risk factors of postoperative pulmonary complications in patients with asthma and COPD. *BMC Pulm Med*. 2018;18(1):4.

15. Wang Y, Bellomo R. Cardiac surgery-associated acute kidney injury: risk factors, pathophysiology and treatment. *Nat Rev Nephrol*. 2017;13:697-711.

16. Oprea AD, del Rio JM, Cooter M, et al. Pre- and postoperative anemia, acute kidney injury, and mortality after coronary artery bypass grafting surgery: a retrospective observational study. *Can J Anesth*. 2018;65(1):46-59.

17. Karkouti K, Wijeysundera DN, Beattie WS. Risk associated with preoperative anemia in cardiac surgery: a multicenter cohort study. *Circulation*. 2008;117(4):478-484.

18. Kloeser R, Buser A, Bolliger D. Treatment strategies in anemic patients before cardiac surgery. *J Cardiothorac Vasc Anesth*. 2023;37:266-275.

19. Mistry R, Upchurch C, Locantore-Ford P. Hemoglobin optimization prior to cardiac surgery results in improved patient outcomes. *Blood*. 2019;134(Suppl. 1):4989.

20. Galindo RJ, Fayfman M, Umpierrez GE. Perioperative management of hyperglycemia and diabetes in cardiac surgery patients. *Endocrinology and Metabolism Clinics of North America*. 2018;47(1):203−222. doi:10.1016/j.ecl.2017.10.005.

21. Reddy P. Blood glucose management in the patient undergoing cardiac surgery: a review. *World J Cardiol*. 2014;6(11):1209.

22. Duggan EW, Carlson K, Umpierrez GE. Perioperative hyperglycemia management: an update. *Anesthesiology*. 2017;126:547-560.

23. Berentsen S, Barcellini W. Autoimmune hemolytic anemias. Longo DL, ed. *N Engl J Med*. 2021;385(15):1407-1419. doi:10.1056/NEJMra2033982

24. Sapatnekar S, Figueroa PI. Cold antibodies in cardiovascular surgery: is preoperative screening necessary? *Am J Clin Pathol*. 2016;145(6):789-795.

25. Crawford TC, Carter MV, Patel RK, et al. Management of sickle cell disease in patients undergoing cardiac surgery. *J Card Surg*. 2017;32:80-84.

26. Teppone-Martin OL, Zhao M, Norris TE. von Willebrand disease and cardiopulmonary bypass: a case report. *AANA J*. 2013;81(1):60-64. www.aana.com/aanajournalonline

27. Pishko AM, Cuker A. Heparin-induced thrombocytopenia in cardiac surgery patients. *Semin Thromb Hemost*. 2017;43(7):691-698.

28. Pishko AM, Cuker A. Heparin-induced thrombocytopenia and cardiovascular surgery. http://ashpublications.org/hematology/article-pdf/2021/1/536/1851441/536pishko.pdf

29. Ringaitienė D, Gineitytė D, Vicka V, et al. Preoperative risk factors of malnutrition for cardiac surgery patients. *Acta Med Litu*. 2016;23(2):99-109.

30. Ringaitiene D, Gineityte D, Vicka V, et al. Concordance of the new ESPEN criteria with low phase angle in defining early stages of malnutrition in cardiac surgery. *Clin Nutr*. 2018;37(5):1596-1601.

31. Lomivorotov VV, Efremov SM, Boboshko VA, et al. Evaluation of nutritional screening tools for patients scheduled for cardiac surgery. *Nutrition*. 2013;29(2):436-442.

32. Stoppe C, Goetzenich A, Whitman G, et al. Role of nutrition support in adult cardiac surgery: a consensus statement from an International Multidisciplinary Expert Group on Nutrition in Cardiac Surgery. *Crit Care*. 2017;21(1):131.

33. Brown JK, Singh K, Dumitru R, Chan E, Kim MP. The benefits of enhanced recovery after surgery programs and their application in cardiothoracic surgery. *Methodist Debakey Cardiovasc J*. 2018;14(2):77. https://journal.houstonmethodist.org/article/10.14797/mdcj-14-2-77/

34. Patel V, Jimenez E, Cornwell L, et al. Cardiac surgery during the coronavirus disease 2019 pandemic: perioperative considerations and triage recommendations. *J Am Heart Assoc*. 2020;9(13):e017042.

35. Atti V, Narayanan MA, Patel B, et al. A comprehensive review of mechanical circulatory support devices. *Heart Int*. 2022;16(1):37-48.

36. Edwards FH, Engelman RM, Houck P, Shahian DM, Bridges CR. The society of thoracic surgeons practice guideline series: antibiotic prophylaxis in cardiac surgery, part I: duration. *Ann Thorac Surg*. 2006;81(1):397-404.

37. Engelman R, Shahian D, Shemin R, et al. The Society of Thoracic Surgeons practice guideline series: antibiotic prophylaxis in cardiac surgery, part II: antibiotic choice. *Ann Thorac Surg*. 2007;83(4):1569-1576.

38. Van Schoonevelt T, Rupp M. Mediastinitis. In: Bennet J, Raphael D, Blaser M, eds. *Mandell, Douglas and Bennet's Principles of Infectious Diseases*. 8th ed. Elsevier Saunders; 2015:1080-1090.

39. Lepelletier D, Maillard JY, Pozzetto B, Simon A. Povidone iodine: properties, mechanisms of action, and role in infection control and *Staphylococcus aureus* decolonization. *Antimicrob Agents Chemother*. 2020;64(9):e00682. doi:10.1128/AAC

40. Sousa-Uva M, Head SJ, Milojevic M, et al. 2017 EACTS guidelines on perioperative medication in adult cardiac surgery. *Eur J Cardiothorac Surg*. 2018;53(1):5-33.

41. Douketis JD, Spyropoulos AC, Murad MH, et al. Executive summary: perioperative management of antithrombotic therapy: an American College of Chest Physicians Clinical Practice Guideline. *Chest*. 2022;162(5):1127-1139.

42. Chai-Adisaksopha C, Hillis C, Siegal DM, et al. Prothrombin complex concentrates versus fresh frozen plasma for warfarin reversal. A systematic review and meta-analysis. *Thromb Haemost.* 2016;116(5):879-890.
43. Practice advisory for the perioperative management of patients with cardiac implantable electronic devices: pacemakers and implantable cardioverter-defibrillators. 2011. http://pubs.asahq.org/anesthesiology/article-pdf/114/2/247/658689/0000542-201102000-00013.pdf
44. Engelman DT, Ben Ali W, Williams JB, et al. Guidelines for perioperative care in cardiac surgery: enhanced recovery after surgery society recommendations. *JAMA Surg.* 2019;154:755-766.
45. McCann M, Stamp N, Ngui A, Litton E. Cardiac prehabilitation. *J Cardiothorac Vasc Anesth.* 2019;33:2255-2265.
46. Koh LY, Hwang NC. Frailty in cardiac surgery. *J Cardiothorac Vasc Anesth.* 2019;33:521-531.
47. Shanker A, Upadhyay P, Rangasamy V, Muralidhar K, Subramaniam B. Impact of frailty in cardiac surgical patients—assessment, burden, and recommendations. *Ann Card Anaesth.* 2021;24:133-139.
48. Subramaniam B, Shankar P, Shaefi S, et al. Effect of Intravenous acetaminophen vs placebo combined with propofol or dexmedetomidine on postoperative delirium among older patients following cardiac surgery. *JAMA.* 2019;321(74):686.
49. Kharasch ED, Clark JD, Kheterpal S. Perioperative gabapentinoids: deflating the bubble. *Anesthesiology.* 2020;133:251-254.

11

Structural Heart and Electrophysiology

Kiran Belani and Richard D. Sheu

KEY POINTS

1. "Structural heart disease" is an overarching term that encompasses the spectrum of noncoronary cardiac disease processes that are linked with abnormalities or defects that weaken the heart's structure. Structural interventions are the associated transcatheter and interventional therapeutic techniques for these pathologies.

2. The site-specific transseptal puncture (TSP) is the first and most critical step to the performance of a successful left-sided transcatheter procedure and is conducted with simultaneous transesophageal echocardiographic (TEE) and fluoroscopic guidance.

3. Mitral transcatheter edge-to-edge repair (TEER) techniques can be utilized in patients with degenerative (primary) or functional (secondary) mitral regurgitation (MR) that are not surgical candidates, and increasingly challenging anatomic characteristics can be addressed with this technology at higher-volume centers.

4. The balloon-expandable SAPIEN valve (Edwards Lifesciences, Irvine CA) is currently the only U.S. Food and Drug Administration (FDA)-approved transcatheter mitral valve replacement (TMVR) device approved for valve-in-valve (ViV) and valve-in-ring (ViR) therapies and is deployed via a transseptal approach.

5. Left atrial appendage (LAA) occlusion devices can be utilized for device-based stroke prevention in patients in whom long-term anticoagulation is contraindicated or not tolerated.

6. TEE, and mainly three-dimensional (3D) TEE, is the primary modality by which prosthetic paravalvular defects (PVDs) are diagnosed, localized, and evaluated for treatment options.

7. Although straightforward patent foramen ovale (PFO) closures can be done under conscious sedation and intracardiac echocardiography (ICE), complex atrial septal defect (ASD) closures often require general anesthesia and TEE for characterization and sizing of the defect, as well as confirmation of anatomic characteristics that allow the defect to be closed in transcatheter manner.

8. Procedures in the electrophysiology (EP) laboratory can utilize the full spectrum of anesthetic techniques (from monitored anesthesia care to general anesthesia), and the anesthesiologist's full understanding of the arrhythmia and treatment mechanisms will dictate the correct choice of anesthetic and allow for adequate monitoring for procedure-specific complications.

I. Introduction

Over the past few decades, we have seen major advancements in catheter-based interventions that aim to alleviate conditions related to both heart structure and rhythms. The term "structural heart disease" was first coined in 1999 and describes any abnormality or defect that weakens the heart's structure.[1] These procedures are typically reserved for patients who are at high or prohibitive surgical risk, as a viable option for correction of pathology and symptom relief. The success of these procedures is reliant on a multidisciplinary heart team to ensure optimal patient selection, appropriate preprocedural screening, meticulous intraprocedural hemodynamic management and imaging guidance, and close postprocedural follow-up. The transcatheter therapies utilized in the electrophysiology (EP) space also require similar degrees of preprocedural planning and are more reliant on variations in intraprocedural anesthetic techniques to identify, localize, and treat any rhythm disturbances that are the initial triggers for patient presentation. Due to the nature of these minimally invasive procedures, where procedural steps cannot always be well visualized, compared to the mainstay of our practice in open cardiac surgery, it is critical for the cardiothoracic anesthesiologist to have a thorough background knowledge of the procedures, potential complications, and an appreciation for the need for constant vigilance at all procedural stages in order to provide the highest level and safest care for these tenuous patient populations.

II. Transcatheter Aortic Valve Replacement

Transfemoral transcatheter aortic valve replacement (TAVR) has been widely accepted as the preferred treatment modality for patients who are at high or prohibitive surgical risk. A recent randomized controlled study also showed a significant mortality and morbidity benefit in low-risk patients undergoing TAVR compared to surgical aortic valve replacements (SAVR).[2] Societal guidelines now view TAVR as an appropriate alternative to SAVR for aortic stenosis (AS) management in any symptomatic patients who are ≥65 years.[3] With the exponential growth of TAVR volume over the course of the past decade, exceeding the total number of SAVRs per year in 2019,[4] it is crucial for the cardiac anesthesiologist to be familiar with all of the TAVR procedural elements. Refer to "Aortic Valve Replacement" section (Chapter 13) in this textbook for further details on this specific procedure.

III. The Transseptal Puncture: Principles and Imaging

A. Introduction

The core and mainstay of left-sided transcatheter procedures is the transseptal puncture (TSP), which is the technique of percutaneously gaining access from the right atrium to the left atrium (LA) through the thin fossa ovalis. The TSP can be guided by simultaneous utilization of fluoroscopy and transesophageal echocardiography (TEE). During this time, a clear communication between the echocardiographer and the interventionalist is critical. The success of several left-sided transcatheter procedures is often based on the accuracy of a site-specific TSP (Figure 11.1A), as it changes the ease of delivering instruments percutaneously to an exact location. This precision in the TSP also allows for avoidance of complications, such as pericardial effusion, atrial wall injury, or perforation.

B. Procedural Techniques and Principles

Femoral venous access is obtained by the interventionalist, and the transseptal sheath and needle are advanced up toward the superior vena cava (SVC). The system is then withdrawn from the SVC to the level of the fossa ovalis and carefully positioned at the predetermined traversal site with the assistance of both fluoroscopy and TEE. Once the puncture site is confirmed in multiple views, a needle is extended from the sheath and advanced into the LA. Septal crossing is confirmed on the available imaging modalities. Immediate scan on TEE should be performed to exclude the presence of a new or developing pericardial effusion, and patient hemodynamics should also be closely monitored. At this point, therapeutic heparin should administered for the target activated clotting time (ACT) that is dependent on the type of procedure and device.

C. Echocardiographic Imaging Considerations

There are three main 2D TEE views that are utilized in visualization of the TSP:

1. The mid-esophageal (ME) bicaval view (90-110°) (Figure 11.1B), where the superior portion of the fossa ovalis is visualized in association with the SVC, and the inferior portion is seen associated with the inferior vena cava (IVC).
2. The ME aortic valve (AV) short-axis view (30-60°) (Figure 11.1C) displays the anterior portion of the interatrial septum and fossa ovalis near the AV, and the posterior portion of the fossa is directly opposite this and close to where the domes of the LA and right atrium meet.
3. The ME four-chamber view (0-15°) (Figure 11.1D) is utilized for the assessment of adequate "height" of the TSP above the atrioventricular valves and specifically for mitral valve (MV) interventions.

The acquisition of these views can be done with either quick omniplane angle switches between 2D views or utilization of the simultaneous orthogonal plane imaging functions for concurrent visualization of a bicaval view and an AV short-axis view. The desired mode of image display should be communicated and confirmed with all team members for facilitation of the intraprocedural steps.

The portion of the puncture that should be visible before transseptal crossing is known as "tenting" of the fossa ovalis, or a deliberate deformation of the fossa with the transseptal system. Confirmation of a safe and desired location of the "tenting" in multiple views will then allow for crossing into the LA.

CLINICAL PEARL

A combination of 2D TEE views, including the ME bicaval view, AV short-axis view, and the four-chamber view, can provide the necessary information and guidance for a site-specific TSP.

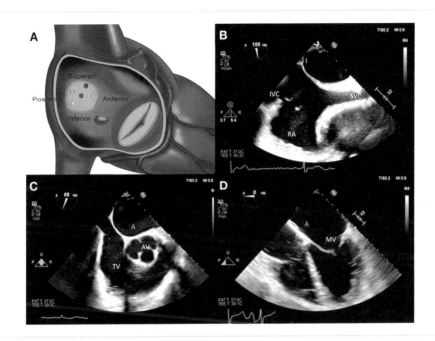

FIGURE 11.1 **(A)** Several site-specific locations for transseptal puncture in the interatrial septum. Yellow: MitraClip, paravalvular leak closure. Purple: Patent foramen ovale closure. Red: Percutaneous left ventricular assist device placement via transseptal approach, and other hemodynamic monitoring. Blue: Left atrial appendage closure. Green: Pulmonary vein interventions. (Adapted from Alkhouli M, Rihal CS, Holmes DR Jr. Transseptal techniques for emerging structural heart interventions. *JACC Cardiovasc Interv.* 2016;9(24):2465-2480, original figure by Lisa Huang, MD.). **(B)** Mid-esophageal bicaval view demonstrating the superior portion of the septum and fossa associated with the SVC, and the inferior portion associated with the IVC. **(C)** Mid-esophageal AV short-axis view demonstrating the anterior portion of the septum close to the AV, and the posterior portion of the septum directly opposing this, close to the point where the domes of the left and right atria meet. **(D)** Mid-esophageal four-chamber view demonstrating anterior and posterior points on the septum and a reference view to assess height of a transseptal puncture above the MV annulus. A, anterior; AV, aortic valve; I, inferior; IVC, inferior vena cava; MV, mitral valve; P, posterior; RA, right atrium; S, superior; SVC, superior vena cava; TV, tricuspid valve.

D. **Site-Specific Transseptal Puncture**

A site-specific TSP is required for procedural precision.[5] It is important to note that a more posterior puncture will allow for the greatest possible height to be obtained above the MV upon entry to the left side of the heart. The classic site-specific locations for each left-sided transcatheter procedure is listed, with the first being the position in the superior-inferior direction and the second being the position in the anterior-posterior direction:

1. **Mitral transcatheter edge-to-edge repair (mitral TEER):** Superior-posterior
2. **Transcatheter MV replacement:** Mid-mid
3. **Mitral paravalvular defect closure:** Site dependent
4. **Left atrial appendage (LAA) occlusion:** Inferior-posterior
5. **Pulmonary vein interventions:** Anterior[5] (see Figure 11.1A)

E. **Complications**

Complications with the TSP can arise if the tenting and crossing is conducted without proper visualization. It is generally not advised to cross through a patent foramen ovale (PFO), which is in a superior and anterior location in the fossa and lies very close to the AV and aortic root, where damage to these structures could inadvertently occur. In addition, it is not recommended to cross through the thick portion of the septum secundum, as traversing through layers of infolding extra-atrial tissue may lead to the rapid development of a pericardial effusion. Finally, crossing at a site in the fossa other than what is recommended for the specific left-sided pathology may lead to procedural failure, simply due to the inability to access the pathology.

IV. **Mitral Valve Transcatheter Edge-to-Edge Repair**

A. **Introduction**

Mitral TEER was first performed in 2003 to treat severe degenerative mitral regurgitation (MR). Since then, procedural feasibility, device safety, and treatment efficacy have been established by various multicenter trials.[6-8] Recent studies further demonstrated its benefits in managing functional MR in addition to goal-directed medical therapy.[8] This resulted in the exponential growth of TEER seen to date.

B. **Patient Selection**

Current guidelines include TEER as a reasonable treatment option for those with chronic severe (≥3+) degenerative or functional MR who are symptomatic and at high or prohibitive surgical risk.[3] TEER devices are designed to percutaneously approximate the MV anterior and posterior leaflets, similar to the surgical Alfieri stitch, thereby reducing the regurgitant orifice and flow. As various intracardiac structures directly interact with the device and its delivery system, preprocedural TEE is critical to determine the MV anatomic suitability, anticipate potential challenges, and exclude contraindications.[9] Optimal valvular morphology is largely based on initial study inclusion criteria and summarized in Table 11.1.

C. **Available Devices**

As of 2022, two different TEER devices, the MitraClip (Abbott) and the PASCAL device (Edwards Lifesciences), are U.S. Food and Drug Administration (FDA) approved and commercially available for degenerative MR (Figure 11.2A). Currently, only MitraClip is approved for functional MR. The two devices share similar valvular repair strategies, yet feature unique designs that may each best suit a specific patient anatomy or pathology. Both devices rely on capturing individual MV leaflets with side arms before bringing them together to form a tissue bridge. However, the PASCAL device has an additional center spacer to help close a large coaptation gap. The newest generation MitraClip comes in four sizes with different combinations of side-arm widths and lengths, whereas the PASCAL comes in two sizes with the larger one (10 mm width) greater than the largest MitraClip (6 mm width).

D. **Contraindications**

With aggregated operator experience and newer device designs, most previously considered anatomic contraindications for mitral TEER are now only deemed challenging procedural targets. Absolute cardiac anatomic contraindications include a short or perforated MV leaflet, severe grasping zone calcification, small MV area, and a large coaptation gap. Those with active endocarditis, a large intracardiac thrombus, hypersensitivity to device components, or who cannot tolerate blood thinners are also not the candidates for mitral TEER.

E. **Procedural Techniques**

Intracardiac access is achieved through the femoral vein. Device guide and delivery catheters are advanced through the interatrial septum via precise TSP. After navigating past the pulmonary veins and LAA, the device is steered down toward the MV and is brought into the left

TABLE 11.1 Mitral Valve Morphology for TEER Therapy

Optimal Morphology	Challenging Morphology
Central A2/P2 lesion	Peripheral A1/P1, A3/P3, or commissural lesions
Posterior leaflet length >10 mm	Short posterior leaflet length 7-10 mm
Tenting height <11 mm	Tenting height ≥11 mm
Coaptation length >2 mm	Coaptation length ≤2 mm or noncoapting leaflets
Flail gap <10 mm	Flail gap ≥10 mm
Flail width <15 mm	Flail width ≥15 mm
Calcification absent	Calcification present in non-grasping zones
MV area >4 cm²	MV area <4 cm² but >3 cm²

MV, mitral valve; TEER, transcatheter edge-to-edge repair.

Reprinted from Nyman CB, Mackensen GB, Jelacic S, Little SH, Smith TW, Mahmood F. Transcatheter mitral valve repair using the edge-to-edge clip. *J Am Soc Echocardiogr*. 2018;31(4):434-453. © 2018 by the American Society of Echocardiography. With permission.

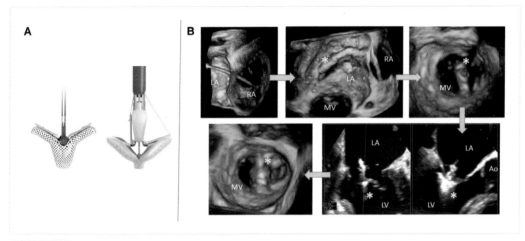

FIGURE 11.2 **(A)** Commercially available transcatheter edge-to-edge leaflet repair devices, MitraClip (**A** (top left): MitraClip is trademark of Abbott or its related companies. Reproduced with permission of Abbott, © 2023. All rights reserved.) and PASCAL (Courtesy of Edwards Lifesciences LLC, Edwards, Edwards Lifesciences, the stylized E logo, PASCAL, PASCAL Ace are trademarks of Edwards Lifesciences Corporation.). **(B)** Transesophageal echocardiographic guidance of transcatheter MV edge-to-edge repair procedure, including crossing interatrial septum, advancing delivery sheath into the LA, positioning and orienting device, capturing mitral leaflets, and deploying device. Asterisk (*) denotes transcatheter device. Ao, aorta; LA, left atrium; LV, left ventricle; MV, mitral valve; RA, right atrium.

ventricle (LV). The MV leaflets are then captured by the device arms in the LV under continuous TEE visualization (Figure 11.2B). Once the device arms are closed with the leaflets securely inserted, reduction of MR is confirmed via a combination of indices, such as improved TEE parameters, decreased LA pressures, and increased systemic pressure. If MR reduction is not satisfactory, the MV leaflets can be released and recaptured after reorienting or repositioning of the device before full deployment. Additional devices may be placed after device deployment to address any residual MR if necessary and if anatomically feasible.

CLINICAL PEARL

Procedural success with mitral TEER is gauged by a combination of several improved and acceptable TEE parameters, decreased LA pressures on invasive measurement, and increased systemic pressures.

F. **Potential Complications**

Key procedural steps such as the TSP, device maneuvering around the LAA, and delivery system withdrawal after device deployment could all result in unintentional cardiac perforation, pericardial effusion, or tamponade. Other potential complications include single leaflet detachment of the device, procedure-induced mitral stenosis (MS), and persistent right-to-left shunting from an iatrogenic atrial septal defect (ASD). The most common complication, however, comes from uncontrolled venous access site bleeding.[10] Finally, esophageal injury from intraprocedural TEE is not uncommon, presumably due to the prolonged examination time and extensive transducer maneuvering. Studies looking at post-mitral TEER esophagogastroduodenoscopy showed longer procedural time and suboptimal imaging quality were both associated with increased risk for esophageal lesions.[11,12]

G. **Periprocedural Anesthetic Management**

1. **Hemodynamic goals**

Although patients who present for mitral TEER tend to be frail with multiple comorbidities, acute hemodynamic instability does not frequently occur during the procedure. Strategies to address significant MR are utilized during the induction and maintenance of anesthesia. It is important to recognize the effects of anesthesia on the severity of MR, as graded by various TEE parameters. Deliberate adjustments of patient preload, afterload, and heart rate to match baseline physiologic state may be needed to assess residual MR and determine procedural end point.

2. **Monitoring and lines**

Arterial pressure monitoring is helpful during the procedure not only to detect intracardiac injuries promptly but also to appreciate the improvement of systemic forward perfusion and cardiac output after device placement. Historically, a dedicated central venous introducer was traditionally placed in order to accommodate pulmonary artery catheter for pulmonary artery wedge pressure measurement before and after TEER. With newer generation device delivery catheters that allow real-time LA pressure measurement, this practice is no longer required. Nowadays, central venous access for intravenous (IV) medication administration is often obtained from the procedural catheter side port, thereby reducing the number of needle punctures and increasing procedural efficiency. After gaining access to the LA, ACT is monitored closely to achieve a value ≥250 seconds throughout the procedure.

Intraprocedural TEE is critical for the success of the procedure. It is used to confirm the preprocedural diagnosis, plan procedural approaches, and exclude any contraindications that may have developed since last clinic visit.[13] Moreover, it is required to safely guide catheter, wire, sheath, and device movement in cardiac chambers to target precise regurgitant locations. Various echocardiographic parameters are used to assess MR severity before and after device placement.[14] Finally, intraprocedural TEE can be used to quickly exclude any iatrogenic complications in real time.

3. **Anesthetic technique**

Although ultrasound imaging modalities such as transthoracic echocardiography (TTE) and intracardiac echocardiography (ICE) have been used to guide the procedure, TEE is still considered the gold standard for its superior imaging quality, noninvasiveness, and low cost. However, since intraprocedural TEE guidance tends to be prolonged and extensive, general anesthesia with endotracheal tube (ETT) placement is typically the anesthetic of choice for patient overall safety and comfort. Furthermore, controlled ventilation is often advantageous for certain challenging cases.

As operators gain experience and reduce overall procedural time, both deep and moderate sedation without airway protection have been utilized. Compared to general anesthesia, no differences in technical success, short-term outcome, major cardiac events, or bleeding complications, all while having lower incidences of hypotension and shorter hospital stays, were observed with sedation.[15,16]

V. Transcatheter Mitral Valve Replacement

A. **Introduction**

Transcatheter mitral valve replacement (TMVR) addresses high-risk patients with severe MR who may have anatomic contraindications to or are not eligible for transcatheter MV repair. Moreover, it has also emerged as an acceptable treatment option for those with symptomatic MS.[17] TMVRs have been successfully performed in degenerated bioprosthetic MVs (valve-in-valve or ViV), mitral annular rings (valve-in-ring or ViR), and native mitral annular calcification (ViMAC). As more data demonstrate the feasibility and safety of TMVR, case volumes are expected to rise rapidly.

B. **Patient Selection**

TMVR is currently reserved for high-risk patients who are symptomatic due to severe mitral disease. It is important to consider the suitability of patient cardiac anatomy before determining candidacy. Implanting commercially available transcatheter heart valve (THV) in the native mitral position poses several challenges as the mitral annulus is not only "D-shaped" but also dynamic in nature during the cardiac cycle. Furthermore, there is generally a lack of a reliable landing zone for THVs with conventional anchoring mechanisms. Finally, the newly implanted mitral THV is predisposed to embolization due to the large pressure difference between the LA and LV. When compared to a calcified native mitral annulus, either a preexisting mitral annuloplasty ring or bioprosthetic valve provides a more circular and secure landing zone. It is, therefore, not surprising that early clinical outcomes for ViR and ViV have been significantly better than ViMAC TMVR.[18]

Comprehensive imaging workup is mandatory before the procedure. TTE and/or TEE are used to assess baseline pathology and severity.[19] Diastolic function is also assessed as those with advanced diseases may not benefit from TMVR. Unlike the mitral TEER preprocedural workup, multidetector computed tomography (MDCT) is crucial in TMVR cases to delineate the morphology of the proposed landing zone, including annular dimension, area, shape, severity, and thickness of calcification and completeness and rigidity of the preexisting prosthesis. It is also used extensively to evaluate for potential complications, such as valve migration, paravalvular regurgitation, and LV outflow tract (LVOT) obstruction (Figure 11.3A). THV size selection is primarily based on preprocedural MDCT.

C. **Available Devices**

Although numerous MV-specific THVs are being developed and investigated, currently, only the balloon-expandable SAPIEN (Edwards Lifesciences) THV, originally designed for TAVR, is FDA approved for ViV and ViR TMVR. Off-label ViMAC TMVR is performed for high-risk patients with limited options at experienced centers. The durability of THVs implanted in the mitral position is unknown, although it is presumed to be comparable to those implanted for TAVRs.

D. **Contraindications**

Absolute contraindications to TMVR include active systemic infection, lack of adequate landing zone (too large or too small, lack of calcification, prosthesis dehiscence, etc), excessive risk for LVOT obstruction, and procedural futility.[20]

E. **Procedural Techniques**

Most TMVRs are now performed via transfemoral venous access, as opposed to the traditional transapical route, due to its less invasive nature. Hybrid transatrial TMVR via a sternal access is another option, although a brief period of cardiopulmonary bypass (CPB) is required and, therefore, requires surgical candidacy.

The transfemoral approach involves TSP to access the MV via an antegrade manner, similar to that of mitral TEER procedures. The interatrial septum and stenotic MV are often balloon

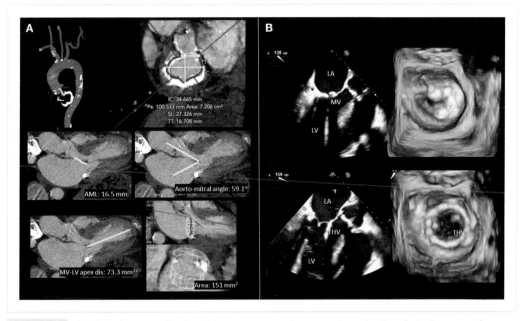

FIGURE 11.3 **(A)** Typical preprocedural multidetector computed tomography evaluation of mitral apparatus for transcatheter MV replacement. **(B)** Severe mitral stenosis due to calcified MV **(top panels)** treated by THV **(bottom panels)**. LA, left atrium; LV, left ventricle; MV, mitral valve; THV, transcatheter heart valve.

dilated in preparation to accommodate the large THV delivery system. Once the THV is advanced into the MV annulus, rapid pacing is commenced by a right ventricular (RV) temporary wire to achieve relative cardiac standstill. The precise position (most often 20%-30% atrial and 70%-80% ventricular) and angulation of the THV is adjusted during the slow and controlled THV deployment (Figure 11.3B). Further ventricular flaring of the THV by repeat balloon dilatation may be needed after deployment to ensure secure seating.

F. Potential Complications

Life-threatening LVOT obstruction, due to anterior mitral leaflet displacement from THV stents, is the most feared complication after TMVR. Risk factors include small preprocedural LVOT area, long anterior mitral leaflet, thick interventricular septum, small LV cavity, ventricular implantation of THV, and a perpendicular aorto-mitral angle.[21] With new MDCT software, THV placement can be simulated preprocedure and the "neo-LVOT" (residual LVOT after the implantation of the mitral THV) estimated to assess overall LVOT obstruction risk. Strategies to alleviate LVOT obstruction include preemptive or rescue alcohol septal ablation, intentional percutaneous laceration of the anterior mitral leaflet to prevent outflow obstruction (LAMPOON procedure), percutaneous septal scoring along the midline endocardium (SESAME procedure), radiofrequency septal ablation, and a kissing balloon bailout technique.[22] Surgical resection of the anterior mitral leaflet via the hybrid transatrial approach may be the most effective method to prevent LVOT obstruction.

Excessive radial force exerted by a THV too large for the mitral annulus may cause circumflex coronary artery compression and ventricular dysfunction. On the other hand, too small of a THV may result in poor apposition of the THV to the landing zone, leading to valvular embolization or paravalvular regurgitation. An embolized THV can be retrieved percutaneously or surgically despite the high risk. Paravalvular defects (PVDs), especially medial and lateral to the THV, are not uncommon and may call for percutaneous closure should they result in clinically significant regurgitation or hemolysis.

Because of the large delivery sheath and THV size, the risk of intracardiac perforation or rupture can occur during TMVR. Maneuvering the THV within the LA and around the LAA should be exercised with great caution. Signs of pericardial effusion and tamponade should be monitored vigilantly. Large iatrogenic ASDs are created during the procedure and frequently require percutaneous closure to prevent acute hypoxemia, cerebral embolic events, or worsening heart failure. Similar to TAVRs, access site bleeding is of concern and crossmatched blood should be readily available.

CLINICAL PEARL

Case planning for a TMVR involves careful assessment of the anatomy and residual area of the LVOT, as "neo-LVOT" obstruction is the most feared complication after the procedure.

G. Periprocedural Anesthetic Management

1. Hemodynamic goals

Depending on the underlying mitral pathology (regurgitation, stenosis, or mixed disease), patient's baseline volume status, heart rate, and systemic vascular resistance can be adjusted pharmacologically to optimize forward cardiac output and systemic perfusion.

2. Monitoring and lines

An arterial line is helpful during the procedure to closely monitor blood pressure and rapidly diagnose complications. A dedicated radial arterial line is ideal, but measurements can also be transduced from a femoral arterial line used for the procedure. During rapid pacing for valve deployment, moments of reduced mean arterial pressure and pulsatility are expected.

As with any transcatheter procedure, external defibrillator pads are required should malignant arrhythmias be induced unintentionally by wires or catheters.

Central venous access is often needed for emergency drug and volume administration. A pulmonary artery catheter is less important as the LA pressure can be directly measured and pulmonary artery pressure estimated by TEE during the procedure.

TEE is critical to guide the TSP, intracardiac maneuvering of the device, and placement of the THV in the mitral position. Postprocedural assessment of the THV function, interatrial shunt direction, and any complications from the procedure should also be performed with TEE.[14]

3. **Anesthetic technique**

General anesthesia with ETT placement is often utilized for the procedure, even for the least invasive transfemoral/transseptal route due to the need for intraprocedural TEE. Preemptive airway control may be more desirable should life-threatening complications after TMVR, such as LVOT obstruction, occur. A minimalist approach utilizing monitored anesthetic care for ViV or ViR TMVR with only ICE use may be considered at highly experienced centers in selected patients.

For a transapical TMVR, lung isolation may be temporarily necessary during surgical access via thoracotomy. Regional anesthesia techniques, such as a paravertebral block, may complement general anesthesia and provide better postprocedural pain control. Risks and benefits of a thoracic epidural may be weighed due to the need for procedural systemic heparinization and postprocedural anticoagulation needs.

A transatrial TMVR will require a sternotomy and is, therefore, treated similar to a standard cardiac surgical case in terms of anesthetic management.

VI. Left Atrial Appendage Occlusion Devices

A. Introduction

Atrial fibrillation (AFib) is a major cardiac risk factor for embolic stroke, and the LAA is the most common site of intracardiac thrombus in patients with nonvalvular AFib. The 5-year outcomes of the pivotal LAA occluder (LAAO) trials with the Watchman device (Boston Scientific), PROTECT AFib and PREVAIL, demonstrated stroke prevention in nonvalvular AFib that was comparable to warfarin therapy.[23]

B. Patient Selection

Patients who have contraindications to the long-term use of oral anticoagulants due to a personal history of bleeding or significant bleeding risk, documented noncompliance with oral medications, or simply a desire to avoid oral anticoagulation with CHA_2DS_2VASc scores ≥ 2 may be the candidates for LAAO therapies.[13,24]

A full anatomic analysis of the LAA can be conducted with multimodality imaging. A preprocedural MDCT scan can provide information regarding the LAA size, shape, and presence of accessory lobes. This information can also be confirmed on intraprocedural TEE or ICE.

C. Available Devices

The FDA-approved devices in the United States for LAAO are the Watchman device family and the Amulet device (Abbott) (see Figure 11.4A). These occluders are available in a variety of sizes depending on the dimensions of the device landing zone and the assessment of the LAA anatomy.

D. Contraindications

The major contraindication to the implantation of an LAAO device in the periprocedural period is the presence of an intracardiac mass, namely, LAA thrombus. True organized thrombus in the LAA remains grounds for procedural cancellation, and this is the first element that should be assessed on the intraprocedural study. Other possible contraindications may include the presence of an atrial septal occluder device that may prevent the performance of a successful TSP, vascular anatomy issues, relevant patient hypersensitivities to device components, or active infections.

CLINICAL PEARL

A major contraindication to placement of an LAAO device is the presence of intracardiac thrombus. Despite thorough preprocedural imaging and planning, thrombus should be ruled out with echocardiography immediately before the start of the procedure.

E. **Procedural Techniques**

Femoral venous access is obtained, and a TSP is conducted with concomitant TEE/ICE and fluoroscopic guidance. Access is gained into the LA, and the device delivery sheath is advanced toward the LAA. The device is positioned into the LAA landing zone and initially deployed without being fully released. After initial deployment, subsequent checks are utilized to assess device size (Figure 11.4B), position, stability, and lack of residual blood flow into the appendage and around the device. Adequate preprocedural LAA sizing is critical in the prevention of para-device leaks. Before full release, the devices can be repositioned and redeployed. Once the criteria have been met for device release, the LAAO is fully deployed, device delivery components are returned to the right atrium and removed from the patient.

F. **Potential Complications**

As with other transcatheter procedures, complications from LAAO can include the development of a pericardial effusion or tamponade, LAA rupture, device embolization, or vascular access complications. Longer term complications of device-related thrombus or device erosion/infection are also possible.

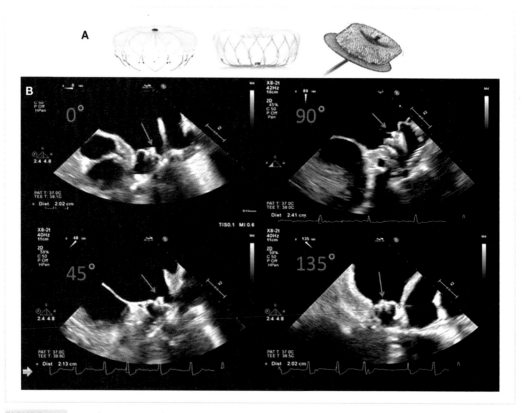

FIGURE 11.4 (**A**) The available left atrial appendage occlusion devices, from left to right, including the Watchman Generation 2.5 (**A** (top left and middle): ©2023 Boston Scientific Corporation or its affiliates. All rights reserved.), Watchman FLX (middle, © 2023 Boston Scientific Corporation or its affiliates. All rights reserved.), and the Amulet device (**A** (top right): Amplatzer, Amulet, Amplatzer Amulet are trademarks of Abbott or its related companies. Reproduced with permission of Abbott, © 2023. All rights reserved.). (**B**) Visualization of final size and device compression after deployment of a Watchman FLX device in the four classic TEE views utilized for appendage and device assessment: 0, 45, 90, and 135. The arrows denote the central threaded insert, which must be present in the view to accurately note the size of the compressed device and prevent device foreshortening.

G. **Periprocedural Anesthetic Management**

1. **Hemodynamic goals**

Direct LA pressures will be monitored with procedural device catheters. If LA pressures are low, this will allow for the careful administration of IV fluids and volume as necessary to ensure that the anatomy of the LA and LAA, in turn, is congruent with the patient's baseline status. Other parameters, such as blood pressure and heart rate, should be noted and maintained over the course of the procedure.

2. **Monitoring and lines**

Femoral venous access is obtained by the interventionalist for the procedure, and as such, additional central venous access may be available for utilization by the anesthesiology team. A radial arterial line can be utilized for monitoring at the anesthesiologist's discretion, given the patient's comorbidities.

3. **Anesthetic technique**

Institutions around the United States are taking one of the following two approaches: (1) general anesthesia with intraprocedural TEE for LAAO or (2) monitored anesthesia care with ICE for the intraprocedural imaging. The outcomes of these two strategies are currently being studied. Hemodynamic goals, as well as monitoring, and access strategies remain the same with both anesthetic techniques.

VII. Transcatheter Prosthetic Paravalvular Defect Closures

A. **Introduction**

A prosthetic PVD can occur after surgical valve replacement due to implant errors, suture failure, annular disruption, or endocarditis. It is also commonly seen after transcatheter valvular replacement because of the lack of annular debridement and poor tissue apposition. Traditionally, these PVDs are addressed by repeat surgery if not responsive to conservative medical therapy. However, percutaneous options for PVD closure have become increasingly more desirable in the past decade, as they avoid repeat sternotomy and also minimize mortality and morbidity associated with surgery in these symptomatic patients.[25]

B. **Patient Selection**

PVDs come in various sizes and shapes and must be distinguished from transvalvular regurgitation. Large PVDs result in severe regurgitation and ultimately heart failure symptoms. Smaller PVDs, although not necessarily hemodynamic significant, can cause intractable hemolysis of erythrocytes from turbulent flow patterns. Clinical sequelae include anemia and renal failure and ultimately recurrent transfusions and, possibly, dialysis.

Echocardiography is the primary imaging modality to diagnose PVD, pinpoint the location, and assess the regurgitation severity (Figure 11.5A).[14] Adjunctive imaging modalities such as MDCT or cardiac magnetic resonance imaging (MRI) can be considered during workup for more complex lesions. The most recent American College of Cardiology/American Heart Association (ACC/AHA) valvular heart disease guidelines recommend percutaneous repair of PVD in symptomatic patients who are at high or prohibitive surgical risks with features suitable for transcatheter closure.[3]

C. **Available Devices**

A plethora of devices, including those originally designed for vascular occlusion, are utilized for PVD closure. Device selection depends on institutional preference, device availability, and PVD features. In the United States, the Amplatzer vascular plug types II and IV (Abbott Vascular) are commonly used in an off-label manner to eliminate the defect (Figure 11.5B). Other septal or ductal occluders have also been utilized.

D. **Contraindications**

If evidence of infective endocarditis is present, risks and benefits of urgent surgical PVD repair or valve replacement should be considered. Should timing allow, completion of antibiotic treatment is preferred before transcatheter PVD closure.

E. **Procedural Techniques**

Aortic PVDs are approached in retrograde manner via the femoral artery. Once the wire is threaded across the PVD, a guide catheter is advanced into the LV and positioned for device placement. Depending on the specific device, some occlude the PVD by retention disks on

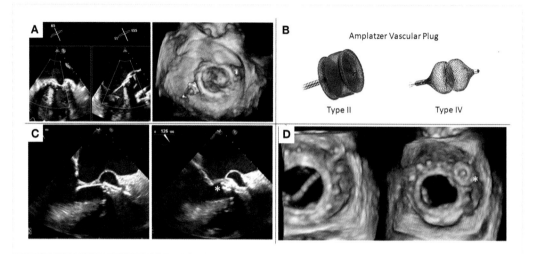

FIGURE 11.5 **(A)** Posterior aortic paravalvular defect at the 12 o'clock location when viewed in standard aortic valve short-axis view **(left)** and mitral prosthetic valve paravalvular defect at 2 and 8 o'clock locations when viewed in standard 3D enface view **(right)**. **(B)** Amplatzer vascular plug used off-label for paravalvular defect occlusion. **(C)** Wire through para-aortic defect and occluder device placement. **(D)** Wire through paramitral defect and occluder device placement. Asterisk (*) denotes transcatheter occlude device.

either side of the PVD, whereas others plug the PVD entirely within the defect (Figure 11.5C). Regardless, leaflet impingement and residual regurgitation must be assessed before the release of the device. If the device is placed in close proximity to the coronary arteries, angiography should also be performed to exclude inadvertent coronary impingement or occlusion.

Mitral PVDs are preferably closed from the LA via femoral venous and TSP in an ante-grade manner. A steerable guide catheter is used to direct a wire through the PVD. Medial or posterior PVDs are generally more difficult to access due to the location and need for acute angulation of the guide catheter. Adjusting TSP sites more posteriorly and superiorly may pro-vide better trajectory in those cases. Transcatheter rails, created by snaring and externalizing a wire through the PVD, are occasionally needed in the challenging locations to facilitate guide catheter placement. The occluder device is eventually released after careful TEE assessment (Figure 11.5D).

F. Potential Complications

Injury to intracardiac structures could occur with advancement, threading, and positioning of guide wires and catheter. Stiff wires may even create additional PVDs unintentionally during attempts to traverse the preexisting lesion. Tension from transcatheter wire rails may dam-age prosthetic leaflets, entangle chordal structures, or cause bradycardia from atrioventricular nodal compression.

Accurate sizing of PVDs for device selection, regardless of the location, is inherently chal-lenging due to their varying shape and course. Instead of circular and cylindrical, most PVDs are irregularly shaped at their orifice and zigzag along the prosthetic valve. The diameter of the PVD often changes along the course, as well. Small PVDs also are more prone to measuring errors, regardless of the imaging modality. Occluder devices selected that are too small may increase the risk for embolism. On the other hand, too large of a device may interfere with valve leaflet function, resulting in iatrogenic transvalvular regurgitation or stenosis. Therefore, crescent-shaped PVDs may best be treated by multiple small devices, deployed side by side, instead of the placement of a single large plug. If the PVDs occupy significant circumferential length, transcatheter ViV deployment could be considered as the THV fabric skirt may seal all PVDs at once.

G. **Periprocedural Anesthetic Management**

1. **Hemodynamic goals**

Patients with PVDs, regardless of the location, predominantly present with flow regurgitation. These patients require normal-to-high heart rates, normal-to-high ventricular filling, and normal-to-low systemic vascular resistance to optimize forward cardiac output.

2. **Monitoring and lines**

Since percutaneous PVD closure procedures do not induce large hemodynamic swings, dedicated arterial lines are not routinely placed for monitoring purposes, unless indicated by other patient comorbidities. During an AV PVD closure procedure performed femoral arterial access, an invasive arterial blood pressure can often be obtained from the femoral sheath side port used for the procedure. However, false readings from dampened pressure tracing may occur when a large device delivery system is inserted into the lumen of a small sheath and a small femoral vessel. If invasive arterial monitoring is needed during a mitral PVD closure procedure where only femoral venous access is planned, the acquisition of a dedicated invasive arterial line for use in the intraprocedural period can be discussed with the interventionalist.

Central venous access, although also not required, may be helpful during the procedure for reliable vasoactive medication infusion.

TEE is utilized for most transcatheter PVD closures to locate the lesion, assess the severity, direct the device, and exclude any complications in real time.[25] It is especially helpful for MV PVDs as the imaging resolution is often superb from the viewpoint of the LA. AV PVD closure, on the other hand, may be performed without TEE support, especially if fluoroscopic angles to access the defect are predetermined by preprocedural MDCT. AV PVDs are also frequently shadowed from prosthetic material and are much more difficult to pinpoint than MV PVDs by TEE. Fusion imaging, with the overlay of live TEE images on fluoroscopy, may be used to facilitate localization of lesion and placement of devices.[26]

3. **Anesthetic technique**

General anesthesia with ETT placement is used for all procedures requiring TEE for comfort reasons during the extensive imaging process. Although monitored anesthesia care can be used for cases without the need of TEE, it must be recognized that transcatheter PVD closures are challenging procedures that may take several hours to complete.

VIII. **Complex Atrial Septal Defect Closures**

A. **Introduction**

Defects in the interatrial septum can take one of two forms: either a PFO or an ASD. PFOs and ASDs can be closed by either surgery or transcatheter devices, with transcatheter devices increasingly being utilized in higher risk patients. After adequate patient prescreening, PFO closures can typically be performed with the utilization of minimal conscious sedation and TTE/ICE. Here, we discuss specific patient considerations for complex ASDs that require more in-depth intraprocedural imaging guidance.

B. **Patient Selection**

The type of ASD that is the most amenable to transcatheter closure is the ostium secundum ASD. Typically, consideration is given to ASD repair if a patient has a significant left-to-right shunt (Qp:Qs >1.5) and right heart enlargement with volume overload, regardless of the presence of symptoms.[27] Small defects with right-to-left shunting that predispose patients to hypoxemia or paradoxical embolism should also be addressed and closed.[28] For definitive transcatheter closure, preprocedural imaging should confirm the presence of adequate (>5 mm) superior/SVC, aortic, atrioventricular valve, inferior/IVC, posterior, and right upper pulmonary vein rims of the defect in order to ensure the stability of the transcatheter device and minimize the chance of embolization.

C. **Available Devices**

Separate devices are available specifically for PFO closure, as the anatomy of a PFO tunnel is different than that of a true secundum ASD. Three ASD closure devices, including the Amplatzer Septal Occluder (Abbott), Gore CARDIOFORM ASD Occluder (Gore), and the Gore CARDIOFORM Septal Occluder, are FDA approved.[28] The Amplatzer Cribriform Occluder

(Abbott), a variation on the other devices, can be utilized to close a fenestrated or complex defect with multiple orifices.

D. Contraindications

Patients with large defects (>38 mm), above the size and diameter of the available devices, and those with defects with deficient rims (<5 mm) cannot be closed with the available transcatheter devices and should be referred for surgery. Patients found to have anomalous pulmonary venous drainage in association with an ASD should also be referred for surgical consultation. A major contraindication to either transcatheter or surgical ASD closure is severe and irreversible pulmonary hypertension (pulmonary vascular resistance >8 Woods units), where the ASD is critical as a "pop-off" mechanism for right heart offloading.[27]

E. Procedural Techniques

Femoral venous access is obtained, and the defect is traversed with the necessary wires, catheters, and sheaths. Sizing of the defect can be performed with either imaging guidance (2D and 3D TEE/ICE) or utilization of a catheter-based compliant sizing balloon. During the procedure, the LA portion of the device will be generally be deployed first, withdrawn to the level of the interatrial septum, before the right atrial portion of the device is deployed. The septum will be interrogated for any residual interatrial shunt. Minimal intradevice flow may still be present but should improve over time as the device endothelializes.

F. Potential Complications

Short-term complications can include residual shunts, device embolization, atrial arrhythmias, and cardiac perforation. Longer term complications include device-related thrombus and cardiac erosion.

G. Periprocedural Anesthetic Management

1. Hemodynamic goals

Any degree of preexisting right heart dysfunction or pulmonary hypertension should be noted and accounted for during the induction of anesthesia and throughout the procedure, with the initiation of infusions or bolus doses of inotropic medications as necessary.

2. Monitoring and lines

Due to the presence of an ASD from the beginning of the procedure, consideration should be given to placing an in-line filter on any venous lines where medications and fluids will be returning to the patient in order to minimize the amount of air that could traverse the defect and enter the systemic circulation. In the presence of significant right heart dysfunction or pulmonary hypertension, consideration can be given to intraprocedural monitoring with a radial arterial line.

3. Anesthetic technique

Aside from straightforward transcatheter PFO closures that can be done with conscious sedation and ICE, more complex ASD closures are typically performed with the assistance of general anesthesia and TEE. TEE can be used to size the defect (along with balloon sizing) and precisely characterize the defect that is being covered (eg, fenestrations, multiple defects, rim sizes).

IX. Electrophysiology Procedures: Anesthetic Considerations

A. Introduction and Preoperative Assessment

Procedures performed in the EP laboratory require special attention from anesthesiologists due to the broad scope and variety of procedures, patient comorbidities, unique anesthetic considerations, and the potential for procedure-specific complications.

At a minimum, preoperative assessment of the patient presenting for a procedure in the EP laboratory should include an assessment and review of patient functional status, results of obstructive sleep apnea screening, pulmonary comorbidities and pulmonary status (eg, home oxygen requirement), available baseline echocardiography data, and a recent or day-of-procedure electrocardiography (ECG). In particular, assessment of a patient's LV and RV function can give the anesthesiologist an idea of the degree of hemodynamic stability or instability that may be encountered during induction of anesthesia or during incitement of a particular rhythm disturbance over the course of the procedure.[29] In addition, if applicable, a review of oral anticoagulant medication therapy and compliance should be conducted by both the electrophysiologist and the anesthesiologist in order to ensure that the procedure can be conducted safely. TEE may need to be conducted preprocedurally to exclude the presence of LAA thrombus before the introduction of intracardiac catheters and wires if an interruption in anticoagulation is discovered before AFib ablation or pulmonary vein isolation.

The appropriate choice of anesthetic technique may depend on the nature of the procedures as described earlier and, as such, monitored anesthesia care, general anesthesia with laryngeal mask airway (LMA), or general anesthesia with ETT may each be warranted in specific procedural situations.

It is important to note that significant volume and crystalloid administration occurs via the electrophysiologists' catheter and sheaths by the procedural team during the majority of these procedures. Therefore, careful volume administration by the anesthesiologist must be conducted throughout.[30]

B. Atrial Flutter and Atrial Fibrillation Ablations

The anatomic origin of the arrhythmia is important to note and discuss with the electrophysiologist in order to determine the most appropriate mode of sedation for the procedure. Typical atrial flutter originates in the right atrium and does not require the performance of TSP for access to left-sided lesions or targets. As such, the procedural time may be shorter.[29] Monitored anesthesia care or general anesthesia with LMA may be appropriate for these typical atrial flutter cases.

Atypical atrial flutter or AFib cases typically have targets that need to be addressed in the LA, requiring a TSP and longer procedural duration. In addition, precision in arrhythmia mapping requires minimal patient movement. For atypical atrial flutter and AFib ablation/pulmonary vein isolation procedures, general anesthesia with ETT is preferred. This strategy should be utilized with minimal muscle relaxant or depolarizing muscle relaxant alone for intubation, as needs may arise during the procedure to pace the diaphragm in order to monitor for phrenic nerve injury. Institutional variation exists on the utilization of ventilation strategies (standard vs high-frequency jet ventilation) and associated anesthetic techniques.[29] These preferences should be discussed before the procedure. Considerations should be given to patient factors related to tolerance of high-frequency jet ventilation (eg, body habitus, preexisting pulmonary obstructive disease) before initiation of this technique.

AFib ablation and pulmonary vein isolation procedures involve the ablation of the pulmonary veins in the posterior portion of the LA, which are close to the esophagus. Vigilant esophageal temperature monitoring should be conducted during the procedure in order to avoid the development of esophageal injury, or more fatally, an atrio-esophageal fistula.[29,30] Rapid rises in temperature during the ablation portion of the procedure should be immediately communicated to the electrophysiologist, and the procedure should be temporarily paused.

This monitoring may involve the utilization of an esophageal temperature probe with a special sensor that can be detected on the electrophysiologist's map. The visualization of the temperature probe on the map allows the proceduralist to ask for adjustment of the position of the probe in association with ablation target locations to precisely detect any temperature derangements over the course of the ablation.

CLINICAL PEARL

Monitoring for phrenic nerve injury and esophageal injury are two critical elements of an atrial fibrillation ablation procedure conducted under general anesthesia.

C. Supraventricular Tachycardia Ablations

The utilization of deep sedation or general anesthesia for supraventricular tachycardia (SVT) ablations often runs the risk of significant arrhythmia suppression, especially with the utilization of higher doses of benzodiazepines, opiates, and propofol. Therefore, these cases involve a balance between obtaining patient comfort for the initial access and targeted lesion therapy and minimizing drug-related blunting of the arrhythmia. A spectrum of sedation level can be utilized during the procedure—first with deep sedation for venous groin access, and subsequently a lighter level of sedation for the identification of the excitable anatomic targets. Deeper sedation may need to be reinitiated during the treatment and ablation phase. If the anesthesiologist feels that it is indicated for either airway protection or patient-specific purposes, utilization of general anesthesia with either LMA or ETT from the beginning of the procedure must be discussed with the electrophysiologist before the start of the case.

D. Ventricular Tachycardia Ablations

Ventricular tachycardia (VT) ablations are often long, complex procedures that are performed on patients with poor functional status and those who have limited cardiopulmonary reserve. The incitement of a malignant arrhythmia that could cause prolonged periods of hemodynamic instability warrants the team's consideration of utilization of temporary mechanical circulatory support (MCS) for the procedural duration.[29] Risks versus benefits of temporary MCS must be weighed for each patient. Either monitored anesthesia care (MAC) or general anesthesia can be utilized for these procedures with appropriate hemodynamic monitoring capabilities. These include arterial line access for continuous invasive blood pressure monitoring and large-bore central venous access (can be provided via femoral access from the electrophysiologist) for patient resuscitation purposes. TEE or ICE may need to be utilized in the event of a cardiac arrest for diagnostic and therapeutic purposes.

E. Device Implants: Pacemakers and Implantable Cardioverter-Defibrillators

The full spectrum of anesthetic techniques (local/regional, monitored anesthesia care, general anesthesia with LMA or ETT) can be utilized as deemed appropriate with respect to patient factors for device implantations. Specific attention must be paid to the administration of antibiotic prophylaxis before incision. The newer leadless pacemakers can be implanted with MAC anesthesia.

In implantable cardioverter-defibrillator (ICD) implantation, the role and value of defibrillation testing has been highly debated over the past several years, but current practice is to avoid routine testing upon ICD implantation unless the device that is being implanted is a subcutaneous ICD. If testing is warranted, this may prompt a choice of brief induction of general anesthesia for the patient to tolerate the energy delivery.[30] General anesthesia with adjunct regional anesthesia is typically indicated for implantation of a subcutaneous ICD due to the need for extensive procedural dissection and device tunneling.

F. Lead Extractions

Lead extractions can typically be performed with laser sheath technologies. The risk of the extraction increases with the length of the time that the lead has been in place, given the amount of scarring and fibrosis that has likely occurred in the upper extremity vessels surrounding the leads. These procedures require invasive arterial line monitoring, large-bore peripheral or central venous access for potential volume resuscitation, and also real-time TEE imaging for monitoring of the development of a pericardial effusion. Intraprocedural TEE can also be used to rule out tricuspid valve leaflet damage or increase in tricuspid regurgitation (TR). Baseline documentation and changes should be noted with respect to the presence or absence of an effusion and the degree of TR, in addition to the rest of the complete TEE examination. Cardiac surgical support should be readily available depending on the risk profile of the patient and procedure.

X. Conclusions

Minimally invasive transcatheter procedures being utilized to treat structural heart disease are steadily increasing, and it is important for the cardiac anesthesiologist to be familiar and facile with these procedures. The success of these procedures is reliant on a multidisciplinary heart team to ensure optimal patient selection, appropriate preprocedural screening with multimodality imaging techniques, precision in intraprocedural management in terms of selection of catheter-based techniques as well as intraprocedural imaging and echocardiographic guidance, continuous monitoring for the development of complications, and incredibly close postprocedural follow-up.

REFERENCES

1. Steinberg DH, Staubach S, Franke J, et al. Defining structural heart disease in the adult patient: current scope, inherent challenges, and future directions. *Eur Heart J Suppl.* 2010;12(Suppl. E):E2-E9.
2. Mack MJ, Leon MB, Thourani VH, et al. Transcatheter aortic-valve replacement with a balloon-expandable valve in low-risk patients. *N Engl J Med.* 2019;380(18):1695-1705.

3. Otto CM, Nishimura RA, Bonow RO, et al. 2020 ACC/AHA guideline for the management of patients with valvular heart disease: executive summary: a report of the American College of Cardiology/American Heart Association Joint Committee on Clinical Practice Guidelines. *Circulation.* 2021;143(5):e35-e71.

4. Carroll JD, Mack MJ, Vemulapalli S, et al. STS-ACC TVT registry of transcatheter aortic valve replacement. *J Am Coll Cardiol.* 2020;76(21):2492-2516.

5. Alkhouli M, Rihal CS, Holmes DR. Transseptal techniques for emerging structural heart interventions. *JACC Cardiovasc Interv.* 2016;9:2465-2480.

6. Feldman T, Wasserman HS, Herrmann HC, et al. Percutaneous mitral valve repair using the edge-to-edge technique: six-month results of the EVEREST phase I clinical trial. *J Am Coll Cardiol.* 2005;46(11):2134-2140.

7. Feldman T, Kar S, Elmariah S, et al. Randomized comparison of percutaneous repair and surgery for mitral regurgitation: 5-year results of EVEREST II. *J Am Coll Cardiol.* 2015;66(25):2844-2854.

8. Asch FM, Grayburn PA, Siegel RJ, et al. Echocardiographic outcomes after transcatheter leaflet approximation in patients with secondary mitral regurgitation: the COAPT trial. *J Am Coll Cardiol.* 2019;74(24):2969-2979.

9. Nyman CB, Mackensen GB, Jelacic S, et al. Transcatheter mitral valve repair using the edge-to-edge clip. *J Am Soc Echocardiogr.* 2018;31(4):434-453.

10. Schnitzler K, Hell M, Geyer M, et al. Complications following MitraClip implantation. *Curr Cardiol Rep.* 2021;23(9):131.

11. Ruf TF, Heidrich FM, Sveric KM, et al. ELMSTREET (Esophageal Lesions during MitraClip uSing TRansEsophageal Echocardiography Trial). *EuroIntervention.* 2017;13(12):e1444-e1451.

12. Freitas-Ferraz AB, Bernier M, Vaillancourt R, et al. Safety of transesophageal echocardiography to guide structural cardiac interventions. *J Am Coll Cardiol.* 2020;75(25):3164-3173.

13. Hahn RT, Saric M, Faletra FF, et al. Recommended standards for the performance of transesophageal echocardiographic screening for structural heart intervention: from the American Society of Echocardiography. *J Am Soc Echocardiogr.* 2022;35(1):1-76.

14. Zoghbi WA, Asch FM, Bruce C, et al. Guidelines for the evaluation of valvular regurgitation after percutaneous valve repair or replacement: a report from the American Society of Echocardiography Developed in Collaboration with the Society for Cardiovascular Angiography and Interventions, Japanese Society of Echocardiography, and Society for Cardiovascular Magnetic Resonance. *J Am Soc Echocardiogr.* 2019;32(4):431-475.

15. Horn P, Hellhammer K, Minier M, et al. Deep sedation vs. general anesthesia in 232 patients undergoing percutaneous mitral valve repair using the MitraClip® system. *Catheter Cardiovasc Interv.* 2017;90(7):1212-1219.

16. Ates I, Okutucu S, Kose G, et al. Evaluation of effectiveness and safety of transcatheter mitral valve repair under moderate conscious sedation. *J Invasive Cardiol.* 2020;32(6):206-210.

17. Baumgartner H, Falk V, Bax JJ, et al. 2017 ESC/EACTS guidelines for the management of valvular heart disease. *Eur Heart J.* 2017;38(36):2739-2791.

18. Eleid MF, Whisenant BK, Cabalka AK, et al. Early outcomes of percutaneous transvenous transseptal transcatheter valve implantation in failed bioprosthetic mitral valves, ring annuloplasty, and severe mitral annular calcification. *JACC Cardiovasc Interv.* 2017;10(19):1932-1942.

19. Mackensen GB, Lee JC, Wang DD, et al. Role of echocardiography in transcatheter mitral valve replacement in native mitral valves and mitral rings. *J Am Soc Echocardiogr.* 2018;31(4):475-490.

20. Urena M, Vahanian A, Brochet E, et al. Current indications for transcatheter mitral valve replacement using transcatheter aortic valves: valve-in-valve, valve-in-ring, and valve-in-mitral annulus calcification. *Circulation.* 2021;143(2):178-196.

21. Reid A, Ben ZS, Turaga M, et al. Neo-LVOT and transcatheter mitral valve replacement: expert recommendations. *JACC Cardiovasc Imaging.* 2021;14(4):854-866.

22. Lisko J, Kamioka N, Gleason P, et al. Prevention and treatment of left ventricular outflow tract obstruction after transcatheter mitral valve replacement. *Interv Cardiol Clin.* 2019;8(3):279-285.

23. Reddy VY, Doshi SK, Kar S, et al. 5-year outcomes after left atrial appendage closure: from the PREVAIL and PROTECT AF trials. *J Am Coll Cardiol.* 2017;70(24):2964-2975.

24. Vainrib AF, Harb SC, Jaber W, et al. Left atrial appendage occlusion/exclusion: procedural image guidance with transesophageal echocardiography. *J Am Soc Echocardiogr.* 2018;31(4):454-474.

25. Cruz-Gonzalez I, Rama-Merchan JC, Rodríguez-Collado J, et al. Transcatheter closure of paravalvular leaks: state of the art. *Neth Heart J.* 2017;25(2):116-124.

26. Zorinas A, Zakarkaitė D, Janušauskas V, et al. Technical recommendations for real-time echocardiography and fluoroscopy imaging fusion in catheter-based mitral valve paravalvular leak and other procedures. *J Clin Med.* 2022;11(5):1328.

27. Fraisse A, Latchman M, Sharma S-R, et al. Atrial septal defect closure: indications and contra-indications. *J Thorac Dis.* 2018;10(Suppl. 24):S2874-S2881.

28. Turner ME, Bouhout I, Petit CJ. Transcatheter closure of atrial and ventricular septal defects: JACC focus seminar. *J Am Coll Cardiol.* 2022;79(22):2247-2258.

29. Alvarez CK, Zweibel S, Stangle A, et al. Anesthetic considerations in the electrophysiology laboratory: a comprehensive review. *J Cardiothorac Vasc Anesth.* 2023;37(1):96-111.

30. Anderson R, Harukuni I, Sera V. Anesthetic considerations for electrophysiologic procedures. *Anesthesiol Clin.* 2013;31(2):479-489.

12

Myocardial Revascularization

John Steven McNeil, Angela M. Taylor, and Erik Strauss

1. Coronary artery disease (CAD) is a leading cause of morbidity and mortality in the United States, with concerning racial disparities in mortality in patients who undergo coronary artery bypass grafting (CABG).
2. CABG remains the preferred intervention for complex CAD, with a lower overall mortality and less risk for revascularization than percutaneous coronary intervention (PCI) but with a greater risk of stroke.
3. Transesophageal echocardiography (TEE) is safe and may reduce morbidity and mortality in CABG and can be used to rapidly detect intraoperative ischemia.
4. The patient in cardiogenic shock may benefit from earlier, rather than later, revascularization with CABG.
5. Intra-aortic balloon pumps (IABPs) and extracorporeal circulation devices decompress the left ventricle (LV) and provide myocardial protection in addition to circulatory support and should be considered for patients in cardiogenic shock before emergent CABG or PCI.

I. Background on Coronary Artery Disease

A. Prevalence and Economic Impact: Cardiovascular disease remains the leading cause of death for Americans. According to the most recent data from the Centers for Disease Control and Prevention (CDC), 20.1 million adults aged ≥20 years have coronary artery disease (CAD).[1] Every year, 805,000 people in the United States experience a myocardial infarction (MI) and 382,820 die from CAD.[1] Angina affects over 10 million people in the United States. The average annual cost of heart disease is $228.7 billion, lagging behind only osteoarthritis, mental disorders, diabetes mellitus, and cancer.[2,3]

B. Symptoms and Progression of Coronary Artery Disease: CAD has two main presentations: stable ischemic heart disease and acute coronary syndromes. CAD is a progressive disease, and to date, therapies have been able to slow progression but rarely regress disease. This section focuses only on the most prevalent mechanisms of disease development and progression. As coronary disease progresses and plaque buildup increases, luminal compromise eventually occurs, resulting in stable angina. Stable angina represents a mismatch between myocardial oxygen supply and demand in the setting of a stressor, such as physical activity, and it is relieved with rest or nitroglycerin. The acute coronary syndromes comprise a spectrum of disorders that result in an abrupt decrease in myocardial blood flow and myocardial injury. This most commonly implies development of thrombus at the site of a ruptured plaque. The syndrome ranges from unstable angina and non–ST-segment elevation myocardial infarction (NSTEMI) in which the thrombus is not occlusive to an ST-elevation myocardial infarction (STEMI) where the thrombus is occlusive. Importantly, plaques with thin-capped fibroatheromas are more prone to rupture, and these plaques are often <50% occlusive.[4,5] Symptoms of angina can manifest as chest pain, chest pressure, shortness of breath, fatigue, nausea, jaw pain, or arm pain. On average, 20%-30% of MIs are silent, and these are more common in patients with diabetes.[6]

C. Historical Perspective of Coronary Artery Bypass Grafting: Coronary artery bypass grafting (CABG) as an accepted procedure evolved over several decades. Robert Goetz, at the Albert Einstein College of Medicine, performed the first successful CABG surgery in 1960 by anastomosing the right internal thoracic artery to the right coronary artery (RCA).[7] Despite being a successful operation, this was the only bypass surgery performed by Goetz and his team. Several surgeons performed limited procedures over the subsequent years without reporting data. The first surgeon to perform and report his data was Vasilii Kolessov in 1964 when he published the outcomes of 12 CABG procedures.[8] Finally, George Green performed the first left internal thoracic artery to left anterior descending (LAD) anastomosis in 1968.[9] Saphenous vein grafts (SVGs) were the most favored conduits in the early years, and it was not until the mid-1980s that the superiority of the internal thoracic artery was demonstrated.[10] Other arterial grafts have also been used, with the radial artery being the most popular, pioneered by Alain Carpentier in 1971; however, successful use of this graft was not mastered until the early 1990s.[11]

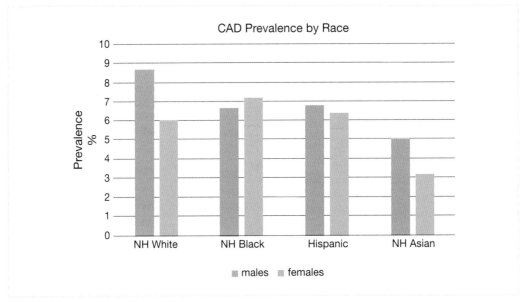

FIGURE 12.1 Coronary artery disease (CAD) prevalence by race and sex. NH, non-Hispanic.

D. **Racial Differences in Risk of Coronary Artery Disease and Need for Coronary Artery Bypass Grafting:** Prevalence of CAD differs by race and gender[1] (Figure 12.1). While the prevalence of angina is roughly equal between males and females (4.5% vs 4.0%), Black and Hispanic females are more likely to experience angina than their male counterparts (Blacks: 4.7% females vs 3.3% males; Hispanics: 4.3% females vs 3.5% males).[12] Age-adjusted CAD death rates vary based on race (Figure 12.2); however, after adjustment for cardiovascular risk factors and social determinants of health, Black males and females have a similar risk for fatal CAD as White males and females.[13] Men, compared with women, and White patients, compared with Black patients, had higher CABG utilization rates.[14] In patients undergoing CABG, Black patients undergoing CABG have a higher mortality than White patients (odds ratio

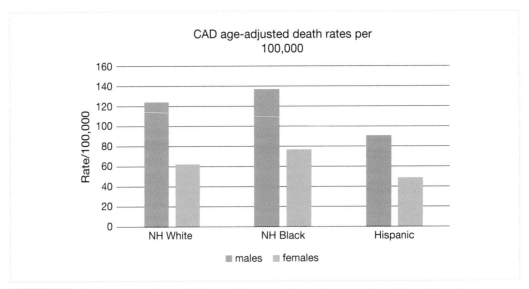

FIGURE 12.2 Coronary artery disease (CAD) age-adjusted death rates by race and sex. NH, non-Hispanic.

[OR] 1.1 [1.05-1.18]). Females also have a higher mortality than males after CABG (OR 1.26 [1.21-1.30]).[15] After controlling for patient factors, non-White patients retain a 33% higher mortality rate.[16]

E. **Evaluating Risk of Morbidity and Mortality After Surgery:** It is important to estimate a patient's risk for CABG preoperatively. Two of the most common risk scores for evaluating the risk of morbidity and mortality perioperatively are the Society for Thoracic Surgeons (STS) Cardiac Surgery Risk Model and the European System for Cardiac Operative Risk Evaluation (EuroSCORE II), though several others exist.[17] Models vary based on the components included in the model and the weights assigned to each component. Common variables include left ventricular (LV) function, age, weight, sex, urgency of surgery, concomitant valve surgery, diabetes, renal function, and immunosuppression.[18]

F. **Effectiveness of Coronary Artery Bypass Grafting as a Therapeutic Option:** Coronary revascularization in patients with multivessel disease is associated with a significant decrease in mortality, regardless of the method of revascularization.[19] Long-term survival is better with CABG than percutaneous coronary intervention (PCI) in patients with intermediate to high complexity disease as defined by a SYNTAX score >23. CABG resulted in fewer MIs and repeat revascularizations in these higher risk groups.[20] In the subset of patients with left main disease, there remains debate as the two largest randomized trials to date produced opposite conclusions.[21,22] Consistent across many trials is that stroke is higher in patients undergoing CABG while repeat revascularization is higher in patients undergoing PCI.

II. Myocardial Oxygen Demand and Supply

A. **Introduction:** Myocardial oxygen consumption, or the actual amount of oxygen consumed per minute, is dependent on the magnitude of coronary blood flow (CBF) and the oxygen-carrying capacity of the blood. Myocardial oxygen consumption at rest is 8-13 mL/100 g/min and can increase to as much as 90 mL/100 g/min in states of maximum contractility.[23] The myocardium maximally extracts most (about 75%) of the oxygen delivered by the coronary arteries at rest. Thus, there is little to no oxygen extraction reserve. Upon exertion or hemodynamic stress, the only way to increase oxygen supply acutely to match increased myocardial demand is by increasing CBF.

B. **Coronary Artery Anatomy:** The heart is supplied by two major coronary arteries, the RCA and the left coronary artery (LCA). Arterial dominance is determined by the blood supply to the inferior wall via the posterior descending artery. Eighty percent of the time, this is supplied by the RCA (right dominant), with the remaining 20% by the circumflex artery, a branch of the LCA (left dominant). When imaging the coronary system, two orthogonal views of the RCA and four orthogonal views of the LCA are generally taken (see Figure 12.3A-F).

C. **Determinants of Myocardial Oxygen Supply**

1. **Oxygen content:** Oxygen content can be calculated using the following formula:

    Oxygen content = (hemoglobin) (1.34) (% saturation) + (0.003) (PO_2)

    The maximum volume of oxygen that can be carried when blood is fully saturated is referred to as the *oxygen-carrying capacity*. In the presence of a normal hemoglobin (Hgb) and saturation, this is, on average, 20 mL/100 mL of blood.[24]

2. **Coronary blood flow:** The main determinant of CBF is myocardial oxygen consumption. Many factors exert an effect on actual CBF.

3. **Heart rate:** Increases in heart rate result in predominantly a decrease in diastolic time and thus less time for CBF to occur.

4. **Coronary perfusion pressure:** The majority of CBF occurs during diastole when the myocardium is relaxed. Coronary perfusion pressure (CPP) can be calculated as the difference between aortic diastolic pressure and left ventricular end-diastolic pressure (LVEDP). CBF varies directly with this pressure differential. Flow is autoregulated by recruitment and de-recruitment of resistance vessels, mainly comprised of nondilatory vessels distal to the arterioles. Flow is independent of CPP between 50 and 150 mm Hg (Figure 12.4). CPP plays a larger role outside this range. To optimize CPP, one should aim for a low heart rate, low LVEDP, and relatively high diastolic blood pressure.[25]

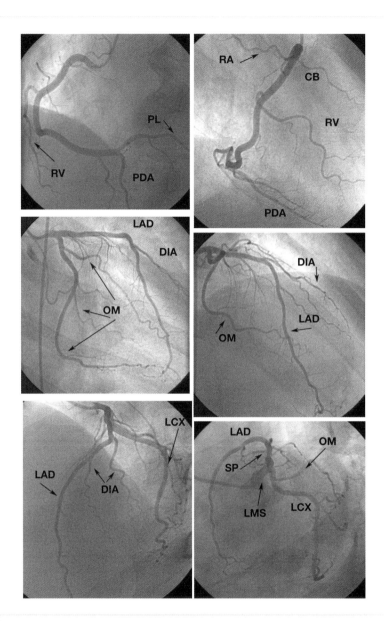

FIGURE 12.3 **(A)** Left anterior oblique projection of the right coronary artery. **(B)** Right anterior oblique projection of the right coronary artery. **(C)** Right anterior oblique caudal projection of the left coronary artery. The circumflex is best seen in this view. **(D)** Right anterior oblique cranial projection of the left coronary artery. The LAD is best seen in this view. **(E)** Left anterior oblique cranial projection of the left coronary artery. The LAD is well seen in this view but may be foreshortened. **(F)** Left anterior oblique caudal projection of the left coronary artery. Also referred to as the "spider view." CB, conus branch; DIA, diagonal branch; LAD, left anterior descending artery; LMS, left main segment; OM, obtuse marginal branch; PDA, posterior descending artery; PL, posterolateral branch; RA, right atrial branch; RV, right ventricular branch.

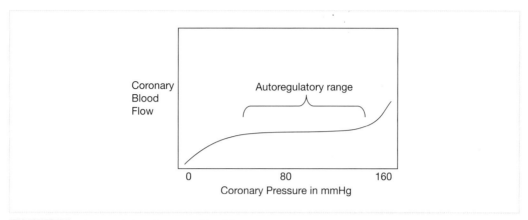

FIGURE 12.4   Autoregulation of coronary blood flow.

5. **Coronary vascular resistance:** Vasomotor tone, and thus vessel diameter, is predominantly a function of the endothelium through release of vasoactive substances. CBF varies indirectly with coronary vascular resistance (CVR). The determinants of CVR are as follows[25,26]:

   a. **Metabolic factors:** Hypoxia, a decrease in CO_2, or an increase in lactate results in vasoconstriction and an increase in CVR. Adenosine release results in vasodilation of the resistance vessels.

   b. **Autonomic factors:** Autonomic effects on the coronary system are relatively weak compared to metabolic influences. Epicardial blood vessels primarily have α receptors, which mediate coronary vasoconstriction. Vasodilation is mediated primarily by $\beta2$ receptors on the intramuscular and subendocardial vessels.

   c. **Humoral factors:** The renin-angiotensin axis exerts the greatest humoral effect on CVR. Angiotensin II induces vasoconstriction predominantly through enhancing calcium influx and stimulating endothelin release. Antidiuretic hormone (vasopressin) can also cause vasoconstriction in patients under myocardial stress. Several factors contribute to endothelium-mediated vasodilation, though to a relatively mild degree, including angiotensin-converting enzyme–induced bradykinin, atrial natriuretic peptide, vasoactive intestinal peptide, and calcitonin gene–related peptide.

   d. **Vascular endothelium:** The vascular endothelium synthesizes and secretes several vasoactive substances that affect contractility of the arterial smooth muscle. Nitric oxide, prostacyclin, endothelium-derived relaxing factor, and bradykinin serve as vasodilators, while endothelin and thromboxane promote vasoconstriction.

   e. **Anatomic factors:** Capillaries, where oxygen and nutrients are exchanged, do not have smooth muscle and, therefore, cannot vasodilate. At rest, capillaries provide one quarter of total resistance. During maximum hyperemia, however, they represent three quarters of total resistance. Arteriolar and venous vasodilation compensate for this and lower resistance. The increase in CBF above the resting state during maximal recruitment of the resistance vessels and capillary network is known as *coronary flow reserve*.

6. **Coronary stenosis:** Resting blood flow is affected by a diameter stenosis of ≥80%. Stenoses of ≥50% may affect response to hyperemia. The degree of reduction in CBF is dependent on the degree and length of the stenosis, the location of the stenosis, the presence of sequential lesions, the presence of collateral vessels, and the presence of coexisting pathologies, such as LV hypertrophy or heart failure. Since CBF is reduced in proportion to the fourth power of the vessel diameter, a 50% diameter decrease in lumen size decreases flow to 1/16th of its initial value, which is hemodynamically consistent with symptoms of angina on exertion. With a progressive coronary stenosis, pressure will drop across the stenosis but resting flow will be maintained because of autoregulation. This is accomplished by recruitment of coronary resistance vessels. When stenosis severity exceeds a critical level, autoregulation is exhausted, with flow becoming dependent on pressure and resting flow decreasing with more advanced stenosis (see Figures 12.5-12.7).

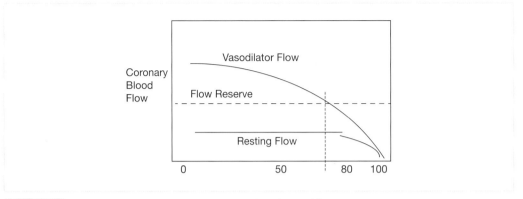

FIGURE 12.5   Relation of stenosis severity to coronary blood flow and flow reserve.

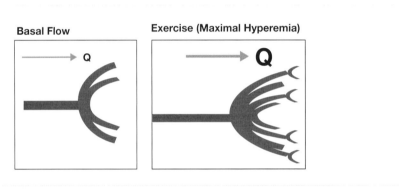

FIGURE 12.6   Coronary blood flow in the absence of a stenosis. Resistance vessels are recruited at maximal hyperemia.

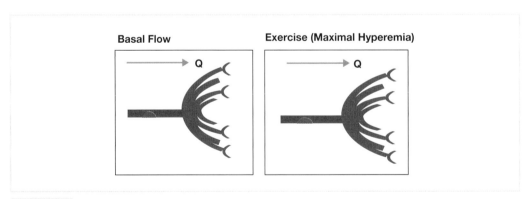

FIGURE 12.7   Coronary blood flow in the presence of a stenosis. Resistance vessels are recruited in the basal state. Further recruitment during hyperemia does not occur.

7. **Hypertension and heart failure:** In the presence of LV hypertrophy, an increase in intramyocardial pressure results in decreased subendocardial flow. A decreased capillary-to-myocyte ratio results in decreased capillary density. In addition, hypertrophied tissue demonstrates an impaired vasodilatory response to hypoxia. This all results in decreased CBF.[25] Increased LVEDP in heart failure similarly decreases blood flow by decreasing subendocardial flow and CPP.

D. **Determinants of Myocardial Oxygen Demand**
   1. **Heart rate:** Increases in heart rate result in an increase in myocardial oxygen requirement. In addition, an increase in heart rate results in a decrease in diastolic cycle time. The majority of myocardial perfusion occurs in diastole; thus, the time for perfusion decreases as does oxygen supply. As heart rate increases, there are small increases in contractility, further increasing oxygen demand. Because of this, a doubling in heart rate results in more than a 2-fold increase in oxygen demand. Heart rate is a critical determinant of myocardial oxygen balance because it has effects on both myocardial oxygen supply and demand.
   2. **Contractility:** A highly contractile heart uses a greater amount of oxygen. It is clinically difficult to quantify the degree of LV contractility. The rate of rise of LV pressure (dp/dt, the pressure difference divided by the time difference) has been proposed to approximate contractility. Contractility can also be approximated in a load-independent manner using LV pressure-volume loops and measuring the slope of the end-systolic pressure-volume relationship. Unfortunately, these methods are not readily clinically available. Contractility can be measured clinically with echocardiography using the rate of rise of a mitral regurgitation jet. Loading conditions and chamber compliance significantly affect the acceleration of the jet, making this method not very reliable.[27] As a result, in the clinical setting, we rely on qualitative assessments using visual estimation of LV ejection fraction as a surrogate for contractility.
   3. **Wall stress:** Ventricular wall stress impacts both myocardial oxygen demand and ventricular workload. An increase in ventricular wall stress increases oxygen demand while also decreasing oxygen supply by impairing filling of resistance vessels. Quantification of stress relies on afterload, preload, and wall thickness using La Place's law.[28]

   $$\text{Wall stress} = \text{pressure (afterload)} \times \text{radius (preload)}/2x \text{ wall thickness}$$

   4. **Pressure (afterload):** The true measure of chamber pressure is the difference between the intrathoracic pressure and the ventricular cavity pressure. Often referred to as *afterload*, pressure is often simplified as the load the LV must eject against. This is typically described by the systolic blood pressure or systemic vascular resistance (SVR). While afterload approximates pressure, the true pressure seen by the LV is much more complex.
   5. **Preload:** Preload is a measure of LV end-diastolic volume; thus, chamber size (radius) is used as a surrogate measure. Volume varies by radius cubed; therefore, preload has a more modest effect on wall stress than pressure, which demonstrates a 1:1 relationship with increases in wall stress. Preload is determined clinically using LVEDP, an indirect reflection of volume that is easily measured. Increases in ventricular volume are beneficial as increased stretch results in increased contractility until the optimal fiber length of the myocardium is exceeded. In dilated ventricles, this ability to enhance myocardial performance with preload increases is attenuated.
   6. **Wall thickness:** Wall thickness is indirectly proportional to wall stress. While increased wall thickness may decrease wall stress initially, as thickness continues to increase, CBF decreases as a result of decreased capillary density.
   7. **Summary:** Many factors affect myocardial oxygen supply and demand. A thorough understanding of coronary and ventricular physiology is necessary for providing optimal care and prevention of ischemia and its consequences.

III. **Monitoring for Myocardial Ischemia**
   A. **Introduction:** Monitoring for CABG surgery requires, at a minimum, standard American Society of Anesthesiologists (ASA) monitors and invasive arterial blood pressure monitoring. The most recent (2010) ASA/SCA (Society for Cardiovascular Anesthesiologists) practice

guidelines recommend that transesophageal echocardiography (TEE) be *considered* for all CABG patients unless probe placement is contraindicated. The use of pulmonary artery (PA) catheters for routine CABG remains controversial, and usage varies widely across centers despite some retrospective evidence of reduction in morbidity.[30] Detection and treatment of intraoperative ischemia is critically important because intraoperative ischemia is an independent predictor of postoperative MI.[29] Only half of intraoperative ischemic events are related to a hemodynamic perturbation, and none can be detected by the presence of angina in anesthetized patients. Reduced or negative lactate extraction in a regional myocardial circulatory bed, while diagnostic of ischemia, cannot be routinely measured. Thus, we seek clues that ischemia leaves in its wake: changes on the electrocardiography (ECG), PA pressure changes, and myocardial wall motion abnormalities (or worsening mitral regurgitation) on TEE.

B. **Electrocardiogram Monitoring:** Despite the ability of TEE to rapidly detect of regional wall motion abnormalities (RWMAs), continuous multilead ECG monitoring remains one of the most important intraoperative monitors for ischemia in CABG patients. ECG monitoring is safe, inexpensive, easy to interpret, can be automated, and is available continuously. ECG changes are often delayed: They occur later in the temporal cascade of events that follow myocardial ischemia, especially with lesser degrees of coronary supply/demand mismatch. Observing the ECG monitor during off-pump coronary artery bypass (OPCAB) may reveal real-time improvement in ischemic signs as coronary vessels are reperfused.

1. **ST-segment analysis:** Depression of the ST segment of the ECG denotes endocardial ischemia, and elevation denotes transmural ischemia. **ST-segment changes typically occur at least 60-120 seconds after the start of ischemia**. The reference for the ST segment is usually taken as 80 milliseconds after the J-point, which is the end of the QRS wave (Figure 12.8). Significant changes are usually defined as 0.1 mV or 1 mm of ST-segment elevation or depression at normal gain in two or more anatomically contiguous leads. ECG monitoring systems include automated real-time ST-segment analysis. Unfortunately, many rhythm disturbances frequently seen in patients undergoing revascularization, such as intraventricular conduction delays, bundle branch blocks, and ventricular pacing, can render ST-segment analysis inaccurate.

2. **Differential diagnosis of ST-segment changes:** ST-segment elevation (Figure 12.8) may arise from transmural ischemia (secondary to atherosclerotic disease, coronary vasospasm, or intracoronary air), pericarditis, or ventricular aneurysm. The differential should also

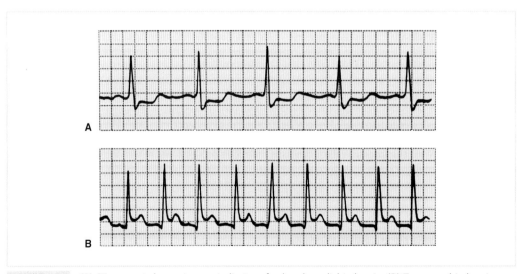

FIGURE 12.8 **(A)** ST-segment depression, an indicator of subendocardial ischemia. **(B)** Transmural ischemia, one cause of ST-segment elevation, produces the pattern appearing in the lower tracing.

include improper lead placement, particularly reversal of limb and leg leads, and improper electronic filtering settings (Figure 12.8).

3. **T-wave changes:** New T-wave alterations (inverted or flattened) may indicate ischemia. These may not be detected by viewing the ST segment alone. Likewise, pseudonormalization of the ST segment or T wave (an ischemic sign that then disappears) may indicate the new onset of ischemia and should be investigated.

4. **Multilead electrocardiogram monitoring:** Simultaneous observation of an inferior lead (II, III, or aVF) and an anterior lead (V5: fifth intercostal space, anterior axillary line) provides detection superior to single-lead monitoring, together detecting approximately 90% of ischemic events. Ischemia limited to the posterior segments of the LV is difficult to detect with standard ECG monitoring. Modified chest leads are often necessary to avoid interference with the surgical field.

C. **Pulmonary Artery Pressure Monitoring**

1. **Indications for a pulmonary artery catheter for revascularization procedures:** PA catheters provide central delivery of infusions (typically via a side port introducer or a proximal lumen in the catheter), measurement of blood temperature and chamber pressures, and calculations of cardiac output and vascular resistance. Some catheters also continuously measure mixed venous oxygen saturation and cardiac output. If TEE is performed, the utility of a PA catheter may be reduced intraoperatively, but postoperative intensive care unit (ICU) management may still benefit from the information provided. In this case, the catheter should ideally be placed in the operating room to maximize sterility and for maximal safety during insertion. Decreased function, pulmonary hypertension, concomitant valvular pathology, and expected long cardiopulmonary bypass (CPB) duration are some factors that may favor PA catheter insertion.

2. **Detection of ischemia with pulmonary artery tracing:** Pulmonary hypertension, whether primary or secondary to chronic ischemia, hypertension, or valvular heart disease, is common in cardiac surgery. PA pressures or pulmonary capillary wedge pressures (PCWPs) can be elevated due to chronic obstructive pulmonary disease (COPD), dependent catheter locations in the lung, or mitral stenosis, making elevated PA pressures and PCWPs less reliable in the diagnosis of ischemia. The shape of the transduced pressure waveform, however, is more predictive. Appearance of a new V wave on the PCWP waveform may indicate new functional mitral regurgitation, which, in a CABG patient, could be caused by acute ischemic papillary muscle dysfunction. This can occur before or even in the absence of ECG changes. However, detection of changes on the pulmonary capillary occlusion waveform requires frequent balloon advancing and inflation (wedging), introducing additional risk of vessel rupture and making it nearly impossible to perform in the busy cardiac operating room.

D. **Transesophageal Echocardiography**

1. **General indications for transesophageal echocardiography during revascularization procedures:** TEE can confirm venous location of the central line wire, assess ventricular preload and contractility, detect myocardial ischemia–induced RWMA, evaluate the aortic cannulation site, detect concomitant valve pathology, detect the presence and pathophysiologic effect of pericardial effusion, aid the placement and positioning of intra-aortic balloon pumps (IABPs) and coronary sinus catheters, and detect the presence of ventricular aneurysms and ventricular septal defects. Intraoperative TEE may provide more benefit in CABG patients with decreased function or with unstable hemodynamics and less benefit in stable outpatients with normal preoperative transthoracic echocardiograms. Thus, TEE utilization for CABG in the United States is highly variable, with one large retrospective study finding 43% of patients between 2013 and 2015 undergoing isolated CABG did not receive TEE monitoring.[31] Reassuringly, no increased risk of esophageal perforation was found in patients who received TEE compared to non-TEE CABG patients.[31] Retrospective, propensity-matched data suggest there may be lower 30-day mortality and lower incidence of stroke in CABG patients monitored with TEE, and a greater chance of an unplanned concomitant valve intervention.[32] In addition to the routine post-CPB TEE-guided

management (presence of air, function, volume status), assessment for new or unchanged RWMAs before the sternum is closed can significantly alter management. The difficult decision to revise a graft or to perform immediate postoperative cardiac angiography may be prompted by TEE. See Chapter 4 for a more detailed review of intraoperative TEE.

2. **Detection of myocardial ischemia with transesophageal echocardiography regional wall motion abnormalities:** The heart **develops abnormal motion <1 minute following perfusion defects.**[33] RWMAs resulting from myocardial ischemia temporally precede ECG changes. TEE can simultaneously interrogate regions of the heart representative of all three major coronary arteries, including the posterior wall, which is not easily monitored with ECG. The best view for this is the transgastric short-axis midpapillary muscle view. However, some ischemia, confined to regions not visualized with this view, such as the apex, will escape detection unless one performs a comprehensive examination with multiple planes and probe depths.

3. **Limitations of monitoring regional wall motion abnormalities**
   a. **Tethering:** Nonischemic tissue adjacent to ischemic tissue may move abnormally because it is attached to poorly moving tissue, potentially exaggerating the size of an RWMA.
   b. **Pacing/bundle branch blocks:** Abnormal ventricular depolarization sequences not only affect ST-segment analysis but also alter wall motion and can mimic RWMA.
   c. **Interventricular septum:** Normal septal motion depends on appropriate ventricular loading conditions, the presence of pericardium, and normal electrical conduction.
   d. **Stunned myocardium:** Adequately perfused myocardium may exhibit RWMA if recovering from recent ischemia, thus prompting inappropriate therapeutic intervention.
   e. **Diastolic left ventricular filling patterns:** Unfortunately, ventricular filling patterns depend on ventricular loading conditions and the site of Doppler interrogation within the ventricular inflow tract, limiting its utility as a monitor for ischemia.

4. **Detection of infarction complications:** TEE can detect complications of ischemia/infarction, such as acute mitral insufficiency, ventricular septal defect, pericardial effusion, and decreased function.

IV. Anesthetic Agents Used During Cardiac Revascularization Surgery
Cardiac pathophysiology and myocardial oxygen supply and demand must be considered in tailoring anesthetic induction and maintenance for each patient. With this consideration, no specific anesthetic agent, induction regimen, or maintenance plan has shown strong evidence of superiority in affecting outcomes related to morbidity and mortality,[34,35] and numerous techniques and agents can be safely used. The severity of coronary disease burden and the degree of ventricular impairment must be assessed before induction of anesthesia to synthesize and execute a safe anesthetic plan with extreme vigilance in monitoring for myocardial ischemia.

A. **Induction Agents and Hypnotics**
   1. **Propofol:** Propofol is frequently used for induction and postoperative maintenance of anesthesia for cardiac surgery. It decreases SVR and causes a limited decrease in cardiac contractility at clinical doses. Cardiac oxygen consumption and myocardial blood flow both decrease.[36]
   2. **Ketamine:** It is primarily an NMDA receptor antagonist but has activity at numerous receptors, producing a dose-dependent increase in sympathetic tone, myocardial oxygen demand, and cardiac work. Induction doses are not typically used for coronary revascularization surgery, but lower dose boluses (≈0.5 mg/kg) and infusions (≈0.5 mg/kg/h) have been administered in an effort to decrease early postoperative opioid consumption.[37]
   3. **Etomidate:** Induction doses of etomidate (0.2-0.3 mg/kg) do not alter heart rate or cardiac output, although mild peripheral vasodilation may lower blood pressure slightly. Thus, it is an ideal drug for rapid induction of anesthesia in patients with ischemic heart disease. Etomidate offers little protection from the increases in heart rate and blood pressure that accompany intubation. Supplement etomidate with other agents (eg, opioids, benzodiazepines, volatile agents, β-blockers, nitroglycerin) in order to control the hemodynamic profile and prevent myocardial oxygen supply/demand imbalance. A single dose of etomidate

may decrease cortisol levels for <24 hours but does not significantly decrease endogenous catecholamine levels or increase postoperative vasopressor requirements.[38]

4. **Benzodiazepines:** Benzodiazepines are compatible with the goal of maintaining hemodynamic stability, as negative inotropic effects are inconsequential. In the past, midazolam (0.2 mg/kg) or diazepam (0.5 mg/kg) was used, but such high doses are now avoided due to concerns for delayed emergence and postoperative delirium. Since practice has changed, benzodiazepines are typically administered at smaller doses as an adjunct, with the goal of preventing intraoperative awareness and decreasing anxiety. Multicenter analysis shows that close to 90% of patients undergoing cardiac surgery from 2014 to 2019 received a benzodiazepine during the perioperative period (typically midazolam with a median intraoperative total dose of 4 mg).[39] Research is ongoing, but there is evidence that at low doses (midazolam equivalent of 4-5 mg), benzodiazepines do not increase adverse outcomes related to delirium after cardiac surgery.[40]

5. **α2-Adrenergic medications:** Centrally acting α2-adrenergic agonists result in a reduction in stress-mediated neurohumoral responses and, therefore, are associated with decreases in heart rate and blood pressure. These agents are typically used during maintenance of anesthesia or postoperatively. Preoperative oral clonidine reduces perioperative myocardial ischemia in patients undergoing CABG surgery but occasionally results in significant intraoperative hypotension. Dexmedetomidine administered as an infusion possesses greater α2-selectivity than clonidine. Both agents have sedative and antinociceptive properties. The use of α2-adrenergic agonists may be associated with a reduced opioid requirement compared to propofol,[41] and α2-adrenergic agonists do not cause respiratory depression. Intraoperative dexmedetomidine infusions are frequently used by many anesthesiologists, but retrospective analysis of the STS Adult Cardiac Surgery Database suggests that there may be an association between dexmedetomidine administration and postoperative delirium.[42]

B. **Volatile Agents and Effect on Myocardial Function:** Volatile agents are commonly used during cardiac revascularization surgery. These agents have a dose-dependent effect on depressing SVR and contractility that can decrease both myocardial supply and demand. The goal is maintain an adequate supply and demand, but this balance can be disturbed by the hemodynamic profile that prevails at the time of administration.

1. **Heart rate:** In preclinical studies, isoflurane has a dose-dependent effect on heart rate by producing a slight increase at low doses (<1.0 minimum alveolar concentration) and a decrease in heart rate and cardiac function at higher doses (>1.0 minimum alveolar concentration).[43] In the steady state, the cardiovascular actions of desflurane are similar to those of isoflurane, but high or rapidly increasing desflurane concentrations similar to those needed for inhalation induction may cause a significant increase in heart rate, systemic pressure, and PA pressure. Junctional rhythms may occur with any volatile agent; they deprive the heart of an atrial "kick," leading to decreased stroke volume and cardiac output and reverses any beneficial effect of a low heart on myocardial oxygen demand.

2. **Contractility:** All volatile anesthetics decrease contractility, lowering O_2 demand. Any change causing an increase in volatile anesthetic concentration over time will cause a decrease in LV pressure: dP/dt. Contractility may be indirectly affected by the decrease in CPP (systemic diastolic pressure − LV diastolic pressure) since increasing isoflurane concentration decreases the load-independent end-systolic pressure-volume relationship.[39]

3. **Afterload:** Decreases in cardiac output and SVR with volatile anesthesia result in decreased systemic blood pressure. All volatile anesthetics vasodilate and decrease O_2 supply and O_2 demand.

4. **Preload:** Volatile agents do cause peripheral vasodilation but do not significantly change LVEDP. Therefore, CPP (diastolic aortic pressure minus LVEDP) may decrease during volatile anesthesia.[43]

5. **Coronary steal:** Coronary steal is a phenomenon where physiologic or pharmacologic vasodilation of a myocardial segment's vasculature "steals" blood from another myocardial segment because it is affected by significant proximal coronary artery stenosis with fully vasodilated distal coronary arteries. Steal-prone anatomy may exist in 23% of the patients

undergoing CABG.[44] Coronary steal has been observed in canine models of steal-prone coronary anatomy with isoflurane administration under circumstances in which collateral flow is pressure dependent. It is doubtful that isoflurane-induced coronary steal is clinically significant in patients undergoing coronary revascularization surgery as long as hypotension and consequent pressure-dependent coronary artery perfusion are avoided. Coronary steal has not been reported with halothane, enflurane, or desflurane.

6. **Preconditioning:** Volatile anesthetics may confer a degree of preconditioning-like protective effect against ischemia-reperfusion injury in human myocardial tissue. Some meta-analyses suggest that volatile agents reduce mortality. Animal studies show inhaled anesthetics reduce infarct size and reduce biomarkers of myocardial injury. However, a recent major randomized prospective multicenter trial showed no difference between use of volatile anesthetic and total intravenous (IV) anesthesia in mortality at 30 days and 1 year, MI, length of ICU stay, and length of hospital stay.[34] A clinically beneficial effect of volatile agents via preconditioning cannot be ruled out, but currently, the evidence is equivocal.

C. **Opioids**

1. **Heart rate:** All opioids, except meperidine, decrease heart rate by centrally mediated vagotonia. The dose of drug and speed of injection affect the degree of bradycardia. The result is decreased O_2 demand. By releasing histamine, morphine or meperidine may elicit a reflex tachycardia that decreases O_2 supply and increases O_2 demand.

2. **Contractility:** Opioids have little effect on contractility in clinical doses.

3. **Afterload:** In compromised patients, who often depend on elevated sympathetic tone to maintain cardiac output and systemic resistance, the loss of sympathetic tone associated with opioid induction of anesthesia may result in a sudden drop in blood pressure and consequent decreases in both O_2 supply and demand. Concomitant midazolam use augments the decreased SVR with opioid induction.

4. **Preload:** Despite a lack of histamine-releasing properties, fentanyl and sufentanil reduce preload when administered in either moderate (25 µg/kg for fentanyl) or larger doses by decreasing intrinsic sympathetic tone. Oxygen demand is decreased.

5. **Use in cardiac surgery:** In the past, higher doses of opioids were regularly administered during cardiac surgery to blunt the sympathetic response to surgery. Currently, more prudent administration of opioids has been preferred at most centers to facilitate extubation within a few hours of ICU arrival.

CLINICAL PEARL

Prudent administration of opioids and benzodiazepines may facilitate early postoperative emergence and extubation.

D. **Muscle Relaxant and Reversal:** With a focus on fast-track cardiac anesthesia, the use intermediate- and short-acting neuromuscular blockers and the plan for reversal should be considered.

1. **Succinylcholine:** The depolarizing neuromuscular blocker has well-described potential side effects and should not be used in patients with a concern for hyperkalemia, myopathy, extensive denervation of skeletal muscle, malignant hyperthermia, and possible muscarinic receptor activation. Succinylcholine provides profound muscle relaxation with rapid onset and short duration that facilitates airway placement. Succinylcholine continues to have a role for emergent intubations and for patients with a possible difficult airway if the combination of rocuronium and high-dose sugammadex is not readily available.

2. **Rocuronium:** The rapid-onset nondepolarizer provides faster muscle relaxation than all other relaxants, except succinylcholine. Rocuronium's mild vagolytic action is typically clinically insignificant. Rocuronium may cause histamine release, resulting in hypotension, rash, and tachycardia. Relaxation lasts an intermediate length of time and can be readily reversed with sugammadex, which facilitates fast-track cardiac anesthetics.

3. **Vecuronium:** Vecuronium has a flat cardiovascular profile that is ideal with a low- or moderate-dose opioid anesthetic supplemented by a volatile agent. Bradycardia occurs when it accompanies the rapid injection of high doses of the highly lipid-soluble opioids. Vecuronium can be reversed by sugammadex.

4. **Cisatracurium:** Cisatracurium lacks significant cardiovascular effects. The majority of metabolism is via Hofmann elimination, with ester hydrolysis making a minor contribution.

5. **Reversal agents:** Neostigmine was the typical agent for reversal of nondepolarizing blockade for decades. The muscarinic effects, including bradycardia, were inhibited by the co-administration of the anticholinergic glycopyrrolate. The effectiveness of this regimen is overshadowed by the new reversal agent sugammadex, which can rapidly bind and reverse the effects of rocuronium and vecuronium.

V. Perioperative Approach for Myocardial Revascularization Procedures
Team members must coordinate their goals and priorities to optimize outcomes and shepherd patients safely through the perioperative period. Anesthesiologists influence outcomes through management decisions made before, during, and after revascularization surgery.

A. Preoperative Assessment: Anesthesiologists need to consider a patient's history, physical, and diagnostic tests to form a risk assessment for potential concerning outcomes and synthesize an appropriate anesthetic plan. Several modifiable conditions need to be considered and possibly addressed if sufficient time and resources are available. Potentially modifiable preoperative conditions that affect outcomes after myocardial revascularization surgery include anemia, hyperglycemia, continued tobacco use, uncontrolled hypertension, and worsening pulmonary disease.

1. **Anemia:** Preoperative Hgb levels <11 g/dL are associated with increased risk of poor renal and cerebrovascular outcomes post-CABG, which may be related to anemia or subsequent transfusion of allogenic blood products. Higher rates of cardiac-specific morbidity is also associated with anemia in patients with EuroSCORE >4.[45] Preoperative iron infusions and erythropoiesis-stimulating agents may increase Hgb before surgery, but further studies are needed to investigate their effect on outcomes.[46]

2. **Hyperglycemia:** Preoperative HbA1C >8% is associated with a higher incidence of major adverse cardiac events after CABG, including death, MI, unstable angina, and repeat revascularization. Lowering HbA1C may require several weeks, but evidence suggests that treating hyperglycemia at any phase in the perioperative course will have a beneficial effect, particularly if hyperglycemia management begins before surgery and continues long into the postoperative period. Evidence suggests that a reasonable target of 140 mg/dL is effective in decreasing the incidence of complications after CABG and provides a buffer to avoid hypoglycemia.[47]

3. **Tobacco use:** Smoking cessation before CABG surgery has been shown to decrease the risk of pulmonary complications and potentially increase SVG patency rates after CABG.[48,49]

4. **Hypertension:** Elevated blood pressure and increased vascular stiffness with pulse pressure >80 mm Hg are associated with adverse cerebral and cardiac outcomes in cardiac revascularization.[50]

5. **β-Blockers:** Administration of a β-blocker within 24 hours of incision for isolated CABGs, presumably to reduce the risk of postoperative atrial fibrillation, remains a closely scrutinized quality metric for CABG outcomes despite limited to no evidence of clinical benefit.[51] Most important is that patients already on β-blockers continue their therapy in the perioperative period.

CLINICAL PEARL

After a detailed preoperative assessment, a discussion with the surgery team about the surgical plan is essential for devising the optimal anesthetic plan. Discussion should include off-CPB versus on-CPB, the need for an aortic cross-clamp, need for radial artery versus saphenous vein harvesting, and any other concerns related to the patient (ie, significant aortic regurgitation, ascending aortic atherosclerosis, or need for IABP).

B. **Intraoperative Approach:** For primary CABG procedures, the anesthetic should include techniques for fast-track cardiac anesthesia that facilitates extubation to be safely and consistently achieved within 6 hours of surgery end. The plan can be adjusted if intraoperative complications, hemodynamic instability, or airway concerns occur. Fast-track anesthesia commonly includes prudent administration of opioids, limited benzodiazepines, use of nonopioid adjunctive medications and regional techniques for postoperative pain control, and reversal of neuromuscular blockade. More complex surgeries such as reoperations and concurrent valve and/or aortic interventions may require a different approach, and fast-track plans may need to become a secondary concern.

1. **Hemodynamic goals:** The intraoperative events during CABG can produce abrupt changes in hemodynamics. Hypovolemia, decreased contractility, arrhythmia, vasodilation, and surgical manipulation are all common sources of hypotension. Surgical stimulation, inadequate analgesia, and the increased vascular tone of patients with chronic hypertension can cause elevated blood pressure and worsen surgical bleeding and myocardial ischemia. Extreme vigilance, quick diagnosis, and treatment are necessary to keep systemic pressure within an appropriate range (mean arterial pressure [MAP] 65-80 mm Hg). Inotropic (eg, epinephrine, dobutamine), vasoconstricting (eg, norepinephrine, vasopressin), and vasodilating (nitroglycerin, nicardipine) medications are commonly used to achieve the appropriate hemodynamic range. During arterial cannulation/decannulation, controlled hypotension (systolic pressure ≤100 mm Hg) may decrease the risk of iatrogenic aortic dissection.

2. **Temperature control:** Monitoring and maintaining satisfactory core temperature after CPB is crucial for planned early extubation. Hypothermia complicates postoperative care by causing arrhythmia, coagulopathy, shivering, increased myocardial oxygen consumption, and slowing drug metabolism.[52] During CABG, temperature should be monitored with probes in the nasopharynx and bladder. Hypothermia for myocardial protection may be intentional if effective cardioplegia cannot be administered. CPB circuit heat exchanger provides the best means of restoring body temperature before separation from CPB. To avoid cerebral hyperthermia, the arterial outlet temperature should be <37 °C while warming to a bladder temperature >35.5 °C to reduce hypothermic "rebound." Forced hot air convective warming helps during OPCAB, despite the minimal body surface available. Maintaining a warm operating room temperature, as can be reasonably tolerated by operative personnel, prevents heat loss after rewarming.[53]

3. **Intraoperative awareness:** Intraoperative awareness occurs in 0.3% of fast-track patients, similar to that observed in general surgery.[54] Processed EEG monitoring such as bispectral index (BIS, Medtronic) has been used to monitor the depth of anesthesia. in an effort not only to avoid awareness but also to coordinate the depth of anesthesia at the end of surgery to facilitate early extubation. The current evidence suggests that anesthetic guidance using processed EEG does not significantly decrease the time to tracheal extubation more than standard end-tidal anesthetic concentration monitoring,[55] but burst suppression recorded intraoperatively has been shown to have a key association with the incidence of postoperative cognitive dysfunction.[56]

4. **Blood conservation and hemostasis:** Multimodal approach to blood conservation is important in decreasing transfusion rates, which occurs in about one-third of CABG patients during the perioperative period. Intraoperative red blood cell (RBC) transfusion increases expense, exposes patients to a risk of transfusion reaction, and has been associated with an increased risk of a healthcare-associated infection.[57] Without signs of compromised end-organ perfusion (low SvO_2, higher base deficit, rising lactate) using a restrictive transfusion protocol Hgb <7.5 g/dL, minimizing hemodilution with retrograde autologous priming, and utilizing cell salvage can significantly decrease intraoperative RBC transfusion rates.[58] To improve perioperative hemostasis, administer lysine analogs and guide decisions related to hemostasis with point-of-care viscoelastic and platelet function tests.

C. **Nonopioid Analgesic Management and Regional Techniques**

1. **Nonopioid Analgesics:** Traditional approach to perioperative analgesia includes opioids typically in the form of IV fentanyl and hydromorphone, but a number of nonopioid

medication adjuncts have been investigated in prospective trials, including acetaminophen, nonsteroidal anti-inflammatory drugs (NSAIDs), ketamine and dexmedetomidine infusions, and gabapentin.[59] There is some evidence for effectiveness of these adjuncts as part of a multimodal approach if the concern for potential side effects does not outweigh the potential benefit.

2. **Neuraxial analgesia:** Neuraxial techniques with local anesthetics and/or opioids can be used to provide analgesia and decrease the sympathetic surge upon emergence and increase myocardial oxygen delivery. Preservative-free morphine 300-500 µg administered intrathecally through a 25G spinal needle to decrease the risk of hematoma can provide improved postoperative analgesia but has not been shown to affect other outcomes, such as the time to extubation, ICU stay, morbidity, or mortality. Thoracic epidural administration with catheter dosing has shown to decrease the time to extubation and improve analgesia, but results are not consistent among studies. Epidural hematomas have been reported. Sympathectomy by neuraxial administration of local anesthetics has not been shown to reliably improve outcomes related to myocardial ischemia.[60]

3. **Fascial plane blocks:** Anatomy of chest wall and location of fascial plane blocks are shown in Figure 12.9. Postoperative pain from median sternotomy can be treated with bilateral deep (transverse thoracic-intercostal plane) and superficial (pecto-intercostal plane) parasternal blocks performed post skin closure at multiple rib spaces with ultrasound guidance using 20 mL of 0.25% bupivacaine or ropivacaine. Small prospective and randomized double-blind studies have shown moderate but significantly less postoperative opioid administration in the local anesthetic group. Internal mammary harvest disrupts the continuity of the endothoracic fascia and may thwart the effectiveness of deep parasternal blocks on that side. Bilateral single-shot and continuous catheter erector spinae plane blocks with 3 mg/kg of ropivacaine have shown improved postoperative pain scores and decreased morphine consumption after median sternotomy, but more studies are needed to determine effectiveness. At least, one small randomized controlled trial (RCT) supports the effectiveness of serratus anterior plane blocks in decreasing postoperative fentanyl administration and improving pain scores after mini-thoracotomy for minimally invasive direct coronary artery bypass (MIDCAB).[61]

D. **Off-Pump Versus On-Pump Coronary Artery Bypass Grafting:** Off-pump revascularization (OPCAB) gained popularity in the 1990s, with the expectation that perioperative transfusion, stroke, organ failure, and ICU stay would decrease. OPCAB requires stabilization of the target coronary artery and lifting/manipulating of the heart for exposure of the anastomotic site. Vasoactive infusions such as norepinephrine (0.02-0.1 µg/kg/min), phenylephrine (40-180 µg/min), and vasopressin (0.01-0.06 U/min) can be used to maintain the MAP during cardiac manipulation.

1. **Coronary artery bypass grafting procedural anticoagulation:** On-pump CABG requires a higher level of anticoagulation for cannulation and to prevent clot formation in the pump circuit. Heparin (300-400 units/kg) is typically administered as a bolus IV, and anticoagulation is quantified with an activated clotting time (ACT) assay with a goal of >480 seconds before initiation of CPB.

2. **Off-pump coronary artery bypass procedural anticoagulation:** Typically, an initial bolus of 100-200 units/kg is required for a goal ACT of 250-300 seconds and repeat measuring/administration to keep anticoagulation within that range during the creation of the surgical anastomoses. The decreased anticoagulation requirement makes OPCAB useful for instances of heparin-induced thrombocytopenia (HIT) since bivalirudin (0.75 mg/kg bolus, 1.75 mg/kg/h infusion) can be used in place of heparin.

3. **Short-term outcomes of off-pump coronary artery bypass versus coronary artery bypass grafting:** OPCAB has short-term benefits in comparison to CABG. RCTs have provided evidence for reduced duration of mechanical ventilation, neurocognitive deterioration, length of hospital and ICU stay, transfusion requirements, and short-term costs for OPCAB. Smaller studies show reduced inflammation but no strong evidence for reduced MI in the immediate postoperative period and no evidence for reduced rates of stroke.

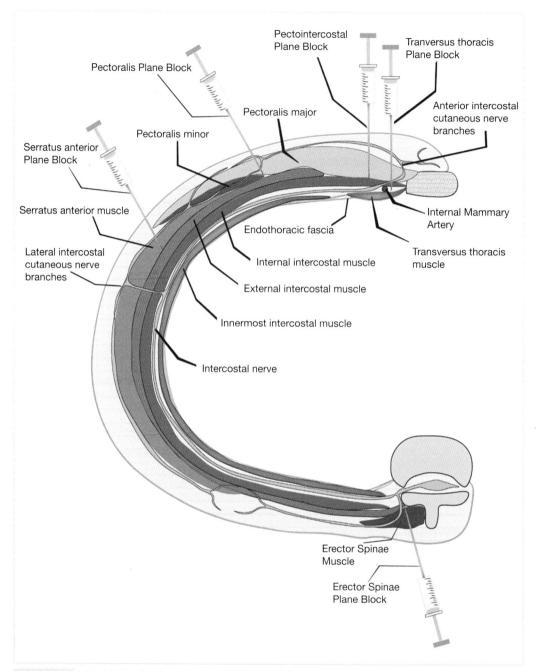

FIGURE 12.9 Fascial plane blocks and thoracic anatomy at T4 level.

4. **Long-term outcomes of off-pump coronary artery bypass versus coronary artery bypass grafting:** Benefits appear to favor CABG over OPCAB. RCTs show that CABG provides improved revascularization, especially in the circumflex distribution, and a higher number grafts per patient. The lower effectiveness in OPCAB revascularization leads to an increased need for repeat surgery and mitigates the short-term decrease in cost. The quality of revascularization appears to be highly dependent on the experience of the surgeon.[62]

The ideal OPCAB candidate would have one or two anteriorly located coronary arteries in need of revascularization.

E. **Special Circumstances**

   1. **Radial artery conduits:** Confirm before inserting arterial catheters whether or not the surgeon intends to utilize radial artery as a conduit. Some protocols call for diltiazem infusions as prophylaxis against arterial spasm in the radial graft; systemic vasodilation is likely in this scenario.

   2. **Port access surgery:** This approach utilizes a small thoracotomy incision, endoscopic instruments inserted through small ports, and TEE-guided placement of endovascular devices to facilitate CPB, including endoaortic clamp, coronary sinus catheter, and PA vent.

   3. **Minimally invasive direct coronary artery bypass:** MIDCAB is a variation of OPCAB that involves harvesting the left internal mammary artery (IMA) either directly or with a surgical robot and anastomosing to the LAD coronary artery without CPB through a small thoracotomy incision. Serratus anterior fascial plane block can reduce postoperative pain from the incision.

   4. **Urgent coronary artery bypass surgery:** Patients who present for urgent coronary artery bypass surgery usually have ongoing ischemia, including actively infarcting tissue, frequently with hemodynamic instability. Discuss with the surgical team whether an IABP to support hemodynamics through induction is indicated. Consider starting inotropic infusion before induction, and be ready to immediately administer anticoagulation in case of emergent cannulation and initiation of CPB. Patients on a heparin infusion may have heparin resistance, so antithrombin III or fresh-frozen plasma should be readily available.

   5. **Coronary artery bypass grafting for patients previously treated with antiplatelet medications:** Recent administration of potent antiplatelet agents, including platelet glycoprotein receptor antagonists and P2Y12 receptor antagonists, may cause significant perioperative coagulopathy. Table 12.1 includes important details for these antiplatelet medications, including average time to recovery of platelet function. It is important to note that platelet transfusion may be needed to treat coagulopathy related to these medications, but the residual circulating reversible P2Y12 antagonist, ticagrelor, and its metabolite may inhibit freshly transfused platelets, and platelet transfusion may not be effective.

TABLE 12.1   Common Antiplatelet Medications Used in Coronary Artery Disease

Route of Administration	Medication	Mechanism of Action	Recovery of Platelet Function on Assay	Point-of-Care Testing	Perioperative Recommendation
Oral	Aspirin	COX-1 inhibitor	7-10 d	Yes (not common)	Continue until surgery
	Clopidogrel	Irreversible P2Y12 receptor antagonist	5-10 d	Yes	Stop 5 d before surgery
	Prasugrel	Irreversible P2Y12 receptor antagonist	7-10 d	Yes	Stop 7 d before surgery
	Ticagrelor	Reversible P2Y12 receptor antagonist	3-5 d	Yes	Stop 3 d before surgery
Intravenous	Cangrelor	Reversible P2Y12 receptor antagonist	1-2 h	Not commonly used due to short half-life	Stop 1-2 h before surgery
Intravenous	Tirofiban	Competitive GP IIb/IIIa receptor inhibitor	2-4 h	Not common	Stop 2 h before surgery
	Eptifibatide	Competitive GP IIb/IIIa receptor inhibitor	2-4 h	Not common	Stop 2 h before surgery
	Abciximab	Antibody to GP IIb/IIIa receptor	12-24 h	Not common	Stop 12 h before surgery

6. **Redo coronary artery bypass grafting procedures:** Repeat CABG is challenging due to bleeding and difficulty of surgical exposure. Coronary grafts, the aorta, and/or the right ventricle may be adhered to the sternum, and occlusion or transection of prior grafts may cause significant ischemia and rapid bleeding. Apply external cutaneous defibrillator pads before induction and ensure blood product availability. Cardioplegia will be less effective in patients with prior internal thoracic to coronary artery grafts, and myocardial protection may require systemic cooling to 24-32 °C (Table 12.2).

VI. **Causes and Treatment of Perioperative Myocardial Ischemia**

A. **Intraoperative Period Before Coronary Artery Intervention or Manipulation**

1. **Hemodynamics:** Myocardial ischemia in the pre-CPB period is largely due to hemodynamic abnormalities; thus, avoiding tachycardia, hypotension, and hypertension is essential. Many intraoperative events precipitate hemodynamic changes, including induction, intubation, changes in the depth of anesthesia, application of cold surgical prepping solutions, incision/sternotomy, and surgical retraction/cannulation. Closely monitor for ECG depressions/elevations and changes in wall motion abnormalities on TEE. Arrhythmias (bradycardia, ventricular tachycardia/fibrillation, etc) may be caused by myocardial ischemia or infarction and may further worsen or enlarge the ischemic area by increasing oxygen demand and/or decreasing supply. Rapid identification and treatment with cardioversion/defibrillation, administration of inotropic medications to support hemodynamics, or initiation of extracorporeal support is vital.

2. **Coronary spasm:** Spasm of coronary arteries and arterial grafts is a concern and may cause infarction and complete cardiovascular collapse.

3. **Plaque rupture:** Atherosclerotic plaque rupture may occur and cause acute thrombosis of a coronary artery, leading to myocardial ischemia or infarction. Plaque rupture has been observed during cardiac catheterization and stent placement and could occur during surgical manipulation or retraction.[63]

B. **During Coronary Artery Intervention With or Without Cardiopulmonary Bypass:** The previously described causes of myocardial ischemia remain, and additional causes must be considered. Air or other microparticles may embolize down the coronary artery grafts or through open coronary artery incisions and be identified by inferior lead ST changes on ECG since air embolization is likely to affect the anteriorly situated RCA in a supine patient.

1. **Aortic cross-clamping:** The protection from cardioplegia may be inadequate, and the potential for ischemic injury increases with cross-clamp time. Washout of cardioplegia solutions may occur with in situ coronary grafts that are not attached to cardioplegia or excluded by cross-clamp (prior internal thoracic artery to coronary artery graft). Systemic cooling and retrograde cardioplegia may aid in the protection of the myocardium.

TABLE 12.2   Perioperative Management of Reoperation for Myocardial Revascularization Patients

Perioperative Problem	Cause	Management
Bleeding	Pericardial adhesions, recent antiplatelet or anticoagulant medication	Large-bore IV access; blood readily available and checked in the OR; femoral area exposed and ready for emergency cannulation; anticipated need for clotting factors and platelets in the post bypass period; availability of blood salvage equipment (cell saver); prophylactic antifibrinolytic medications
Ischemia or infarction; pump failure after bypass	Long period before bypass instituted, thrombus in vein grafts embolize to native vessels; interruption of vein graft flow, longer bypass, and cross-clamp ties; increased amount of noncoronary collateral flow causing ineffective cardioplegia	Close monitoring of ischemia (ECG, PA catheter, two-dimensional TEE); expeditious treatment of ischemia once detected; careful manipulation of vein grafts; retrograde cardioplegia; minimal cross-clamp time; consider use of hypothermia 24-32°, anticipate need for IV inotropic and mechanical support during CPB separation

CPB, cardiopulmonary bypass; IV, intravenous; OR, operating room.

2. **Surgical complications:** With myocardial electrical silence during CPB, surgical complications can only be perceived by direct observation. After reperfusion, monitor for ECG and wall motion abnormalities closely.

   a. **Coronary artery dissection:** Injury to the coronary artery back or sidewall may cause coronary artery dissection.

   b. **Vein graft complications:** Vein grafts can become occluded by twisting or kinking and improper handling, and preservation may lead to thrombus formation.

   c. **Anastomotic complications:** Both arterial and venous distal anastomoses can be occluded by poor-quality grafts with sutures that close the lumen. Hematomas adjacent to the anastomosis may also occlude the graft.

3. **Immediately postrevascularization and reperfusion:** Identification and assessment of myocardial ischemia should be done by monitoring for ECG changes and wall motion abnormalities on TEE after cardioplegia is washed out. Post-CPB causes of myocardial ischemia include the previously described hemodynamic and surgical factors in addition to incomplete revascularization (poor distal targets, mislocated graft site, or too few coronary grafts).

C. **Treatment of Myocardial Ischemia:** Appropriate treatment depends on considering all causes of myocardial ischemia and providing appropriate medical, surgical, and extracorporeal support.

1. **Hemodynamic abnormalities:** Tachycardia, hypotension, and hypertension can upset the balance of oxygen delivery and demand. Consider increasing or decreasing anesthetic depth. Administer vasodilators or vasopressors when SVR is either high or low, respectively, assuming euvolemia. Administer esmolol, which has a short half-life, to treat tachycardia.

2. **Rhythm disturbances:** Slow junctional rhythm or complete heart block can be treated with atrioventricular sequential pacing, either transcutaneously, via epicardial lead, or via temporary transvenous pacemaker.

3. **Pump failure:** Use inotropes for ventricular failure, diagnosed by decreased cardiac output and increased ventricular filling pressures or with TEE. Pump failure leads to severe decreases in CPP because diastolic blood pressure is decreased and LVEDP is increased.

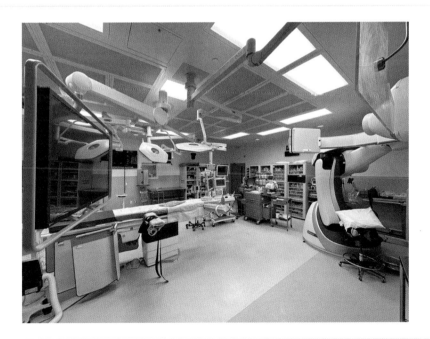

FIGURE 12.10   A hybrid cardiac operating room at the University of Virginia Health System.

Indiscriminate use of inotropes may aggravate ischemia. Therefore, preload and heart rate and rhythm should be optimized before using inotropes.

4. **Ischemia/instability upon CPB separation:** If heparin has not yet been neutralized, consider resuming CPB for a short period to facilitate myocardial recovery and/or to facilitate initiation of circulatory support with an inotrope or IABP.

5. **Correction of surgical complications and mechanical problems:** Avoid overinflation of the lungs when an IMA graft is present. Increasing systemic blood pressure with a vasoconstrictor such as phenylephrine can push intracoronary air through the vasculature and restore blood flow to regions not perfused because of the intravascular air lock.

6. **Treatment of coronary spasm:** IV nitroglycerin, diltiazem, and nicardipine can treat coronary spasm.

7. **Mechanical support:** IABPs are often the first-line support of mechanical support considered when difficulty with weaning off CPB is encountered (see later). Veno-arterial extracorporeal membrane oxygenation (VA-ECMO) can also be used to rest the heart after unsuccessful attempt(s) in separating from CPB before planning for a subsequent support device (left ventricular assist device [LVAD] or right ventricular assist device [RVAD]).

D. **Other Clinical Challenges in Myocardiac Revascularization Surgery**

1. **Improving outcomes due to ischemic heart failure with an intra-aortic balloon pump:** IABPs increase CPP and decrease LV afterload, which improves oxygen delivery and decreases demand. Despite significant theoretical and anecdotal benefits, evidence of a definitive improvement in outcomes with IABP remains elusive in the literature. The IABP-SHOCK II trial randomized 600 patients with ischemia awaiting revasularization (either surgical or percutaneous) to IABP or no IABP, with no reduction in 30-day mortality in the IABP group.[64] A smaller RCT that was predominantly (>90%) CABG patients also found no 30-day mortality benefit.[65] For elective CABG in high-risk patients, a meta-analysis did find a reduction in both perioperative and 30-day mortality, but half of the studies included were considered low quality.[66] IABPs themselves can cause significant injury to the vasculature and, if not timed correctly or positioned appropriately, can worsen ischemia.

2. **Issues with conduit:** Currently, the use of saphenous vein as conduit is more common than the use of a radial artery, but that may soon change. Recent American College of Cardiology/American Heart Association (ACC/AHA) guidelines suggest that the radial artery should be preferred to saphenous vein conduit based on evidence of greater long-term patency and a meta-analysis reporting decreased mortality.[67] Thus, more cardiac surgeons may change practice and communication with the surgical team before arterial line cannulation will become essential to avoid damaging a potential graft. When saphenous vein is harvested endoscopically, CO_2 is used for insufflation, and embolus can occur. There are multiple case reports of massive and life-threatening embolus, and it is important to consider this as a cause for any decompensation during vein harvesting.[68] The diagnosis may be confirmed with evidence of bubbles in the inferior vena cava (IVC) or the right side of the heart on TEE.

3. **Issues with internal thoracic artery harvest:** The majority of myocardial revascularization surgeries will involve internal thoracic artery harvest, which can be a source of complications. The left pleural space will be opened and require a chest tube to drain any collection of blood or air in the postoperative course. During harvest, the surgeon may require pauses in ventilation or low-tidal volumes, which can cause significant right ventricular strain from hypoxia or hypercarbia. In addition, the site may bleed, especially while anticoagulated for CPB, and can cause gradual signs of hypovolemia or sudden hypovolemia to those who are not circumspect and watching for an accumulating hemothorax. Before removal of the TEE probe, both pleural spaces should be examined for evidence of new or worsening effusion.

4. **Patients who present in cardiogenic shock:** This patient population is very challenging, with short-term mortality estimates ranging from 20% to 50%.[69]

   a. **Intervene rapidly or to stabilize first?** Recent evidence beginning to favor rapid intervention, rather than "waiting and stabilizing."

b. **CABG versus PCI:** One study found no difference in mortality between the two despite the CABG cohort having more comorbidities.[70] Many centers favor CABG for patients with diabetes, significant left main CAD, or multivessel disease. With a higher risk for structural abnormalities, valvular abnormalities, and difficulty weaning from CPB, TEE is of high value in this patient population. In addition, having groin catheters in femoral vessels (arterial and venous) as placeholders before induction allows for rapid intervention if there is further decompensation.

c. **Left ventricular decompression:** More centers are beginning to emphasize both circulatory support and LV protection via decompression with IABP, a percutaneous ventricular assist device, or VA-ECMO.

d. **Perioperative risk:** Salvage CABG, with active cardiac arrest and cardiopulmonary resuscitation, likely carries the highest risk of in-hospital mortality, but a substantial percentage of patients will have meaningful survival.[69]

5. **Postoperative opioid requirements, delirium, and length of intensive care unit stay:** Delirium is a major cause of increased length of ICU stay, morbidity, and mortality. Incidence and severity of delirium is associated with multiple factors, including postoperative sedation and analgesic regimens. Dexmedetomidine, when compared to propofol for sedation after CABG, shows mixed results for decreasing outcomes related to opioid use and delirium. For older patients, administration of IV acetaminophen in combination with dexmedetomidine or propofol infusion appears to improve outcomes related to delerium, breakthrough pain, and length of ICU stay.[70]

CLINICAL PEARL

The patient in cardiogenic shock needing emergent CABG or PCI may benefit from both circulatory support and LV protection via decompression.

VII. **Anesthesia for Hybrid Cardiac Procedures**
A. **Introduction/Background:** An anterior thoracotomy incision permits access for harvesting of the left IMA and its anastomosis to the LAD coronary artery without CPB. Although this is technically a variation on OPCAB, typically, it is called *minimally invasive direct coronary artery bypass* (MIDCAB). Most patients requiring coronary revascularization can now be treated with nonsurgical interventions, thanks to advances in stent design, stent drug elution, oral antiplatelet drug therapy, and interventional access techniques. However, anatomic and other technical factors still render complex lesions better managed surgically. Many cardiac centers have hybrid operating rooms combining the space, lighting, monitoring, and supplies of a cardiac surgical suite with that of an imaging-equipped interventional cardiology laboratory (Figure 12.10). These facilities allow combined surgical anastomosis and catheter-based interventions within one suite. Typically, the LAD artery is revascularized surgically, based on data indicating better patency, while other grafts may be individualized to either surgical or catheter approaches based on patient-specific factors. Despite theoretical benefits, hybrid revascularization remains a niche procedure at a small number of centers, and most small RCTs and observational studies have not found a significant difference in outcomes compared to traditional CABG.[71] The Hybrid Coronary Revascularization trial, a phase 3, large-scale, randomized trial designed to compare multivessel PCI with hybrid coronary surgery in patients with disease of the LAD and ≥1 additional stenoses, was terminated early because of low enrollment (ClinicalTrials.gov identifier: NCT03089398). Thus, the 2021 ACC/AHA/SCAI (Society for Cardiovascular Angiography & Interventions) guidelines do not provide any recommendation about hybrid approaches, stating the evidence is unclear.[67]

B. **Coronary Artery Bypass Grafting in a Hybrid Room**
1. **Overview:** Hybrid facilities permit both surgical bypass and endovascular stenting in the same suite and can also provide excellent anesthetizing conditions for open heart, structural heart, vascular endograft, electrophysiology, neurovascular, and other procedures.

2. **Rationale:** Hybrid procedures allow for immediate correction of graft occlusion. Graft failure before discharge from the hospital occurs in 5%-20% of patients. These failures arise from vein valves impeding flow, IMA dissections, vein graft kinking, or incorrect graft placement. About 6% of grafts imaged immediately after surgery have problems that should be addressed by interventional techniques, minor adjustments, or surgical revision. A case-control study compared 141 consecutive hybrid patients with disease not amenable to CABG alone or PC) alone to matched CABG and PCI cohorts. The hybrid patients underwent LAD surgical grafting using the left IMA followed by PCI of other lesions. After 3 years, repeat revascularization occurred in six hybrid, three CABG, and 18 PCI patients and death in one, four, and five patients, respectively.[72] The markedly different anatomic and physiologic states of the cases relative to the selected controls limit clinical inference from this study. Other potential advantages include avoidance of aortic manipulation, fewer transfusions, and, especially compared to OPCAB, less hemodynamic compromise. Patients who may benefit from hybrid CABG include those with limitations to traditional CABG (such as a heavily calcified proximal aorta or poor surgical target vessels, but amenable to PCI), a lack of suitable graft conduits, or unfavorable LAD for PCI (excessive tortuosity or chronic occlusion).

CLINICAL PEARL

Consider hybrid revascularization approach in patients with limitations to traditional CABG, (such as a heavily calcified proximal aorta or poor surgical target vessels, but amenable to PCI), a lack of suitable graft conduits, or unfavorable LAD for PCI (excessive tortuosity or chronic occlusion).

Avoidance of a full median sternotomy and shorter duration of CPB may allow early extubation, so the anesthetic should be designed with rapid recovery in mind. Some centers are performing preoperative morphine spinals in robotic CABG with better analgesia and reduced opioid consumption 48 hours after surgery.[73]

REFERENCES

1. Tsao CW, Aday AW, Almarzooq ZI, et al. Heart disease and stroke statistics—2022 update: a report from the American Heart Association. *Circulation.* 2022;145(8):e153-e639.
2. Agency for Healthcare Research and Quality. Medical Expenditure Panel Survey (MEPS): household component summary tables: medical conditions, United States. Accessed April 8, 2021. https://meps.ahrq.gov/data_files/publications/st471/stat471.pdf
3. Centers for Disease Control and Prevention, National Center for Health Statistics. National Vital Statistics System: public use data file documentation: mortality multiple cause-of-death micro-data files. Accessed April 8, 2021. https://www.cdc.gov/nchs/nvss/mortality_public_use_data.htm
4. Ambrose JA, Dangas G. Unstable angina: current concepts of pathogenesis and treatment. *Arch Intern Med.* 2000;160(1):25-37.
5. Fuster V, Chesebro JH. Antithrombotic agents in coronary artery disease. *N Engl J Med.* 1986;315:1023-1025.
6. Burgess DC, Hunt D, Li L, et al. Incidence and predictors of silent myocardial infarction in type 2 diabetes and the effect of fenofibrate: an analysis from the Fenofibrate Intervention and Event Lowering in Diabetes (FIELD) study. *Eur Heart J.* 2010;31(1):92-99.
7. Goetz RH, Rohman M, Haller JD, Rosenak SS. Internal mammary-coronary artery anastomosis. A nonsuture method employing tantalum rings. *J Thorac Cardiovasc Surg.* 1961;41:378-386.
8. Kolessov VI. Mammary artery-coronary artery anastomosis as method of treatment for angina pectoris. *J Thorac Cardiovasc Surg.* 1967;54(4):535-544.
9. Melly L, Torregrossa G, Lee T, et al. Fifty years of coronary artery bypass grafting. *J Thorac Dis.* 2018;10(3)1960-1967.
10. Loop FD, Lytle BW, Cosgrove DM, et al. Influence of the internal-mammary-artery graft on 10-year survival and other cardiac events. *N Engl J Med.* 1986;314(1):1-6.
11. Acar C, Jebara VA, Portoghese M, et al. Revival of the radial artery for coronary artery bypass grafting. *Ann Thorac Surg.* 1992;54(4):652-659; discussion 659-660.
12. Colantonio LD, Gamboa CM, Richman JS, et al. Black-White differences in incident fatal, nonfatal, and total coronary heart disease. *Circulation.* 2017;136(2):152-166.
13. Conrad Z, Rehm CD, Wilde P, et al. Cardiometabolic mortality by Supplemental Nutrition Assistance Program participation and eligibility in the United States. *Am J Public Health.* 2017;107(3):466-474.

14. Angraal S, Khera R, Wang Y, et al. Sex and race differences in the utilization and outcomes of coronary artery bypass grafting among medicare beneficiaries, 1999-2014. *J Am Heart Assoc.* 2018;7(14):e009014.

15. Enumah ZO, Canner JK, Alejo D, et al. Persistent racial and sex disparities in outcomes after coronary artery bypass surgery: a retrospective clinical registry review in the drug-eluting stent era. *Ann Surg.* 2020;272(4):660-667.

16. Randgrass G, Ghaferi AA, Dimick JB. Explaining racial disparities in outcomes after cardiac surgery: the role of hospital quality. *JAMA Surg.* 2014;149(3):223-227.

17. He G, Taggart DP. Antispastic management in arterial grafts in coronary artery bypass grafting surgery. *Ann Thorac Surg.* 2016;102(2):573-579.

18. Nilsson J, Algotsson L, Höglund P, et al. Comparison of 19 pre-operative risk stratification models in open-heart surgery. *Eur Heart J.* 2006;27(7):867-874.

19. Min JK, Berman DS, Dunning A, et al. All-cause mortality benefit of coronary revascularization vs. medical therapy in patients without known coronary artery disease undergoing coronary computed tomographic angiography: results from CONFIRM (COronary CT Angiography EvaluatioN For Clinical Outcomes: an InteRnational Multicenter Registry). *Eur Heart J.* 2012;33(24):3088-3097.

20. Serruys PW, Morice MC, Kappetein AP, et al. Percutaneous coronary intervention versus coronary-artery bypass grafting for severe coronary artery disease. *N Engl J Med.* 2009;360(10):961-972.

21. Makikallio T, Holm NR, Lindsay M, et al. Percutaneous coronary angioplasty versus coronary artery bypass grafting in treatment of unprotected left main stenosis (NOBLE): a prospective, randomised, open-label, non-inferiority trial. *Lancet.* 2016;388(10061):2743-2752.

22. Stone GW, Sabik JF, Serruys PW, et al. Everolimus-eluting stents or bypass surgery for left main coronary artery disease. *N Engl J Med.* 2016;375(23):2223-2235.

23. Hoffman JI, Buckberg GD. The myocardial oxygen supply: demand index revisited. *J Am Heart Assoc.* 2014;3(1):e000285.

24. Collins JA, Rudenski A, Gibson J, Howard L, O'Driscoll R. Relating oxygen partial pressure, saturation and content: the haemoglobin-oxygen dissociation curve. *Breathe (Sheff).* 2015;11(3):194-201.

25. Ramanathan T, Skinner H. Coronary blood flow. *Contin Educ Anaesth Crit Care Pain.* 2005;5:61-64.

26. Kaul S, Jayaweera AR. Myocardial capillaries and coronary flow reserve. *J Am Coll Cardiol.* 2008;52(17):1399-1401.

27. Bargiggia GS, Bertucci C, Recusani F, et al. A new method for estimating left ventricular dP/dt by continuous wave Doppler-echocardiography. *Circulation.* 1989;80(5):1287-1292.

28. Westerhof N, Stergiopulos N, Noble MIM, Westerhof BE. *Snapshots of Hemodynamics An Aid for Clinical Research and Graduate Education.* Springer; 2019.

29. Shaw AD, Mythen MG, Shook D, et al. Pulmonary artery catheter use in adult patients undergoing cardiac surgery: a retrospective, cohort study. *Perioper Med (Lond).* 2018;7:24.

30. Slogoff S, Keats AS. Does perioperative myocardial ischemia lead to postoperative myocardial infarction? *Anesthesiology.* 1985;62(2):107-114.

31. MacKay EJ, Zhang B, Heng S, et al. Association between transesophageal echocardiography and clinical outcomes after coronary artery bypass graft surgery. *J Am Soc Echocardiogr.* 2021;34(6):571-581.

32. Metkus TS, Thibault D, Grant MC, et al. Transesophageal echocardiography in patients undergoing coronary artery bypass graft surgery. *J Am Coll Cardiol.* 2021;78(2):112-122.

33. Shanewise JS. How to reliably detect ischemia in the intensive care unit and operating room. *Semin Cardiothorac Vasc Anesth.* 2006;10(1):101-109.

34. Landoni G, Lomivorotov VV, Nigro NC, et al. Volatile anesthetics versus total intravenous anesthesia for cardiac surgery. *N Engl J Med.* 2019;380(13):1214-1225.

35. Pisano A, Torella M, Yavorovskiy A, Landoni G. The impact of anesthetic regimen on outcomes in adult cardiac surgery: a narrative review. *J Cardiothorac Vasc Anesth.* 2021;35(3):711-729.

36. Stephan H, Sonntag H, Schenk HD, et al. Effects of propofol on cardiovascular dynamics, myocardial blood flow and myocardial metabolism in patients with coronary artery disease. *Br J Anaesth.* 1986;58(9):969-975.

37. Cameron M, Tam K, Al Wahaibi K, et al. Intraoperative ketamine for analgesia post-coronary artery bypass surgery: a randomized, controlled, double-blind clinical trial. *J Cardiothorac Vasc Anesth.* 2020;34(3):586-591.

38. Yao YT, He LX, Fang NX, Ma J. Anesthetic induction with etomidate in cardiac surgical patients: a PRISMA-compliant systematic review and meta-analysis. *J Cardiothorac Vasc Anesth.* 2021;35(4):1073-1085.

39. Janda AM, Spence J, Dubovoy T, et al. Multicentre analysis of practice patterns regarding benzodiazepine use in cardiac surgery. *Br J Anaesth.* 2022;128(5):772-784.

40. Spence J, Belley-Côté E, Jacobsohn E, et al. Restricted versus liberal intraoperative benzodiazepine use in cardiac anaesthesia for reducing delirium (B-Free Pilot): a pilot, multicentre, randomised, cluster crossover trial. *Br J Anaesth.* 2020;125(1):38-46.

41. Subramaniam B, Shankar P, Shaefi S, et al. Effect of intravenous acetaminophen vs placebo combined with propofol or dexmedetomidine on postoperative delirium among older patients following cardiac surgery: the DEXACET Randomized Clinical Trial. *JAMA.* 2019;321(7):686-696.

42. Pal N, Abernathy JH III, Taylor MA, et al. Dexmedetomidine, delirium, and adverse outcomes: analysis of the Society of Thoracic Surgeons Adult Cardiac Surgery database. *Ann Thorac Surg.* 2021;112(6):1886-1892.

43. Yang C-F, Yu-Chih CM, Chen T-I, Cheng C-F. Dose-dependent effects of isoflurane on cardiovascular function in rats. *Tzu Chi Med J.* 2014;26(3):119-122.

44. Buffington CW, Davis KB, Gillispie S, et al. The prevalence of steal-prone coronary anatomy in patients with coronary artery disease: an analysis of the Coronary Artery Surgery Study Registry. *Anesthesiology.* 1988;69(5):721-727.

45. Nashef SA, Roques F, Hammill BG, et al. Validation of European System for Cardiac Operative Risk Evaluation (EuroSCORE) in North American cardiac surgery. *Eur J Cardiothorac Surg.* 2002;22(1):101-105.

46. Tankard KA, Park B, Brovman EY, Bader AM, Urman RD. The impact of preoperative intravenous iron therapy on perioperative outcomes in cardiac surgery: a systematic review. *J Hematol.* 2020;9(4):97-108.
47. Turgeon RD, Koshman SL, Youngson E, et al. Association between hemoglobin A1c and major adverse coronary events in patients with diabetes following coronary artery bypass surgery. *Pharmacotherapy.* 2020;40(2):116-124.
48. Benedetto U, Albanese A, Kattach H, et al. Smoking cessation before coronary artery bypass grafting improves operative outcomes. *J Thorac Cardiovasc Surg.* 2014;148(2):468-474.
49. Bahar R, Hermansen SE, Dahl-Eriksen Ø, et al. The risk factors for radial artery and saphenous vein graft occlusion are different. *Scand Cardiovasc J.* 2022;56(1):127-131.
50. Fontes ML, Aronson S, Mathew JP, et al. Pulse pressure and risk of adverse outcome in coronary bypass surgery. *Anesth Analg.* 2008;107(4):1122-1129.
51. da Graca B, Filardo G, Sass DM, et al. Preoperative β-blockers for isolated coronary artery bypass graft. *Circ Cardiovasc Qual Outcomes.* 2018;11(12):e005027.
52. Leslie K, Sessler DI. The implications of hypothermia for early tracheal extubation following cardiac surgery. *J Cardiothorac Vasc Anesth.* 1998;12(6):30-34; discussion 41-44.
53. Engelman R, Baker RA, Likosky DS, et al. The Society of Thoracic Surgeons, The Society of Cardiovascular Anesthesiologists, and The American Society of ExtraCorporeal Technology: clinical practice guidelines for cardiopulmonary bypass—temperature management during cardiopulmonary bypass. *J Cardiothorac Vasc Anesth.* 2015;29(4):1104-1113.
54. Dowd NP, Cheng DC, Karski JM, Wong DT, Munro JA, Sandler AN. Intraoperative awareness in fast-track cardiac anesthesia. *Anesthesiology.* 1998;89(5):1068-1073; discussion 9A.
55. Lewis SR, Pritchard MW, Fawcett LJ, et al. Bispectral index for improving intraoperative awareness and early postoperative recovery in adults. *Cochrane Database Syst Rev.* 2019;9(9):Cd003843.
56. Pedemonte JC, Plummer GS, Chamadia S, et al. Electroencephalogram burst-suppression during cardiopulmonary bypass in elderly patients mediates postoperative delirium. *Anesthesiology.* 2020;133(2):280-292.
57. Mazzeffi MA, Holmes SD, Taylor B, et al. Red blood cell transfusion and postoperative infection in patients having coronary artery bypass grafting surgery: an analysis of the Society of Thoracic Surgeons Adult Cardiac Surgery database. *Anesth Analg.* 2022;135(3):558-566.
58. Salenger R, Mazzeffi MA. The 7 pillars of blood conservation in cardiac surgery. *Innovations.* 2021;16(6):504-509.
59. Nazarnia S, Subramaniam K. Nonopioid analgesics in postoperative pain management after cardiac surgery. *Semin Cardiothorac Vasc Anesth.* 2021;25(4):280-288.
60. Chaney MA. Intrathecal and epidural anesthesia and analgesia for cardiac surgery. *Anesth Analg.* 2006;102(1):45-64.
61. Hargrave J, Grant MC, Kolarczyk L, et al. An expert review of chest wall fascial plane blocks for cardiac surgery. *J Cardiothorac Vasc Anesth.* 2023;37(2):279-290.
62. Shaefi S, Mittel A, Loberman D, Ramakrishna H. Off-pump versus on-pump coronary artery bypass grafting—a systematic review and analysis of clinical outcomes. *J Cardiothorac Vasc Anesth.* 2019;33(1):232-244.
63. Gonzalo N, Tearney GJ, van Soest G, et al. Witnessed coronary plaque rupture during cardiac catheterization. *JACC Cardiovasc Imaging.* 2011;4(4):437-438.
64. Thiele H, Zeymer U, Neumann FJ, et al. Intraaortic balloon support for myocardial infarction with cardiogenic shock. *N Engl J Med.* 2012;367(14):1287-1296.
65. Rocha FGS, de Almeida JP, Landoni G, et al. Effect of a perioperative intra-aortic balloon pump in high-risk cardiac surgery patients: a randomized clinical trial. *Crit Care Med.* 2018;46(8):e742-e750.
66. Zangrillo A, Pappalardo F, Dossi R, et al. Preoperative intra-aortic balloon pump to reduce mortality in coronary artery bypass graft: a meta-analysis of randomized controlled trials. *Crit Care.* 2015;19(1):10.
67. Lawton JS, Tamis-Holland JE, Bangalore S, et al. 2021 ACC/AHA/SCAI Guideline for coronary artery revascularization: executive summary: a report of the American College of Cardiology/American Heart Association Joint Committee on Clinical Practice Guidelines. *Circulation.* 2022;145(3):e4-e17.
68. Strauss E, Taylor B, Mazzeffi M, et al. The auscultation of a carbon dioxide embolization event during endoscopic vein harvest. *Case Rep Anesthesiol.* 2016;2016:6947679.
69. Ibrahim M, Spelde AE, Gutsche JT, et al. Coronary artery bypass grafting in cardiogenic shock: decision-making, management options, and outcomes. *J Cardiothorac Vasc Anesth.* 2021;35(7):2144-2154.
70. Mehta RH, Lopes RD, Ballotta A, et al. Percutaneous coronary intervention or coronary artery bypass surgery for cardiogenic shock and multivessel coronary artery disease? *Am Heart J.* 2010;159(1):141-147.
71. Lowenstern A, Wu J, Bradley SM, Fanaroff AC, Tcheng JE, Wang TY. Current landscape of hybrid revascularization: a report from the NCDR CathPCI Registry. *Am Heart J.* 2019;215:167-177.
72. Shen L, Hu S, Wang H, et al. One-stop hybrid coronary revascularization versus coronary artery bypass grafting and percutaneous coronary intervention for the treatment of multivessel coronary artery disease: 3-year follow-up results from a single institution. *J Am Coll Cardiol.* 2013;61(25):2525-2533.
73. Dhawan R, Daubenspeck D, Wroblewski KE, et al. Intrathecal morphine for analgesia in minimally invasive cardiac surgery: a randomized, placebo-controlled, double-blinded clinical trial. *Anesthesiology.* 2021;135(5):864-876.

Aortic Valve Repair and Replacement

Nishank P. Nooli and Matthew M. Townsley

KEY POINTS

1. All valvular lesions can potentially lead to changes in cardiac loading conditions, and a well-planned anesthetic should account for this through the manipulation of several hemodynamic variables. Most importantly, these include heart rate and rhythm, preload, afterload, and cardiac contractility.

2. During transcatheter aortic valve replacement (TAVR), there may be periods of acute hemodynamic instability due to the device occluding the valve orifice, the creation of acute aortic regurgitation (AR) during balloon valvuloplasty, massive bleeding from aortic root injury, aortic dissection, pericardial tamponade, complete heart block, TAVR valve embolization, or acute occlusion of a coronary ostium.

3. Because atrial contraction contributes up to 40% of left ventricular (LV) filling in patients with aortic stenosis (AS) and hypertrophic cardiomyopathy (HCM), the maintenance of sinus rhythm and aggressive treatment of dysrhythmias is critical in both conditions.

4. In patients with AS, early use of α-adrenergic agonists (ie, phenylephrine) is indicated to prevent hypotension that can quickly escalate to severe hemodynamic compromise and cardiac arrest.

5. The dynamic left ventricular outflow tract (LVOT) obstruction caused by systolic anterior motion (SAM) of the mitral valve occurs proximal to the aortic valve (ie, subaortic) in mid-to-late systole. The degree of obstruction is directly proportional to LV contractility and inversely proportional to LV preload (end-diastolic volume) and afterload. Specifically, decreases in systemic vascular resistance (SVR) and preload, as well as increases in contractility and heart rate will precipitate or worsen SAM/LVOT obstruction.

6. Patients with severe, acute AR are not capable of maintaining sufficient forward stroke volume and often develop sudden and severe dyspnea, hemodynamic instability, and rapid clinical deterioration. Patients with chronic AR may be asymptomatic for many years.

7. The hemodynamic requirements for combined AS and mitral regurgitation (MR) are contradictory. Because AS is more likely to cause severe cardiac instability, it should be given priority when managing hemodynamic parameters.

I. Introduction

The management of patients with valvular heart disease continues to evolve, with continuing advancements in both catheter-based and surgical interventions. This is especially true for aortic valve disease, as transcatheter aortic valve replacement (TAVR) has revolutionized the surgical approach to aortic stenosis (AS), which is the most common valvular heart lesion in the United States. The role of the anesthesiologist also continues to evolve and expand with these advancements. In particular, the less invasive nature of TAVR, as compared to surgical aortic valve replacement (SAVR), has changed the landscape of patients presenting for AVR. The growing older population and those with significant comorbidities, who would not previously have been operative candidates, are now presenting for valve replacement. Thus, the cardiac anesthesiologist is now increasingly called upon to provide care for a more complicated and challenging patient population with aortic valve disease. With results of the PARTNER 3 and Evolut Low-Risk trials proving noninferiority of TAVR to SAVR when looking at outcomes of stroke and death, a broadened use of TAVR, even in low-risk patient populations, is becoming more common. Importantly, advancements in these catheter-based techniques also involve modifications of the anesthetic technique, as many centers perform TAVR procedures with moderate anesthesia care or no sedation at all.

Regardless of the procedural approach, the goal of aortic valve intervention is to improve symptoms and survival, in addition to minimizing the risk of complications, such as irreversible ventricular dysfunction, stroke, pulmonary hypertension, and dysrhythmias.[1] The anesthetic management of aortic valve disease is often challenging, as both AS and aortic regurgitation (AR) lead to pathophysiologic changes in the heart with profound hemodynamic consequences. All valvular lesions can lead to changes in cardiac loading conditions (ie, volume and/or pressure overload), and a well-planned anesthetic must compensate for this through the manipulation of several hemodynamic variables.[2] Most importantly, these variables include heart rate and rhythm, preload, afterload, and cardiac contractility. In addition, it is essential to consider the time course of the disease, as the clinical presentation and management considerations vary dramatically in the setting of acute versus chronic valvular disorders.

II. Stenotic Versus Regurgitant Lesions

A. Valvular Stenosis

Obstruction of flow through a cardiac valve translates into an increase in blood flow velocity as it approaches the stenotic valve orifice. The pattern of blood flow is distinctly different in the regions proximal and distal to a stenotic valve. The high-velocity flow proximal to the stenosis is laminar and organized, while distal to the stenosis, it becomes turbulent and disorganized. In addition, this high-velocity flow results in an increase in the pressure gradient across the valve. The simplified Bernoulli equation helps explain this relationship:

$$\Delta P = 4v^2$$

where ΔP represents the pressure gradient, and v represents peak blood flow velocity.

The simplified Bernoulli equation converts blood flow velocities measured by Doppler echocardiography into pressure gradients that may be used to quantify the severity of valvular stenosis.

Valvular obstruction occurs in two primary forms: fixed versus dynamic. In a fixed obstruction (ie, true valvular AS, subaortic membrane), the degree of obstruction to blood flow remains constant throughout the cardiac cycle. With dynamic obstruction (ie, hypertrophic obstructive cardiomyopathy [HOCM] with dynamic subaortic stenosis), obstruction is only present for part of the cardiac cycle, primarily occurring in mid-to-late systole. The degree of dynamic obstruction is highly dependent on loading conditions, varying in severity as loading conditions change.

B. Valvular Regurgitation

Regurgitant lesions lead to volume overload, with eventual chamber dilatation and eccentric hypertrophy (wall thickness increases in proportion to the increase in left ventricular [LV] chamber size). Initially, this chamber remodeling allows the LV to compensate for an increased volume load; however, it will eventually lead to a decline in LV systolic function that may result in irreversible LV failure. Effective perioperative management of valvular regurgitation is facilitated by understanding how preload, afterload, and heart rate each affect the contributions of the forward stroke volume (flow reaching the peripheral circulation) and regurgitant stroke volume (retrograde flow back across the valve) to the overall total stroke volume of the ventricle.[3] Hemodynamic management aims to optimize forward stroke volume, while minimizing the amount of regurgitant stroke volume.

III. Structural and Functional Response to Valvular Heart Disease

A. Cardiac Remodeling includes changes in the size, shape, and function of the heart in response to an acute or chronic cardiac pathology. In valvular heart disease, this pathology is primarily caused by alterations in ventricular loading conditions. Depending on the nature of the valvular pathology, the ventricle will be subject to either volume or pressure overload, leading to remodeling in the form of chamber dilation or ventricular hypertrophy, respectively. In addition to mechanical stress, cardiac remodeling results from the activation of neurohumoral factors, enzymes (such as angiotensin II), ion channels, and oxidative stress. Intended initially as an adaptive response to maintain cardiac performance, remodeling eventually leads to deterioration in ventricular performance.

Ventricular hypertrophy is defined as increased LV mass and can be either concentric or eccentric. Pressure overload results in concentric ventricular hypertrophy, meaning that ventricular mass is increased by myocardial thickening while ventricular volume is not increased. Concentric versus eccentric hypertrophy can be determined using echocardiography. LV mass index >95 g/m^2 for women and >115 g/m^2 for men define hypertrophy. If relative wall thickness is >0.42, the hypertrophy is concentric. If relative wall thickness is <0.42, the hypertrophy is eccentric. Recall the law of Laplace to understand how this compensatory hypertrophy results in reduced wall stress, where:

$$\text{LV wall stress} = (\text{LV pressure} \times \text{LV radius})/(2 \times \text{LV wall thickness})$$

AS is a fixed obstruction at the level of the aortic valve, which increases LV afterload and intracavitary pressure. Concentric hypertrophy has the beneficial effect of reducing LV wall stress and avoiding a significant decline in LV systolic function. The cost of LV hypertrophy, however, is a reduction in LV compliance. This leads to diastolic dysfunction, with an increase in LV end-diastolic pressure (LVEDP) and greater risk for subendocardial ischemia.

Volume overload, on the other hand, leads to eccentric hypertrophy, where the increase in ventricular mass is associated with ventricular cavity dilatation. In this scenario, myocardial thickness increases in proportion to the increase in ventricular chamber radius.

B. Ventricular Function

To anticipate the effects of valvular lesions on ventricular function, it is helpful to separate ventricular function into its two distinct components[2]:

1. **Systolic function** represents the ventricle's ability to eject blood into the systemic circulation.

   a. **Contractility** is defined as the intrinsic ability of the myocardium to contract and generate force. Contractility itself is independent of preload and afterload. Normal contractility means that a ventricle of normal size and normal preload can generate sufficient stroke volume at rest and during exercise.
   b. **Preload** is defined as the load placed on the myocardium before contraction. This load results from a combination of diastolic volume and filling pressure and is expressed as end-diastolic wall stress.
   c. **Afterload** is the load placed on the myocardium during contraction. This load results from the combination of arterial blood pressure and systemic vascular resistance (SVR). The generated pressure is expressed as end-systolic wall stress.
2. **Diastolic function** represents the ventricle's ability to accept inflowing blood. Diastolic function consists of a combination of relaxation and compliance. In general, normal diastolic function means that the ventricle accepts normal diastolic volume at normal filling pressure. When diastolic dysfunction occurs, maintaining a normal ventricular diastolic volume requires an elevated ventricular filling pressure. Both systolic and diastolic function are energy-dependent processes and are compromised by ventricular ischemia.

IV. Pressure-Volume Loops
The pressure-volume loops are useful aids for illustrating LV function and performance. These loops are constructed by plotting ventricular pressure (*y*-axis) versus ventricular volume (*x*-axis) over the course of a complete cardiac cycle (Figure 13.1). The presence of valvular heart disease alters the normal pressure-volume loop, representing changes in ventricular physiology and loading conditions imposed by valvular pathology. The ventricle adapts differently to each valvular lesion, and characteristic patterns of the pressure-volume loops demonstrate these changes.

V. Aortic Stenosis
   A. **Natural History**
      1. **Etiology:** The normal adult aortic valve has three cusps, with an aortic valve area (AVA) of 2.6-3.5 cm^2 (representing a normal aortic valve index of 2 cm^2/m^2) (▶ **Video 13.1**). AS may result from congenital or acquired valvular heart disease.

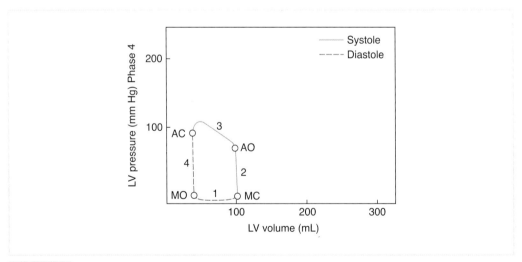

FIGURE 13.1 Normal pressure-volume loop. The first segment of the ventricular pressure-volume loop (phase 1) represents diastolic filling of the LV. The next two segments represent the two stages of ventricular systole: isovolumic contraction (phase 2) and ventricular ejection (phase 3). The final segment of the loop corresponds to isovolumic relaxation of the LV, which precedes ventricular filling and the start of the next cardiac cycle. The isovolumic relaxation and ventricular filling phases constitute the two phases of diastole. Both end-systolic volume at the time of aortic valve closure (AC) and end-diastolic volume at the time of mitral valve closure (MC) are represented as distinct points on the loop. AO, aortic valve opening; LV, left ventricle; MO, mitral valve opening. (Based on Jackson JM, Thomas SJ, Lowenstein E. Anesthetic management of patients with valvular heart disease. *Semin Anesth*. 1982;1:240.)

Congenital AS is classified as valvular, subvalvular, or supravalvular based on the anatomic location of the stenosis. Subvalvular (⊙ **Video 13.2**) and supravalvular AS are usually caused by a membrane or muscular band. Congenital valvular AS may occur with a unicuspid, bicuspid, or a tricuspid aortic valve with partial commissural fusion. Aortic valves with supernumerary cusps (>3 cusps) have also been reported. A congenitally bicuspid aortic valve occurs in −1%-2% of the general population, making it the most common congenital valvular malformation (⊙ **Video 13.3**). Calcification of a congenitally bicuspid valve results in the early onset of AS and represents the most common cause of AS among patients younger than 70 years.[4] Bicuspid aortic valve disease accounts for ~50% of all valve replacements for AS in the United States and Europe.[5] Commonly associated findings include abnormalities of the aorta, including proximal ascending aortic aneurysm, aortic coarctation, aortic root dilatation, and an increased risk of aortic dissection.

Of the acquired AS, senile degeneration is the most common etiology in the developed world. Aortic sclerosis describes fibrotic and calcific changes in the aortic valve before the onset of stenosis. Its incidence may be as high as 25% of individuals aged >65 years and 50% of individuals aged >85 years. Epidemiologic data suggest that the incidence of severe AS may be as high as 3.4% in individuals aged >75 years in developed countries.[6] The calcification in senile degeneration of the aortic valve also appears to have an inflammatory component, similar to that observed with coronary artery disease (CAD). While rheumatic AS is rarely seen in the developed world, it remains an important cause of AS in developing countries. However, senile calcific disease is the most prevalent etiology of AS worldwide. Less frequent causes of AS include atherosclerosis, end-stage renal disease, and rheumatoid arthritis.

A characteristic finding of senile valvular degeneration is progression of calcification from the base of the valve toward the edge, as opposed to rheumatic degeneration in which calcification spreads from the edge toward the base.

2. **Symptoms:** Unicuspid AS usually presents in infancy. Patients with rheumatic AS may be asymptomatic for ≥40 years. Congenital bicuspid aortic valves in the majority of cases must undergo calcific degeneration to become stenotic. The time of onset and speed of progression of calcific degeneration vary from patient to patient. Therefore, patients with congenitally bicuspid aortic valves may develop symptomatic AS at any point between the ages of 15 and 65 years (or even later in life). Degenerative stenosis of a tricuspid aortic valve typically develops in the seventh or eighth decade of life. Asymptomatic patients with AS have an excellent prognosis. Patients with severe AS may remain asymptomatic for many years. However, the onset of any one of the following triad of symptoms is an ominous sign, indicating a life expectancy of <5 years:

   a. **Angina pectoris:** Angina is the initial symptom in approximately two-thirds of patients with severe AS. Angina and dyspnea secondary to AS alone initially occur with exertion.[7] Life expectancy following the development of angina is ~5 years.

   b. **Syncope;** Syncope is the first symptom in 15%-30% of patients. Once syncope appears, the average life expectancy is 3-4 years.

   c. **Congestive heart failure:** Once signs of LV failure occur, the average life expectancy is only 1-2 years.

B. Pathophysiology

1. **Cardiac remodeling:** As stenosis progresses, the maintenance of normal stroke volume requires an increased systolic pressure gradient between the LV and the aorta. The LV systolic pressure (LVSP) may increase to as much as 300 mm Hg, whereas the aortic systolic pressure and stroke volume remain relatively normal. This pressure gradient results in a compensatory concentric LV hypertrophy. Occasionally, as stenosis progresses, eccentric LV hypertrophy may develop and result in impaired LV systolic function.

2. **Hemodynamic changes**

   a. **Arterial pressure:** In severe AS, the arterial pulse pressure is often reduced to <50 mm Hg. The systolic pressure rise is delayed, with a late peak and a prominent anacrotic notch. As stenosis increases in severity, the anacrotic notch occurs lower in the ascending arterial pressure trace. The dicrotic notch is relatively small or absent.

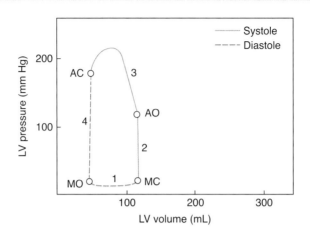

FIGURE 13.2 Pressure-volume loop in aortic stenosis. In comparison to the normal loop, note the elevated peak systolic pressure necessary to generate a normal stroke volume in the face of the elevated pressure gradient through the aortic valve. Also, end-diastolic pressure is elevated with a steeper diastolic slope, reflecting diastolic dysfunction with altered LV compliance. Phase 1, diastolic filling; phase 2, isovolumic contraction; phase 3, ventricular ejection; phase 4, isovolumic relaxation. AC, aortic valve closure; AO, aortic valve opening; LV, left ventricle; MC, mitral valve closure; MO, mitral valve opening. (Based on Jackson JM, Thomas SJ, Lowenstein E. Anesthetic management of patients with valvular heart disease. *Semin Anesth.* 1982;1:240.)

   b. **Pulmonary arterial wedge pressure:** Because of the elevated LVEDP, which stretches the mitral valve annulus, a prominent V wave can be observed, but with progression of the disease and the development of left atrial hypertrophy, a prominent A wave becomes the dominant feature.
 3. **Pressure-volume loop in aortic stenosis** (Figure 13.2)
C. **Preoperative Evaluation and Assessment of Severity**
 1. **Echocardiographic evaluation** (Table 13.1)
   Echocardiography is the standard modality for quantifying the severity of AS. Quantification methods include measurement of peak blood flow velocity and mean gradient across the aortic valve and determination of AVA. The AVA can be measured by the two-dimensional (2D) or three-dimensional (3D) planimetry, as well as the continuity equation methods. The pressure gradient is measured using a simplified Bernoulli equation (Figure 13.3).
   Transesophageal echocardiography (TEE) is particularly useful in patients with poor transthoracic windows or in patients with complex cardiac pathology (eg, a combination of subaortic and valvular stenoses). It is also useful when precise planimetry of the AVA is

TABLE 13.1 Assessment of AS Severity With Echocardiography

Measurement	AS	Mild AS	Moderate AS	Severe AS
Aortic valve area (cm²)	2.6-3.5	>1.5	1.0-1.5	<1.0
Mean gradient (mm Hg)	<10	<20	20-40	>40
Indexed aortic valve area (cm²/m²)	2.0	>0.85	0.60-0.85	<0.6
Peak velocity of blood flow through aortic valve (m/s)	<2.6	2.6-3.0	3-4	>4

AS, aortic stenosis.
Adapted from Baumgartner H, Hung J, Bermejo J, et al. Echocardiographic assessment of valve stenosis: EAE/ASE recommendations for clinical practice. *J Am Soc Echocardiogr.* 2009;22(1):1-23. © 2009 Elsevier. With permission.

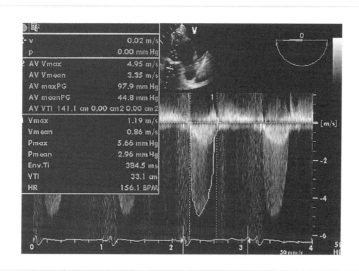

FIGURE 13.3   Severe aortic stenosis (AS), showing determination of the aortic valve (AV) gradient using the Bernoulli equation. This image displays a deep transgastric long-axis transesophageal echocardiography view with a continuous-wave Doppler beam aligned through the left ventricular outflow tract (LVOT) and AV. Tracing 2 on the spectral display (outer traced envelope) represents blood flow through the severely stenotic AV, with a mean velocity (AV Vmean) of 3.35 m/s and mean AV pressure gradient (AV mean PG) of 44.8 mm Hg. A mean PG ≥40 mm Hg is consistent with severe AS. (Reprinted with permission from Perrino AC, Reeves ST, eds. *A Practical Approach to Transesophageal Echocardiography*. 2nd ed. Wolters Kluwer Health/Lippincott Williams & Wilkins; 2008:246.)

necessary or when infective endocarditis is suspected. Supplemental ⊙ **Videos 13.4, 13.5,** and **13.6** demonstrate TEE images of a severely stenotic trileaflet aortic valve, with 2D imaging, 3D imaging, and color-flow Doppler, respectively.

2. Most patients with severe AS will have a mean transvalvular gradient >40 mm Hg and peak velocity >4 m/s. However, up to 30% of patients with an AVA <1 cm² may have transvalvular gradients and velocities less than the cutoffs for severe stenosis.[6]

   a. Classic low-flow, low-gradient severe AS describes a scenario in which a patient has diminished LV ejection fraction (LVEF), resulting in a low-flow state (defined as stroke volume index <35 mL/m²) and mean gradient <40 mm Hg, peak velocity <4 m/s, and AVA <1 cm². In this scenario, dobutamine stress echocardiography (DSE) should be performed. If the addition of inotropic support results in a mean gradient >40 mm Hg and the calculated AVA remains <1 cm², the diagnosis of true severe AS is confirmed. If the mean gradient remains <40 mm Hg, but the calculated AVA increases to >1 cm², then a diagnosis of pseudo-severe AS is made. Pseudo-severe AS is primarily an issue of LV dysfunction, and AVR is not indicated.

   b. Paradoxical low-flow, low-gradient severe AS describes a scenario in which a patient with normal LVEF has an AVA <1 cm², mean gradient <40 mm Hg, and peak velocity <4 m/s. In this case, the patient has a low-flow state (stroke volume index <35 mL/m²) because of small stroke volumes secondary to concentric remodeling and impaired diastolic filling. Low-dose DSE may be useful in confirming this diagnosis as well.

   c. However, if DSE fails to increase the flow across the aortic valve and the discordant values remain, it is possible to calculate a projected AVA based on normal flow. For patients who fail to increase the stroke volume by 20% with dobutamine, the mortality for surgical AVR is high. In addition, multidetector computed tomography (CT) can be used to quantify the calcification of the aortic valve, and a calcium score can be used to predict the risk of stenosis progression.

CLINICAL PEARL

In the patient with AS and low LVEF, the pressure gradients generated with echocardiography may not suggest criteria for severe AS. However, patients with low-flow, low-gradient AS represent a high-risk population.

3. If cardiac catheterization data are utilized, the mean pressure gradient may be measured from a direct transaortic measurement, and the AVA may be calculated using the Gorlin formula.

D. **Timing and Type of Intervention**

1. The timing of intervention is based upon the stage of the disease, which takes into account not only the severity determined by echocardiography but also the presence or absence of symptoms. Table 13.2 summarizes indications for valve replacement.

2. Due to the high risk of sudden death and limited life expectancy, symptomatic patients should undergo AVR. Asymptomatic patients with severe AS may be monitored closely until symptoms develop. However, the risk of waiting should be carefully weighed against the risk of the procedure. For example, before elective noncardiac surgery under general or neuraxial anesthesia, asymptomatic patients with severe AS should be considered for AVR.

3. Patients with moderate AS should have aortic valve surgery if they happen to require another cardiac operation, such as coronary artery bypass grafting (CABG), because the rate of progression of AS is −0.1 cm² per year and the risk of having to redo cardiac surgery is substantially higher than the risk of the primary operation. Similarly, if a patient undergoing aortic valve surgery has significant CAD, CABG should be performed simultaneously. In patients over age 80 years, the risk of AVR alone is approximately the same as the risk of combined AVR and CABG.[8]

4. A commissural incision or balloon aortic valvuloplasty may be the first procedure performed in young patients with severe noncalcific aortic valve stenosis, even if they are asymptomatic.[7] This operation frequently results in some residual AS and AR. Eventually, most patients require a subsequent prosthetic valve replacement. In older adult patients with calcific AS, valve replacement is the primary operation. In young adults, a viable

TABLE 13.2   Recommendations for Timing of AVR in Aortic Stenosis

Class I indications

Symptomatic patients with severe high-gradient AS who have symptoms by history or on exercise testing

Asymptomatic patients with severe AS and LVEF <50%

Severe AS when undergoing other cardiac surgery

Class IIa indications

Asymptomatic patients with very severe AS (aortic velocity ≥5 m/s) and low surgical risk

Asymptomatic patients with severe AS and decreased exercise tolerance or a fall in blood pressure with exercise

Asymptomatic patients with low-flow/low-gradient severe AS with reduced LVEF with low-dose dobutamine stress study showing an aortic velocity ≥4 m/s (mean pressure gradient ≥40 mm Hg) with a valve area ≤1 cm² at any dobutamine dose

Symptomatic patients who have low-flow/low-gradient severe AS who are normotensive and have an LVEF ≥50% if clinical, hemodynamic, and anatomic data support valve obstruction as the most likely cause of symptoms

Patients with moderate AS (aortic velocity 3-3.9 m/s) who are undergoing other cardiac surgery

Class IIb indication

Asymptomatic patients with severe AS and rapid disease progression and low surgical risk

AS, aortic stenosis; AVR, aortic valve replacement; LVEF, left ventricular ejection fraction.

Adapted from Nishimura RA, Otto CM, Bonow RO, et al. 2014 AHA/ACC guideline for the management of patients with valvular heart disease: executive summary: a report of the American College of Cardiology/American Heart Association Task Force on Practice Guidelines. *J Am Coll Cardiol.* 2014;63(22):2438-2488. © 2014 American Heart Association, Inc., and the American College of Cardiology Foundation. With permission.

alternative to AVR may be the Ross procedure in which the diseased aortic valve is replaced with the patient's normal pulmonary valve and the pulmonary valve is replaced with a pulmonary homograft. This more complex procedure avoids the need for systemic anticoagulation and extends the time until reoperation is required by several decades.

5. **Balloon aortic valvuloplasty** in adults with advanced disease often results in significant AR and early restenosis. It is typically reserved for patients with severe comorbidities.

6. **Transcatheter aortic valve replacement:** Over the past decade, TAVR has revolutionized the treatment of symptomatic severe AS. It was initially used in inoperable and high-risk patients; however, over time, its use has been broadened to include intermediate- and low-risk patient populations. Compared to the traditional SAVR, TAVR is a less invasive alternative performed without cardiopulmonary bypass (CPB), in which a bioprosthetic valve is implanted within the native aortic valve via a catheter introduced through a major artery. This technique requires brief cessation of the patient's cardiac output via rapid ventricular pacing during positioning of the device. Hemodynamic instability is not uncommon and necessitates prompt recognition and treatment. The 30-day all-cause mortality has significantly improved and is at 2.2%, while at 1-year post-TAVR, the stroke rate is 1%-3% and the overall mortality is 1%-2.4%.[9]

    a. There are several TAVR valves currently available, and among them, two of the most widely used ones include:

    (1) **SAPIEN 3 Ultra (Edwards Lifesciences):** Transfemoral or transaortic or transapical deployment. This valve requires rapid ventricular pacing during deployment and is expanded with a balloon. Thus, the cardiac output is near zero during deployment.

    (2) **Evolut FX System (Medtronic):** Transfemoral deployment. This valve is self-expanding and requires a lower rate of rapid ventricular pacing to deploy. The LV continues to eject during deployment.

    b. **Contraindications:** Potential contraindications include acute myocardial infarction within 1 month, infective endocarditis, congenital unicuspid or bicuspid valve, pure aortic valvular regurgitation, hypertrophic cardiomyopathy (HCM), LVEF <20%, native aortic annulus size outside the manufacturer's recommended range, severe vascular disease precluding safe placement of the introducer sheath (for the transfemoral approach), cerebrovascular event within 6 months, and need for emergency surgery.

    c. **Hybrid operating room**[10]**:** Cardiovascular hybrid surgery, which includes TAVR, is a rapidly evolving field where less invasive surgical approaches are combined with interventional cardiology techniques in the same setting. Such procedures require a combination of high-quality imaging modalities found in a cardiac catheterization suite (fluoroscopy, navigation systems, postprocessing capabilities, high-resolution invasive monitoring, intracardiac and intravascular ultrasound, echocardiography, etc), in addition to the ability to perform open surgery under general anesthesia, including the use of CPB. These procedures require close collaboration and communication among multidisciplinary teams, including interventional cardiologists, surgeons, anesthesiologists, perfusionists, technicians, and nursing staff, some of whom may be distant from the operating field. Thus, the presence of multiple monitor panels in areas visible to all and advanced communication systems are critical. Large amounts of space and careful planning of room layout are crucial for all equipment to be readily accessible and to allow unobstructed access to the patient. In addition, both the radiation safety requirements of the cardiac catheterization suite and the hygienic standards of the operating room must be met. These many demands have led to the creation of specialized hybrid operating rooms (Figure 10.7).

    d. Surgical approaches (Figure 13.4)[11-13]

    (1) Retrograde or transfemoral approach

    (a) The femoral artery is accessed for device deployment. The femoral vein is used for transvenous pacer placement and preparation for emergent CPB.

    (b) Heparin (100-150 units/kg) is given intravenously, titrating therapy to an activated clotting time (ACT) of about 300 seconds.

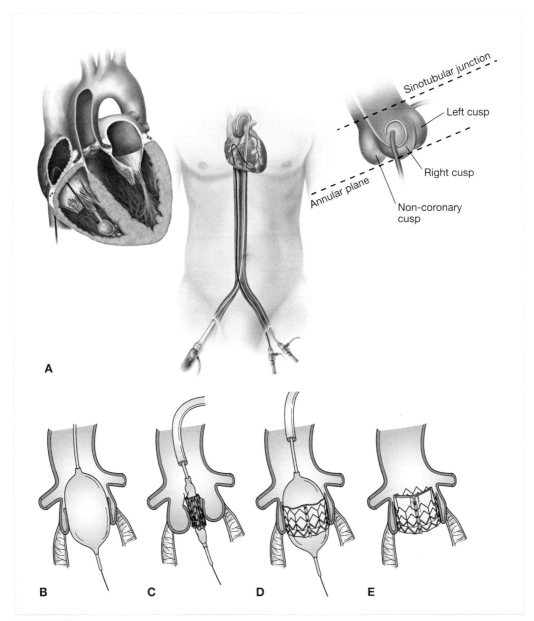

FIGURE 13.4 Surgical approaches to aortic valve replacement. **A.** Transcatheter aortic valve replacement through the transfemoral approach is facilitated by a temporary pacemaker placed in the right ventricle and a pigtail catheter in the aortic root to identify the aortic annulus radiographically. Typically, both femoral arteries are accessed, with one accommodating the valve delivery sheath and the other a much smaller sheath for catheter access in the aortic root. The artery can be controlled with percutaneous preclosure devices. (Reprinted with permission from Sarin EL, Thourani VH. Transcatheter Aortic Valve Replacement. In: Grover FL, Mack MJ, eds. Cardiac Surgery. Wolters Kluwer; 2017:13-28. Figure 2.1.) **B-E.** Schematic diagram of percutaneous aortic valve replacement. B: Balloon valvuloplasty. C: Balloon catheter with valve in the native diseased valve. D: Balloon inflation to secure the valve. E: Valve in place. (Reprinted with permission from Burns DJP, Wierup P, Gillinov AM. Valvular Heart Disease. In: Dimick JB, Upchurch GR Jr, Alam HB, Pawlik TM, Hawn MT, Sosa JA, eds. Mulholland & Greenfield's Surgery: Scientific Principles & Practice. 7th ed. Wolters Kluwer; 2022:1397-1408. Figure 82.7.)

13. Aortic Valve Repair and Replacement **275**

   (c) A guidewire is advanced across the aortic valve, and the balloon angioplasty catheter is advanced over the wire.

   (d) Ventricular pacing at about 140-180 beats/min (bpm) creates a low cardiac output state for valve deployment (Figure 13.5).

   (e) The device is positioned using fluoroscopy and TEE (in cases done under general anesthesia). Rapid ventricular pacing and apnea are used during valve deployment.

   (f) Fluoroscopy and transthoracic echocardiography (TTE) or TEE are used to assess valve position and function and to check for leak.

(2) Antegrade transapical approach

   (a) This more invasive approach is reserved for patients with peripheral arterial disease, which would not accommodate the introducer and valve deployment systems.

   (b) The left femoral artery and vein are accessed as mentioned earlier.

   (c) The LV apex is exposed via left anterolateral thoracotomy. TEE may facilitate identification of the apex.

   (d) Heparin is given with the same ACT targets described earlier.

   (e) A needle is inserted through the LV apex, through which a guidewire is passed through the aortic valve under fluoroscopic and TEE guidance.

   (f) A balloon valvuloplasty catheter is introduced over the guidewire and positioned in the aortic valve. Similar to the retrograde approach, rapid ventricular pacing and apnea are initiated to create a motionless field during inflation.

   (g) The valvuloplasty sheath is then replaced by the device introducer sheath through which the prosthetic valve is deployed in a similar manner.

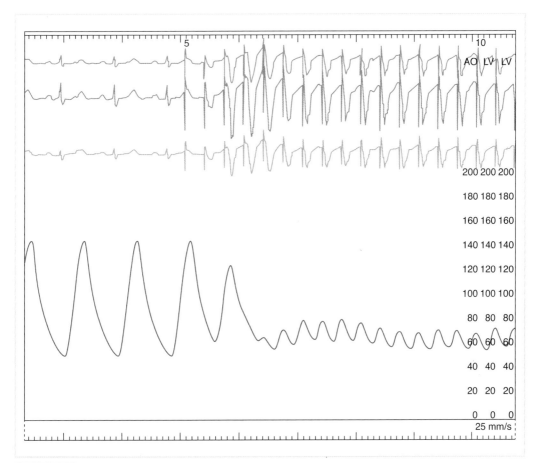

FIGURE 13.5 Hemodynamics during rapid ventricular pacing. The bottom waveform is taken from the arterial catheter. AO, aorta; LV, left ventricle.

(3) Other approaches

    (a) A transaxillary approach is an alternative for patients with severe iliofemoral arterial disease.[14] Preoperative CT imaging is obtained to ensure that the vasculature is suitable for this approach. Access is obtained via surgical cutdown, and the valve is deployed similar to the retrograde (transfemoral approach).

    (b) Transaortic approach via suprasternal access has also been reported. In the authors' institution, this is the most commonly used alternative approach when peripheral vascular disease prevents a transfemoral technique.

    (c) Recently, a transcarotid approach has been used in patients who are not the candidates for other approaches.

e. Anesthetic considerations

    (1) In addition to standard monitors, large-bore venous access and invasive arterial blood pressure monitoring are essential. TEE is helpful as a monitor and guide for valve placement, but TTE or fluoroscopy alone may be used in patients having the procedure done via the retrograde transfemoral approach, using local anesthesia and sedation.

    (2) Blood should be readily available, as massive hemorrhage from arterial injury can occur acutely.

    (3) Radiolucent defibrillation pads should be placed before draping the patient in case the need arises for cardioversion or defibrillation.

    (4) With the transapical and transaortic approaches, general anesthesia is necessary. Lung isolation may be helpful for surgical exposure but is not absolutely needed. For the retrograde approach, local or regional anesthesia with monitored anesthesia care (MAC) may be adequate, but each patient should be assessed on an individual basis. The advantages of using local/regional anesthesia with sedation include the ability to assess neurologic status, avoidance of airway manipulation, and a more rapid recovery. However, general anesthesia may be more comfortable for the patient, provide immobility during valve deployment, and provide a secure airway in the event of complications and the need for emergent CPB.[15-17] General anesthesia is especially helpful when TEE is used, and some clinicians see this as the "tipping point" for its selection. With either method of anesthesia, the goal is for the patient to recover rapidly. Shorter acting anesthetic agents along with other adjuncts, such as intercostal nerve blocks performed under direct vision by the surgical team (transapical approach), will help accomplish this goal.

    (5) During the procedure, there may be periods of acute hemodynamic instability as a result of the device occluding the already narrow valve, the creation of acute AR during valvuloplasty, massive bleeding from dissection of major vasculature, damage to the LV or mitral valve, or acute occlusion of a coronary ostium. Arrhythmias are common during insertion of guidewires and catheters into the LV. Clear communication with the surgical team is of the utmost importance in order to treat appropriately and to avoid "overshooting" with vasopressors. Sometimes, the solution is as simple as repositioning the catheter.

CLINICAL PEARL

Acute, dramatic hemodynamic changes are common during TAVR, for both patient- and procedure-related causes, making it essential to communicate with the surgical team so that they can contribute to diagnosis and treatment of these changes.

    (6) Normothermia should be actively maintained with the use of forced air warming blankets and fluid warmers as needed.

    (7) TEE/TTE are used to assess global cardiac function, measure the aortic root for sizing of the prosthesis, screen for aortic disease, facilitate proper valve positioning, and identify complications of the procedure such as paravalvular leak (● **Video 13.7**), tamponade, or coronary occlusion.[9,18]

   f. **Complications**[19,20]: Major complications of TAVR include stroke, vascular damage including dissection, rupture of the aortic root, occlusion of coronary ostia, cardiac conduction abnormalities, damage to other cardiac structures such as the mitral valve, embolization of the prosthesis requiring emergent surgical retrieval, and massive blood loss from vascular damage or rupture of the LV. Paravalvular leak is more common after TAVR than open surgery, probably because diseased, calcified tissue that may hinder optimal valve deployment is not removed. Paravalvular leaks may be treated with balloon reinflation to better appose the stented prosthesis to the aortic annulus.

   g. **Outcomes**[8,21]: For nonsurgical candidates, TAVR has been associated with an improvement of symptoms and mortality at 1 year as compared to medical management. For patients at too high risk for SAVR, TAVR has transformed the management and led to significant reductions in mortality. The success of TAVR in this population has led to considerable interest in its use for lower risk patients. However, paravalvular regurgitation remains a limitation with TAVR, and even mild residual postoperative paravalvular leak may increase mortality. In addition, there appears to be a higher incidence of heart block, stroke, and major vascular complications with TAVR. Recently, results of PARTNER III and Evolut Low-Risk trials have led to expansion of TAVR valve use in low-risk patients as well. We look forward to more long-term outcomes data as the procedure becomes more common.

7. **Surgical (open) aortic valve replacement**
   a. Patients who require AVR and who do not qualify for (or sometimes who do not choose) TAVR require a traditional open AVR, which is most often performed using a median sternotomy and CPB.
   b. Anesthetic considerations and goals of perioperative management are as generally the same as previously discussed for TAVR.
   c. Types of valves are discussed in Section IX.

E. Goals of Intraoperative Management
   1. **Hemodynamic profile** (Table 13.3)
      a. **Left ventricular preload:** Due to the decreased LV compliance as well as the increased LVEDP and LV end-diastolic volume (LVEDV), preload augmentation is necessary to maintain a normal stroke volume.
      b. **Heart rate:** Extremes of heart rate are not tolerated well. A high heart rate can lead to decreased coronary perfusion. A low heart rate can limit cardiac output in these patients with a fixed stroke volume. If a choice must be made, however, low heart rates (50-70 bpm) are preferred to rapid heart rates (>90 bpm) to allow time for systolic ejection across a stenotic aortic valve. Because atrial contraction contributes up to 40% of LV filling, due to decreased LV compliance and impaired early filling during diastole, it is essential to maintain a sinus rhythm. Supraventricular dysrhythmias should be treated aggressively, if necessary, with synchronized direct current shock because both tachycardia and the loss of effective atrial contraction can lead to rapid reduction of cardiac output.
      c. **Contractility:** Stroke volume is maintained through preservation of a heightened contractile state. β-Blockade is not well tolerated and can lead to an increase in LVEDV and a decrease in cardiac output significant enough to induce clinical deterioration.
      d. **Systemic vascular resistance:** Most of the afterload to LV ejection is caused by the stenotic aortic valve itself and thus is fixed. Systemic blood pressure reduction does

TABLE 13.3 Hemodynamic Goals for Management of AS

	LV Preload	Heart Rate	Contractility	SVR	Pulmonary Vascular Resistance
AS	↑	↓ (sinus)	Maintain constant	↑	Maintain constant

AS, aortic stenosis; SVR, systemic vascular resistance.

little to decrease LV afterload. In addition, patients with hemodynamically significant AS cannot increase cardiac output in response to a drop in SVR. Thus, arterial hypotension may rapidly develop in response to the majority of anesthetics. Finally, when hypotension develops, the hypertrophied myocardium of the patient with AS is at a greater risk for subendocardial ischemia because coronary perfusion depends on the maintenance of an adequate systemic diastolic perfusion pressure. Therefore, the early use of α-adrenergic agonists such as phenylephrine is indicated to prevent drops in blood pressure that can lead quickly to sudden death.

4

  e. **Pulmonary vascular resistance:** Except for end-stage AS, pulmonary artery (PA) pressures remain relatively normal. Special intervention for stabilizing pulmonary vascular resistance is not necessary.

2. An experienced cardiac surgeon should be present, and perfusionists should be prepared before induction of anesthesia, should rapid cardiovascular deterioration necessitate emergency use of CPB.

3. **Placement of external defibrillator pads** should be considered to allow for rapid defibrillation if cardiovascular collapse occurs on induction or before sternotomy.

4. **Preinduction arterial line placement** is standard practice at most institutions and is generally well tolerated with light premedication and local anesthetic infiltration. Invasive blood pressure monitoring facilitates early recognition and intervention if any hemodynamic instability occurs during induction.

5. During induction of anesthesia, in order to maintain hemodynamic stability, medications should be carefully titrated to a fine line between a reasonable depth of anesthesia and hemodynamic stability.

CLINICAL PEARL

During induction of general anesthesia for the patient with AS (or any other valvular lesion), it is less important to focus on the use of specific anesthetic agents or vasopressor drugs, as it is to proceed with a regimen/plan that aims to achieve and optimize specific hemodynamic goals (ie, related to choosing a drug regimen based on overall optimization of heart rate/rhythm, SVR, or inotropy).

6. During the maintenance stage of anesthesia, anesthetic agents causing myocardial depression, vasodilation, tachycardia, or dysrhythmias can lead to rapid deterioration. A narcotic-based anesthetic is usually chosen for this reason. Low concentrations of volatile anesthetics are usually safe.

7. If the patient develops signs or symptoms of ischemia, nitroglycerin should be used with caution because its effect on preload or arterial pressure may actually make things worse.

8. **Thermodilution cardiac output:** Pulmonary artery catheters (PACs) may be helpful in evaluating the cardiac output of high-risk patients before repair/replacement of the aortic valve. The pulmonary capillary wedge pressure (PCWP), however, may overestimate preload of a noncompliant LV. Mixed venous oxygen saturation monitoring via an oximetric PAC may be used to provide a continuous index of cardiac output. However, because the post-bypass management is not likely to be marked by myocardial failure or low output states, this technique may be best reserved for other patients who may be at higher risk of post-bypass hemodynamic complications.

9. There is a small risk of life-threatening arrhythmias leading to drug-resistant hypotension during passage of a PAC through the right atrium and ventricle. In the absence of preexisting left bundle branch block or tachyarrhythmias, a PAC may be placed under continuous rhythm monitoring, perhaps, after placement of transcutaneous pacing electrodes. In the presence of preexisting abnormal rhythms or conduction disturbances, however, the most conservative approach dictates leaving the catheter tip in a central venous position until the chest is open, when internal defibrillator pads can be easily applied and CPB can be initiated within a few minutes, if necessary.

10. TEE is useful for intraoperative monitoring of LV function, preload, and afterload. TEE can predict prosthetic aortic valve size based on the aortic annulus width. It is also very helpful in the detection of air and facilitating de-airing before/after weaning from CPB. TEE is the method of choice for the post-bypass assessment of a prosthetic valve for paravalvular regurgitation and prosthetic valve stenosis. It is important to remember that Doppler-derived blood flow velocities and pressure gradients must be interpreted in light of the altered loading conditions seen in the dynamic operating room setting.

11. In the presence of myocardial hypertrophy, adequate myocardial preservation with cardioplegic solution during bypass is a challenging task. A combination of antegrade cardioplegia administered via aortic root or coronary ostia and retrograde cardioplegia via the coronary sinus has an important role in preserving myocardial integrity.

12. In the absence of preoperative ventricular dysfunction and associated coronary disease, inotropic support is often not required after CPB because valve replacement decreases ventricular afterload.

F. Postoperative Care

After a sharp drop in the aortic valve gradient, PCWP and LVEDP immediately decrease and stroke volume rises. Myocardial function improves rapidly, although the hypertrophied ventricle may still require an elevated preload to function normally. Over a period of several months, LV hypertrophy regresses. It must be remembered that a properly sized and functional prosthetic aortic valve may cause an elevated mean pressure gradient (ie, ~7-19 mm Hg).

1. TAVR patients who receive general anesthesia are often usually extubated in the operating room.

2. Patients undergoing open AVRs are less often extubated in the operating room but may be fast-tracked if conditions permit.

VI. Hypertrophic Cardiomyopathy

A. Natural History

1. **Etiology and classification:** HCM is a relatively common genetic cardiac disorder, affecting ~0.2% of the general population worldwide. This equates to roughly one case in every 500 births, with some estimates now suggesting an even greater prevalence of HCM, with increased awareness and screening. Nomenclature and classification schemes related to HCM have historically been confusing, with several different names being used to describe this disease state (ie, idiopathic hypertrophic subaortic stenosis [IHSS], asymmetric septal hypertrophy, muscular subaortic stenosis). Since ventricular hypertrophy may occur in several different patterns (and not just confined to the ventricular septum), HCM is recognized as the preferred term for describing this disorder. In addition, despite the classic association of HCM with dynamic obstruction to systolic outflow through the LV outflow tract (LVOT), only ~25% of patients with HCM exhibit subvalvular obstruction. The term *hypertrophic obstructive cardiomyopathy* is used to refer to this subset of patients with HCM.

   HCM is a familial disease, inherited in an autosomal dominant manner with variable penetrance. Mutations in a number of different genes encoding various components of cardiac sarcomere proteins have been identified as a cause for HCM. Most common are mutations involving the β-myosin heavy chain, myosin-binding protein C, troponin T, troponin I, and tropomyosin α-1 chain.

2. **Symptoms:** Patients with HCM may present with a wide range of symptoms, with many having no symptoms at all. The most common presenting symptom is dyspnea on exertion, with poor exercise tolerance. Patients may also experience syncope, presyncope, chest pain, fatigue, and palpitations. While LVOT obstruction may cause symptoms, there is no clear relationship between the degree of LVOT obstruction and the occurrence or severity of symptoms. Other equally important causes of symptoms include diastolic dysfunction, dysrhythmias, mitral regurgitation (MR), and an imbalance of myocardial oxygen supply and demand. Unfortunately, the initial presenting symptom in many patients is sudden cardiac death, usually due to ventricular fibrillation. While all patients with HCM are at

risk for sudden death, the highest-risk groups include those with a family history of HCM and young patients undergoing significant physical exertion. This has led to increased and improved measures to screen for HCM in young athletes and patients with a family history of the disorder.

B. **Pathophysiology**

By definition, HCM involves an abnormal thickening of the myocardium without a clearly identifiable cause for the hypertrophy (ie, chronic hypertension, AS). There is an absence of chamber dilation and, in most cases, normal-to-hyperdynamic LV systolic function. In addition, there are important histologic derangements, including abnormal cellular architecture and disarray of the cardiac myocytes, interstitial fibrosis, increased connective tissue, and patchy myocardial scarring. These cellular abnormalities contribute to problems with diastolic filling, including decreased chamber compliance and impaired relaxation. Even more importantly, these histopathologic abnormalities lead to a derangement in the electrophysiology of the heart and are capable of inducing potentially catastrophic dysrhythmias. Patients with HCM are prone to both atrial and ventricular dysrhythmias, with ventricular fibrillation representing the most common cause of sudden death.

In the subset of patients with outflow tract obstruction, systolic anterior motion (SAM) of the anterior mitral valve leaflet (AML) is the underlying cause of dynamic outflow tract obstruction. Severe hypertrophy of the ventricular septum results in narrowing of the LVOT, whose borders are formed by the septum and the anterior leaflet of the mitral valve. During systole, further narrowing of the LVOT occurs due to septal thickening with ventricular contraction. This leads to an increase in the blood flow velocity (and pressure gradient) through the narrowed outflow tract. An important distinction between this condition and AS is that the preexisting ventricular hypertrophy leads to the elevated pressure gradient in HCM, as opposed to the stenotic orifice leading to ventricular hypertrophy in AS.

Basal septal hypertrophy results in a decreased physical distance between the AML and the septum. In addition, patients with HCM tend to have hypertrophied, anteriorly displaced papillary muscles along with elongated mitral valve leaflets. This shifts the mitral apparatus toward the septum, causing the posterior mitral valve leaflet (PML) to coapt closer to the base of the AML, when the two valve leaflets oppose one another during systole. The result of this altered coaptation is excess, slack AML tissue extending beyond the coaptation point. Rapid blood flow creates hydraulic forces (Venturi effect) capable of pulling this slack anterior mitral leaflet tissue into the LVOT. Although the Venturi effect has long been hypothesized as the primary mechanism of SAM, it is likely that a drag force generated by LV contraction pulls the anteriorly displaced, slack leaflet tissue into the LVOT in early systole. In fact, this drag force (ie, pushing/sweeping of the mitral valve leaflet) into the outflow tract is now believed to be the predominant cause of SAM. SAM leads to dynamic obstruction, in which the degree of obstruction varies based upon cardiac loading conditions and contractility. Specifically, the extent of LVOT obstruction is a function of the mitral valve leaflet physically contacting the septum in order to obstruct flow. Therefore, the degree of obstruction correlates directly with the onset, extent, and duration of mitral-septal contact. The obstruction occurs proximal to the aortic valve (subaortic) in mid-to-late systole, with the degree of obstruction directly proportional to LV contractility and inversely proportional to LV preload (end-diastolic volume) and afterload. Specifically, decreases in SVR and preload, as well as increases in contractility and heart rate will precipitate or worsen SAM/LVOT obstruction.

A further consequence of SAM is a posteriorly directed jet of MR that results from the abnormal mitral valve leaflet motion. During SAM, the distal portion of the AML remains in the LVOT during systole, as opposed to coapting with the PML in systole. This creates a funnel, formed by the distal portions of both mitral valve leaflets, directing regurgitant flow posteriorly through this channel. In this scenario, MR occurs after the onset of SAM, with its severity primarily related to the degree of LVOT obstruction. Therefore, maneuvers to alleviate LVOT obstruction will also lead to improvement or resolution of the MR. In addition to LVOT obstruction, dynamic midcavitary obstruction may also occur in patients with HCM. This typically occurs in patients with concentric hypertrophy most pronounced at the mid-LV level. Intracavitary obstruction is affected by the same hemodynamic conditions as dynamic LVOT obstruction.

While dynamic LVOT obstruction is seen in only a subset of patients with HCM, most all will exhibit diastolic dysfunction secondary to ventricular hypertrophy, as well as hypertrophy and disarray of the myocytes. Early diastolic filling is impaired secondary to this poor diastolic compliance, making atrial contraction, and thus maintenance of sinus rhythm, critical for adequate diastolic filling. Mismatch of oxygen supply and demand is a frequent occurrence in HCM, predisposing to ischemia. The hypertrophied myocardium represents a large muscle mass, with increased oxygen demand associated with elevated ventricular pressures and wall tension.

C. **Preoperative Evaluation and Assessment of Severity**
Echocardiography allows for assessment of the location and severity of hypertrophy and helps determine the necessity and feasibility of potential surgical intervention. When patients with HOCM present for surgical myectomy, the baseline intraoperative TEE examination is a critical component of the procedure. The extent of basal septal hypertrophy is assessed in a mid-esophageal long-axis (ME LAX) view at end diastole (Figure 13.6). In addition, a non-standard ME five-chamber view may also be used. While normal LV thickness is ≤1 cm, many patients will often present with severe basal septal hypertrophy in excess of 2 cm. The diameter of the LVOT, as well as the distance from mitral coaptation point to the septum (C-sept distance) is also measured. Both a narrow LVOT (≤2.0 cm) and small C-sept distance (≤2.5 cm) have been identified as risk factors for the development of hemodynamically significant SAM. Both of the abovementioned views may be used to evaluate for the presence of SAM (◉ **Video 13.8**). In the presence of SAM, color-flow Doppler will demonstrate high-velocity, turbulent flow (aliasing) in the LVOT. In addition, a posteriorly directed jet of MR is also frequently observed as a consequence of the SAM, resulting in a characteristic "Y-shaped" color-flow Doppler (CFD) pattern (◉ **Video 13.9**).

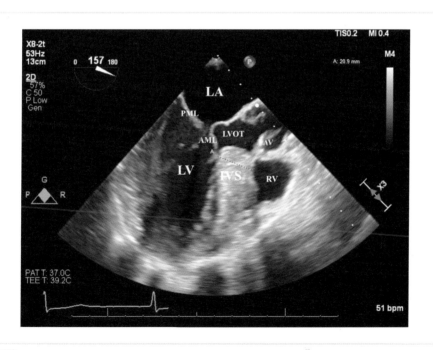

FIGURE 13.6 Basal septal hypertrophy in a patient with hypertrophic cardiomyopathy. Caliper measurement of the basal septum (dotted white and black lines) demonstrates severe hypertrophy (20.9 mm) visualized in a mid-esophageal long-axis transesophageal echocardiography view. AML, anterior mitral valve leaflet; AV, aortic valve; IVS, interventricular septum; LA, left atrium; LV, left ventricle; LVOT, left ventricular outflow tract; PML, posterior mitral valve leaflet; RV, right ventricle.

Continuous-wave Doppler (CWD) measurements of the peak LVOT velocity and pressure gradient, in either a deep transgastric LAX or transgastric LAX view, quantify the severity of subaortic obstruction. With dynamic LVOT obstruction, the Doppler profile demonstrates a late peaking, "dagger-shaped" envelope of high-velocity flow due to the onset of obstruction in mid-to-late systole (Figure 13.7). A mean gradient of ≥30 mm Hg is considered significant. In addition to the mitral coaptation defect associated with SAM, the mitral apparatus itself may be abnormal in patients with HCM and should be thoroughly examined. LV systolic function is typically normal or hyperdynamic, and diastolic function is almost always abnormal.

D. **Timing and Type of Intervention**

The mainstay of medical therapy for HCM involves treatment with β-blockers, which help reduce LVOT obstruction due to their negative inotropic effects and reduction in heart rate. Calcium channel blockers are also frequently utilized for their favorable effect on diastolic compliance. The most critical intervention in patients identified as high risk for malignant dysrhythmias is placement of an automated implantable cardioverter-defibrillator. Other non-surgical approaches to decrease outflow obstruction include dual-chamber pacing and ethanol ablation of the ventricular septum. Surgical treatment involves removal of septal muscle tissue to widen the LVOT via septal myectomy and may occasionally involve modification of the mitral valve apparatus or mitral valve repair/replacement. Following myectomy, the intraoperative TEE examination allows for immediate assessment of the adequacy of surgical

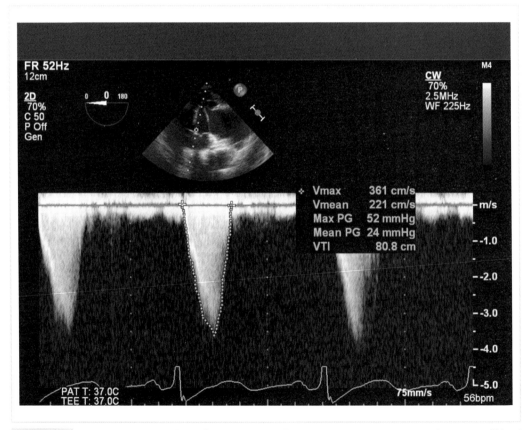

FIGURE 13.7 Dynamic left ventricular outflow tract (LVOT) obstruction. Continuous-wave Doppler tracing of blood flow through the LVOT in a patient with hypertrophic cardiomyopathy demonstrating a high-velocity Doppler flow profile with a delayed peak ("dagger shaped"), consistent with dynamic LVOT obstruction peaking in mid-to-late systole. The peak gradient (max PG) is significantly elevated at 52 mm Hg. (Reprinted with permission from Hymel BJ, Townsley MM. Echocardiographic assessment of systolic anterior motion of the mitral valve. *Anesth Analg*. 2014;118(6):1197-1201. © 2014 International Anesthesia Research Society.)

intervention. Expected findings are a significant reduction in the LVOT gradient by CWD, as well as thinning of the septum/widening of the LVOT and resolution of SAM.

E. Goals of Perioperative Management

1. Hemodynamic profile

a. Left ventricular preload: Any condition that leads to a decrease in LV cavity size can potentially exacerbate dynamic LVOT obstruction, as this places the septum and anterior mitral leaflet in closer proximity, narrowing the outflow tract and increasing the potential for SAM and obstruction. In this regard, preload augmentation is essential to help maintain ventricular volume. In addition, similar to AS, diastolic dysfunction will lead to decreased LV compliance with increased LVEDP, which will necessitate adequate preload to maintain a normal stroke volume. Treatment with nitroglycerin, or other vasodilators, should be avoided, as it may dangerously reduce cardiac output.

b. Heart rate: It is essential to avoid tachycardia in patients with HCM because it leads to a reduction in ventricular volume, exacerbation of dynamic LVOT obstruction, and increased oxygen demand. A decrease in heart rate is beneficial, as this prolongs diastole and allows more time for ventricular filling. Maintenance of sinus rhythm and the atrial contraction component of ventricular filling are critical due to reduced early diastolic filling because of reduced LV compliance.

c. Contractility: Decreases in myocardial contractility help reduce outflow obstruction. β-Blockade, volatile anesthetics, and avoidance of sympathetic stimulation are all potentially beneficial. The use of intraoperative inotropic agents can increase contractility, worsen LVOT obstruction, and lead to severe hemodynamic instability. Thus, they should be avoided.

CLINICAL PEARL

HOCM is one of the few clinical scenarios in which agents with positive inotropic effects can lead to clinical deterioration.

d. Systemic vascular resistance: Decreases in afterload must be promptly and aggressively treated with vasopressors, such as phenylephrine or vasopressin. Hypotension can be especially detrimental in this population because diastolic dysfunction leads to increased LVEDP, requiring an increased blood pressure to provide adequate coronary perfusion pressure (CPP):

$$CPP = \text{aortic diastolic pressure} - LVEDP$$

e. Pulmonary vascular resistance: PA pressures remain relatively normal in most patients. Specific intervention for stabilizing pulmonary vascular resistance is typically not necessary.

2. Anesthetic technique

a. Premedication: Many of these patients are on maintenance therapy with β-blockers or calcium channel blockers, which should be given on the day of surgery and continued throughout the perioperative period.

b. Induction and maintenance of anesthesia: During induction and laryngoscopy, careful attention is required to avoid decreases in afterload, as well as sympathetic stimulation leading to increases in heart rate and contractility. Adequate preload must be maintained, and all blood or fluid losses should be aggressively replaced. The direct myocardial depressant effect of volatile anesthetics is potentially advantageous.

c. Patients with HCM are at risk for atrial and ventricular tachyarrhythmias during surgery. Preparation must be in place for immediate cardioversion or defibrillation.

d. Intraoperative TEE, like preoperative echocardiography, allows visualization of the location and extent of hypertrophy in the septum, the degree of SAM and LVOT obstruction, and quantification of the degree of MR. It is customary to measure the thickness of the septum at the point of contact with the anterior leaflet, as this information is helpful to the surgeon. Since central venous pressure (CVP) and PCWP measurements will overestimate true volume status, TEE is the most reliable means of accurately assessing volume. The ability to monitor LV systolic function and wall motion is useful, as the oxygen supply-demand relationship is tenuous in these patients, making them prone to ischemia. The adequacy of surgical repair and any postrepair complications can also be immediately assessed.

e. **Postoperative care:** Potential complications in the immediate postoperative period following septal myectomy include residual LVOT obstruction, residual SAM, residual MR, complete heart block, and the creation of a ventricular septal defect (VSD). Unroofing of septal perforator vessels is an expected TEE finding after septal myectomy and should not be confused with an iatrogenic VSD.

VII. **Aortic Regurgitation**

A. **Natural History**

1. **Etiology:** AR may be caused by abnormalities of either the aortic valve leaflets or the aorta itself. Problems with the valve leaflets may occur from degenerative, inflammatory, infectious, traumatic, iatrogenic, or congenital etiologies. Specific examples include calcific valve disease, rheumatic disease, endocarditis, a congenitally bicuspid aortic valve, myxomatous valve disease, and systemic inflammatory disorders. Aortic root dilatation, leading to separation and incomplete apposition of the aortic valve leaflets in diastole, can be caused by degenerative aortic dilation, syphilitic aortitis, Marfan syndrome, and aortic dissection. Acute AR is usually caused by aortic dissection, trauma, or aortic valve endocarditis.

   A helpful approach to understanding the underlying cause of AR is based upon a modification of the well-established classification scheme used in mechanisms for MR (Carpentier classification). With this approach, three types of AR morphology are described, based upon the motion of the aortic valve leaflets. Type I is associated with normal aortic valve leaflet motion, type II with excessive valve leaflet motion (ie, leaflet prolapse), and type III with restricted valve leaflet motion (ie, thickening and/or calcification of leaflets). Type I AR may be further divided into four additional subtypes based upon pathology of the aortic root and aortic valve. Type Ia involves sinotubular junction enlargement and dilatation of the ascending aorta, type Ib involves dilatation of the sinuses of Valsalva and sinotubular junction, type Ic involves dilation of the aortic valve annulus, and type Id involves perforation of the aortic valve leaflet.[22]

2. **Symptoms:** Patients with chronic AR may be asymptomatic for many years. However, although they remain asymptomatic, many patients will be undergoing progressive ventricular dilatation with the development of impaired myocardial contractility. Symptoms such as shortness of breath, palpitations, fatigue, and angina usually develop only after significant dilatation and dysfunction of the LV myocardium have occurred. The 10-year mortality for asymptomatic AR varies between 5% and 15%. Once symptoms develop, however, patients progressively deteriorate and have an expected survival around 10 years. Patients with severe acute AR, due to the lack of long-standing compensation, are not capable of maintaining sufficient forward stroke volume. These patients are likely to develop sudden and severe dyspnea, significant pulmonary edema, and refractory heart failure and may deteriorate rapidly due to cardiovascular collapse.

B. **Pathophysiology**

1. **Pathophysiology and natural progression**

   a. **Acute aortic regurgitation:** The sudden occurrence of acute AR places a major volume load on the LV. The immediate compensatory mechanism for the maintenance of adequate forward flow is increased sympathetic tone, producing tachycardia and an increased contractile state. Fluid retention increases preload. However, the combination of increased LVEDV, along with increased stroke volume and heart rate, may not be sufficient to maintain a normal cardiac output. Rapid deterioration of LV function can occur, necessitating emergency surgical intervention.

6

CLINICAL PEARL

The patient with acute-onset, severe AR represents an especially high-risk patient population, and the perioperative plan must include preparations to manage sudden cardiac collapse.

b. **Chronic aortic regurgitation:** Chronically, AR leads to LV systolic and diastolic volume overload. LV wall tension also increases, precipitating the replication and lengthening of cardiac sarcomeres. This causes the wall thickness to increase in proportion to the increase in LV chamber size in a pattern of eccentric ventricular hypertrophy. Because the LVEDV increases slowly, the LVEDP remains relatively normal. Forward flow is aided by the presence of chronic peripheral vasodilation, which occurs along with a large stroke volume. As the LV dilatation progresses, coronary perfusion finally decreases, leading to irreversible LV myocardial tissue damage and dysfunction. The onset of LV dysfunction is followed by an increase in PA pressure with symptoms of dyspnea and congestive heart failure. As a compensatory mechanism for the poor cardiac output and poor coronary perfusion, sympathetic constriction of the periphery occurs to maintain blood pressure, which, in turn, leads to further decreases in cardiac output.

2. **Pressure wave disturbances**
   a. **Arterial pressure:** Incompetence of the aortic valve leads to regurgitant blood flow from the aorta back into the LV during diastole. This causes a pronounced decline in aortic diastolic blood pressure, translating into a wide pulse pressure. Patients with AR, therefore, show a wide pulse pressure with a rapid rate of rise, a high systolic peak, and a low diastolic pressure. The pulse pressure may be as great as 80-100 mm Hg. The rapid upstroke is due to the large stroke volume, and the rapid downstroke is due to the rapid flow of blood from the aorta back into the ventricle and then into the dilated peripheral vessels. The occurrence of a double peaked, or bisferiens pulse trace, is not unusual due to the occurrence of a "tidal" or back wave. It is this wide pulse pressure that leads to the presence of the many eponymous clinical signs associated with AR.
   b. **Pulmonary capillary wedge trace:** Stretching of the mitral valve annulus may lead to functional MR, a prominent V wave, and a rapid Y descent. In patients with acute AR associated with poor ventricular compliance, LV pressure may increase fast enough to close the mitral valve before end diastole. In this situation, AR raises the LVEDP above left atrial pressure, and the PCWP can significantly underestimate the true LVEDP.
3. **Pressure-volume loop in aortic regurgitation** (Figure 13.8)
C. **Preoperative Evaluation and Assessment of Severity**
   1. Historically, the amount of AR was estimated based on angiographic clearance of dye injected into the aortic root. Currently, echocardiography is the method of choice for qualitative, semiquantitative, and quantitative assessment of AR.

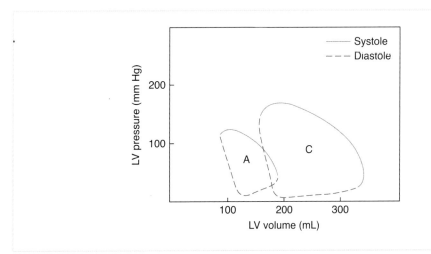

FIGURE 13.8 Pressure-volume loop in acute and chronic aortic regurgitation (AR). Note the rightward shift of the loop in chronic AR (C), reflecting elevated left ventricular (LV) volume without a dramatic elevation in filling pressure. In acute AR (A), LV volumes are also increased; however, the ventricle has not adapted to accommodate the increased volumes without elevation of filling pressures. (Based on Jackson JM, Thomas SJ, Lowenstein E. Anesthetic management of patients with valvular heart disease. *Semin Anesth.* 1982;1:247.)

TABLE 13.4 Hemodynamic Goals for Management of Dynamic Subaortic Stenosis

	LV Preload	Heart Rate	Contractility	SVR	Pulmonary Vascular Resistance
Dynamic subaortic stenosis	↑	↓	↓	↑	Maintain constant

LV, left ventricle; SVR, systemic vascular resistance.

 a. Echocardiographic assessment of aortic regurgitation (Table 13.4)
  ▶ **Videos 13.10** and **13.11** demonstrate the appearance of AR as seen on TEE in both LAX and short-axis views, respectively. The severity of AR can be assessed with echocardiography by several techniques (Table 13.5). Qualitative assessment includes the 2D analysis of the aortic valve anatomy, with particular attention to any structural abnormalities of the leaflets. The aortic root and LV cavity should be closely examined for evidence of dilation. CFD allows for visualization of the regurgitant jet, originating at the aortic valve and extending back into the LVOT in diastole. An experienced echocardiographer can often accurately estimate the degree of regurgitation with this initial observation; however, quantitative measurements are made to assess the severity more accurately. The vena contracta is, perhaps, the most widely utilized measurement. It represents the narrowest point of the regurgitant jet and corresponds to the size of the regurgitant orifice. It is a relatively easy-to-obtain measurement and is also unaffected by changes in preload or afterload (Figure 13.9). Severity of regurgitation can also be estimated by measuring the extent in which the regurgitant jet occupies the LVOT. The ratio of jet width to LVOT width, or jet area to LVOT area, has been found to correlate well with angiographic assessment (Figure 13.10).

TABLE 13.5 Assessment of AR Severity With Echocardiography

	Mild	Moderate		Severe
Left ventricular size	Normal[a]	Normal or dilated		Usually dilated[b]
Jet deceleration rate/ pressure half-time (msec)[c]	Slow (>500)	Medium (500-200)		Steep (<200)
Diastolic flow reversal in descending thoracic aorta	Brief, early diastolic reversal	Intermediate		Prominent holodiastolic reversal
Vena contracta width (cm)	<0.3	0.3-0.6		>0.6
Grade	**Mild (1+)[d]**	**Mild-moderate (2+)**	**Moderate-severe (3+)**	**Severe (4+)**
Jet width/LVOT width (%)	<25	25-45	46-64	≥65
Jet CSA/LVOT CSA (%)	<5	5-20	21-59	≥60
Regurgitant volume (mL/beat)	<30	30-44	45-59	≥60
RF (%)	<30	30-39	40-49	≥50
EROA (cm²)	<0.10	0.10-0.19	0.20-0.29	≥3.0

AR, aortic regurgitation; CSA, cross-sectional area; EROA, effective regurgitant orifice area; LVOT, left ventricular outflow tract; RF, regurgitant fraction.
[a]Unless there are other reasons for LV dilation.
[b]The LV is usually dilated in chronic AR. In acute AR, the LV size is often normal since the ventricle has not had time to dilate.
[c]Pressure half-time is shortened with increasing LV diastolic pressure and vasodilator therapy. It may be prolonged with chronic adaptation to severe AR.
[d]Note that there are several echocardiographic parameters that can subclassify regurgitation severity into mild, mild-moderate, moderate-severe, and severe. These subclassifications correspond to the angiographic grades of 1+, 2+, 3+, and 4+, respectively.
Adapted from Zoghbi WA, Adams D, Bonow RO, et al. Recommendations for noninvasive evaluation of native valvular regurgitation: a report from the American Society of Echocardiography developed in collaboration with the Society for Cardiovascular Magnetic Resonance. *J Am Soc Echocardiogr.* 2017;30(4):303-371. © 2017 by the American Society of Echocardiography. With permission.

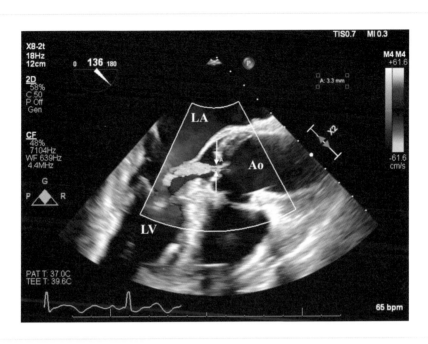

FIGURE 13.9 Vena contracta. Caliper measurement of the narrowest portion of the aortic regurgitant jet, which corresponds to an approximation of the regurgitant orifice area. Ao, aorta; LA, left atrium; LV, left ventricle.

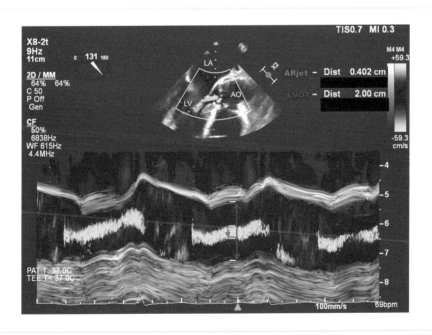

FIGURE 13.10 Color M-mode assessment of aortic regurgitation (AR). Utilizing an ME aortic long-axis view, the width of the regurgitant jet (pink arrow) and the LVOT (red arrow) are measured. The ratio of jet width to LVOT width can be used to estimate the severity of the AR. Ao, aorta; LA, left atrium; LV, left ventricle; LVOT, left ventricular outflow tract; ME, mid-esophageal.

CWD can be used to measure the deceleration rate of the regurgitant jet and the pressure half-time. These measurements are based on the rate of equilibration between aortic and LV pressures. As the severity of AR increases (ie, regurgitant orifice becomes larger), the more quickly these pressures will equilibrate. Thus, significant AR corresponds to a steep slope of the jet deceleration rate and a short pressure half-time. Severe AR may also be associated with holodiastolic flow reversal in the descending thoracic aorta seen on a pulsed-wave Doppler (PWD) examination.

    b. **Quantitative assessment of AR—calculation of regurgitant volume and regurgitant fraction:** A quantitative estimate of the severity of AR may be obtained by calculating the regurgitant volume and regurgitant fraction (RF). The total stroke volume in a patient with AR is the regurgitant volume plus the forward stroke volume actually ejected into the circulation. The regurgitant volume is the amount of blood that flows back through the incompetent aortic valve during diastole. It is quantified as the difference between the total stroke volume flowing through the aortic valve and the total *forward* stroke volume through a different valve. This reference valve is most commonly the mitral valve, with Doppler echocardiography being used to calculate the transmitral stroke volume. Total LV stroke volume can be determined with Doppler echocardiography measurement of flow through the LVOT, or it may be derived from the left ventriculogram on cardiac catheterization. The RF, or fraction of each stroke volume flowing back into the LV, equals the ratio of the right ventricle (RV) to the total stroke volume through the regurgitant aortic valve.

D. Timing and Type of Intervention

    1. **Acute aortic regurgitation:** Urgent surgical intervention is often indicated in acute AR due to a high incidence of hemodynamic instability. Inotropic support is frequently needed to maintain cardiac output.

    2. **Chronic aortic regurgitation:** AVR is recommended for the symptomatic patient with chronic, severe AR, regardless of LV systolic function. Asymptomatic patients with chronic AR and LV systolic function (EF <50%) should also undergo AVR. The asymptomatic patient with normal LV function should be closely followed for the onset of clinical symptoms and with serial echocardiographic examination. These patients should have surgical intervention at the earliest sign of LV dysfunction, as overall outcomes are significantly improved when surgery is performed before deterioration of ventricular function. In addition, evidence of ventricular dilatation (LV end-diastolic diameter >65 mm, LV end-systolic diameter >50 mm) should prompt consideration for surgery, even in the presence of normal LV function.[1]

    3. **Surgical intervention:** The most frequent approach to surgical treatment of AR is AVR. Experience with aortic valve repair has been limited to only a few highly specialized centers, and the durability of aortic valve repair remains unproven. Although enthusiasm for valve repair in certain patient populations (ie, young patients with bicuspid aortic valves) has resulted in advances in the technique, the American Heart Association/American College of Cardiology (AHA/ACC) guidelines only recommend aortic valve repair in specialized centers with proven experience and expertise.[1] In cases in which AR is secondary to aortic root and/or ascending aortic dilatation, valve-sparing replacement of the aorta may effectively resolve AR if there is no significant underlying aortic valve pathology.

E. Goals of Perioperative Management

    1. **Hemodynamic management** (Table 13.6)

TABLE 13.6 Hemodynamic Goals for Management of AR

	LV Preload	Heart Rate	Contractile State	SVR	Pulmonary Vascular Resistance
AR	↑	↑	Maintain	↓	Maintain

AR, aortic regurgitation; SVR, systemic vascular resistance.

    a. **Left ventricular preload:** Due to the increased LV volumes, maintenance of forward flow depends on preload augmentation. Pharmacologic intervention producing venous dilation has the potential to impair cardiac output in these patients by reducing preload.

    b. **Heart rate:** Patients with AR show a significant increase in forward cardiac output with an increase in heart rate. Decreased time spent in diastole, as occurs with a faster heart rate, results in a decrease in RF. Actual improvement in subendocardial blood flow is observed with an increased heart rate, owing to a higher systemic diastolic pressure and a lower LVEDP. This explains why a patient who is symptomatic at rest may show an improvement in symptoms with exercise. A heart rate of around 90 bpm seems to be optimal, improving cardiac output while not inducing ischemia.

    c. **Contractility:** LV contractility must be maintained. In patients with impaired LV function, the use of pure β-agonists or phosphodiesterase inhibitors can increase stroke volume through a combination of peripheral dilation and increased contractility ("inodilation").

    d. **Systemic vascular resistance:** The forward flow can be improved with afterload reduction. Increases in LV afterload result in increased stroke work and can significantly increase the LVEDP.

    e. **Pulmonary vascular resistance:** Pulmonary vascular pressure remains relatively normal, except in patients with end-stage AR associated with severe LV dysfunction.

2. **Anesthetic technique**

    a. **Premedication:** Light premedication is recommended if needed.

    b. **Induction and maintenance:** Serious hemodynamic instability during induction of general anesthesia is less likely with severe AR than with severe AS because arterial vasodilation, which is a major effect of most of the induction drugs, is beneficial in AR, and transient hypotension is usually well tolerated. However, the importance of careful titration of induction agents in combination with adequate hydration should not be underestimated. Particular caution is warranted with acute AR, where ventricular decompensation is more likely to occur. The hemodynamic goals for induction and maintenance of anesthesia should be directed at preserving the patient's preload and contractility, maintaining the peripheral arterial dilation, and avoiding bradycardia. Careful attention should be paid to avoiding profound bradycardia/asystole in the period after aortic cannulation and onset of CPB, since the LV is especially prone to distend due to the presence of the AR. Until it is vented surgically, the LV must, therefore, vent itself via systolic ejection.

    c. In high-risk patients, a PAC may be helpful in evaluating the cardiac output of patients before repair of the aortic valve and especially in the post-bypass period for monitoring and optimizing preload and myocardial function.

    d. Intraoperative TEE is beneficial for monitoring LV function and assessment of the severity of regurgitation before valve surgery. Specific pathology of the aortic valve leaflets and aortic root can be easily assessed. It is also useful in predicting the appropriate size of a prosthetic valve based on the diameters of the aortic annulus and LVOT. If aortic valve repair is performed, TEE is valuable for providing immediate feedback concerning the integrity of valvular function. In AVR, TEE allows for immediate assessment of any perivalvular regurgitation, as well as the pressure gradient across the newly placed prosthetic valve.

    e. Use of an intra-aortic balloon pump is contraindicated in the presence of significant AR because augmentation of the diastolic pressure will increase the amount of regurgitant flow.

    f. Weaning from CPB may be complicated by LV dysfunction secondary to suboptimal myocardial protection and coronary air embolism. AVR leads to a mild transvalvular gradient because most prosthetic valves have a degree of inherent stenosis. An elevated transvalvular gradient, in combination with a significantly dilated LV, may result in increased afterload and low cardiac output and may contribute to LV dysfunction. Inotropic support may be indicated in order to maintain cardiac output and avoid further LV dilation and dysfunction. Preload augmentation must be continued to maintain filling of the dilated LV.

3. **Postoperative care:** Immediately following AVR, the LVEDP and LVEDV decrease. However, the LV dilation and eccentric hypertrophy persist. In the early postoperative period, a decline in LV function may necessitate inotropic or intra-aortic balloon pump support. If surgical intervention is delayed until significant LV dysfunction has occurred, the prognosis for long-term survival is poor. The 5-year survival rate for patients whose hearts do not return to a relatively normal size within 6 months following surgical repair is only 43%. If surgery is performed early enough, the heart will return to relatively normal dimensions, and a long-term survival rate of 85%-90% after 6 years can be expected.[2]

VIII. Mixed Valvular Lesions

For all mixed valvular lesions, management decisions emphasize the most severe or the most hemodynamically significant lesion.

A. Aortic Stenosis and Mitral Stenosis

Pathophysiologically, the progression of the disease follows a course similar to that seen in patients with pure mitral stenosis with development of pulmonary hypertension and, eventually, RV failure. Symptoms are primarily referable to the pulmonary circulation, including dyspnea, hemoptysis, and atrial fibrillation. This combination of valvular heart disease may lead to underestimation of the severity of the AS because the aortic valve gradient may be relatively low owing to low aortic valvular flow. Such a combination of lesions can be extremely serious because of the limitation of blood flow at two points. Intraoperative management should focus on maintaining adequate preload, preserving sinus rhythm, and avoiding tachydysrhythmias in order to optimize ventricular filling. SVR and systemic blood pressure must be preserved in order to avoid ventricular ischemia.

B. Aortic Stenosis and Mitral Regurgitation

MR is not an uncommon finding in the setting of severe AS. With progression of the stenotic lesion, the LVSP increases to overcome the flow obstruction. MR flows from the LV during systole into the left atrium (LA). Elevated LVSP results in a larger gradient between the LV and the LA and a subsequent increase in MR. Compensatory ventricular remodeling can further worsen MR, as the mitral valve annulus is distorted. MR may improve after the aortic valve is replaced as the LVSP decreases, and this has led to controversy in the surgical management of moderate, functional MR in the setting of severe AS. In managing these patients, the hemodynamic requirements for AS and MR are contradictory. Because AS is more likely to cause cardiovascular collapse, it should be given priority when managing the hemodynamic variables.

C. Aortic Stenosis and Aortic Regurgitation

The combination of AR and AS is not well tolerated because it leads to severe LV pressure and volume overload. These stresses lead to major increases in myocardial oxygen consumption (MVO_2), and as might be expected, angina pectoris is an early symptom with this combination. Once symptoms develop, the prognosis is similar to that of pure AS.

D. Aortic Regurgitation and Mitral Regurgitation

The combination of AR and MR occurs frequently, and this combination can cause rapid clinical deterioration. The hemodynamic requirements of AR and MR are similar. The primary problem is providing adequate forward flow into the systemic circulation. The development of acidosis, leading to peripheral vasoconstriction and increased impedance to LV outflow, can lead to rapid clinical deterioration. Therefore, keeping the SVR relatively low while maintaining an adequate perfusion pressure is the goal until CPB can be initiated.

E. **Multivalve Surgical Procedures**

   While the surgical management of multivalve disease has continued to improve, these patients still represent a significantly higher risk group than patients presenting for surgery on a single valve.

IX. **Prosthetic Valves**

The decision regarding which prosthetic valve should be used for a particular patient is based upon a variety of factors, including the expected longevity of the patient (mechanical prostheses last longer), the ability of the patient to comply with anticoagulation therapy (mechanical prostheses require ongoing anticoagulation), the anatomy and pathology of the existing valvular disease, and the experience of the operating surgeon.[23]

A. **Essential Characteristics of Prosthetic Heart Valves**

   An ideal prosthetic heart valve mimics the characteristics of the native valve and has excellent hemodynamics; is nonthrombogenic, durable, and chemically inert; preserves blood elements; and allows physiologic blood flow. The large number of different prosthetic valves that have been developed means that no ideal valve has yet been found and that each valve has its own inherent limitations.[24]

B. **Types of Prosthetic Valves**

   1. **Mechanical:** Current mechanical prosthetic valves are durable but thrombogenic. At present, all patients with mechanical prosthetic valves require anticoagulation therapy for the remainder of their lives. Normally, anticoagulation is provided with warfarin sodium, administered at a dose that will elevate the prothrombin time to 1.5-2 times control. There are four basic types of mechanical prosthetic valves, the caged ball, caged disc, single tilting disc, and bileaflet tilting disc valves. Of these, the bileaflet tilting disc valves are in common use today. This valve design is less bulky than its predecessors and provides improved central laminar blood flow.

      a. **Bileaflet tilting disc valve prosthesis (Figure 13.11):** In 1977, a bileaflet St. Jude cardiac valve was introduced as a low-profile device to allow central blood flow around two semicircular discs that pivot on supporting struts. When the leaflets open, the opening angle relative to the leaflets ranges from 75° to 90°. Three orifices are present within the valve when open: a smaller central orifice between two larger semicircular orifices on the lateral edges.[24] Due to these size differences, higher flow velocities occur within the smaller central orifice as compared to the two larger outer orifices of the valve. The valve is designed to have an inherent (but small) degree of regurgitant flow originating from backflow from the motion of the occluders and leakage through the components of the prosthesis. This purposeful regurgitant flow is included in the valve to provide "washing jets" to minimize blood stasis and thrombus formation on the valve components.[24] The St. Jude bileaflet tilting disc valve can be placed in the aortic, mitral, or tricuspid positions. These valves produce low resistance to blood flow and have a lower incidence of thromboembolic complications, though anticoagulation is still necessary. The most popular bileaflet tilting disc is still

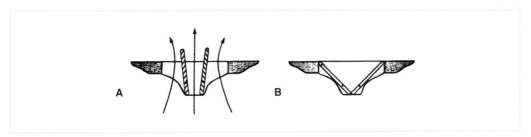

FIGURE 13.11   Bileaflet valve prosthesis showing discs in open **(A)** and closed **(B)** positions.

the St. Jude Medical (Saint Paul, MN). Other bileaflet tilting disc valve prostheses include the CarboMedics (Sorin Group), On-X (MRCI), and Advancing the Standard (ATS) Medtronic valves.

2. **Bioprosthetic valves:** The Hancock porcine aortic bioprosthesis (now the Medtronic Hancock II stented porcine bioprosthesis) was introduced in 1970, followed by the Ionescu-Shiley bovine pericardial prosthesis in 1974, and the Carpentier-Edwards porcine aortic valve bioprosthesis in 1975. In contrast to modern mechanical prostheses, current bioprostheses are not only less durable but also less thrombogenic. Long-term anticoagulation is not necessary for a bioprosthetic valve. Bioprosthetic valves in the aortic position last longer than in the mitral position. Because durability is an issue and because their life span is longer in older patients, bioprosthetic valves are usually used for patients older than 60 years and when anticoagulation is not a desirable option (eg, when pregnancy is anticipated).

Bioprosthetic valves fall into two types: stented and stentless.

a. Stented bioprosthetic valves constructed from porcine aortic valves or bovine pericardium are placed on a polypropylene stent, which is attached to a silicone sewing ring covered with Dacron. These valves allow for improved central annular flow and less turbulence, but the stent does cause some obstruction to forward flow, thereby leading to a residual pressure gradient across the valve. The effective orifice areas of bioprosthetic valves (for a given annulus size) are typically smaller than for bileaflet mechanical valves. A small amount of central regurgitant flow is common in most bioprosthetic valves. Most valves in current production are treated with glutaraldehyde to reduce antigenicity and anticalcification agents or processes.[27] Examples of stented bioprosthetic valves that can be found in clinical use today include the Inspiris Resilia, Carpentier-Edwards Perimount, Magna, and S.A.V. valves (Edwards Lifesciences); Epic (St. Jude Medical); Biocor (St. Jude Medical); Hancock II (Medtronic); Mitroflow (Sorin Group); Mosaic (Medtronic); and Trifecta (St. Jude Medical).

b. **Stentless bioprostheses:** Stentless valves were developed in order to provide improved hemodynamic characteristics and durability as compared to stented bioprostheses. These valves are constructed from intact porcine aortic valves or bovine pericardium. Stentless bioprosthetic valves are technically more difficult to place and are used almost exclusively in the aortic position. Modern stentless bioprosthetic valves are often used when aortic root replacement is also necessary. The first generation of stentless bioprostheses includes Medtronic Freestyle, Toronto SPV (St. Jude Medical), and Prima-Edwards (Edwards Lifesciences). Newer generations include the Shelhigh Super Stentless aortic valve (Shelhigh Inc) and Sorin Pericarbon Freedom valve (Sorin Group), which are easier to implant since they only require one layer of suture for implantation.[24]

3. **Sutureless bioprosthetic valves:** Stent-mounted sutureless valves have recently been designed for AVR involving sutureless positioning and anchoring at the site of implantation. These sutureless valves can be used for replacement of either a diseased native valve or dysfunctional prosthetic valve. A primary advantage of these valves lies in the fact that they can be implanted more quickly than other valves, with a significant reduction in aortic cross-clamp and bypass time. Examples include the Perceval (Sorin Group), 3F Enable valve (Medtronic), and Intuity (Edwards Lifesciences).[24]

4. **Human valves:** The first use of a bioprosthesis taken from a cadaver occurred in 1962. However, techniques such as irradiation or chemical treatment used to sterilize and preserve the early homografts for implantation led to a shortened life span. More recently, antibiotic solutions have been used to sterilize human valves, which then are frozen in liquid nitrogen until implantation. Using these techniques, weakness of the prosthesis leading to cusp rupture occurs infrequently, with >75% of prostheses lasting for >10 years, regardless of patient age. The incidence of prosthetic valve endocarditis and hemolysis resulting from blood flow

through the homograft is very low. Anticoagulation is usually not required. Homografts are predominately used in the aortic position, especially when aortic root replacement is necessary and for pulmonary valve replacement during Ross procedure. Homografts may be most useful in patients younger than 35 years and in patients with native valve endocarditis.

5. **Transcatheter valves:** Valves utilized in the TAVR procedure have been introduced and discussed earlier in this chapter. The classification of TAVR valves falls into two main categories/types: balloon-expandable valves and self-expanding valves. The Edwards valves initially used for the procedure were balloon-expandable valves mounted in a steel frame, available in either 23-mm or 26-mm size. The newer generation of valve is the Edwards SAPIEN 3 Ultra (Edwards Lifesciences), which is made of bovine pericardium mounted in a cobalt chromium frame. This valve is available in 20-, 23-, 26-, and 29-mm sizes and is implanted using either 14-Fr or 16-Fr delivery catheter. Of note, it appears that balloon-expandable valves typically have larger effective orifice areas and lower gradients compared to surgical bioprosthetic valves. As previously discussed, however, paravalvular regurgitation is a more frequent issue with TAVR valves.[24]

CoreValve systems (Medtronic) first introduced for this procedure were self-expanding valves made from bovine pericardium in a nitinol, self-expanding frame. Subsequent modifications of this valve have occurred, most notably to allow for true supra-annular placement of the valve. The current, fourth-generation CoreValve labeled as Evolut FX is available in 23-, 26-, 29-, and 34-mm sizes and is implanted using a 14-Fr or 18-Fr delivery catheter. It appears as though the CoreValve results in larger effective orifice areas and lower gradients than the SAPIEN valves, but there is a higher risk of complete heart block after the CoreValve implantation.[24]

C. **Echocardiographic Evaluation of Prosthetic Valves in the Aortic Position**
   1. **Evaluation for aortic prosthetic valve stenosis**
      a. The 2D examination should focus on the sewing ring and valve leaflets. Doppler interrogation should determine the mean transvalvular gradient, peak velocity, contour of the jet velocity, acceleration time (AT), Doppler velocity index (DVI), and the effective orifice area of the prosthesis.
      b. The following findings are suggestive of significant stenosis: mean gradient >35 mm Hg, peak velocity >4 m/s, rounded symmetrical contour of the Doppler velocity profile index (as opposed to early peaking triangular shape), AT >100 msec, and DVI <0.25.
      c. Occasionally, there are normal prosthetic valves with elevated peak velocities. Figure 13.12 presents a useful algorithm for determining if the conflicting data are due to a high-flow state, measurement error, or patient-prosthesis mismatch.
   2. **Evaluation for aortic prosthetic valve regurgitation**
      a. The same criteria in determining the severity of native aortic valve regurgitation can be applied to prosthetic aortic valves.
      b. The 2D evaluation focuses on the sewing ring and valve leaflet motion. Doppler interrogation allows determination of jet width in the LVOT, pressure half-time, the presence of holodiastolic flow reversal in the descending thoracic aorta, and calculation of regurgitant volume and RF.
      c. TTE has limited ability to evaluate for posterior paravalvular regurgitation, and TEE may add incremental value if pathology is suspected in this location.

CLINICAL PEARL

When performing TEE or TTE for TAVR procedures, it is especially important to assess for the presence and location of paravalvular regurgitation, as this is a common complication of the procedure that may need to be immediately addressed with percutaneous or surgical intervention following initial valve deployment.

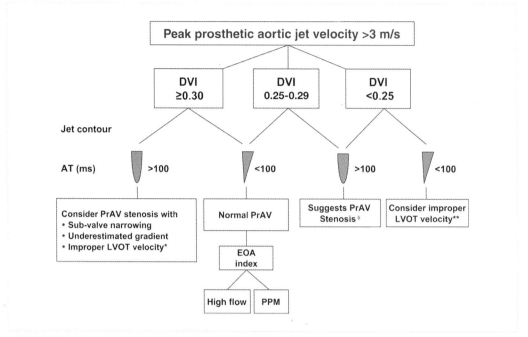

FIGURE 13.12 Algorithm for the echocardiographic evaluation of elevated peak velocities in prosthetic valves in the aortic position. AT, acceleration time; DVI, Doppler velocity index; EOA, effective orifice area; LVOT, left ventricular outflow tract; PPM, patient-prosthesis mismatch; PrAV, prosthetic aortic valve. *Pulsed-wave Doppler sample too close to the valve (particularly when jet velocity by continuous-wave Doppler is ≥4 m/s. **Pulsed-wave Doppler sample too far (apical) from the valve (particularly when jet velocity is 3-3.9 m/s). ⁺Stenosis further substantiated by effective orifice area derivation compared with reference values if valve type and size are known. (Reprinted from Zoghbi WA, Chambers JB, Dumesnil JG, et al. Recommendations for evaluation of prosthetic valves with echocardiography and doppler ultrasound: a report from the American Society of Echocardiography's Guidelines and Standards Committee and the Task Force on Prosthetic Valves, developed in conjunction with the American College of Cardiology Cardiovascular Imaging Committee, Cardiac Imaging Committee of the American Heart Association, the European Association of Echocardiography, a registered branch of the European Society of Cardiology, the Japanese Society of Echocardiography and the Canadian Society of Echocardiography, endorsed by the American College of Cardiology Foundation, American Heart Association, European Association of Echocardiography, a registered branch of the European Society of Cardiology, the Japanese Society of Echocardiography, and Canadian Society of Echocardiography. *J Am Soc Echocardiogr*. 2009;22(9):975-1084. © 2009 Elsevier. With permission.)

X. Prophylaxis of Bacterial Endocarditis

When an invasive procedure puts the patient with valvular heart disease at risk for bacteremia, precautions should be taken to prevent seeding of an abnormal or artificial valve with bacteria that, once present, are very hard to eradicate. Practically, this concern translates into (a) a strict aseptic technique for all procedures performed in patients with valvular heart disease; (b) elimination of existing sources of infection before implantation of a prosthetic valve; and (c) in selected cases, antibiotic prophylaxis. Guidelines from AHA/ACC on the prevention of infective endocarditis limit antibiotic prophylaxis to cardiac conditions associated with the highest risk of infective endocarditis.[25] These conditions include patients with prosthetic cardiac valves (including transcatheter-implanted prostheses and homografts) or material used in heart valve repair (ie, annuloplasty rings and chords), previous infective endocarditis, unrepaired cyanotic congenital heart disease or repaired congenital heart disease with residual shunts or defects in the proximity of the site of a prosthetic patch or device, and cardiac transplant recipients with valvular disease. Endocarditis prophylaxis is recommended only for "dental procedures that involve manipulation of gingival tissue or the periapical region of teeth or perforation of the oral mucosa." There is no evidence to support the administration of antibiotic prophylaxis in gastrointestinal or genitourinary procedures if there is no known active infection. Guidelines for antibiotic prophylaxis, to be begun 1 hour before a procedure, are shown in Table 13.7.

TABLE 13.7   Antibiotic Recommendations for Prophylaxis of Bacterial Endocarditis

	Agent	Adult Dose (30-60 min Before Procedure)	Pediatric Dose[a]
Standard general prophylaxis	Amoxicillin	2 g PO	50 mg/kg/PO
Patients unable to take oral medications	Ampicillin	2 g IV or IM	50 mg/kg IV or IM
Penicillin- and amoxicillin-allergic patients	**Cephalexin[b] or clindamycin or azithromycin or clarithromycin**	**2 g PO** **600 mg PO** 500 mg PO	**50 mg/kg PO** **20 mg/kg PO** 15 mg/kg PO
Penicillin- and amoxicillin-allergic patients unable to take oral medications	Clindamycin or cefazolin[b] or ceftriaxone[b]	600 mg IV or IM 1 g IV or IM	**20 mg/kg IV or IM** **50 mg/kg IV or IM**

IM, intramuscular; IV, intravenous; PO, oral.
[a]Total pediatric dose should not exceed the adult dose.
[b]Cephalosporins should not be used in patients with immediate-type hypersensitivity reaction (urticaria, angioedema, or anaphylaxis) to penicillins.
Based on Nishimura RA, Otto CM, Bonow RO, et al. 2017 AHA/ACC focused update of the 2014 AHA/ACC guideline for the management of patients with valvular heart disease: a report of the American College of Cardiology/American Heart Association Task Force on Clinical Practice Guidelines. *J Am Coll Cardiol.* 2017;70(2):252-289.

REFERENCES

1. Nishimura RA, Otto CM, Bonow RO, et al. 2014 AHA/ACC guideline for the management of patients with valvular heart disease: executive summary: a report of the American College of Cardiology/American Heart Association Task Force on Practice Guidelines. *J Am Coll Cardiol.* 2014;63(22):2438-2488.
2. Cook DJ, Housmans PR, Rehfeldt KH. Valvular heart disease: replacement and repair. In: Kaplan JA, Reich DL, Savino JS, eds. *Kaplan's Cardiac Anesthesia: The Echo Era,* 6th ed. Elsevier Saunders; 2011:570-614.
3. Otto CM. *Textbook of Clinical Echocardiography.* 4th ed. Elsevier Saunders; 2009:259-325.
4. Roberts WC, Ko JM. Frequency by decades of unicuspid, bicuspid, and tricuspid aortic valves in adults having isolated aortic valve replacement for aortic stenosis, with or without associated aortic regurgitation. *Circulation.* 2005;111(7):920-925.
5. Baumgartner H, Hung J, Bermejo J, et al. Echocardiographic assessment of valve stenosis: EAE/ASE recommendations for clinical practice. *J Am Soc Echocardiogr.* 2009;22(1):1-23.
6. Lindman BR, Clavel MA, Mathieu P, et al. Calcific aortic stenosis. *Nat Rev Dis Primers.* 2016;2:16006.
7. Otto CM, Bonow RO. Valvular heart disease. In: Bonow RO, Mann DL, Zipes DP, et al., eds. *Braunwald's Heart Disease: A Textbook of Cardiovascular Medicine.* 9th ed. Elsevier; 2011:1468-1530.
8. Maslow A, Casey P, Poppas A, et al. Aortic valve replacement with or without coronary bypass graft surgery: the risk of surgery in patients ≥80 years old. *J Cardiothorac Vasc Anesth.* 2010;24(1):18-24.
9. Anwaruddin S, Desai ND, Vemulapalli S, et al. Evaluating out-of-hospital 30-day mortality after transfemoral transcatheter aortic valve replacement: an STS/ACC TVT analysis. *JACC Cardiovasc Interv.* 2021;14(3):261-274.
10. Kpodonu J. Hybrid cardiovascular suite: the operating room of the future. *J Card Surg.* 2010;25(6):704-709.
11. Singh IM, Shishehbor MH, Christofferson RD, et al. Percutaneous treatment of aortic valve stenosis. *Cleve Clin J Med.* 2008;75(Suppl. 11);805-812.
12. Billings FT IV, Kodali SK, Shanewise JS. Transcatheter aortic valve implantation: anesthetic consideration. *Anesth Analg.* 2009;108(5):1453-1462.
13. Heinze H, Sier H, Schafer U, et al. Percutaneous aortic valve replacement: overview and suggestions for anesthetic management. *J Clin Anesth.* 2010;22(5):373-378.
14. Fraccaro C, Napodano M, Taratini G, et al. Expanding the eligibility for transcatheter aortic valve implantation the trans-subclavian retrograde approach using: the III generation CoreValve revalving system. *JACC Cardiovasc Interv.* 2009;2(9):828-833.
15. Covello RD, Maj G, Landoni G, et al. Anesthetic management of percutaneous aortic valve implantation: focus on challenges encountered and proposed solutions. *J Cardiothorac Vasc Anesth.* 2009;23(3):280-285.
16. Dehedin B, Guinot PG, Ibrahim H, et al. Anesthesia and perioperative management of patients who undergo transfemoral transcatheter aortic valve implantation: an observational study of general versus local/regional anesthesia in 125 consecutive patients. *J Cardiothorac Vasc Anesth.* 2011;25(6):1036-1043.
17. Covello RD, Ruggeri L, Landoni G, et al. Transcatheter implantation of an aortic valve: anesthesiological management. *Minerva Anestesiol.* 2010;76(2):100-108.
18. Chin D. Echocardiography for transcatheter aortic valve replacement. *Eur J Echocardiogr.* 2009;10:21-29.

19. Krishnaswamy A, Tuczu EM, Kapadia SR. Update on transcatheter aortic valve replacement. *Curr Cardiol Rep.* 2010;12(5):393-403.
20. Abdel-Wahab M, Zahn R, Horack M, et al. Aortic regurgitation after transcatheter aortic valve implantation: incidence and early outcome. Results from the German transcatheter aortic valve interventions registry. *Heart.* 2011;97(11):899-906.
21. Smith CR, Leon MB, Mack MJ, et al. Transcatheter versus surgical aortic-valve replacement in high-risk patients. *N Engl J Med.* 2011;364(23):2187-2198.
22. Zoghbi WA, Adams D, Bonow RO, et al. Recommendations for noninvasive evaluation of native valvular regurgitation: a report from the American Society of Echocardiography developed in collaboration with the Society for Cardiovascular Magnetic Resonance. *J Am Soc Echocardiogr.* 2017;30(4):303-371.
23. Rahimtoola SH. Choice of prosthetic heart valve in adults: an update. *J Am Coll Cardiol.* 2010;55(22):2413-2426.
24. Mahjoub H, Dumesnil JG, Pibarot P. Classification of prosthetic valve types and fluid dynamics. In: Lang RM, Goldstein SA, Kronzon I, et al., eds. *ASE's Comprehensive Echocardiography.* 2nd ed. Elsevier Saunders; 2016:542-549.
25. Nishimura RA, Otto CM, Bonow RO, et al. 2017 AHA/ACC focused update of the 2014 AHA/ACC guideline for the management of patients with valvular heart disease. *J Am Coll Cardiol.* 2017;70(2):252-289.

Mitral, Tricuspid, and Pulmonic Valves

Rabia Amir, Feroze Mahmood, and Aidan Sharkey

KEY POINTS

1. With an aging population and an increase in life expectancy, the burden of valvular heart encountered in the perioperative period is increasing.
2. Knowledge of these effects is imperative for the safe management of these patients undergoing both cardiac and noncardiac surgery.
3. Each valvular lesion will result in unique structural, functional, and hemodynamic effects on the upstream and downstream heart chambers.
4. Stenotic lesions are generally associated with pressure overload proximal to the affected valve, whereas regurgitant lesions that result in volume overload are associated with chamber dilation and eccentric hypertrophy in the originating chamber.
5. Mixed valvular lesions pose a particular challenge as management and treatment needs to consider the severity and impact of each valve disease on the patient's overall cardiac function.
6. The increasing utilization of intraoperative transesophageal echocardiography (TEE) has greatly expanded the role of the cardiac anesthesiologist in managing patients with valvular heart disease undergoing both cardiac and noncardiac surgery.

I. Introduction

The prevalence of valvular heart disease continues to increase in industrialized countries due to an aging population. Valvular heart interventions account for up to 20% of all cardiac surgical procedures in the United States, and there has been a significant increase in recent years in the number of patients undergoing percutaneous valvular interventions. A comprehensive understanding of the pathophysiology and clinical progression associated with the valvular heart disease is required for optimal perioperative care for those undergoing both cardiac and noncardiac surgery. Hemodynamic variables such as heart rate, rhythm, preload, afterload, and contractility should be tailored for each valvular lesion for physiologic optimization.

Intraoperative transesophageal echocardiography (TEE) has expanded the role of the cardiac anesthesiologist for patients with valvular heart disease undergoing both cardiac and noncardiac surgery and provides an enhanced physiologic perspective through the dynamic display of anatomy. In addition, intraoperative TEE provides real-time diagnostic interpretation to guide surgical decision-making.

II. Stenotic Versus Regurgitant Lesions

Valvular lesions result in unique structural, functional, and hemodynamic consequences on the upstream and downstream heart chambers and/or vessels.

A. Valvular Stenosis

Stenotic valvular lesions are associated with structural, functional, and hemodynamic consequences related to pressure overload in the cardiac chamber proximal to the stenosis.

The narrowed valvular orifice obstructs blood flow across the valve (during systole in aortic and pulmonary valves; during diastole in mitral [MV] and tricuspid valves), resulting in an increased pressure in the proximal cardiac chamber. As the stenotic valvular lesion progresses, there is flow convergence as blood reaches the stenotic valve with increased velocity. As blood is ejected through the stenotic orifice, there is a simultaneous drop in pressure, resulting in a consequent increase in the pressure gradient across the valve.

There are two types of valvular obstruction:

1. **Fixed obstruction:** The degree of obstruction to blood flow is constant throughout the cardiac cycle.
2. **Dynamic obstruction:** The degree of obstruction is variable and is dependent on the stage of the cardiac cycle.

B. Valvular Regurgitation

Regurgitant lesions are associated with volume overload, resulting in chamber dilatation and eccentric hypertrophy. Left-sided lesions such as mitral (MR) and aortic regurgitation result in backflow of blood toward the left ventricle (LV), resulting in ventricular dilation and increased wall stress. The ventricles initially compensate for the increased volume load with increased stroke volume, but eventually, ventricular function declines and heart failure occurs. The hemodynamic management of these patients focuses on maximizing forward stroke volume and minimizing regurgitant stroke volume.

Right-sided lesions such as tricuspid (TR) and pulmonic regurgitation (PR) result in blood flow back toward the chamber that receives blood from the veins, resulting in an increase in the volume of blood within the chamber. Over time, there is chamber dilation and increased wall stress, leading to right ventricular (RV) hypertrophy, decreased contractility, and heart failure. Right-sided regurgitant lesions tend to progress more slowly than left-sided lesions and may not result in symptoms until they become severe.

Mixed and multiple valvular heart lesions are becoming more prevalent. Mixed valvular disease refers to the presence of both stenotic and regurgitant lesions in one or more heart valves. Multiple valvular disease refers to the presence of significant valvular lesions involving two or more heart valves. The management of mixed and multiple valvular lesions is complex, and various individual patient factors, such as loading conditions, innate ventricular systolic and diastolic function, and the type and number of valvular lesions present along with the timing of onset and severity of individual lesions must be considered when managing these patients.

III. Structural and Functional Response to Valvular Heart Disease

Valvular cardiac lesions will result in specific structural and functional changes in response to changes in pressure and volume brought on as a result of the cardiac lesion.

A. Cardiac Remodeling

Cardiac remodeling is an important adaptive response in valvular heart disease and includes changes in the size, shape, structure, and function of the heart in response to changes in pressure and/or volume within the heart chambers. Initially, remodeling is an adaptive and compensatory measure; however, it ultimately results in decompensation and deterioration in ventricular function. Neurohumoral factors and enzymes, such as angiotensin-II, ion channels, and oxidative stress, also contribute to cardiac remodeling.

Ventricular hypertrophy, defined as increased ventricular mass, can be concentric or eccentric. Pressure overload results in concentric ventricular hypertrophy where ventricular mass is increased by myocardial thickening and the ventricular volume stays constant. Conversely, volume overload results in eccentric ventricular hypertrophy where increased ventricular volume raises ventricular mass without changing myocardial wall thickness and results in a more spherically shaped heart.

B. Ventricular Function

Valvular heart disease results in changes to both systolic and diastolic ventricular performance. Initial reductions in systolic ventricular performance are initially countered by activation of the Frank-Starling mechanism. Activation of neurohumoral systems results in increased fluid retention and an increase in LV pressure. This increase in LV pressure generates an increase in ventricular performance by increasing sarcomere length and contractility. This adaptive response is limited when as the sarcomere becomes overstretched and the number of crossbridges that can form is reduced. Eventually, LV pressure increases to a point where further increases in LV filling pressures lead to minimal increases in cardiac output. As valvular heart disease progress, there is an upward shift in the end-diastolic pressure-volume (PV) relationship. Development of diastolic dysfunction with resultant impaired LV filling results in the onset of heart failure symptoms.

C. Pressure-Volume Loops

PV loops are used to illustrate ventricular function and performance, with ventricular pressure plotted on the y-axis and the ventricular volume plotted on the x-axis for one cardiac cycle. In a normal PV loop, the volume of blood in the ventricles increases during diastole and then decreases during systole as the ventricles empty. The pressure in the ventricles increases during systole and then decreases during diastole as the ventricles fill again (Figure 14.1). In valvular heart disease, the PV loop may be altered depending on the type and severity of the cardiac lesion.

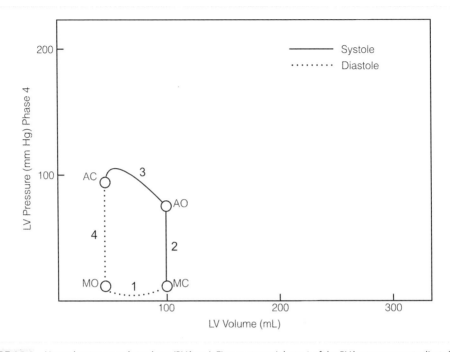

FIGURE 14.1 Normal pressure-volume loop (PV loop). First segment/phase 1 of the PV loop represents diastolic filling of the left ventricle (LV). Phase 2 represents isovolumetric contraction and phase 3 represents ventricular ejection, and both these phases constitute ventricular systole. Phase 4 represents the isovolumetric relaxation of the LV and, along with phase 1, constitutes ventricular diastole. AC, aortic valve closure at end systole; AO, aortic valve opening; MC, mitral valve closure at end diastole; MO, mitral valve opening. (Based on Jackson JM, Thomas SJ, Lowenstein E. Anesthetic management of patients with valvular heart disease. *Semin Anesth.* 1982;1:240.)

IV. **Echocardiography and Valvular Heart Disease**

6

Echocardiography is routinely used in the diagnosis, quantification and monitoring of valvular heart disease. In addition to assessing a particular valvular pathology, echocardiography can also provide information about mixed and multiple valvular disease as well as chamber assessment.

Transthoracic echocardiography (TTE) has the advantage of being noninvasive and does not require the need for sedation or anesthesia. TTE is also more widely available, better tolerated by patients, less time-consuming and expensive than TEE. TEE has the advantage of improved image quality, better visualization of intracardiac pathologies such as vegetations and thrombi, accurate assessment of valvular anatomy and function in multiple planes as well as being able to provide real-time monitoring during cardiac and noncardiac surgery.

Three-dimensional (3D) echocardiography has opened another dimension of imaging by allowing more comprehensive and accurate visualization of cardiac structures, enabling better visualization of complex anatomy and spatial relationships between structures. Multiplanar reconstruction allows simultaneous visualization of structures in multiple planes and allows for more accurate measurements.

V. **Mitral Valve Stenosis**

A. **Etiology**

Mitral stenosis (MS) is the most common valvular sequela of rheumatic heart disease, which is a widespread problem in developing countries.[1] In developed countries, early detection and treatment of streptococcal pharyngitis has resulted in a reduced incidence of rheumatic heart disease. Rheumatic heart disease more commonly affects females, and the MV is primarily affected, although other valves can also be affected, resulting in multiple valvular disease.

Valvular lesions that occur as a result of rheumatic heart disease may be pure stenotic or mixed stenotic and regurgitant in nature. Other causes of MS include congenital MS, calcific MV disease, radiation-associated valve disease, carcinoid syndrome, left atrial (LA) myxoma causing functional MS, rheumatoid arthritis, systemic lupus erythematous (SLE), and iatrogenic MS after MV repair surgery.

Calcific MV disease is associated with aging, female gender, high blood pressure, diabetes, chronic kidney disease, and a history of smoking. It is a progressive disease and is often associated with calcific aortic valve disease. Untreated MS results in complications, such as atrial fibrillation (AF), pulmonary hypertension, heart failure, and eventual death.

B. **Symptoms**

Patients with MS from rheumatic heart disease may be asymptomatic for more than two decades after the initial insult of rheumatic carditis. Symptoms begin to appear with the development of valvular stenosis. Dyspnea and reduced exercise tolerance are generally the primary symptoms that develop. Other symptoms include pulmonary edema, hemoptysis, chest pain, ascites, and lower extremity edema, which occur as a result of changes in LA pressure, pulmonary pressures, pulmonary vascular resistance (PVR), and cardiac output.

Atrial enlargement can result in the onset of AF and may cause hoarseness if the dilated LA compresses the recurrent laryngeal nerve. Patients with MS are at high risk of thromboembolism, with thrombi developing due to blood stasis in the LA as well as the high incidence of AF. Symptoms associated with MS are exacerbated by high output states and with the development of AF.

C. **Pathophysiology**

1. **Natural progression**
   a. The normal adult mitral valve area (MVA) is 4.0-6.0 cm^2 (mitral valve index: 4-4.5 cm^2/m^2). The symptoms of MS manifest with progressive decreases in valve area and generally become apparent when the valve area is <2 cm^2. Initially, dyspnea may occur with moderate exertion and, as the valve area further decreases, symptoms become evident on mild exertion and eventually at rest when the valve area is <1 cm^2.
   b. As MS progresses, there is enlargement of the LA with consequent increase in LA volume, which may lead to the onset of AF. The onset of AF may result in exacerbation of symptoms, with the loss of atrial contraction contributing to ventricular filling. High LA pressures also contribute to increased PVR and subsequent pulmonary hypertension secondary to chronic venous backflow. This can result in RV dilation and failure with left-sided bowing of the interventricular septum, further reducing LV size, limiting stroke volume, impairing cardiac output, and resulting in TR with further dilation. The degree of pulmonary hypertension is also a marker of the global hemodynamic consequences of MS, and severe pulmonary hypertension is associated with increased mortality.

2. **Intracardiac hemodynamics and cardiac remodeling**
   a. Significant MS is characterized by a reduced left ventricular end-diastolic volume (LVEDV) and left ventricular end-diastolic pressure (LVEDP) as the blood flow from the LA to the LV is restricted. Reduced filling of the LV decreases stroke volume, and LV contractility may also decrease due to chronic LV deconditioning.

3. **Pressure wave disturbances**
   a. PV loops have a characteristic appearance in patients with MS. Stroke volume is reduced due to decreased LV filling pressures and low end-diastolic and end-systolic volumes (Figure 14.2).

D. **Echocardiography in Mitral Stenosis**

Echocardiographic assessment of patients with MS includes both a qualitative and quantitative assessment.

1. **Qualitative examination**
   a. Characteristic findings in patients with rheumatic MS include thickening, fibrosis, and calcification of the leaflet cusps; fusion of leaflet commissures as well as thickening and shortening of leaflet commissures. Restricted motion of the anterior MV leaflet

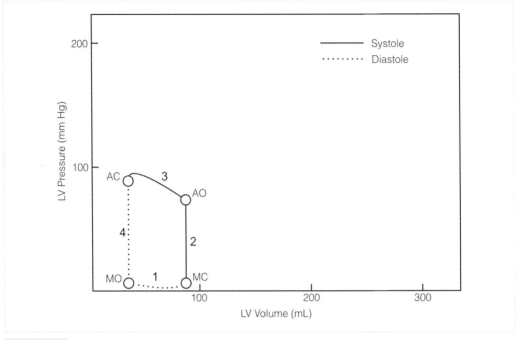

FIGURE 14.2 Pressure-volume loop (PV loop) in mitral stenosis (MS). Due to the reduction in end-diastolic and end-systolic volumes and LV filling pressure, the stroke volume is decreased in MS. AC, aortic valve closure; AO, aortic valve opening; MC, mitral valve closure; MO, mitral valve opening. Phase 1, ventricular filling; phase 2, isovolumetric contraction; phase 3, ventricular ejection; phase 4, isovolumetric relaxation. (Based on Jackson JM, Thomas SJ, Lowenstein E. Anesthetic management of patients with valvular heart disease. *Semin Anesth.* 1982;1:244.)

in diastole shows "diastolic doming" and is described as having a "hockey-stick" appearance (Figure 14.3A). There is restricted leaflet motion in diastole and systole with commissural fusion (Figure 14.3B). The posterior leaflet may also be identified as immobile with echocardiography. LA enlargement with spontaneous echo contrast is associated with a low-flow state and should prompt exclusion of thrombi, especially in the LA appendage.

b. Mixed and multiple valvular heart disease can also be qualitatively assessed with echocardiography. Assessment of morphologic features with 2D echocardiography can be used for scoring systems, such as the Wilkins score where features such as leaflet mobility, leaflet thickening, leaflet calcification, and subvalvular thickening are graded on a scale of 1-4, yielding a maximal score of 16.[2,3]

c. Echocardiographic grouping follows the echocardiographic and fluoroscopic (calcification) evaluation of the following characteristics: valve mobility, fusion of the subvalvular apparatus, and the amount of leaflet calcification. These scores are used to grade MV pathology and determine suitability for treatment options.[4]

2. Quantitative assessment

a. The severity of MS should not be described by a single value but should be evaluated using a multimodality approach that establishes valve areas, mean Doppler gradients, and pulmonary pressures.[5] These can be calculated using echocardiography and/or cardiac catheterization. The different methods for grading MS severity along with advantages and disadvantages of each modality are summarized in Table 14.1.

b. Interpretation of results obtained by echocardiography must be done in the context of other valvular lesions, high output states, or coexisting pathologies, such as diastolic dysfunction, which may lead to inaccurate and discordant data.

c. Routine assessment of the severity of MS involves the combination of mean gradient using the pressure half-time (PHT) method and planimetry, respectively. However, the

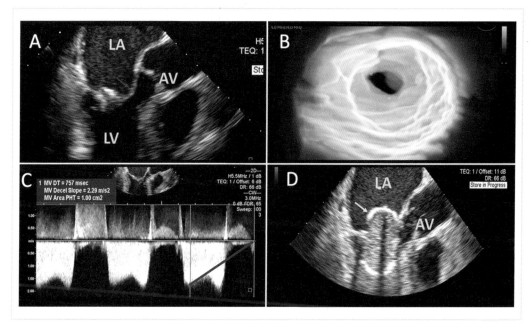

FIGURE 14.3 **(A)** Mid-esophageal long-axis view showing rheumatic valve with characteristic thickening of leaflet tips and diastolic doming or hockey-stick shape of the anterior mitral valve leaflet (red arrow). **(B)** Three-dimensional en face view of a rheumatic mitral valve depicting characteristic commissural fusion. **(C)** Continuous-wave Doppler through a stenotic rheumatic valve showing prolongation of the pressure half-time (purple line). **(D)** Balloon valvuloplasty (yellow arrow) of a stenotic rheumatic mitral valve. AV, aortic valve; LA, left atrium; LV, left ventricle.

mean gradient and systolic pulmonary artery pressure (PAP) cannot be considered as surrogate markers of the severity of MS as they are largely supportive signs.

d. The most commonly used method in assessing the severity of MS is the PHT method (Figure 14.3C). PHT measures the time interval in milliseconds between the maximal mitral gradient in early diastole and the time point where the gradient is half the maximal value. A normal PHT is relatively short and correlates to the rapid early diastolic filling of the LV and the associated rapid fall in the LA-to-LV pressure gradient during this early filling phase. Since the LA-to-LV pressure gradient is increased for a longer period in MS, the PHT will become more prolonged as the degree of stenosis worsens.

e. Planimetry involves the direct tracing of the MV orifice area during mid-diastole and can be done with both TTE and TEE in the parasternal and transgastric basal short-axis views, respectively. 3D imaging of the MV with multiplanar reconstruction has the advantage of viewing the valve at different planes and ensuring the measurement is made at the leaflet tips.[6]

f. The continuity equation uses the principle of the conservation of mass but requires a series of measurements that increase the impact of errors of measurements. It is difficult to use for MS severity since it cannot be used in the presence of AF or significant MR or aortic regurgitation.

g. The proximal isovelocity surface area (PISA) method allows the estimation of mitral volume flow by dividing mitral volume flow by the maximum velocity of diastolic mitral flow as assessed by continuous-wave Doppler (CWD) interrogation. While it is technically demanding, it is independent of flow conditions and can be used in the presence of significant regurgitation.

h. Measurement of transmitral pressure gradients is a quick and easy measurement of MS severity; however, this measurement is significantly influenced by hemodynamic variables, such as cardiac output and heart rate, so caution must be taken when interpreting this result.

TABLE 14.1 Grading the Severity of Chronic MR by Echocardiography

Measurement	Units	Formula/Method	Concept	Advantages	Disadvantages
Valve area					
• Planimetry by 2D echo	cm²	Tracing mitral orifice using 2D echo	Direct measurement of anatomic MVA	• Accuracy • Independence from other factors	• Experience required • Not always feasible (poor acoustic window, severe valve calcification)
• Pressure half-time	cm²	$220/T_{1/2}$	Rate of decrease of transmitral flow is inversely proportional to MVA	Easy to obtain	Dependence on other factors (AR, LA compliance, LV diastolic function…)
• Continuity equation	cm²	$MVA = (CSA_{LVOT})\,(VTI_{Aortic})/VTI_{Mitral}$	Volume flows through mitral and aortic orifices are equal	Independence from flow conditions	• Multiple measurements (sources of errors) • Not valid if significant AR or MR
• PISA	cm²	$MVA = \pi(r^2)\,(V_{aliasing})/\text{peak}\,V_{mitral}\cdot\alpha/180°$	MVA assessed by dividing mitral volume flow by the maximum velocity of diastolic mitral flow	Independence from flow conditions	Technically difficult
Mean gradient	mm Hg	$\Delta P = \Sigma 4v^2/N$	Pressure gradient calculated from velocity using the Bernoulli equation	Easy to obtain	Dependent on heart rate and flow conditions
Systolic pulmonary artery pressure	mm Hg	$sPAP = 4V^2_{Tricuspid} + RA\ pressure$	Addition of RA pressure and maximum gradient between RV and RA	Obtained in most patients with MS	• Arbitrary estimation of RA pressure • No estimation of pulmonary vascular resistance
Mean gradient and systolic pulmonary artery pressure at exercise	mm Hg	$\Delta P = \Sigma 4v^2/N$ $sPAP = 4V^2_{Tricuspid} + RA$ pressure	Assessment of gradient and sPAP for increasing workload	Incremental value in assessment of tolerance	• Experience required • Lack of validation for decision-making

Level of recommendations: (1) appropriate in all patients (yellow); (2) reasonable when additional information is needed in selected patients (green); and (3) not recommended (blue).

AR, aortic regurgitation; CSA, cross-sectional area; DFT, diastolic filling time; LA, left atrium; LV, left ventricle; LVOT, left ventricular outflow tract; MR, mitral regurgitation; MS, mitral stenosis; MVA, mitral valve area; MV_{res}, mitral valve resistance; N, number of instantaneous measurements; ΔP, gradient; PISA, proximal isovelocity surface area; r, the radius of the convergence hemisphere; RA, right atrium; RV, right ventricle; sPAP, systolic pulmonary artery pressure; $T_{1/2}$, pressure half-time; v, velocity; VTI, velocity time integral.

Reprinted from Baumgartner H, Hung J, Bermejo J, et al. Echocardiographic assessment of valve stenosis: EAE/ASE recommendations for clinical practice. J Am Soc Echocardiogr. 2009;22(1):1–23. [published correction appears in J Am Soc Echocardiogr. 2009;22(5):442; J Am Soc Echocardiogr. 2023;36(4):445]. © 2009 Elsevier. With permission.

E. **Timing and Type of Intervention**

1. Intervention is recommended for all patients with symptomatic severe MS as well as as-ymptomatic severe MS with systolic PAP >50 mm Hg.[7] For those with mild-to-moderate MS, conservative management with regular clinical and echocardiographic examinations is recommended.

2. The type of intervention to be undertaken ultimately depends on individual patient charac-teristics, taking into account comorbid disease, the presence of mixed and multiple valvular lesions as well as the presence of any thrombi in the LA.

3. Balloon mitral valvuloplasty is a percutaneous intervention procedure routinely performed in the cardiac catheterization laboratory under general anesthesia or conscious sedation to increase MVA in patients with rheumatic MS (Figure 14.3D).

4. This procedure involves balloon dilation across the MV with subsequent fracture of the commissures. Suitability for this procedure is determined by echocardiography, and pa-tients must have commissural fusion, a Wilkins score <8-9, and no more than moder-ate regurgitation. In addition, this procedure is not suitable for patients with concomitant coronary artery disease requiring surgical intervention, multiple severe valvular disease, and the presence of thrombi in the LA.

5. Balloon mitral valvuloplasty results in an immediate increase in MVA, thus lowering the severity of stenosis; however, restenosis is common, and patients must be followed with serial echocardiograms to assess for restenosis (Figure 14.3D). For many patients, surgical intervention is eventually required after balloon mitral valvuloplasty as the valve becomes stenotic again overtime.

6. Surgical intervention with MV replacement is performed for patients who are unsuitable for balloon mitral valvuloplasty or patients who wish to have a definitive intervention for their MS.[7]

7. For patients with calcific MV disease, balloon mitral valvuloplasty is not an option, and management involves medical optimization and surgical intervention if severe stenosis is present. Open and closed mitral commissurotomy are older procedures that are no longer performed as balloon mitral valvuloplasty has been shown to have equal or better success rates with fewer complications.

F. **Goals of Perioperative Management**

1. **Hemodynamic management**

   a. **Left ventricular preload**

   Given the elevated LA pressures and pulmonary vascular congestion associated with MS, patients are sensitive to abrupt changes in preload. TEE is the ideal modality used to monitor volume status intraoperatively. Adequate preload is necessary to facilitate forward flow across the stenotic valve, and fluids must be titrated carefully to maintain chamber filling while not exacerbating symptoms including acute pulmonary edema brought on by excessive fluid administration.

   b. **Heart rate**

   Maintenance of sinus rhythm and avoidance of tachycardia are the hallmarks of heart rate control in patients with MS. While in theory, bradycardia assists hemodynamic stability in MS, stroke volume generally cannot match excessively low heart rates; there-fore, heart rate must be at a rate that ensures adequate cardiac output. Atrioventricular pacing may be challenging, and a long PR interval will prevent declines in diastolic flow that could decrease cardiac output. Induction of tachycardia should be avoided.

   c. **Contractility**

   End-stage MS may be marked by reduced biventricular function. Atrial filling may also be limited by RV contractility. Both these factors can lower cardiac output, which may be hazardous during surgery. Inotropic support may be required to maintain cardiac output; however, careful titration should be done so as not to induce a hyperdynamic state, which may exacerbate symptoms further.

    d. Systemic vascular resistance

      Owing to the relatively fixed cardiac output associated with MS, any reduction in systemic vascular resistance can result in reduced coronary blood flow; therefore, afterload maintenance is crucial in these patients.

    e. Pulmonary vascular resistance

      Pulmonary vasoconstriction should be prevented as much as possible by avoiding hypoxia, inadequate anesthesia, hypercapnia, or acidosis.

2. Perioperative management

    a. Premedicate with caution in these patients to avoid sudden decreases in preload or exacerbation of preexisting pulmonary hypertension via a slow respiratory drive and concomitant hypoxia and hypercapnia.

    b. If there is onset of new AF, consider cardioversion.

    c. Proceed cautiously while inserting pulmonary artery catheters in these patients due to the risk of pulmonary artery rupture. Also, it should be noted that wedge pressures are often inaccurate and do not reflect actual LVEDP.

    d. PAPs should be monitored carefully as they may rise suddenly due to hypoxia, hypercarbia, and acidosis.

    e. Perioperative TEE is mandatory for these patients undergoing MV replacement for both monitoring and diagnostic purposes. Monitoring of preload, biventricular function, and cardiac output are continuously performed throughout the procedure, while diagnosis of multiple valvular disease and evaluation of the prosthetic valve after implantation are also performed with TEE.

    f. After valve replacement, preload should be maintained, and excessive afterload avoided to promote forward flow.

    g. LV support may be required owing to the effects of open-heart surgery, cross-clamping with cardioplegia, and surgical alterations to the mitral annulus, resulting in how the left heart contracts.

    h. RV support in the form of inotropy, and pulmonary vasodilation may also be required to optimize hemodynamics.

3. Postoperative course

    A successful postoperative surgical course is evident as early as postoperative day 1 by a robust cardiac output accompanied by reduced PAP and LA pressure. PVR continues to decrease in most patients; however, careful monitoring of these patients is essential as the failure of PAP to decrease is usually a sign of irreversible pulmonary hypertension, which can signal poor prognosis.

VI. Mitral Valve Regurgitation

    A. Natural History: MR is a common valvular disorder that may be acute or chronic in nature. MR can occur because of abnormalities of any part of the MV apparatus (Figure 14.4).

    1. Acute mitral regurgitation

      Myocardial ischemia leading to papillary muscle dysfunction and/or rupture is the most common cause of acute MR. Other potential causes of acute MR include rupture of chordae tendineae due to myxomatous disease, fibroelastic disease, acute rheumatic fever, leaflet destruction secondary to infective endocarditis, post balloon valvuloplasty, or penetrating chest trauma.

    2. Chronic mitral regurgitation

      Chronic MR is due to a primary abnormality of one or more components of the MV apparatus or can also occur secondary to another cardiac disease. Common causes of chronic MR include:

      a. Mitral annulus dilatation occurs secondary to LV dilation as a result of cardiomyopathy (dilated or ischemic) or concomitant valvular disease, such as aortic insufficiency. It can also develop from LA enlargement in patients with diastolic dysfunction from pathologies such as systemic hypertension or aortic stenosis. Finally, mitral annulus dilatation will eventually exacerbate MR of other etiologies secondary to LA and LV enlargement with subsequent stretching and flattening of the annulus. This annular flattening can be expressed as an increased nonplanarity angle, which is defined as the angle between the mitral anterior annulus and the posterior annulus planes.[8]

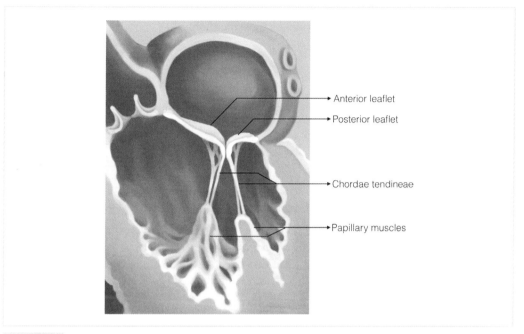

FIGURE 14.4   An illustration of the mitral valve apparatus demonstrating the anterior and posterior leaflets along with the suspension network which is comprised of chordae tendineae and papillary muscles.

    b. Disorders of the MV leaflets include MV prolapse, which may be idiopathic or caused by rheumatic fever; myxomatous degeneration; mitral leaflet damage caused by infective endocarditis; and restrictive changes secondary to thickening or calcification from any inflammatory or degenerative processes. Valvular restriction resulting in complete valve closure can also occur due to the disproportionate enlargement of the LV in relation to the papillary muscles and chordae tendineae, as is frequently the case in ischemic MR.

    c. Disorders of the subvalvular apparatus: MR can also occur secondary to rupture or elongation of the chordae tendineae. Depending on the type and number of chordae ruptured, the resulting MR can range from acute to chronic and from mild to severe. Rupture or elongation of chordae tendineae can occur in myxomatous degeneration or fibroelastic deficiency. Similarly, rheumatic heart disease can not only lead to chordae tendineae rupture and thickening but also result in MR from deposition of calcium in the subvalvular apparatus.

3. Functional mitral regurgitation

MR that occurs in the setting of normal leaflets and chordal structures is frequently due to functional MR. This phenomenon occurs as a result of global LV dysfunction, causing disruption of the normal geometric relationship between the MV leaflets, papillary muscles, and the LV. The LV dysfunction results in ventricular and annular dilatation and a more spherical appearance of the LV, which ultimately disrupts the normal structure and function of the entire mitral apparatus.

4. Carpentier classification

This classification scheme divides MR into three types based on leaflet motion—normal leaflet motion, excessive leaflet motion, and restricted leaflet motion (Figure 14.5).[9]

B. Pathophysiology

1. Acute mitral regurgitation

Sudden development of MR leads to a rapid and marked rise in LA volume. Because the LA has normal compliance, this sudden increase in LA volume leads to a rapid rise in LA pressure that is passed on to the pulmonary circuit, resulting in elevated PAPs, pulmonary

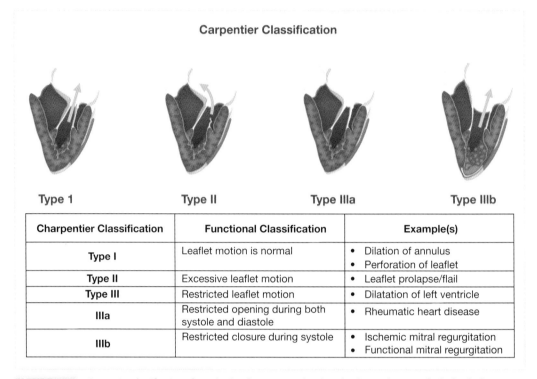

Carpentier Classification

Type 1   Type II   Type IIIa   Type IIIb

Charpentier Classification	Functional Classification	Example(s)
Type I	Leaflet motion is normal	• Dilation of annulus • Perforation of leaflet
Type II	Excessive leaflet motion	• Leaflet prolapse/flail
Type III	Restricted leaflet motion	• Dilatation of left ventricle
IIIa	Restricted opening during both systole and diastole	• Rheumatic heart disease
IIIb	Restricted closure during systole	• Ischemic mitral regurgitation • Functional mitral regurgitation

FIGURE 14.5 Carpentier classification of mitral valve disease is used to describe the mechanism of valvular dysfunction. In type 1 dysfunction, there is normal leaflet motion and regurgitation is due to annular dilation, or leaflet perforation. In type 2 dysfunction, there is excessive leaflet motion with the free edge of one or more leaflets above the plane of the annulus during systole. In type 3 dysfunction, there is restricted leaflet motion. Type 3 dysfunction is further classified into type 3a, where there is restricted leaflet motion during both diastole and systole, and type 3b, where there is restricted leaflet motion in systole only.

edema, and RV failure. The forward stroke volume is reduced as a result of regurgitant flow, and as a compensatory measure, there is sympathetic modulation, causing tachycardia and an increase in ventricular contractility. In addition, the LV functions on a higher portion of the Frank-Starling curve owing to increased LV volume. Owing to this increased LV volume, the LVEDP is also increased, which, in combination with tachycardia, can cause ischemia and LV dysfunction. With acute MR affecting both the right and left heart, patients often present with biventricular failure.

2. **Chronic mitral regurgitation:** LA dilatation and eccentric hypertrophy mark the gradual development of chronic MR. Despite a rise in LV volume, a relatively normal LVEDP is maintained, primarily due to LV dilation. Cardiac output is maintained by an increase in heart rate and also an increase in forward stroke volume brought on by an improved contractility. However, once LV dilatation and hypertrophy can no longer meet the necessary forward stroke volume to maintain cardiac output, LV dysfunction ensues and symptoms of heart failure manifest. Despite a normal ejection fraction, much of the blood ejected is ejected back into the low-pressure pulmonary system. LA dilatation also causes widening of the mitral annulus, thereby worsening regurgitation and contributing to elevated PAPs, pulmonary congestion, and, ultimately, RV dysfunction and failure.

C. **Intracardiac Hemodynamics and Cardiac Remodeling**

In acute MR, there is a rapid rise in LVEDP to dilate the LA and maintain stroke volume. In chronic MR, LA and LV dilation occurs more gradually, and the LVEDP may remain relatively normal until the disease is more advanced. Forward stroke volume is maintained by an overall increase in total stroke volume that occurs due to eccentric hypertrophy.

3. **Pressure wave disturbances**

The compliance of the LA, the compliance of the pulmonary vasculature, the amount of pulmonary venous return, and the regurgitant volume all collectively determine the size of the regurgitant wave ("giant V wave") on pulmonary capillary wedge tracing. V waves develop in patients with acute MR and are absent in patients with chronic disease due to increased atrial compliance.

4. **Pressure-volume loop in mitral regurgitation**

In chronic MR, LVEDV is elevated without significant elevation of LV filling pressures. In contrast, with acute MR, LVEDV is increased, but accompanied by an increase in LV filling pressure (Figure 14.6).

D. **Transesophageal Echocardiography Examination**

The TEE examination should follow a stepwise approach, which includes (a) identifying the presence and severity of MR, (b) identifying the mechanism of regurgitation and the pathophysiology of the responsible mechanism, (c) excluding contraindications to repair, and (d) assessing suitability and establishing predictors of repair failure.[6]

1. **Identifying the presence and severity of mitral regurgitation:** Identifying the presence of MR is performed qualitatively using color-flow Doppler as well as supportive signs on echocardiography. Quantification of the severity of MR should be based on the American Society of Echocardiography (ASE) guidelines for comprehensive assessment of valvular regurgitation.[10] The severity of MR is often underestimated under the altered loading conditions of general anesthesia, and so it is more appropriate to grade the severity of MR using the preoperative echo examination. Alternatively, preload and afterload augmentation to match awake state hemodynamics can be performed to evaluate the severity of MR. It is important to confirm the severity using multiple criteria as set out by the ASE guidelines, and the limitations of each method should be appreciated. The most common methods used to quantify the severity of MR in the operating room include vena contracta, jet area, pulmonary venous flow patterns, 3D vena contracta, and PISA[6,10] (Table 14.2 and Figure 14.7).

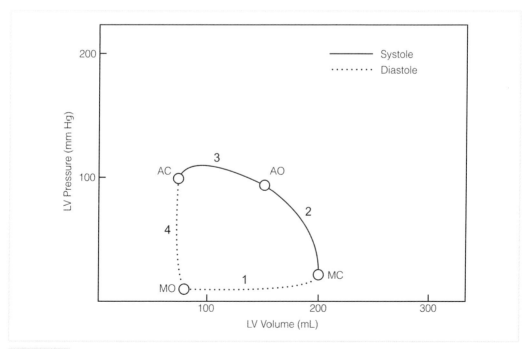

FIGURE 14.6 Pressure-volume loop (PV loop) in acute and chronic mitral regurgitation (MR). In chronic MR, there is an increase in end-diastolic volume without significant increase in LV filling pressures. Whereas in acute MR, the increase in end-diastolic volume is associated with an increase in LV filling pressure. AC, aortic valve closure; AO, aortic valve opening; MC, mitral valve closure; MO, mitral valve opening. Phase 1, ventricular filling; phase 2, isovolumetric contraction; phase 3, ventricular ejection; phase 4, isovolumetric relaxation. (Modified from Jackson JM, Thomas SJ, Lowenstein E. Anesthetic management of patients with valvular heart disease. *Semin Anesth.* 1982;1:248.)

TABLE 14.2   Grading the Severity of Chronic TR by Echocardiography

	MR Severity		
	Mild	**Moderate**	**Severe**
Structural			
MV morphology	**None or mild leaflet abnormality** (eg, mild thickening, calcifications or prolapse, mild tenting)	Moderate leaflet abnormality or moderate tenting	**Severe valve lesions** (primary: flail leaflet, ruptured papillary muscle, severe retraction, large perforation: secondary: severe tenting, poor leaflet coaptation)
LV and LA size[a]	Usually normal	Normal or mild dilated	Dilated[b]
Qualitative Doppler			
Color-flow jet area[c]	**Small, central, narrow, often brief**	Variable	Large central jet (>50% of LA) or eccentric wall-impinging jet of variable size
Flow convergence[d]	**Not visible, transient or small**	Intermediate in size and duration	**Large throughout systole**
CWD jet	Faint/partial/parabolic	Dense but partial or parabolic	Holosystolic/dense/triangular
Semiquantitative			
VCW (cm)	<0.3	Intermediate	≥0.7 (>0.8 for biplane)[e]
Pulmonary vein flow[f]	**Systolic dominance** (may be blunted in LV dysfunction or AF)	Normal or systolic blunting[f]	Minimal to no systolic flow/systolic flow reversal
Mitral inflow[g]	**A-wave dominant**	Variable	E-wave dominant (>1.2 m/s)
Quantitative[h]			
EROA, 20 PISA (cm^2)	<0.20	0.20-0.29	0.30-0.39	≥0.40 (may be lower in secondary MR with elliptical ROA)
RVol (mL)	<30	30-44	45-59[g]	≥60 (may be lower in low-flow conditions)
RF (%)	<30	30-39	40-49	≥50

CWD, continuous-wave Doppler; EROA, effective regurgitant orifice area; LA, left atrium; LV, left ventricular; MR, mitral regurgitation; MV, mitral valve; PISA, proximal isovelocity surface area; RF, regurgitant fraction; VCW, vena contracta width.
[a]This pertains mostly to patients with primary MR.
[b]LV and LA can be within the "normal" range for patients with acute severe MR or with chronic severe MR who have small body size, particularly women, or with small LV size preceding the occurrence of MR.
[c]With Nyquist limit 50-70 cm/second.
[d]Small flow convergence is usually <0.3 cm, and large is ≥1 cm at a Nyquist limit of 30-40 cm/second.
[e]For average between apical two- and four-chamber views.
[f]Influenced by many other factors (LV diastolic function, atrial fibrillation, LA pressure).
[g]Most valid in patients >50 years old and is influenced by other causes of elevated LA pressure.
[h]Discrepancies among EROA, RF, and RVol may arise in the setting of low or high flow states.
[i]Quantitative parameters can help subclassify the moderate regurgitation group.
Reprinted from Zoghbi WA, Adams D, Bonow RO, et al. Recommendations for noninvasive evaluation of native valvular regurgitation: a report from the American Society of Echocardiography developed in collaboration with the Society for Cardiovascular Magnetic Resonance. *J Am Soc Echocardiogr.* 2017;30(4):303-371. © 2017 by the American Society of Echocardiography. With permission.

2. **Identifying the mechanism of regurgitation and pathophysiology of the responsible mechanism of regurgitation:** The mechanism of MR should be classified according to Carpentier classification system (Figure 14.5). Subsequently, the underlying pathophysiology should be identified, such as myxomatous degeneration, fibroelastic disease, ischemic heart disease, rheumatic heart disease, and infective endocarditis.
3. **Exclude contraindications to repair:** A thorough examination of the structure and function of the MV leaflets is critical, as is close examination of the subvalvular apparatus and LV function and shape in order to exclude contraindications to repair.[6] Contraindications to repair such as preexisting MS, severe mitral annular calcification, and active infective endocarditis with leaflet destruction should be excluded.

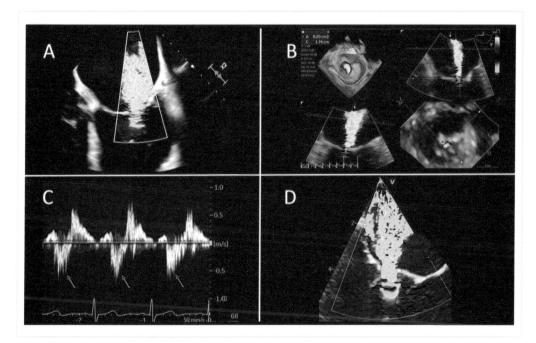

FIGURE 14.7 Various quantitative methods to measure severity of mitral regurgitation. **(A)** Vena contracta. **(B)** Three-dimensional effective regurgitant orifice area. **(C)** Pulmonary vein systolic flow reversal (red arrows). **(D)** Proximal isovelocity surface area.

4. **Assess suitability and establish predictors of repair failure**
   a. If there are no contraindication to MV repair, then suitability of repair should be under-taken. 3D imaging has allowed precise geometric measurements to be made that aid in clinical decision-making with regard to repairing or replacing the MV. The 3D LA en face view of the MV also easily allows any structural abnormalities, such as flail and prolapsed portions of the anterior and posterior leaflets, to be easily visualized[11] (Figure 14.8).

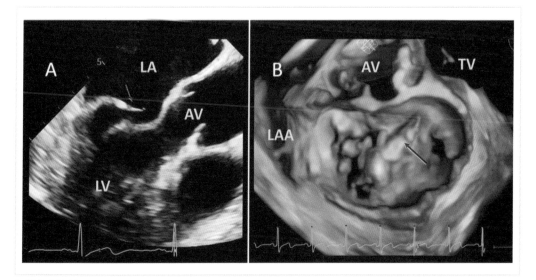

FIGURE 14.8 **(A)** Mid-esophageal long-axis view showing a flail segment of the posterior mitral valve leaflet (red arrow). **(B)** Three-dimensional en face view of the mitral valve showing the flail P2 segment of the mitral valve (red arrow). AV, aortic valve; LA, left atrium; LAA, left atrial appendage; LV, left ventricle.

b. In general, easily reparable MV lesions include leaflet perforation, MV annulus dilatation, and excessive motion of MV leaflets. Isolated lesions of the posterior leaflet such as flail and prolapse are more amenable to repair than bileaflet or multiple scallop disease.

c. The most common reason for immediate repair failure includes residual regurgitation, iatrogenic stenosis, and dynamic left ventricular outflow tract (LVOT) obstruction due to systolic anterior motion (SAM) of the MV.

d. The risk of SAM should be routinely evaluated. Measurements are performed in the mid-esophageal five-chamber view or mid-esophageal long-axis view and include the length of the posterior and anterior MV leaflets, the ratio of anterior and posterior leaflet heights measured at end systole from the MV annulus to the coaptation point, the end-systolic distance from the coaptation point perpendicular to the interventricular septum (C-sept distance), and the angle between the MV and aortic valve planes[12,13] (Figure 14.9).

e. Indices of remodeling in ischemic MR should also be undertaken to assess for durable repair in these patients. Specific geometric measurements that should be routinely evaluated in patients with ischemic MR include measurement of tenting height, tenting area, posteromedial scallop (P3) tenting angle, and LV dimensions in systole and diastole.[14]

f. The presence of geometric measurements that predict repair failure should prompt consideration for MV replacement over repair. Measurement of the anterior and posterior MV leaflet heights, which are measured in factors that may predict postrepair SAM of the anterior MV leaflet leading to LVOT obstruction and hemodynamic instability as well as geometric indices that may predict repair failure, will determine whether the MV is to be replaced or repaired.

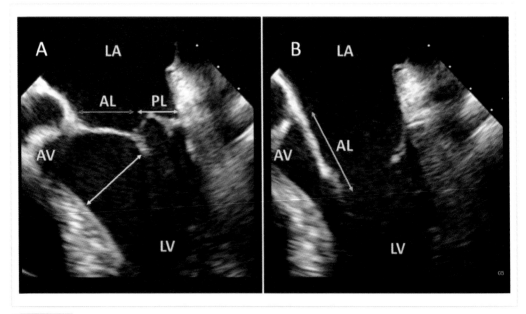

FIGURE 14.9   Routine geometric measurements used to predict the risk of SAM post mitral valve repair. **(A)** In the mid-esophageal five-chamber view, following measurements are made in systole: (1) AL/PL ratio is the ratio of the heights of the AL (double ended red arrow) and PL (double ended green arrow) measured in early systole. The height for each leaflet is the distance from the mitral annulus to the coaptation point for each leaflet. (2) C-sept distance (double ended yellow arrow) is the distance from the coaptation point to the closest part of the ventricular septum measured in early systole. **(B)** In the mid-esophageal five-chamber view, the AL length (double ended blue arrow) is measured. The AL length is the distance from the mitral annulus to the tip of the leaflet when measured in diastole. AL, anterior leaflet; AV, aortic valve; LA, left atrium; LV, left ventricle; PL, posterior leaflet.

E. **Surgical Intervention**

1. MV intervention involves either MV repair or replacement and is determined by multiple factors, including etiology of MR, echocardiographic parameters, patient factors, and surgical expertise. If possible, MV repair is preferable to MV replacement. Benefits of MV repair over replacement include avoidance of chronic anticoagulation (with mechanical valves) and future reoperation for prosthetic valve failure (with bioprosthetic valves). Perhaps more importantly, LV function is better preserved following valve repair.

2. The MV support apparatus is a critical structural and functional component to the LV, and any disruption of this apparatus, as can occur during MV replacement, can lead to LV dysfunction. Since MV repair leaves the mitral apparatus intact, this cause of LV failure can be avoided.

3. Timing of surgical intervention is critical in preventing irreversible complications associated with MR. In symptomatic patients with New York Heart Association (NYHA) class II heart failure and/or chronic or recurrent AF resulting from MR, surgical intervention is strongly endorsed. In asymptomatic patients, the decision to wait or go ahead for surgery depends on the presence of LV enlargement, dysfunction, and pulmonary hypertension, with the onset of LV dysfunction being the most important indicator for surgery in these patients.

4. A stress echo can be done to search for latent LV dysfunction. If chances of repair are good, early surgery is recommended because good long-term results are likely and anticoagulation is not needed. If coronary artery bypass grafting (CABG) is indicated and at least moderate ischemic MR is present, MV repair/replacement at the same time as CABG is beneficial.[7]

F. **Transcatheter Intervention**

Transcatheter edge-to-edge repair (TEER) of the MV is an evolving minimally invasive treatment option for patients with both primary and functional MR. TEER approximates the anterior and posterior MV leaflets by grasping them with a clipping device in an approach similar to the surgical Alfieri stitch–based edge-to-edge repair (Figure 14.10). For patients with primary MR, TEER is an option in patients who are high-risk surgical candidates with favorable MV anatomy. For patients with functional MR, selection for TEER is for patients with severe MR who remain symptomatic despite optimal guideline-directed medical therapy and have favorable anatomic, geometric, and functional parameters for successful TEER.[15]

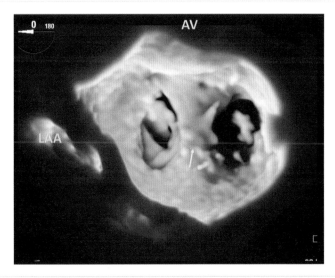

FIGURE 14.10 Three-dimensional view of the mitral valve showing the characteristic tissue bridge (yellow arrow) and double orifice created after transcatheter edge-to-edge repair. AV, aortic valve; LAA, left atrial appendage.

G. **Goals of Perioperative Management**
   1. **Hemodynamic management**
      a. **Left ventricular preload**

         Preload augmentation and maintenance is frequently helpful to ensure adequate forward stroke volume. The need for and degree of preload augmentation are largely patient specific and can be effectively gauged by assessing the patient's clinical and hemodynamic response to a fluid bolus. Preload augmentation should be done with extreme caution as this intervention can also result in worsening of regurgitant fraction and thus reduced forward stroke volume.

      b. **Heart rate**

         Heart rate should be maintained in the normal to elevated range for these patients. Bradycardia should be avoided as it can lead to an increase in LV volume, reduction in forward stroke volume, and an increase in regurgitant fraction. AF is common in these patients due to LA dilation.

      c. **Contractility**

         Maintenance of systolic function is critical in promoting forward stroke volume. Depression of myocardial contractility can result in major LV dysfunction and clinical deterioration. Patients who present with an ejection fraction of <50% are at the later stages of the disease process and are particularly sensitive to change in LV function. Inotropic agents, therefore, play a key role in management by augmenting forward flow and diminishing regurgitation via mitral annular constriction.

      d. **Systemic vascular resistance**

         Afterload reduction is desired since increased afterload leads to an increase in regurgitant fraction and consequently a reduction in forward stroke volume.

      e. **Pulmonary vascular resistance**

         Elevated pulmonary pressure is often seen in patients with severe MR and is due to increased PVR, as well as elevated LA pressure. Situations that may lead to pulmonary constriction, such as hypercapnia, hypoxia, nitrous oxide, and inadequate anesthesia in patients with high PVR, should be avoided as much as possible.

H. **Anesthetic Management**
   1. **Premedication**

      Premedication with a shorter acting benzodiazepine is usually appropriate. In patients with advanced disease and RV strain, there should be judicious use of these medications to avoid hypoxia and hypercarbia.

   2. **Induction and maintenance of general anesthesia**

      The hemodynamic goals for induction and maintenance of anesthesia should be directed at maximizing forward stroke volume. Heart rate should be maintained close to 90 beats/min, contractility should be preserved, and systemic vascular resistance should be reduced. Cautious use of volatile anesthetics, narcotics, and anxiolytics should be titrated to effect. Periods of intense stimulation should be anticipated, and sympathetic response blunted as any sudden rise in arterial blood pressure will increase regurgitant fraction and may lead to acute pulmonary edema or RV strain.

   3. **Pulmonary artery catheters**

      Pulmonary artery catheters are routinely used in MV surgery and serve as monitoring devices as well as aiding in directing clinical care. Pulmonary artery catheters aid in guiding fluid management as well as the need for inotropes and/or vasopressors. Sudden increases in PAPs that may occur because of LV ischemia or arterial vasoconstriction leading to an increase in regurgitant fraction can be readily identified and treated accordingly before causing significant hemodynamic effects. Therapies aimed at reducing PAPs, such as nitric oxide, inhaled epoprostenol, and systemic or inhaled phosphodiesterase-3 inhibitors, can be titrated to effect with pulmonary artery catheters.

   4. **Weaning from cardiopulmonary bypass**

      LV function is often compromised after MV surgery for a multitude of reasons. First, there is always an element of myocardial stunning after cardiopulmonary bypass (CPB) that may compromise LV function, but most importantly once the MV has been repaired or replaced, the LV must eject a full stroke volume into the high-pressure systemic system without the protection of a low-pressure pop-off system into the LA. This results in an increase in LV wall tension that can cause LV dysfunction. Post CPB, LV dysfunction should be anticipated in all patients undergoing MV surgery but is particularly evident in those patients with a presurgery ejection fraction of <50% as well as patients undergoing MV replacement as opposed to repair. Those who undergo MV replacement are more prone to LV dysfunction as some of the subvalvular apparatus, which helps maintain LV structure and function, is resected during this surgery. Inotropic support is often used prophylactically in these patients and can be quickly weaned if not required. In some cases, insertion of an intra-aortic balloon pump may be required to prevent LV dilation and failure. Maintenance of sinus rhythm is also important in these patients, and amiodarone is often used if the surgery was combined with a MAZE procedure.

5. **Transesophageal echocardiography**

Post bypass, TEE is essential for the assessment of an MV that has been repaired or replaced. 2D, 3D, and Doppler interrogation should be performed in multiple views. For an MV repair, it is essential to interrogate for any residual regurgitation, and any more than mild regurgitation should warrant return to CPB for further repair or MV replacement. Because MV repair with restrictive annuloplasty results in an immediate and continued reduction in MVA, the newly repaired valve should be assessed for iatrogenic stenosis. Return to bypass for MV replacement should be considered for repaired valves that have a mean transmitral gradient of >5 mm Hg or a valve area of <1.5 cm^2. SAM of the anterior MV leaflet causing LVOT obstruction is a common complication of MV repair and should be evaluated for post MV repair.[12] Confirmation of significant SAM includes 2D evaluation demonstrating septal contact of the anterior MV leaflet during systole along with evidence of flow acceleration, elevated gradients in the LVOT, and, classically, a posteriorly directed jet of MR (Figure 14.11). Only after confirmation of no more than mild regurgitation, no

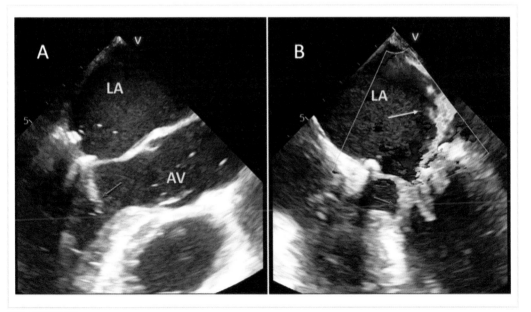

FIGURE 14.11 **(A)** Mid-esophageal long-axis view showing systolic anterior motion of the anterior mitral valve leaflet post mitral valve repair. **(B)** Mid-esophageal five-chamber view with color flow Doppler showing systolic anterior motion of the anterior mitral valve leaflet post mitral valve repair and the characteristic posteriorly directed jet of mitral regurgitation.

evidence of iatrogenic stenosis or significant SAM causing LVOT obstruction should prot-amine be considered. For patients undergoing MV replacement, the post-CPB examina-tion should focus on ensuring the new valve is well seated and that there is no valvular or paravalvular leak. It should be demonstrated that all leaflets or discs or the newly placed valve are adequately opening and closing symmetrically and that there is no significant transmitral pressure gradient.

6. **Postoperative course**

Following MV repair or replacement, LA pressure and PAP should decline over time. Pa-tients with advanced disease at the time of surgery may continue to need an elevated LA pressure for maintenance of adequate forward stroke volume.

VII. Tricuspid Valve Stenosis

A. **Natural History**

1. **Etiology**

Tricuspid stenosis (TS) is an uncommon valvular lesion in developed countries. Rheumatic heart disease is the most common etiology when TS is encountered and is commonly as-sociated with TR as this lesion almost never exists in isolation. When TS does occur be-cause of rheumatic heart disease, the MV is almost always also involved. Congenital TS not previously diagnosed in childhood, endocardial fibroelastosis, SLE, infective endocarditis, hypereosinophilic syndromes, carcinoid syndrome, and right atrial (RA) tumors causing functional TS are other etiologies of this disease.

2. **Symptoms**

The tricuspid valve (TV) is the largest cardiac valve, and as a result, symptoms are slow to progress with a long asymptomatic period before symptom onset. When valvular stenosis develops, the RA pressure increases, dilates, and, as a result, forward blood flow decrease. Patients subsequently develop symptoms associated with systemic venous congestion, which include jugular venous distension, ascites, and peripheral edema. Shortness of breath and fatigue may also occur as a result of obstruction of tricuspid flow, which limits cardiac output. Because TS rarely occurs in isolation, the symptoms and signs of concomitant val-vular lesions may be more prominent.

B. **Pathophysiology**

1. **Natural progression**

Composed of three leaflets (anterior, posterior, and septal), the TV is the largest cardiac valve with a normal area of 7-9 cm^2 in the typical adult. The normal gradient across the TV is only 1 mm Hg. By the time the valve opening decreases to <1.5 cm^2, the TV has endured significant degradation and has severely impaired forward blood flow in addition to RA dilation and increased RA pressures. A mean gradient of 3 mm Hg across the TV typically correlates to a valve area of 1.5 cm^2.

C. **Calculation of Severity**

Cardiac catheterization and echocardiography can be used to grade the severity of TS by cal-culating orifice area and pressure gradient. Severe stenosis is indicated in a gradient of 5 mm Hg across the TV and TV area of ≤1 cm^2.

D. **Transesophageal Echocardiography**

Patients with rheumatic TS will demonstrate thickened leaflets with restricted motion and diastolic doming, often accompanied by fusion of the commissures. For functional TS, such as those caused by intracardiac masses, an RA mass is apparent on imaging that is responsible for the obstruction of RV inflow. CWD can be used to assess the pressure gradients for the valve and subsequently grade the severity of the stenosis.[7]

E. **Medical and Surgical Therapy**

Medical therapy centers around managing symptoms associated with TS, with loop diuretics being the mainstay of treatment. If TS is the result of medical conditions such as SLE, then medical therapy should be directed toward this pathology. In advanced cases, surgical inter-vention is usually required.[7] Depending on the pathology causing the TS as well as patient characteristics, intervention may be in the form of percutaneous valvulotomy, TV repair with open commissurotomy, or TV replacement. Because TS almost never occurs in isolation, other concomitant valvular surgeries are usually warranted at the time of TV surgery. It must be noted that the operative mortality for isolated TS surgery is significant and increases if performed with other valvular surgery.

F. **Goals of Perioperative Management**
   1. **Hemodynamic management**
      a. **Right ventricular preload**
         Adequate preload is key to maintaining forward flow across the stenotic TV.
      b. **Heart rate**
         Normal sinus rhythm should be maintained in patients with TS. Both supraventricular tachyarrhythmias and bradycardia can be harmful. The former can cause rapid cardiac deterioration and should be controlled with immediate cardioversion or pharmacologic intervention, while the latter can reduce total forward flow and should be treated pharmacologically or via pacing.
      c. **Contractility**
         RV filling is impeded by TS; however, adequate cardiac output is maintained by an increase in RV contractility. Sudden deterioration in RV contractility should be avoided as any decrease in function can severely limit cardiac output, elevate RA pressure, and exacerbate symptoms.
      d. **Systemic vascular resistance**
         In patients with limited blood flow through the stenotic TV, systemic vasodilation can exacerbate hypotension, so normal-to-high systemic vascular resistance is desirable.
      e. **Pulmonary vascular resistance**
         Reducing PVR has little benefit in improving forward flow since the limitation to forward flow is mechanical and found at the level of the TV. Maintaining PVR in the normal range is adequate.
   2. **Anesthetic management**
      a. In patients with isolated TS, the anesthetic goals include maintenance of high preload, high afterload, and adequate contractility.
      b. Insertion of a pulmonary artery catheter through the stenotic TV can be challenging and is not always clinically warranted. Often, the catheter can be kept in the superior vena cava (SVC) until after bypass and then advanced by the surgeon after completion of the surgery or floated after weaning from CPB.
      c. During CPB, because no flow into the RA is allowed and SVC pressure completely depends on the adequate drainage of the SVC by the SVC cannula, attention must be paid to the SVC drainage in order to avoid elevated SVC pressure, reduced cerebral perfusion pressure, and irreversible brain damage. Central venous pressure monitoring above the SVC tie, as well as intermittent assessment of the patient's head for any signs of edema, is indicated. No drug infusions should be given through any pulmonary artery accessory port since it is isolated from the blood flow during CPB.
      d. Preload augmentation must be continued during the post-CPB period, and inotropic support may be warranted if RV dysfunction becomes apparent.

VIII. **Tricuspid Valve Regurgitation**
   A. **Natural History**
      Isolated TR is uncommon and often associated with TV endocarditis, carcinoid syndrome, Ebstein anomaly, connective tissue disorders leading to leaflet prolapse, or rarely, from chest trauma. Functional TR (FTR) is more common and develops secondary to RV failure, pulmonary hypertension, or left-sided cardiac disease, such as aortic stenosis or MS. With left-sided disease, there is elevated PAPs that lead to RV strain, pressure, and volume overload. TR subsequently develops as a result of TV annular dilatation. RV dilatation that often occurs can also lead to tethering of the TV leaflets, which restricts their mobility and exacerbates the regurgitation. Implantable leads can also cause chronic or acute TR from geometric changes in the tricuspid annulus from chronic pacing, direct contact of the leads with leaflets, leaflet inflammation, infective endocarditis, and thrombosis.[16]

B. **Pathophysiology**

1. **Natural progression**

TR is associated with increased RA volume secondary to systolic regurgitant flow through the incompetent valve. Since the RA and inferior vena cava (IVC) are compliant, large volumes can be accommodated without a significant increase in RA pressure, even in the presence of large regurgitant volumes. As TR becomes severe, RA pressure and venous pressures will increase and result in signs and symptoms of RV failure. Since RV can compensate for volume overload, isolated TR is generally well tolerated. Most TR symptoms occur from increased RV afterload. Therefore, when TR is associated with pulmonary hypertension, the impedance to RV ejection produces significant deterioration secondary to decreased cardiac output. AF is also a common concurrent issue in patients with TR due to distension of the RA.

C. **Transesophageal Echocardiography Evaluation and Grading of Severity of Tricuspid Regurgitant**

TEE examination of FTR shows dilatation of the RV and subsequently the tricuspid annulus, accompanied by leaflet restriction due to tethering. Different TR etiologies will have characteristic TEE appearances. In the setting of infective endocarditis, vegetations and valvular perforations may be seen (Figure 14.12A). With rheumatic heart disease, findings will include thickened leaflets with commissural fusion and probable MV and/or aortic valve involvement. Patients with carcinoid heart disease will have diffuse leaflet thickening, leading to both stenosis and regurgitation with TS and pulmonic valve involvement. In Ebstein anomaly, the tricuspid leaflets are displaced into the RV cavity, reducing its size and forcing the leaflets toward the RV apex. Quantification of the severity of TR should encompass multiple parameters, including jet area calculation, vena contracta, PISA radius calculation, regurgitant volume, 3D effective regurgitant orifice area (EROA) calculation, and hepatic vein flow patterns (Table 14.3 and Figure 14.12B,C).

D. **Pressure Wave Abnormalities**

Although central venous pressure tracings may show the presence of giant V waves, other factors, including the compliance of the RA, filling of the RA, and regurgitant volume, determine the size of the regurgitant wave.

E. **Medical and Surgical Intervention**

1. Medical therapy should be directed at treating the underlying cause of the FTR. In addition, medical therapy aimed at reducing symptoms is the mainstay of medical therapy. Medications aimed at treating pulmonary hypertension may also improve symptoms in some patients.

2. Isolated surgical intervention for patients with FTR is rarely performed; however, consideration for intervention should be undertaken at the time of left-sided surgery and/or coronary revascularization surgery.

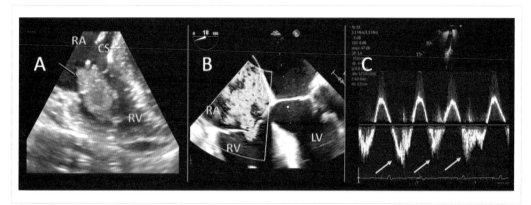

FIGURE 14.12 **(A)** Mid-esophageal four-chamber view focused on the right side showing a large tricuspid valve vegetation. **(B)** Mid-esophageal four-chamber view with color-flow Doppler showing severe tricuspid regurgitation **(C)** Hepatic vein systolic flow reversal (yellow arrows). CS, coronary sinus; RA, right atrium; RV, right ventricle.

TABLE 14.3   Grading the Severity of Chronic TR by Echocardiography

Parameters	Mild	Moderate	Severe
Structural			
TV morphology	**Normal or mildly abnormal leaflets**	Moderately abnormal leaflets	**Severe valve lesions** (eg, flail leaflet, severe retraction, large perforation)
RV and RA size	Usually normal	Normal or mild dilatation	Usually dilated[a]
Inferior vena cava diameter	Normal <2 cm	Normal or mildly dilated 2.1-2.5 cm	Dilated >2.5 cm
Qualitative Doppler			
Color-flow jet area[b]	**Small, narrow, central**	Moderate central	**Large central jot** or eccentric wall-impinging jet of variable size
Flow convergence zone	**Not visible, transient or small**	Intermediate in size and duration	**Large throughout systole**
CWD jet	**Faint/partial/parabolic**	Dense, parabolic, or triangular	Dense, often triangular
Semiquantitative			
Color-flow jet area (cm^2)[b]	Not defined	Not defined	>10
VCW (cm)[b]	<0.3	0.3-0.69	≥0.7
PISA radius (cm)[c]	≤0.5	0.6-0.9	>0.9
Hepatic vein flow[d]	Systolic dominance	Systolic blunting	**Systolic flow reversal**
Tricuspid inflow[d]	**A-wave dominant**	Variable	E-wave >1.0 m/s
Quantitative			
EROA (cm^2)	<0.20	0.20-0.39[e]	≥0.40
RVol (2D PISA) (mL)	<30	30-44	≥45

CWD, continuous-wave Doppler; EROA, effective regurgitant orifice area; RA, right atrium; RV, right ventricle; TR, tricuspid regurgitant; TV, tricuspid valve; VCW, vena contracta width.
[a]RV and RA size can be within the "normal" range in patients with acute severe TR.
[b]With Nyquist limit >50-70 cm/second.
[c]With baseline Nyquist limit shift of 28 cm/second.
[d]Signs are nonspecific and are influenced by many other factors (RV diastolic function, atrial fibrillation, RA pressure).
[e]There are little data to support further separation of these values.
Reprinted from Zoghbi WA, Adams D, Bonow RO, et al. Recommendations for noninvasive evaluation of native valvular regurgitation: a report from the American Society of Echocardiography developed in collaboration with the Society for Cardiovascular Magnetic Resonance. *J Am Soc Echocardiogr.* 2017;30(4):303-371. © 2017 by the American Society of Echocardiography. With permission.

3. For patients with primary TR, the timing of surgical intervention should be when their symptoms are no longer responsive to medical therapy, preferably before the onset of significant RV dysfunction and organ failure.[7]

4. Percutaneous interventions on the TV are evolving as a potential treatment option for patients with FTR. Edge-to-edge repair, transcatheter TV replacement, and heterotopic caval valve implantation are percutaneous interventions that are currently under investigation for the treatment of patients with severe FTR.

F. **Goals of Perioperative Management**

1. **Hemodynamic management**

a. **Right ventricular preload**

Since a drop in central venous pressure can severely limit RV stroke volume, preload augmentation is useful for adequate forward flow.

b. **Heart rate**

Normal-to-high heart rates are beneficial in these patients to sustain forward flow and prevent peripheral congestion.

c. **Contractility**

RV failure is the primary cause of clinical deterioration in patients with TR. Since the RV is designed geometrically to accommodate volume but not acute increases in pressure, positive-pressure ventilation, elevated PVR, or suppression of myocardial contractility can all lead to RV failure. Consequently, care must be given to avoid acute changes in RV pressure and avoid myocardial depressants that may induce RV failure.

d. **Systemic vascular resistance**

In the absence of aortic or MV lesions, variations in systemic afterload have little effect on TR.

e. **Pulmonary vascular resistance**

Decreases in PVR improve RV function and forward blood flow. Hyperventilation can be helpful in reducing PVR by producing hypocarbia. However, when ventilating these patients, high airway pressures and agents that increase PAP should be avoided. Agents that dilate the pulmonary vasculature are especially useful if inotropic support is necessary. Dobutamine, isoproterenol, and milrinone are excellent in this regard. In addition, inhaled nitric oxide and epoprostenol will reduce PVR in isolation. Vasopressin is also useful since it increases SVR without significant effects on PVR.

2. **Anesthetic technique**

a. In patients with coexisting MV and/or aortic valve disease, the anesthetic management is usually dictated by the lesion, causing the most significant hemodynamic effect.

b. Passage of a pulmonary artery catheter through the regurgitant TV may prove difficult due to the tendency of the regurgitant jet to push the catheter in the opposite direction. In addition, cardiac output calculations may be inaccurate in the presence of TR since the cold injectate is ejected retrograde into the atrium rather than the pulmonary artery.

c. Similar to TS, during CPB, close attention must be paid to the SVC drainage, given the risk of SVC syndrome.

d. Residual TS can occur if a prosthetic valve is placed since the prosthesis is often smaller than the native valve and post-CPB preload augmentation may be needed. In addition, post valve repair or replacement, the entirety of the RV stroke volume is ejected against a higher PVR without the protection of a low-pressure pop-off system into the RA, leading to increased RV strain. Accordingly, RV failure requiring inotropic support may occur and should be anticipated.

IX. Pulmonic Stenosis

A. **Etiology**

Pulmonic stenosis (PS) is primarily found in the pediatric population and is congenital in over 95% of cases. About 80% of PS is isolated, while the remainder occurs with other congenital cardiac anomalies. Other etiologies include rheumatic heart disease, malignant carcinoid, or extrinsic compression by a tumor or sinus of Valsalva aneurysm.[17]

B. **Symptoms**

Most patients with PS are asymptomatic for years and frequently live past the age of 70 without surgical intervention. As PS worsens from mild or moderate to severe, patients are unable to augment pulmonary flow, particularly during exertion, and start to develop signs and symptoms of right heart failure, such as dyspnea, hepatomegaly, and peripheral edema. Physical findings may include a systolic crescendo-decrescendo murmur, which is best auscultated at the upper left border and may radiate to the suprasternal notch and left neck, a left parasternal heave with an RV systolic impulse, and, occasionally, an ejection click or ejection sound that decreases in intensity with inspiration.

C. **Quantification and Classification**

Quantitative assessment of PS is primarily based on the transpulmonary pressure gradient. A transpulmonary peak gradient of <36 mm Hg is classified as mild PS, a peak gradient of between 36 and 64 mm Hg is classified as moderate PS, and a peak gradient of >64 mm Hg is classified as severe PS. Estimation of RV systolic pressure in patients with PS is another useful index of severity.

PS is almost always congenital in nature and can be classified based on the level of obstruction as (1) valvular (eg, carcinoid disease), (2) subvalvular (RV hypertrophy, infiltrative processes, tumor), or (3) supravalvular (membrane above the valve).

D. **Natural Progression**

As PS progresses, RV hypertrophy occurs, leading to increased pressure within the RV and, eventually, RV pressure overload. As subendocardial blood flow in the RV occurs in diastole, there is an increasing risk of RV ischemia with continued hypertrophy. Therefore, coronary perfusion pressure must be maintained to provide an adequate RV subendocardial coronary blood supply.

E. **Pressure Wave Abnormalities**

The PAP upstroke is delayed, and there is a late systolic peak owing to impedance to blood flow through the stenotic pulmonary valve. A prominent A wave is frequently found in the central venous pressure trace.

F. **Transesophageal Echocardiography**

Given the anterior location of the pulmonic valve, TEE interrogation of the valve can be challenging. Valvular anatomy, location of stenosis, as well as assessment of the severity and associated pathologies can be evaluated with echocardiography. Severity is assessed based on transpulmonic velocity for calculation of the transvalvular pressure gradient.

G. **Surgical Intervention**

Surgical intervention should be considered for patients experiencing severe symptoms, a peak systolic gradient >80 mm Hg, or peak RV systolic pressure of 100 mm Hg. Surgical approaches include valvulotomy, balloon valvuloplasty, and, rarely, replacement of the pulmonic valve. Alternative percutaneous options include a transluminal balloon angioplasty and percutaneous valve implantation.

H. **Goals of Perioperative Management**

1. **Hemodynamic management**

The mainstay of hemodynamic management of patients with PS includes maintaining contractility and SVR while increasing heart rate, increasing RV preload, and decreasing PVR as well.

2. **Right ventricular preload**

RV function relies heavily on adequate RV preload to generate an appropriate RV stroke volume. This is not possible if there are decreases in central venous pressure that lead to inadequate filling of the RV and decreased RV stroke volume.

3. **Heart rate**

Adequate RV filling also becomes increasingly dependent on the atrial contraction as PS progresses. This is complicated, however, by RA dilation and development of AF secondary to TR that frequently occurs from worsening RV function because of severe PS. Tachycardia is beneficial in patients with PS since blood flow across the stenotic pulmonary valve occurs primarily during ventricular systole. Rarely, RV hypertrophy in combination with angina symptoms dictates the need for a slower heart rate to allow adequate time in diastole for subendocardial coronary blood flow

4. **Contractility**

RV hypertrophy secondary to pressure overload occurs with severe PS. RV dysfunction is not uncommon, and further decreases in contractility can lead to RV failure and hemodynamic deterioration. Therefore, contractility should be maintained, and pharmacologic agents that can depress RV function should be avoided.

5. **Systemic vascular resistance**

SVR should be maintained to obtain adequate coronary perfusion to the hypertrophied RV that can be at risk of subendocardial ischemia.

6. **Pulmonary vascular resistance**

Forward blood flow in PS is not affected by PVR since the obstruction is mechanical. However, especially in patients with mild or moderate PS, major increases in PVR can potentially harm forward blood flow and lead to RV dysfunction. Therefore, PVR should be kept in the low-normal range.

X. Pulmonic Regurgitation

A. **Etiology**

PR can be categorized as physiologic, primary, or secondary.

While physiologic PR is common and clinically inconsequential, primary PR is most often associated with congenital valve deformities or is iatrogenic occurring secondary to surgical procedures to correct these deformities. Less common etiologies of primary PR include connective tissue disorders, trauma, carcinoid syndrome, infective endocarditis, and rheumatic fever. Patients with secondary or acquired PR have annular dilatation that may or may not be secondary to pulmonary hypertension of various etiologies.

B. Symptoms

Patients with PR without pulmonary hypertension are usually asymptomatic. However, patients with pulmonary hypertension are especially prone to developing RV dilatation, RV dysfunction, and, eventually, RV failure. FTR is also common in these patients. As RV function worsens, patients develop a low cardiac output state and exhibit symptoms of congestive heart failure, such as dyspnea on exertion and fatigue.

C. Transesophageal Echocardiography

TEE is extremely useful in diagnosing and determining the mechanism, etiology, and severity of PR. Similarly, 2D and 3D echocardiography can be used to assess RV function and associated TR and to measure the hemodynamic effects of the valvular lesion.

D. Surgical Intervention

Surgical or percutaneous intervention for PR consists of pulmonary valve replacement or repair and should always be considered for patients with symptomatic, severe PR.

It should also be considered in asymptomatic patients who have RV dilatation with worsening RV dysfunction that is mild or moderate, particularly if patients are starting to develop exercise intolerance.

E. Anesthetic Management

1. Intraoperative management of patients with PR is directed by the degree of pulmonary hypertension and RV dilatation and dysfunction.[18]
2. The use of invasive monitoring such as pulmonary artery catheters and intraoperative TEE to guide hemodynamic is recommended.
3. Ideally, RV contractility and function should be optimized without significant increases in PAP.
4. This can be accomplished by using ionodilators, like milrinone and dobutamine. PVR can be reduced by using inhaled epoprostenol and inhaled nitric oxide.

XI. Prosthetic Valves

Prosthetic valves can be broadly characterized as either mechanical or bioprosthetic. The decision regarding which prosthetic valve to implant is patient specific and depends on various factors, including the expected longevity of the patient, the ability of the patient to comply with anticoagulation therapy, the anatomy and pathology of the existing valvular disease, and the experience of the operating surgeon. Mechanical prostheses have the benefit of increased longevity; however, they require ongoing anticoagulation and subsequently have an increased risk of bleeding.

A. Essential Characteristics of Prosthetic Valves

1. An ideal prosthetic valve is nonthrombogenic, chemically inert, nonobstructive, nonregurgitant, durable, preserves blood elements, and allows physiologic blood flow.
2. The evolution of prosthetic valves has evolved significantly in recent years and has been driven by the desire to reduce proximal pressure to open the valve, increase central flow, provide a larger effective orifice area, and reduce the likelihood of thromboembolism.

B. Types of Prosthetic Valves

1. **Mechanical**

Although durable, current mechanical valves are thrombogenic and so patients with mechanical prosthetic valves require anticoagulation therapy indefinitely. Anticoagulation is normally provided with warfarin sodium, administered at a dose that will elevate the prothrombin time to 1.5-2 times control. There are four basic types of mechanical prosthetic valves: the caged ball, caged disc, monocuspid tilting disc, and bicuspid tilting disc valves. The bicuspid tilting disc valves are the most common owing to their streamlined design as well as improved laminar blood flow.

a. **Bileaflet tilting disc valve prosthesis**
   (1) In 1977, a bileaflet St. Jude cardiac valve was introduced as a low-profile device to allow central blood flow through two semicircular discs that pivot on supporting struts.
   (2) These valves have a central narrow orifice and two lateral orifices. In the closed position, the leaflets are at 30° angles with the valve orifice and tilt 70-90° when they are fully open.
   (3) To prevent stasis and to reduce thromboembolic potential, a small amount of retrograde flow is built into the valve assembly system known as washing jets.[19]
   (4) These valves can be placed in the aortic, mitral, or tricuspid positions and produce low resistance to blood flow and thus have a lower incidence of thromboembolic complications, though anticoagulation is still necessary.

2. **Bioprosthetic valves**
   The Hancock porcine aortic bioprosthesis (now the Medtronic Hancock II stented porcine bioprosthesis) was introduced in 1970, followed by the Ionescu-Shiley bovine pericardial prosthesis in 1974 and the Carpentier-Edwards porcine aortic valve bioprosthesis in 1975. Bioprosthetic valves are beneficial because they usually do not require long-term anticoagulation therapy and are less thrombogenic; however, they are less durable as well. Because of lower durability and because these valves last longer in older patients, they are usually recommended for older patients and when anticoagulation is contraindicated. These valves tend to last longer in the aortic position than in the mitral position. Bioprosthetic valves fall into two categories: stented and nonstented.
   a. **Stented bioprosthetic valves**
      (1) These valves are constructed from porcine aortic valves or bovine pericardium and are placed on a polypropylene stent attached to a silicone sewing ring covered with polyethylene terephthalate (Dacron).
      (2) These valves allow for improved central annular flow and less turbulence, but the stent does cause some obstruction to forward flow, thereby leading to a residual pressure gradient across the valve.
      (3) Stented valves that can be found in clinical use today include the Carpentier-Edwards perimount, Medtronic Mosaic, Carpentier-Edwards porcine, Hancock porcine, and Medtronic intact porcine.
   b. **Stentless bioprostheses**
      (1) Porcine valves fixed in a pressure-free glutaraldehyde solution and without the use of a stent make up the category of stentless bioprostheses.
      (2) The primary types of valves clinically encountered in this category include the St. Jude Medical Toronto SPV stentless porcine, Edwards Prima Plus stentless bioprosthesis, and Medtronic Freestyle stentless porcine.
      (3) Stentless bioprosthetic valves are used almost exclusively in the aortic position and often when aortic root replacement is also necessary. They have excellent hemodynamic characteristics but technically are more difficult to place.

3. **Human valves**
   a. The first use of a bioprosthesis taken from a cadaver occurred in 1962. However, techniques such as irradiation or chemical treatment used to sterilize and preserve homografts decreased life span.
   b. Antibiotic solutions are used to sterilize human valves that are then frozen in liquid nitrogen until implantation. This method allows >75% of prostheses to last >10 years, regardless of patient age, as cusp ruptures from weakness of the prostheses are minimized.
   c. Anticoagulation is often unnecessary, and the incidence of prosthetic valve endocarditis and hemolysis from blood flow through the homograft is low.
   d. Homografts are primarily used for aortic or pulmonary valve replacement.
   e. These are most useful in patients younger than 35 years and those with native valve endocarditis.

REFERENCES

1. Chandrashekhar Y, Westaby S, Narula J. Mitral stenosis. *Lancet*. 2009;374(9697):1271-1283.
2. Makinae H, Daimon M, Tambara K, et al. Reconsiderations of mitral stenosis: rheumatic mitral valve repair and the Wilkins score. *J Echocardiogr*. 2010;8(4):106-111.
3. Wilkins GT, Weyman AE, Abascal VM, Block PC, Palacios IF. Percutaneous balloon dilatation of the mitral valve: an analysis of echocardiographic variables related to outcome and the mechanism of dilatation. *Br Heart J*. 1988;60(4):299.
4. Iung B, Cormier B, Ducimetière P, et al. Immediate results of percutaneous mitral commissurotomy: a predictive model on a series of 1514 patients. *Circulation*. 1996;94(9):2124-2130.
5. Nishimura RA, Otto CM, Bonow RO, et al. 2017 AHA/ACC focused update of the 2014 AHA/ACC guideline for the management of patients with valvular heart disease: a report of the American College of Cardiology/American Heart Association Task Force on Clinical Practice Guidelines. *J Am Coll Cardiol*. 2017;70(1):252-289.
6. Mahmood F, Sharkey A, Maslow A, et al. Echocardiographic assessment of the mitral valve for suitability of repair: an intraoperative approach from a mitral center. *J Cardiothorac Vasc Anesth*. 2022;36(7):2164-2176.
7. Writing Committee Members, Otto CM, Nishimura RA, et al. 2020 ACC/AHA guideline for the management of patients with valvular heart disease: a report of the American College of Cardiology/American Heart Association Joint Committee on Clinical Practice Guidelines. *J Thorac Cardiovasc Surg*. 2021;162(2):e183-e353.
8. Khabbaz KR, Mahmood F, Shakil O, et al. Dynamic 3-dimensional echocardiographic assessment of mitral annular geometry in patients with functional mitral regurgitation. *Ann Thorac Surg*. 2013;95(1):105-110.
9. Stewart WJ, Currie PJ, Salcedo EE, et al. Evaluation of mitral leaflet motion by echocardiography and jet direction by Doppler color flow mapping to determine the mechanisms of mitral regurgitation. *J Am Coll Cardiol*. 1992;20(6):1353-1361.
10. Zoghbi WA, Adams D, Bonow RO, et al. Recommendations for noninvasive evaluation of native valvular regurgitation: a report from the American Society of Echocardiography Developed in Collaboration with the Society for Cardiovascular Magnetic Resonance. *J Am Soc Echocardiogr*. 2017;30(4):303-371.
11. Mahmood F, Warraich HJ, Shahul S, et al. En face view of the mitral valve. *Anesth Analg*. 2012;115(4):779-784.
12. Jiang L, Shakil O, Montealegre-Gallegos M, et al. Systolic anterior motion of the mitral valve and three-dimensional echocardiography. *J Cardiothorac Vasc Anesth*. 2015;29(1):149-150.
13. Maslow AD, Regan MM, Haering JM, Johnson RG, Levine RA. Echocardiographic predictors of left ventricular outflow tract obstruction and systolic anterior motion of the mitral valve after mitral valve reconstruction for myxomatous valve disease. *J Am Coll Cardiol*. 1999;34(7):2096-2104.
14. Mahmood F, Knio ZO, Yeh L, et al. Regional heterogeneity in the mitral valve apparatus in patients with ischemic mitral regurgitation. *Ann Thorac Surg*. 2017;103(4):1171-1177.
15. Feldman T, Foster E, Glower DD, et al. Percutaneous repair or surgery for mitral regurgitation. *N Engl J Med*. 2011;364(15):1395-1406.
16. Arsalan M, Walther T, Smith RL, Grayburn PA. Tricuspid regurgitation diagnosis and treatment. *Eur Heart J*. 2017;38(9):634-638.
17. Almeda FQ, Kavinsky CJ, Pophal SG, Klein LW. Pulmonic valvular stenosis in adults: diagnosis and treatment. *Catheter Cardiovasc Interv*. 2003;60(4):546-557.
18. Shillcutt SK, Tavazzi G, Shapiro BP, Diaz-Gomez J. Pulmonic regurgitation in the adult cardiac surgery patient. *J Cardiothorac Vasc Anesth*. 2017;31(1):215-228.
19. Mahmood F, Matyal R, Mahmood F, Sheu RD, Feng R, Khabbaz KR. Intraoperative echocardiographic assessment of prosthetic valves: a practical approach. *J Cardiothorac Vasc Anesth*. 2018;32:823-837.

Right Heart Disease Assessment and Management

Etienne J. Couture, Lars Grønlykke, Lachlan F. Miles, Juan C. Bianco, and André Y. Denault

KEY POINTS

1. Right ventricular (RV) dysfunction and failure are associated with increased morbidity and mortality.
2. Signs of dysfunction of the brain, liver, kidney, and gastrointestinal system are prognostic and can be recognized at the bedside with ultrasound.
3. The diagnosis of RV dysfunction can be obtained using history, physical examination, laboratory data, pressure waveform analysis, cardiac and extracardiac imaging modalities, (particularly ultrasound), and direct RV visualization intraoperatively.
4. Right heart failure will lead to impaired left ventricular (LV) filling. The combination of reduced cardiac output, reduced arterial pressure, and elevated venous pressure will lead to tissue organ dysfunction and worsening of RV function.
5. Continuous monitoring of RV function is feasible using combined RV pressure and pulmonary artery pressure (PAP) monitoring. It allows diagnosis of RV dysfunction, RV failure, RV outflow tract obstruction, and titration of pharmacologic therapy.
6. Echocardiography is an essential diagnostic modality for RV function with a multitude of cardiac and extracardiac parameters existing to quantify RV function and the impact of venous congestion.
7. It is recommended to use a multiview and multiparametric approach to evaluate RV systolic function. Simple or single parameters are insufficient in the evaluation.
8. Normal range values in the context of cardiac surgery still need validation. Following cardiac surgery, the RV shows a decrease in longitudinal contraction and an increase in transverse contraction. This should be accounted for when choosing modality.
9. The single most important element in the management of RV dysfunction is identification and correction of the cause.
10. Treatment of RV dysfunction is based on the maintenance of systemic arterial perfusion pressure, restoration of atrioventricular synchrony, RV afterload reduction and preload optimization, increased RV contractility, and, finally, mechanical support.

I. Importance of Right Ventricular Function in Cardiac Surgery

A. Overview

Perioperative right ventricular (RV) dysfunction and pulmonary hypertension (PH) are significant contributors to morbidity and mortality in both cardiac and noncardiac surgery, and in the critical care unit. The incidence of acute refractory RV failure varies from 0.1% after cardiotomy to 30% after left ventricular assist device (LVAD) implantation.[1] In cardiac surgery, acute refractory RV failure increases the risk of perioperative mortality (up to 75% in high-risk patients), as well as other adverse outcomes, including increased intensive care unit length of stay, prolonged duration of mechanical ventilation, renal and hepatic failure, and hospital readmissions. Multiple factors may lead to a significant reduction in RV function after cardiopulmonary bypass (CPB), such as RV ischemia or infarction, poor myocardial preservation during CPB, coronary air embolism, volume overload, and PH aggravated by lung reperfusion injury or protamine. Perioperative RV failure in cardiac surgery is a major concern because of its challenging diagnosis and treatment[2] (Figure 15.1; ⦿ **Video 15.1**). In this chapter, we highlight the current definitions of RV dysfunction and failure, review the RV perioperative evaluation (using clinical, hemodynamic, and sonographic assessment), and, finally, discuss the pharmacologic and mechanical management of RV dysfunction and failure.

B. Definitions

1. **Right ventricular dysfunction:** In cardiac surgery, abnormal RV function can be recognized on visual inspection of the heart in an open chest (⦿ **Videos 15.2-15.4**), interpretation of the right atrial pressure (RAP) and waveform, RV pressure and pulmonary artery pressure (PAP) waveform, the echocardiographic features, and the amount of pharmacologic support required to maintain cardiac function. Thus, RV dysfunction can be defined as isolated echocardiographic or hemodynamic abnormalities of the RV without repercussions for other organs (notably the brain and abdominal viscera).[3]

2. **Right ventricular failure:** Generally, RV failure refers to RV dysfunction that has negative effects on the function of other organs, such as the brain, kidney, liver, and intestines. RV failure can be defined as a rapidly progressive state of systemic congestion secondary to increased RV filling pressure and impaired RV antegrade flow.[4] RV failure usually presents as intraoperative hemodynamic instability requiring significant inotropic or mechanical circulatory support, difficult separation from CPB, and postoperatively as low cardiac output syndrome and multiorgan dysfunction. There are several mechanisms of RV failure, and several definitions using various criteria have been proposed. This generates variability in the prevalence of the disease, making study more difficult in large populations as well as in different contexts.

3. **Intraoperative right ventricular failure in cardiac surgery** is defined as (a) the presence of (1) difficult separation from CPB requiring both vasopressors and inotropes and/or inhaled vasodilators or (2) more than one attempt to wean from CPB as a result of RV failure or (3) the requirement for mechanical support to facilitate weaning right ventricular assist device (RVAD) or intra-aortic balloon pump and (b) anatomic impaired or absent RV function by (1) direct visualization in an open chest (⦿ **Video 15.3**) or (2) >20% reduction in right ventricular fractional area change (RVFAC) on intraoperative transesophageal echocardiography (TEE).[1]

4. **Postoperative right ventricular failure in cardiac surgery** is defined as the (a) presence of RAP >15 mm Hg and cardiac index <1.8 mL/min/m^2 and (b) absence of elevated left atrial pressure and pulmonary capillary wedge pressure (PCWP) >18 mm Hg, tamponade, pneumothorax causing hemodynamic compromise, and (c) RV stroke work index <4 g/m/m^2 (normal = 7-12 g/m/m^2).[1]

5. **Right ventricular failure related to LVAD based on the Mechanical Circulatory Support Academic Research Consortium** is defined as early acute, early postimplant, and late (>30 days) RV failure. It implies the (a) need for RVAD and/or (b) inability to wean inotropes and nitric oxide (NO) within 14 days.[1]

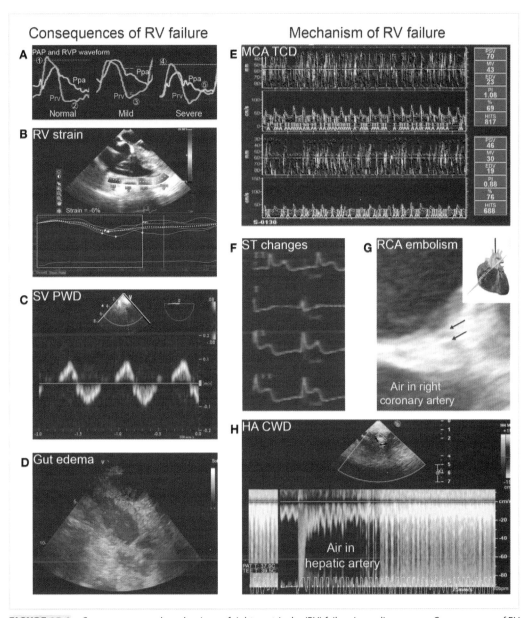

FIGURE 15.1   Consequences and mechanisms of right ventricular (RV) failure in cardiac surgery. Consequences of RV failure include **(A)** RV performance evaluation using RV pressure waveform. (A-1) Normal RV pressure (Prv) waveform with rapid systolic pressure changes. (A-2) Normal horizontal RV diastolic filling characterized by a pressure difference between the beginning and end of diastole of <4 mm Hg. (A-3) Abnormal RV diastolic slope >4 mm Hg in the presence of RV diastolic dysfunction. (A-4) Severe RV systolic dysfunction with RV pulsus tardus. (A-5) Square root sign with diastolic equalization between the Prv and the diastolic pulmonary artery pressure (Ppa). **(B)** Reduction in RV strain. **(C)** Splenic vein (SV) pulsed-wave Doppler (PWD) flow reversal associated with portal hypertension and **(D)** gut edema. Possible mechanisms of RV failure include **(E)** air embolization detected through middle cerebral artery (MCA) microembolism seen on transcranial Doppler (TCD) leading to **(F)** RV ischemia or infarction with ST changes **(G)** right coronary artery (RCA) air embolism and **(H)** hepatic artery (HA) air embolism using continuous-wave Doppler (CWD). EDV, end-diastolic velocity; HITS; high-intensity transient signals; MV, mean velocity; PAP, pulmonary artery pressure; PI, pulsatility index; PSV, peak systolic velocity; RVP, right ventricular pressure. (Reprinted from Denault A, Haddad F, Lamarche Y, Bouabdallaoui N, Deschamps A, Desjardins G. Postoperative right ventricular dysfunction-Integrating right heart profiles beyond long-axis function. *J Thorac Cardiovasc Surg*. 2020;159(5):e315-e317. Adapted from Denault A, Vegas A, Lamarche Y, Tardif J, Couture P. *Basic Transesophageal and Critical Care Ultrasound*. CRC Press; 2018. © 2018 by Taylor and Francis Group, LLC. Reproduced by permission of Taylor and Francis Group, LLC, a division of Informa plc.)

CLINICAL PEARL

Intraoperative RV failure is defined as difficult separation from CPB, requiring pharmacologic or mechanical support, and conclusive evidence of RV contractile dysfunction.

CLINICAL PEARL

Postoperative RV failure diagnosis is based on hemodynamic criteria on arrival to intensive care unit, including elevated RAP, reduced cardiac index, and low RV stroke work index.

II. **Preoperative Evaluation**
  A. **Overview**

Preoperative evaluation of a patient undergoing cardiac surgery includes a detailed history and a focused physical examination, as well as a comprehensive review of diagnostic studies and preoperative tests. Since RV dysfunction is frequently present in patients with PH, it is essential in the preoperative consultation to assess the severity of the patient's PH and RV dysfunction, functional status, and any modifiable factors that would improve the condition of the patient. Considering that patients' medical conditions should be optimized before elective procedures, all attempts should be made to reduce pulmonary vascular resistance (PVR) and improve RV function before the procedure, including optimizing medical treatment for PH and heart failure and avoiding conditions that could result in critical worsening.

  B. **History and Physical Examination**
    1. **Venous congestion:** History of weight gain, expanding abdomen circumference, appetite reduction or early satiety, and the onset of edema in dependent organs (extremities or presacral) may indicate RV congestion. The liver is frequently enlarged and sensitive, and ascites may be present in patients with advanced RV dysfunction. In addition, a pulsatile liver denotes severe tricuspid regurgitation that can be related to tricuspid annular dilation and leaflet tethering in the setting of RV dysfunction.
    2. **Pulmonary hypertension—clinical manifestations:** Signs and symptoms of PH are nonspecific; symptoms range from exertional dyspnea, general fatigue, and chest pain to syncope in advanced PH. New York Heart Association functional class is an important predictor of survival in these patients. Patients may also present with signs and symptoms of the causative diseases of PH (eg, left heart failure, chronic lung disease, connective tissue disorders). Syncope and other signs of low cardiac output, including hypoxemia and metabolic acidosis, are ominous indicators that portend a poor prognosis in PH.
    3. **Jugular venous pressure:** Assessment of the height of the jugular venous pulsation is utilized to estimate RAP. RV failure causes an increase in central venous pressure, reflected in jugular venous distention, and often associated with large V waves that indicate severe tricuspid regurgitation. Venous pulsations above the clavicle with the patient in the sitting position are clearly abnormal, because the distance from the right atrium (RA) is at least 10 cm. With inspiration, the normal venous pressure should decrease by at least 3 mm Hg. An increase in venous pressure with inspiration (Kussmaul sign), or its failure to diminish, is associated with RV failure, as well as constrictive pericarditis and restrictive cardiomyopathy. Moreover, a positive abdominojugular reflux sign is observed in RV failure, which shows the inability of the RV to accommodate an augmented venous return.
    4. **Palpation of the heart:** A left parasternal lift indicates RV pressure or volume overload.
    5. **Auscultation of the heart:** A right-sided third heart sound (S_3) indicative of RV failure, a tricuspid regurgitation systolic murmur, and an intensification of P_2 relative to A_2 of the second heart sound are all indicative of PH and may be detected during physical examination.
    6. **Signs of low cardiac output:** In decompensated RV failure, ventricular interdependence leads to decreased left ventricular (LV) filling, a reduction in LV stroke volume, and, ultimately, a decrease in systemic cardiac output. Systemic hypotension, tachycardia, cold extremities, oliguria, severe functional limitations, and/or changes in mental status are common signs in low cardiac output state.

C. **Preoperative Testing**

Routine preoperative studies include electrocardiography, chest radiography, laboratory studies, echocardiography, and consideration of right heart catheterization. Further studies should be considered if the etiology of PH has not yet been determined, in order to guide perioperative management, including blood gas analysis, pulmonary function tests, ventilation/perfusion (V/Q) scan to rule out thromboembolic disease, and serologic studies for connective tissue disorders and the human immunodeficiency virus.

1. **Electrocardiogram:** The electrocardiogram may reveal signs of RV hypertrophy and enlargement. Common findings include R/S ratio >1 or R wave >0.5 mV in lead V_1, right-axis deviation, and right bundle branch block. P-wave amplitude >2.5 mm in II, III, and aVF or >1.5 mm in V_1 is indicative of RA enlargement. An S1Q3T3 pattern (initial S deflection in I, initial Q deflection in III, and inverted T in III) may suggest a pulmonary embolism. Atrial arrhythmias, such as atrial fibrillation and flutter, are common in RV dysfunction.

2. **Chest radiograph:** Findings include RA and RV enlargement; in coexistent PH, the main PA will be dilated, and peripheral branches may appear "pruned."

3. **Echocardiography:** Transthoracic echocardiography (TTE) is one of the most useful and readily available bedside tools with which to evaluate the right heart. Echocardiography can determine the RV size and function, find RA enlargement, estimate systolic PAP with tricuspid regurgitation, and evaluate RAP by measuring the diameter and respiratory variation of the inferior vena cava. Associated findings such as intracardiac shunt or pulmonary emboli may help determine the etiology of PH (see "Echocardiographic Assessment of Right Heart Function" section).

4. **Right heart catheterization:** Right heart cardiac catheterization for hemodynamic assessment of disease severity should be considered before surgery in patients who suffer more than mild PH based on history and/or noninvasive evaluation to guide and optimize perioperative care. Right heart catheterization can be done weeks in advance to facilitate the appropriate treatment and prepare the patient for the cardiac surgery, depending on the urgency of the procedure and the severity of the disease. Otherwise, a pulmonary artery catheter (PAC) should be inserted before the beginning of the surgery to guide intraoperative and postoperative treatment.

   The diagnosis and type of PH are determined by right heart catheterization, which also provides important information about the severity of PH and right heart function. In addition, right heart catheterization enables the distinction between precapillary and postcapillary vascular abnormalities, which is crucial to comprehend the pathophysiology of PH. Precapillary PH is caused by an increase in pulmonary arterial blood flow resistance proximal to pulmonary capillaries that can be typically seen in pulmonary arterial hypertension. Preoperative vasoreactivity testing may also be helpful in predicting the effectiveness of pulmonary vasodilators for perioperative planning in pulmonary arterial hypertension. Postcapillary PH is due to an increase in pulmonary venous pressure and is commonly seen in left-sided heart disease.

5. **Other imaging modalities:** Computed tomography, magnetic resonance imaging, coronary angiography, and nuclear imaging are other cardiovascular imaging modalities that can offer helpful information to help direct the care of right heart diseases.

CLINICAL PEARL

All attempts should be made to reduce PVR and improve RV function before the procedure, including optimizing medical treatment for PH and heart failure and avoiding conditions that could result in critical worsening.

III. **Hemodynamic Assessment**

A. **Pressure-Volume Loop**

The gold standard of invasive RV hemodynamic evaluation is by using pressure-volume loops obtained using a conductance catheter by varying the preload using a balloon within the inferior vena cava. The slope of the end-systolic point of the pressure-volume loop is defined by the ventricular elastance at end systole (E_{es}). E_{es} describes contractility independently of preload and afterload. The pressure-volume loop of the RV is more trapezoid in response to the very compliant pulmonary vascular tree, compared to that of the LV, which is rather rectangular. The slope joining the end-systolic and end-diastolic pressure-volume point describes the arterial elastance (E_a). E_a is independent of the ventricular condition and strongly associated with the arterial load or the PVR[5] (Figure 15.2A). The main limitation of the conductance catheter to assess the RV lies in the complexity of its use. Mainly used in research, its clinical use remains limited. Despite these limitations, its great advantage remains the ability to combine pressure measurements and robust preload variations. The use of a conductance catheter to measure E_{es} and E_a allows a better understanding of the relation between RV function and PAP. In fact, the RV can be functioning normally after hypertrophying to adapt to states of chronic high PAP, whereas the same high PAP can be deleterious to a patient with a nonadapted RV.

Acute RV dysfunction or failure may be secondary to increased afterload, increased preload, or direct impairment of contractility. In any case, the main factor limiting its adaptability and thus the antegrade flow from the right heart to the left will be an increase in RV afterload. The RV does not have the architecture allowing it to cope with rapid preload and afterload increases. As a result, it has two adaptation mechanisms: heterometric and homeometric mechanism.[6] Heterometric autoregulation occurs during an acute change of preload or afterload. An increase in preload will produce an increase in end-diastolic volume and an increase in stroke volume of the same order to restore end-systolic volume without affecting end-systolic pressure or inotropy, based on the Frank-Starling concept. This mechanism is dependent on a change in the length of the myocardial fibers in order to optimize the positioning of the actin-myosin complex. Homeometric autoregulation relies on an increase in inotropy in response to an increase in afterload without altering preload. In a situation of rapidly increasing afterload, a rapid heterometric adaptation takes place, allowing the RV to accommodate the increase in RV pressure by shifting these working conditions to larger volumes. As soon as the homeometric adaptive mechanism becomes effective, the increase in contractility allows a normalization of the end-diastolic volume. In a case where the RV fails to hypertrophy sufficiently or reaches its limit, ventricular dilation remains the main effective adaptive mechanism in the face of an increased afterload condition.

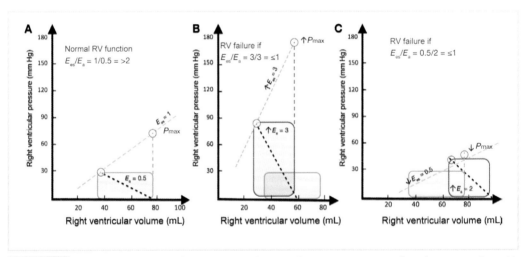

FIGURE 15.2 Pressure-volume loop of the right ventricle (RV). Schematic RV pressure-volume loop in a patient with **(A)** normal RV function, **(B)** RV dysfunction from pressure overload, and **(C)** RV dysfunction from volume overload. A normal RV elastance (E_{es}) to arterial elastance (E_a) ratio should be >1. Abnormal ventriculo-arterial coupling is present when the E_{es}/E_a ratio is ≤1. (Panel B adapted from Pinsky MR. The right ventricle: interaction with the pulmonary circulation. *Crit Care.* 2016;20(1):266. http://creativecommons.org/licenses/by/4.0/)

Consideration of RV-to-PA coupling illustrates the nature of the interrelationship between RV performance and PAP. It represents the mechanical efficiency or the optimal balance between the mechanical work of the RV and its oxygen consumption, according to the vascular conditions to which it is subjected.[7] This measurement is obtained from the pressure-volume loops by calculating the ratio E_{es}/E_a. Cardiac efficiency or normal ventriculo-arterial coupling would be reached when E_{es}/E_a is between 1 and 2. Progressive decoupling manifests as an E_{es}/E_a <0.5.[7] The concept of right ventriculo-arterial coupling helps better conceptualize the relation between RV function and PAP (Figure 15.2B-C).

B. **Pulmonary Artery Catheter**
In acute care settings such as the operating room and intensive care unit, hemodynamic or catheter-based assessment of RV function relies on the PAC. Invasive hemodynamic monitoring using a PAC is indicated for presumed cardiogenic shock and severe clinical heart failure decompensation requiring escalation of vasoactive medication, especially when mechanical circulatory support is being considered. The use of a PAC has significantly decreased over the past two decades, but its popularity appears to be once again increasing, particularly in cases of acute cardiogenic shock in an era of more frequent use of mechanical circulatory support.[8]

The hemodynamic variables made available by the PAC are extensive. Many of these variables do not have clear normality thresholds for cardiac surgical patients as they have been studied essentially in pathologic contexts such as PH or during implantation of LVAD.[9] Cardiac output can be measured using Fick method (the current gold standard) or by continuous or intermittent thermodilution. Different iterations of the original PAC are available, including catheters capable of measuring continuous mixed venous oxygen saturation, right ventricular ejection fraction (RVEF), and RV pressure monitoring.

Intraoperatively, the use of the PAC remains the gold standard for real-time measurement of cardiac output, RV pressure, and mixed venous oxygen saturation.[9,10] It is largely used in high-risk patients with PH, heart failure, or severe valvular disease, and its utility in adult low-risk cardiac surgery is debated. Even with the emergence of noninvasive devices, the PAC is still the preferred monitoring modality among cardiac anesthesiologists for multiple reasons, including cost savings from the reduction of cardiopulmonary complications. Obtaining a complete hemodynamic profile including systolic and diastolic PAP and PCWP with mixed venous oxygen saturation in addition to RAP before mechanical circulatory support initiation has been associated with improved outcomes when compared to incomplete assessment.[11]

The use of a pressure transducer on the RV opening of the PAC, originally designed to accommodate a cardiostimulation probe, allows continuous monitoring of RV pressure in order to track its systolic and diastolic function and also RV outflow tract obstruction.[12] A visual assessment of RV dysfunction can be made from the RV pressure waveform. Normally, the pressure difference between the beginning and end of diastole is <4 mm Hg. In the presence of mild RV diastolic dysfunction, this difference will increase, and the RV end-diastolic pressure will be increased. As diastolic dysfunction progresses, a proto-diastolic notch will appear. Finally, in advanced RV failure, the maximum rate of rise of the RV pressure change (dP/dt) will be decreased and the RV end-diastolic pressure increased above the diastolic PAP, leading to a diastolic opening of the pulmonic valve (Figure 15.3). Elevated RV end-diastolic pressure tracked using the RV port of a thermodilution PAC has been associated with difficult separation from CPB.[13]

CLINICAL PEARL

The RV can be functioning normally after hypertrophying to adapt to states of chronic high PAP, whereas the same high PAP can be deleterious to a patient with a nonadapted RV.

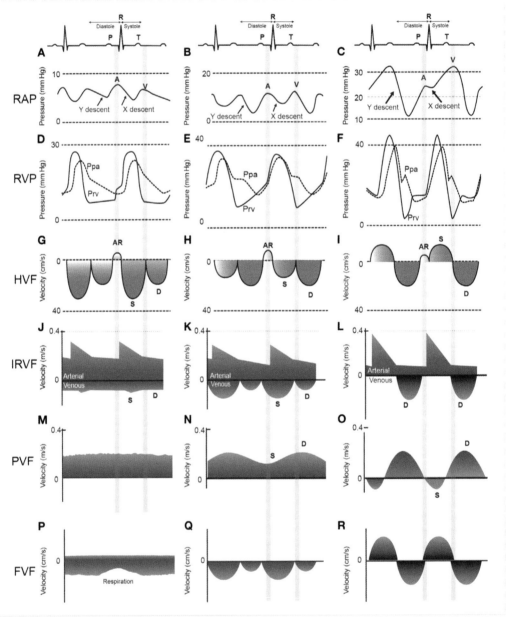

FIGURE 15.3 Evaluation of the right ventricular function using central hemodynamic waveforms and Doppler vein flow analysis. Right atrial pressure (RAP) waveform, right ventricular pressure (RVP) waveform, hepatic venous flow (HVF), interlobar renal venous flow (IRVF), portal venous flow (PVF), and femoral venous flow (FVF) in normal patients **(A, D, G, J, M, P)**. Typical patterns commonly observed in patients with mild **(B, E, H, K, N, Q)** and severe **(C, F, I, L, O, R)** right ventricular dysfunction. AR, atrial reversal Doppler velocity; D, diastolic Doppler velocity; Ppa, pulmonary artery pressure; Prv, right ventricular pressure; S, systolic Doppler velocity. (Reprinted with permission from Couture EJ, Grønlykke L, Denault AY. New developments in the understanding of right ventricular function in acute care. *Curr Opin Crit Care.* 2022;28(3):331-339.)

IV. Echocardiographic Assessment of Right Heart Function
   A. Cardiac Assessment of Right Heart Function

Echocardiography is a cornerstone of evaluating RV function, and a multitude of both quantitative and qualitative parameters exist. A full report of RV function should include several different parameters and acoustic views to be complete, and a multiparametric approach is recommended.[14] Physicians involved in the evaluation and treatment of RV dysfunction should be aware of the pitfalls and difficulties associated with each parameter.

   1. Right heart size: Quantification of the RV and RA size is essential when evaluating the right heart. Current guideline consensus on normative reference values using TTE is that abnormal values are RV basal diameter ≥42 mm.[15] RV hypertrophy is defined as RV free wall thickness >5 mm.[14] Because of the complex crescent shape wrapped around the LV, it can be difficult to get a full overview of the RV. The shape of the RV does not resemble any simple geometric shape, which makes volumetric assumptions difficult. Under normal circumstances, the RV is two-thirds of the size of the LV. In case of RV volume overload, it will manifest as RV dilation with septal flattening in end diastole, whereas in pressure overload, it will show as RV dilation with septal flattening in end systole[16] (Figure 15.4). Right heart size estimation can be performed using TEE; however, specific recommendations on right heart size obtained from TEE have not been endorsed by scientific societies.

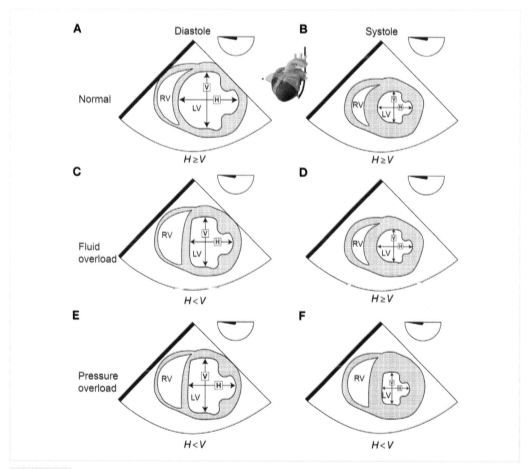

FIGURE 15.4 Eccentricity index. Using the transgastric mid short-axis view, the eccentricity index (EI) corresponds to the ratio of the vertical (*V*) and horizontal (*H*) diameter of the left ventricle (LV). **(A, B)** In normal loading condition, the interventricular septal curvature is preserved and the EI is ≤1. **(C, D)** In fluid overload, the horizontal diameter is smaller than the vertical diameter, especially at end diastole. **(E, F)** In pressure overload, the horizontal diameter remains smaller than the vertical diameter in both systole and diastole. RV, right ventricle. (Derived from Haddad F, Couture P, Tousignant C, Denault AY. The right ventricle in cardiac surgery, a perioperative perspective: I. Anatomy, physiology, and assessment. *Anesth Analg.* 2009;108(2):407-421.)

2. **Right ventricular systolic function:** In the normal RV, the longitudinal contraction from base to apex accounts for up to 80% of the RV output. Simple measures of longitudinal contraction have a reasonable correlation with RV stroke volume in most situations. However, following CPB, there is a shift in contraction pattern to more radial contribution, which will resemble RV dysfunction on longitudinal measures without necessarily meaning a reduced RV output. Change in contraction pattern must be kept in mind when evaluating RV function postoperatively or in heart transplant patients.[17]

   a. **Tricuspid annular plane systolic excursion:** Tricuspid annular plane systolic excursion (TAPSE) is one of the most used measures of RV systolic function. It measures the distance that the tricuspid annulus travels toward the apex, and its normal value is considered to be >17 mm.[14] On TTE, it is usually measured in M-mode and is a robust measure with low interobserver and intraobserver variability. On TEE, it is usually not possible to get a good (ie, parallel) alignment for M-mode, although a valid alternative with correction for angle of interrogation does exist (Figure 15.5). TAPSE only evaluates longitudinal contraction and can underestimate RV function following CPB and after both heart and lung transplantation.[18]

   b. **Peak systolic velocity of the tricuspid annulus using tissue Doppler imaging (TDI S'):** TDI S' is measured by applying TDI to the tricuspid annulus (Figure 15.6). TDI S' measures myocardial deformation and thereby assesses longitudinal systolic function.[15] The reference normal value is >10 cm/s.[14] The modality is well established with a good

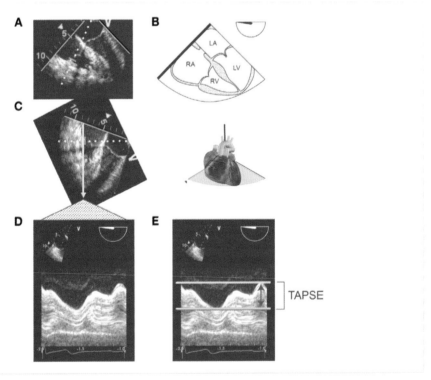

FIGURE 15.5 Tricuspid annular plane systolic excursion (TAPSE). **(A-E)** Steps in the measurement of the TAPSE using anatomic M-mode are shown. **(A, B)** First, a mid-esophageal four-chamber view is acquired and then **(C)** the M-mode cursor is positioned along the plane of the TAPSE motion to obtain the M-mode image of this displacement **(D)**. The lower point corresponds to the maximal systolic excursion, and the upper point is the atrial contraction. **(E)** The TAPSE is equal to the total systolic displacement of the tricuspid annulus, which is normally higher that 17 mm. LA, left atrium; LV, left ventricle; RA, right atrium; RV, right ventricle. (From Denault AY, Vegas A, Lamarche Y, Tardif J-C, Couture P, eds. *Basic Transesophageal and Critical Care Ultrasound.* Taylor and Francis; 2018:74. Figure 5.13. © 2018 by CRC Press. Reproduced by permission of Taylor & Francis Group.)

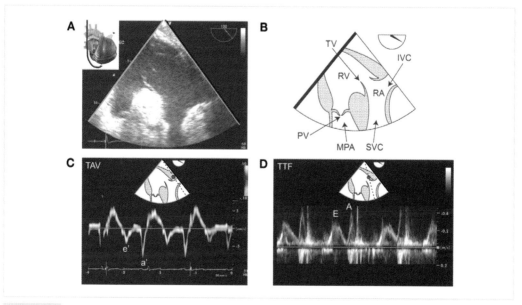

FIGURE 15.6 Tissue Doppler imaging (TDI). **(A, B)** Transgastric right ventricle (RV) inflow/outflow long-axis view can evaluate both the pulsed-wave Doppler interrogation of the tricuspid valve (TV) and TDI of the tricuspid annulus along the dotted line. **(C)** The TDI signal is obtained at the base of the tricuspid annulus and shows e' and a' waves. **(D)** Trans tricuspid flow (TTF) can be assessed using PW Doppler from this TG view to show E (early filling) and A (atrial contraction) waves. a', TDI peak late diastolic tricuspid annular velocity (TAV); e', TDI peak early diastolic TAV; IVC, inferior vena cava; MPA, main pulmonary artery; PV, pulmonic valve; RA, right atrium; SVC, superior vena cava. (From Denault AY, Vegas A, Lamarche Y, Tardif J-C, Couture P, eds. *Basic Transesophageal and Critical Care Ultrasound*. Taylor and Francis; 2018:206. Figure 12.3. © 2018 by CRC Press. Reproduced by permission of Taylor & Francis Group.)

correlation to RV stroke volume. In postoperative cardiac surgery patients, TDI S' suffers from the same shortcomings as TAPSE by only quantifying the longitudinal function and thereby fails to accurately depict RV stroke volume after CPB.[19]

c. **Right ventricular fractional area change:** RVFAC is defined as the percentage area change between end diastole and end systole. It is measured by tracing the endocardium excluding the trabeculae in end systole and end diastole. The normal value is >35%.[14] RVFAC has a good correlation with cardiac magnetic resonance imaging–derived RVEF.

d. **Strain and strain rate:** Strain is measured using either tissue Doppler or speckle tracking to measure local myocardial deformation (strain) or the rate of deformation (strain rate) through the cardiac cycle in both two-dimensional (2D) (Figure 15.1B; ⏺ **Video 15.5**) and three-dimensional (3D) echocardiography. The advantage of speckle tracking over tissue Doppler is that speckle tracking is angle independent, but the disadvantage is that speckle tracking requires good image quality and can be affected by image artifacts. The most common measure of RV strain in the literature is RV global longitudinal strain, which usually refers to the average strain value of either the free wall alone or both the free wall and septum.[15] The specific cutoff value for strain differs in different studies according to the software used. Strain is a load-dependent measure, whereas strain rate is a load-independent measure of systolic function. This is especially important considering the RV sensitivity to load changes.

e. **Right ventricular ejection fraction from three-dimensional echocardiography:** Because of the difficulties in assessing RV function, caused by its complex anatomy and contraction pattern, 3D echocardiography can overcome the limitations from 2D echocardiography. 3D echocardiography can measure RV end-diastolic volume and RV end-systolic volume and calculate RVEF and RV stroke volume from an RV-focused four-chamber view obtained with TTE or TEE. 3D RV echocardiography is still not as widely used as 2D echocardiography, most likely because it is more time-consuming and requires specific training. After cardiac surgery, 3D echocardiography more accurately tracks changes in stroke volume than 2D echocardiography when compared to PAC measurements.[19]

B. **Extracardiac Assessment of Right Heart Function**

RV dysfunction and failure are associated with hypoperfusion of various organs through venous congestion and arterial hypoperfusion.[20] RV dilatation increases pericardial pressure and reduces LV dimension through negative diastolic interaction. The increased leftward septal shift will increase LV end-diastolic pressure, left atrial pressure, and PAP, leading to an increase in RV afterload. In addition, leftward septal shift will reduce LV preload. Both the increase in RV afterload and decrease in LV preload will lead to a reduction in stroke volume, cardiac output, and arterial pressure. The increase in wall tension and RV end-diastolic pressure leads to decreased RV coronary blood flow and has the potential to induce subendocardial ischemia, which again can lead to RV ischemia, further reducing cardiac output. RV dilatation and dysfunction are associated with an increase in RAP and peripheral venous pressure. Elevated filling pressures of the right heart also cause coronary sinus congestion, which reduces coronary blood flow and can accentuate RV ischemia. The reduction in arterial pressure and increase in venous pressure from RV dysfunction tend to reduce the perfusion pressure of the brain, liver, kidneys, and intestines. Signs of venous congestion at different levels can be seen and quantified using bedside ultrasound and the venous excess ultrasound score (VExUS).[21,22] These venous Doppler signs are generated by an increase in RAP and consequently correlate with progressive RV dysfunction and failure that can be confirmed through analysis of the RAP and RV pressure waveforms[21,23] (Figure 15.3).

CLINICAL PEARL

After CPB, there is a shift in contraction pattern to a more radial contribution, which may resemble RV dysfunction on longitudinal measures without necessarily meaning a reduced RV output.

CLINICAL PEARL

Using echocardiography, venous Doppler flow alteration generated by an increase in RAP can be identified. These signs consequently correlate with progressive RV dysfunction that can be suspected through analysis of the RAP and RV pressure waveforms.

V. **Management of Right Ventricular Dysfunction**

A. **General Principles**

Successful management of acute RV dysfunction hinges on early recognition, addressing, and excluding reversible causes (coronary air embolism, outflow tract obstruction, acute ischemia, pulmonary embolism, etc) and providing supportive care until recovery. Supportive care involves maintenance of sinus rhythm and optimal mean arterial pressure (MAP) to ensure adequate coronary perfusion pressure in the first instance, followed by optimizing preload, usually requiring fluid removal, reducing RV afterload, and maintaining inotropy. If these measures fail, temporary RV mechanical circulatory support has advanced considerably in the past decade, with multiple percutaneous devices now on the market. Successful use, such as patient survival and eventual device explantation, relies on early recognition of the failure of medical management. Delayed recognition and implantation of mechanical circulatory support is still associated with high mortality due to irreversible end-organ dysfunction despite restoration of adequate hemodynamics.

B. **Preload**

1. **Principles of therapy:** Patients with RV decompensation are preload dependent. Inappropriate infusion of intravenous fluid to correct hypotension exacerbates RV dysfunction by

right-side chamber dilatation that increases wall tension, aggravates ventricular interdependence, impairs LV filling, and, ultimately, reduces cardiac output and myocardial perfusion; this further exacerbates the crisis. This pressure and volume overload of the RV manifests as right shift of the RV pressure-volume loop along the end-diastolic pressure-volume relationship and is frequently accompanied by depression of the RV end-systolic pressure-volume relationship (ie, depressed systolic function) (Figure 15.2C). Initial recognition of RV volume overload and management can be guided by both hemodynamic pressure waveform analysis and both cardiac and extracardiac echocardiographic parameters. Primary objective of RV volume overload management is displacement of venous capacitance volume away from the right heart.

2. **Loop diuretics:** Intravenous loop diuretics remain the mainstay of acute treatment in the intraoperative and acute care environments. Loop diuretics decrease right-sided pressures by facilitating natriuresis and diuresis, and acutely increasing venous capacitance—both actions lower RAP. Increase in venous capacitance is presumably prostaglandin mediated and requires intact kidneys. Intravenous dosing is highly individualized. Efficacy may be impaired by reductions in renal blood flow and glomerular filtration due to low cardiac output and venous congestion, or previous chronic kidney injury. The starting dose of furosemide should be determined by renal function and previous diuretic use. For patients with previous exposure to loop diuretics, previous chronic kidney disease, or marked renal congestion, higher doses may be needed. Repeated and increased dosing may be required if patient remains fluid overloaded with suboptimal diuretic response. Titrated, continuous infusion may be contemplated to reach the desired fluid balance.

3. **Ultrafiltration:** Early institution of ultrafiltration should be considered when there is a poor response to diuresis; persistently elevated RAP with signs of systemic venous congestion seen with, for example, ongoing portal venous pulsatility; and lack of clinical improvement. Ultrafiltration removes isotonic plasma water by machine generation of a gradient across a semipermeable membrane. It requires peripheral insertion of a hemodialysis catheter, which is associated with a certain risk of complications. It can also be done while the patient is on CPB. Ultrafiltration has the benefit of managing metabolic complications of cardiogenic shock, such as hyperkalemia, metabolic acidosis, and uremia. Rate of fluid removal may be limited by hemodynamic instability, which requires constant reassessment of volume status.

C. **Afterload**
1. **Principles of therapy:** Acute increases in RV afterload are caused by increased PVR due to chemical (ie, hypoxia, hypercapnia, acidemia, etc) or mechanical (ie, pulmonary embolism, excessive positive end-expiratory pressure (PEEP)) factors. It manifests as a right shift in RV E_a (Figure 15.2). This can be supported up to a point by the RV, after which depression of the end-systolic pressure-volume relationship and systolic function supervene. Reduction in RV afterload can be facilitated by vasodilation of the pulmonary circulation to encourage ventricular emptying and increase stroke volume.

2. **Mechanical ventilation:** Mechanical ventilation can be both harmful and beneficial in RV dysfunction. Increasing PEEP reduces venous return to the right heart and may reduce preload, whereas increasing tidal volume is linearly associated with increase in RV afterload. No mechanical ventilation strategy is necessarily superior due to competing physiologic priorities; PEEP and tidal volume should be manipulated to prevent overdistention, hypercapnia, and hypoxemia to avoid an increase in PVR.

3. **Pulmonary vasodilators:** Systemically administered pulmonary vasodilator therapies, such as epoprostenol and milrinone, are frequently associated with systemic vasodilation and hypotension. In addition, systemic epoprostenol is a potent platelet inhibitor. Loss of perfusion pressure from systemic hypotension that worsens RV ischemia, thereby worsening RV function and increasing V/Q mismatch, can be prevented by concomitantly starting vasopressors alongside, such as vasopressin or angiotensin-II (AT-II). Inhaled pulmonary vasodilator therapies are preferred to reduce PVR in RV dysfunction as they spare the systemic circulation. Inhaled agents such as NO and epoprostenol (prostaglandin I_2 or PGI_2)

should be used with caution in severe LV systolic dysfunction as the left heart may not be able to compensate for increased filling from the reduction in RV afterload. This will manifest as elevated left atrial pressure and acute pulmonary edema.

   a. **Inhaled nitric oxide:** Basal vasodilator tone in the pulmonary circulation is dependent on a constant supply of inhaled NO that induces localized pulmonary vasodilation, reduces RV afterload, and enhances V/Q matching. Systemic effects are limited due to rapid inactivation within red blood cells as its affinity for hemoglobin is 1,500-fold that of oxygen. Inhaled NO is normally delivered in a dose that ranges from 20 to 80 parts per million (ppm). The lowest effective dose to achieve the desired result should be used. Despite being rare in clinical practice, inhaled NO is contraindicated in patients with known methemoglobin reductase deficiency as NO oxidizes Fe^{2+} to Fe^{3+}, resulting in methemoglobinemia. Methemoglobin concentrations should thus be monitored during therapy.

   b. **Inhaled epoprostenol:** This analog of PGI_2 acts to reduce pulmonary vasomotor tone by inducing cyclic adenosine monophosphate (cAMP) and decreasing endothelin-1. It can theoretically inhibit platelets but has not been shown to increase the risk of bleeding complications after cardiac surgery when used as an inhaled therapy. Inhaled PGI_2 can be administered directly into the breathing circuit using an ultrasonic or vibrating mesh nebulizer after being reconstituted from a glycine diluent that may cause ventilator malfunction. In fact, heat and moisture exchanger filters should be attached to the proximal inspiratory and expiratory limbs in order to protect the anesthetic machine. Saturation of the filters by buffer solution may manifest as increased resistance to flow. The normal dose range for continuous therapy via nebulizer is 0.01-0.05 μg/kg/min. Intermittent therapy with dosage of 20-60 μg can be administered safely over 15 minutes to obtain RV afterload reduction with minimal systemic effects. Inhaled PGI_2 is less expensive than inhaled NO and has similar efficacy and outcome.

   c. **Inhaled milrinone:** This phosphodiesterase type III inhibitor is commonly used in its intravenous form for its inodilator capabilities. It works by preventing cAMP degradation, which leads to increase in Ca^{2+} influx and release from cell stores to increase cardiac output and promote smooth muscle relaxation. In total, 4-5 mg intermittent inhaled milrinone therapy can be administered over 20-30 minutes using a nebulizer, and this will isolate the effects to the pulmonary vasculature, reduce PVR, decrease RV afterload, and increase both LV and RV contractility without affecting systemic vascular resistance. It can also be administered directly into the tracheal tube in an emergency. The maximal effect takes place 20 minutes after initiation of the inhalation with a shorter interval when the tracheal route is chosen. Inhaled milrinone can be administered in combination with inhaled PGI_2, which increases the response rate up to 80% by acting on both afterload reduction and increase in contractility.[24]

D. **Contractility and Right Ventricular Perfusion**
   1. **Principles of therapy:** Impaired RV excitation-contraction coupling and decreased systolic function can be treated with inotropes. Poor systolic function depresses the RV end-systolic pressure-volume relation and is frequently accompanied by a right shift in the end-diastolic pressure-volume relation from volume overload (Figure 15.2). In general, β-agonists increase myocardial oxygen consumption and may worsen ischemia. These agents should be used in combination with RV afterload and preload reduction where appropriate. The failing RV is particularly vulnerable to ischemia. Maintenance of coronary perfusion pressure with vasopressors, targeting an MAP ≥ 65 mm Hg, even in low cardiac output state, while other measures are brought to bear, is vital to prevent further deterioration. Ideally, a combination of inotropes, vasopressors, and inhaled vasodilators should aim to improve RV-to-PA coupling, increase RV contractility, and decrease PVR, while minimizing decreases in systemic vascular resistances.

   2. **Inotropes**
      a. **Epinephrine** is a naturally occurring catecholamine and has α- and β-adrenoceptor agonist capabilities. Its pharmacodynamic effects vary according to dose; at low doses, β effects predominate to increase contractility, heart rate, myocardial oxygen demand,

and coronary vasodilation while reducing arrhythmia threshold. Doses can range from 0.01 to 0.5 µg/kg/min with adjustment to cardiac output optimization. It is rapidly reversible due to its short half-life of 2 minutes due to rapid metabolism within mitochondria, liver, kidneys, and blood.

  b. **Dobutamine** is a synthetic isoprenaline derivative that predominately has β_1 effects, leading to increased cardiac rate, contractility, and myocardial oxygen consumption. Doses can range from 0.5 to 20 µg/kg/min intravenously. It has a short half-life of 2 minutes and is metabolized by liver and excreted in urine.

  c. **Milrinone** is a phosphodiesterase type III inhibitor that works by prevention of cAMP degradation in smooth muscle and increases intracellular Ca^{2+} concentrations. This increases cardiac contractility and causes vasodilation in systemic and pulmonary vasculature. High loading and infusion doses frequently cause systemic hypotension that needs to be offset by vasopressors. Common loading dose ranges from 12.5 to 75 µg/kg over 10 minutes, whereas continuous infusion doses range between 0.125 and 0.75 µg/kg/min. Milrinone undergoes extensive plasma protein binding (70%) and has a half-life of 1-2.5 hours, which explains the extended duration of its effect after cessation. It is predominately (80%) excreted unchanged in the urine.

  d. **Levosimendan** sensitizes troponin, independent of Ca^{2+} and cAMP to increase contractility. As intracellular Ca^{2+} does not change, myocardial oxygen consumption is not increased. It also opens ATP-gated K^+ channels in smooth muscle to cause vasodilation. It may also increase the risk of atrial fibrillation. Dosing ranges from 6 to 12 µg/kg as a loading dose over 10 minutes, followed by 0.05-2 µg/kg/min. This drug is reduced to multiple active metabolites with a biological half-life of 1.5 hours. The active metabolites, and thus clinical effects, have an elimination half-life of 70-80 hours. It has not conferred a mortality benefit in several clinical trials but may be useful to avoid or wean from mechanical support.

3. **Vasopressors**
  a. **Norepinephrine** is a naturally occurring catecholamine and is both an α- and β-adrenoceptor agonist. Effects vary according to dose; at low doses, α_1 effects predominate with systemic and pulmonary vasoconstriction, decreased renal blood flow, and reflex bradycardia; thus, it is generally considered to be a vasopressor. The increased LV and RV afterload will increase myocardial work and oxygen consumption. Increased venous return is then a consequence of reduction in venous capacitance and attendant effective increase in stressed volume. Dosing generally ranges from 0.05 to 0.5 µg/kg/min intravenously to reach therapeutic goal. It undergoes similar metabolism to epinephrine within mitochondria, blood, kidney, and liver to inactive metabolites and then is excreted in the urine. Roughly, 25% is also taken up into lung tissue. It has a short half-life of 1-2 minutes.

  b. **Vasopressin** is a synthetic form of antidiuretic hormone. It acts on V_{1a}-receptors to cause vasoconstriction and V_2-receptors to cause increased free water absorption in the renal medullary collecting ducts. It is useful to offset vasodilation from systemic milrinone while reducing RV afterload, or to augment the effects of norepinephrine. Its dosing ranges from 0.01 to 0.04 units/min intravenously. It is metabolized in liver and kidney with minimal renal excretion. Its half-life is between 10 and 20 minutes. It is particularly useful for the management of RV dysfunction because of the relative paucity of V_1 receptors in the pulmonary circulation.

  c. **Angiotensin-II** is a synthetic form of the peptide hormone. It acts via G-protein–coupled type 1 AT-II receptors on smooth muscle to stimulate Ca^{2+}/calmodulin-dependent phosphorylation of myosin and smooth muscle contraction. Its dosing ranges from 1 to 40 ng/kg/min intravenously and may be higher in septic shock. It is converted to AT-III and AT-I in plasma, red blood cells, and visceral organs. Its half-life is under 1 minute. There are limited data available from cardiac surgical populations.

E. **Temporary Mechanical Support**
RV mechanical circulatory support acts by displacing volume from the RV into either the PA (RVAD) or the systemic circulation (veno-arterial extracorporeal membrane oxygenation

[VA-ECMO]). The RV pressure-volume loop is shifted to the left along the end-diastolic pressure-volume relationship, decreasing ventricular distension, myocardial work, and myocardial oxygen consumption. Reduction in RAP decreases venous congestion of the abdominal viscera and thus improves systemic perfusion pressure (MAP-RAP). Intra-aortic balloon counterpulsation is generally not recommended for RV failure as diastolic augmentation of coronary blood flow and reduction in afterload preferentially benefit the LV. However, some centers do occasionally place an IABP in order to improve RV perfusion, usually in the setting of a competent aortic valve but compromised LV function. Timing of mechanical support is crucial. If placed too early, the patient may be unnecessarily exposed to the surgical risks of implantation; if too late, the end-organ dysfunction may not be reversible. The decision to initiate mechanical circulatory support is usually based on ongoing or worsening biochemical and hemodynamic derangement despite optimal medical therapy. Development of transaminitis and/or an elevated international normalized ratio (INR) is particularly concerning. Decline in serum lactate over 6-8 hours, with or without ultrafiltration, after instituting mechanical circulatory support is associated with improved survival. All currently available devices require anticoagulation for institution of therapy (Table 15.1).

CLINICAL PEARL

Successful management of RV dysfunction begins with early recognition.

CLINICAL PEARL

Mechanical ventilation can be both beneficial and harmful for RV dysfunction. Recognize that hypoxia and hypercapnia both increase PVR, similar effects can be seen with increase in tidal volume.

CLINICAL PEARL

The use of inhaled pulmonary vasodilators in biventricular failure may precipitate pulmonary edema if LV dysfunction is undertreated.

CLINICAL PEARL

Late institution of mechanical circulatory support after multiorgan failure has supervened is associated with poor outcome. Treatment should be rapidly escalated if biochemical or clinical evidence of end-organ impairment becomes evident.

TABLE 15.1 Mechanical Circulatory Device Options in Right Ventricular Failure

Device	Device Characteristics				Hemodynamic Effects			
	Inflow	Outflow	Flow (LPM)	Oxygenator	RAP	MPAP	PCWP	SVR
Protek Duo	RA	PA	2-4	+	↓	↑	↑	↔
Impella RP	RA	PA	2-4	−	↓	↑	↑	↔
CentriMag RVAD	RA, RV	PA	≤10	+ or −	↓	↑	↑	↔
VA-ECMO	RA, FV	Ao, FA	2-6	+	↓	↔/↑	↓	↑↑

Ao, aorta; ECMO, extracorporeal membrane oxygenation; FA, femoral artery; FV, femoral vein; LPM, liters per minute; MPAP, mean pulmonary artery pressure; PA, pulmonary artery; PCWP, pulmonary artery capillary wedge pressure; RA, right atrium; RAP, right atrial pressure; RP, right percutaneous; RV, right ventricle; RVAD, right ventricular assist device; SVR, systemic vascular resistance; VA, veno-arterial.

VI. Summary

RV dysfunction and failure are associated with increased morbidity and mortality. Multimodal hemodynamic monitoring and echocardiography are essential diagnostic tools to quantify systolic and diastolic function and the impact of venous congestion using a multitude of cardiac and extracardiac parameters. RV failure leads to impaired LV filling that, in combination with elevated venous pressure, reduced cardiac output and reduced arterial pressure will lead to end-organ malperfusion. Following cardiac surgery, a decrease in longitudinal contraction and an increase in transverse RV contraction should be accounted for when choosing a modality to evaluate systolic function. The most important element in the management of RV dysfunction is to identify the etiology and correct it as soon as possible. Treatment of RV dysfunction should be based on the maintenance of end-organ perfusion pressure, improved atrioventricular synchrony, RV afterload reduction and preload optimization, and increased RV contractility.

REFERENCES

1. Jabagi H, Nantsios A, Ruel M, et al. A standardized definition for right ventricular failure in cardiac surgery patients. *ESC Heart Fail.* 2022;9:1542-1552.
2. Denault A, Haddad F, Lamarche Y, et al. Postoperative right ventricular dysfunction—integrating right heart profiles beyond long-axis function. *J Thorac Cardiovasc Surg.* 2020;159:e315-e317.
3. Lahm T, Douglas IS, Archer SL, et al. Assessment of right ventricular function in the research setting: knowledge gaps and pathways forward. An Official American Thoracic Society Research Statement. *Am J Respir Crit Care Med.* 2018;198:e15-e43.
4. Harjola VP, Mebazaa A, Celutkiene J, et al. Contemporary management of acute right ventricular failure: a statement from the Heart Failure Association and the Working Group on pulmonary circulation and right ventricular function of the European Society of Cardiology. *Eur J Heart Fail.* 2016;18:226-241.
5. Vonk Noordegraaf A, Westerhof BE, Westerhof N. The relationship between the right ventricle and its load in pulmonary hypertension. *J Am Coll Cardiol.* 2017;69:236-243.
6. Bellofiore A, Chesler NC. Methods for measuring right ventricular function and hemodynamic coupling with the pulmonary vasculature. *Ann Biomed Eng.* 2013;41:1384-1398.
7. Vonk-Noordegraaf A, Haddad F, Chin KM, et al. Right heart adaptation to pulmonary arterial hypertension: physiology and pathobiology. *J Am Coll Cardiol.* 2013;62:D22-D33.
8. Saxena A, Garan AR, Kapur NK, et al. Value of hemodynamic monitoring in patients with cardiogenic shock undergoing mechanical circulatory support. *Circulation.* 2020;141:1184-1197.
9. Bootsma IT, Boerma EC, Scheeren TWL, et al. The contemporary pulmonary artery catheter. Part 2: measurements, limitations, and clinical applications. *J Clin Monit Comput.* 2022;36:17-31.
10. Bootsma IT, Boerma EC, de Lange F, et al. The contemporary pulmonary artery catheter. Part 1: placement and waveform analysis. *J Clin Monit Comput.* 2022;36:5-15.
11. Garan AR, Kanwar M, Thayer KL, et al. Complete hemodynamic profiling with pulmonary artery catheters in cardiogenic shock is associated with lower in-hospital mortality. *JACC Heart Fail.* 2020;8:903-913.
12. Raymond M, Gronlykke L, Couture EJ, et al. Perioperative right ventricular pressure monitoring in cardiac surgery. *J Cardiothorac Vasc Anesth.* 2019;33:1090-1104.
13. Grønlykke L, Couture EJ, Haddad F, et al. Preliminary experience using diastolic right ventricular pressure gradient monitoring in cardiac surgery. *J Cardiothorac Vasc Anesth.* 2020;34:2116-2125.
14. Rudski LG, Lai WW, Afilalo J, et al. Guidelines for the echocardiographic assessment of the right heart in adults: a report from the American Society of Echocardiography endorsed by the European Association of Echocardiography, a registered branch of the European Society of Cardiology, and the Canadian Society of Echocardiography. *J Am Soc Echocardiogr.* 2010;23:685-713; quiz 786-788.
15. Lang RM, Badano LP, Mor-Avi V, et al. Recommendations for cardiac chamber quantification by echocardiography in adults: an update from the American Society of Echocardiography and the European Association of Cardiovascular Imaging. *J Am Soc Echocardiogr.* 2015;28:1-39.e14.
16. Haddad F, Couture P, Tousignant C, et al. The right ventricle in cardiac surgery, a perioperative perspective: I. Anatomy, physiology, and assessment. *Anesth Analg.* 2009;108:407-421.
17. Gronlykke L, Ihlemann N, Ngo AT, et al. Measures of right ventricular function after transcatheter versus surgical aortic valve replacement. *Interact Cardiovasc Thorac Surg.* 2017;24:181-187.
18. Raina A, Vaidya A, Gertz ZM, et al. Marked changes in right ventricular contractile pattern after cardiothoracic surgery: implications for post-surgical assessment of right ventricular function. *J Heart Lung Transplant.* 2013;32:777-783.
19. Gronlykke L, Korshin A, Holmgaard F, et al. Severe loss of right ventricular longitudinal contraction occurs after cardiopulmonary bypass in patients with preserved right ventricular output. *Int J Cardiovasc Imaging.* 2019;35:1661-1670.
20. Konstam MA, Kiernan MS, Bernstein D, et al. Evaluation and management of right-sided heart failure: a scientific statement from the American Heart Association. *Circulation.* 2018;137:e578-e622.

21. Couture EJ, Grønlykke L, Denault AY. New developments in the understanding of right ventricular function in acute care. *Curr Opin Crit Care*. 2022;28:331-339.

22. Beaubien-Souligny W, Rola P, Haycock K, et al. Quantifying systemic congestion with point-of-care ultrasound: development of the venous excess ultrasound grading system. *Ultrasound J*. 2020;12:16.

23. Deschamps J, Denault A, Galarza L, et al. Venous Doppler to assess congestion: a comprehensive review of current evidence and nomenclature. *Ultrasound Med Biol*. 2023;49:3-17.

24. Elmi-Sarabi M, Jarry S, Couture EJ, et al. Pulmonary vasodilator response of combined inhaled epoprostenol and inhaled milrinone in cardiac surgical patients. *Anesth Analg*. 2022;136:282-294. doi:10.1213/ANE.0000000000006192

Anesthetic Considerations for Surgical Myectomy in Patients With Hypertrophic Cardiomyopathy

Elena Ashikhmina Swan, Jeffrey B. Geske, and Hartzell V. Schaff

KEY POINTS

1. Obstructive hypertrophic cardiomyopathy (HCM) is manifested by fatigue, dyspnea, chest pain, and syncope exacerbated by dynamic obstruction of the left ventricular outflow tract or left ventricular cavity, systolic anterior motion of the mitral valve, mitral regurgitation, diastolic dysfunction, and postcapillary pulmonary hypertension.

2. Transaortic septal myectomy, or a combination of transaortic and apical myectomy depending on the distribution of myocardial hypertrophy is indicated for patients with limiting symptoms despite medical treatment.

3. The anesthetic management of surgical myectomy for HCM is often challenging. Pronounced hemodynamic swings precipitating low cardiac output related to decreased systemic vascular resistance and worsening of outflow obstruction due to sympathetic stimulation should be anticipated and avoided by careful selection of anesthetic and analgesic agents. Their potential side effects should be mitigated by vasopressors and volume administration.

4. Intraoperative direct left ventricle (LV) to aorta gradient monitoring with simultaneous transesophageal echocardiography to assess the degree of the LV outflow obstruction and MR is key for successful myectomy. It may be necessary to resume cardiopulmonary bypass for additional myectomy if residual gradient of >25 mm Hg is present.

5. Surgical myectomy for HCM is commonly a relatively short procedure with cardiopulmonary bypass time averaging <45 minutes. Patients usually do not require inotropic support. Fast-track recovery pathway should be considered.

I. Introduction

Hypertrophic cardiomyopathy (HCM) is the most common genetic cardiac disease, with a prevalence of 1 in 200-500 adults.[1,2] It is defined as left ventricular (LV) hypertrophy without an underlying cause, such as systemic hypertension or valvular aortic stenosis.[3] In the obstructive form of HCM, a combination of septal hypertrophy and abnormal systolic anterior motion (SAM) of the mitral valve produce left ventricular outflow tract (LVOT) obstruction and mitral valve regurgitation (MR). The distribution of LV hypertrophy is variable in patients with HCM, and in some patients, it is more prominent at the mid-ventricular or apical level.[4]

343

LVOT obstruction is common in HCM and frequently is a driver of symptoms. Transaortic septal myectomy is most often indicated in patients with obstructive HCM who continue to have limiting symptoms despite medical treatment (ie, β-blockade, calcium antagonists, disopyramide, mavacamten). The anesthetic management of surgical myectomy for HCM may be challenging due to labile loading conditions leading to blood pressure swings. This chapter reviews the physiologic implications of HCM and the practical approach to the perioperative management of these patients.

II. Hypertrophic Cardiomyopathy

A. Epidemiology, Morphology, Histopathology, Genetics

1. Epidemiology

Epidemiologic studies indicate that HCM affects ~600,000-700,000 individuals in the United States alone; many people, such as asymptomatic family members, remain undiagnosed; therefore, the true prevalence of HCM in the general population might be underestimated. HCM is a global disease, particularly prevalent in Asia (China and Japan), Western Europe, and North America.[5]

2. Morphology

Asymmetric septal hypertrophy is the most common form of HCM, often manifesting with a sigmoid septum, wherein the basal interventricular septum is the thickest opposite to the anterior leaflet of the mitral valve in its open position. This results in subaortic obstruction, which may be limited to the immediate subaortic area (Figures 16.1B, 16.2A) or may extend

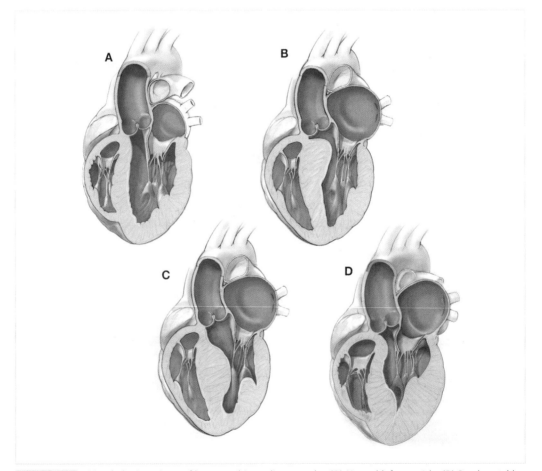

FIGURE 16.1 Morphologic variants of hypertrophic cardiomyopathy. **(A)** Normal left ventricle. **(B)** Basal septal hypertrophy. **(C)** Midventricular septal hypertrophy. **(D)** Apical hypertrophy. (From Kotkar KD, Said SM, Dearani JA, Schaff HV. Hypertrophic obstructive cardiomyopathy: the Mayo Clinic experience. *Ann Cardiothorac Surg.* 2017;6(4):329-336. Figure 1. Used with permission of Mayo Foundation for Medical Education and Research. All rights reserved.)

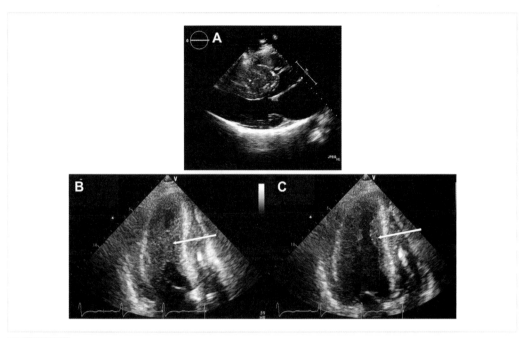

FIGURE 16.2 Transthoracic echocardiography demonstrates different variants of myocardial hypertrophy distribution. **(A)** Massive basal interventricular septal hypertrophy. **(B)** Arrow points to near obliteration of left ventricular cavity in patient with midventricular HCM in systole. **(C)** Arrow points to near obliteration of left ventricular cavity in patient with midventricular HCM in diastole. HCM, hypertrophic cardiomyopathy.

to the mid-ventricle (Figures 16.1C, 16.2B, C). Hypertrophy of the free wall of the LV is variable. There may be isolated obstruction in the mid-ventricle where hypertrophy of the septum leads to contact with the papillary muscles, producing obstruction to the ejection of blood; in other patients, there may be an apical distribution of hypertrophy (Figure 16.1D). The HCM phenotype and severity of hypertrophy do not correlate with the genotype. Indeed, multiple ventricular morphologic appearances may be found in the same family.

In obstructive HCM, as blood is ejected through a narrow LVOT with high velocity, turbulent flow results in a drag force effect on the mitral valve, resulting in systolic anterior mitral apparatus movement into LVOT, further narrowing the LVOT (Figure 16.3A). Displacement of the valve leaflets in systole, described as SAM, may lead to variable degrees of MR (Figure 16.3A, B). The MR jet is typically, but not always, directed posteriorly.[4] It is important to recognize that LVOT obstruction is often dynamic, and provocative maneuvers, such as Valsalva, repetitive squat-to-stand exercise, and adrenergic stimulation, may be necessary to elicit SAM, MR, and LVOT obstruction.[6]

3. **Histopathology**

Myocyte hypertrophy, myocardial disarray, and interstitial fibrosis are histopathologic findings that are characteristic of, but not specific to, HCM. Myocardial disarray may be present in any condition with ventricular pressure overload.[7] Interstitial fibrosis of variable degrees is another important histologic feature of the myocardium of patients with HCM[8] that contributes to diastolic dysfunction. Late gadolinium enhancement on cardiac magnetic resonance imaging (MRI) provides assessment of myocardial fibrosis burden, associated with an increased risk of sudden death.[9]

4. **Genetics**

The disorder of the cardiac muscle in HCM is caused by autosomal dominant mutations in one of several genes encoding both the thin and thick myofilaments of the sarcomere as well as nonsarcomeric proteins. The most common mutation involves the gene encoding cardiac myosin–binding protein C; however, there is considerable genetic heterogeneity, and at least 15 other genes have been identified with >1,000 distinct mutations.[10]

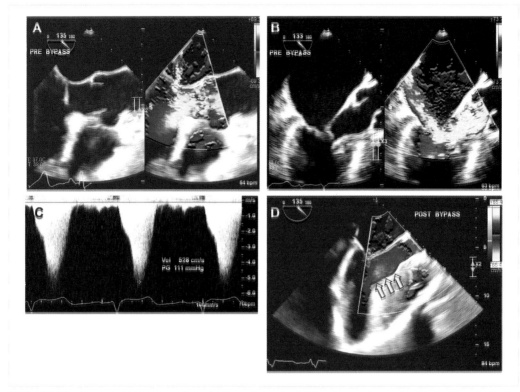

FIGURE 16.3   Intraoperative transesophageal echocardiography. **(A)** Systolic anterior motion (SAM) of the mitral valve into left ventricular outflow tract causing mitral insufficiency. **(B)** SAM and severe mitral regurgitation with posteriorly directed jet. **(C)** High-velocity, late peaking, "dagger-shaped" continuous-wave Doppler signal demonstrating an obstruction of left ventricular outflow tract. **(D)** Postoperative result demonstrating normal laminal flow in left ventricular outflow tract and interventricular septum post myectomy (yellow arrows).

The familial form comprises ~60%-80% of the HCM population, but patients who develop HCM sporadically with de novo mutations in genes have similar characteristics as those with the familial form of HCM.[11]

Genetic testing is available clinically; however, only approximately 34% of patients with HCM might have an identifiable gene mutation. In addition to finding pathogenic mutations, a significant proportion of patients will have a variant of uncertain significance.[12] The relationship between a specific mutation and clinical outcome or prognosis has yet to be established.[13] Thus, the clinical use of genetic testing is confined mainly to screening at-risk phenotype-negative family members of a patient with definitive HCM.

CLINICAL PEARL

Phenotypical features of HCM and severity of hypertrophy cannot be inferred from the genotype. Genetic testing is available clinically; however, only about one-third of patients with HCM will have an identifiable gene mutation. The disorganized whirling of muscle fibers and myocardial disarray are characteristics, but not specific, of HCM. Late gadolinium enhancement suggesting myocardial fibrosis on cardiac MRI has been associated with an increased risk of sudden cardiac death.

B. **Pathophysiology**

Patients with HCM have diastolic dysfunction driven by reduced LV compliance due to LV hypertrophy and fibrosis. This results in increased left atrial and pulmonary venous pressures, which contribute to dyspnea on exertion and limited aerobic capacity. LVOT obstruction lengthens ejection time and reduces LV stroke volume. With worsening LVOT obstruction and diastolic dysfunction, LV filling becomes more dependent on atrial contraction. Atrial arrhythmias, especially atrial fibrillation (AF), may cause an acute decrease in cardiac output and exacerbation of symptoms.

Dynamic LVOT obstruction is an important cause of symptoms in ~70% of patients with HCM. Accelerated blood flow near the hypertrophied basal septum leads to SAM of the mitral valve. Thus, leaflet coaptation is reduced, producing variable degrees of MR characteristically directed posteriorly (Figure 16.3A, B). An anteriorly directed color jet on Doppler echocardiography should raise the possibility of primary mitral valve diseases, such as a flail or prolapsing segment. MR is an important pathophysiologic component of HCM that contributes to the symptoms of dyspnea and fatigue.

C. **Clinical Presentation and Diagnosis**

The clinical course of HCM is variable, but the onset of symptoms (dyspnea, fatigue, chest pain, syncope) often correlates with the development of LVOT obstruction, an independent predictor of heart failure, stroke and death. It is uncertain why initially asymptomatic patients without obstruction may develop obstruction in adulthood. AF occurs in nearly one in five patients with HCM, and the onset of AF can precipitate symptoms and predispose to systemic thromboembolism.[14] Infective endocarditis rarely occurs with HCM, with a reported incidence of 1.4 cases per 1,000 person-years.[15]

1. **Echocardiography**

   Two-dimensional and Doppler transthoracic echocardiography (TTE) is the primary imaging modality for diagnosing HCM, providing information on ventricular morphology, hemodynamics, and valve function. 15 mm septal wall thickness is a commonly used threshold for the diagnosis of HCM. In 5-10% of patients, LV wall thickness is massively increased, measuring >30 mm (up to 50 mm). Morphology of the septum varies, with the most common being the sigmoid configuration (Figure 16.1B). On continuous-wave Doppler echocardiography, LVOT obstruction is seen as a high-velocity, late peaking, "dagger-shaped" signal (Figure 16.3C). In patients with a low velocity at rest (<3 m/s), Valsalva maneuver (decreases venous return), squat-to-stand (decreases preload and afterload), inhalation of amyl nitrite (vasodilator), exercise or isoproterenol administration (vasodilation and tachycardia) may unveil latent obstruction. The presence and severity of MR can be determined by Doppler color-flow imaging. It is essential to differentiate the true outflow tract velocity from the MR jet, which can be challenging given spatial proximity and similar timing. MR that results from SAM is eccentric and classically directed posterolaterally during late systole (Figure 16.3B). A centrally or anteriorly directed jet should raise suspicion of a primary leaflet abnormality. Outpatient preoperative transesophageal echocardiography (TEE) is unnecessary in most patients, but TEE is important in assessing the extent of hypertrophy and the results of myectomy in the operating room.

2. **Cardiac magnetic resonance imaging**

   Cardiac MRI is synergistic with echocardiographic imaging. Cardiac MRI helps identify regions of LV hypertrophy not easily recognized by TTE, like the anterolateral free wall and the apex. A unique feature of cardiac MRI is the ability to detect the presence, distribution, and severity of late gadolinium enhancement (myocardial fibrosis), which can play a role in sudden cardiac death risk stratification.

3. **Cardiac catheterization**

   In current practice, cardiac catheterization is rarely necessary to diagnose HCM. Coronary angiography is indicated for patients with symptoms of angina and in patients at risk for coronary artery disease (CAD) who undergo myectomy. A hemodynamic study with isoproterenol provocation can help identify patients with occult labile obstruction that cannot be elicited during echocardiography.

CLINICAL PEARL

The development of dynamic LVOT obstruction, MR, and/or diastolic dysfunction frequently precipitates fatigue, dyspnea, and syncope in HCM.

D. Natural History

In contemporary series of HCM, survival is similar to individuals without disease with an annual mortality rate of ~1%. However, certain subgroups have an increased risk of cardiac death. The greatest risk factor for sudden death is a personal history of prior cardiac arrest or sustained ventricular tachycardia. Other major risk factors include a family history of sudden death due to HCM, massive ventricular hypertrophy (wall thickness >30 mm), unexplained syncope, LV systolic dysfunction (ejection fraction <50%), and apical aneurysm. Both non-sustained ventricular tachycardia on ambulatory monitoring and extensive late gadolinium enhancement on cardiac MRI may also portend arrhythmogenic risk.[16]

An implantable cardioverter-defibrillator (ICD) is strongly recommended for secondary prevention of sudden cardiac death in patients with prior cardiac arrest or sustained ventricular tachycardia. Although primary prevention risk stratification can be complex, an ICD should be considered in patients with a major risk factor.

E. Surgical Treatment

Septal myectomy is indicated for patients with limiting symptoms despite medical treatment. Surgical treatment of HCM was introduced at Mayo Clinic in 1958 by J. Kirklin, who described a simple myotomy without actual muscle resection. Surgical management further evolved and has been replaced by the more predictable and complete transaortic extended myectomy.[17] Operation is performed through a median sternotomy utilizing normothermic cardiopulmonary bypass established with a single, two-stage venous cannula. After aortic cross-clamping, cold blood cardioplegia (1,000-1,200 mL) is infused through the aortic needle vent to arrest the heart. An oblique aortotomy is made slightly closer to the sinotubular ridge than is usual for aortic valve replacement, and the incision is carried through the midpoint of the noncoronary aortic sinus of Valsalva to a level ~1 cm above the valve annulus. Exposure of the distal septum can be improved by depressing the right ventricle to rotate the septum posteriorly. The incision in the septum begins just to the right of the nadir of the right aortic sinus and continues upward and to the left to a point near the attachment of the anterior leaflet of the mitral valve. Scissors are used to complete the excision of this initial portion of the myocardium. The area of septal excision is then deepened and lengthened toward the apex to remove hypertrophied septum beyond the endocardial scar. A typical septal myectomy usually yields 3-12 g of muscle.

In some patients with apical HCM, the small volume of LV cavity impairs ventricular filling, causing progressive diastolic heart failure. Such patients respond poorly to medical therapy. For most, cardiac transplantation has been the only surgical option. However, apical myectomy can enlarge the LV cavity and improve stroke volume (Figure 16.4). At operation with cardioplegic arrest, the apex of the heart is delivered anteriorly, and a left ventriculotomy is made lateral and parallel to the left anterior descending coronary artery. Hypertrophied muscle from the septum is excised with special care to avoid injury to the papillary muscles, and, if greatly hypertrophied, the papillary muscles may be shaved to further increase LV volume. The myectomy is extended proximally, beyond the midventricular level. If an apical aneurysm is present, the outpouching is resected completely. The ventriculotomy is closed using a two-layer approximation over strips of Teflon felt. Survival of patients following apical myectomy is similar to those who received heart transplants for apical HCM and better than those on the waiting list for transplant. In addition to improved survival, 76% of patients had significant improvements in functional capacity.[18]

Both operative mortality and complications, such as complete heart block, iatrogenic ventricular septal defect, injury to aortic and mitral valves, and incomplete relief of obstruction, are related to the surgical team's experience. In a nationwide survey, overall perioperative mortality following septal myectomy was 2.6%, but only 0.9% in centers

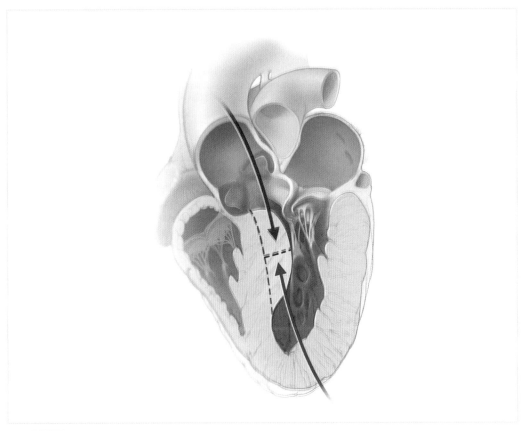

FIGURE 16.4 Complex long-segment septal hypertrophy may require both a transaortic approach (red arrow) and transapical approach (blue arrow). (From Hang D, Schaff HV, Ommen SR, Dearani JA, Nishimura RA. Combined trans-aortic and transapical approach to septal myectomy in patients with complex hypertrophic cardiomyopathy. *J Thorac Cardiovasc Surg*. 2018;155(5):2096-2102. Figure 2. Used with permission of Mayo Foundation for Medical Education and Research. All rights reserved.)

performing >10 procedures per year. And in multivariable analysis, the lowest annual case volume (average <1 case per year) was associated with greater early mortality (odds ratio [OR] 5.4, $P < .001$), greater risk of ventricular septal defects (OR 9.3, $P < .001$), increased incidence of complete heart block (OR 2.0, $P < .001$), and a higher likelihood of mitral valve replacement (OR 9.4, $P < .001$).[19]

III. Anesthetic Considerations

A. Preoperative Encounter

Patients are usually admitted to the hospital in the morning of surgery. At the time of their preoperative appointment, a few days before the surgical date, they should be instructed not to skip their morning β-blocker or calcium channel blocker dose. Adequate hydration, even in the morning of surgery with clear liquids, is permitted and encouraged up until 2 hours before anesthesia[20] Some patients will have automatic ICD with pacing capabilities in place. These devices should be interrogated, and antitachycardia therapy should be disabled. If this is not feasible, placing a magnet over the ICD will disable the antitachycardia functionality and eliminate the risk of internal defibrillation related to the use of cautery. If the patient is pacemaker dependent, the device should be switched to asynchronous mode as needed. Of note, faster than usual heart rate might worsen LVOT obstruction. Patients should be monitored after pacemaker settings changes. Heart rate might have to be adjusted if non-invasive blood pressure decreases from baseline or there are other signs of systemic hypoperfusion. After peripheral intravenous (IV) is inserted, it is reasonable to start IV fluids in the preoperative area at a maintenance rate. Many patients undergoing surgical myectomy are young and nervous, and anxiolytic such as midazolam 1-2 mg IV should be offered. However, anxiolysis can downregulate catecholamine excess and provoke hypotension, exacerbating LVOT obstruction, so careful monitoring after premedication is recommended. Preinduction arterial line placement should be performed for patients with particularly severe LVOT gradients, severe pulmonary hypertension, and a history of arrhythmias.

B. **Intraoperative Management**

1. **General considerations**

Surgical myectomy for HCM is usually a relatively short procedure, with cardiopulmonary bypass time <45 minutes. Patients with HCM can exhibit swings in blood pressure in response to anesthetic agents, positioning, and surgical stimulation. Thus, emergency drugs, such as phenylephrine, vasopressin, and esmolol should be available to use. Goals of intraoperative management include maintenance of LV preload and afterload, avoidance of tachycardia, and suppression of myocardial hypercontractility as needed.

Ultimately, whatever mix of anesthetics and analgesics is selected, it should be tailored to enhance preload and afterload and only result in a mild decrease in contractility. Inhalation anesthetics reduce myocardial contractility and potentially could reduce dynamic LVOT gradient, but these agents may also reduce peripheral vascular resistance, which, conversely, might increase the dynamic LVOT outflow gradient. The net effect would depend on the relative balance between these two effects and would be influenced by the use of vasopressors to offset the vasodilatory effect of volatile agents. Preoperative fasting and relative hypovolemia, typically offset by the infusion of fluids, are among other factors that might affect the venous return and change cardiac chamber dimensions compared to preoperative measurements. These processes reduce cardiac output and might shift the equilibrium between "forward" cardiac output and SAM-related MR. Autologous perioperative blood collection in patients with HCM is not routinely performed as it can cause intravascular volume shifts, which are poorly tolerated. Commonly used narcotics such as fentanyl and sufentanil have vagotonic effects that will reduce heart rate, increase diastolic time, and improve LV filling.

2. **Induction and maintenance of anesthesia**

A commonly used technique is balanced IV induction with fentanyl 1-2 μg/kg, ketamine 1 mg/kg, propofol 0.5-1 mg/kg, and rocuronium 1-1.2 mg/kg. A bolus of phenylephrine 50-100 μg/kg is usually administered with the induction drugs to prevent an acute drop in systemic vascular resistance and hypotension. After endotracheal intubation, anesthesia is maintained with 1 MAC (minimum alveolar concentration) of isoflurane.

3. **Separation from cardiopulmonary bypass**

Typically, patients with HCM separate from cardiopulmonary bypass without difficulty. However, it is important to vent the LV of air before separation from bypass. Transient right ventricular dysfunction can occur from air bubbles entering right coronary artery located superiorly. Full cardiopulmonary bypass support or partial bypass with higher mean arterial pressure can drive air out of coronary circulation and restore contractility. Inotropic support is usually not required. Once hemodynamic conditions have stabilized, TEE should be performed to confirm normalization of ventricular function. An augmentation of systemic vascular resistance with boluses of phenylephrine and/or ephedrine helps to separate from bypass. Care should be taken to return blood from the cardiopulmonary bypass to provide adequate preload so that the assessment of residual gradients and MR is performed in the state as close as possible to the physiologic conditions with normal arterial and central venous pressures. Post-bypass TEE should rule out potential iatrogenic complications (including ventricular septal defect and aortic valve injury), and the mitral valve should be assessed to determine whether SAM is still present as well as the severity of residual MR. TEE should also confirm the absence of turbulent flow in LVOT (Figure 16.3D), with care taken to assess both the LVOT and the mid-LV for the presence of obstruction. It is prudent to remeasure the gradient (or rather its absence) between the aorta and the LV to confirm surgical success. While some patients have elevated pulmonary pressures typically related to postcapillary pulmonary hypertension, we rarely initiate milrinone intraoperatively because it can decrease systemic vascular resistance and exacerbate SAM. Post-cardiopulmonary bypass coagulopathy is uncommon, and blood product transfusion is rarely required.

CLINICAL PEARL

Goals of intraoperative management include maintenance of LV preload and afterload, avoidance of tachycardia, and suppression of myocardial hypercontractility as needed. Hemodynamic swings in response to anesthesia and surgery are not uncommon. Emergency drugs, such as phenylephrine, vasopressin, esmolol, and calcium chloride should be ready to use. Careful de-airing is recommended before separation from bypass.

C. **Intraoperative Monitoring**

In addition to standard monitors recommended by the American Society of Anesthesiology, invasive blood pressure monitoring and central venous access are required. A pulmonary artery catheter allows an assessment of pulmonary artery pressure, which is frequently elevated. Many patients have decreased cardiac output at baseline; both parameters are expected to improve after a successful myectomy.

TTE and TEE are essential in identifying the distribution of LV hypertrophy, MR and LVOT gradient severity, mitral valve anatomy, and the presence of SAM (Figures 16.2, 16.3). TEE imaging should be performed preceding cardiopulmonary bypass in all cases. At some centers, direct needle measurements of the gradient between the LV and the aorta are checked before and after cardiopulmonary bypass to assess the adequacy of relief of LVOT obstruction. Of note, it is not uncommon to observe some discrepancy in hemodynamic values characterizing LVOT obstruction preoperatively and in the operating room under general anesthesia.[21] Before the institution of cardiopulmonary bypass, a 2.5-inch, 22-G spinal needle is inserted into the aorta near the inflow cannula, and a 3.5-inch, 22-G spinal needle is inserted through the right ventricle and septum into the LV (Figure 16.5A). Simultaneous pressures at both locations are measured to calculate the gradient. The surgeon then induces a premature ventricular contraction by gently tapping the heart to accentuate any transaortic gradient, the Brockenbrough-Braunwald-Morrow response (Figure 16.5B).[22,23] In some patients, we use a bolus of isoproterenol 4-12 µg IV to unmask a latent gradient. It is useful to have IV esmolol

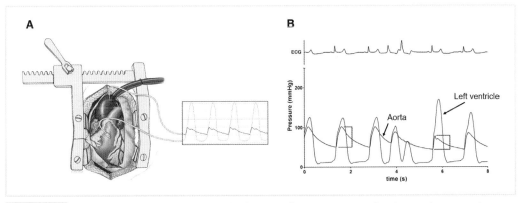

FIGURE 16.5 Intracavitary gradients determined by direct needle measurements of peak-to-peak pressures between the aorta and the left ventricle. **(A)** Positioning of the needles in left ventricle and aorta. **(B)** Arterial and left ventricular pressure tracing. Note two important changes after induced premature ventricular contraction: a decline in a pulse pressure on arterial pressure tracing and increase in a gradient between the left ventricle and the aorta. (Used with permission of Mayo Foundation for Medical Education and Research. All rights reserved.)

available to stabilize the hemodynamics by slowing the heart rate down after the isoproterenol test is completed. Baseline and stimulated gradient measurements are repeated after cardiopulmonary bypass discontinuation to assess a relief of obstruction. Cardiopulmonary bypass should be resumed to remove additional septal muscle if the maximal residual LVOT gradient exceeds 25-30 mm Hg.

D. Early Postoperative Care

The majority of patients with HCM are eligible for fast-track recovery. For postoperative pain control, bilateral pecto-intercostal facial plane blocks can be performed after chest closure utilizing 0.25% bupivacaine 0.5-1 mL/kg. Patients with uncomplicated intraoperative courses are usually extubated within 2-4 hours after intensive care unit (ICU) admission. Patients with no significant comorbidities and smooth intraoperative course can be extubated in the operating room.

IV. Surgical Subgroups and Anesthetic Considerations

A. Apical Myectomy

In a subset of patients with HCM, hypertrophy is primarily localized at the apex of the LV. These patients can have progressive, drug-refractory diastolic heart failure with limiting symptoms related to low cardiac output, even absent left ventricular obstruction. Previously heart transplantation was the only surgical therapy available for such patients. Apical myectomy to enlarge the LV cavity and improve diastolic dysfunction is now one of the therapeutic options for symptomatic patients with HCM.[24] The ventricle is opened at the apex, and excessive muscle is excised during this procedure. In contrast to patients having transaortic septal myectomy for subaortic obstruction, patients with apical HCM undergoing ventricular enlargement by apical myectomy usually require low-dose inotropic support (epinephrine 0.03 μg/kg/min) during discontinuation of cardiopulmonary bypass. Unlike patients with cardiomyopathy due to systolic dysfunction who are managed with afterload reduction, patients with apical HCM require normal or slightly higher than normal peripheral resistance both before and after the operation.

CLINICAL PEARL

Patients undergoing apical myectomy might require inotropic support after cardiopulmonary bypass because of ventriculotomy.

B. Pulmonary Hypertension

Some degree of pulmonary hypertension is present in ~50% of patients undergoing septal myectomy, and almost 15% have moderate-to-severe pulmonary hypertension (systolic pulmonary artery pressure ≥50 mm Hg). Preoperative pulmonary hypertension is independently associated with late mortality following septal myectomy.[25] Intraoperatively, pulmonary pressure is monitored with pulmonary artery catheter, and elevated pulmonary artery pressure is expected to improve following relief of LVOT obstruction; post-bypass use of pulmonary inodilator milrinone or inhaled nitric oxide is uncommon.

C. Hypertrophic Cardiomyopathy in Children

HCM is a common genetic disorder in adults; it is often well tolerated in pediatric populations, which may reduce the rates of pediatric diagnosis.[26] Similar to adult patients, presentation in early childhood is usually associated with dynamic LVOT obstruction and various degrees of MR related to SAM. Children often appear less symptomatic than adults, possibly because their activities are self-limited. However, the progression of LV hypertrophy may be more rapid in children than in adults. Further, the reported incidence of sudden cardiac death in children with HCM may be as high as 6% compared to 1%-3% in adults. Surgical myectomy should be considered for symptomatic children when the resting or provoked LVOT gradient is >50 mm Hg. Surgery may also be advised in children who are asymptomatic or mildly symptomatic with high gradients of between 75 and 100 mm Hg at rest or when there is severe concomitant MR.

Although the operation is technically more challenging in children because of the difficulty of exposure of the smaller structures, there is a role for surgery in the pediatric group with similarly acceptably low-risk and good late results. Late survival after myectomy is improved compared to the natural history of this disease without surgery. Anesthetic management of surgical myectomy for HCM in children, particularly induction of general anesthesia, is more challenging than in adults. Preoperative hydration is essential. Some experts recommend admission of children to the hospital for IV hydration before the day of surgery. Placement of preinduction arterial lines in children is seldomly possible. Also, inhalation induction with a higher dose of volatile agent common in pediatric practice might compromise cardiac output due to decreased systemic vascular resistance and exacerbation of LVOT obstruction. Larger doses of oral premedication (midazolam 0.5-1 mg/kg, ketamine 3-5 mg/kg) may help before induction. IV induction is utilized when peripheral IV can be placed without upsetting the child. Otherwise, gentle inhalation induction with sevoflurane not exceeding 4% can facilitate peripheral IV placement. IV fluids and phenylephrine should be readily available to maintain preload and vascular resistance during and after induction. The rest of anesthetic management is similar to the adult population. Pecto-intercostal fascial nerve blocks can be used for teenagers or older children, alternatively younger children receive wound local anesthetic infiltration by the surgeon.

D. Right Ventricular Hypertrophy

Right ventricular hypertrophy may rarely occur with HCM,[27] and some young patients may present with both LVOT and right ventricular outflow tract obstruction. Right ventricular enlargement and dysfunction are associated with worse prognosis.[28] Patients with right ventricular obstruction may require right ventricular myectomy and outflow patch augmentation in addition to LV myectomy. In these patients, inotropic support might be necessary early postoperatively following bilateral ventriculotomy.

V. Summary

Extended septal myectomy can be performed in symptomatic patients with HCM with very low mortality and excellent relief of symptoms. Early significant reductions in LVOT obstruction and degree of MR are maintained at late follow-up in the majority of patients. Anesthetic management of surgical myectomy is challenging but rewarding. While severe hemodynamic swings are common, they usually respond well to maneuvers, alleviating dynamic LVOT obstruction. At the end of the myectomy operation, the immediate result can be appreciated with the direct measurements of absent or minimal LVOT gradient and improvement of pulmonary pressure.

REFERENCES

1. Maron BJ, Gardin JM, Flack JM, Gidding SS, Kurosaki TT, Bild DE. Prevalence of hypertrophic cardiomyopathy in a general population of young adults. Echocardiographic analysis of 4111 subjects in the CARDIA Study. Coronary Artery Risk Development in (Young) Adults. *Circulation*. 1995;92(4):785-789.
2. Semsarian C, Ingles J, Maron MS, Maron BJ. New perspectives on the prevalence of hypertrophic cardiomyopathy. *J Am Coll Cardiol*. 2015;65(12):1249-1254.
3. McKenna WJ, Maron BJ, Thiene G. Classification, epidemiology, and global burden of cardiomyopathies. *Circ Res*. 2017;121(7):722-730.
4. Sun D, Schaff HV, Nishimura RA, Geske JB, Dearani JA, Ommen SR. Transapical septal myectomy for hypertrophic cardiomyopathy with midventricular obstruction. *Ann Thorac Surg*. 2021;111(3):836-844.
5. American College of Cardiology Foundation/American Heart Association Task Force on Practice, American Association for Thoracic Surgery, American Society of Echocardiography, et al. 2011 ACCF/AHA guideline for the diagnosis and treatment of hypertrophic cardiomyopathy: a report of the American College of Cardiology Foundation/American Heart Association Task Force on Practice Guidelines. *J Thorac Cardiovasc Surg*. 2011;142:e153-e203.
6. Peng L, Burczak DR, Newman DB, Geske JB. Repetitive squat-to-stand provocation of dynamic left ventricular outflow tract obstruction in hypertrophic cardiomyopathy. *J Am Soc Echocardiogr*. 2022;35(3):323-326.
7. Maron BJ, Roberts WC. Hypertrophic cardiomyopathy and cardiac muscle cell disorganization revisited: relation between the two and significance. *Am Heart J*. 1981;102(1):95-110.
8. Tanaka M, Fujiwara H, Onodera T, Wu DJ, Hamashima Y, Kawai C. Quantitative analysis of myocardial fibrosis in normals, hypertensive hearts, and hypertrophic cardiomyopathy. *Br Heart J*. 1986;55(6):575-581.

9. Chan RH, Maron BJ, Olivotto I, et al. Prognostic value of quantitative contrast-enhanced cardiovascular magnetic resonance for the evaluation of sudden death risk in patients with hypertrophic cardiomyopathy. *Circulation.* 2014;130(6):484-495.

10. Roma-Rodrigues C, Fernandes AR. Genetics of hypertrophic cardiomyopathy: advances and pitfalls in molecular diagnosis and therapy. *Appl Clin Genet.* 2014;7:195-208.

11. Marian AJ, Roberts R. The molecular genetic basis for hypertrophic cardiomyopathy. *J Mol Cell Cardiol.* 2001;33:655-670.

12. Bos JM, Will ML, Gersh BJ, Kruisselbrink TM, Ommen SR, Ackerman MJ. Characterization of a phenotype-based genetic test prediction score for unrelated patients with hypertrophic cardiomyopathy. *Mayo Clin Proc.* 2014;89(6):727-737.

13. Maron BJ, Maron MS, Semsarian C. Genetics of hypertrophic cardiomyopathy after 20 years: clinical perspectives. *J Am Coll Cardiol.* 2012;60:705-715.

14. Siontis KC, Geske JB, Ong K, Nishimura RA, Ommen SR, Gersh BJ. Atrial fibrillation in hypertrophic cardiomyopathy: prevalence, clinical correlations, and mortality in a large high-risk population. *J Am Heart Assoc.* 2014;3(3):e001002.

15. Oberoi M, Schaff HV, Nishimura RA, Geske JB, Dearani JA, Ommen SR. Surgical management of hypertrophic cardiomyopathy complicated by infective endocarditis. *Ann Thorac Surg.* 2022;114(3):744-749.

16. Geske JB, Ommen SR, Gersh BJ. Hypertrophic Cardiomyopathy: Clinical Update. *JACC Heart Fail.* 2018;6(5):364-375.

17. Said SM, Schaff HV. Surgical treatment of hypertrophic cardiomyopathy. *Semin Thorac Cardiovasc Surg.* 2013;25(4):300-309.

18. Nguyen A, Schaff HV, Nishimura RA, et al. Apical myectomy for patients with hypertrophic cardiomyopathy and advanced heart failure. *J Thorac Cardiovasc Surg.* 2019;159(1):145-152.

19. Holst KA, Schaff HV, Smedira NG, et al. Impact of hospital volume on outcomes of septal myectomy for hypertrophic cardiomyopathy. *Ann Thorac Surg.* 2022;114(6):2131-2138.

20. Practice guidelines for preoperative fasting and the use of pharmacologic agents to reduce the risk of pulmonary aspiration: application to healthy patients undergoing elective procedures: an updated report by the American Society of Anesthesiologists Task Force on Preoperative Fasting and the Use of Pharmacologic Agents to reduce the risk of pulmonary aspiration. *Anesthesiology.* 2017;126:376-393.

21. Carvalho JL, Ashikhmina E, Abel MD, et al. Hypertrophic obstructive cardiomyopathy: discrepancy between hemodynamic measurements in the cardiac laboratory and operating room is to be expected. *J Cardiothorac Vasc Anesth.* 2022;36(2):422-428.

22. Ashikhmina EA, Schaff HV, Ommen SR, Dearani JA, Nishimura RA, Abel MD. Intraoperative direct measurement of left ventricular outflow tract gradients to guide surgical myectomy for hypertrophic cardiomyopathy. *J Thorac Cardiovasc Surg.* 2011;142:53-59.

23. Cui H, Nguyen A, Schaff HV. The Brockenbrough-Braunwald-Morrow sign. *J Thorac Cardiovasc Surg.* 2018;156(4):1614-1615.

24. Schaff HV, Brown ML, Dearani JA, et al. Apical myectomy: a new surgical technique for management of severely symptomatic patients with apical hypertrophic cardiomyopathy. *J Thorac Cardiovasc Surg.* 2010;139(3):634-640.

25. Ahmed EA, Schaff HV, Al-Lami HS, et al. Prevalence and influence of pulmonary hypertension in patients with obstructive hypertrophic cardiomyopathy undergoing septal myectomy. *J Thorac Cardiovasc Surg.* 2022:S0022-5223(22)00915-1.

26. Arghami A, Dearani JA, Said SM, O'Leary PW, Schaff HV. Hypertrophic cardiomyopathy in children. *Ann Cardiothorac Surg.* 2017;6(4):376-385.

27. Zhang Y, Zhu Y, Zhang M, et al. Implications of structural right ventricular involvement in patients with hypertrophic cardiomyopathy. *Eur Heart J Qual Care Clin Outcomes.* 2022;9(1):34-41.

28. Wen S, Pislaru C, Ommen SR, Ackerman MJ, Pislaru SV, Geske JB. Right ventricular enlargement and dysfunction are associated with increased all-cause mortality in hypertrophic cardiomyopathy. *Mayo Clin Proc.* 2022;97(6):1123-1133.

17

Adult Congenital Heart Disease (Basics)

Ravi V. Joshi, Tiffany Williams, and Ingrid Moreno-Duarte

KEY POINTS

1. In adult congenital heart disease (ACHD), a clinically relevant classification of lesions divided into three categories is useful: (1) "complete" surgical correction, (2) partial surgical correction or palliation, and (3) uncorrected congenital heart disease (CHD).
2. Over one million patients with CHD have reached adulthood in the United States. Adults with CHD now clearly outnumber the population of children with CHD.
3. Improvements in surgical techniques have allowed 90% of children with CHD to survive to adulthood with relatively normal functionality.

4. Ventricular and atrial arrhythmias are extremely common in ACHD, accounting for nearly 50% of emergency hospitalizations.
5. Patients with ACHD have an incidence of pulmonary arterial hypertension (PAH) as high as 10%.
6. Patients with PAH have a high surgical mortality rate (4%-24%).
7. For both cyanotic (right-to-left shunts) and left-to-right shunts, there are general principles that affect anesthetic management.
8. Patients with complicated residual lesions requiring medium- to high-risk surgery should be managed at centers of excellence with physicians and staff trained in adult congenital disease.

I. Introduction

The adult patient with congenital heart disease (CHD) offers a unique challenge to the cardio-thoracic anesthesiologist. CHD encompasses a wide spectrum of cardiac anomalies, each with their own specific pathophysiology. Because each individual patient undergoes a series of palliative procedures and reconstructive repairs tailored to their respective cardiac defects in childhood, the physician is often presented with an adult who has multiple layers of medical and surgical complexity requiring specialized anesthetic management in the perioperative setting. *Rarely, these repairs are considered curative, and as these patients age into young adulthood, the chronic sequelae of disease (such as heart failure [HF], arrhythmias, or pulmonary hypertension) begin to manifest.* Essential to the proper anesthetic care for the adult congenital heart disease (ACHD) patient is a thorough understanding of the underlying cardiopulmonary physiology dictated by the patient's altered cardiac anatomy. This chapter serves as a primer for the perioperative care of patients with ACHD intended for the cardiothoracic anesthesiology fellow, practicing cardiothoracic anesthesiologist, or other physician.

A. Definition: The term *congenital heart disease* covers a wide spectrum of cardiac abnormalities such that prevalence, mortality, and survival data vary depending on the definition used by specific epidemiology studies. In this chapter, we restrict the definition of ACHD as per Mitchell et al (1971): "a gross structural abnormality of the heart and intrathoracic great vessels that is actually or possibly of functional significance."[1] In practice, this definition excludes some common congenital cardiac malformations, such as bicuspid aortic valves, persistent left-sided superior vena cava (PL-SVC), congenital arrhythmias, Marfan syndrome, mitral valve prolapse, and inherited forms of cardiomyopathy. These conditions and their anesthetic implications are discussed elsewhere in this textbook.

B. Epidemiology

1. Prevalence

a. CHD is one of the most common classes of births defects, with an estimated worldwide birth prevalence of ~0.8%-1.2% of live births.[2] In the United States, based on data of infants born in the Atlanta metropolitan area between 1998 and 2005, the observed prevalence of CHD was determined to be 81.4 in 10,000 of all live births,[3] consistent with the incidence in other developed nations.[2] The most common defect by far was the presence of muscular ventricular septal defects (VSDs), followed by perimembranous VSDs and atrial septal defects (ASDs), that in total make up ~30% of all CHD lesions diagnosed. The prevalence of severe congenital heart lesions including cyanotic disease is ~1.5 per 1,000 live births or 0.15%.[4] Since the 1950s, where childhood mortality reached nearly 90% for complex congenital lesions, major surgical and medical advances over the past half-century have now reduced childhood mortality to where 85% of infants with CHD are predicted to reach adulthood.[5]

b. In 2000, the prevalence of ACHD was estimated to be about 3,000 per million to that of the adult population.[6] This correlated to an estimated 790,000 adult patients in the United States, with 420,000 living with moderate or severe congenital lesions in 2000.[7] A more recent Canadian study indicates even higher prevalence of ACHD at 6.2 cases per 1,000 adult patients in 2010, nearly twice that estimated in 2000.[8] Current estimates

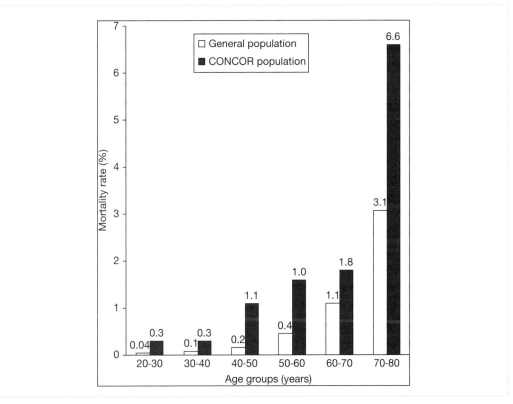

FIGURE 17.1 Increasing mortality of adult patients with complex congenital defects (black bars) compared to the age-matched general population (white bars). (From Verheugt CL, Uiterwaal CS, van der Velde ET, et al. Mortality in adult congenital heart disease. *Eur Heart J.* 2010;31(10):1220-1229. Reproduced by permission of European Society of Cardiology.)

place the population of patient with ACHD in the United States at more than one million. Although more patients with CHD with moderate or complex disease are surviving into adulthood, the mortality of these patients is nearly 2-7 times that of the general population, particularly in the fourth and fifth decades (Figure 17.1). The median age of death for patients of ACHD is estimated to be at 57 years.[6,9]

2

    c. Recent population analyses have demonstrated that the prevalence of childhood CHD has increased by 10% from 2000 to 2010, while the number of adult patients living with severe congenital heart disease (ACHD) increased by over 50% in a decade.[10] The current number of adult patients living with CHD exceeds the number of children living with CHD, and the proportion of patients with ACHD continues to increase in North America and in the Europe Union, with more patients reaching the sixth decade of life[11] (Figure 17.2).

3

    d. A study looking at the percentage of patients with ACHD admitted for noncardiac surgery compared to all admissions for noncardiac surgery between 2002 and 2009 demonstrates a 2.6× increase in the percentage of patients with ACHD over the 7-year study period[12] (Figure 17.3). Many women with CHD are also reaching a childbearing age, increasing the population of obstetrical patients with CHD. Current trends indicate encountering adult patients with moderate or severe congenital heart disease (ACHD) for noncardiac surgery obstetrical procedures will become more commonplace.

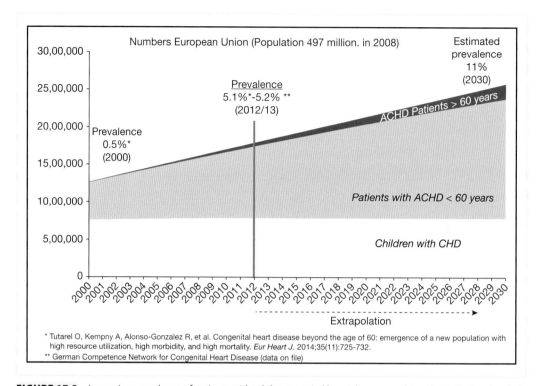

FIGURE 17.2 Increasing prevalence of patients with adult congenital heart disease reaching the sixth decade of life. (From Baumgartner H. Geriatric congenital heart disease: a new challenge in the care of adults with congenital heart disease? *Eur Heart J.* 2014;35(11):683-685. Reproduced by permission of European Society of Cardiology.)

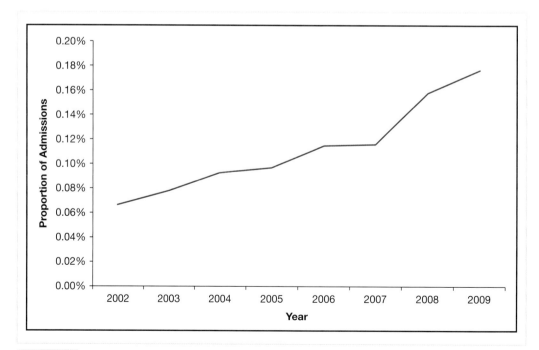

FIGURE 17.3 Increasing incidence of patients with adult congenital heart disease as percent of admissions for noncardiac surgery admissions over 2002-2009. (Reprinted with permission from Maxwell BG, Wong JK, Kin C, Lobato RL. Perioperative outcomes of major noncardiac surgery in adults with congenital heart disease. *Anesthesiology.* 2013;119(4):762-769. © 2013 American Society of Anesthesiologists.)

CLINICAL PEARL

- The epidemiologic data demonstrate a growing population of adult patients living with CHD repaired, palliated, or unrepaired.
- This population of patients has a decreased life expectancy and increased mortality than the general public.
- Adult patients with moderate or complex congenital lesions are also increasing and are at higher risk for perioperative morbidity and mortality.
- The increasing number of ACHD is accompanied by the increasing number of noncardiac surgical procedures performed on these patients as they age.

C. **Providing Health Care Access**

  1. Patients with ACHD have lower mortality when treated at medical facilities with specialized care in CHD.[13] It is recommended that patients with moderate or complex lesions (II or III, A-D) or those with simple lesions with severe physiologic sequelae (IB-D) should be treated at medical facilities offering specialized care in ACHD.[14]

  2. In addition, patients with ACHD have lower mortality and better outcomes when undergoing cardiac procedures at ACHD specialized medical centers. The American College of Cardiology/American Heart Association (ACC/AHA) guidelines recommend that patients with ACHD undergoing cardiac surgery, interventional cardiac procedures, and electrophysiologic (EP) procedures should be cared for by physicians and providers with knowledge and proficiency in congenital heart lesions in consultation with an ACHD cardiologist.[14]

D. **Role of the Cardiothoracic Anesthesiologist:** Patients with severe congenital cardiac lesions have a lower mortality when cared for at specialized medical centers with expertise in ACHD. An important component is the expertise of the perioperative team in ACHD, including the ACHD cardiologist, cardiac anesthesiologists, interventional cardiologists, cardiac surgeons, physician consultants (eg, pulmonology, nephrology, radiology), and supporting staff. *The 2018 ACC/AHA guidelines recommend the involvement of a cardiac anesthesiologist for patients with ACHD undergoing invasive procedures requiring anesthesia, particularly those patients with moderate or severe disease (Class II or III, A-D) or simple disease (Class IB-D) with significant physiologic sequelae.*[14] Examples include the patient with a perimembranous VSD with ≥moderate shunt (I-C) or cyanosis (I-D) or the stable patient with single ventricle and Fontan physiology (Class IIIA). Unfortunately, specific training pathways for anesthesiologists in the care of patients with ACHD are not currently available. Current recommendations are for primarily physicians subspecialized in adult cardiac anesthesiology, pediatric anesthesiology, or pediatric cardiac anesthesiology to obtain training through mentoring and practice experience.

E. **Nomenclature for Congenital Heart Disease:** Although there are multiple systems of nomenclature to describe congenital cardiac lesions, the Van Praagh notation is the most commonly used schema. The Van Praagh nomenclature uses three elements to describe a congenital condition: (1) the *situs* or the orientation of thoracoabdominal viscera and cardiac atria, (2) looping (either D or L) or orientation of the morphologic right ventricle (RV), and (3) the relationship of the aorta and pulmonary artery (PA).[15] Proper terminology is determined by answering the following questions in a stepwise manner:

  1. What is the *situs* of the organ in the chest and abdomen?
  2. What is the position of the morphologic RV and left ventricle (LV)?
  3. What are the positions and relations of the great vessels?
     The last two questions establish atrioventricular (AV) concordance (or discordance) and ventriculo-arterial concordance (or discordance), respectively.
  4. What are the connections between the atria and the ventricles?
  5. What are the connections between the ventricles and the great arteries?

The notation use a three-element bracket with the first element as the situs (S, I, or A), the second as the looping (D, L, X), and the great vessel arrangement (S, I, D/L-MGA, or D/L-TGA) (see Figure 17.4).

F. Classification of Severity of Congenital Disease: Procedural risk and mortality are directly related to the severity of CHD; thus, classification of ACHD by burden of disease is valuable to the cardiothoracic anesthesiologist for perioperative planning and intraoperative decision-making. Since 2001, stratification of ACHD severity was primarily based on the anatomic complexity of the native lesion. Nevertheless, due to the variability of surgical repairs and differing hemodynamic consequences in patients with the same lesion, actual severity of disease did not correlate well with just anatomic complexity. The majority of congenital cardiac

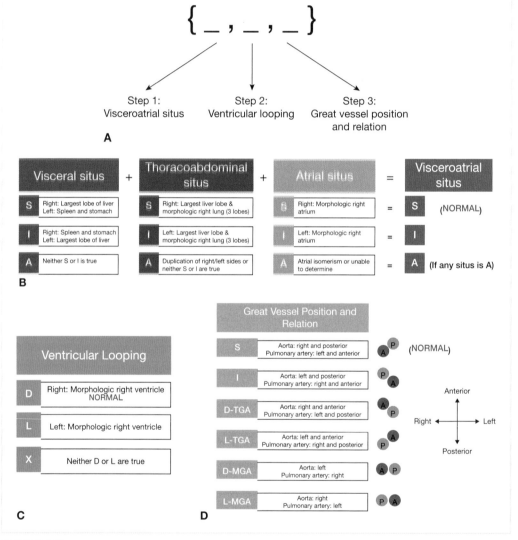

FIGURE 17.4 The Van Praagh nomenclature for congenital heart disease. The shorthand notation for the anatomic arrangement for a congenital lesion is shown **(A)**. The initial step to determine the first element (visceroatrial situs) by **(B)** assessing visceral, thoracoabdominal, and atrial orientation. Next element is the ventricular looping **(C)** by determining the position of the morphologic right ventricle. And final element is the position of the great vessels (aorta and pulmonary artery) to each other **(D)**.

surgical procedures are often not curative but palliative in nature with functional consequences that can lead to significant morbidity in adulthood (eg, HF in patients with single ventricle physiology). Certain late physiologic sequelae including the development of pulmonary hypertension, HF, ventricular arrhythmias, or even Eisenmenger syndrome have important implications for perioperative outcomes.

1. **American College of Cardiology/American Heart Association Classification 2018[14]:** In the most recent 2018 ACC/AHA guidelines on ACHD, a new ACHD-AP classification was presented and attempts to include these three main factors in determining the severity of disease: (1) anatomic complexity, (2) surgical repair, and (3) physiologic stage. Physiologic stage is defined by the presence and severity of common sequelae of ACHD. These variables influence prognosis of patient with ACHD and have important implications for the management of the disease. The inclusion of these variables in risk stratification may better reflect the perioperative risk for a given patient with ACHD (Figure 17.5; Table 17.1).

CLINICAL PEARL

- Patients with ACHD have a lower mortality at specialized care centers. Adult patients with moderate or complex congenital lesions or those with significant sequelae should be treated at centers specialized in the treatment of CHDs.
- A cardiac anesthesiologist should be involved in the care of the patient with ACHD with ≥ moderate disease or simple disease with significant sequelae.
- The Van Praagh terminology system is commonly used to describe the anatomic orientation and segmental elements of congenital heart lesions. Perioperative risk and mortality are directly correlated to the severity of disease. The ACHD-AP classification system is useful in perioperative risk stratification.

II. Perioperative Considerations for Patients With Adult Congenital Heart Disease

   A. Preoperative History and Physical: Surgery for patients with ACHD spans the gamut of procedures from simple surgeries (eg, hernia repair) to heart transplants. *In general, patients with ACHD have higher perioperative morbidity and mortality than the age-matched general population.*[9,16] Thorough preoperative evaluation of patients with ACHD for noncardiac and cardiac surgery is essential to optimize perioperative outcomes. Patients with simple, repaired lesions and good functional status may be treated like the general population. Moderate defects, high-risk lesions, or poor functional status mandate an individualized approach with input from the ACHD cardiologist and surgeon. The preoperative history should include the following key elements to determine the perioperative anesthetic plan and estimate perioperative risk:

   1. **Original type of congenital defect and anatomy**
   2. **History of repair or palliative surgeries:** Prosthetic material, closure devices, sternotomies
   3. **Class of congenital defect (I-III):** Simple/moderate/complex
   4. **Patient's functional status (A-D) or New York Heart Association (NYHA) class**
   5. **Presence of residual or native shunt:** Location, magnitude, direction, shunt fraction (Q_p/Q_s)
   6. **AV valve dysfunction:** Degree and mechanism of regurgitation/stenosis
   7. **Arrhythmia history:** Antiarrhythmic drugs, history of ablations, presence of permanent pacemaker/implantable cardioverter-defibrillators (PPM/ICDs)
   8. **Anticoagulation regimen:** Prior deep vein thrombosis (DVT)/paradoxical embolus, Fontan, atrial arrhythmia
   9. **High-risk populations:** See section that follows
   10. **Associated congenital defects or collateral lesions**

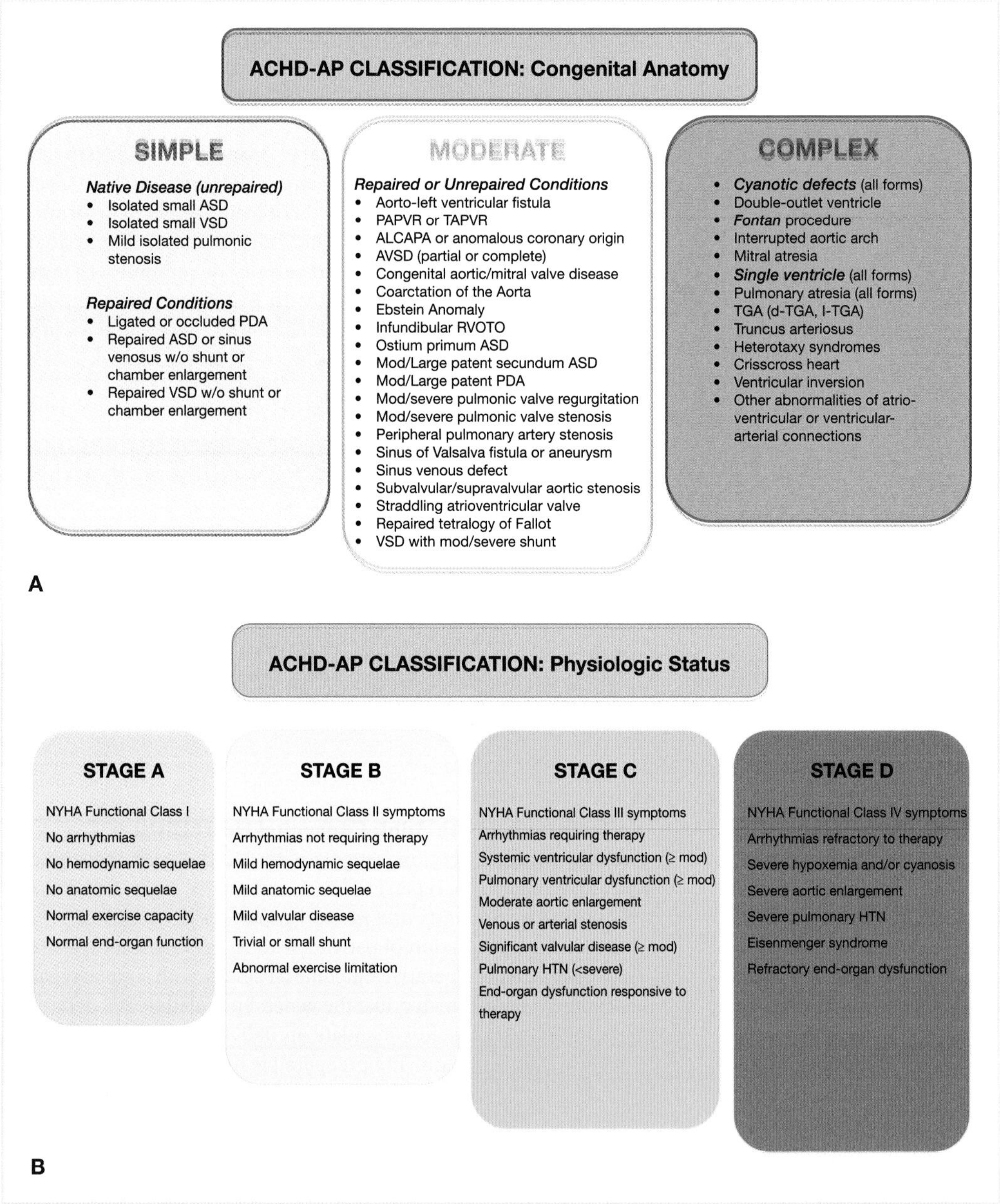

ACHD-AP CLASSIFICATION: Congenital Anatomy

SIMPLE

Native Disease (unrepaired)
- Isolated small ASD
- Isolated small VSD
- Mild isolated pulmonic stenosis

Repaired Conditions
- Ligated or occluded PDA
- Repaired ASD or sinus venosus w/o shunt or chamber enlargement
- Repaired VSD w/o shunt or chamber enlargement

MODERATE

Repaired or Unrepaired Conditions
- Aorto-left ventricular fistula
- PAPVR or TAPVR
- ALCAPA or anomalous coronary origin
- AVSD (partial or complete)
- Congenital aortic/mitral valve disease
- Coarctation of the Aorta
- Ebstein Anomaly
- Infundibular RVOTO
- Ostium primum ASD
- Mod/Large patent secundum ASD
- Mod/Large patent PDA
- Mod/severe pulmonic valve regurgitation
- Mod/severe pulmonic valve stenosis
- Peripheral pulmonary artery stenosis
- Sinus of Valsalva fistula or aneurysm
- Sinus venous defect
- Subvalvular/supravalvular aortic stenosis
- Straddling atrioventricular valve
- Repaired tetralogy of Fallot
- VSD with mod/severe shunt

COMPLEX

- *Cyanotic defects* (all forms)
- Double-outlet ventricle
- *Fontan* procedure
- Interrupted aortic arch
- Mitral atresia
- *Single ventricle* (all forms)
- Pulmonary atresia (all forms)
- TGA (d-TGA, l-TGA)
- Truncus arteriosus
- Heterotaxy syndromes
- Crisscross heart
- Ventricular inversion
- Other abnormalities of atrioventricular or ventricular-arterial connections

A

ACHD-AP CLASSIFICATION: Physiologic Status

STAGE A

NYHA Functional Class I
No arrhythmias
No hemodynamic sequelae
No anatomic sequelae
Normal exercise capacity
Normal end-organ function

STAGE B

NYHA Functional Class II symptoms
Arrhythmias not requiring therapy
Mild hemodynamic sequelae
Mild anatomic sequelae
Mild valvular disease
Trivial or small shunt
Abnormal exercise limitation

STAGE C

NYHA Functional Class III symptoms
Arrhythmias requiring therapy
Systemic ventricular dysfunction (≥ mod)
Pulmonary ventricular dysfunction (≥ mod)
Moderate aortic enlargement
Venous or arterial stenosis
Significant valvular disease (≥ mod)
Pulmonary HTN (<severe)
End-organ dysfunction responsive to therapy

STAGE D

NYHA Functional Class IV symptoms
Arrhythmias refractory to therapy
Severe hypoxemia and/or cyanosis
Severe aortic enlargement
Severe pulmonary HTN
Eisenmenger syndrome
Refractory end-organ dysfunction

B

FIGURE 17.5 **(A)** ACHD-AP classification. Anatomic and defect classification is separated into simple, moderate, or complex lesions. **(B)** Physiologic status is staged from **A to D:** Normal to worsening physiology and impairment of end-organ function. ASD, atrial septal defect; HTN, hypertension; NYHA, New York Heart Association; PAPVR, partial anomalous pulmonary venous return; PDA, patent ductus arteriosus; RVOTO, right ventricular outflow tract obstruction; TAPVR, total anomalous pulmonary venous return; TGA, transposition of the great arteries; VSD, ventricular septal defect. (Based on Stout KK, Daniels CJ, Aboulhosn JA, et al. 2018 AHA/ACC guideline for the management of adults with congenital heart disease: a report of the American College of Cardiology/American Heart Association Task Force on Clinical Practice Guidelines. *Circulation*. 2019;139(14):e698-e800.)

TABLE 17.1 Physiologic Variables as Used in ACHD-AP Classification

Variable	Description
Aortopathy	Aortic enlargement is common in some types of CHD and after some repairs. Aortic enlargement may be progressive over a lifetime. There is no universally accepted threshold for repair, nor is the role of indexing to body size clearly defined in adults, as is done in pediatric populations. For purposes of categorization and timing of follow-up imaging:
	Mild aortic enlargement is defined as maximum diameter 3.5-3.9 cm
	Moderate aortic enlargement is defined as maximum diameter 4.0-4.9 cm
	Severe aortic enlargement is defined as maximum diameter ≥5.0 cm
Arrhythmia	Arrhythmias are very common in patients with ACHD and may be both the cause and consequence of deteriorating hemodynamics, valvular dysfunction, or ventricular dysfunction. Arrhythmias are associated with symptoms, outcomes, and prognosis; thus, they are categorized based on the presence and response to treatment.
	No arrhythmia: No documented clinically relevant atrial or ventricular tachyarrhythmias
	Arrhythmia not requiring treatment: Bradyarrhythmia, atrial or ventricular tachyarrhythmia not requiring antiarrhythmic therapy, cardioversion, or ablation
	Arrhythmia controlled with therapy:
	Bradyarrhythmia requiring pacemaker implantation
	Atrial or ventricular tachyarrhythmia requiring antiarrhythmic therapy, cardioversion, or ablation
	AF and controlled ventricular response
	Patients with an ICD
	Refractory arrhythmias:
	Atrial or ventricular tachyarrhythmia currently unresponsive to or refractory to antiarrhythmic therapy or ablation
Concomitant VHD	Severity defined according to the 2014 VHD guideline.
	Mild VHD
	Moderate VHD
	Severe VHD
End-organ dysfunction	Clinical and/or laboratory evidence of end-organ dysfunction including:
	Renal (kidney)
	Hepatic (liver)
	Pulmonary (lung)

(continued)

TABLE 17.1 Physiologic Variables as Used in ACHD-AP Classification (*continued*)

Variable	Description
Exercise capacity	Patients with ACHD are often asymptomatic notwithstanding exercise limitations demonstrated as diminished exercise capacity when evaluated objectively.[S2.2-12-S2.2-14] Thus, assessment of both subjective and objective exercise capacity is important (see NYHA classification system below). Exercise capacity is associated with prognosis.
	Abnormal objective cardiac limitation to exercise is defined as an exercise maximum ventilatory equivalent of oxygen below the range expected for the specific CHD anatomic diagnosis.
	Expected norms for CPET values should take into account age, sex, and underlying congenital diagnosis. Published studies with institution-specific norms can be used as guides, bearing in mind variability among institutional norms and ranges.
Hypoxemia/hypoxia/cyanosis	Hypoxemia is defined as oxygen saturation measured by pulse oximetry at rest ≤90%.
	Severe hypoxemia is defined as oxygen saturation at rest <85%.
	In patients with normal or high hemoglobin concentrations, severe hypoxemia will be associated with visible cyanosis (which requires ≥5 g/L desaturated hemoglobin to be appreciated).
	The terms *cyanosis* and *hypoxemia (or hypoxia)* are sometimes used interchangeably. Such interchangeability would not apply; however, in the presence of anemia, severe hypoxemia can be present without visible cyanosis.
NYHA functional classification system[S2.2-19]	**Class** **Functional Capacity**
	I Patients with cardiac disease but resulting in no limitation of physical activity. Ordinary physical activity does not cause undue fatigue, palpitation, dyspnea, or anginal pain.
	II Patients with cardiac disease resulting in slight limitation of physical activity. They are comfortable at rest. Ordinary physical activity results in fatigue, palpitation, dyspnea, or anginal pain.
	III Patients with cardiac disease resulting in marked limitation of physical activity. They are comfortable at rest. Less than ordinary activity causes fatigue, palpitation, dyspnea, or anginal pain.
	IV Patients with cardiac disease resulting in inability to carry on any physical activity without discomfort. Symptoms of HF or the anginal syndrome may be present even at rest. If any physical activity is undertaken, discomfort increases.
Pulmonary hypertension	*Pulmonary hypertension* is a broad term that encompasses pulmonary arterial hypertension, which is pulmonary hypertension with increased pulmonary vascular resistance. This document defines PH and PAH as they are used in the field of pulmonary hypertension.
	Pulmonary hypertension is defined as:
	Mean PA pressure by right heart catheterization ≥25 mm Hg
	PAH is defined as:
	Mean PA pressure by right heart catheterization ≥25 mm Hg and a pulmonary capillary wedge pressure ≤15 mm Hg and pulmonary vascular resistance ≥3 Wood units

Shunt (hemodynamically significant shunt)	An intracardiac shunt is hemodynamically significant if:
	There is evidence of chamber enlargement distal to the shunt
	And/or evidence of sustained $Q_p:Q_s \geq 1.5:1$
	An intracardiac shunt not meeting these criteria would be described as small or trivial.
Venous and arterial stenosis	Aortic recoarctation after CoA repair
	Supravalvular aortic obstruction
	Venous baffle obstruction
	Supravalvular pulmonary stenosis
	Branch PA stenosis
	Stenosis of cavopulmonary connection
	Pulmonary vein stenosis

ACHD, adult congenital heart disease; AF, atrial fibrillation; AP, anatomic and physiologic; CHD, congenital heart disease; CoA, coarctation of the aorta; CPET, cardiopulmonary exercise test; HF, heart failure; ICD, implantable cardioverter-defibrillator; NYHA, New York Heart Association; PA, pulmonary artery; PAH, pulmonary arterial hypertension; $Q_p:Q_s$, pulmonary-systemic blood flow ratio; VHD, valvular heart disease.

Reprinted from Stout KK, Daniels CJ, Aboulhosn JA, et al. 2018 AHA/ACC guideline for the management of adults with congenital heart disease: a report of the American College of Cardiology/American Heart Association Task Force on Clinical Practice Guidelines. *J Am Coll Cardiol.* 2019;73(12):e81-e192. © 2019 by the American College of Cardiology Foundation. With permission.

B. **Extracardiac Organ System Involvement**[17]

1. **Pulmonary:** Approximately >40% of patients with ACHD have evidence of restrictive lung disease on pulmonary function testing, particularly those with tetralogy of Fallot (TOF) repair and Fontan palliation. Hemoptysis and pulmonary hemorrhage are more common in patients with Eisenmenger syndrome. Pulmonary hypertension is discussed in the section that follows.

2. **Renal:** Impaired kidney function is prevalent among ~50% of patients with ACHD and increased among cyanotic patients. Congenital renal anomalies may be associated with CHD, including patients with VACTERL and CHARGE syndromes.

3. **Hepatic:** Liver disease from congestive hepatopathy is common in patients with Fontan physiology (see later) and may present in other congenital syndromes or patients with right-sided HF. Alagille syndrome is associated with cholestatic liver disease.

4. **Hematologic:** Several hematologic perturbations may occur in CHD. Anemia may be prevalent in the HF population. Coagulation abnormalities and passive venous stasis are associated with Fontan palliation and significantly increase the risk of DVT and thrombosis, necessitating anticoagulation. Cyanotic patients including Eisenmenger syndrome can present with secondary erythrocytosis, which can be complicated by hyperuricemia, gout, and hyperviscosity syndrome (see later).

5. **Immune/Infectious:** Patients with heterotaxy syndromes may present with asplenia, increasing susceptibility to encapsulated organisms. Preventative measures including vaccination history should be addressed. Pneumonia is currently the most common noncardiac cause of death in patients with CHD.

C. **Preoperative Imaging, Testing, and Laboratories:** Patient history, physical examination, and input from ACHD specialists should tailor the basic preoperative workup for patients with ACHD undergoing cardiac and noncardiac surgery. Basic laboratory workup should include the following:

1. Essential
   a. Recent chest x-ray
   b. Electrocardiogram
   c. Basic metabolic panel, including glucose and creatinine
   d. Complete blood count (w/ or w/o differential)
   e. Coagulation tests, including prothrombin time/international normalized ratio (PT/INR), partial thromboplastin time (PTT)
   f. Recent echocardiogram (TTE or transesophageal echocardiography [TEE]) defining ventricular and valvular function, the presence of residual shunts or fenestrations, and status of repairs (eg, baffle patency)
   g. Further workup may be indicated in special ACHD populations with complex lesions. Patients may need cardiopulmonary testing to determine functional status. Cardiac catheterization may be required to define circulatory anatomy including coronaries, estimate shunt fraction, and evaluate for pulmonary hypertension. Input from the ACHD cardiologist is essential for determining the proper testing or imaging to calculate perioperative risk.

2. Additional
   a. Liver function tests
   b. Ferritin and iron levels
   c. Complete metabolic panel, including serum calcium, magnesium
   d. Computed tomography (CT) scan or cardiac magnetic resonance imaging (cMRI)
   e. Cardiac left and right heart catheterization with or without coronary angiography
   f. **Cardiopulmonary testing:** 6-minute walk test, nuclear medicine studies, stress testing
   g. A recommended algorithm provided by the AHA for preoperative evaluation for patients with ACHD undergoing noncardiac surgery is shown in Figure 17.6.[17]

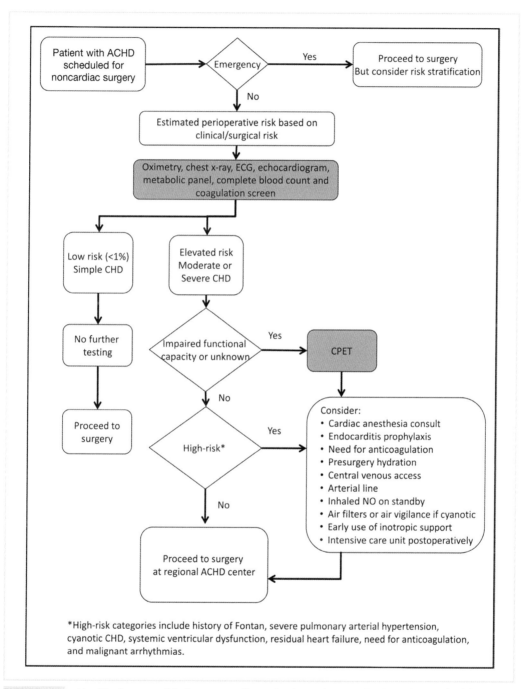

FIGURE 17.6 Algorithmic approach to the preoperative evaluation and preparation for patients with adult congenital heart disease (ACHD) undergoing noncardiac surgery. CHD, congenital heart disease; ECG, electrocardiography. (Reprinted with permission from Lui GK, Saidi A, Bhatt AB, et al. Diagnosis and management of noncardiac complications in adults with congenital heart disease: a scientific statement from the American Heart Association. *Circulation.* 2017;136(20):e348-e392. Figure 2. © 2017 American Heart Association, Inc.)

D. **Intraoperative Monitoring and Access:** Vascular access and intraoperative monitors will be determined by the type of anesthesia (general, regional, neuraxial, or sedation), the type of procedure (eg, early graft dysfunction [EGD] vs heart transplant), and the patient disease (eg, simple ASD vs Fontan).

1. **General monitors:** In all patient types and situations, basic standard American Society of Anesthesiologists (ASA) monitors (noninvasive blood pressure, 5-lead EKG, ETCO$_2$, SpO$_2$, temperature) are the minimum required monitors. Pulse oximetry has particular importance in patients with ACHD with shunt lesions, as the magnitude and direction of shunt can be inferred from hemoglobin saturation.

2. **Invasive monitoring:** Invasive monitors are useful in more complex procedures or complicated patients. Invasive arterial blood pressuring monitoring is highly recommended in patients with complex lesions (Class II-III) or poor physiologic status (B-D). Central venous monitoring may be helpful in complex patients for measuring filling pressures and for central venous access. The anesthesiologist should be aware of the following considerations:

   a. **Prior Blalock-Thomas-Taussig shunts:** The use of a subclavian artery for palliation by Blalock-Thomas-Taussig (BTT) shunt may affect the blood pressure measured in that side. Alternative sites such as the contralateral arm or lower extremities should be used for noninvasive or invasive blood pressure monitoring.

   b. **Glenn shunts, Fontan palliation:** In single ventricle palliation, the central venous circulation is connected directly to the pulmonary tree. Central venous pressures (CVPs) are reflective of left-sided (systemic) filling pressures, and relative pulmonary vascular resistance (PVR).

   c. **Pulmonary artery catheters:** Pulmonary artery catheters (PACs) should be used judiciously in most patients with ACHD. PACs can cause several major complications, including inducing arrhythmia. In certain patient types, right heart catheterization would be difficult or contraindicated (eg, Senning, Mustard, PL-SVC) due to anatomic considerations.

   d. **Transesophageal echocardiography:** Echocardiography is an invaluable tool to visualize cardiac structures, monitor function, and evaluate percutaneous interventions or surgical repairs for patients with ACHD. The 2018 AHA/ACC guidelines consider TEE monitoring standard of care in structural heart disease procedures, such as ASD closure.[14] TEE should be used in all major cardiac surgeries or structural heart interventions involving patients with ACHD unless absolutely contra-indicated (ie, esophageal disease).

3. **Vascular access:** Based on the type of procedure, simple intravenous (IV) venous cannulation many be sufficient. Central venous access is recommended in complex procedures, for moderate- to high-risk lesions, or patients with poor functional status for delivery of inotropes and vasoactive medications. Important vascular access considerations in patients with ACHD are as follows:

   a. **Previous access:** Due the multiple procedures in childhood and teenage years, patients with significant CHD lesions may have occluded radial or femoral arteries. Prior extracorporeal membrane oxygenation (ECMO) cannulation in children may have sacrificed the right carotid artery and internal jugular vein. It is prudent to review IV contrast CTs or angiograms to help define adequate vessels for central cannulation. Ultrasound-guided cannulation is recommended.

   b. **Altered venous anatomy:** Systemic venous anatomy and blood return are significantly altered in a variety of lesions, repairs, or palliative surgeries. Glen shunts, Mustard baffles, or patients with heterotaxy syndrome are examples of patients with unique systemic venous anatomy. Prior imaging (eg, IV contrast CT, cardiac catheterization/angiography, cMRI) should be reviewed to map the best site for venous cannulation. Difficult access sites may require fluoroscopic-guided cannulation.

E. **General Considerations for Redo Sternotomies:** Many of the patients with moderate or complex ACHD have undergone one or more surgical palliations/repairs in childhood or adolescence. As with repeat sternotomies in non-CHD adults, the reentry into the sternum carries increased perioperative risk due to adhesion of cardiac structures to the sternum, alteration of normal anatomic planes, and neovascularization. Difficulty in central cannulation for emergency cardiopulmonary bypass (CPB) adds to the complexity of the operation. In addition, patients with ACHD often have critical prosthetic grafts or conduits that be damaged upon reentry. Preoperative planning is essential for redo sternotomies in ACHD, and several considerations include the following:

1. **Alternative cardiopulmonary bypass cannulation site:** Reviewing available imaging (CT, MRI) and discussion with the surgical team to plan for emergency CPB cannulation. In many cases, femoral vessels can be accessed and guidewires placed for easy cannulation before chest dissection in case of emergency.

2. **External defibrillation pads:** Due to difficulty of dissection, defibrillation paddles often cannot be used. External pads are critical in the event of an arrhythmia during sternotomy.

3. **Risk of hemorrhage:** This risk is much greater due injury to major structures such as the aorta or RV on reentry. Blood products (ie, $\geq$6-8 units red blood cells [RBCs], 4-6 fresh-frozen plasma [FFP], 1-2 platelets, 10-pack cryoprecipitate) and hemostatic agents should be available in the operating room before incision.

4. **Vascular access:** Placement of multiple large-bore IV, large central venous cannula, or a rapid infusion catheter is required in the case of catastrophic hemorrhage. The availability of a rapid infusion device or pump is recommended.

F. **Air Emboli and Air Vigilance Prophylaxis:** There is a risk of paradoxical air embolus from introduction of air via IV access, even in patients with left-to-right shunts, as shunt reversal can occur in brief periods during the cardiac cycle.[18] Proper vigilance to removal of air bubbles in all vascular (arterial and venous) catheters and tubing is recommended. Air filters are also recommended on all IV access sites.

G. **Endocarditis Prophylaxis:** Antibiotic prophylaxis should be used in procedures for cyanotic patients, patients with previous infectious endocarditis, prosthetic valves, and patients with known residual shunts, especially if there is remaining prosthetic material. Patients with surgeries using prosthetic graft material should have antibiotic prophylaxis for up to 6 months postrepair.[14]

H. **Arrhythmias and Electrophysiologic Devices:** Arrhythmias are a common and occur in ~25% of patients with ACHD. Patients with ACHD with arrhythmias are also more likely to have other comorbid conditions and a higher mortality. The risk of ventricular arrhythmias is nearly 100 times greater in the ACHD population, and arrhythmias are one of the most common causes of sudden cardiac death in patients with ACHD.[19,20] The types of arrhythmias are often dependent on the specific lesion or surgical procedure; common examples include the following:

1. **Sinoatrial node dysfunction:** Atrial switch procedures (Mustard/Senning)
2. **Atrial tachyarrhythmias:** Fontan repair, Ebstein anomaly, venous baffle (Mustard/Senning)
3. **AV node dysfunction and AV block:** Atrioventricular septal defect (AVSD), congenitally corrected transposition of the great arteries (cc-TGA)
4. **AV nodal reentry or Wolff-Parkinson-White (WPW):** Ebstein anomaly
5. **Ventricular arrhythmias:** D-Transposition of the great arteries (D-TGA), cc-TGA, TOF, repaired VSDs

Unless specifically contraindicated, antiarrhythmic medication should be continued through the perioperative period. Many patients with adult congenital heart have implanted pacemakers for AV block or defibrillators as primary or secondary prevention for sudden cardiac death. In specific situations, switching to a nonsensing pacing mode (ie, DOO), increasing the baseline rate for pace-dependent individuals, or deactivating tachyarrhythmia therapies may be desirable. Discussion with the ACHD cardiologist may be warranted in these situations. All devices should be interrogated before procedures as recommended in perioperative guidelines by the Heart Rhythm society.[21]

I. **Anticoagulation:** Patients with ACHD presenting for surgery may be on systemic anticoagulation as either secondary prevention to prevent recurrent thrombosis and thromboembolism prophylaxis for mechanical valves or primary prevention as in atrial arrhythmias (atrial fibrillation or flutter), which are common in this population. The use of anticoagulation in patients with Eisenmenger or cyanotic patients as primary prophylaxis is controversial and not currently recommended. Patients with ACHD with Fontan palliation are at an increased risk for thrombosis and thromboembolism and often on systemic anticoagulation.[17] Holding anticoagulation should be weighed against the bleeding risk from impending procedure. Discussion with ACHD cardiologist and surgeon is vital to determine halting anticoagulation before surgery and the timing of when to restart the anticoagulation. In certain cases (eg, mechanical valves in the mitral position), bridging with low-molecular-weight heparin or unfractionated heparin may be warranted.

J. **High-Risk Populations**

1. **Single ventricle physiology and Fontan palliation:** Patients with single ventricles and Fontan palliation are a special population of patients with ACHD (see "Fontan Physiology and Anesthetic Management" section) with perioperative complication rates as high as 31% for noncardiac surgery.[22] Consideration should be given for the presence of BTT or Glenn shunts for central access and invasive monitoring. Atrial arrhythmias are common in this population, and many patients require anticoagulation for the increased risk of thromboembolism. Protein-losing enteropathy (PLE) can occur in Fontan patients and carries potential higher perioperative risk. Fontan-associated liver disease (FALD) is progressive liver cirrhosis that develops several years post palliation and is associated with the development of hepatocellular carcinoma.

2. **Pulmonary hypertension and right heart failure:** Patients with pulmonary hypertension with or without right heart dysfunction have a high perioperative risk, with a mortality as high as 18%.[23] Care of these patients requires multidisciplinary team involvement to optimize perioperative anesthetic management.

3. **Unrepaired cyanotic heart disease and Eisenmenger syndrome:** Eisenmenger syndrome arises from a persistent communication between the right and left heart coupled with severe pulmonary hypertension, leading to right-to-left shunting and mixing of venous with arterial blood. The resulting physiologic effects are cyanosis and chronic hypoxemia. The systemic consequences include secondary erythrocytosis complicated by hyperviscosity syndrome and iron deficiency, increased risk for both bleeding and thrombosis, increased risk of infection, increased risk of sudden cardiac arrest (SCD) from malignant arrhythmia, and HF. Patients with Eisenmenger have among the highest perioperative mortality rates for noncardiac surgery, ranging as high as 25% in some studies.[24] Preoperative preparation should be based on multidisciplinary discussion among all physicians, including the anesthesiologist, surgeon, and ACHD specialist. Patients undergoing surgery should have iron repletion, correction of coagulation abnormalities and thrombocytopenia, and adequate hydration. Hemodynamic management may be complex, including the use of pulmonary vasodilators and systemic vasopressors. Realize that decreasing shunt magnitude in these patients may result in a severe reduction in cardiac output.

4. **Systemic heart failure or residual heart failure:** HF is the number one cause of mortality in ACHD, followed by arrhythmia. It can occur as early as the third decade of life in repaired or palliated patients. The causes of HF in patients with ACHD are varied, including the consequences of surgical palliation, residual shunt and volume overload, severe pulmonary hypertension, severe valvular regurgitation, and even ischemic heart disease. The development of HF increases over time with differing rates, dependent on lesion[25,26] (see Figure 17.7). Specific populations with highest rates of HF include patients with single ventricles (Fontan), systemic RVs, TGA with atrial switch procedure, cc-TGA, and TOF with pulmonic insufficiency. The presence of both diastolic and systolic HF increases perioperative risk and is a key consideration in the evaluation of ACHD for noncardiac and cardiac surgery.

K. **Collateral Circulation:** Physiologic changes in patients with CHD can prompt the development of compensatory circulatory pathways that may be both beneficial and deleterious for the patient.

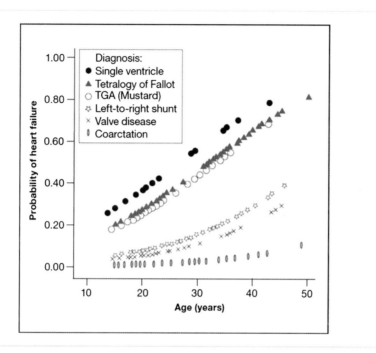

FIGURE 17.7   Graph demonstrating the increasing incidence of heart failure for moderate and complex congenital heart defects with increasing age. Heart failure occurs with great frequency and at a younger age in patients with morphologic right systemic ventricles or in patients with single ventricular physiology. TGA, transposition of the great arteries. (Reprinted from Norozi K, Wessel A, Alpers V, et al. Incidence and risk distribution of heart failure in adolescents and adults with congenital heart disease after cardiac surgery. *Am J Cardiol.* 2006;97(8):1238-1243. © 2006 Elsevier. With permission.)

1. **Aortopulmonary collateral arteries:** Aortopulmonary collaterals are connections from the systemic arteries to pulmonary channels. These vessels may arise from any major thoracic artery, including the aorta, subclavian arteries, or intercostal arteries. The collaterals often develop in patients with cyanotic syndromes (eg, TOF with pulmonary atresia) and single ventricles with Fontan circulation. Aortopulmonary vessels can interfere with normal pulmonary blood flow-limiting oxygenation and can result in volume overload of the systemic ventricle due to increased pulmonary venous return. The presence of significant aortopulmonary vessels may make transplantation prohibitive in select patients with ACHD due to bleeding risk.[27]

2. **Mediastinal collateral arteries:** Patients with long-standing coarctation of the aorta or occlusion of the subclavian arteries may develop bilateral collateral arteries arising from the internal thoracic and intercostal artery network, producing the "rib-notching" sign on chest radiographs. In cases of interruption of the descending thoracic aorta, mediastinal collateral arteries may be the only arterial connection to the distal aorta. Enlarged mediastinal collateral arteries increase the risk of perioperative bleeding in sternotomy or thoracotomies.

L. **Common Surgical Palliations (Figure 17.8)**

1. **Blalock-Taussig-Thomas shunt:** The BTT shunt is performed in infants or children with cyanotic heart disease due to inadequate pulmonary blood flow. The BTT shunt consists of direct anastomosis or placement of a graft conduit between either right or left subclavian artery to the ipsilateral PA branch in order to increase pulmonary blood flow and blood oxygenation. BTT shunts allow for sufficient increase in oxygenation to allow for growth until a more durable palliation or corrective surgery can be performed.

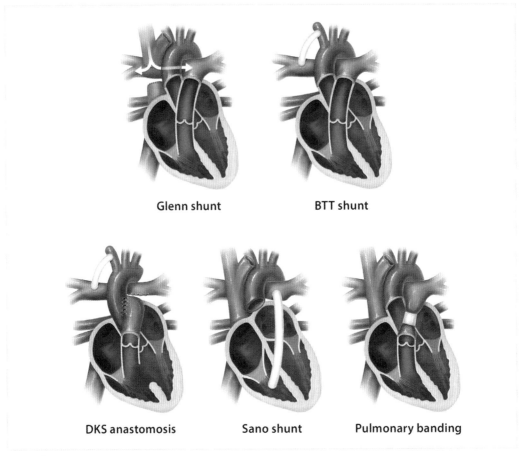

FIGURE 17.8 Palliative procedures. Surgical repairs commonly used for palliation in childhood or infancy of various congenital heart defects. These palliations may still exist well into adulthood. BTT, Blalock-Thomas-Taussig; DKS, Damus-Kaye-Stansel. (Illustration by Townsend Majors and courtesy of Ravi V. Joshi, UT Southwestern.)

2. **Bidirectional Glenn shunt:** This surgical palliation involves the anastomosis of the SVC to the right PA branch to allow venous return from the upper body to drive pulmonary blood flow and improve oxygenation in cyanotic patients. The Glenn shunt is commonly performed as the second stage palliation in patients with single ventricle physiology. It is also performed as a replacement for the BTT shunt in older infants or children who require more pulmonary blood flow.

3. **Damus-Kaye-Stansel procedure:** The Damus-Kaye-Stansel (DKS) procedure is performed in congenital heart lesions with single ventricle physiology and obstruction to systemic flow. The procedure involves the anastomosis of the main PA trunk to the proximal aorta to allow for increased systemic circulation. Pulmonary blood flow requires concomitant Glenn or BTT shunt placement.

4. **Sano shunt:** The Sano shunt is an extracardiac graft conduit connection between the RV and the PA. The Sano shunt is used as a modification to the Norwood procedure for single ventricle anomalies (see later). Because pulmonary blood flow is provided in systole, the Sano shunt avoids the coronary steal phenomenon that can occur with the BTT shunt during diastole.

5. **Pulmonary banding:** This procedure involves the placement of an external band on main PA to limit pulmonary blood flow. The technique is used to prevent pulmonary overcirculation and the development of pulmonary arterial hypertension (PAH) in patients with excessive left-to-right shunting. It also can reduce the blood flow steal phenomenon from the systemic circulation in patients with double outlet physiology.

CLINICAL PEARL

- Patients with ACHD have higher perioperative morbidity and mortality compared to age-matched general population.
- Perioperative management of patients with ≥moderate lesions or simple defects with ≥B physiologic status should involve a multidisciplinary approach involving the anesthesiologist, surgeon, and the ACHD cardiology specialist.
- High-risk populations include patients with single ventricular physiology, Fontan repair, pulmonary hypertension, HF, and/or Eisenmenger syndrome.

III. Shunt Lesions

    A. Atrial Septal Defects

        1. Definition: An ASD is an abnormal malformation of the interatrial septum that allows persistent communication between the right atrium (RA) and left atrium (LA), leading to shunting of blood between the pulmonary and systemic circulations. ASDs are one of the most common cardiac defects and are found in about one-third of adults with CHD. There is a greater occurrence in women than in men in a ratio of about 3:1. ASDs are common cardiac lesions observed in a variety of congenital syndromes (eg, Holt-Oram syndrome, Lutembacher syndrome, Ebstein anomaly).

        2. Classification: There are four main types of ASDs (see Figure 17.9).

            a. The *ostium primum* defect is a failure of the endocardial cushion and the inferior portion of atrial septum to meet, forming a communication above the AV valves. Ostium primum defect is the second most common type and accounts for 15% of ASDs.[28] Because it involves the malformation of the endocardial cushion with the AV canal, it is often considered the simplest of the AVSDs, which are further discussed later. Ostium primum ASDs are often associated with other cardiac defects, most commonly the cleft anterior mitral valve leaflet. Primum ASDs can also be found in patients with Down syndrome (trisomy 21), DiGeorge syndrome, and Ellis-Van Creveld syndrome.

            b. A defect in the central portion of the septum around the *fossa ovalis* in the original position of the *foramen ovale* is called an *ostium secundum* defect. Despite the name, the primary defects in secundum ASDs occur in the embryologic *septum primum*. This is the most commonly encountered type, making up about 75% of all ASDs.[28] Iatrogenic ostium secundum ASDs may occur after interventional cardiac procedures requiring trans-septal atrial puncture to cross from the RA to the LA.

            c. **The sinus venous:** This ASD occurs between the cavoatrial junction and the LA. Most sinus venous defects are a communication between the SVC and the LA, but they can occur at the level of the inferior vena cava (IVC). The sinus venosus ASD is often associated with partial or total anomalous pulmonary venous return (PAPVR or TAPVR) and makes up about 10% of all ASDs[28] (see Figure 17.10).

            d. The *coronary sinus septal defect* or the *"unroofed" coronary sinus* is the rarest form, making up <1% of all ASDs.[29] This congenital anomaly arises from a fenestration or complete absence of the common wall between the coronary sinus and the LA. The unroofed coronary sinus can be very challenging to detect with multiple imaging modalities, including echocardiography. Often, saline contrast is needed to identify the defect. Coronary sinus septal defects are commonly associated with a PL-SVC and anomalous pulmonary venous return (PAPVR or TAPVR).

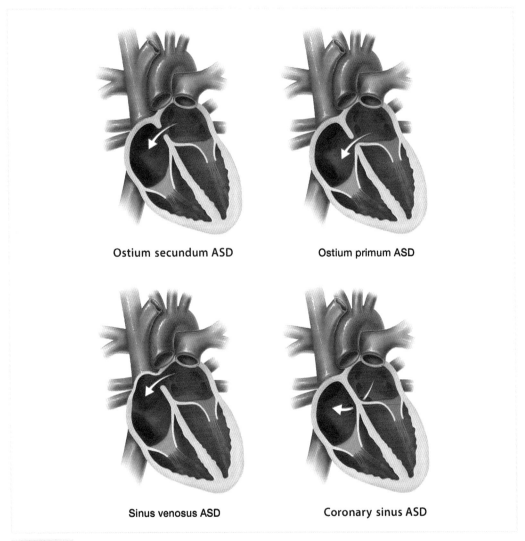

Ostium secundum ASD   Ostium primum ASD

Sinus venosus ASD   Coronary sinus ASD

FIGURE 17.9   Atrial septal defect (ASD) subtypes. (Illustration by Townsend Majors and courtesy of Ravi V. Joshi, UT Southwestern.)

3. **Pathophysiology of atrial septal defects:** The primary clinical consequences of ASD depend on the magnitude and direction of interatrial shunting of blood (left-to-right or right-to-left). Shunting arises in both systole and diastole, but the vast majority of shunting occurs during diastole. The magnitude or volume rate (flow) of shunting is directly determined by the size of the atrial communication (resistance) and by the relative interatrial pressure differential (gradient) due to LV and RV compliances.

ASD size is based on diameter measurements on cardiac imaging, usually echocardiography. Small ASDs of ≤5 mm are classified as "restrictive" ASDs and usually have insignificant shunt flows, whereas large ASDs of >25 mm are classified as "unrestrictive" and permit passage of large shunt volumes. Patients with ASDs of <10 mm rarely present with many of the long-term sequelae, although the risk for paradoxical embolus is still present.

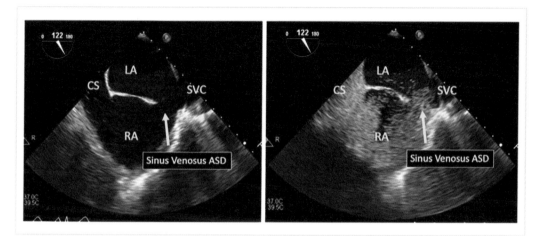

FIGURE 17.10 Sinus venosus atrial septal defect (ASD) visualized (left panel) by transesophageal echocardiography in the bicaval view at a multiplane angle of 122°. Notice the enlarged coronary sinus (CS) indicative of a persistent left-sided superior vena cava (PL-SVC). An agitated saline contrast study (right panel) from a left arm I.V. confirms the presence of a PL-SVC and demonstrates shunting between the right atrium (RA) and left atrium (LA) through the ASD.

Because the relative pressures of each atria are determined in diastole while equilibrating with their respective ventricles, the interatrial pressure gradient is established by differing compliances (or elastances) of the corresponding ventricle. In most cases, the LV compliance is lower (higher elastance) than the RV, leading to elevated LV diastolic pressures. Consequently, mean LA pressures are greater than RA pressures, resulting in predominantly left-to-right shunting of blood.

The degree of shunting is given by the ratio of pulmonary blood flow (Q_p) to systemic blood flow (Q_s) or the shunt fraction (Q_p/Q_s). In a normal patient without shunting, pulmonary blood flow is equal to systemic cardiac output; thus, Q_p/Q_s is 1:1. If some level of left-to-right shunt exists, pulmonary blood flow will exceed systemic blood flow and Q_p/Q_s >1. Conversely, if a right-to-left shunt exists, systemic blood flow surpasses pulmonary flow, then Q_p/Q_s <1. A significant left-to-right shunt fraction, defined as a Q_p/Q_s ratio of ≥1.5, is one major indicator for closure of an ASD.

4. **Natural history of the unrepaired atrial septal defects:** The natural history of an unrepaired ASD depends on several factors, but the key determinants of shunt fraction are the size of the ASD and relative ventricular compliances of the left and right heart. Small restrictive ASDs rarely cause problems at early ages, due to hemodynamically insignificant shunting. As patients age, LV compliance decreases, increasing the magnitude of shunting leading to long-term sequelae. Consequently, patients with an ASD often become symptomatic by their fourth and fifth decades. The common physiologic sequelae from unrepaired ASDs are as follows:

   a. **Right heart chamber enlargement:** Significant left-to-right shunting increases the pulmonary circulatory flow, leading to volume overloading of the right heart and progressive chamber dilatation. Excessive RV dilatation can lead to systolic dysfunction and right HF. Evidence of RV dilatation is the main indication for ASD closure in adults.

   b. **Arrhythmias:** The progressive dilatation of the atria from excessive left-to-right interatrial shunting leads to stretching of the atrial conduction system, leading to primarily atrial fibrillation and atrial flutter. Arrhythmias are much more common in older patients (>40 years) with ASDs.

c. **Paradoxical emboli and stroke:** Although the bulk of shunt flow is left to right in ASDs, transient right-to-left shunting occurs in almost all ASDs, regardless of size, allowing passage of venous emboli (thrombus or air) to the systemic circulation. The exact incidence of stroke in patients with an ASD is unknown. Aside from paradoxical emboli, the presence of atrial arrhythmias such as atrial fibrillation also increases the risk of stroke in these patients.

d. **Pulmonary hypertension:** Significant left-to-right shunting augments pulmonary circulation, which may lead to PAH overtime. Fortunately, the majority of patients with ASDs do not develop PAH. The incidence of PAH is estimated between 6% and 15% of patients with an ASD.[30] Severe PAH leads to elevated right heart filling pressures and can reverse shunt direction to right to left. An admixture of venous and arterial blood entering into the systemic circulation leads to cyanosis and Eisenmenger syndrome.

5. **Closure of atrial septal defects**

   a. **Indications:** Management of symptomatic adult patients with ASDs involves the decision for ASD closure. There is good evidence that ASD closure improves functional status, reduces the incidence of atrial arrhythmias, and may reduce chamber remodeling of the RV and LV. There are few small studies demonstrating better outcomes with closure in adults; however, robust clinical data on long-term morbidity and mortality are lacking. The main indications for ASD closure are as follows[14]:

      (1) Evidence of RA or RV chamber enlargement in the absence of PAH coupled with an ASD of >10 mm or significant shunt fraction $Q_p/Q_s \geq 1.5{:}1$.

      (2) Reduced functional status on exercise testing (NYHA II-IV)

      (3) Sequelae of paradoxical embolus (eg, stroke)

      (4) Cyanosis with exercise in the absence of PAH

      (5) Risk of paradoxical embolus from procedure (eg, hip replacement surgery)

   b. **Minimally invasive closure:** Amendable only to *secundum* ASDs of <36 mm in size due the requirement for a sufficient rim of tissue surrounding the ASD for device engagement. This involves the use of various closure device systems via percutaneous and transvenous delivery (eg, Amplatzer). The anterior, posterior, superior, and inferior tissue rims must all be ≥5 mm in length. Very large secundum ASDs of >36 mm in diameter or ASDs with inadequate tissue rims (<5 mm) preclude the use of transcutaneous closure devices and require surgical patch closure. Patients with multiple defects in the interatrial septum or those with an aneurysmal septum are also difficult to close by transcatheter devices and may require a surgical approach.

   c. **Intraoperative transesophageal echocardiography guidance:** The AHA/ACC considers the use of intraprocedural TEE guidance for device placement *as standard of care.*[14] TEE is used to (1) evaluate ASD size and the shunt fraction, (2) assess sufficient tissue rim for device deployment, (3) rule out pulmonary venous anomalies, (4) rule out LA appendage thrombus, (5) evaluate deployed device, (6) assess for residual shunt, and (7) rule out postprocedural pericardial effusion.

   d. **Surgical closure:** Ostium primum, sinus venosus, rare coronary sinus ASDs, and large secundum ASDs (>36 mm) with small tissue rims must be closed via open-heart surgery requiring CPB. In addition, surgery allows repair of associated congenital anomalies (eg, anomalous pulmonary venous return, cleft anterior mitral valve leaflet). Small secundum ASD lesions are directly sutured closed, while larger lesions often require a pericardial patch repair. Ostium primum defects are also closed by patch repair and often require repair of the anterior mitral leaflet cleft. Sinus venosus ASDs with anomalous pulmonary venous return are repaired via a two-patch technique or the Warden procedure. Coronary sinus ("unroofed") ASDs are simply patch repaired or "roofed" in the LA floor to allow drainage into the RA.

   e. **Contraindications to atrial septal defects closure:** Closure of an ASD may not be benign in a certain select group of patients with advanced disease. The ACC/AHA guidelines present an example decision algorithm for secundum ASD repair. Although the decision to close an ASD is based on the total clinical picture, three major groups of patients where ASD closure may be detrimental are as follows[14]:

(1) **Chronic pulmonary hypertension and right ventricular dilatation** can preclude closure of the ASD. Closure of an ASD in such patients may lead to increased RV strain, decreased pulmonary flow, and decreased pulmonary venous return. In turn, this will decrease systemic cardiac output, leading to failure, hypotension, and/or shock. Typically, patients with PVR >1/3 system vascular resistance (SVR) and/or pulmonary artery systolic pressure (PASP) ≥50% systolic blood pressure (SBP) should be approached cautiously for ASD closure with consultation with the ACHD team.

(2) **Severe left ventricular dysfunction** with elevated filling pressures, as left-to-right shunting can alleviate elevated LA pressures (pop-off valve). Closure may lead to rapid increases in LA and pulmonary venous pressures, leading to pulmonary edema.

(3) *Atrial septal defects with pulmonary arterial hypertension and cyanosis (right-to-left shunt) or Eisenmenger syndrome* are contraindicated for closure. At this level of PAH, the LV receives a significant portion of its venous return through the right-to-left shunt as opposed through the pulmonary venous system. The shunt also serves as a pop-off valve for elevated filling pressures in the right heart. Closure of the ASD can lead to systemic shock from either or both right HF and underfilled LV.

B. Ventricular Septal Defect

1. **Definition:** A ventricular septal defect is a congenital malformation of the interventricular septum (IVS), resulting in a communication between RV and LV of the heart. Much like the ASD, the VSD allows for mixing of blood between the deoxygenated pulmonary (venous) circulation and the oxygenated systemic circulation. VSDs are the most common congenital defect arising in infancy; however, the majority of isolated VSDs are often small and spontaneously close in young childhood. Acquired VSDs that occur as a serious complication of myocardial infarction, surgical interventions (eg, septal myectomy), or mechanical erosion from device placement are discussed elsewhere.

2. **Classification:** In adult hearts, the IVS consists of a muscular section that makes up the majority of the shared septal wall and a fibrous membranous septum that sits in a central position at the confluence of several important cardiac structures. The muscular septum can be anatomically split into inlet, trabecular, and infundibular subdivisions. The membranous septum is located just behind the septal leaflet of the tricuspid valve on the right side and the underneath right coronary cusp (RCC) of the aortic valve in the left ventricular outflow tract (LVOT). The membranous septum can be further divided into the AV and interventricular component septa. The AV component lies at the attachment of the tricuspid septal leaflet and separates the *RA* from the *LV*. It is of great importance as the AV conduction systems travel through this portion of the membranous septum.

There are five main anatomic types of congenital VSDs that correspond to these subdivisions of the IVS (see Figure 17.11):

a. **Type I:** Subpulmonic, supracristal, subarterial, infundibular, doubly committed, or outlet VSDs are synonymous with a communication in the superior infundibulum division of the IVS between the LVOT and the right ventricular outflow tract (RVOT), just below annuli of the aortic and pulmonic valves. They make up about 5% of VSDs.[28] The position of the membranous septum to the RCC and noncoronary cusp (NCC) of the aortic valve and the high-velocity shunting seen in small, restrictive VSDs can result in aortic valve prolapse (usually the RCC) by Venturi effect (Laubry-Pezzi syndrome) and significant aortic regurgitation (AR) with progressive dilatation of the aortic root. In addition, subpulmonic VSDs are also associated with the development of sinus of Valsalva aneurysms (SOVAs). The subpulmonic VSD is seen more frequently in East Asian populations (30% of VSDs).[31]

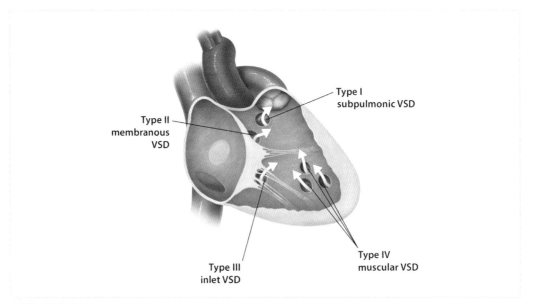

FIGURE 17.11 Subtypes of ventricular septal defects (VSDs). Relative positions of the different types of VSDs seen from the right ventricular side. (Illustration by Townsend Majors and courtesy of Ravi V. Joshi, UT Southwestern.)

  b. **Type II:** The membranous VSD, as the name implies, is a communication in the membranous septum between the LV and RV (see Figure 17.12). Membranous VSDs compromise the vast majority of VSDs encountered (~80%).[30] Type II VSD jets have been implicated in the development of tricuspid regurgitation by inhibiting proper leaflet coaptation. Membranous VSDs can also cause AR due to aortic valve prolapse as described earlier, although less commonly than type I defects. Due to its proximity to the membranous septum, the tricuspid septal leaflet may seal over a membranous VSD, resulting in closure of the defect overtime. In rare instances, the leaflet tissue extension can expand, creating an aneurysm of the membranous IVS that may also be associated with tricuspid regurgitation due to an adherent septal leaflet. Lastly, about 10% of patients with membranous VSDs often develop a double-chambered right ventricle (DCRV).[32]

  c. **Type III:** Inlet or AV VSDs are typically found in the inlet or posterior septum in proximity to the AV canal and make up about 8% of all VSDs.[31] Inlet VSDs can be an isolated defect or a component of larger AVSD (or AV "canal" defects; see in the section that follows).

  d. **Type IV:** Muscular VSDs are defects arising in the trabecular subdivision of the muscular IVS. Small muscular VSDs are commonly discovered in infancy and often spontaneously close within the first several years of life. Muscular VSD defects make up about 20% of VSDs encountered at birth.[28,31] Due to the rate of spontaneous closure in early childhood, isolated muscular VSDs in adults are less common.

  e. **The Gerbode ventricular septal defects:** As a very rare abnormality, the Gerbode defect arises in the AV component of the membranous septum, resulting in a communication and shunt between the LV and *RA*.

3. **Pathophysiology of ventricular septal defects:** Similar to the ASD, the physiology and pathologic consequences of the VSD arise from the magnitude and direction of shunt flow between the LV and RV. In contrast to the ASD, the shunting happens at the ventricular level and predominantly in systole. The LV stroke volume, therefore, has an alternate pathway through the VSD into the RV, a lower pressure compartment, rather than through the

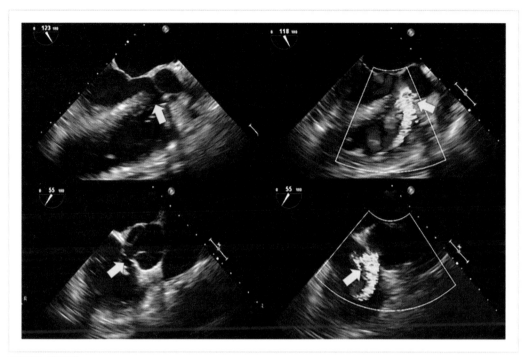

FIGURE 17.12   Type II (membranous) ventricular septal defects visualized by transesophageal echocardiography in the ME long-axis (left and right upper panels) and ME AoV short-axis (left and right lower panels) with and without color-flow Doppler imaging. Doppler imaging demonstrates left-to-right shunting. AoV, aortic valve; ME, mid-esophageal.

LVOT and aorta. The shunt (flow) is then determined by the size of the defect (resistance) and the pressure differential between both ventricular chambers (gradient) in systole. Therefore, the differential between LV and RV systolic blood pressures (SBP and PASP) will govern the degree of shunting for a given VSD size.

The clinical physiologic consequences of VSDs shunting are 2-fold. The effect of splitting the LV stroke volume between systemic circulation and pulmonary circulation reduces overall cardiac output, especially for moderate and large VSDs. Compensatory mechanisms for reduced effective circulating volume are activated, resulting in more volume loading of the left heart and progressive chamber dilatation. Patients may develop both elevated filling pressures and left HF. The second consequence is pulmonary overcirculation and pressure overload of the right heart. The increased flow in the left-to-right shunt is transmitted through the pulmonary circuit, leading to LA volume overload and increasing PAH. Pressure overload of the right heart may lead to right ventricular hypertrophy (RVH) initially and then, as PAH and volume overload worsen, to RV dilatation, systolic dysfunction, and right HF. Reversal of shunt direction to right to left leads to hypoxemia, cyanosis, and Eisenmenger syndrome.

The VSD size is graded based on comparison to the patient's aortic valve annular diameter. Small or "restrictive" VSDs have diameters $\leq 25\%$ of the aortic valve annulus. Moderate-sized VSDs are $>25\%$ to $\leq 75\%$ and large or "nonrestrictive" VSDs are $>75\%$ of the aortic valve annular diameter.

As in the case of ASDs, the degree of shunting for VSDs is given by the shunt fraction (Q_p/Q_s). Normally, the shunt fraction (Q_p/Q_s) is 1:1, indicating no shunt exists. A left-to-right shunt results in a shunt fraction (Q_p/Q_s) >1. Conversely if a right-to-left shunt exists, then Q_p/Q_s is <1. Again, a significant left-to-right shunt fraction is defined as a Q_p/Q_s ratio of $\geq 1.5:1$ and is one major indicator for closure of a VSD.

4. **Natural history of unrepaired ventricular septal defects:** VSDs are the most common congenital abnormality found in infancy, but many of these (especially muscular VSDs) tend to close spontaneously with growth. VSDs are also very commonly associated with many congenital syndromes, including TOF and D-TGA. Isolated VSDs in adults are less common but still make up about 10% of congenital defects.[33] The clinical consequences of VSDs for adult patients depend on the size of the lesion. Patients with small persistent VSDs may be asymptomatic throughout life as the shunt fraction is too small to cause hemodynamic consequence. Whereas patients with moderate or large VSDs can progress to significant HF and even shunt reversal, resulting in cyanosis and Eisenmenger syndrome. The common sequelae or complications from unrepaired VSDs are as follows:

   a. **Endocarditis:** The presence of a high-velocity shunt flow in VSDs increases the risk of endocarditis, even in patients with small unrepaired VSDs. The incidence of endocarditis in patients with VSDs (~0.2%) is nearly 25 times greater than the general public (~0.008%).[33,34]

   b. **Aortic valve regurgitation:** Significant aortic valve regurgitation can develop in patients with subpulmonic or membranous VSDs due to prolapse of an aortic valve cusp, most commonly the RCC. AR is more than twice as likely seen in subpulmonic VSDs as in membranous VSDs. Progression to severe AR can lead to left-sided HF.

   c. **Sinus of Valsalva aneurysm:** Subpulmonic VSDs also predispose patients to an aneurysm of the right sinus of Valsalva with dilation of the aortic root. The presence of an SOVA is often associated with aortic cusp prolapse and AR. Rupture of the aneurysm may be fatal.

   d. **Paradoxical emboli and stroke:** Due to the high-pressure left-to-right systolic shunting seen in the majority of VSDs, the risk of paradoxical stroke is very low. In situations where there is shunt flow reversal such as in elevated pulmonary hypertension or Eisenmenger syndrome, the risk of stroke increases as a right-to-left shunt promotes passage of venous emboli (thrombus or air) into the systemic circulation.

   e. **Double-chamber right ventricle:** The DCRV develops in the presence of a membranous VSD. The exposure to the high-pressure VSD shunt incites hypertrophy of the trabecular muscle from the supraventricular crest of the RV to create a thickened band of tissue, causing RVOT obstruction (RVOTO) in systole. The resultant obstruction creates a high-pressure distal chamber at the RV inlet and a lower pressure RV chamber below the pulmonic valve just past the obstruction. The clinical result is increasing exercise intolerance and right HF.

   f. **Heart failure:** Progressive increase in left-to-right VSD shunting at the ventricular level decreases systemic stroke volume and results in volume loading by compensatory mechanisms to maintain cardiac output. Over time, this results in left-sided volume overload, LA enlargement, and LV dilatation with decreasing systolic function. This can also develop due to severe AR associated with the VSD.

   g. **Pulmonary hypertension and Eisenmenger syndrome:** The high pulmonary flows through moderate to large VSDs lead to worsening PAH. High PVR leads to pressure overload, RVH, and elevation in PA pressures. RV dysfunction and HF may also occur in the setting of severe PAH. Once pulmonary systolic pressures exceed systemic systolic pressures, shunt reversal ensues and right-to-left flow predominates, leading to hypoxemia and cyanosis. Eisenmenger syndrome heralds a reduced survival.

5. **Repair of ventricular septal defects**

   a. **Indications:** The indications for closure of a VSD are dependent upon the size of the defect, the shunt magnitude, and sequelae of disease. Small restrictive VSDs do not require closure as the 25-year survival of patients is 87%. In these patients, nonshunt complications such infective endocarditis (IE) or AR are usually indications to close a restrictive VSD. Moderate or large VSDs have significant shunt flow, often leading to clinical syndromes ending in HF. Moderately restrictive or nonrestrictive VSDs with normal or mildly elevated pulmonary pressures are candidates for VSD repair. The following are a list of common indications for repair[14]:

(1) **Hemodynamically significant left-to-right shunt:** Shunt fraction ($Q_p/Q_s \geq 1.5:1$) without substantial pulmonary hypertension, defined as PASP <50% of systemic pressure or PVR <1/3 of SVR.

(2) **Aortic regurgitation (≥moderate):** In the case of membranous or subpulmonic VSDs, the presence of significant progressive AR may be an indication for aortic valve repair/replacement. The VSD should also be repaired concomitantly.

(3) **History of infective endocarditis:** IE occurs in VSDs more frequently than the general population, and previous episode increases the risk of repeat IE. VSD closure or repair may be warranted in these patients.

(4) **Left ventricular enlargement:** Left heart chamber dilatation and/or symptoms of left HF are indications for repair.

b. **Contraindications:** Patients with nonrestrictive VSDs who have severe pulmonary hypertension (defined as PASP ≥50% of systemic pressures or a PVR >1/3 of SVR) but still left-to-right shunting may not benefit from VSD closure and may still continue to have persistent PAH with a poor prognosis. An alternate strategy is preoperative treatment with pulmonary vasodilator therapy and improvement in hemodynamics before VSD closure. This option has been successful in a select group of patients.[14] VSDs associated with right-to-left shunt and Eisenmenger syndrome should not be closed. Via right-to-left shunting, the VSD acts as a release valve for a stressed RV and provides LV preload. VSD closure in patients with Eisenmenger results in RV failure with a decrease in systemic cardiac output and carries a very high mortality.

c. **Surgical patch repair:** Repair of a VSD depending on anatomic pattern and size can be either a direct primary closure with suture or patch closure with prosthetic material or tissue graft from the patient. This requires median sternotomy and CPB.

d. **Minimally invasive repair:** Percutaneous closure of VSDs using a septal occluder device is becoming a more common option for select cases. Again, intraoperative TEE can be used in conjunction with fluoroscopy to evaluate the lesion and guide placement.

e. **Complications of ventricular septal defect repairs**

(1) **Aortic root dilatation:** Progressive dilatation of the ascending aorta and aortic root may occur in about 10%-30% patients with surgically repaired subpulmonic VSDs.[35] Surgical repair may be appropriate based on current guidelines for aortic aneurysms.

(2) **Valvular regurgitation:** (1) AR: A small portion of repaired VSDs may lead to progressive AR, particularly for type I VSDs, which often involve aortic cusp prolapse. (2) Tricuspid regurgitation: Due to the proximity of type II VSDs to the tricuspid valve annulus, a VSD repair may be complicated by tricuspid valve regurgitation from traumatic or iatrogenic injury to the septal leaflet.

(3) **Arrhythmias:** Conduction system disease is frequently found after surgical repair, especially the right bundle branch block (RBBB), although complete heart block is rare (~2%).[36] Ventricular arrhythmias including premature ventricular contractions (PVCs) and ventricular tachycardia are also common after VSD repair. The incidence of ventricular arrhythmia increases with increasing NYHA functional status, older age of surgery, and the presence of elevated pulmonary pressures.[37]

(4) **Residual ventricular septal defect shunt:** Both percutaneous device closure and surgical patch repair may leave a residual VSD shunt in 2%-3% of patients undergoing repair.[33] Since the residual VSD shunt flows are typically insignificant, reoperation is rarely necessary. *The presence of a residual VSD and prosthetic material is a nidus for infection, requiring antibiotic prophylaxis for increased risk of endocarditis.*

C. **Atrioventricular Septal Defects**

1. **Definition:** AVSD is a constellation of defects that all arise from abnormal fusion of the developing atrial and ventricular septum with the endocardial cushion in the AV canal. The term "AV canal defect" is synonymous with AVSD. AVSDs occur in about 0.2%-0.3% of live births and account for 3% of all congenital lesions.[38] Isolated *primum* ASDs, unroofed coronary sinuses, and inlet VSDs can be considered simple forms of AV canal defects. More complex lesions often involve malformation of the AV valves or complete lack of

an atrial septum ("common atria"). AVSDs are often associated with genetic or congenital syndromes, especially with trisomy 21 (Down syndrome). AVSDs are also linked with left or right isomerism (heterotaxy) syndromes, particularly those with asplenia or polysplenia. Other associated congenital lesions include pulmonary vein stenosis, patent ductus arteriosus (PDA), narrowing of the aortic isthmus, and PAPVR/TAPVR.

2. **Classification** (see Figure 17.13)
   a. **Partial or incomplete atrioventricular septal defect:** The presence of separate, distinguishable right and left heart AV valves (eg, tricuspid and mitral) at the AV orifice is the hallmark of a partial AVSD. The congenital defect is a partial fusion of embryologic septa with the endocardial cushion, resulting in a combination of a *primum* ASD with a cleft mitral valve and an inlet VSD.

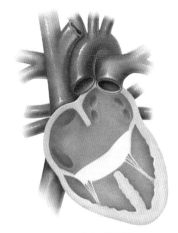

complete AVSD

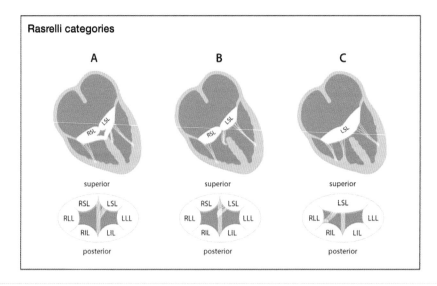

FIGURE 17.13 Atrioventricular septal defect (AVSD) or AV "canal" defect. Inlet shows the Rastelli classification for AVSD variants. LIL, left inferior leaflet; LLL, left lateral leaflet; LSL, left superior leaflet; RIL, right inferior leaflet; RLL, right lateral leaflet; RSL, right superior leaflet. (Illustration by Townsend Majors and courtesy of Ravi V. Joshi, UT Southwestern.)

    b. **Complete atrioventricular septal defect:** The complete AVSD is failure of fusion of the endocardial cushion with the septa. The key characteristic for a complete defect is a single (common) AV valve that spans the entire AV orifice and both ventricles. Based on the appearance of the common AV valve anterior (or superior) leaflet and chordae, AVSD can be further categorized using the *Rastelli classification*[38]:

      (1) **Type A:** The anterior (superior) bridging leaflet can be separated into left and right portions with chordal attachments to the IVS. This is the most common form of complete AVSDs.

      (2) **Type B:** The anterior bridging leaflet spans across the IVS with a left medial chordal attachment to an RV papillary muscle. This is the rarest form of complete AVSDs.

      (3) **Type C:** The anterior bridging leaflet spans across the IVS without any medial chordal attachments and is considered a free-floating leaflet. Type C defects are often associated with other more severe congenital anomalies.

      (4) **Unbalanced complete atrioventricular septal defect:** A more severe form of AVSD that involves malalignment of the AV valve, hypoplasia of one ventricle (either right or left), and hypoplasia of the respective outflow valve due to low flow.

3. **Pathophysiology:** The presence of AVSDs permits significant mixing of the pulmonary and systemic circulations. Clinical signs of cyanosis or hypoxemia will arise based on the direction and magnitude of *dependent* shunting determined by the afterload or impedance of the respective outflow tracts. Elevated systemic afterload will increase left-to-right shunting, while any pulmonary stenosis (PS) or pulmonary hypertension will result in shunt reversal and cyanosis. In partial AVSDs, the attachments of both AV valves to the IVS limit shunting through the VSD; thus, primary shunting often occurs through the *primum* ASD. The presence of a cleft mitral valve or a common AV valve results in significant AV valve regurgitation. The pressures in the LV are much greater than in the RV or the atria so that mitral regurgitation predominates. With the presence of a communication between the atria such as an ASD, severe mitral regurgitation can cause *obligatory* left-to-right shunting that is independent of pulmonary afterload.[39] As in other shunting lesions, excessive left-to-right shunt leads to volume and pressure overload of the right heart, leading to congestion and HF. Prolonged pulmonary overcirculation leads to pulmonary hypertension.

4. **Natural history of atrioventricular septal defects:** The natural history of AVSDs is dependent on the type of defect. Patients with partial AVSD may not present with symptoms in childhood unless complicated by severe left AV valve (LAVV) regurgitation or other associated lesions. Over time, patients with partial AVSD develop symptoms similar to unrestricted ASDs with RV volume overload, HF, and pulmonary hypertension. In contrast, clinical symptoms of complete AVSDs present in early infancy, and if not immediately treated, progress quickly to HF. Unrepaired complete AVSDs have a high childhood mortality in relation to the complexity of the lesion.[30] If associated with increased left-to-right shunt as in AV valve regurgitation or a systemic obstructive lesion (eg, aortic stenosis [AS], coarctation), these patients develop HF and pulmonary hypertension (and possibly Eisenmenger syndrome) more rapidly. Early surgical correction in childhood is critical for complete AVSDs. Unbalanced lesions may require conversion to single ventricle palliation.

5. **Repair of atrioventricular septal defects**

    a. **Indications:** Partial AVSDs are repaired as symptoms arise as in ASDs (see earlier discussion). Complete AVSDs carry a large mortality and disease burden and are almost always surgically repaired in infancy or early childhood depending on the individual and complexity of the lesion. Current prognosis after surgery is good demonstrating a ≥85% 15-year survival rate. Perioperative mortality has decreased to about 3% since the 1990s. About 10% of patients with repaired AVSD return for reoperation due to complications of the primary repair.[40]

    b. **Surgical repair:** Surgical repair is the only current option. Partial AVSDs are repaired with patch closure of the *primum* ASD and inlet VSD with left AV (mitral) valvuloplasty. Balanced AVSDs are repaired with a two-patch technique and valvuloplasty, whereas unbalanced AVSDs may undergo single ventricle palliation (eg, Fontan) depending on the anatomy of the lesion. Pulmonary banding is no longer standard for these patients.[40,41]

   c. **Complications from atrioventricular septal defect repair:** Reoperation is common in patients with repaired AVSDs in adulthood. The most common reasons for reoperation are as follows:

     (1) **Left (mitral) atrioventricular valvular regurgitation:** Valve repair or replacement for severe regurgitation of the LAVV is a common cause for reoperation and usually occurs in early adulthood.

     (2) **Left ventricular outflow tract obstruction:** In many cases, the position of the aortic valve and LVOT is anteriorly displaced, creating a goose-neck conformation with LVOT narrowing. Obstruction or further narrowing leads to LVOTO by various mechanisms, including impingement of a patch repair or valvuloplasty, development of septal hypertrophy, position of the anterolateral muscle bundle, and fibromuscular stenosis.

     (3) **Residual shunts:** The presence of significant residual shunts with prosthetic material is a risk for endocarditis and possible paradoxical emboli. Significant residual shunts from patch dehiscence will lead to symptoms similar to other shunt lesions, such as pulmonary congestion and HF.

     (4) **Arrhythmias:** Patients with AVSD are prone to the development of complete AV block postrepair and may require pacemaker insertion.

D. Patent Ductus Arteriosus

   1. **Definition:** The *ductus arteriosus* is a communication bridging the fetal main PA and fetal aorta at the aortic isthmus. In fetal circulation, the *ductus arteriosus* allows relatively oxygenated blood returning from the placenta through the right heart to be shunted across the PA to the systemic circulation. Typically, the *ductus arteriosus* closes in the first week of life with exposure to elevated blood oxygen levels. Failure to close leads to a *PDA* and long-standing left-to-right shunt. Adult patients with a PDA may progress to left HF, pulmonary hypertension, and Eisenmenger syndrome. PDAs are found in 1 in 2,000 live births, or 5%-10% of all congenital disease.[42] Prematurity and Rubella infection in pregnancy are factors that predispose for the development of a PDA.

   2. **Classification:** PDAs are classified by their anatomic configuration (Krichenko Class A-E)[42] seen on angiography.

   3. **Pathophysiology and natural history:** Unrepaired PDAs follow a similar pattern of disease as VSDs, although the shunting occurs at the aortopulmonary level. Excessive left-to-right shunting leads to left heart volume overload and dilatation, leading to systolic failure. High pulmonary flows cause changes in the PA tree, leading to pulmonary hypertension. As with ASDs and VSDs, the size of the communication and the magnitude of shunt are responsible for the clinical sequelae. Patients with small restrictive PDAs may be asymptomatic. Moderate-sized lesions may cause exercise intolerance and congestive HF in later decades of life. Large unrestricted PDAs can lead to severe PAH, shunt reversal, and, ultimately, Eisenmenger syndrome. Realize that cyanosis may not present in the head or upper extremities in cases of right-to-left shunting as the PDA insertion site is generally distal to the left subclavian artery origin.

   4. **Indications for patent ductus arteriosus closure:** Indications for closure of a PDA depend heavily on patient clinical symptoms, cardiac imaging, and invasive catheterization measurements, as shunt fraction is difficult to measure. The presence of left chamber dilation and the degree of pulmonary hypertension help determine the level of intervention.[43]

     a. Current ACC/AHA recommendations suggest PDA closure in symptomatic patients with left-to-right shunting and chamber dilatation of the LA and/or ventricle, PA pressures <50% of systemic pressures, and PVR <1/3 systemic.

     b. PDA closure can be *considered* in select symptomatic patients with PA pressures >50% of systemic and/or PVR >1/3 systemic vascular resistance (SVR).

     c. PDA closure should be *avoided* in patients with PA pressures >2/3 systemic pressures and/or PVR >2/3 systemic.

   5. **Patent ductus arteriosus closure**

     a. **Percutaneous catheter-based device:** The preferred method of closure is the transcatheter delivery of an occlusive device or coil. Small PDAs are suitable for deployment of an occlusive coil. Moderate or larger PDAs will require an expansive septal occluder device. Successful closure rates exceed 90% using these types of devices. Device embolization is a rare complication.

b. **Surgical ligation or closure:** PDAs not amendable to transcatheter closure devices may require surgical ligation. This is often done through a left thoracotomy incision or by video-assisted thoracoscopy. In rare instances, patch closure of the PDA is required, necessitating sternotomy and CPB support.

E. **Partial Anomalous Pulmonary Venous Return**

1. **Definition:** This is a rare congenital lesion occurring in about 0.7% of population at autopsy.[34] PAPVR involves the incorrect drainage of one or more of the pulmonary veins into the central venous circulation and RA. Central venous drainage includes pulmonary vein drainage to the SVC (type I: most common), the IVC (type II), brachiocephalic veins (type III), coronary sinus (type IV), and azygous vein. PAVPRs are commonly associated with sinus venosus ASD defects (Figure 17.14).

2. **Variants**

a. **Total anomalous pulmonary venous return** is the serious condition where all four pulmonary veins drain into the central venous circulation, leading to a cyanosis at birth. TAPVR with and without obstruction requires surgical correction in infancy and is rarely ever seen unrepaired in adults.

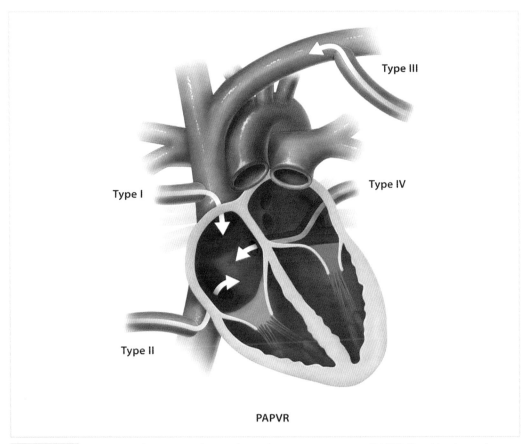

PAPVR

FIGURE 17.14   Anatomic subtypes partial anomalous pulmonary venous return (PAPVR). Type I involves pulmonary venous attachment to the superior vena cava. Type II shows anomalous pulmonary vein insertion into the inferior vena cava. Type III demonstrates pulmonary venous drainage into the left brachiocephalic (innominate) vein. Type IV is a pulmonary venous connection to the coronary sinus system. (Illustration by Townsend Majors and courtesy of Ravi V. Joshi, UT Southwestern.)

b. **Scimitar syndrome** involves right pulmonary venous drainage connects to the IVC via a single "scimitar" vein seen on chest radiography. Due to the anomalous venous drainage, the affected lung may be hypoplastic. In certain cases, the large scimitar vein may cause sequestration of the lower lobes of the affected lung.

c. **Sinus venosus ASD–associated PAPVR** arises from the "unroofing" of a right pulmonary vein and RA wall such that it can drain into the LA, RA, and SVC.

3. **Pathophysiology and natural history:** The addition of partial pulmonary drainage into the RA results in a constant left-to-right shunt, leading to the common pattern of right heart chamber dilatation and excessive pulmonary circulation. As with other shunt lesions, the magnitude of the defect determines clinical sequelae. The effect of small anomalous veins is inconsequential to cardiac function, and patients are typically asymptomatic. The consequence of large venous drainage is similar to large, unrestricted ASDs and can include RV dilation, right HF, and pulmonary hypertension. It should be noted that PAPVRs are not subject to reversal of shunt flow, so cyanosis is not commonly seen (unlike TAPVR). Obstruction of the drainage vessels can lead to pulmonary venous occlusion, leading to pulmonary hypertension as well.

4. **Repair of partial anomalous pulmonary venous return**
   a. **Indications:** Based on current ACC/AHA guidelines, PAPVR repair is recommended in symptomatic adults who have a shunt fraction (Q_p/Q_s) $\geq$1.5:1, evidence of right chamber dilatation, and PA pressures less than half systemic pressures or a PVR <1/3 systemic. Repair should also be considered in asymptomatic individuals with RV overload and similar shunt fractions without significant pulmonary hypertension.[14]
   b. **Surgical repair:** Surgical repair involves creating patch repair and baffle to direct flow into the LA. In other situations, the anomalous vein is removed from the central vein and directly implanted into the LA. PAPVRs with associated sinus venosus defects are repaired in combination via a Warden procedure.

F. **Anesthetic Management for Shunt Lesions**
   1. **Preoperative evaluation**
      a. **Patient history** (assess for)
         (1) Defect type and associated anomalies
         (2) **Physiologic status:** NYHA functional class, exercise symptom
         (3) **Repair or palliation history:** Presence of prosthetic material or closure device, number of redo sternotomies
         (4) **Native/residual shunt:** Magnitude, direction, and if shunt fraction (Q_p/Q_s) $\geq$1.5:1
         (5) **Anticoagulation:** Regimen, atrial arrhythmias, history of thrombosis or embolism
         (6) **Arrhythmia history:** Ablations, antiarrhythmic medication, PPM, or ICDs
         (7) **High-risk sequelae:** HF, pulmonary hypertension, Fontan/single ventricle, Eisenmenger syndrome (cyanosis)
      b. **Laboratory studies**
         (1) Baseline blood pressures (all four extremities), O_2 saturation (SpO_2), heart rate
         (2) Baseline metabolic panel, creatinine, glucose, lactate
         (3) Complete blood count
         (4) Coagulation studies including PT/INR, PTT, fibrinogen, thromboelastography
      c. **Imaging and functional studies**
         (1) Essential
            (a) **Electrocardiogram:** Baseline morphology, detect atrial arrhythmias, pacing, or PVCs
            (b) **Echocardiography:** TTE or TEE imaging to survey cardiac anatomy and function
            (c) Chest x-ray
         (2) Additional
            (a) **Cardiac catheterization:** For patients with residual shunts, PAH, and HF
            (b) CT scan or cMRI for complex lesions or associated anomalies
            (c) **Cardiopulmonary testing if available:** 6-minute walk test, stress testing, nuclear medicine studies in patients with poor functional class (NYHA III or IV)

2. **Air emboli prophylaxis** (see "Perioperative Considerations for Patients With Adult Congenital Heart Disease" section)
3. **Circulation and shunt fraction (Q_p:Q_s)**
    a. **Definition:** The pulmonary circulation (Q_p) must be close to equal to that of the systemic circulation (Q_s) to provide optimal oxygen delivery. The ratio of the pulmonary circulation to the systemic circulation is known as the shunt fraction Q_p:Q_s, ideally equal to 1. An unbalanced may suggest overcirculation in the pulmonary vasculature (Q_p:Q_s > 1) and undercirculation of the systemic flow or vice versa (Q_p:Q_s <1). Consequently, Q_p:Q_s affects end-organ oxygen delivery. Overcirculation may cause chamber dilation and dysfunction, while undercirculation may cause multiorgan atrophy and lack of growth.
    b. **Calculation of Q_p:Q_s:** The Fick equation utilizes the oxygen consumption and the arteriovenous difference to estimate flow:

$$Q_s = \frac{VO_2}{CaO_2 - CmvO_2}$$

$$Q_p = \frac{VO_2}{CpvO_2 - CpaO_2}$$

$CpvO_2$ = oxygen content in the pulmonary veins. $CpaO_2$ = oxygen content in the PA. CaO_2 = arterial oxygen content in the systemic arterial system. CvO_2 = mixed venous oxygen content.

As VO_2 and the hemoglobin oxygen carrying capacity are constant, the equation can be further simplified to:

$$\frac{Q_p}{Q_s} = \frac{CaO_2 - CmvO_2}{CpvO_2 - CpaO_2} = \frac{SaO_2 - SmvO_2}{SpvO_2 - SpaO_2}$$

$CpvO_2$ = oxygen content in the pulmonary veins. $CpaO_2$ = oxygen content in the PA. CaO_2 = arterial oxygen content in the systemic arterial system. CvO_2 = mixed venous oxygen content. $SpvO_2$ = Oxygen content in the pulmonary veins. $SpaO_2$ = Oxygen content in the PA. SaO_2 = Arterial oxygen content in the systemic arterial system. SvO_2 = Mixed venous oxygen content.

$SpvO_2$ is close to 100% in patients with healthy lungs. The values for SaO_2, $SmvO_2$, and $SpaO_2$ result from arterial, central venous, and PA blood samples. For biventricular hearts with no shunts, the Q_p:Q_s is 1:1, as the pulmonary flow equals the systemic flow. Realize the Q_p:Q_s is variable for univentricular, unrepaired hearts as the single ventricle simultaneously pumps blood to the systemic and pulmonary circulations. The systemic flow decreases when the pulmonary flow increases, and vice versa. The best oxygen delivery for single ventricle physiology occurs at any given cardiac output with Q_p:Q_s ratios of 0.5-1:1.[44,45]

4. **Dependent shunt hemodynamics:** The magnitude and flow direction of shunting are determined by the pressure differential at the level of the defect in question (eg, interventricular pressure gradient for VSDs, aortopulmonary gradient for PDAs). Manipulation of the SVR and PVR can, therefore, determine shunt direction and magnitude by influencing the net pressure differential. The SVR/PVR ratio should be kept >1 to maintain left-to-right shunting. It is important to understand that to avoid cyanosis, PVR should be minimized by avoiding hypoxia, hypercapnia, and using low ventilation pressures/positive end-expiratory pressure (PEEP). Avoid hypotension (low SVR), which can also precipitate shunt reversal. Realize moderate or severe hypertension (high SVR) can lead to excessive left-to-right shunting and decrease systemic cardiac output. Systemic blood pressures should be kept at or slightly above the patient's baseline blood pressure. Vasopressin is an ideal agent to maintain SVR as it has very little effect on the pulmonary vasculature. Phenylephrine and, to a larger extent, norepinephrine can both increase PVR due to the α_1-adrenergic activation and should be used judiciously.

   c. **Exceptions**

     (1) Patients with *Eisenmenger or right-to-left* shunt may depend on the shunt flow to contribute to systemic cardiac output. Decreasing PVR may result in less right-to-left shunt, reducing cardiac output in these individuals.

     (2) Patients with PAPVR do not experience shunt reversal unless accompanied by a sinus venosus ASD. Intracardiac pressures may not affect PAPVR draining directly from pulmonary veins to the central venous circulation, consequently SVR changes will have limited effect on shunt magnitude.

     (3) AVSDs or primum ASDs with severe mitral (or LAVV) regurgitation may experience *obligate left-to-right shunting* as SBPs and elevated LA pressures drive the gradient for interatrial shunting of the regurgitant jet. Excessive hypertension will lead to severe shunting and reduce cardiac output.[39]

5. **Anesthetic agents:** In general, most anesthetic agents can be used safely in induction and maintenance of general anesthesia in patients with simple shunt lesions keeping in mind the hemodynamic goals. The use of nitrous oxide (N_2O) should be avoided; however, due to the risk of worsening pulmonary hypertension and risk of volume expansion of any entrained IV air. Remember with left-to-right shunts, inhalation agents have a rapid onset due to the increased pulmonary circulation, while IV agents will take longer to induce the patient. The opposite is true for right-to-left shunts. In noncardiac surgery, patients with complex disease may benefit from regional or neuraxial techniques if applicable. Again, the same hemodynamic goals of maintaining systemic blood pressure should determine the type of technique (eg, epidural vs spinal).

6. **Heart (left) failure:** Patients with left or right heart failure should continue HF medications up to the day of surgery medications. Typically, renin-angiotensin-aldosterone system (RAAS) pathway inhibitors and diuretics are held the day of surgery. Perioperative β-blockade is recommended unless significant hypotension or bradycardia is present. Intraoperative management may require the use of inotropic support. Dobutamine, milrinone, and epinephrine are common options for left heart support. In more complex situations, mechanical support (eg, IABP, Impella, ECMO) may be required.

7. **Pulmonary hypertension and right heart failure:** Medical therapies for pulmonary hypertension (PDE inhibitor/endothelin antagonist/guanylate cyclase stimulator/ prostacyclin) should generally be continued throughout the perioperative period. Management of patients with significant pulmonary hypertension or RV dysfunction are as follows:

   a. **Ventilation strategies:** Minimize hypoxia, hypercarbia, avoid high PEEP, and use low inspiratory pressures or maintain patient spontaneous (negative pressure ventilation)

   b. **Pulmonary vasodilators:** Preoperative or intraoperative use to reduce PVR, reduce right-to-left shunting, and decrease RV afterload

   c. **Inotropic support:** Intraoperative use to support right heart function, including dobutamine, milrinone, and epinephrine

   d. **Mechanical support:** Temporary use of VA-ECMO/ECLS to support right heart function and systemic circulation. Severe precapillary pulmonary hypertension is a contraindication to support with other devices, such as RVAD.

   e. **Palliative procedures for pulmonary hypertension:** Select patients with severe pulmonary hypertension and decreased RV function will not respond to medications and require interventional or surgical procedures to alleviate elevated right-sided pressures.

     (1) **Atrial septostomy:** Incision on the interatrial septum can create communication between the atria. Alternatively, balloon catheter septostomy can also be performed to create an interatrial communication via percutaneous approach. Any communication will increase right-to-left shunt, improving cardiac output but increasing cyanosis.

     (2) **Pulmonary artery ballooning:** In patients with PA stenosis, balloon arterioplasty can alleviate the obstruction and decrease pulmonary pressures. Risks include PA rupture, a possible fatal complication.

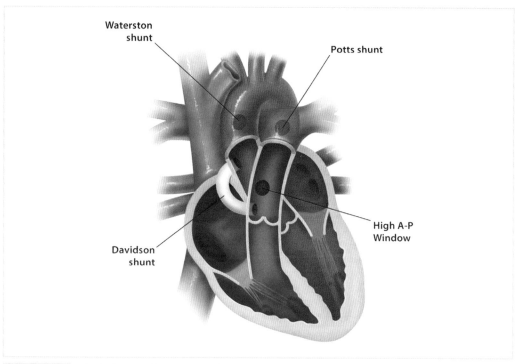

FIGURE 17.15   Surgical aortopulmonary (A-P) shunts. Used for palliation of pulmonary hypertension and to improve cardiac output with the drawback of increasing venous admixture. High A-P windows are a congenital defect that resemble patent ductus arteriosus in physiology and effect. (Illustration by Townsend Majors and courtesy of Ravi V. Joshi, UT Southwestern.)

(3) **Surgical aortopulmonary shunts:** Surgical communication between the aorta and the PA can alleviate right-sided pressures, increase cardiac output, but increase venous admixture and cyanosis. A Davidson shunt involves placement of graft conduit between the ascending aorta and the main PA. The Potts shunt is a side-to-side anastomosis from the left PA to the descending aorta. Likewise, the Waterson shunt connects the right PA and the ascending aorta (Figure 17.15).

CLINICAL PEARL

- The physiologic impact of simple shunt lesions is based on the direction and magnitude of shunt flow. Significant shunts have high shunt fractions (Q_p:Q_s ≥1.5), and closure may be indicated to avoid late-term complications.
- Left-to-right shunting leads to pulmonary overcirculation and volume overload of the receiving chambers. Excessive pulmonary circulation leads to pulmonary hypertension in later years.
- Anesthetic hemodynamic management of dependent shunt lesions requires balancing the SVR/PVR ratio to prevent hypoxemia from right-to-left shunting and maximize cardiac output by minimizing left-to-right shunting.
- Adult patients with congenital shunt defects may have specific late-term complications arising from the location of the shunt or residual effects from a previous repair.

IV. Obstructive Lesions

A large class of congenital defects with moderate severity are congenital obstructive lesions. Obstruction at every cardiac level can lead to significant functional sequelae. Lesions include valvular stenosis, conduit or great vessel narrowing, and muscular hypertrophy of outflow tracts, all resulting in increased ventricular workload to produce an effective stroke volume and maintain adequate cardiac output. Elevated afterload results in compensatory changes in the ventricular myocardium, leading to wall thickening and resulting in reduce diastolic compliance, elevated filling pressures, and venous congestion. Many complications of these lesions present in infancy and early childhood, but a subset of defects may persist undiagnosed until adulthood. A summary of common obstructive lesions and their respective anesthetic management is found in Table 17.2.

A. **Cor triatriatum:** A *cor triatriatum* is a fibromuscular membrane that divides either the RA or the LA into two compartments. The *cor triatriatum* is thought to be the remnant of the common pulmonary vein, which, due to incomplete absorption into the LA during development, results in a partially obstructive atrial membrane. It is a rare congenital abnormality with a general incidence of 0.4% among congenital lesions.[46]

There are two general types:

1. **Dexter (R):** The fibromuscular membrane divides the RA.
   Cor triatriatum is associated with other defects, including RV hypoplasia, pulmonary valve atresia, pulmonary valve stenosis, and Ebstein anomaly.[47,48]

2. **Sinister (L):** The fibromuscular membrane divides the LA and is the most common form of cor triatriatum. The pulmonary veins drain to an upper chamber (proximal compartment) that connects to a lower section (distal compartment) via a small orifice or a channel. Obstructed pulmonary drainage leads to physiology similar to mitral stenosis (MS).

   Cor triatriatum is commonly associated with other defects, including secundum ASDs, patent foramen *ovale* (PFO), persistent left SVC, PAPVR, mitral valve regurgitation, isolated PA stenosis, TOF, and double outlet right ventricle (DORV).[47,48]

   a. **Natural history of disease:** The atrial obstruction by *cor triatriatum* leads to venous congestion, pulmonary hypertension (in *sinister* type), and HF often presenting in infancy. In the rare presentation in adults, symptoms resemble those of severe mitral (*sinister*) or tricuspid (*dextra*) stenosis. The *cor triatriatum* membrane is incomplete, and the overall transmembrane gradient reflects lesion severity. These patients are extremely susceptible to atrial rhythm disturbances, especially the development of atrial fibrillation, which can be catastrophic. Venous congestion increases the risk of DVT and pulmonary embolus, and many patients are maintained on systemic anticoagulation for thromboprophylaxis. Definitive treatment is surgical excision of the membrane and should be performed in patients with symptoms or considerable transmembrane mean gradient (≥8 mm Hg).[14]

B. **Congenital Left-Sided Outflow Obstruction:** Left-sided outflow lesions occur due to narrowing or stenosis at the level of the aortic valve, at the LVOT, above the aortic valve, or in the aorta or arch. All these lesions lead to significant left-sided outflow obstruction and reduction of systemic cardiac output. Elevated afterload leads to compensatory ventricular changes, including significant LV concentric hypertrophy, reduced diastolic compliance, and increased LV filling pressures. Ventricular wall thickening will lead to decreasing diastolic compliance, elevated left-sided diastolic pressures, and pulmonary venous congestion or edema. Aortic coarctation also has the effect of altered collateral circulation (see section that follows).

1. **Congenital aortic stenosis:** The three types of congenital AS are as follows:
   a. **Subvalvular:** Subvalvular obstruction can occur as luminal narrowing of the LVOT, as a discrete fibromuscular membrane in the LVOT, or due to hypertrophic cardiomyopathy resulting in turbulent flow and elevated transaortic pressure gradient. Due to turbulent flow characteristics, many patients develop clinically significant aortic insufficiency. Subvalvular obstruction is commonly associated with *Shone syndrome.*

TABLE 17.2 Anesthetic Considerations for Obstructive Congenital Lesions

Defect Variable	Cor triatriatum	Congenital Aortic Stenosis (AS)	Aortic Coarctation	Congenital Mitral Stenosis (MS)	Congenital Pulmonic Stenosis (PS)	Pulmonary Atresia	Severe Pulmonary Insufficiency (PR)
Rate	Normal to low	Normal to low	Normal to low	Normal to low	Normal to low	Normal to low, except in patients with pulmonary valve insufficiency who can tolerate mildly elevated heart rates	Normal to high
Rhythm	Sinus rhythm is essential to permit flow to the distal chamber and to maintain cardiac output. Avoid atrial fibrillation	Sinus rhythm is essential as atrial contraction may contributed to 40% of LV filling	Sinus rhythm	Sinus rhythm is essential	Sinus rhythm is essential	Sinus rhythm is essential. Some of these patients may have severe atrial dilation and refractory arrhythmias	Sinus rhythm
Preload (volume status)	Normal. High risk of fluid overload and pulmonary hypertension	Normal to high	Maintain within normal parameters	Norma -to high	Normal. Caution with fluids in patients with RV dysfunction	Normal to high. Very preload dependent. Stenosed conduit with RV dysfunction and dilation. Try to avoid volume overload	RV dilation, judicious fluid administration to avoid further dilation
Contractility	Normal to mildly increased for right ventricular support	Normal. Then ventricle is usually hyperdynamic—caution with epinephrine	Maintain within normal parameters. Patients with reduced ventricular function may need inotropic support	Normal	Normal to high	Normal. Beware hyperdynamic episodes may compromise coronary circulation in patients with RV-dependent circulation. Presence of RV dysfunction/failure with need inotropic support	Normal to high

(continued)

TABLE 17.2 Anesthetic Considerations for Obstructive Congenital Lesions *(continued)*

Defect Variable	Cor triatriatum	Congenital Aortic Stenosis (AS)	Aortic Coarctation	Congenital Mitral Stenosis (MS)	Congenital Pulmonic Stenosis (PS)	Pulmonary Atresia	Severe Pulmonary Insufficiency (PR)
Afterload (SVR)	Normal to mildly increased to maintain coronary perfusion	Normal to high to maintain coronary perfusion. Phenylephrine is an excellent choice	Normal to low. Consider clevidipine, nicardipine, or esmolol. Blood pressure should be measured in the right arm	Normal to high for maintenance coronary perfusion. Severe increases in afterload may not be well tolerated, especially with concomitant mitral regurgitation	Normal to mildly increased to maintain coronary perfusion	Normal to mildly increased to maintain coronary perfusion	Normal. Be mindful of coronary perfusion
PVR	Maintain normal values. Avoid hypoxia or hypercapnia. Consider using a pulmonary artery catheter in patients with *cor triatriatum sinister*	Maintain normal values. Avoid hypoxia or hypercapnia	Maintain within normal values. Avoid hypoxia or hypercapnia	Maintain normal values. Avoid hypoxia or hypercapnia	Maintain normal values. Avoid hypoxia or hypercapnia	Maintain normal values. Avoid hypoxia or hypercapnia	Low PVR. Avoid hypothermia, hypercarbia, acidosis, hypoxia, and high ventilator pressures. Consider nitric oxide (NO) or inhaled prostacyclin
Special notes	IV medications may have their onset of action delayed due to the accumulation of blood in the large right atrium	IV medications may have their onset of action delayed due to the accumulation of blood in the large right atrium	See "late-term complications" table	Low Spo$_2$ is a sign of right-to-left shunting. After repair, high risk of PI in adulthood. See "late-term complications" table	General considerations for redo sternotomy: (1) high risk of bleeding. (2) review previous imaging to determine relationship between sternum and cardiac structures including coronaries, (3) consider preoperative insertion of femoral wires for emergent cannulation, (4) large-bore central and peripheral access (difficult IV access)	See "late-term complications" table	Commonly associated with DiGeorge syndrome. Check calcium levels. See "late-term complications" table

IV, intravenous; LV, left ventricle; RV, right ventricle; SVR, system vascular resistance.

Indications for surgery resection of the membrane or myectomy include symptomatic patients with a mean gradient ≥50 mm Hg, symptomatic patients with ischemia or HF, and asymptomatic with a mean gradient ≥50 mm Hg plus mild AR.

b. **Valvular:** Congenital obstruction at the aortic valve is due to incomplete development of the leaflets or the annulus. The pathophysiology is identical to acquired AS. The bicuspid valve is the most common cause of congenital AS.[47] Surgical treatment involves aortic valve replacement (AVR) or repair on CPB. The use of percutaneous interventions such as TAVR approaches is becoming more prevalent. Indications are identical to acquired aortic valvular stenosis. Some patients may have a hypoplastic aortic annulus that may require an additional aortic annular enlargement procedure.

c. **Supravalvular:** This obstruction is narrowing at or above the level of the sinotubular junction. This condition is associated with *Williams syndrome* and homozygous familial hypercholesteremia. *Williams syndrome* is also associated with narrowing of the PAs and coronary anomalies, including coronary ostial obstruction. Patients with mild obstruction (<20 mm Hg) may be monitored.[49] More severe obstruction causing significant symptoms including angina are indications for surgical repair. Percutaneous interventions are not recommended due to the proximity to the aortic valve and coronary ostia. Patients with coronary obstruction should undergo coronary artery bypass grafting (CABG) as well.[14]

2. **Complications from childhood aortic stenosis repair presenting in adulthood**
   a. Subvalvular stenosis can recur after repair.
   b. Bicuspid valves can become stenotic, requiring balloon valvuloplasty or surgical replacement.
   c. Patients with a previous Ross procedure can present with graft decay, manifesting as stenosis or regurgitation.
   d. Risk for aneurysms, ventricular dysfunction, and endocarditis years after repair

3. **Aortic coarctation:** Aortic coarctation involves narrowing of the proximal thoracic aorta just distal to the takeoff of the left subclavian artery near the junction of the ductus arteriosus. The incidence of coarctation is about 5%-8% of patients with CHD.[49] It is commonly associated with several syndromes, including Shone abnormality and Turner syndrome. Around 50%-85% of coarctations also present with a bicuspid aortic valve. The presence of a coarctation creates a situation with altered circulation proximal and distal to the lesion. The upper aortic vessels are perfused normally being proximal to the lesion, whereas organs distal to the narrowing experience reduced circulation. This activates the neurohormonal response (RAAS, antidiuretic hormone [ADH]) to increase blood volume and pressure, resulting in severe hypertension in the upper body. This results in elevated afterload and LV hypertrophy in these individuals. Collateral flow channels from the upper arterial tree (eg, intercostal and internal thoracic arteries) will develop to help reduce upper circulation congestion and pressure.

4. **Natural history of aortic coarctation:** Clinical signs vary according to the patient's age, primarily manifesting as asymptomatic hypertension and blood pressure differences between the upper and lower extremities. The high upper body blood pressures lead to the development of cerebral artery aneurysms, coronary artery disease, HF, postcoarctation aneurysms, and aortic dissections. Patients with coarctations have an increased risk of mortality. The average age of survival for an unrepaired coarctation is 35 years.[49] Patients with severe aortic coarctation may also develop an extensive collateral burden, which increases surgical bleeding risk.

5. **Indications and interventions:** A significant pressure differential across a coarctation is defined as a mean >20 mm Hg by echocardiography or peak-to-peak gradient by catheterization in current guidelines.[14] Intervention is indicated in patients with significant pressure gradients or symptoms. Management of significant coarctation can be treated by percutaneous balloon dilation with or without stent placement or by surgical repair (either thoracotomy or sternotomy approach).

C. **Congenital Mitral Stenosis:** Congenital mitral stenosis is defined as narrowing or obstruction at the level of the mitral valve or any components (annulus, valve leaflets, cords, papillary muscles). The flow is obstructed and increases pressure in the LA. Over time, this will cause atrial dilation, pulmonary venous congestion, pulmonary hypertension, and RV function. A supravalvular mitral ring and parachute mitral valve resulting in MS is commonly associated with Shone complex. In adults, the presentation of congenital MS parallels that of acquired MS, including elevated pulmonary pressures, pulmonary hypertension, and right HF in extreme cases. Surgical mitral valve replacement or repair (MVR) is the definitive treatment. Balloon valvuloplasty is often not effective in congenital MS. Indications for surgery are the same as for acquired MS.

D. **Congenital Right-Sided Obstruction**

1. **Congenital pulmonary stenosis:** PS presents as narrowing or obstruction at the level of, below (subvalvular), or above the pulmonic valve (supravalvular).[47] Depending on the severity of obstruction, adults presenting with significant RV outflow obstruction often develop RVH from pressure overload, increased right-side filling pressures with decreased compliance, and congestive right HF.[47] Elevations in RV pressures lead to diminished coronary blood flow and increase the risk of ischemia. Patients with mild obstruction or distal PA obstruction may have milder symptoms or be asymptomatic. Severity of RVOTO is determined by peak RVOT gradients[14]:

RVOTO Severity	Peak Gradient (mm Hg)	Velocity (m/s)
Mild	<36	<3
Moderate	≥36 and <64	3-4
Severe	>64 (or mean >35)	>4

   a. **Subvalvular pulmonary stenosis (double-chamber right ventricle):** Subvalvular PS can occur in either isolated forms or associated with other congenital abnormalities, such as a membranous VSD. It arises due to hypertrophy of a muscular band surrounding the infundibulum or RVOT leading to RVOT outflow during systole. Medical management includes reducing heart rate and contractility using β-blockers or calcium channel blockers. Symptomatic patients with moderate or severe obstruction should undergo myectomy of the muscular band with RVOT patching.

   b. **Valvular pulmonary stenosis:** Pulmonary valvular stenosis often occurs due to dysplasia or abnormal development. It is one of the most commonly encountered congenital anomalies, with an incidence of approximately 7% of children with CHD.[14,49] It is commonly associated with Noonan syndrome, a dilated main PA, stenosed branch PAs, and dysplastic cusps. Patients with mild obstruction often do not require intervention and may be asymptomatic. Moderate PS has a variable presentation but may progress overtime to severe PS by adulthood. Severe PS is often detected in childhood and has a good prognosis with intervention.[14] Indications for intervention include symptomatic patients with moderate or severe valvular obstruction. The standard therapy for these individuals is balloon valvuloplasty if appropriate, and surgical replacement if there are other conditions.

   c. **Supravalvular pulmonary stenosis:** Supravalvular PS involves narrowing of the PA above the pulmonic valve. It is associated with teratogenic effects of rubella or toxoplasmosis as well as other congenital syndromes (eg, *Noonan syndrome*). Narrowing of the main PA creates the same physiology as valvular PS; therefore, anesthetic management is similar. Balloon dilation and stenting of supravalvular PS is an acceptable therapy; however, it presents with lower rates of success.[49] Surgical resection of the stenosed segment is the definitive treatment.

d. **Post-valvulotomy pulmonary regurgitation:** Many adult patients with PS have had prior balloon valvuloplasty or surgical valvulotomy, resulting in pulmonary regurgitation (PR). Although well tolerated, progressive PR develops overtime and can cause RV dilation and systolic dysfunction in late adulthood. Symptomatic moderate or severe PR with evidence of RV chamber enlargement is a Class I indication for pulmonic valve replacement.[14] In extreme cases, patients with PR and right HF benefit from inotropic support, diuresis, and afterload reduction with pulmonary vasodilators.

2. **Pulmonary atresia:** Pulmonary atresia is the absence of communication between the RV and the PAs. In addition, the pulmonary vascular anatomy may be abnormal (hypoplastic, nonconfluent, supplied by collaterals from the aorta, etc). After birth, these patients are classified into two groups: (1) pulmonary atresia with an intact ventricular septum or (2) atresia with a VSD. Most of these patients will undergo biventricular repair with an RV-to-PA conduit or a pulmonary valvotomy. Patients with a hypoplastic ventricle will go through single ventricle palliation and completion Fontan. Still, others may not be amenable to repair due to their complex anatomy and require a heart transplant.[50] These patients present with a high incidence of RV dysfunction, arrhythmias, and hypoxia during adulthood. Patients with an RV-to-PA conduit may present with conduit dysfunction, either with severe stenosis or with insufficiency, requiring surgical replacement. As with PS, patients with a history of pulmonary valvotomy will develop pulmonary insufficiency overtime and may need a valvular replacement.

CLINICAL PEARL

- Obstructive lesions often occur from malformation either of the AV inflow apparatus or in the ventriculo-arterial outflow. The lesions can be isolated defects or part of a constellation of abnormalities in a congenital syndrome.
- Obstruction in the ventriculo-arterial outflow can be either below the valve in the respective outflow tract, above the valve in the great vessel, or at the level of the semilunar valves.
- Most adult patients with obstructive lesions have had either palliation using percutaneous approaches such as balloon valvulotomy or surgical interventions in early childhood.
- Adult patients with previous pulmonary valvulotomy may have residual PR that can lead to RV overload. Definitive treatment is pulmonic valve replacement with or without RVOT reconstruction.

V. Complex Lesions

As adult patients with complex congenital cardiac lesions are surviving into later decades of life, they pose a considerable challenge to the cardiothoracic anesthesiologist throughout the perioperative period. Complex defects often consist of a combination of AV or ventriculo-arterial discordance, hypoplasia of cardiac chambers, obstructive lesions, and great vessel misalignments. In cases of heterotaxy, infants with CHD may have other organs affected, such as the abdominal viscera. All too often, complex lesions are not compatible with life and require palliation or surgical correction. Despite corrective procedures, these patients still suffer from the short- and late-term complications from their corrective procedures as well as their disease. Many of these complex lesions are rare and unique; thus, perioperative care needs to be individualized. These patients pose the highest perioperative risk (see Section I.B. "Introduction: Epidemiology"). Consultation with the ACHD cardiologist is essential for understanding the underlying physiology to optimize perioperative management. The following section reviews several of the more common complex lesions, but it should be recognized that each individual patient may have varied anatomic or functional features (or even variations in surgical correction) from the typical presentation that can impact perioperative management.

A. **Ebstein Anomaly:** First described in 1868, Ebstein anomaly is a rare malformation of the tricuspid valve, which occurs in <1% of all patients with CHD. The combination of leaflet tethering, "sail-like" anterior leaflet, and downward displacement of the tricuspid annulus creates an "atrialized" area of the RV that does not contribute to RV cardiac output (Figure 17.16). The degree of dysplastic valvular function and annular displacement is on a continuum from minimal to severe. Ebstein anomaly is strongly associated with ASDs (secundum ASD), PFO, and conduction abnormalities, such as WPW syndrome. Other CHD lesions found concurrently with Ebstein anomaly include VSDs, pulmonary atresia/stenosis, and cardiomyopathy (LV noncompaction). The presence of an atrial communication leads to right-to-left shunting with elevation in right-sided filling pressures and increases the risk of paradoxical emboli. The anatomic abnormalities and pathophysiology commonly lead to right-sided HF, arrhythmias, cyanosis, and sudden death. The severity of the anatomic abnormality and functional changes will determine the age at presentation for surgical treatment.

1. **Atrial septal defect or patent foramen ovale closure:** Patients with episodes of right-to-left shunting and hypoxemia may undergo transcatheter closure of the ASD/PFO. Important criteria include the RA pressures <15 mm Hg with balloon occlusion of the shunt. Patients in whom RA pressures exceed 15 mm Hg may require right-to-left shunting for the maintenance of adequate systemic cardiac output.[51]

2. **Surgical intervention:** Indications for primary surgical intervention or reoperation include objective worsening of exercise capacity, progressive RV systolic dysfunction, or HF

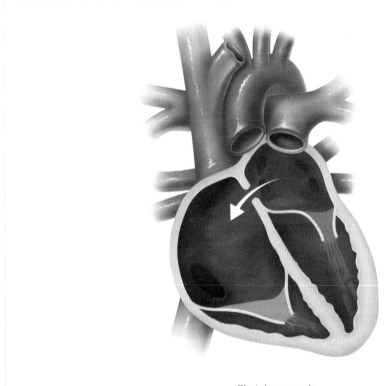

Ebstein anomaly

FIGURE 17.16 Ebstein anomaly. Give specific attention to the apical displacement of tricuspid valve septal insertion and the "atrialization" of the right ventricular wall. (Illustration by Townsend Majors and courtesy of Ravi V. Joshi, UT Southwestern.)

symptoms. In pediatric patients, surgery options include biventricular repair with valve repair versus replacement, 1.5 ventricular repair (*Glenn shunt* with valve repair/replacement), or, lastly, single ventricle palliation. In adults undergoing primary intervention, the choice of surgery is valvular repair or replacement, while reoperation usually involves valvular replacement. Valvular repair can include tricuspid annuloplasty or the *da Silva cone* procedure, which involves surgical delamination of leaflets, plication of "atrialized" RV with annulus reduction, and leaflet reattachment.

3. **Arrhythmias:** Supraventricular tachyarrhythmias are common in patients with Ebstein anomaly due to the presence of one or more accessory bypass pathways. Both pediatric and adult patients frequently undergo EP studies with possible radiofrequency ablation therapy for symptomatic arrhythmias.

Ebstein Anomaly	Late-Term Complications
Unrepaired	Tricuspid regurgitation, arrhythmias, RV failure, hepatic congestion, stroke and paradoxical emboli
Repaired	Worsening tricuspid regurgitation, tricuspid endocarditis, RV failure, hepatic congestion

B. **Shone Complex:** Shone complex, also known as Shone anomaly or syndrome, is a congenital heart defect affecting left-sided cardiac structures and has multilevel obstructive pathophysiology. It is a constellation of lesions, including aortic coarctation, aortic arch hypoplasia, subaortic stenosis, valvular AS with bicuspid valve, LV hypoplasia, mitral valve pathology (supravalvular mitral ring, congenital MS, or parachute mitral valve), and *cor triatriatum* (see earlier section above). The multilevel obstructive lesions result in a hypoplastic LV and potentially hypoplastic aorta. Importantly, the Shone complex is *not* part of the hypoplastic left heart syndrome spectrum (see "Single Ventricle Defects" section). The degree of obstruction across the LV inflow and LV outflow will determine the severity of symptoms and age at presentation.

1. **Surgical intervention:** Repair is focused on the specific lesions and can include mitral or aortic balloon valvuloplasty, resection of *cor triatriatum*, subaortic stenosis resection, mitral or aortic valve repair versus replacement, Ross-Konno procedure with RV-to-PA conduit, and arch augmentation. The type of surgical intervention depends upon the age at presentation and degree of obstruction.

Shone Complex	Late-Term Complications
Unrepaired or repaired Shone complex	MS, LVOT obstruction, AS, restenosis of coarctation

C. **Tetralogy of Fallot:** The TOF is a common complex lesion consisting of four defects: a VSD, an overriding aorta, subpulmonic stenosis, and RVH (Figure 17.17). During embryologic development, an anterior misaligned VSD creates obstruction in the RVOT with subsequent RVH and an overriding aorta. TOF can be associated with an ASD as well (so-called Pentalogy of Fallot). Patients with unrepaired TOF have variable presentation based on the degree of RVOTO, which can vary from mild to severe (pulmonary atresia). Patients with TOF with mild pulmonary obstruction will have adequate pulmonary blood flow and few symptoms. Increasing obstruction or resistance to pulmonary flow will result in more venous blood shunting across the VSD, resulting in cyanosis, particularly during exertion ("Tet" spells). In severe TOF, patients will have pulmonary atresia and may have blood supply to the lungs supplied by arteries originating from the aorta, so-called major aortopulmonary collateral arteries (MAPCAs). An adult with an unrepaired TOF may present with significant limitation to exercise, severe hypoxemia, and polycythemia. Patients with unrepaired TOF are

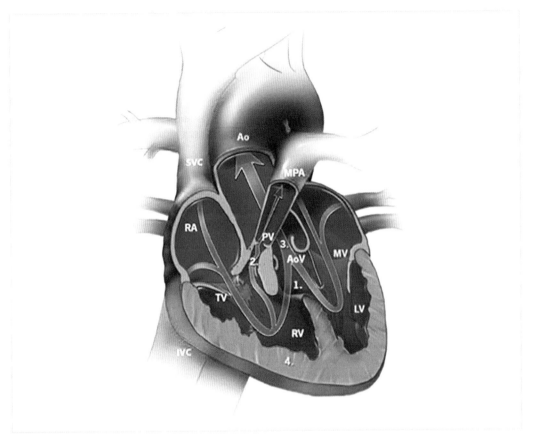

FIGURE 17.17   Tetralogy of Fallot (TOF). Elements of TOF include **1.** a large ventricular septal defect, **2.** pulmonic outflow narrowing or stenosis, **3.** an overriding aorta (Ao), and **4.** right ventricular (RV) hypertrophy. AoV, aortic valve; IVC, inferior vena cava; LV, left ventricle; MPA, main pulmonary artery; MV, mitral valve; PV, pulmonary valve; RA, right artery; SVC, superior vena cava; TV, tricuspid valve. (Adapted from public domain illustrations of the Centers for Disease Control and Prevention, National Center on Birth Defects and Developmental Disabilities. https://www.cdc.gov/ncbddd/heartdefects/facts.html)

at increased risk for complications of cyanosis, hemoptysis, and development of cerebral abscess.[51]

1. **Surgical intervention:** TOF surgical repair is commonly performed in childhood and involves relief of the RVOTO and closure of the VSD. Pediatric patients with TOF with pulmonary atresia become cyanotic in the first weeks of life and require the placement of an RV-to-PA conduit.

2. **Issues post tetralogy of Fallot repair:** Although surgical repair has increased the number of long-term survivors of TOF, adults with TOF repairs are still at higher risk of morbidity and mortality in early adulthood than in the general population.[25] Later term complications include aortic root dilation and aortic insufficiency, PA conduit stenosis, or residual VSD shunt. One common concern is pulmonic valve regurgitation (PR) from prior valvulotomy during TOF repair. Patients with severe PR will develop severe RV overload and dysfunction, leading to exercise intolerance. Symptomatic patients may undergo pulmonic valve replacement with or without RVOT reconstruction. Due the high frequency of arrhythmias

and the increased risk for SCD in patients with TOF, ICD insertion is often considered for SCD prevention.[14]

TOF	Late-Term Complications
Repaired	Aortic valve regurgitation, aortic dilation, VSD patch leak, PR, pulmonary endocarditis, RVOT stenosis, arrhythmias
Unrepaired	Cyanosis, hemoptysis, cerebral thromboembolism, cerebral abscess, arterial thrombosis, right HF

D. **Transposition of the Great Arteries:** TGA, present in 5%-7% of all patients with CHD, is both the most frequent cyanotic lesion and the most frequent neonatal diagnosis.[51] There are two forms of TGA known as L-TGA or cc-TGA and D-TGA. There terms D- (or dextro-) and L- (or levo-) arise from the position of the aorta to the pulmonary trunk.

1. **Congenitally corrected transposition of the great arteries (or L-TGA):** In cc-TGA, the ventricular looping (L-looping) of the heart occurs in the opposite orientation during fetal development. This results in the morphologic RV in the LV position as the systemic ventricle with AV discordance (inflow connection to the LA) and ventriculo-arterial discordance (outflow connection to the aorta). The morphologic LV is connected to the RA and PA trunk. The aorta sits anterior and to the left of the PA. Patients with cc-TGA are physiologically normal as systemic and pulmonary circulations are correctly in series. Children with cc-TGA are often asymptomatic, and the condition can be undiagnosed until later in adulthood. As patients with cc-TGA age, the weaker RV (as the systemic ventricle) begins to progressively dilate, leading to severe AV valve insufficiency and congestive HF. For adults with cc-TGA and systemic RV dysfunction, HF therapies are the mainstay treatments with heart transplantation as the final solution. Since ~45% of patients with cc-TGA develop HF, valvular regurgitation, and death within 20 years of diagnosis, the *double switch repair* has become a more desirable treatment option in children with cc-TGA.[52] AV heart block is common in patients with cc-TGA and is treated by pacemaker implantation. Patients with cc-TGA may present with pulmonary hypertension or Eisenmenger syndrome from lifelong pulmonary overcirculation due to left-to-right shunting via an ASD or VSD.

2. **D-Transposition of the great vessels:** In contrast to cc-TGA, D-TGA arises from malformation of the conotruncal septum where the aorticopulmonary segment does not spiral during formation of the great arteries.[53] This results in ventriculo-arterial discordance, where the aorta is connected to the RV and the PA is connected to the LV (Figure 17.18). D-TGA is not compatible with life owing to the isolated parallel pulmonary and systemic circulations. The presence of the PDA or other communication (eg, VSD) allows for some mixing of pulmonary and systemic blood flow and is critical to life. Infants born with D-TGA are typically operated on in the first several weeks of life. There are two major repairs for D-TGA, each with their respective complications that may arise in adulthood.

3. **Atrial switch (Senning/Mustard):** The atrial switch procedure was developed in the 1950s (Senning 1958) and 1960s (Mustard 1964) redirected central venous blood flow to the subpulmonic (left) ventricle and pulmonary venous return to the system (right) ventricle by creating an intracardiac baffle connecting the IVC and SVC to the mitral valve and LV. The interatrial septum is removed to allow the pulmonary venous return to drain from the LA into the RV. The atrial switch converts a D-TGA to a cc-TGA (or L-TGA) circulatory pathway. Late complications include, as with cc-TGA, congestive HF due a systemic RV and development of severe AV regurgitation. A significant percentage (~40%) of repaired patients with D-TGA with atrial switch have sinus node dysfunction and atrial tachyarrhythmias.[51] Finally, patients with D-TGA may develop stenosis or leak of the venous baffle, necessitating transcatheter ballooning or baffle stenting (Figure 17.19, left panel).

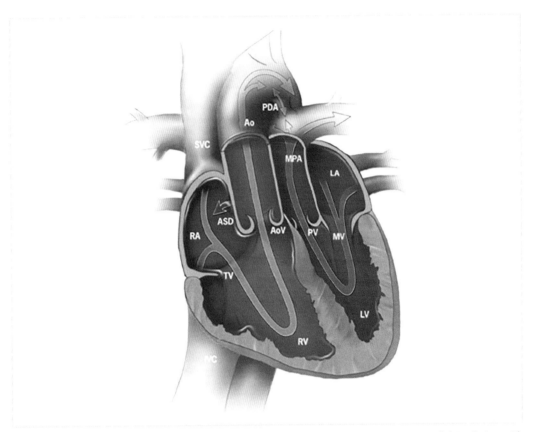

FIGURE 17.18   D-Transposition of the great vessels (D-TGA). Infants born with D-TGA have two parallel circulations with a single communication via the PDA, which provides insufficient pulmonary blood flow and oxygenation to allow for survival past the first initial weeks of life. AoV, aortic valve; ASD, atrial septal defects; IVC, inferior vena cava; LA, left artery; LV, left ventricle; MPA, main pulmonary artery; MV, mitral valve; PDA, patent ductus arteriosus; PV, pulmonary valve; RA, right artery; RV, right ventricle; SVC, superior vena cava; TV, tricuspid valve. (Adapted from public domain illustrations of the Centers for Disease Control and Prevention, National Center on Birth Defects and Developmental Disabilities. https://www.cdc.gov/ncbddd/heartdefects/facts.html)

4. **Arterial switch (Jatene procedure):** Advancements in microvascular surgery allowed for the development of the arterial switch operation where the aorta and PAs removed from the native roots and attached to the opposite root. Because the coronary arteries arise from the native aortic root attached to the RV, they are removed and implanted into the native pulmonary root along with the ascending aorta. The procedure reestablishes the systemic-to-pulmonary in-series circulatory pathway and normal cardiac physiology. The survival rate is >90% at 10 years, and many children have no limitations in physical activity.[51] Later complications include coronary stenosis or obstruction, progressive dilation of the neo-aortic root, and AR (from native pulmonary valve) (Figure 17.19, right panel).

D-Transposition of Great Arteries	Late-Term Complications
Arterial switch (Jatene procedure)	Coronary obstruction, AR, aortic aneurysm, arrhythmias, residual shunt
Atrial switch (Senning/Mustard procedure)	Baffle stenosis or leak, arrhythmias, ventricular failure

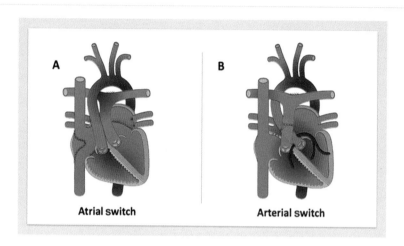

A   Atrial switch

B   Arterial switch

FIGURE 17.19   Repairs for D-transposition of the great vessels. The atrial switch repair **(A)** involves creating a baffle from the central venous circulation to the subpulmonary left ventricle to provide pulmonary blood flow. The arterial switch repair **(B)** corrects the underlying defect to provide the normal circulatory pathway, including reimplantation of the coronary arteries into the neo-aortic root. (Adapted from illustrations from https://www.chd-diagrams.com. Illustrations are licensed under Creative Commons Attribution-NonCommercial-NoDerivatives 4.0 International License by the New Media Center of the University of Basel. Reprinted with permission from New Media Center of the University of Basel.)

E. Persistent Truncus Arteriosus: Persistent truncus arteriosus (TA) is a rare congenital defect, with an incidence of 7 per 100,000 live births.[54] During development, a single arterial trunk (TA) arises from both ventricles and later divides to form the aorta and PA. In persistent TA, the arterial trunk does not septate, resulting in a common ventricular outflow tract shared by both ventricles. There is a single semilunar valve, which can be bicuspid, tricuspid, or quadricuspid, and an outlet VSD connecting the RV and LV. One-third of patients with TA will have DiGeorge syndrome, deletion at 22q11.2, and may have associated hypocalcemia, cleft palates, autoimmune diseases, and impaired cognitive development. If left untreated, death in infancy is the norm. Surgical intervention creates two outflow tracts with an RV-to-PA conduit and closure of the VSD. The truncal valve becomes the neo-aortic valve and may need future repair or replacement for regurgitation. Patients outgrow the initial RV-to-PA conduit and will need subsequent procedures to replace the conduit.

The anesthetic management for specific complex congenital lesions can be found in Table 17.3.

Truncus Arteriosus	Late-Term Complications
Neo-aorta reconstruction and RV-to-PA conduit	Neo-aortic valve regurgitation, VSD patch leak, RVOT conduit stenosis, endocarditis, PA stenosis

CLINICAL PEARL

- Patients with ACHD with complex lesions have commonly undergone palliative procedures to reestablish sufficient cardiopulmonary circulation for viability.
- Long-term complications include arrhythmias, endocarditis, severe valvular regurgitation, residual shunt, thromboembolism, and HF.
- Patients with complex congenital heart demonstrate great variation in the constellation of presenting defects; thus, care should be individualized for each patient. Consultation with the ACHD specialist is essential for perioperative management.

TABLE 17.3 Anesthetic Management of Complex Congenital Lesions

Defect Variable	Ebstein Anomaly/Tricuspid Regurgitation	Ebstein Anomaly/Tricuspid Stenosis	Shone Complex/Mitral Stenosis/Aortic Stenosis	Tetralogy of Fallot (Unrepaired)/Pulmonic Valve Stenosis	D-Transposition of the Great Arteries (TGA) s/p Arterial or Atrial Switch	L-Transposition of the Great Arteries (TGA) (Unrepaired) or s/p Double Switch	Persistent Truncus Arteriosus (TA) s/p Repair
Rate	Normal to high to decrease tricuspid regurgitant fraction	Normal to low to increase diastolic filling time	Normal to low to augment diastolic filling time	Normal to low	Normal to low	Normal to low	Normal to low
Rhythm	Keep in sinus rhythm. High risk for supraventricular arrhythmias. Accessory conduction pathways common, preexcitation syndromes, WPW	Keep in sinus rhythm. High risk for supraventricular arrhythmias. Accessory conduction pathways common, preexcitation syndromes, WPW	Keep in sinus rhythm	Keep in sinus rhythm, increased risk of ventricular arrhythmias	Keep in sinus rhythm. High risk for supraventricular arrhythmias/sinus node dysfunction. Pacemakers/ICDs common	Keep in sinus rhythm. High risk for supraventricular arrhythmias/AV node dysfunction. Pacemakers/ICDs common	Keep in sinus
Preload (volume status)	Normal. Aim for euvolemia and be mindful with fluids. RV dysfunction is common. Right atrium is dilated at baseline	Normal. Aim for euvolemia and be mindful with fluids. Right atrium is dilated at baseline	Normal. Aim for euvolemia and be mindful with fluids. Patients at risk of RV dysfunction	Normal to high, keep RV full, avoid hypovolemia to prevent RVOT obstruction	Normal. Aim for euvolemia and be mindful with fluids. Patients at risk of RV dysfunction, particularly if baffle obstruction/leak also present	Increased at baseline, avoid dilation of the systemic ventricle. Aim for euvolemia. Patients at risk of RV dysfunction, particularly if baffle obstruction/leak also present	Increased at baseline, avoid dilation of the systemic ventricle. Aim for euvolemia
Contractility	Normal to increased for RV support	Normal to increased for RV support	Normal to increased for RV support	Normal to mildly low. High contractility may cause RVOT obstruction	Normal to increased to support the systemic ventricular. Systemic ventricular failure (RV failure) is common	Normal to increased to support the systemic ventricular. Systemic ventricular failure (RV failure) is common if unrepaired	Normal or increased

Afterload (SVR)	Normal to mildly high to optimize coronary perfusion	Normal to mildly high to optimize coronary perfusion	Normal to mildly high to optimize coronary perfusion	Normal to mildly high to optimize coronary perfusion and to keep LVOT open	Systemic failing RV in atrial switch may require mild afterload reduction. Risk of coronary artery stenosis after arterial switch	Normal to mildly high to optimize coronary perfusion	Keep at baseline values as possible
PVR	Normal to low to decrease RV afterload and to reduce the regurgitant fraction. Consider pulmonary vasodilators (eg, inhaled nitric oxide)	Normal to low	Normal to low to decrease RV afterload	Normal to low to decrease RV afterload, although flow will be limited by pulmonary stenosis	Normal to low to decrease RV afterload	Normal to low to decrease RV afterload	Normal to low to decrease RV afterload
Special notes	Intravenous medications may have their onset of action delayed due to the accumulation of blood in the large right atrium	Intravenous medications may have their onset of action delayed due to accumulation of blood in the large right atrium	See "late-term complications" table	Low SpO2 is a sign of right-to-left shunting. After repair, high risk of PI in adulthood. See "late-term complications" table	General considerations for redo sternotomy	See "late-term complications" table	Commonly associated with DiGeorge syndrome. Check calcium levels. See "late-term complications" table

AV, atrioventricular; ICD, implantable cardioverter-defibrillator; LVOT, left ventricular outflow tract; PVR, pulmonary vascular resistance; RV, right ventricle; RVOT, right ventricular outflow tract; SVR, systemic vascular resistance; WPW, Wolff-Parkinson-White.

VI. Single Ventricle Defects

Several complex congenital disorders present with a single functional ventricle due to hypoplasia or the absence of the opposite ventricle or due to the absence of a dividing septum. Although each situation is unique, palliation or corrective surgery results in a single ventricle, whether the morphologic LV or RV, that *simultaneously pumps blood through the pulmonary and systemic circulation.* Common congenital disorders with single ventricle physiology include (Figure 17.20)[55] the following:

- Tricuspid atresia or hypoplastic right heart syndrome (HRHS)
- Hypoplastic left heart syndrome (HLHS)
- Pulmonary atresia without VSD
- DORV
- Double inlet RV or LV
- Unbalanced AVSD or AV canal defects

Viabilty for an individual with a single ventricle must meet three physiologic principles to work appropriately and deliver adequate oxygenation (see Figure 17.21):

- Adequate, unobstructed *PA* blood flow
- Unobstructed *pulmonary venous* blood flow
- Unobstructed *systemic (arterial)* blood flow

In order to establish proper cardiopulmonary function in complex congenital lesions in infancy, corrective surgeries occur in staged procedures or palliations to achieve each of the aforementioned three physiologic principles.

A. Surgical Stages of Palliation

1. **First stage of palliation—the Norwood procedure:** The first stage of palliation provides four major physiologic goals:

   a. Adequate systemic venous return

   b. Source of unobstructed PA flow

   c. Limit pulmonary overcirculation and excessive pressure

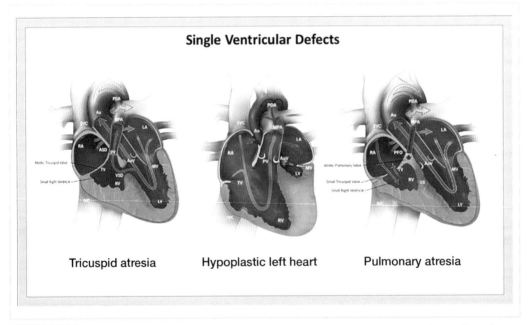

FIGURE 17.20   Congenital defects with single ventricular physiology. Examples of various defects with single ventricles amendable to repair to establish pulmonary and systemic circulation in series. AoV, aortic valve; ASD, atrial septal defects; IVC, inferior vena cava; LA, left artery; LV, left ventricle; MPA, main pulmonary artery; MV, mitral valve; PDA, patent ductus arteriosus; PV, pulmonary valve; RA, right artery; RV, right ventricle; SVC, superior vena cava; TV, tricuspid valve. (Adapted from public domain illustrations of the Centers for Disease Control and Prevention, National Center on Birth Defects and Developmental Disabilities. https://www.cdc.gov/ncbddd/heartdefects/facts.html)

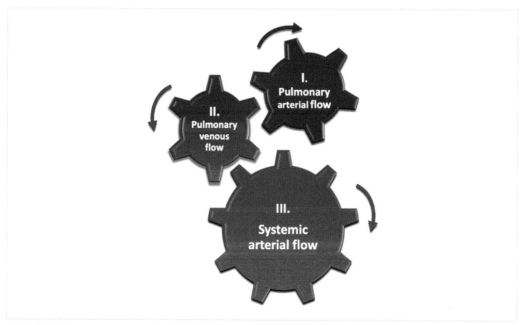

FIGURE 17.21 Physiologic principles underpinning single ventricular circulation.

d. Establish unobstructed systemic forward flow, a stable source of unobstructed pulmonary flow, and good systemic venous return, to establish free systemic outflow and to limit pulmonary flow and PA pressure.[44] A common first stage palliation surgery for various complex congenital lesions with a single ventricle is the *Norwood procedure* (Figure 17.22, left panel). The Norwood involves the establishment of a systemic outflow tract by creating a neo-aorta from the PA main trunk, which is detached from the right

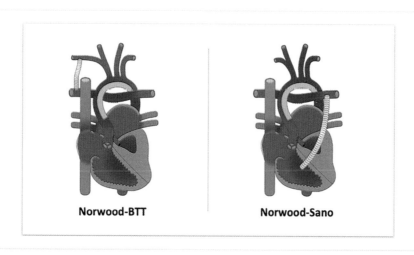

FIGURE 17.22 The Norwood procedure and palliation for single ventricular congenital lesions. The Norwood-BTT uses a BTT shunt for pulmonary blood flow (left panel) and the Norwood-Sano uses an RV-to-PA conduit to provide pulmonary flow (right panel). BTT, Blalock-Thomas-Taussig; PA, pulmonary artery; RV, right ventricle. (Adapted from illustrations from https://www.chd-diagrams.com. Illustrations are licensed under Creative Commons Attribution-NonCommercial-NoDerivatives 4.0 International License by the New Media Center of the University of Basel. Reprinted with permission from New Media Center of the University of Basel.)

and left branches. The neo-aorta root and systemic semilunar valve are open to the functional ventricle depending on the original patient anatomy. An atrial septectomy allows unobstructed pulmonary venous flow from the pulmonary veins, and a *BTT shunt* (see "Collateral Circulation" section II.K, Figure 17.8) is created to provide PA blood flow. Systemic diastolic blood pressures <30 mm Hg with a BTT shunt may compromise coronary perfusion. In this instance, a Sano shunt (see Figure 17.22, right panel) can be placed from the ventricle to the branch PAs to establish flow without an effect on diastolic blood pressure.[56] Another procedure for first stage palliation is *pulmonary banding* to limit elevated pulmonary blood flow and pressure as well as to shunt blood flow through the aorta as in a patient with DORV. Patients with pulmonary banding should have the three other requirements for first stage palliation already established with native anatomy (see "Collateral Circulation" section II.K, Figure 17.8).

2. **Second stage—bidirectional Glenn shunt:** The second stage of palliation aims to provide continuous pulmonary blood flow via the SVC and the superior systemic venous circulation. The most common procedure performed for second stage palliation is the *bidirectional Glenn shunt* (see "Collateral Circulation" section II.K, Figure 17.8). The Glenn shunt involves removing the SVC from the RA to create an anastomosis to the right PA. Pulmonary blood flow is now dependent on venous return from the upper body through the SVC. The Q_p:Q_s ratio is now 0.5:1 as the pulmonary flow is determined by half of the venous return from the upper body.

   a. **Transpulmonary gradient:** The *transpulmonary gradient (TPG)* becomes more important in determining adequate pulmonary flow and oxygenation. *TPG* is the pressure differential between the PAs and the atrial pressure, and a normal TPG is 5-10 mm Hg. An elevated TPG is indicative of increased PVR or PA obstruction, whereas a low TPG is indicative of hypovolemia, ventricular dysfunction, AV valvular regurgitation, or presence of aorto-pulmonary collaterals. Previous BTT shunts may be taken down or ligated at this time to allow for proper limb development. Older versions of this procedure include the "classic Glenn" and the Hemi-Fontan.

3. **Third stage—Fontan palliation:** The third stage of palliation completes the surgical interventions to establish a stable cardiopulmonary circuit. The last stage of palliation involves diverting the remainder of the systemic venous return to the PAs. The most common procedure is the *Fontan procedure*, which attaches the IVC to the PA. There are several variations of the Fontan procedure, the most common being the extracardiac and the lateral tunnel anastomoses (Figure 17.23).

B. **Fontan Physiology and Anesthetic Management**

1. **Hemodynamic management:** The adult patient with a single ventricle and completion Fontan imparts a unique physiology that creates several challenges to the cardiac anesthesiologist (Figure 17.24). Regardless of the original congenital defect, the repaired patient now has a single ventricle that drives *both* systemic and pulmonary flow. The single ventricle is highly preload dependent. Critical to optimal function is unimpeded pulmonary flow and pulmonary venous return, such that pulmonary flow (Q_p) is 1:1 with systemic flow (Q_s). Without the presence of a subpulmonary ventricle, pulmonary blood flow (and oxygenation) is passive and fully dependent on the TPG. Ideally, the TPG should be 5-10 mm Hg and can be measured as the difference between CVP and common atrial pressure (CAP).[57] Elevations in TPG indicate obstruction or increased PVR, while low TPG is indicative of hypovolemia. Realize that TPG is a *pressure* differential and *not* a measure of *flow*. Normal TPGs can exist in low-flow situations, such as elevations in ventricular filling pressures or pulmonary vein obstruction. In contrast, low filling pressures and TPGs (<5 mm Hg) indicate hypovolemia and should be treated with judicious use of intravascular fluids. During intraoperative management, the anesthesiologist should endeavor to achieve maximal pulmonary flow and oxygenation with minimizing PVR and optimizing ventricular filling pressures. PVR is heavily influenced by pH and gas exchange; thus, avoiding intraoperative acidosis, hypoxemia, and hypercapnia is vital. If appropriate, spontaneous (negative) pressure ventilation is preferred. Excessive positive pressure ventilation

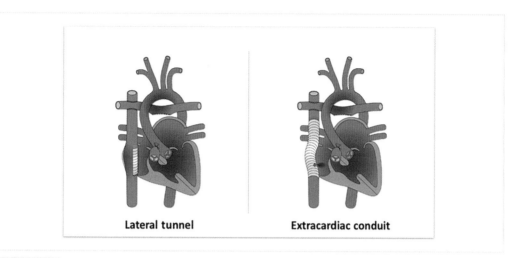

Lateral tunnel   **Extracardiac conduit**

FIGURE 17.23   The Fontan palliation in patients with tricuspid atresia (hypoplastic right heart syndrome) with the intracardiac lateral tunnel (left panel) and the more common alternative extracardiac conduit (right panel) with a fenestration. (Adapted from illustrations from https://www.chd-diagrams.com. Illustrations are licensed under Creative Commons Attribution-NonCommercial-NoDerivatives 4.0 International License by the New Media Center of the University of Basel. Reprinted with permission from New Media Center of the University of Basel.)

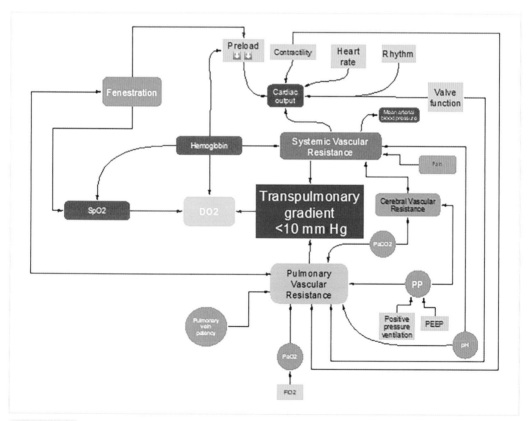

FIGURE 17.24   Physiologic determinants of oxygen delivery after completion Fontan. The Fontan diverts the inferior vena cava flow to the pulmonary artery with a graft. Along with the bidirectional Glenn shunt, the entire systemic venous return drains directly into the pulmonary arteries, resulting in nearly 100% of the venous return will be oxygenated in the lungs, establishing a $Q_p:Q_s$ of 1:1. In this situation, the transpulmonary gradient becomes more relevant. Obstruction of pulmonary flow will directly affect oxygen delivery.

and PEEP can also impair pulmonary blood flow; thus, pressure-controlled ventilation with low inspiratory pressures and minimal PEEP (4-5 cm H_2O) to prevent aveolar collapse is warranted. In addition, inadequate analgesia can lead to increased sympathetic outflow, leading to elevations in PVR. Many adult patients with Fontan physiology present with reduced ejection fractions and HF, particularly those with a morphologic RV.[25] As poor systolic function, impaired diastolic function, or severe AV valve regurgitation can all result in increased atrial pressure, mild afterload reduction and inotropes may be required to help reduce elevated filling pressures, reduce volume overload, increase systemic output, and consequently improve pulmonary blood flow. This may be challenging in patient with coronary stenosis or anomalies who may require elevated systemic pressures to preserve coronary blood flow.

2. **Fenestrated Fontans:** The presence of a Fontan fenestration in certain patients adds another challenge to the hemodynamic management of these patients. The fenestration is a deliberate communication surgically placed between the cavopulmonary conduit and the common atrium. The role of the fenestration was to reduce CVPs and to return the volume (increase preload) to the systemic circulation at the expense of some venous admixture and arterial desaturation. Fenestrations generally behave similar to atrial-level communications, such as ASDs. Fenestrated Fontans present with the added risk of thromboembolism and increased right-to-left shunting with possible cyanosis. Moderate or severe hypotension will exacerbate the right-to-left shunting and increase hypoxemia. Excessive shunting can also precipitate volume overload in patients with heart failure with reduced ejection fraction (HFrEF). These patients are often on anticoagulation (see earlier), which may need to be discontinued perioperatively. Fortunately, long-term outcomes for fenestrated conduits as compared to nonfenestrated Fontans are not significantly different.[58]

CLINICAL PEARL

- Single ventricle patients require unobstructed pulmonary blood flow to function.
- Palliative surgery connects the central venous circulation to the pulmonary tree, establishing a 1:1 relationship between pulmonary flow and cardiac output.
- In Fontan patients, monitoring the TPG is useful in determining the cause of systemic hypotension and poor peripheral perfusion.
- There is an increased risk of thromboembolism and cyanosis from patients with fenestrated Fontan conduits.

VII. Conclusion

Improvements in the management of pediatric patients with congenital heart defects have led to an ever-increasing population of adult patients living with the later sequelae of CHD. Although they are living longer, the perioperative risk for patients with ACHD is higher than the general population. An interdisciplinary approach that engages all involved physicians (cardiothoracic anesthesiologist, ACHD specialist, surgeon, intensivist) and other members of the perioperative team is essential to successful outcomes for these complicated patients. Patients with ACHD with complex disease or impaired functional status should be referred to regional medical centers experienced in the care of adults with CHD. As a key physician involved in the perioperative care for these patients, the cardiothoracic anesthesiologist must be aware of the perioperative risk, hemodynamic derangements, and complications arising from the respective congenital cardiac lesions. This chapter introduces the general classifications of congenital cardiac lesions, the pathophysiology of the most commonly encountered lesions, and guidelines for anesthetic management for each respective heart defect. The chapter also describes the common later term complications from CHD and the common surgical repairs or palliations the cardiac anesthesiologist may encounter.

REFERENCES

1. Mitchell SC, Korones SB, Berendes HW. Congenital heart disease in 56,109 births. Incidence and natural history. *Circulation.* 1971;43(3):323-332.
2. Wu W, He J, Shao X. Incidence and mortality trend of congenital heart disease at the global, regional, and national level, 1990-2017. *Medicine (Baltimore).* 2020;99(23):e20593.
3. Reller MD, Strickland MJ, Riehle-Colarusso T, et al. Prevalence of congenital heart defects in metropolitan Atlanta, 1998-2005. *J Pediatr.* 2008;153(6):807-813.
4. van der Bom T, Bouma BJ, Meijboom FJ, et al. The prevalence of adult congenital heart disease, results from a systematic review and evidence based calculation. *Am Heart J.* 2012;164(4):568-575.
5. Moodie D. Adult congenital heart disease: past, present, and future. *Tex Heart Inst J.* 2011;38(6):705-706.
6. van der Bom T, Zomer AC, Zwinderman AH, et al. The changing epidemiology of congenital heart disease. *Nat Rev Cardiol.* 2011;8(1):50-60.
7. Warnes CA, Liberthson R, Danielson GK, et al. Task force 1: the changing profile of congenital heart disease in adult life. *J Am Coll Cardiol.* 2001;37(5):1170-1175.
8. Marelli AJ, Ionescu-Ittu R, Mackie AS, et al. Lifetime prevalence of congenital heart disease in the general population from 2000 to 2010. *Circulation.* 2014;130(9):749-756.
9. Verheugt CL, Uiterwaal CS, van der Velde ET, et al. Mortality in adult congenital heart disease. *Eur Heart J.* 2010;31(10):1220-1229.
10. Alshawabkeh LI, Opotowsky AR. Burden of heart failure in adults with congenital heart disease. *Curr Heart Fail Rep.* 2016;13(5):247-254.
11. Baumgartner H. Geriatric congenital heart disease: a new challenge in the care of adults with congenital heart disease? *Eur Heart J.* 2014;35(11):683-685.
12. Maxwell BG, Wong JK, Kin C, et al. Perioperative outcomes of major noncardiac surgery in adults with congenital heart disease. *Anesthesiology.* 2013;119(4):762-769.
13. Mylotte D, Pilote L, Ionescu-Ittu R, et al. Specialized adult congenital heart disease care: the impact of policy on mortality. *Circulation.* 2014;129(18):1804-1112.
14. Stout KK, Daniels CJ, Aboulhosn JA, et al. 2018 AHA/ACC guideline for the management of adults with congenital heart disease: a report of the American College of Cardiology/American Heart Association Task Force on Clinical Practice Guidelines. *Circulation.* 2019;139(14):e698-e800.
15. Van Praagh R. Terminology of congenital heart disease. Glossary and commentary. *Circulation.* 1977;56(2):139-143.
16. Tutarel O, Kempny A, Alonso-Gonzalez R, et al. Congenital heart disease beyond the age of 60: emergence of a new population with high resource utilization, high morbidity, and high mortality. *Eur Heart J.* 2014;35(11):725-732.
17. Lui GK, Saidi A, Bhatt AB, et al. Diagnosis and management of noncardiac complications in adults with congenital heart disease: a scientific statement from the American Heart Association. *Circulation.* 2017;136(20):e348-e392.
18. Yen P. ASD and VSD flow dynamics and anesthetic management. *Anesth Prog.* 2015;62(3):125-130.
19. Silka MJ, Hardy BG, Menashe VD, Morris CD. A population-based prospective evaluation of risk of sudden cardiac death after operation for common congenital heart defects. *J Am Coll Cardiol.* 1998;32(1):245-251.
20. Loomba RS, Buelow MW, Aggarwal S, et al. Arrhythmias in adults with congenital heart disease: what are risk factors for specific arrhythmias? *Pacing Clin Electrophysiol.* 2017;40(4):353-361.
21. Crossley GH, Poole JE, Rozner MA, et al. The Heart Rhythm Society (HRS)/American Society of Anesthesiologists (ASA) Expert Consensus Statement on the perioperative management of patients with implantable defibrillators, pacemakers and arrhythmia monitors: facilities and patient management this document was developed as a joint project with the American Society of Anesthesiologists (ASA), and in collaboration with the American Heart Association (AHA), and the Society of Thoracic Surgeons (STS). *Heart Rhythm.* 2011;8(7):1114-1154.
22. Gerardin JF, Earing MG. Preoperative evaluation of adult congenital heart disease patients for non-cardiac surgery. *Curr Cardiol Rep.* 2018;20(9):76.
23. Price LC, Martinez G, Brame A, et al. Perioperative management of patients with pulmonary hypertension undergoing non-cardiothoracic, non-obstetric surgery: a systematic review and expert consensus statement. *Br J Anaesth.* 2021;126(4):774-790.
24. Arvanitaki A, Gatzoulis MA, Opotowsky AR, et al. Eisenmenger syndrome: JACC state-of-the-art review. *J Am Coll Cardiol.* 2022;79(12):1183-1198.
25. Norozi K, Wessel A, Alpers V, et al. Incidence and risk distribution of heart failure in adolescents and adults with congenital heart disease after cardiac surgery. *Am J Cardiol.* 2006;97(8):1238-1243.
26. Dinardo JA. Heart failure associated with adult congenital heart disease. *Semin Cardiothorac Vasc Anesth.* 2013;17(1):44-54.
27. Powell AJ. Aortopulmonary collaterals in single-ventricle congenital heart disease: how much do they count? *Circ Cardiovasc Imaging.* 2009;2(3):171-173.
28. Brickner ME, Hillis LD, Lange RA. Congenital heart disease in adults. First of two parts. *N Engl J Med.* 2000;342(4):256-263.
29. Murli L, Ranjit MS, Shah P. Unroofed coronary sinus: an unusual interatrial communication and a rare childhood entity. *Ann Pediatr Cardiol.* 2019;12(1):64-65.
30. Sommer RJ, Hijazi ZM, Rhodes JF Jr. Pathophysiology of congenital heart disease in the adult: part I: shunt lesions. *Circulation.* 2008;117(8):1090-1099.
31. Dakkak W, Oliver TI. Ventricular septal defect. *StatPearls [Internet].* StatPearls Publishing; 2022.
32. Simpson WF Jr, Sade RM, Crawford FA, et al. Double-chambered right ventricle. *Ann Thorac Surg.* 1987;44(1):7-10.
33. Connolly HM, Ammash NM. Management and prognosis of ventricular septal defect in adults. In: Greutmann M, ed. *UpToDate.* UpToDate; 2019.

34. Ammash NM, Seward JB, Warnes CA, et al. Partial anomalous pulmonary venous connection: diagnosis by transesophageal echocardiography. *J Am Coll Cardiol.* 1997;29(6):1351-1358.

35. Saito C, Fukushima N, Fukushima K, et al. Factors associated with aortic root dilatation after surgically repaired ventricular septal defect. *Echocardiography.* 2017;34(8):1203-1209.

36. Mongeon FP, Burkhart HM, Ammash NM, et al. Indications and outcomes of surgical closure of ventricular septal defect in adults. *JACC Cardiovasc Interv.* 2010;3(3):290-297.

37. Wolfe RR, Driscoll DJ, Gersony WM, et al. Arrhythmias in patients with valvular aortic stenosis, valvular pulmonary stenosis, and ventricular septal defect. Results of 24-hour ECG monitoring. *Circulation.* 1993 Feb;87(2 Suppl):89-101.

38. Ahmed I, Anjum F. Atrioventricular septal defect. *StatPearls [Internet].* StatPearls Publishing; 2022.

39. Rudolph AM. *Congenital Diseases of the Heart: Clinical-Physiological Considerations.* 3rd ed. Wiley-Blackwell; 2009:538 p.

40. Chauhan S. Atrioventricular septal defects. *Ann Card Anaesth.* 2018;21(1):1-3.

41. Vida VL, Tessari C, Castaldi B, et al. Early correction of common atrioventricular septal defects: a single-center 20-year experience. *Ann Thorac Surg.* 2016;102(6):2044-2051.

42. Schneider DJ, Moore JW. Patent ductus arteriosus. *Circulation.* 2006;114(17):1873-1882.

43. Rychik J, Atz AM, Celermajer DS, et al. Evaluation and management of the child and adult with Fontan circulation: a scientific statement from the American Heart Association. *Circulation.* 2019;140(6):e234-e284. doi:10.1161/CIR0000000000000696

44. Schwartz SM, Dent CL, Musa NL, Nelson DP. Single-ventricle physiology. *Crit Care Clin.* 2003;19(3):393-411.

45. Barnea O, Austin EH, Richman B, Santamore WP. Balancing the circulation: theoretic optimization of pulmonary/systemic flow ratio in hypoplastic left heart syndrome. *J Am Coll Cardiol.* 1994;24(5):1376-1381.

46. Gatzoulis MA, Webb GD, Daubeney PEF. *Diagnosis and Management of Adult Congenital Heart Disease.* 3rd ed. Elsevier; 2018:xiv, 721 p.

47. Stout KK, Daniels CJ, Aboulhosn JA, et al. 2018 AHA/ACC guideline for the management of adults with congenital heart disease: a report of the American College of Cardiology/American Heart Association Task Force on Clinical Practice Guidelines. *J Am Coll Cardiol.* 2019;73(12):e81-e192.

48. Jha AK, Makhija N. Cor triatriatum: a review. *Semin Cardiothorac Vasc Anesth.* 2017;21(2):178-185.

49. Rhodes JF, Hijazi ZM, Sommer RJ. Pathophysiology of congenital heart disease in the adult, part II. Simple obstructive lesions. *Circulation.* 2008;117(9):1228-1237.

50. Montanaro C, Merola A, Kempny A, et al. The outcome of adults born with pulmonary atresia: high morbidity and mortality irrespective of repair. *Int J Cardiol.* 2019;280:61-66.

51. Sommer RJ, Hijazi ZM, Rhodes JF. Pathophysiology of congenital heart disease in the adult: part III: complex congenital heart disease. *Circulation.* 2008;117(10):1340-1350.

52. Barron DJ, Guariento A. Strengthening the argument for the double switch: but where is the limit? *Circ Cardiovasc Interv.* 2021;14(7):e010888.

53. Szymanski MW, Moore SM, Kritzmire SM, Goyal A. Transposition of the great arteries. *StatPearls [Internet].* StatPearls Publishing; 2022.

54. Bhansali S, Phoon C. Truncus arteriosus. *StatPearls [Internet].* StatPearls Publishing; 2022.

55. Lee M, Shahjehan RD. Fontan completion. *StatPearls [Internet].* StatPearls Publishing; 2022.

56. Mair R, Tulzer G, Sames E, et al. Right ventricular to pulmonary artery conduit instead of modified Blalock-Taussig shunt improves postoperative hemodynamics in newborns after the Norwood operation. *J Thorac Cardiovasc Surg.* 2003;126(5):1378-1384.

57. Eagle SS, Daves SM. The adult with Fontan physiology: systematic approach to perioperative management for noncardiac surgery. *J Cardiothorac Vasc Anesth.* 2011;25(2):320-334.

58. Daley M, Buratto E, King G, et al. Impact of Fontan fenestration on long-term outcomes: a propensity score-matched analysis. *J Am Heart Assoc.* 2022;11(11):e026087.

18

Pericardial Disease and Tamponade

J. Bradley Meers and Matthew M. Townsley

KEY POINTS

1. The manifestations of pericardial disease are primarily expressed as pericardial inflammation, constriction, and fluid accumulation (effusion). A unifying theme is impaired cardiac filling, with the severity of symptoms dependent upon the degree to which filling is impaired.

2. Constrictive pericarditis (CP) is a diagnosis encompassing a wide spectrum of disease, from acute and subacute cases that may resolve spontaneously, or with medical therapy, to the classic chronically progressive form of CP that may require surgical pericardiectomy.

3. A relatively small amount of fluid (50-100 mL) that accumulates rapidly within the closed pericardial space is sufficient to dramatically increase intrapericardial pressure and interfere with cardiac filling. Conversely, a chronic increase in pericardial fluid will typically result in hemodynamic instability only after a large volume of fluid accumulation, perhaps as great as a liter.

4. The right heart is most vulnerable to pericardial compression, due to its thinner walls and lower chamber pressures, as compared to the left heart.

5. Pulsus paradoxus (an abnormally high drop in systolic pressure >20 mm Hg during inspiration) occurs secondary to ventricular septal shift crowding the left ventricle (LV) during right ventricular (RV) filling. The opposite occurs during expiration. This phenomenon is described as enhanced ventricular interdependence.

6. Diastolic chamber collapse lasting more than one-third of diastole, as demonstrated with echocardiography, is a highly specific finding for cardiac tamponade.

7. Cardiovascular collapse may quickly ensue with induction of general anesthesia in a patient with cardiac tamponade. If pericardiocentesis cannot be performed in a hemodynamically compromised patient before surgical intervention, the patient should be prepped and draped before anesthetic induction so that surgery may proceed immediately following intubation. Volume loading before general anesthetic induction, as well as inotropic and vasopressor support, is often required. Expect further deterioration after positive pressure ventilation is initiated.

I. Introduction

Diseases of the pericardium may be acute or chronic entities that present with a wide spectrum of signs and symptoms, ranging from asymptomatic incidental findings to life-threatening emergencies. Common pericardial disease syndromes include congenital or acquired pericardial defects, pericarditis, myopericarditis, constrictive pericarditis (CP), pericardial effusion, and cardiac tamponade. Although the etiologies of pericardial disorders are quite variable—including infectious, inflammatory, autoimmune, and malignant states—common themes arise, allowing the anesthesiologist to safely approach the patient presenting with pericardial disease. Regardless of the underlying etiology, hemodynamic effects most often present as impaired cardiac filling, with the severity of symptoms dependent upon the degree to which filling is impaired. The altered physiology of these disease states presents numerous challenges to safe perioperative management.

Diagnosing pericardial disease requires a detailed history and physical examination along with electrocardiographic (ECG) and multimodal imaging, ranging from echocardiography to cardiac magnetic resonance (CMR) imaging. Although imaging modalities such as computed tomography (CT) and CMR are increasingly used to characterize pericardial disease, transthoracic echocardiography (TTE) remains the first-line diagnostic tool, given its noninvasive and relatively inexpensive nature.[1] In addition, echocardiography allows for rapid recognition of life-threatening pericardial tamponade in the perioperative setting.

This chapter reviews the normal structure and function of the pericardium, as well as the most common causes of pericardial disease. The most clinically relevant pericardial disorders—pericarditis, CP, pericardial effusion, and cardiac tamponade—are discussed in detail, focusing on pertinent anesthetic management considerations.

II. Pericardial Anatomy and Physiology

A. The normal pericardium is a dual-enveloped sac surrounding the heart and great vessels (Figure 18.1). It is composed of two layers: the parietal pericardium and the visceral pericardium. The parietal pericardium is a thick, fibrous outer layer composed primarily of collagen and elastin. The inner visceral pericardium rests on the surface of the heart. It is composed of a single layer of mesothelial cells, which adhere to the pericardium. Normal pericardial thickness is 1-2 mm.

B. The pericardium has attachments to the sternum anteriorly, the parietal pleura laterally, the diaphragm inferiorly, and to the mainstem bronchi, esophagus, and descending aorta posteriorly.

C. The space between the visceral and parietal pericardium normally contains 20-60 mL of plasma ultrafiltrate. This transudative fluid originates from epicardial capillaries and is cleared by lymphatic vessels within the parietal pericardium.

D. Two distinct sinuses are formed at points where the pericardium appears to fold onto itself. The oblique sinus forms posteriorly, between the left atrium and the pulmonary veins, and is a common location for blood to collect after cardiac surgery (⊙ **Video 18.1**). The transverse sinus also forms posteriorly behind the left atrium, situated behind the aorta and pulmonary artery (⊙ **Video 18.2**).

E. Normal cardiac function can still occur in the absence of the pericardium, making it nonessential for survival. However, the pericardium does provide several useful physiologic functions. It aids in reducing friction between the heart and surrounding structures, limits acute dilatation of cardiac chambers, provides a barrier to infection, optimizes coupling of left (LV) and right ventricular (RV) filling and function, and limits excessive motion of the heart within the chest cavity. The pericardium is also metabolically active, secreting prostaglandins that affect coronary artery tone and cardiac reflexes.

F. Congenital absence of the pericardium is a rare anomaly that may involve the complete or partial absence of the pericardium. Autopsy studies have identified complete absence and left-sided partial defects as more common than right-sided defects.[2] The majority of cases are clinically silent, but there is a risk of cardiac strangulation across a left-sided partial defect. Acquired pericardial defects also carry the risk of potential cardiac herniation.

G. The pericardium is a highly innervated structure. Pericardial inflammation or manipulation may produce severe pain or vagally mediated reflexes.

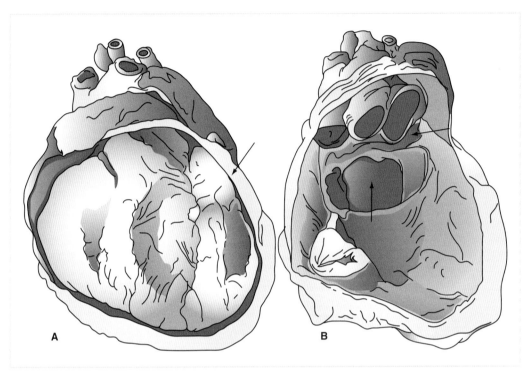

FIGURE 18.1 Anatomy of the pericardium and pericardial sinuses. The left image **(A)** demonstrates the heart in situ with a section of the parietal pericardium cut away. The right image **(B)**, with the heart cut away, demonstrates the oblique sinus (arrow at ~6 o'clock) and the transverse sinus (arrow at ~3 o'clock). (From Lachman N, Syed FF, Habib A, et al. Correlative anatomy for the electrophysiologist, part I: the pericardial space, oblique sinus, transverse sinus. *J Cardiovasc Electrophysiol.* 2010;21(12):1421-1426. © 2010 Wiley Periodicals, Inc. Reprinted by permission of John Wiley & Sons, Inc.)

III. Causes of Pericardial Disease

The etiologies of pericardial disease are numerous and can lead to pericardial inflammation, effusion, or both. Often, the care of these patients must not only consider the underlying pericardial pathology but the manifestations and complications of the underlying condition as well. Pericardial disease can be caused by infection (ie, viral, bacterial, fungal, tuberculosis [TB]), connective tissue disorders (ie, systemic lupus erythematosus, sarcoidosis, rheumatoid arthritis), trauma, uremia, malignancy, post-myocardial infarction (MI) (Dressler syndrome), or following cardiac surgery and other invasive cardiac procedures.

IV. Pericarditis

A. Natural History

1. **Etiology:** Pericarditis is responsible for ~5% of chest pain evaluations in the emergency department that are not attributable to MI.[3] The etiology of pericarditis is often idiopathic. However, establishing the cause as either infectious or noninfectious helps guide therapy. Infectious causes of pericardial disease include viral, bacterial, and fungal etiologies. TB is the most common cause of pericarditis in the developing world, and anti-TB therapy significantly improves survival. However, despite adequate TB therapy, 30%-60% of affected individuals will progress to CP. Most idiopathic cases in areas with low endemic rates of TB are attributed to viral etiology. Noninfectious causes of pericarditis include autoimmune, neoplastic, metabolic, traumatic, iatrogenic, pharmacologic, and congenital processes.[4]

2. **Symptomatology:** Pericarditis presents with a constellation of symptoms and findings. The most classic symptom is pleuritic chest pain, which is attenuated by sitting up and leaning forward. A new or worsening pericardial effusion may be noted, and symptoms such

as fatigue, edema, dyspnea on exertion, and orthopnea may be present depending on the volume and rate of fluid accumulation.

3. **Clinical course:** Pericarditis can be subclassified based on the duration of symptoms and whether the patient experiences subsequent episodes. Acute pericarditis typically resolves over 2-4 weeks with treatment. Incessant pericarditis lasts >4 weeks, but <3 months without remission. Pericarditis lasting >3 months is defined as chronic. Recurrent pericarditis is defined as a recurrence of symptoms after 4-6 weeks of the symptom resolution. The rate of recurrence is ~20%.[5]

B. **Pathophysiology**
   1. Acute pericarditis is characterized by fibrin deposits localized on the pericardial surface.
      a. Serous effusion may accompany the fibrinous inflammation.
      b. The mesothelial cell layer is replaced by a fibrin membrane that has white blood cells scattered throughout.
      c. Pericardial fluid may suggest a bacterial, neoplastic, viral, or inflammatory cause.
   2. Pleuritic chest pain with acute pericarditis is described in the center of the chest radiating to the back and left trapezius muscle.
      a. Pain is often more continuous than the intermittent pain of myocardial ischemia, but this is not diagnostic.
      b. Some degree of dyspnea may be present, and right heart failure can occasionally occur with rapid accumulation of fluid.
   3. Myocardial inflammation
      a. Patients with pericarditis may also have myocardial inflammation.
      b. It is important to identify if the process is primarily pericardial or myocardial in origin.
      c. Pericarditis with associated myocardial inflammation is called myopericarditis.
      d. Diagnosis of myopericarditis requires the same clinical criteria as acute pericarditis in addition to elevated markers of myocardial injury.
      e. Based on expert opinion, coronary angiography should be performed in cases of pericarditis with suspected myocardial involvement to rule out ischemia.
      f. CMR should be performed to confirm the diagnosis of myopericarditis.
      g. After diagnosis is confirmed, patients with myopericarditis should refrain from strenuous activity for 6 months.
      h. Primary myocarditis with pericardial involvement is called perimyocarditis.

CLINICAL PEARL

Perimyocarditis is more likely than myopericarditis to be associated with echocardiographic findings of new-onset focal wall motion abnormalities to significant global LV systolic dysfunction.[6]

C. **Diagnostic Evaluation and Assessment**
   1. **Clinical evaluation**
      a. The diagnostic evaluation of patients with suspected acute pericarditis begins with a detailed history and physical examination. An ECG and markers of myocardial injury (troponins and creatinine kinase [CK]-MB) are obtained, as the evaluation must first rule out myocardial ischemia.
      b. Diagnostic criteria for pericarditis (requires two out of four) include (1) pleuritic chest pain, (2) friction rub, (3) new diffuse ST elevation or PR depression, and (4) new or worsening pericardial effusion.
      c. High-risk features include fever >38 °C, subacute onset, large pericardial effusion, tamponade, failure to improve after 1 week of nonsteroidal anti-inflammatory drug (NSAID) therapy, myopericarditis, immunosuppression, trauma, and anticoagulant use (Table 18.1).
      d. Chest radiography is recommended to evaluate for pleuropericardial involvement.

TABLE 18.1 Acute Pericarditis—Diagnostic Features

Acute pericarditis is diagnosed when at least two of the following criteria are present: 1. Pleuritic chest pain 2. Pericardial friction rub 3. Electrocardiographic changes (ie, diffuse ST-segment elevation) 4. Pericardial effusion **Diagnosis is further supported by the presence of the following:** 1. Elevated C-reactive protein or erythrocyte sedimentation rate 2. Leukocytosis 3. Pericardial inflammation (visualized on computed tomography or cardiac magnetic resonance imaging)	**The following are high-risk features of acute pericarditis (require hospital admission and evaluation for underlying etiology):** 1. Fever >38 °C 2. Subacute onset 3. Large pericardial effusion 4. Cardiac tamponade or hemodynamic instability 5. Immunosuppression 6. Myopericarditis 7. Concurrent anticoagulation therapy 8. Associated trauma 9. Failure to improve following 1 wk of medical therapy

Adapted from Tuck BC, Townsley MM. Clinical update in pericardial diseases. *J Cardiothorac Vasc Anesth.* 2019;33(1):184-199. Table 1. © 2018 Elsevier. With permission.

    e. TTE should be performed on all cases of suspected acute pericarditis to evaluate for the presence of pericardial effusion, cardiac tamponade, and LV wall motion abnormalities.

        (1) TTE may demonstrate pericardial effusion (with or without tamponade), segmental wall motion abnormalities (if there is myocardial involvement), increased brightness of the pericardium, or normal findings.

    f. If the TTE is normal, or yields uncertainty, in a patient with high-risk features, CMR should be performed, given the high sensitivity (94%-100%) for detecting pericardial inflammation, edema, and constrictive physiology. Potential limitations of CMR include cost, availability, and the need for a hemodynamically stable patient for the examination to be performed.[1,4]

    g. Chest CT is an additional second-line imaging modality that may be useful in detecting pericardial inflammation.

D. Treatment

    1. For patients with known etiology, the medical management of acute pericarditis is directed at treating the underlying cause.[1,3,7]

    a. For presumed viral or idiopathic acute pericarditis, pharmacologic therapy includes NSAIDs and colchicine as first-line agents.

    b. Aspirin or ibuprofen is commonly administered 3 times daily for a 1- to 2-week duration and then tapered over a 2- to 4-week period.

    c. Indomethacin and ketorolac have demonstrated efficacy, but patient comorbidities should be considered. Indomethacin may decrease coronary blood flow and should be avoided in patients with coronary artery disease.[8]

    d. Patients with acute pericarditis are instructed to refrain from strenuous physical activity for 3 months or until symptoms have resolved and inflammatory markers, such as C-reactive protein (CRP) or erythrocyte sedimentation rate (ESR), have returned to normal levels due to concern for potential occurrence of sudden cardiac arrest. For competitive athletes, 3 months is considered the minimal period of restricted activity.

    e. Colchicine is an important treatment given in addition to NSAIDs and should be continued for up to 3-6 months. Colchicine binds tubulins and exerts anti-inflammatory effects by disrupting microtubules function within leukocytes.[9,10]

        (1) Gastrointestinal symptoms, such as diarrhea, are common adverse side effects and are frequently cited as a reason for patient cessation of therapy.

        (2) Colchicine is primarily metabolized by the liver and cytochrome P450 pathway. Renal excretion accounts for 10%-20% of metabolism.

        (3) Colchicine may increase sensitivity to central nervous system depressants and exerts respiratory depressant effect.

    f. Corticosteroids rapidly alleviate pericarditis symptoms but are associated with higher rates of recurrence if used during the initial treatment of acute pericarditis.[11]

    g. For patients with recurrent pericarditis refractory to treatment with NSAIDs, colchicine, and corticosteroids, third-line medical therapy includes immunosuppressive agents, such as azathioprine, intravenous (IV) immunoglobulin, or off-label use of anakinra (an interleukin-1 receptor antagonist).[12,13]

    h. For the patient with recurrent pericarditis who fails medical management, surgical pericardiectomy is a safe and effective option. Pericardiectomy in the setting of recurrent pericarditis may be less complicated than when undertaken for constrictive disease because of fewer adhesions and preserved cardiac function.[8]

E. Goals of Perioperative Management

    1. Anesthesiologists may encounter patients with acute pericarditis in situations of malignancy, MI, postcardiotomy syndrome, uremia, or infection.

    2. Thorough preoperative assessment should rule out underlying myocardial ischemia.

    3. Patients may be receiving drug therapy with steroids, anti-inflammatory agents, or other immune-modulating agents as described earlier with perioperative implications and potential drug interactions.

    4. The presence and volume of pericardial fluid should be assessed, along with signs of myocardial compression and cardiopulmonary compromise.

V. Constrictive Pericarditis

    A. Natural History

    1. Etiology: CP is a diagnosis that encompasses a wide spectrum of disease, from acute or subacute cases that may resolve spontaneously (or with medical therapy) to the classic chronic, progressive CP, which is the focus of this section. Other entities include effusive CP, in which patients present with cardiac effusion or tamponade but retain characteristics of CP following drainage of the effusion; localized CP, involving only parts of the pericardium with variable hemodynamic sequelae; and occult CP, in which rapid infusion of IV fluids can provoke the signs and symptoms of the disease.[14] While numerous etiologies have been described, the most common causes are idiopathic, viral, postcardiac surgery, mediastinal radiation, and, in developing countries, TB.

    2. Symptomatology: CP presents most commonly as chronic and progressive fatigue, orthopnea, dyspnea on exertion, peripheral edema, and abdominal distention. Given the nonspecific nature of these findings, care must be taken to differentiate this disease process from other entities, such as hepatic failure, RV failure, tricuspid valve disease, and, in particular, restrictive cardiomyopathy. As the pathophysiology underlying these conditions is markedly different, the medical and surgical management varies considerably as well.

    B. Pathophysiology

    The hallmark of CP is a thickened, calcified, and adherent pericardium. This effectively confines the heart inside a rigid shell. From a pathophysiologic perspective, this has three major consequences[15]:

    1. Impaired diastolic filling: The noncompliant pericardium limits filling of all cardiac chambers, with elevation and near equalization of end-diastolic pressures. Ventricular filling occurs rapidly during early diastole but ceases abruptly as the volume, and thus pressure, in the ventricle, reaches a critical point. This results in the characteristic "dip-and-plateau" or "square-root" sign, noted in ventricular pressure tracings (Figure 18.2). Atrial systole does little to augment LV filling, and cardiac output is maintained by a compensatory increase in heart rate.

    2. Dissociation of intrathoracic pressures: The rigid pericardium isolates the cardiac chambers from the negative pressure generated during inspiration, resulting in a decreased gradient between the pulmonary veins and the left atrium. Consequently, left heart filling, and thus cardiac output, is decreased (Figure 18.3).

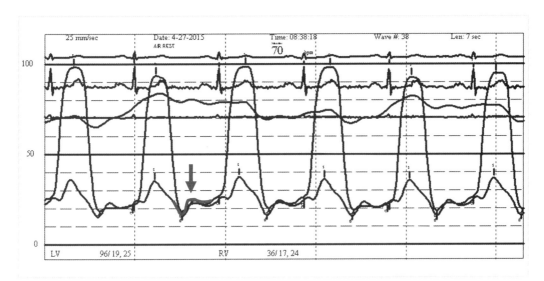

FIGURE 18.2 Hemodynamic profile of constrictive pericarditis. Overlapping left ventricular and right ventricular waveforms demonstrating equalization of diastolic pressure. The square-root sign (highlighted in red) is indicated by the red arrow and reflects rapid diastolic filling. LV, left ventricle; RV, right ventricle. (Reprinted from Tuck BC, Townsley MM. Clinical update in pericardial diseases. *J Cardiothorac Vasc Anesth.* 2019;33(1):184-199. © 2018 Elsevier. With permission.)

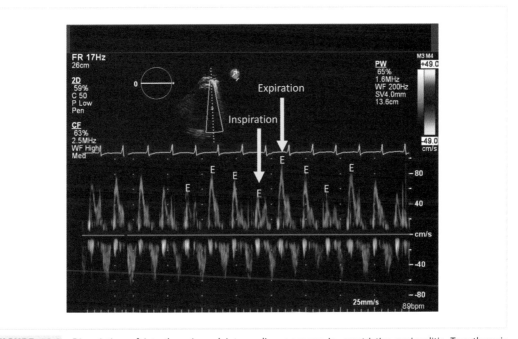

FIGURE 18.3 Dissociation of intrathoracic and intracardiac pressures in constrictive pericarditis. Transthoracic echocardiographic pulsed-wave Doppler transmitral spectral display demonstrating significant respiratory variation in E-wave velocity in a spontaneously breathing patient. (Reprinted from Tuck BC, Townsley MM. Clinical update in pericardial diseases. *J Cardiothorac Vasc Anesth.* 2019;33(1):184-199. © 2018 Elsevier. With permission.)

3. **Ventricular interdependence:** As discussed previously, left and right heart filling are not independent events. Increases in right heart filling may cause a leftward shift in the interventricular septum at the expense of left heart filling. Expiration, as would be expected, reverses this pattern. This phenomenon is known as ventricular interdependence and is exaggerated in CP.

4. One of the most important consequences of pericardial constriction is significant respiratory variation in LV and RV filling patterns. This is an important consideration in the diagnosis of CP and provides the foundation for the diagnostic workup. Of note, this respiratory variation is maintained, but reversed, in patients on mechanical ventilation.[16]

C. **Diagnostic Evaluation and Assessment**
   1. **Clinical evaluation**
      a. The diagnosis of CP is difficult to make on history and physical examination alone but must be considered in patients presenting with the signs and symptoms of venous congestion mentioned previously. On examination, jugular venous distention (JVD) with Kussmaul sign (an increase in JVD on inspiration) and Friedreich sign (a rapid decrease in JVD during early diastole) may be present. Pulsus paradoxus is variably present. On cardiac auscultation, a "pericardial knock" may be noted. This is a high-pitched sound in early diastole that is caused by the sudden cessation of ventricular filling and is a highly specific, but insensitive, clue to the diagnosis. Pulmonary edema is often absent, and pulsatile hepatomegaly may be noted on abdominal examination.
      b. Laboratory investigation may reveal organ dysfunction secondary to the disease process (ie, kidney injury, elevated liver enzymes). Natriuretic peptide levels, which are released in response to myocardial stretch and are increased in many cases of heart failure, are usually normal or only slightly elevated. This is attributed to the rigid pericardium, limiting the amount of potential chamber dilatation.
      c. ECG findings are nonspecific and may include sinus tachycardia, atrial fibrillation, conduction delays, left atrial enlargement (P mitrale), and ST-segment or T-wave changes.
      d. While calcification of the pericardium is not universal, its presence on the lateral chest x-ray may suggest CP. A thickened pericardium (>2 mm) may be appreciated on CT or MRI, and other imaging techniques may demonstrate the pericardium being adherent to the myocardium.
   2. **Catheterization data:** Cardiac catheterization is not always necessary for the diagnosis of CP. However, it may be helpful in the diagnosis of effusive CP, with some suggesting its routine use during the drainage of pericardial effusions. Certain waveform characteristics may be seen during placement of invasive monitors in the operating room. Right atrial (RA) pressure tracings may show "M" or "W" waveforms with a prominent y-descent, the diagnostic equivalent of Friedreich sign. Ventricular pressure tracings may show the characteristic "dip-and-plateau" or "square-root" sign, as previously described. The end-diastolic pressures in all chambers are elevated and nearly equal (≤5 mm Hg difference). RV systolic pressures are usually <50 mm Hg, with an RV end-diastolic to RV end-systolic ratio of ≥1:3. Increased RV stroke volumes during inspiration with simultaneous decrease in LV stroke volumes can be observed during catheterization, suggesting ventricular discordance (Figure 18.4).
   3. **Echocardiography:** Echocardiography is essential for the diagnosis of CP (Table 18.2), and more advanced techniques have become useful in its differentiation from other disease processes. Two-dimensional and M-mode examination may show a thickened, hyperechoic pericardium; diastolic flattening of the LV posterior wall, reflective of the abrupt cessation of ventricular filling; a ventricular septal "bounce," caused by the sudden changes in the trans-septal pressure gradient (Figure 18.5; ▶ **Video 18.3**); atrial tethering (▶ **Video 18.4**); premature closure of the mitral valve and opening of the pulmonic valve, indicative of high chamber pressures; enlarged hepatic veins; and inferior vena cava (IVC) plethora, where the vessel remains dilated and lacks the normal change in diameter during the respiratory cycle. Doppler evaluation of transmitral, transtricuspid, and pulmonary vein flow shows characteristic tracings with profound respiratory variation (often >25%).

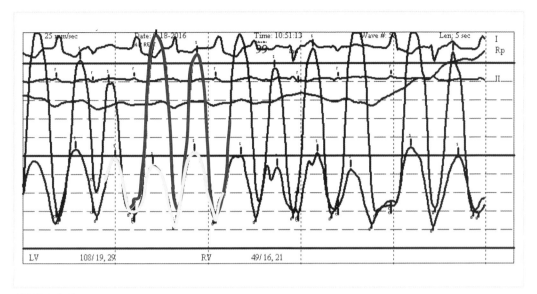

FIGURE 18.4 Ventricular discordance in constrictive pericarditis. During inspiration, right ventricular systolic pressure (yellow) increases as left ventricular systolic pressure decreases (red), caused by increased ventricular interdependence. LV, left ventricle; RV, right ventricle. (Reprinted from Tuck BC, Townsley MM. Clinical update in pericardial diseases. *J Cardiothorac Vasc Anesth.* 2019;33(1):184-199. © 2018 Elsevier. With permission.)

Advanced techniques, such as tissue Doppler imaging (TDI) of the mitral annulus (Figure 18.6) and color Doppler M-mode of transmitral flow propagation velocity (Figure 18.7), allow further characterization and differentiation from restrictive cardiomyopathy (Table 18.3).[17]

D. Treatment

As previously mentioned, some cases of acute constriction may resolve spontaneously or with medical management. The definitive management of chronic CP, however, is usually surgical. Pericardiectomy, or pericardial decortication, is often performed via left thoracotomy or midline sternotomy, depending on the extent of resection necessary. The goal of treatment is total resection of both the visceral and parietal pericardium. While this can often be performed without the use of cardiopulmonary bypass (CPB), its use may be indicated in more difficult dissections. Despite improvements in surgical technique, operative mortality remains as high as 10%, with poor prognostic predictors including prior cardiac surgery, radiation, malignancy, and advanced heart failure on presentation. As opposed to patients with tamponade, where surgical drainage may provide immediate improvement in hemodynamic and clinical status, an immediate improvement in symptoms is not generally observed. The perioperative transesophageal echocardiography (TEE) examination allows for continuous monitoring of chamber size and ventricular function. Particular emphasis should be placed on assessing baseline

TABLE 18.2   Echocardiographic Features of Constrictive Pericarditis

- Pericardial thickening
- Inferior vena cava plethora
- Restrictive pattern of ventricular filling (Doppler echocardiography)
- Ventricular septal bounce
- Medial mitral annular E′ >8
- Annulus reversus: medial mitral annular E′ greater than lateral mitral annular E′
- Transmitral E wave decrease ≥25% with inspiration
- Transtricuspid E wave decrease ≥40% with expiration

Adapted from Tuck BC, Townsley MM. Clinical update in pericardial diseases. *J Cardiothorac Vasc Anesth.* 2019;33(1):184-199. Table 5. © 2018 Elsevier. With permission.

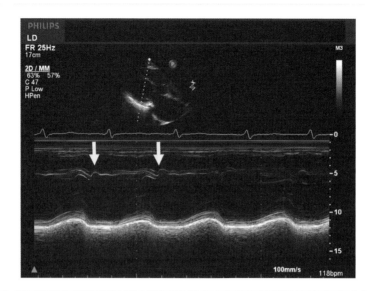

FIGURE 18.5 Septal bounce. On transthoracic echocardiographic examination, this M-mode parasternal left ventricular long-axis view demonstrates characteristic septal bounce (yellow arrow) in a patient with constrictive pericarditis. (Reprinted from Tuck BC, Townsley MM. Clinical update in pericardial diseases. *J Cardiothorac Vasc Anesth.* 2019;33(1):184-199. © 2018 Elsevier. With permission.)

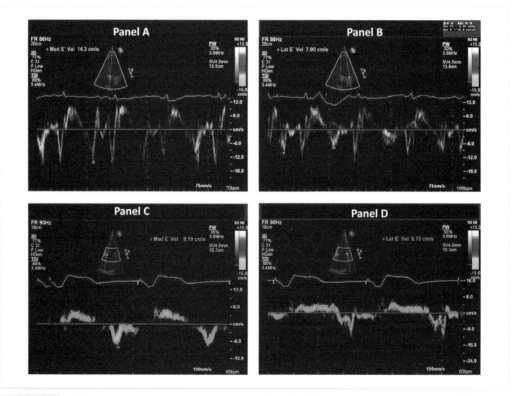

FIGURE 18.6 Mitral annular tissue Doppler in constrictive pericarditis (CP) and restrictive cardiomyopathy (RCM). These transthoracic echocardiographic images taken from the same patient **(panels A and B)** demonstrate annulus reversus, in which the mitral medial annular E′ is greater than the mitral lateral E′. These findings are consistent with the diagnosis of CP. In a different patient with RCM **(panels C and D)**, both mitral medial and lateral E′ are reduced. (Reprinted from Tuck BC, Townsley MM. Clinical update in pericardial diseases. *J Cardiothorac Vasc Anesth.* 2019;33(1):184-199. © 2018 Elsevier. With permission.)

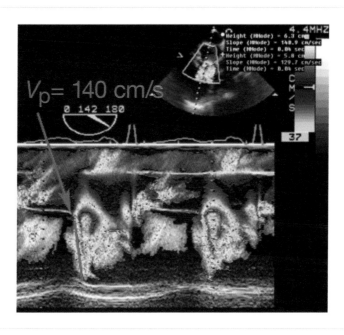

FIGURE 18.7   Transesophageal echocardiographic image of the transmitral color M-mode (propagation velocity, V_p) profile of a patient with constrictive pericarditis. The slope of the first aliasing velocity is used in this determination and is depicted by the pink line. (Reprinted with permission from Avery EG, Shernan SK. Echocardiographic evaluation of pericardial disease. In: Savage RM, Aronson S, Shernan SK, eds. *Comprehensive Textbook of Perioperative Transesophageal Echocardiography.* 2nd ed. Wolters Kluwer Health/Lippincott Williams & Wilkins; 2011:738.)

TABLE 18.3   Clues to the Differentiation of CP and Restrictive Cardiomyopathy

	CP	Restrictive Cardiomyopathy
Pulsus paradoxus	Variable	Absent
Kussmaul sign	Common	Absent
Pericardial knock	Common	Absent
Chest x-ray	Pericardial calcification	No pericardial calcification
CT and MRI	Pericardial thickening (>2 mm)	Normal pericardium
B-type natriuretic peptide	Normal to mildly elevated	Significantly elevated
Catheterization data	LVEDP-RVEDP ≤5 mm Hg PASP <40-50 mm Hg RVEDP:RVSP >1:3	LVEDP-RVEDP >5 mm Hg PASP >40-50 mm Hg RVEDP:RVSP <1:3
Atrial size	Usually normal	Enlarged
Ventricular septal motion	Abnormal: septal "bounce"	Normal
Respiratory variation (Doppler flow patterns)	Exaggerated (often >25%)	Normal/minimal (<10%)
Color M-mode propagation velocity	>100 cm/s	<100 cm/s
Tissue Doppler imaging of mitral annulus	E′ >8 cm/s	E′ <8 cm/s

CP, constrictive pericarditis; CT, computed tomography; LVEDP, left ventricular end-diastolic pressure; MRI, magnetic resonance imaging; PASP, pulmonary artery systolic pressure; RVEDP, right ventricular end-diastolic pressure; RVSP, right ventricular systolic pressure.

valvular function before pericardiectomy, as well as valvular function postprocedure. It is not uncommon for tricuspid regurgitation to worsen following pericardial resection due to acute volume overload of the RV and tricuspid annular dilatation (Figure 18.8).

When pericardiectomy is performed without the use of CPB, it is not uncommon for patients to require significant support with inotropic and/or vasopressor drugs—the anesthetic plan should carefully (and preemptively) plan for the use of these agents.

E. Goals of Perioperative Management

1. If needed, premedication with benzodiazepines or opioids must be titrated judiciously and according to the patient's preoperative hemodynamic status. The sympathetic nervous system plays an important role in maintaining cardiac output, and any inhibition may lead to clinical and hemodynamic deterioration.

2. In addition to standard noninvasive monitors, the intraoperative and postoperative management of patients with CP often requires invasive monitors. An arterial line is beneficial for frequent blood gas analysis (most importantly for cases involving thoracotomy), as well as continuous blood pressure monitoring (especially during cardiac manipulation and when CPB is utilized). The decision to place an arterial line either preoperatively or after induction of anesthesia must take into account the patient's clinical status and the possibility of hemodynamic instability on induction. Adequate IV access must be obtained, given the possibility of marked and precipitous blood loss (cardiac chamber or coronary artery perforation, myocardial injury due to stripping of the pericardium), with central venous access allowing the rapid infusion of IV fluids/blood products and vasoactive drugs, as well as the monitoring of central venous pressure (CVP). Intraoperative TEE provides useful information for both the surgeon and the anesthesiologist, in particular, with regard to ventricular filling and function.

3. Preload must be maintained, and often augmented, to ensure cardiac filling. Reductions in either preload or afterload are usually poorly tolerated. An elevated heart rate plays an important role in the maintenance of cardiac output, and bradycardia can be particularly detrimental. While the atrial "kick" does little to enhance ventricular filling in patients with CP, extreme tachycardia, such as atrial fibrillation with a rapid ventricular rate, may be poorly tolerated. Contractility should be maintained, as significant myocardial depression will adversely affect cardiac output and systemic perfusion.

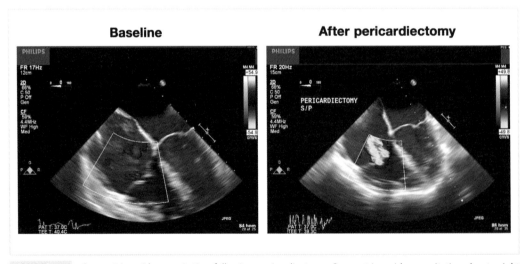

FIGURE 18.8 Severe tricuspid regurgitation following pericardiectomy. Severe tricuspid regurgitation due to right ventricular volume overload and tricuspid annular dilatation may occur after pericardiectomy. Careful analysis of chamber size and valvular assessment should be performed before and immediately after pericardiectomy. (Reprinted from Tuck BC, Townsley MM. Clinical update in pericardial diseases. *J Cardiothorac Vasc Anesth.* 2019;33(1):184-199. © 2018 Elsevier. With permission.)

4. Vasoactive medications must be readily available to offset any perturbations caused by anesthetic agents or surgical manipulations, most notably decreased preload, afterload, contractility, and heart rate. Surgical blood loss and coagulopathy may be significant, necessitating aggressive resuscitation and correction of the underlying coagulopathy.

5. Depending on the extent of surgical dissection, severe surgical bleeding and coagulopathy are common with pericardiectomy.

VI. Pericardial Effusion and Tamponade

A. Natural History

1. **Etiology:** The visceral pericardium is responsible for the production of pericardial fluid, which is an ultrafiltrate of plasma. This fluid provides lubrication to decrease friction between the pericardial layers. The pericardial space normally contains 10-50 mL of fluid, which is drained by the lymphatic system. As previously discussed, many conditions can cause fluid (serous, serosanguineous, and purulent) or blood to accumulate within the pericardial space. The majority of pericardial effusions are not hemodynamically significant and do not progress to tamponade. Tamponade occurs when extrinsic pericardial compression of the heart leads to diminished venous filling and, ultimately, reduced cardiac output. In addition to fluid collection within the pericardium, tamponade may also be caused by the accumulation of clot or air in the pericardial space. Acute, life-threatening tamponade most frequently results from bleeding into the pericardial space after cardiac surgery or other invasive cardiac procedures, following blunt chest trauma, or due to a ruptured ascending aortic aneurysm or aortic dissection.[18] Tamponade may occur in as many as 8.8% of patients presenting for cardiac surgery, although it is more commonly seen after valve surgery than coronary artery bypass grafting (CABG). The onset is typically in the immediate postoperative period but may potentially occur several days following surgery. Frequently, there is localized clot or effusion, which causes non-uniform compression of the cardiac chambers and manifests without the classical clinical features of tamponade. The diagnosis of postcardiac surgery tamponade can, therefore, be challenging, especially when considering the many potential causes of hemodynamic instability during this time period. Unfortunately, morbidity and mortality increase significantly the longer the diagnosis is delayed.

2. **Symptomatology:** Symptoms of cardiac tamponade are usually rapid in onset but depend upon the rate at which pericardial fluid accumulates. A relatively small amount of fluid (50-100 mL) that rapidly accumulates within the closed pericardial space is sufficient to dramatically increase intrapericardial pressure and interfere with cardiac filling. However, a chronic increase in pericardial fluid will produce tamponade only after a large volume (>1 L) is present. A gradual accumulation of fluid stretches the parietal pericardium, allowing larger volumes to be tolerated before symptoms occur. Lack of this pericardial stretch explains the abrupt onset of symptoms and clinical deterioration in the setting of acute tamponade. Figure 18.9 illustrates this pressure-volume relationship in acute versus chronic pericardial effusions. The primary symptoms of cardiac tamponade include dyspnea, orthopnea, diaphoresis, and chest pain. Dyspnea is often the first and most sensitive symptom.[19]

B. Pathophysiology

The primary abnormality in cardiac tamponade is impaired diastolic filling of the heart, caused by elevated intrapericardial pressure that leads to compression of the atria and ventricles. The right heart is most vulnerable to the compression due to its thinner walls and lower chamber pressures as compared to the left heart. Diastolic filling pressures (ie, CVP, left atrial pressure, pulmonary capillary wedge pressure, left and right ventricular end-diastolic pressures [LVEDP and RVEDP]) become elevated and began to equilibrate with one another, as well as the intrapericardial pressure. Physiologic manifestations of pericardial fluid, as previously discussed, are contingent upon the rate and amount of fluid accumulation, with a continuum ranging from clinical insignificance to severe hemodynamic collapse. Cardiac filling is critically reduced, which translates into decreased stroke volume, cardiac output, and systemic blood pressure. Compensatory sympathetic

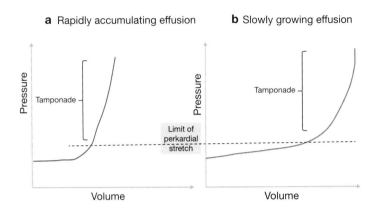

a Rapidly accumulating effusion   **b** Slowly growing effusion

FIGURE 18.9 Pressure-volume relationship in acute versus chronic pericardial effusions. Intrapericardial pressure is contingent upon the change in intrapericardial volume. Pressure is relatively stable until a critical volume occurs. At this point, minimal increases in volume will lead to significant changes in intrapericardial pressure. With chronic effusions, pericardial stretch allows for a greater amount of volume to accumulate before critical increases in pressure occur. The lack of pericardial stretch explains the significant elevations in pressures seen with only small amounts of rapidly accumulating intrapericardial fluid. (Reprinted by permission from Springer: Flint N, Siegel RJ. Echo-Guided Pericardiocentesis: When and How Should It Be Performed? *Curr Cardiol Rep.* 2020;22(8):71. Figure 1. Copyright © 2020 Springer Science Business Media, LLC.)

responses attempt to offset this reduction in stroke volume, with elevated levels of plasma catecholamines resulting in systemic vasoconstriction and tachycardia. This may temporarily maintain cardiac output and systemic perfusion; however, sudden hemodynamic collapse may rapidly occur with depletion of catecholamines and/or continued elevation of intrapericardial pressure.

C. **Diagnostic Evaluation and Assessment**

1. Clinical evaluation

    a. Acute tamponade is often described by Beck triad: muffled heart sounds, JVD (due to increased venous pressure), and hypotension. Other common findings include tachypnea and tachycardia.

    b. Pulsus paradoxus, although not specific for tamponade, may be present. While a modest decrease in systolic arterial blood pressure during inspiration is physiologic, an exaggerated decrease in blood pressure is pathologic. Pulsus paradoxus is defined as a decrease in >10 mm Hg in systolic arterial pressure that occurs with inspiration. Tamponade physiology leads to respiratory variability in ventricular diastolic filling, in which the negative intrathoracic pressure accompanying inspiration leads to enhanced right-sided filling. Since total intracardiac volume is fixed by the pericardial compression, as the RV fills, it will lead to a shift of the interventricular septum toward the LV. This crowding of the LV impedes its filling, decreasing LV stroke volume and resulting in an exaggerated decline in systolic blood pressure seen with inspiration. The opposite is true during expiration, with diminished RV and enhanced LV filling. Pulsus paradoxus is also seen in patients with chronic lung disease, large pleural effusions, RV dysfunction, and CP.

    c. The chest x-ray may show an enlarged, globular, and bottle-shaped cardiac silhouette. The right costophrenic angle is reduced to <90°, and the lung fields are typically clear. Pericardial fat lines in a lateral film are an uncommon, but highly specific, finding.

TABLE 18.4	Cardiac Tamponade—Clinical Manifestations

Hypotension

Tachycardia

Widened mediastinum (on chest x-ray)

Elevation and near equalization of filling pressures

Increasing inotrope requirements

Pulsus paradoxus

Electrical alternans

Initial high output chest tube drainage that abruptly subsides

    d. The ECG is nonspecific but may demonstrate sinus tachycardia, low-voltage QRS, non-specific ST-T wave abnormalities, and electrical alternans. Electrical alternans is due to swinging of the heart within the fluid of the pericardial sac, leading to beat-to-beat changes in the electrical axis.

    e. Table 18.4 summarizes the classic clinical manifestations most commonly described in cardiac tamponade.

  2. Catheterization data: Cardiac tamponade is a clinical diagnosis that cannot be made with catheterization data alone; however, common patterns of intracardiac pressures are usually seen. There is elevation and near equalization of the CVP, RVEDP, pulmonary capillary wedge pressure, left atrial pressure, and LVEDP. Increased CVP and RA pressures are seen with a prominent x-descent and a diminished or absent y-descent (Figure 18.10).

CLINICAL PEARL

When hemodynamic instability occurs within the setting of elevated filling pressures (as demonstrated by CVP and/or pulmonary artery pressure measurements), cardiac tamponade must be immediately included in the differential diagnosis (especially in the postcardiac surgery patient).

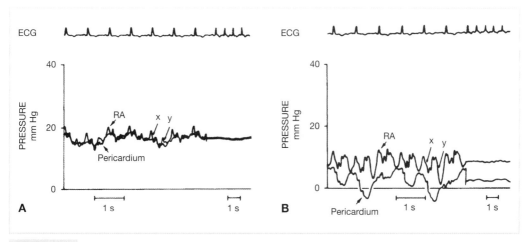

FIGURE 18.10 Right atrial (RA) and pericardial pressures in cardiac tamponade. **(A)** Note equal RA and pericardial pressures and the diminished y-descent of the RA waveform. **(B)** After removal of 100 mL of fluid, the pericardial pressure is lower than RA pressure, and the normal large descent has returned. ECG, electrocardiogram. (Reprinted with permission from Hensley FA, Martin DE, Gravlee GP. *A Practical Approach to Cardiac Anesthesia.* 3rd ed. Lippincott Williams & Wilkins; 2003:475.)

Panel A   Panel B

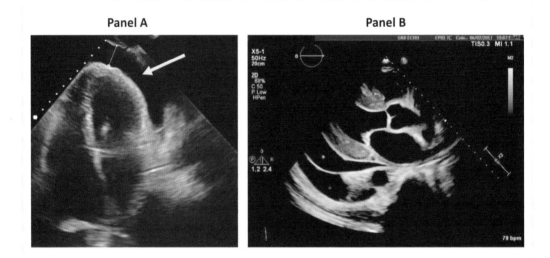

FIGURE 18.11 Pericardial effusions visualized with transthoracic echocardiography (TTE). **Panel A** demonstrates a TTE apical four-chamber view with a large pericardial effusion indicated by the yellow arrow. **Panel B** shows a TTE parasternal long-axis view with a large pericardial effusion (yellow asterisk) and pleural effusion (red asterisk). (Reprinted from Tuck BC, Townsley MM. Clinical update in pericardial diseases. *J Cardiothorac Vasc Anesth.* 2019;33(1):184-199. © 2018 Elsevier. With permission.)

    3. Echocardiography: Echocardiography is the diagnostic modality of choice in evaluating cardiac tamponade. It is the most sensitive tool for making the diagnosis of pericardial effusion. Initial evaluation should focus on the presence, size, and extent (circumferential vs localized/loculated) of the pericardial effusion, which is seen as an echo-free space surrounding the heart (Figures 18.11 and 18.12). Several echocardiographic parameters may be utilized to further characterize the effusion and its severity (Table 18.5).

    Although echocardiography alone cannot definitively diagnose tamponade, in the presence of a pericardial effusion, there are several echocardiographic features consistently

Panel A   Panel B

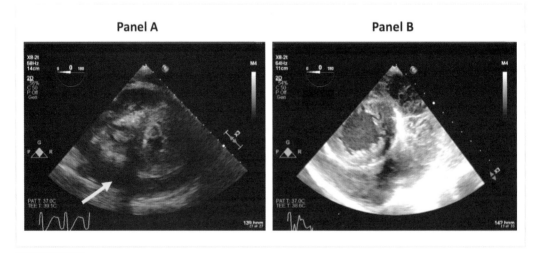

FIGURE 18.12 Pericardial effusions with transesophageal echocardiography (TEE). **Panel A** demonstrates a TEE transgastric left ventricular short-axis view with a large circumferential pericardial effusion indicated by the yellow arrow. **Panel B** shows a TEE transgastric short-axis view demonstrating a large, loculated effusion with fibrin strands. (Reprinted from Tuck BC, Townsley MM. Clinical update in pericardial diseases. *J Cardiothorac Vasc Anesth.* 2019;33(1):184-199. © 2018 Elsevier. With permission.)

TABLE 18.5   Echocardiographic Assessment of Pericardial Effusions

Onset of effusion:
Acute vs chronic

Extent of effusion:
Circumferential vs localized

Hemodynamic effects:
Hemodynamic instability (ie, cardiac tamponade) vs insignificant

Effusion size (measured at end diastole):
Small (50-100 mL): <10 mm
Medium (100-500 mL): 10-20 mm
Large (>500 mL): >20 mm

Adapted from Tuck BC, Townsley MM. Clinical update in pericardial diseases. *J Cardiothorac Vasc Anesth.* 2019;33(1):184-199. Table 2. © 2018 Elsevier. With permission.

associated with tamponade physiology. With tamponade, RA collapse is a sensitive sign, typically beginning in end diastole and continuing through systole (Figure 18.13; ▶ **Video 18.5**). Systolic RA collapse persisting for more than one-third of the cardiac cycle is specific for tamponade. Diastolic RV collapse is also observed and, when lasting for more than one-third of diastole, is even more specific than systolic RA collapse for the identification of tamponade. End-diastolic dimensions of the RV will be reduced, reflective of diminished ventricular filling. Paradoxical motion of the interventricular septum is a frequent finding, reflecting the reciprocal respiratory variability in diastolic filling. These changes are also reflected in Doppler transmitral and transtricuspid inflow velocity profiles (Figure 18.14).

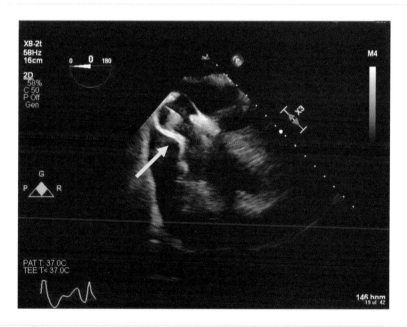

FIGURE 18.13 Cardiac tamponade with right atrial compression. Transesophageal echocardiographic midesophageal four-chamber view with large pericardial effusion causing significant compression of the right atrium (yellow arrow). (Reprinted from Tuck BC, Townsley MM. Clinical update in pericardial diseases. *J Cardiothorac Vasc Anesth.* 2019;33(1):184-199. © 2018 Elsevier. With permission.)

Panel A. Transtricuspid pulsed wave

Panel B. Transmitral pulsed wave

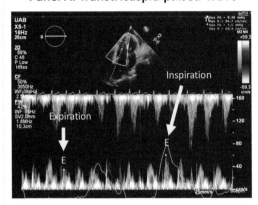 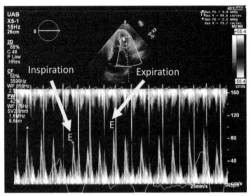

FIGURE 18.14 Respiratory variation in cardiac tamponade noted on transthoracic echocardiography in a spontaneously breathing patient. **Panel A** shows increased tricuspid inflow velocity during inspiration with decreased inflow velocity during expiration. **Panel B** demonstrates decreased transmitral velocity with inspiration and increased velocity during expiration. (Reprinted from Tuck BC, Townsley MM. Clinical update in pericardial diseases. *J Cardiothorac Vasc Anesth.* 2019;33(1):184-199. © 2018 Elsevier. With permission.)

CLINICAL PEARL

If tamponade is suspected, bedside echocardiography can provide immediate information to assist/confirm clinical diagnosis by allowing for visualization of pericardial effusion and/or compression, leading to cardiac chamber collapse.

D. **Treatment**

Definitive treatment of cardiac tamponade is emergent drainage and/or relief of pericardial compression, which may be accomplished through either pericardiocentesis or surgical decompression.

1. **Pericardiocentesis:** Pericardiocentesis may be performed with or without imaging guidance (ie, echocardiography, fluoroscopy). Imaging is often preferred to assist in safely guiding the needle tip through the pericardium to the most optimal location for drainage, as well as assessing the adequacy of fluid removal. Without imaging, there is a significantly higher risk of complications, such as cardiac perforation, puncture of coronary or internal mammary arteries, and pneumothorax. In the setting of severe hemodynamic instability, however, it may be necessary to proceed without imaging due to the significant risk of rapid and profound clinical deterioration. A catheter is frequently left in the pericardial space to allow for continuous drainage. Figure 18.15 demonstrates the most common needle insertion points for pericardiocentesis.

2. **Surgical drainage:** Indications for surgical drainage include unsuccessful pericardiocentesis, localized/loculated effusions, removal of clot, and ongoing intrapericardial bleeding (ie, acute aortic dissection, trauma, following cardiac surgery or percutaneous cardiac procedures). The surgical approach is primarily via subxiphoid pericardial window or a small anterior thoracotomy. The subxiphoid approach is easier to perform but offers a limited exposure, while a thoracotomy provides excellent exposure and is indicated if a larger surgical field is required. Both approaches allow for open exploration, facilitating the removal of clot and fibrinous debris. With hemorrhagic tamponade following cardiac surgery, full mediastinal exploration is often needed to localize the source of bleeding and stabilize the patient. In the setting of malignant effusions, diagnostic pericardial biopsies can be obtained with a surgical approach to drainage.[18] Some patients may continue to experience recurrent pericardial effusions, requiring consideration of pericardiectomy. This is most commonly seen in patients with malignant

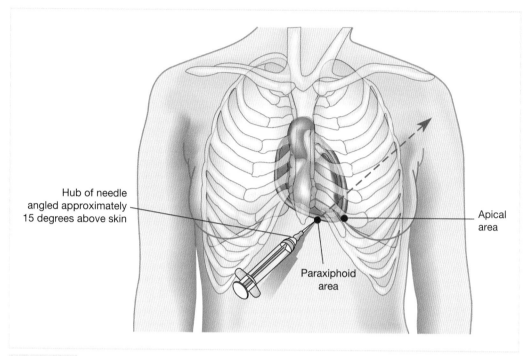

FIGURE 18.15 The most common needle insertion points for pericardiocentesis, including the paraxiphoid and apical approaches. When using the paraxiphoid approach, the needle tip should be directed toward the left shoulder. With the apical approach, the needle tip is aimed internally. (Redrawn from Spodick DH. Acute cardiac tamponade. *N Engl J Med.* 2003;349(7):684–690.)

effusions or uremia. Note that large pleural effusions can yield similar hemodynamic effects as a pericardial effusion and similarly are treated by drainage.[20]

E. Goals of Perioperative Management

The hemodynamic state of the patient will dictate the sequence of anesthesia and surgery. While general anesthesia is frequently used, it may likely contribute to clinical decompensation in the severely compromised patient. Direct myocardial depression, systemic vasodilation, and diminished preload accompanying the induction of general anesthesia can lead to a profound decrease in cardiac output. Potentially life-threatening cardiac collapse may ensue. In this scenario, pericardiocentesis or subxiphoid pericardial window can be performed under local anesthesia to avoid these complications. Frequently, hemodynamic instability is dramatically improved with the removal of only a small amount of fluid. This is due to the steep curve of the pressure-volume relationship of the pericardial contents.[18] Following initial drainage, the patient may become stable enough to tolerate the institution of general anesthesia for the remainder of the procedure.

7

CLINICAL PEARL

In a patient with tamponade, it is important to discuss with the surgeon the feasibility of draining at least a portion of the pericardial effusion before induction in order to relieve cardiac compression and minimize the risk of severe cardiac compromise.

---

1. Premedication with anxiolytics or opioids should be avoided in patients with true cardiac tamponade, as even small doses of these medications can precipitate acute cardiac collapse.
2. To facilitate ventricular filling, preload should be optimized with IV fluids before induction. Any manipulations that decrease venous return should be avoided or minimized as much as possible.
3. In addition to standard noninvasive monitors, an arterial line should be strongly considered before induction to allow for preoperative quantification of pulsus paradoxus and beat-to-beat monitoring of systemic blood pressure. Adequate IV access is needed for volume

replacement and drug administration. Central venous access may be beneficial but is not always essential. In a severely unstable patient, surgical intervention should not be delayed for the placement of lines or monitors.

4. Before proceeding with induction, the patient should be fully prepped and draped, with the surgical team immediately available to make incision in the event of hemodynamic collapse upon induction.

5. The perioperative anesthetic plan should follow the hemodynamic goals outlined in Table 18.6. Reductions in heart rate should be avoided and contractility optimized to preserve cardiac output, as these patients have both a fixed and reduced stroke volume. Adequate preload is essential to promote RV filling. Decreases in systemic vascular resistance are particularly detrimental, as this will reduce RV filling and systemic perfusion pressure.

6. Positive pressure ventilation can cause a dramatic decline in preload and cardiac output. It is, therefore, suggested that patients with tamponade be allowed to breathe spontaneously until the pericardial sac is opened and drained. If spontaneous ventilation is not possible, ventilation with high respiratory rates and low-tidal volumes should be considered to minimize elevation in mean airway pressures.

7. Careful consideration should be given to the selection of induction drugs, with particular attention aimed at minimizing myocardial depression and peripheral vasodilation. Etomidate is a reasonable induction agent, as it produces minimal decreases in contractility and systemic vascular resistance, although hemodynamic instability may still occur in the setting of tamponade physiology. Benzodiazepines are also a reasonable choice. Many advocate the use of ketamine in this setting, relying on the sympathetic stimulation it provides to minimize hemodynamic compromise. It is important to note, however, that in a catecholamine-depleted state, many patients will have a diminished ability to increase their own sympathetic nervous system activity. In these patients, the myocardial depressant properties of ketamine may be unmasked and significant hypotension could occur. Opioids should be given with caution, as vagally mediated bradycardia can significantly diminish cardiac output.

CLINICAL PEARL

Vasopressor and inotropic drugs should be immediately available to administer with general anesthetic induction, and in many cases, it is prudent to begin infusions of vasoactive medications (if not already started before arrival in the operating room) to support the patient's hemodynamics during and following induction.

8. Inotropes (ie, epinephrine, norepinephrine) and vasoconstrictors (ie, phenylephrine, vasopressin) are often needed to maintain cardiac output and peripheral vascular resistance, but serve only as a temporizing measure until tamponade can be definitively treated with drainage.

9. Tamponade is rarely seen in patients presenting for surgical drainage of chronic, recurrent pericardial effusions. In this scenario, however, it is still essential to obtain as much information as possible regarding the clinical significance and severity of the effusion. This should include a review of the preoperative echocardiogram, a thorough discussion with the surgeon, and a detailed history and physical examination, focusing, in particular, on any vital sign abnormalities. A high index of suspicion should be maintained for the potential of perioperative hemodynamic instability.

TABLE 18.6	Hemodynamic Goals in Cardiac Tamponade			
	Heart Rate	**Contractility**	**Preload**	**Systemic Vascular Resistance**
Tamponade	↑	↑	↑	↑

CLINICAL PEARL

While tamponade is not commonly seen in the setting of a chronic pericardial effusion, it is still important to remain vigilant and prepared for the occurrence of hemodynamic instability.

REFERENCES

1. Klein AL, Abbara S, Agler DA, et al. American Society of Echocardiography clinical recommendations for multimodality cardiovascular imaging of patients with pericardial disease: endorsed by the Society for Cardiovascular Magnetic Resonance and Society of Cardiovascular Computed Tomography. *J Am Soc Echocardiogr.* 2013;26(9):965-1012.e15.
2. Lopez D, Asher CR. Congenital absence of the pericardium. *Prog Cardiovasc Dis.* 2017;59(4):398-406.
3. Khandaker MH, Espinosa RE, Nishimura RA, et al. Pericardial disease: diagnosis and management. *Mayo Clin Proc.* 2010;85(6):572-593.
4. Tuck BC, Townsley MM. Clinical update in pericardial diseases. *J Cardiothorac Vasc Anesth.* 2019;33(1):184-199.
5. Imazio M, Gribaudo E, Gaita F. Recurrent pericarditis. *Prog Cardiovasc Dis.* 2017;59(4):360-368.
6. Imazio M, Brucato A, Barbieri A, et al. Good prognosis for pericarditis with and without myocardial involvement: results from a multicenter, prospective cohort study. *Circulation.* 2013;128(1):42-49.
7. Lilly LS. Treatment of acute and recurrent idiopathic pericarditis. *Circulation.* 2013;127(16):1723-1726.
8. Khandaker MH, Schaff HV, Greason KL, et al. Pericardiectomy vs medical management in patients with relapsing pericarditis. *Mayo Clin Proc.* 2012;87(11):1062-1070.
9. Imazio M, Bobbio M, Cecchi E, et al. Colchicine as first-choice therapy for recurrent pericarditis: results of the CORE (COlchicine for REcurrent pericarditis) trial. *Arch Intern Med.* 2005;165(17):1987-1991.
10. Imazio M, Belli R, Brucato A, et al. Efficacy and safety of colchicine for treatment of multiple recurrences of pericarditis (CORP-2): a multicentre, double-blind, placebo-controlled, randomised trial. *Lancet.* 2014;383(9936):2232-2237.
11. Farand P, Bonenfant F, Belley-Côté EP, Tzouannis N. Acute and recurring pericarditis: more colchicine, less corticosteroids. *World J Cardiol.* 2010;2(12):403-407.
12. Brucato A, Imazio M, Gattorno M, et al. Effect of Anakinra on recurrent pericarditis among patients with colchicine resistance and corticosteroid dependence: the AIRTRIP randomized clinical trial. *JAMA.* 2016;316(18):1906-1912.
13. Cantarini L, Lopalco G, Selmi C, et al. Autoimmunity and autoinflammation as the yin and yang of idiopathic recurrent acute pericarditis. *Autoimmun Rev.* 2015;14(2):90-97.
14. Sagrista-Salueda J. Pericardial constriction: uncommon patterns. *Heart.* 2004;90(3):257-258.
15. Myers RB, Spodick DH. Constrictive pericarditis: clinical and pathophysiologic characteristics. *Am Heart J.* 1999;138 (2 pt 1):219-232.
16. Abdalla IA, Murray RD, Awad HE, et al. Reversal of the pattern of respiratory variation of Doppler inflow velocities in constrictive pericarditis during mechanical ventilation. *J Am Soc Echocardiogr.* 2000;13(9):827-831.
17. Rajagopalan N, Garcia MJ, Rodriguez L, et al. Comparison of new Doppler echocardiographic methods to differentiate constrictive pericardial heart disease and restrictive cardiomyopathy. *Am J Cardiol.* 2001;87(1):86-94.
18. O'Connor CJ, Tuman KJ. The intraoperative management of patients with pericardial tamponade. *Anesthesiol Clin.* 2010;28(1):87-96.
19. Gandhi S, Schneider A, Mohiuddin S, et al. Has the clinical presentation and clinician's index of suspicion of cardiac tamponade changed over the past decade? *Echocardiography.* 2008;25(3):237-241.
20. Alam HB, Levitt A, Molyneaux R, et al. Can pleural effusions cause cardiac tamponade? *Chest.* 1999;116(6):1820-1822.

19

Cardiac Masses

Promise Ariyo and Julie A. Wyrobek

KEY POINTS

1. Primary cardiac tumors are rare. Myxomas are the most common benign cardiac tumors that occur in adults. Cardiac sarcomas are the most common malignant tumors that occur in adults.
2. Metastatic cardiac tumors from other sites are more common and often carry worse prognosis.
3. Transesophageal echocardiography (TEE) has a 97% sensitivity of identifying that a patient has a cardiac tumor.
4. Cardiac tumors can not only be asymptomatic but also cause signs and symptoms, such as arrhythmias, pericardial tamponade, heart failure, embolic events, or sudden cardiac death.
5. Anesthetic management should include multidisciplinary discussions and thorough knowledge of tumor anatomy and related physiologic derangements. In some situations, preparing for induction of anesthesia should involve the multidisciplinary team, with patient prepped and possibly cannulated for the possibility of emergency cardiopulmonary bypass (CPB) on induction of anesthesia.
6. Risk factors for poor prognosis from endocarditis include advanced age, prosthetic valve, heart failure, stroke, and *Staphylococcus aureus* infection.
7. The modified Duke criteria consist of major and minor criteria to diagnose endocarditis, though it should not serve as a substitute for high clinical suspicion.
8. The most common complications after endocarditis surgery include septic shock, heart failure, coagulopathy, acute renal failure, and stroke and need for a permanent pacemaker.
9. TEE has imaging sensitivity and specificity approaching 100% for detecting a left atrial appendage (LAA) thrombus. Pulsed-wave Doppler velocities <40 cm/s are associated with an increased risk of thrombus.
10. Anesthetic induction for pulmonary embolism (PE) surgical intervention is associated with a high risk of hemodynamic collapse. It is a common practice to have surgical draping complete before induction and intubation.

There are a number of different etiologies for cardiac masses. This chapter discusses identification and perioperative management for cases with cardiac masses. The descriptions of anesthetic considerations and approaches are grouped first to understand cardiac tumors and then to discuss endocarditis, thrombus, and normal variants.

I. Cardiac Tumors

A. Introduction

Cardiac tumors are quite uncommon, although advances in imaging modalities have led to an increase in the diagnosis of these tumors. The first diagnosis of an intracardiac tumor by echocardiography was in 1959.[1] Patients with cardiac tumors can present with a broad range of signs and symptoms. Definitive diagnosis of the type of cardiac tumor with biopsy can be technically challenging. Therefore, providers may rely on multimodal imaging, including preoperative computed tomography (CT) scan, cardiac magnetic resonance imaging (MRI), echocardiography, and cardiac catheterization to plan tissue diagnosis and possible tumor resection.

B. Epidemiology

Cardiac tumors can be broadly classified as primary or secondary tumors. Primary cardiac tumors are rare, and an autopsy incidence has been reported between 0.001% and 0.28%.[2,3] About 75% of cardiac tumors are benign and about 25% are malignant.[4,5] Secondary or metastatic cardiac tumors are more common, and the heart can be the site of metastases for any kind of tumor. The incidence of secondary cardiac tumors ranges from 2.3% to 18.3%.[6-8] This number has increased in recent years, probably secondary to improved treatment options and life expectancy in patients with cancer.[6]

C. Clinical Presentation

Patients with cardiac tumors may not exhibit any cardiac symptoms at all, and the cardiac tumor may be an incidental finding on imaging obtained for other diagnostic evaluation or discovered on postmortem investigation. Others may present with a myriad of symptoms, including sudden cardiac death. These symptoms may include the following:

1. **Constitutional symptoms:** Fever, fatigue, weight loss, night sweats
2. Tumors that infiltrate the inferior vena cava (IVC) or the superior vena cava (SVC) can impede venous return and cause venous congestion, including lower extremity edema and SVC syndrome, respectively. Other intracavitary lesions can also lead to obstruction of transvalvular flow or ventricular outflow obstruction. Right-sided obstruction can result in peripheral edema, congestive hepatopathy, and ascites. Left-sided obstruction can result in pulmonary edema and low cardiac output. Extensive involvement can cause systolic dysfunction or restrictive diastolic dysfunction and heart failure symptoms.
3. **Embolic symptoms:** Distal embolization of tumor or thrombus can result in pulmonary embolism (PE) for right-sided tumors. Left-sided tumors can cause strokes, mesenteric, or limb ischemia.
4. Electrophysiologic derangements may occur from tumor infiltration and architectural changes of the epicardium and/or myocardium. This can result in atrial or ventricular tachyarrhythmias or a high-degree heart block.
5. The pericardium is the most common location for cardiac metastasis. Pericardial tamponade from pericardial fluid collection (serous or hemorrhagic) results from metastatic disease or direct invasion of breast or lung cancer.
6. Paragangliomas are extra-adrenal catecholamine-secreting neuroendocrine tumors, and patients may have signs consistent with high catecholamine release, such as high blood pressure and tachyarrhythmia.

D. Diagnosis of Cardiac Tumors

Two-dimensional (2D) echocardiography as well as CT or MRI can be used to assess cardiac tumor. Transesophageal echocardiography (TEE) is slightly more sensitive (97%) compared to transthoracic echocardiography (TTE) (93%), although both have finite tissue planes that limit the ability to fully characterize tumor anatomy, including the origin and extent of the mass.[9] Echocardiography with contrast is useful in distinguishing between tumors and thrombus, which are not always mutually exclusive.[10] Cardiac CT scan is noninvasive and readily available and provides useful anatomic details about cardiac tumors, although cardiac MRI can furnish better characterization of the cardiac tumors.[11,12]

E. **Primary Cardiac Tumors: Benign**

1. **Cardiac myxomas:** These are the most common benign tumors in adults. They are more common in women and in the fifth decade of life.[13] Myxomas are usually seen in the left atrium and attached via a pedicle to the intra-atrial septum on the fossa ovalis. However, about 20% of the time, they are in the right atrium.[14] Approximately 90% of myxomas are sporadic, while about 10% are associated with a hereditary condition—**Carney complex**, which is a rare hereditary multiple endocrine neoplasia syndrome and manifests as both cardiac and cutaneous myxomas; cutaneous hyperpigmentation; and endocrine secretory tumors. There are two recognized subtypes of this syndrome—**NAME** (nevi, atrial myxomas, mucocutaneous myxomas, and ephelides) and **LAMB** (lentiginosis, atrial myxomas, myocutaneous myxomas, and blue nevi).[15] Myxomas can cause atrial enlargement, arrhythmias, valvular obstruction with functional valvular stenosis, intra-atrial septal defect, heart failure, and devastating embolization of tumor; therefore, surgical resection is usually recommended.

2. **Lipomas:** Cardiac lipomas are the second most common benign tumors representing about 8%-12% of all benign cardiac masses and are more common in middle-aged adults. These can grow anywhere in the heart where there is adipose tissue, although about 50% occur in the subendocardium.[16] Subpericardial lipomas tend to be large compared to the subendocardial lipomas, which tend to be smaller.[17] On echocardiography, lipomas appear broad and well circumscribed and have been described as hyperechoic in the heart cavities and hypoechoic in the pericardium.[18]

3. **Papillary fibroelastoma:** These tumors are the most common valvular tumors, more common on the aortic valve, followed by mitral valves.[19] They are usually small and can appear round, oval, or irregularly shaped, with a stalk in about 50% of the time.[20,21] When compared to valvular vegetations, papillary fibroelastomas are usually found on the downstream side of the valve, for example, on the aortic side of the aortic valve and the ventricular side of the mitral valve, and they seldom cause valvular dysfunction.[22] They tend to be asymptomatic, but depending on their size and location, they can cause valvular dysfunction or outflow obstruction.[19] In addition, because of their high-flow and pressure locations, they can embolize and cause coronary ostial occlusion and myocardial ischemia. Cerebrovascular accidents are the most common (25%) sequela of this embolization phenomenon. For these reasons, surgical resection is recommended to patients with left-sided lesions that are 1 cm and in whom surgical risks are not prohibitive and asymptomatic right-sided lesions are managed more conservatively.[23] Figure 19.1 shows an image of a fibroelastoma attached to the papillary muscle in the left ventricle (LV).

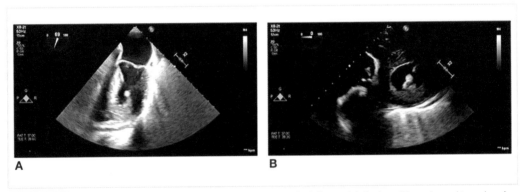

FIGURE 19.1   Fibroelastoma attached to the papillary muscle in the left ventricle in the midesophageal two chamber view **(A)** and transgastric midpapillary view **(B)** via transesophageal echocardiography.

4. **Rhabdomyomas:** These account for >60% of tumors in children.[24] These can be solitary lesions but more often occur as multiple lesions. The multiple lesions are associated with tuberous sclerosis in up to 60%-80% of cases.[25] Patients can be asymptomatic or have symptoms ranging from obstructive symptoms to arrhythmias. Complete resolution may occur in up to 80% of patients in early childhood, so surgery is usually reserved for patients with severe obstruction symptoms or intractable arrhythmias.[26]

5. **Cardiac paragangliomas:** These rare tumors are from the paraganglionic cells located in the great vessels, coronary arteries, or atria. The most common location is the left atrium. These can secrete catecholamines and have symptoms, including tachycardia, tremors, and flushing, like pheochromocytoma. Such patients usually benefit from α- and β-blockage before surgical resection, the definitive treatment.

F. **Primary Cardiac Tumors: Malignant**

Malignant cardiac tumors are very rare and represent about 5%-6% of primary cardiac tumors. Sarcomas are the most common cardiac malignant tumors, representing about 65% of all malignant tumors, followed by lymphomas and mesotheliomas. These are often aggressive tumors with poor prognosis. Cardiac sarcomas include angiosarcomas, leiomyosarcomas, liposarcoma, rhabdomyosarcomas, synovial sarcomas, myxofibrosarcomas, and undifferentiated pleomorphic sarcomas. Figure 19.2 shows images and gross specimen of a synovial sarcoma.

1. **Angiosarcomas:** These are the most common sarcomas, accounting for >30% of cardiac malignant tumors. They occur most frequently in middle-aged men and tend to be predominantly occur in the atrium or pericardium. These are highly vascularized tumors typically having an aggressive course with devastating consequences, such as obstruction and hemorrhagic pericardial effusions.[27]

2. **Leiomyosarcomas** are the second most common types of malignant cardiac tumors. They occur in about 9% of adults and are very aggressive and fatal. They can be seen in all chambers but have a predilection for the left atrium where they are often seen as a sessile mass with a mucoid appearance.[28]

3. **Primary cardiac lymphomas:** These are more commonly diagnosed in immunocompromised patients. Patients present with a myriad of symptoms, ranging from nonspecific constitutional symptoms to heart failure. These tumors favor the right side of the heart where they can appear as homogeneous masses with associated wall thickening and restrictive physiology or nodular structures, especially in the right heart chambers.[29] They are sometimes associated with pericardial effusions, and pericardial fluid sampling can be used in making the diagnosis, in addition to myocardial biopsy. Treatment is usually chemotherapy and antibody based.[30]

4. **Rhabdomyosarcomas:** These are the most common malignant cardiac tumors in the pediatric population and tend to affect valves and cause obstruction symptoms. These tumors are aggressive and often managed with surgery, chemotherapy, and radiation therapy.

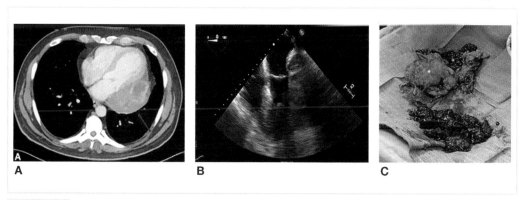

A   **B**   **C**

FIGURE 19.2   **(A)** Computed tomography scan showing mass along the lateral aspect of the left ventricle and left atrium, as indicated by the red arrow. **(B)** Transesophageal imaging showing same mass compressing left atrium and left ventricle. **(C)** Gross specimen of resected synovial sarcoma mass. (Images courtesy of Ahmet Kilic, MD.)

5. **Aortic sarcomas:** These are extremely rare and more common in men, with an average age of 60 years. They are more frequent in the descending thoracic aorta. They are difficult to diagnose with existing imaging modalities and can be confused for mycotic aneurysms. Complete resections of these tumors are challenging, and prognosis is poor.[31]

6. **Pulmonary artery sarcomas** are very rare and tend to grow into the lumen and in the direction of blood flow. They are often misdiagnosed as PE and can cause obstruction of flow and result in right heart strain, right heart failure, or thromboembolic events. CT scan can show a filling defect in the pulmonary arterial (PA) vasculature (Figure 19.3). Echocardiographic findings can include evidence of right heart strain and enlarged PA. Surgical resection is often necessary, but the tumor recurrence rate is unfortunately very high, and there are few reports of heart and lung transplantation as a curative option.[32]

7. **Mesothelioma**: These are rare but aggressive tumors that arise from the pericardial mesothelial layers. They are more common in men and in the middle age. They are typically associated with the pericardium and pericardial effusions, which are the major findings on echocardiogram with or without an associated mass. These are aggressive diseases with poor prognosis. Patients can be offered pericardial window or pericardiectomy, usually as palliative procedure.[33]

G. Metastatic Cardiac Cancer

Metastatic cardiac tumors (secondary cardiac tumors) occur up to 20-40 times more commonly than primary cardiac tumors, and these are spread via blood, the lymphatic system, extensions from the IVC, or direct invasion.[34] The most common type of metastatic tumor to the heart is melanoma.[35] Carcinomas of the lung, breast, and esophagus are the most common metastatic carcinomas to the heart. They can invade structures like pericardium and can cause pleural effusion and/or restrictive pericardial disease. These can also be intracavitary lesions and obstruction of transvalvular blood flow. Leukemias and lymphomas both have a high tendency for cardiac metastasis and can infiltrate the myocardium and cause hemorrhagic pericardial effusions. Management is usually tailored to the primary tumor and extent of cardiac involvement.

H. Cardiac Tumor Imitators

There are intracardiac masses that can mimic cardiac tumors on echocardiography, and distinguishing these is key for the echocardiographer.

1. **Pericardial cysts** are benign lesions of the pericardium, which can be congenital or acquired postinfection or inflammation. They are often incidental findings easily diagnosed on cardiac CT, cardiac MRI, or 2D echocardiography. Echocardiography is helpful in distinguishing a pericardial cyst from a fat pad or ventricular aneurysm.[36]

2. **Lipomatous hypertrophy** of the intra-atrial septum is a condition that is unique to the septum at the level of the fossa ovalis. These are usually composed of adipose and muscle tissues, and they are not true lipomas.[28] On echocardiography, they appear as bilobed

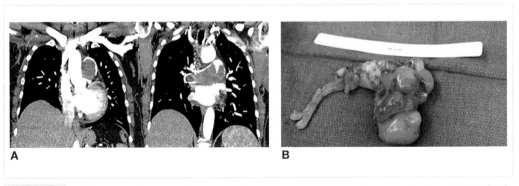

A   B

FIGURE 19.3 **(A)** Computed tomographic angiography showing near occlusion of main pulmonary artery and right pulmonary artery, mimicking a saddle pulmonary embolus. **(B)** En bloc specimen of pulmonary artery sarcoma. (Images courtesy of Ahmet Kilic, MD.)

intra-atrial septum. They are typically asymptomatic, although they have been linked occasionally to atrial arrhythmias and associated with the presence of coronary artery disease.[37]

3. **Lambl excrescences** are filamentous masses found associated with the atrial surface of the mitral and the ventricular surface of aortic valve. These are usually asymptomatic and are incidental findings on echocardiograms. Like papillary fibroelastoma, these can be associated with embolic events and strokes or coronary ischemia; therefore, surgical resection may be requirement if thought to be associated with strokes.

4. **Valvular vegetations** are associated with infective endocarditis. They are more commonly seen on the left side of the heart but sometimes on the right-side valves in patients who are intravenous (IV) drug users. They appear on echocardiography as echogenic, irregular, and mobile masses attached to the valvular surfaces.

5. **Intracardiac thrombus** are the most common intracardiac masses seen on echocardiography, and the presence of spontaneous echo contrast suggests blood stasis and should raise the suspicion for the presence of clots (see "Cardiac Thrombus" section).

I. **Key Anesthetic Considerations and Management**

Surgical resection with the support of cardiopulmonary bypass (CPB) remains the main therapy for most cardiac tumors. Rarely, orthotopic heart transplant is indicated as a curative tool. Anesthesia care for patients with cardiac tumors need to be carefully thought-out. Comprehensive knowledge of the location of tumor and associated complications such as obstruction, valvulopathy, arrhythmogenicity, and the presence of tamponade physiology is important in successful anesthetic management. Regardless of the anesthetic choice, the goal is to maintain adequate preload, ventricular contractility, and adequate mean arterial pressure to maximize systemic and coronary perfusion pressure.

Patients with intra-atrial tumors may present with obstructive physiology and may benefit from augmenting preload with preinduction IV fluids. Defibrillator pads should be in place to promptly manage hemodynamically unstable arrhythmias. Preinduction arterial line is necessary in most clinical scenarios to closely monitor hemodynamic changes with induction of anesthesia. It is also prudent to have the surgical and perfusion teams in the case of hemodynamic collapse with induction of anesthesia with adequate preparation for emergency CPB. With true interatrial masses, preparation for femoral arterial and venous cannulation may be necessary before induction of anesthesia. This is to circumvent catastrophic obstruction to intracardiac flow that may occur in these cases. Preoperative sedation should be minimized especially with right ventricular (RV) dysfunction as this may result in hypoventilation, respiratory acidosis, elevated PA pressures, and worsening right-sided function.

Slow-controlled induction with close attention to hemodynamics is essential. Titration of low-dose vasopressor infusion is a reasonable option in many cases to maintain adequate systemic vascular resistance with induction of anesthesia. Initiation of mechanical ventilation should be handled with care as increased positive pressure can increase pulmonary vascular resistance and RV afterload, leading to compromise in RV stroke volume and RV preload. Careful titration of positive pressure is also relevant in cases of pericardial effusion and tamponade physiology where positive pressure ventilation can impair venous return and cardiac output. Patients with tamponade will benefit from maintenance of contractility and chronotropic with spontaneous breathing when possible.

Central venous catheter (CVC) is helpful for both volume resuscitation and titration of vasoactive medications. The location of placement is important and is ideally guided by echocardiography, especially in right atrial tumors where embolization or worsening obstruction from CVC is a specific risk.

Certain tumors such as paragangliomas can be secretory in nature and behave functionally like extra-adrenal pheochromocytoma. Excess catecholamine can produce lethal arrhythmias, cardiac failure, and pulmonary edema. Diagnosis is with a combination of biochemical confirmation of excessive catecholamines and imaging to localize the tumor. Preoperative optimization usually includes 1-3 weeks of α-blockade titrated to normal hemodynamics (systolic blood pressure [SBP] <135, heart rate [HR] <100). β-Blockers should be avoided until there has been sufficient α-blockade to avoid unopposed α-stimulation.[38,39] In addition, these patients are usually hypovolemic, and careful attention to restoring euvolemia pre-op is essential to avoid dense hypotension during surgery. Deep anesthetic plane and vasoactive infusions to lower blood pressure and control HR should be readily available to mitigate the adrenergic surges, especially with tumor manipulation. The use of TEE is indicated in most cases to assess cardiac function, tumor resection, and integrity of reconstruction.

II. Endocarditis

A. Epidemiology and Natural History

Infective endocarditis is a life-threatening contamination and inflammation of endocardial tissue. Approximately 75% of patients have preexisting structural heart disease, and one-third of cases are attributed to healthcare-acquired infections. **Risk factors** include rheumatic valve disease (highest factor in low-income countries), congenital or degenerative valvular disease, prosthetic valves, cardiovascular implantable electronic devices (CIEDs), IV drug use, and indwelling IV devices and catheters.[40] **Right-sided endocarditis** is associated with younger patients, history of IV drug use, larger vegetations, higher rates of PE, and lower mortality. Risk factors for poor prognosis include advanced age, prosthetic valve, heart failure, stroke, and *Staphylococcus aureus* infection.[41] Heart failure, sepsis, arrhythmias, and cerebral embolism are the leading causes of death in patients with endocarditis.

B. Pathophysiology and Etiology

There are five distinct phases: bacteremia, adhesion (biofilm formation), proliferation, structural damage, and dissemination. *S. aureus* is the most common organism in high-income countries, and *Streptococcus viridans* is the most common in low-income countries.[41] In 10% of cases, no organism is identified as the cause. **Nonbacterial thrombotic endocarditis** (NBTE) is associated with systemic lupus erythematosus, malignancy, antiphospholipid and anticardiolipin antibodies, fulminant sepsis, hypercoagulable states, and burns.

C. Presentation and Diagnosis

Fever and malaise are the most common presenting symptoms. Patients can present with sepsis, stroke, pulmonary edema, and hemodynamic compromise. A new cardiac murmur, petechiae, or splinter hemorrhages should increase suspicion. The **modified Duke criteria**[42] consist of major and minor criteria to diagnose endocarditis, though it should not serve as a substitute for high clinical suspicion.

D. Echocardiographic Assessment

TEE has a higher specificity (91%-100%) and sensitivity (87%-100%) compared to TTE (specificity: 90%-94%, sensitivity: 60%-70%). If no vegetations are seen via TEE and clinical suspicion remains high, it is recommended to repeat imaging in 7-10 days.[43] **Vegetations** are likely to be found on the low-pressure side of the affected valve, often irregularly shaped and heterogeneous in echogenicity (Figure 19.4). A left-sided vegetation ≥10 mm and a right-sided vegetation ≥20 mm are associated with increased mortality.[44]

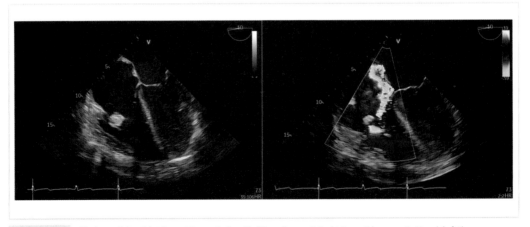

FIGURE 19.4 Endocarditis with tricuspid vegetation **(left)** and associated tricuspid regurgitation **(right)**.

Leaflet prolapse, flail, torn chords, and ruptured papillary muscles can all be present. Areas of regurgitant color-flow Doppler acceleration at a noncommissural leaflet site should increase suspicion of a **leaflet perforation**. Paravalvular leak of the prosthesis can lead to movement and rocking of the valve once 40% of the annulus is involved. **Abscess formation** may begin as a region of periannular thickening and progress to an echolucent pocket. A **pseudoaneurysm** occurs when there is damage to blood vessel with contained bleeding (Figure 19.5) and is most likely to develop in the mitral-aortic intervalvular fibrosa. If blood flow connection is formed to another chamber, it is referred to as an **intracardiac fistula**. An **acquired Gerbode defect** refers to a communication between the LV and the right atria. Fistulas have a >40% risk of mortality despite surgical intervention.[41]

4

E. **Timing and Type of Intervention**

Up to 50% of patients diagnosed with endocarditis undergo surgical correction. There are **three surgical indications**: heart failure due to valve dysfunction, uncontrolled infection, and prevention of emboli. The American Association of Thoracic Surgery (AATS) recommends considering emergent surgery in patients with >10-mm mobile vegetations (Class of Recommendation: IIB, Level of Evidence: B).[45] The American Heart Association/American College of Cardiology (AHA/ACC) recommends surgical intervention during initial hospitalization and not waiting for full course of antibiotic treatment to be completed.[46] Early surgery (<48 hours) was associated with lower mortality than conventional therapy in a small randomized controlled trial.[47] Surgery should not be delayed for embolic stroke, minor ischemic stroke, or subclinical cerebral embolization. Surgery should be delayed for at least 4 weeks if there is evidence of a major ischemic stroke, hemorrhagic stroke, intracranial hemorrhage, or severe neurologic dysfunction.[46]

5

F. **Perioperative Anesthetic Considerations**

Patients may present with septic shock, cardiogenic shock, heart block, and/or severe pulmonary edema. Depending on the urgency of the surgery, medical optimization may be difficult. Existing hypercoagulable state, anticoagulation medications, and high rates of heparin resistance can complicate a patient's coagulation profile. Endocarditis is associated with **higher fibrinogen levels, lower antithrombin III activity,** and **lower fibrinolytic activity**.[40] Increased rates of transfusions and postoperative bleeding are seen in patients with endocarditis.

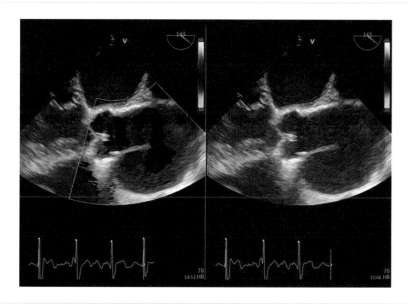

FIGURE 19.5 Aortic pseudoaneurysm with associated type A dissection visualized in the ascending aorta with (left) and without (right) color flow doppler via transesophageal echocardiography.

Viscoelastography can aid in guiding patient-specific care. Despite **increased levels of cytokine and inflammatory mediators** during CPB and increased risk of developing vasoplegia, routine use of perioperative steroids or hemoadsorption is not recommended.[48] Endocarditis is associated with high rates of strokes and intracranial hemorrhage. The highest risk of emboli is thought to be before diagnosis and decreases significantly after initiation of IV antimicrobial treatment.[43] Other associated conditions include congestive heart failure (up to 40%) due to valvular, chordae or papillary muscle damage, arrhythmias, acute renal injury (up to 30%) most commonly due to immune complex–mediated glomerulonephritis, and liver cirrhosis. The most common complications after endocarditis surgery include septic shock, heart failure, coagulopathy, acute renal failure, and stroke. Approximately 13% of patients require a **permanent pacemaker** due to damage of the conduction system. Recurrent infective endocarditis rates are as high as 5%-10%.

6 G. **Summary for Endocarditis Management**

1. Vasopressors should be immediately available as patients with endocarditis are at higher risk of septic shock and vasoplegia.
2. Full evaluation of each valve is imperative as TEE has a much higher sensitivity and specificity than TTE for vegetation detection.
3. TEE evaluation should also include evaluation for possible intracardiac fistulas, pseudoaneurysms, and the degree of pericardial effusion.
4. Quantitative data for coagulation profile including viscoelastic testing can be helpful as patients can present with hypercoagulopathy or hypocoagulopathy.

III. **Cardiac Thrombus**

7 A. **Introduction**

Intracardiac thrombi can found in areas of low flow, blood stasis, or on iatrogenic material with the heart. Thrombus can be of any size and shape, with fresh clot more likely to be mobile, round, and well defined. Visualization of spontaneous echo contrast (smoke) should increase suspicion of a localized thrombus. It is important to image the suspected thrombus at several multiplanar views throughout the cardiac cycle utilizing both 2D and 3D imaging. IV contrast can be used to establish a diagnosis.

8 B. **Left-Sided Cardiac Thrombus**

1. **Left atrium and left atrial appendage**
   a. **Atrial fibrillation** is the most significant risk factor for atrial thrombus. The risk of embolic events without anticoagulation is up to 7%. The $CHADS_2$ and CHA_2DS_2-VASc scores can be used to predict a likelihood of left atrial appendage (LAA) thrombus and embolic risk, but $CHADS_2$ should not be used to exclude an LAA thrombus.[49] Other important risk factors include mitral stenosis and atrial enlargement.
   b. **Echocardiography:** TEE has imaging sensitivity and specificity approaching 100%. Pulsed-wave Doppler velocities <40 cm/s placed in the LAA 1 cm from the orifice are associated with an increased risk of thrombus. Spontaneous echocardiogram contrast in the left atrium has a positive predictive value of 66% and negative predictive value of 84%.[49] It is important to rule out prominent pectinate and possible reverberation artifact from the coumadin ridge within the LAA.
   c. **Management:** Cardioversion, atrial fibrillation ablation, LAA clipping, LAA occlusion device placement, and mitral valvuloplasty are contraindicated procedures in the presence of a thrombus. Anticoagulation should be initiated with resolution of clot before proceeding. If incidentally found during cardiac surgery, the thrombus can be removed via surgical excision (Figure 19.6).
2. **Prosthetic valve thrombosis:** Thrombus can develop on either mechanical or bioprosthetic valves. Evidence of increased pressure gradients across the valve (increase in >50% over baseline or >10 mm Hg increase through an aortic valve) with either restricted leaflet motion or echogenic masses on the valve will be present.[46] For mechanical valve thrombus, the ACC/AHA recommends immediate treatment with either low-dose fibrinolytic therapy or emergency surgery. In those with bioprosthetic valve thrombosis, initial treatment with a vitamin K antagonist is reasonable if the patient is hemodynamically stable.

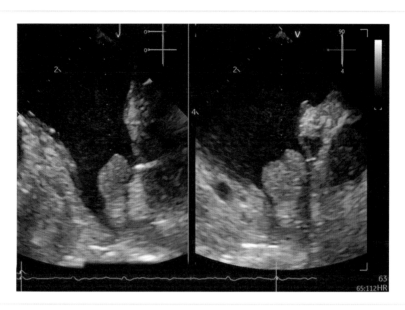

FIGURE 19.6 Left atrial appendage thrombus as an incidental finding during cardiac surgery at 0° (left) and 90° (right) omniplane via transesophageal echocardiography.

3. **Left ventricle:** Risk factors include ischemic heart disease, regional wall motion abnormalities, ventricular aneurysms, pseudoaneurysm, and dilated cardiomyopathy (end-diastole diameter >60 mm). LV thrombus is often seen in the apex and less likely to be mobile compared to other types of thrombi. It appears as an echogenic, avascular, outgrowth that is distinct from the endocardial wall. TTE has been shown to have a much higher sensitivity for apical thrombi. LV thrombi are contraindicated in left-sided mechanical support devices. The patient should be anticoagulated, and neurologic status monitored closely until the resolution of clot before proceeding with elective cases. For those with existing LV assist devices (LVADs), an unexplained increase in power consumption should raise suspicion for thrombus, which should prompt immediate medical and possible surgical intervention.

C. **Right-Sided Cardiac Thrombus**
De novo right-sided thrombi are rare as right-sided thrombi are much more likely to **embolize from the periphery or found on iatrogenic material**. CIED wires, PA catheters, central lines, and peripherally inserted central catheter lines are all potential sources of thrombus.

1. A **pulmonary embolism** is a blockage of the PA vasculature that is usually embolized from a distal venous thromboembolism (VTE).

2. **Risk factors** include lower limb fracture, hip/knee replacement, hospitalization for heart failure or atrial dysrhythmias, major trauma, malignancy, myocardial infection within 3 months, spinal cord injury, or previous deep vein thrombosis.[50]

   a. "Virchow triad" of vessel wall injury, vascular stasis, and hypercoagulability is often used to describe patients at high risk of VTE. Patients may be hypoxemic, tachycardic, and hypocapnic with signs of RV strain on electrocardiogram (ECG), such as S1Q3T3 or a right bundle branch block. The modified Wells and Geneva criteria can be used to determine a pretest probability.

   b. For patients with elevated scores, **CT pulmonary angiography** (CPTA) is more sensitive (96%-100%) and specific (97%-98%) than TEE (70% sensitive and 91% specific) to diagnose a PE. A ventilation-perfusion (V/Q) scan can also be used as an alternative to CPTA.

   c. **Echocardiography:** Thrombus will be seen as a hyperechoic often mobile mass with well-defined boundaries. Migrating thrombi are seen in <10% of confirmed cases of PE[51] (Figure 19.7). A patent foramen ovale (PFO) >4 mm in diameters increases the risk of systemic emboli.[52]

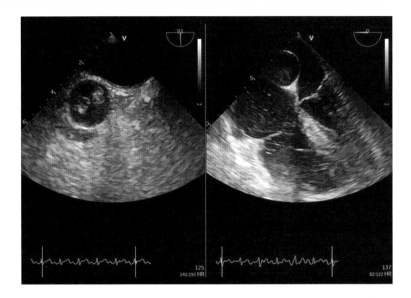

FIGURE 19.7   Thrombus noted in the pulmonary artery **(left)** with associated dilated right ventricle and bowing of the interatrial septum toward the left atrium indicating high right-sided pressures **(right)**.

3. TEE evaluation should also include RV size, strain, and signs of dysfunction. RV/LV end-diastolic diameter ratio of >0.7, apical sparing hypokinesis (McConnell sign), and RV end-diastolic diameter >27 mm are all signs of RV dysfunction. Initial **management** of a PE is IV anticoagulation. According to the American College of Chest Physicians (ACCP) and 2019 European Society of Cardiology (ESC) guidelines, patients presenting with high-risk PE who are hemodynamically unstable should immediately be considered for IV thrombolytics. **Surgical intervention** is considered more beneficial in patients with large, proximal PA clot burden and in-transit thrombus. **Percutaneous thrombectomy** is an emerging therapy that can be an option to avoid sternotomy and possibly general anesthesia.

4. **Anesthetic considerations**: A massive PE significantly increases **alveolar dead space** and V/Q mismatch whereby the $P_{ET}CO_2$ no longer accurately reflects the Pa_{CO_2}. Strict monitoring of arterial blood gases is warranted to avoid acidosis. Thrombus also increases **RV afterload** and can lead to RV strain and dysfunction. In addition to impaired systolic function, tachycardia and decreased preload from positive pressure ventilation can add to significant hemodynamic compromise. Anesthetic induction for surgical intervention is associated with a high risk of hemodynamic collapse. It is a common practice to have arterial line placement, central venous access, and surgical draping complete before induction and intubation. Femoral cannulation for CPB should be performed cautiously as thrombi may be contained within the IVC. Risk factors associated with morality include cancer, congestive heart failure, RV hypokinesis, age >70 years, and systolic hypotension.

D. **Summary for Pulmonary Embolism Management**
1. Place awake arterial line, central venous access, surgical prep, and drape before anesthetic induction and intubation.
2. Have vasopressor and inotrope infusions immediately available in preparation for potential hemodynamic instability.
3. Discuss cannulation strategy with the surgical team to minimize incision to CPB start duration.
4. Avoid hypercarbia, hypoxia, and acidosis to optimize pulmonary vascular resistance.

5. TEE evaluation should include thrombus location, RV size and strain, and the degree of tricuspid regurgitation.
6. Consider inotropes and/or inhaled pulmonary vasodilators if there are signs of persistent RV dysfunction.

IV. Anatomic Variants

A. There are certain cardiac structures that can be falsely interpreted as pathologic masses or thrombi. According to chamber and valve location, these structures should be on the differential when evaluating a cardiac mass:

1. **Right atrium:** Chiari network, eustachian valve, crista terminalis, interatrial septal aneurysm, pectinate muscles, interatrial septal aneurysm, lipomatous hypertrophy, Thebesian valve, CIED wires, IV access lines, interatrial occluder devices
2. **Right ventricle:** Moderator band, papillary muscles, CIED wires, IV access lines
3. **Left ventricle:** Hypertrophic LV outflow tract (LVOT), false tendons, trabeculae, papillary muscles, CIED wires, PA catheter
4. **Left atrium:** LA chords, pectinate muscles in LAA, multilobe LAA
5. **Mitral valve:** Annular calcification, mitral valve interventional clips
6. **Aortic valve:** Lambl excrescences, nodules of Arantius

REFERENCES

1. Effert S, Domanig E. Diagnostik intraaurikularer Tumoren und grosser Thromben mit dem Ultraschall-Echoverfahren [Diagnosis of intra-auricular tumors & large thrombi with the aid of ultrasonic echography]. *Dtsch Med Wochenschr.* 1959;84(1):6-8. doi:10.1055/s-0028-1113531
2. Butany J, Nair V, Naseemuddin A, Nair GM, Catton C, Yau T. Cardiac tumours: diagnosis and management. *Lancet Oncol.* 2005;6(4):219-228. doi:10.1016/s1470-2045(05)70093-0
3. Dhillon G, Rodríguez-Cruz E, Kathawala M, Alqassem N. Primary cardiac myofibroblastic sarcoma, case report and review of diagnosis and treatment of cardiac tumors. *Bol Asoc Med P R.* 1998;90(7-12):130-133.
4. Cooley DA. Surgical treatment of cardiac neoplasms: 32-year experience. *Thorac Cardiovasc Surg.* 1990;38(suppl 2):176-182. doi:10.1055/s-2007-1014063
5. Bakaeen FG, Reardon MJ, Coselli JS, et al. Surgical outcome in 85 patients with primary cardiac tumors. *Am J Surg.* 2003;186(6):641-647; discussion 647. doi:10.1016/j.amjsurg.2003.08.004
6. Butany J, Leong SW, Carmichael K, Komeda M. A 30-year analysis of cardiac neoplasms at autopsy. *Can J Cardiol.* 2005; 21(8):675-680.
7. Silvestri F, Bussani R, Pavletic N, Mannone T. Metastases of the heart and pericardium. *G Ital Cardiol.* 1997;27(12):1252-1255.
8. Manojlović S. Metastatic carcinomas involving the heart. Review of postmortem examination. *Zentralbl Allg Pathol.* 1990;136(7-8):657-661.
9. Meng Q, Lai H, Lima J, Tong W, Qian Y, Lai S. Echocardiographic and pathologic characteristics of primary cardiac tumors: a study of 149 cases. *Int J Cardiol.* 2002;84(1):69-75. doi:10.1016/s0167-5273(02)00136-5
10. Kirkpatrick JN, Wong T, Bednarz JE, et al. Differential diagnosis of cardiac masses using contrast echocardiographic perfusion imaging. *J Am Coll Cardiol.* 2004;43(8):1412-1419. doi:10.1016/j.jacc.2003.09.065
11. Araoz PA, Eklund HE, Welch TJ, Breen JF. CT and MR imaging of primary cardiac malignancies. *Radiographics.* 1999;19(6):1421-1434. doi:10.1148/radiographics.19.6.g99no031421
12. Mousavi N, Cheezum MK, Aghayev A, et al. Assessment of cardiac masses by cardiac magnetic resonance imaging: histological correlation and clinical outcomes. *J Am Heart Assoc.* 2019;8(1):e007829. doi:10.1161/jaha.117.007829
13. Pinede L, Duhaut P, Loire R. Clinical presentation of left atrial cardiac myxoma. A series of 112 consecutive cases. *Medicine (Baltimore).* 2001;80(3):159-172. doi:10.1097/00005792-200105000-00002
14. Azevedo O, Almeida J, Nolasco T, et al. Massive right atrial myxoma presenting as syncope and exertional dyspnea: case report. *Cardiovasc Ultrasound.* 2010;8:23. doi:10.1186/1476-7120-8-23
15. Bertherat J. Carney complex (CNC). *Orphanet J Rare Dis.* 2006;1:21. doi:10.1186/1750-1172-1-21
16. Rajiah P, Kanne JP, Kalahasti V, Schoenhagen P. Computed tomography of cardiac and pericardiac masses. *J Cardiovasc Comput Tomogr.* 2011;5(1):16-29. doi:10.1016/j.jcct.2010.08.009
17. Gaerte SC, Meyer CA, Winer-Muram HT, Tarver RD, Conces DJ Jr. Fat-containing lesions of the chest. *Radiographics.* 2002;22:S61-S78. doi:10.1148/radiographics.22.suppl_1.g02oc08s61
18. Mankad R, Herrmann J. Cardiac tumors: echo assessment. *Echo Res Pract.* 2016;3(4):R65-R77. doi:10.1530/erp-16-0035
19. Gowda RM, Khan IA, Nair CK, Mehta NJ, Vasavada BC, Sacchi TJ. Cardiac papillary fibroelastoma: a comprehensive analysis of 725 cases. *Am Heart J.* 2003;146(3):404-410. doi:10.1016/S0002-8703(03)00249-7
20. Sun JP, Asher CR, Yang XS, et al. Clinical and echocardiographic characteristics of papillary fibroelastomas: a retrospective and prospective study in 162 patients. *Circulation.* 2001;103(22):2687-2693. doi:10.1161/01.cir.103.22.2687
21. Edwards FH, Hale D, Cohen A, Thompson L, Pezzella AT, Virmani R. Primary cardiac valve tumors. *Ann Thorac Surg.* 1991;52(5):1127-1131. doi:10.1016/0003-4975(91)91293-5

22. Capotosto L, Elena G, Massoni F, et al. Cardiac tumors: echocardiographic diagnosis and forensic correlations. *Am J Forensic Med Pathol.* 2016;37(4):306-316. doi:10.1097/paf.0000000000000271

23. Tamin SS, Maleszewski JJ, Scott CG, et al. Prognostic and bioepidemiologic implications of papillary fibroelastomas. *J Am Coll Cardiol.* 2015;65(22):2420-2429. doi:10.1016/j.jacc.2015.03.569

24. Chan HS, Sonley MJ, Moës CA, Daneman A, Smith CR, Martin DJ. Primary and secondary tumors of childhood involving the heart, pericardium, and great vessels: a report of 75 cases and review of the literature. *Cancer.* 1985;56(4):825-836. doi:10.1002/1097-0142(19850815)56:43.0.co;2-7

25. Watson GH. Cardiac rhabdomyomas in tuberous sclerosis. *Ann N Y Acad Sci.* 1991;615:50-57. doi:10.1111/j.1749-6632.1991.tb37747.x

26. Bosi G, Lintermans JP, Pellegrino PA, Svaluto-Moreolo G, Vliers A. The natural history of cardiac rhabdomyoma with and without tuberous sclerosis. *Acta Paediatr.* 1996;85(8):928-931. doi:10.1111/j.1651-2227.1996.tb14188.x

27. Roberts WC. Primary and secondary neoplasms of the heart. *Am J Cardiol.* 1997;80(5):671-682. doi:10.1016/s0002-9149(97)00587-0

28. Sarjeant JM, Butany J, Cusimano RJ. Cancer of the heart: epidemiology and management of primary tumors and metastases. *Am J Cardiovasc Drugs.* 2003;3(6):407-421. doi:10.2165/00129784-200303060-00004

29. Tyebally S, Chen D, Bhattacharyya S, et al. Cardiac tumors: JACC cardiooncology state-of-the-art review. *JACC CardioOncol.* 2020;2(2):293-311. doi:10.1016/j.jaccao.2020.05.009

30. Burke A, Tavora F. The 2015 WHO classification of tumors of the heart and pericardium. *J Thorac Oncol.* 2016;11(4):441-452. doi:10.1016/j.jtho.2015.11.009

31. Seelig MH, Klingler PJ, Oldenburg WA, Blackshear JL. Angiosarcoma of the aorta: report of a case and review of the literature. *J Vasc Surg.* 1998;28(4):732-737. doi:10.1016/s0741-5214(98)70104-1

32. Shanmugam G. Primary cardiac sarcoma. *Eur J Cardiothorac Surg.* 2006;29(6):925-932. doi:10.1016/j.ejcts.2006.03.034

33. Cao S, Jin S, Cao J, et al. Malignes Perikardmesotheliom: Systematische Übersicht über das aktuelle Vorgehen. [Malignant pericardial mesothelioma: a systematic review of current practice]. *Herz.* 2018;43(1):61-68. doi:10.1007/s00059-016-4522-5

34. Goldberg AD, Blankstein R, Padera RF. Tumors metastatic to the heart. *Circulation.* 2013;128(16):1790-1794. doi:10.1161/circulationaha.112.000790

35. Waller BF, Gottdiener JS, Virmani R, Roberts WC. The "charcoal heart;" melanoma to the cor. *Chest.* 1980;77(5):671-676. doi:10.1378/chest.77.5.671

36. Hynes JK, Tajik AJ, Osborn MJ, Orszulak TA, Seward JB. Two-dimensional echocardiographic diagnosis of pericardial cyst. *Mayo Clin Proc.* 1983;58(1):60-63.

37. Zeebregts CJ, Hensens AG, Timmermans J, Pruszczynski MS, Lacquet LK. Lipomatous hypertrophy of the interatrial septum: indication for surgery? *Eur J Cardiothorac Surg.* 1997;11(4):785-787. doi:10.1016/s1010-7940(96)01078-0

38. Guenthart BA, Trope W, Keeyapaj W, et al. Intracardiac paragangliomas: surgical approach and perioperative management. *Gen Thorac Cardiovasc Surg.* 2021;69(3):555-559. doi:10.1007/s11748-020-01503-2

39. Fang F, Ding L, He Q, Liu M. Preoperative management of pheochromocytoma and paraganglioma. *Front Endocrinol (Lausanne).* 2020;11:586795. doi:10.3389/fendo.2020.586795

40. Hermanns H, Eberl S, Terwindt LE, et al. Anesthesia considerations in infective endocarditis. *Anesthesiology.* 2022;136(4):633-656. doi:10.1097/ALN.0000000000004130

41. Cahill TJ, Prendergast BD. Infective endocarditis. *Lancet.* 2016;387(10021):882-893. doi:10.1016/S0140-6736(15)00067-7

42. Li JS, Sexton DJ, Mick N, et al. Proposed modifications to the Duke criteria for the diagnosis of infective endocarditis. *Clin Infect Dis.* 2000;30(4):633-638. doi:10.1086/313753

43. Saric M, Armour AC, Arnaout MS, et al. Guidelines for the use of echocardiography in the evaluation of a cardiac source of embolism. *J Am Soc Echocardiogr.* 2016;29(1):1-42. doi:10.1016/j.echo.2015.09.011

44. Okonta KE, Adamu YB. What size of vegetation is an indication for surgery in endocarditis? *Interact Cardiovasc Thorac Surg.* 2012;15(6):1052-1056. doi:10.1093/icvts/ivs365

45. AATS Surgical Treatment of Infective Endocarditis Consensus Guidelines Writing Committee Chairs, Pettersson GB, Coselli JS, et al. 2016 The American Association for Thoracic Surgery (AATS) consensus guidelines: surgical treatment of infective endocarditis: executive summary. *J Thorac Cardiovasc Surg.* 2017;153(6):1241-1258.e29. doi:10.1016/j.jtcvs.2016.09.093

46. Otto CM, Nishimura RA, Bonow RO, et al. 2020 ACC/AHA guideline for the management of patients with valvular heart disease: executive summary: a report of the American College of Cardiology/American Heart Association Joint Committee on Clinical Practice Guidelines. *Circulation.* 2021;143(5):e35-e71. doi:10.1161/CIR.0000000000000932

47. Kang DH, Kim YJ, Kim SH, et al. Early surgery versus conventional treatment for infective endocarditis. *N Engl J Med.* 28;366(26):2466-2473. doi:10.1056/NEJMoa1112843

48. Diab M, Lehmann T, Bothe W, et al. Cytokine hemoadsorption during cardiac surgery versus standard surgical care for infective endocarditis (REMOVE): results from a multicenter randomized controlled trial. *Circulation.* 2022;145(13):959-968. doi:10.1161/CIRCULATIONAHA.121.056940

49. Zhan Y, Joza J, Al Rawahi M, et al. Assessment and management of the left atrial appendage thrombus in patients with nonvalvular atrial fibrillation. *Can J Cardiol.* 2018;34(3):252-261. doi:10.1016/j.cjca.2017.12.008

50. Konstantinides SV, Meyer G, Becattini C, et al. 2019 ESC guidelines for the diagnosis and management of acute pulmonary embolism developed in collaboration with the European Respiratory Society (ERS). *Eur Heart J.* 2020;41(4):543-603. doi:10.1093/eurheartj/ehz405

51. L'Angiocola PD, Donati R. Cardiac masses in echocardiography: a pragmatic review. *J Cardiovasc Echogr.* 2020;30(1):5-14. doi:10.4103/jcecho.jcecho_2_20

52. Goldhaber SZ. Echocardiography in the management of pulmonary embolism. *Ann Intern Med.* 2002;136(9):691-700. doi:10.7326/0003-4819-136-9-200205070-00012

Chronic Thromboembolic Pulmonary Hypertension and Pulmonary Thromboendarterectomy

Christine Choi and Dalia Banks

KEY POINTS

1. Pulmonary hypertension (PH) is divided into five categories based on common clinical features. Chronic thromboembolic pulmonary hypertension (CTEPH) is a form of precapillary PH.
2. Recurrent pulmonary embolism with incomplete resolution of thrombotic material is the main cause of CTEPH.
3. Gold standard for the diagnosis of CTEPH is through catheter-based pulmonary angiography.
4. Transthoracic or transesophageal echocardiography will provide an assessment on right ventricular (RV) size and function.
5. Pulmonary thromboendarterectomy (PTE) provides definitive treatment for CTEPH. PTE surgery can be performed via standard sternotomy or minimally invasive method.
6. PTE requires deep hypothermic circulatory arrest to provide a completely bloodless surgical field for accurate identification and dissection of surgical plane.
7. Preanesthetic evaluation should focus on RV and left ventricular function, pulmonary artery pressures, right atrial pressure, and underlying coagulopathic disorders.
8. Avoidance of factors that could worsen pulmonary vascular resistance such as hypoxia or hypercarbia is crucial in anesthetic management.
9. Airway bleeding and reperfusion pulmonary edema are the two most feared complications of PTE surgery. These complications are usually managed with conservative therapy.
10. Special considerations for PTE surgery include patients with sickle cell disease, cold agglutinins, and heparin-induced thrombocytopenia.

I. Introduction to Pulmonary Hypertension

A. Classification

The current classification system for pulmonary hypertension (PH) is derived originally from the Evian classification of the Second World Symposium on PH held in 1998.[1] It divides PH into five categories based on common clinical features. The classification system underwent a major update during the Fourth World Symposium in 2008 to better reflect the clinical conditions each category represents (Table 20.1). The hemodynamic definition for PH was revised most recently during the Sixth World Symposium in 2018 by lowering the mean pulmonary artery pressure (mPAP) cutoff from 25 to 20 mm Hg. The definition of precapillary PH, isolated

TABLE 20.1   WHO Classification of Pulmonary Hypertension (PH)

WHO Class	Mechanism of Action	Hemodynamic Definition	Clinical Mechanism
I	Pulmonary arterial hypertension	Precapillary	mPAP >20 mm Hg PAWP ≤15 mm Hg PVR ≥3 WU
II	PH from left heart disease	Isolated postcapillary	mPAP >20 mm Hg PAWP >15 mm Hg PVR <3 WU
		Combined pre- and postcapillary	mPAP >20 mm Hg PAWP >15 mm Hg PVR ≥3 WU
III	PH associated with primary lung pathology or hypoxia	Precapillary	mPAP >20 mm Hg PAWP ≤15 mm Hg PVR ≥3 WU
IV	Chronic thromboembolic pulmonary hypertension	Precapillary	mPAP >20 mm Hg PAWP ≤15 mm Hg PVR ≥3 WU
V	Multifactorial/unclear mechanism	Precapillary	mPAP >20 mm Hg PAWP ≤15 mm Hg PVR ≥3 WU
		Isolated postcapillary	mPAP >20 mm Hg PAWP >15 mm Hg PVR <3 WU
		Combined pre- and postcapillary	mPAP >20 mm Hg PAWP >15 mm Hg PVR ≥3 WU

mPAP, mean pulmonary artery pressure; PAWP, pulmonary artery wedge pressure; PVR, pulmonary vascular resistance; WU, Woods unit.

postcapillary PH, or combined precapillary and postcapillary PH has been updated to incorporate pulmonary vascular resistance (PVR).

Chronic thromboembolic pulmonary hypertension (CTEPH) is a form of precapillary PH that belongs to the World Health Organization (WHO) group 4 category of PH. It is diagnosed by mPAP >20 mm Hg with pulmonary capillary wedge pressure (PCWP) <15 mm Hg and PVR >300 dynes·s/cm^5 on right heart catheterization.

B. Pathophysiology

Acute or recurrent chronic pulmonary embolism (PE) with incomplete resolution of the thrombus is the cause of CTEPH. While most PEs resolve naturally with conventional treatment such as systemic anticoagulation, residual thrombotic material remains in CTEPH. This residual thrombotic material leads to organized fibrosis, fibrin clot formation, and vascular remodeling that yields to endothelialization of those clots. Eventually, this results in increased PVR and subsequent CTEPH. The reason for incomplete resolution of thromboembolic material is unknown. The risk factors for CTEPH include acute PE, presence of ventriculoatrial shunts, infected pacemakers, splenectomy, chronic inflammatory disease or autoimmune conditions such as lupus anticoagulant or antiphospholipid antibodies, hypothyroidism, or a history of malignant disease.[2] Elevated levels of factor VIII and von Willebrand factor and fibrin abnormalities have also been associated with CTEPH, although the overall prevalence of hereditary thrombophilic diseases, such as deficiencies of antithrombin III, protein C, protein S, factor II, and factor V Leiden mutations are similar to that in patients with idiopathic PH.[2]

C. Clinical Manifestations

Not all patients with CTEPH present with a history of PE.[3] The International CTEPH Registry of 2021 demonstrated that only 65.6% of registered patients had a medically confirmed diagnosis of PE and only 35.8% had a confirmed diagnosis of deep vein thrombosis (DVT).[3] Therefore, a high degree of clinical suspicion is necessary in those patients presenting with dyspnea on exertion without evidence of PE or DVTs. During the early stages of the disease, patients will often go through a "honeymoon" period with minimal symptoms. As the degree of CTEPH gets worse with increase in PVR and right ventricle (RV) dilation, right heart failure develops, and patients will start to show progressive exertional dyspnea, presyncope, hepatic congestion and ascites, arrhythmias, and hemoptysis. Nonproductive cough, early satiety, right upper quadrant pain, or chest pain may be present. Pulmonary flow murmurs may be auscultated over the lung fields due to turbulent blood flow across narrowed pulmonary arteries (PAs), which is typically not present with idiopathic PH. With severe right heart failure, dyspnea at rest, hypoxia, syncope, hepatomegaly, visible jugular venous distension, and peripheral edema will be evident. Tricuspid regurgitation murmur and RV gallop may be appreciated on chest auscultation. If the left PA enlargement is severe enough to impinge on the recurrent laryngeal nerve, then vocal cord paralysis and hoarseness of voice may occur.

D. Clinical Diagnosis

Catheter-based pulmonary angiogram is considered the gold standard for the diagnosis of CTEPH. Angiogram is obtained to assess the severity, location, and surgical accessibility of the disease. Common angiographic patterns consistent with the CTEPH include "pouching defects," webs and bands with abrupt narrowing of the PA, complete flow obstruction of PA, and intimal irregularities.[4] Chest radiograph may show RV or PA enlargement in more advanced disease states but will be relatively benign in early stages of the disease. Pulmonary function tests provide nonspecific clues for diagnosis and is utilized more to assess the degree of concomitant airway obstruction and pulmonary flow disease states. Transthoracic echocardiography is useful in assessing RV size and function, degree of tricuspid regurgitation, and the presence of intracardiac shunt, such as a patent foramen ovale (PFO). Ventilation/perfusion (V/Q) scintigraphy is a good screening tool for CTEPH as it has high sensitivity and specificity.[5] Negative V/Q scintigraphy essentially eliminates the diagnosis of CTEPH. Computed tomography (CT) of the chest and magnetic resonance imaging (MRI) are other modalities that aid in surgical planning.

E. Treatment

Surgical treatment with pulmonary thromboendarterectomy (PTE) is the definitive treatment for CTEPH. Those patients with PVR >800 dynes·s/cm[5] are at higher perioperative mortality risk.[6] For those who are not deemed surgical candidates or have recurrent disease despite surgical treatment, medical management with pharmacologic agents is recommended. Prostacyclin/prostaglandin analogs, soluble guanylate cyclase stimulator, phosphodiesterase-5 inhibitors, and endothelin receptor antagonists are commonly used medications. Lifelong anticoagulation is also recommended in those patients under medical management. Percutaneous balloon angioplasty of the PA may be offered to select patients.

II. Pulmonary Thromboendarterectomy

A. History

Surgical treatment for acute PE in the form of embolectomy was first described by Dr Trendelenburg back in 1908. By the late 1920s, chronic PA occlusion from recurrent PE was becoming recognized, and attempts at embolectomy were performed during subsequent decades. Treatment of CTEPH through surgical endarterectomy was first suggested in 1956 by Dr Hollister, and Dr Hurwitt performed the first planned PA endarterectomy in 1957. By the 1960s, the need for a true formal endarterectomy surgery utilizing cardiopulmonary bypass (CPB) was becoming apparent, and Drs Moser and Braunwald worked to establish a formal PTE program at the University of California, San Diego (UCSD), in the 1970s.[7] Over the next decade, PTE with CPB was performed by various surgeons around the world, and the use of median sternotomy rather than lateral thoracotomy became popularized.

B. Surgical Management

1. Standard pulmonary thromboendarterectomy

The surgical procedure follows four basic principles: (1) median sternotomy is the preferred approach for bilateral endarterectomy, (2) correct identification of the dissection plane is crucial, hence (3) the use of CPB and deep hypothermic circulatory arrest (DHCA) is essential, (4) complete dissection down to distal arteries is necessary.[8] Median sternotomy allows for better surgical exposure for bilateral endarterectomy, although, recently, the operation has been performed in a minimally invasive manner through lateral or anterior thoracotomy for select patients. Once surgical exposure of the heart and great vessels is achieved, standard loading dose of intravenous (IV) heparin is given. Hemodynamic instability from cardiac manipulation during cannulation can occur. CPB is initiated after an aortic cannula and two caval cannulas are placed. Cooling of the patient down to 18 °C is started immediately after initiation of CPB through the CPB circuit along with a cooling head wrap (Figure 20.1). Temperature gradient between arterial and bladder/rectal temperature is maintained at <10 °C for even cooling. Cooling time can range from 45 minutes up to 120 minutes. During this cooling period, the surgeons may perform some preliminary dissections, such as mobilization of the PAs and venae cavae. Once cooling is complete, aortic cross-clamp is placed, a cooling jacket is placed around the heart for further cardioprotection, cardioplegia is given to arrest the heart, and DHCA is initiated. As circulatory arrest is initiated, the lungs are inflated and deflated with a Valsalva maneuver 3-4 times using unwarmed room air to ensure complete exsanguination of residual blood in the pulmonary circulation. Circulatory arrest ensures a completely bloodless field for identification and successful removal of the thrombotic material through the correct dissection plane. If the dissection plane is too deep, then the adventitial layer of the PA may be exposed and perforation of the PA may occur. If the dissection plane is too shallow, then clot removal is deemed inadequate with incomplete resolution of the disease. The disease severity is classified (Table 20.2) based on the location and anatomy of the thrombotic material.[9] Level 3 and 4 diseases present a surgical challenge as clots are located in distal hard-to-reach locations, making surgical dissection difficult. Once clots are successfully removed, the patient is rewarmed while the PA is sutured backup. Further surgical procedures such as PFO closure, tricuspid valve repair, or coronary artery bypass grafts (CABGs) are performed during the rewarming phase. Rewarming time ranges from 60 to 120 minutes. With rewarming complete, CPB is terminated, hemostasis is achieved, and surgical closure of the sternotomy ensues. Patients remain intubated and sedated at the conclusion of the case, and they are transported to the intensive care unit (ICU) on a portable transport ventilator to ensure adequate ventilation during transport.

   2. **Minimally invasive pulmonary thromboendarterectomy**

   Minimally invasive PTE surgery can be performed in select patients who have normal body habitus and suitable chest anatomy, lack significant CTEPH disease burden or other comorbidities, and have no need for concomitant cardiac surgery, such as CABG or valve replacements. These patients tend to be of younger age. Surgical exposure of the PA is achieved with bilateral anterior thoracotomy through the second or third intercostal space. CPB can be initiated through central or peripheral cannulation (femoral artery and internal jugular vein). Circulatory arrest times tend to be reduced as the disease is usually not as severe, and overall hospital length of stay tends to be shorter compared to conventional standard PTE technique. The reduction in PVR is comparable to the conventional PTE technique.[10]

C. **Anesthetic Management**
   1. **Preoperative evaluation**

   Right atrial (RA) pressure, PA pressure, and PVR from right heart catheterization are the gold standard used to assess the severity of CTEPH. Patients with preoperative

TABLE 20.2   Chronic Thromboembolic Pulmonary Hypertension (CTEPH) Disease Severity Classification

Level 0	No evidence of CTEPH. Misdiagnosis has occurred
Level 1	Thromboembolic material readily visible in main right and left PA
Level 2	Main PA is unaffected. Thromboembolic disease starts at lobar or intermediate PA branches
Level 3	Thromboembolic disease is present in the segmental vessels only
Level 4	Thromboembolic disease is present in the sub-segmental vessels

PA, pulmonary artery.
Used with permission of Elsevier Science & Technology Journals from Banks DA, Auger WR, Madani MM. Pulmonary thromboendarterectomy for chronic thromboembolic pulmonary hypertension. In: Kaplan JA, ed. *Kaplan's Cardiac Anesthesia: In Cardiac and Noncardiac Surgery*. 7th ed. Elsevier; 2017:994-1021; permission conveyed through Copyright Clearance Center, Inc.

PVR >1,000 dynes·s/cm^5 have a mortality rate around 10% compared to 1.3% in those with PVR <1,000 dynes·s/cm^5.[11] RV and left ventricular dysfunction should be assessed. Underlying coagulopathic disorder and the patient's anticoagulation regimen should be noted. Other comorbidities, functional status, and the use of home oxygen should be noted as well.

2. **Intraoperative management**
   a. Induction and pre-cardiopulmonary bypass period
      Large-bore IV catheters and radial arterial line should be placed before induction. Anxiolytic medications and opioids should be used with caution before induction as respiratory depression can raise PVR and lead to RV dysfunction. These medications should be given judiciously once standard monitors have been applied to the patient in the operating room. Induction agents should be chosen to maintain stable hemodynamic conditions. Typically, a combination of IV induction agents, opioids, and paralytic agents is utilized for induction. Inotropes and vasopressors should be readily available in case hemodynamic instability is encountered. In cases where RV failure is evident with reduced cardiac index <2 L/min/m^2 and elevated RA pressure with elevated PVR, the use of inotropes during induction is beneficial and indicated. Upon induction, rapid control of respiratory effort is achieved with hyperventilation during masking, and swift intubation is performed. Central venous catheter and pulmonary artery catheters (PACs) are placed subsequently after patient is under general anesthesia. Right internal jugular vein is usually chosen for ease of access. Transesophageal echocardiography (TEE) guidance is useful during PAC placement as significant tricuspid regurgitation or RA/RV enlargement may make PAC placement difficult. Femoral arterial line is placed postinduction as radial arterial signal frequently dampens and significant mean arterial pressure (MAP) differences are noted post-DHCA and upon rewarming due to peripheral vasoconstriction. Electroencephalogram and cerebral oxygen saturation monitors are also applied before surgery start. The head is wrapped with a cooling device to ensure adequate even cooling of the brain (Figure 20.1).

      The pre-bypass period is relatively short. TEE is utilized to assess for cardiac function and valvular abnormalities during this period. Once sternotomy is performed and the pericardium is open, loading dose of heparin is given. IV bubble study with TEE and agitated echocardiographic contrast to assess for PFO is performed at this time. Bubble study should only be performed if color-flow Doppler was inconclusive in showing the presence of a PFO. A Valsalva maneuver is held for 10 seconds; then with the release of the Valsalva maneuver, agitated echocardiographic contrast is injected. Movement of the echocardiographic contrast bubbles from the RA to the left atrium (LA) within the first 3-4 heart beats since the release of "pop-off" valve confirms the presence of a PFO. Once cannulation is complete, initiation of CPB ensues and cooling of the patient begins.

   b. Bypass/circulatory arrest/rewarming period
      Cooling through the bypass circuit starts immediately after initiation of CPB. Patient is cooled down to a tympanic membrane temperature <18 °C, bladder and rectal temperatures <20 °C. Temperature is measured at multiple locations to ensure even cooling across the body. Before initiation of circulatory arrest, propofol or fosphenytoin bolus is administered to ensure isoelectric brain activity on electroencephalogram. All stopcocks are turned off to the patient during circulatory arrest to decrease the risk of air entrainment. Circulatory arrest periods are limited to 20 minutes at a time with blood flow restored for 10 minutes in between each arrest to minimize neurologic consequences. Once all thrombotic materials are removed in satisfactory manner, the patient is rewarmed to 36.5 °C. During rewarming, the temperature gradient is again maintained to <10 °C across various temperature measurement sites. Rapid rewarming may promote gas bubble formation in the systemic circulation or cerebral ischemia. Rewarming past 37 °C is not recommended. Low-dose vasodilators such as clevidipine may be infused to promote faster and even rewarming if hemodynamic conditions permit. Once the core temperature reaches around 34 °C, an additional dose of opioids or benzodiazepine

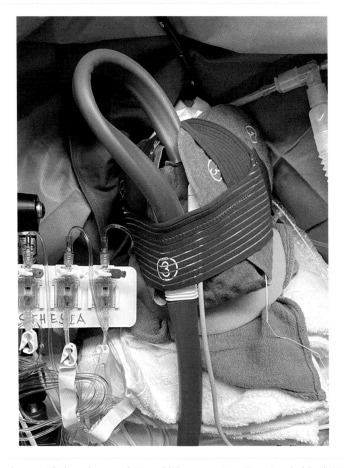

FIGURE 20.1   Head wrap with the polar care glacier cold therapy system. (Breg, Inc, Carlsbad, CA.)

should be administered to ensure adequate amnesia. Furthermore, a soft suction cath-eter (typically 14F) is passed down the endotracheal tube, and the airway is suctioned to monitor for airway bleeding. If bleeding is noted, then a bronchoscopy is performed to identify the location of the bleeding before coming off bypass. High positive end-expiratory pressure (PEEP) or bronchial blocker may be placed depending on the degree of bleeding present (Figure 20.2).

c. Post-bypass period

Once the patient is normothermic, cardiac rhythm has been established, and acid-base balance is normalized, CPB is terminated. Protamine is given to reverse the effects of heparin. Inotropic and vasopressor medication may be needed to maintain adequate hemodynamics. TEE use is critical during and after this process to assess for RV func-tion and valvular abnormalities. Cardiac output and PVR are measured with significant reduction in PVR typically. If PVR reduction is marginal and signs of RV dysfunction persist, then one should consider the use of higher dose of inotropes or addition of sec-ondary inotropes, the use of inodilators such as milrinone, institution of inhaled nitric oxide, and mechanical circulatory support with extracorporeal membrane oxygenator (ECMO). Hemostasis is achieved, and chest closure occurs. The use of blood products is rare unless clinically significant bleeding continues. Upon conclusion of the surgical procedure, patient is transported to the ICU in intubated and sedated condition. The use of a transport ventilator is recommended to ensure proper ventilation.

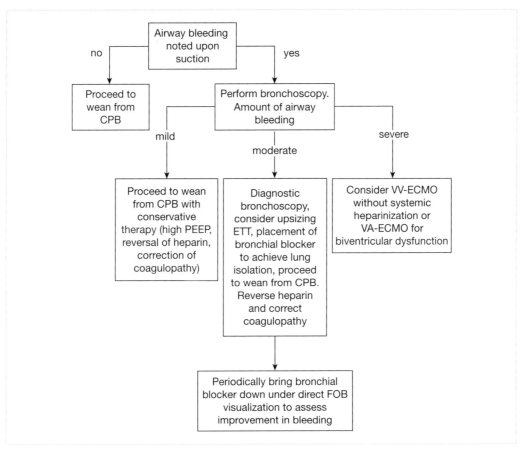

FIGURE 20.2 Airway bleeding algorithm. CPB, cardiopulmonary bypass; ETT, endotracheal tube; FOB, fiberoptic bronchoscope; PEEP, positive end-expiratory pressure; VA-ECMO, venoarterial extracorporeal membrane oxygenator; VV-ECMO, veno-veno extracorporeal membrane oxygenator. (Derived from Cronin B, Maus T, Pretorius V, et al. Case 13-2014: Management of pulmonary hemorrhage after pulmonary endarterectomy with venovenous extracorporeal membrane oxygenation without systemic anticoagulation. *J Cardiothorac Vasc Anesth.* 2014;28(6):1667-1676.)

3. **Postoperative management**

Upon arrival to the ICU, coagulopathy along with transient rise in creatinine and transaminases can be noted likely from hypoperfusion during CPB/DHCA period. Coagulopathy should be monitored and treated with appropriate blood products if indicated. Inotropic and vasopressor support may be continued in the ICU until hemodynamic stability is achieved. Rarely, adrenal insufficiency can cause hypotension and should be treated with administration of corticosteroids. IV prostanoids may be administered for persistently elevated PVR. Temporary use of pacemaker may be needed if sinus node dysfunction occurs. Postoperative delirium and mental status changes may be noted as well related to circulatory arrest. Most patients have routine recovery with typical extubation within 24 hours of surgery and discharge from the ICU within 2-3 days. Significant immediate reduction in PVR will be noted; however, RV strain may be persistent and may take months for the RV to remodel to a normal state.

D. **Complications**

1. **Airway bleeding**

Airway bleeding and reperfusion pulmonary edema (RPE) are the two most significant complications of PTE surgery. While the magnitude of the bleeding is difficult to predict, the difficulty and extent of surgical dissection will help surgeons anticipate the presence of airway bleeding. Before coming off bypass, a soft suction catheter is passed down the endotracheal tube and airway may be suctioned to see if there is blood return. Dark red blood will be noted if there is a breakdown of blood-airway barrier. If blood is noticed on this preliminary screen, then, while letting the heart eject for a brief period of time, a bronchoscopy is performed to determine the exact location of the bleeding. If the bleeding is small, then conservative therapy with high PEEP should suffice followed by swift reversal of heparin with protamine at the time of termination of CPB. If there is a large amount of bleeding, then a bronchial blocker should be placed and the bleeding lung segment should be isolated to prevent contamination of other areas of the lung before coming off bypass.[12] After separation from bypass and reversal of heparin, the degree of bleeding can be assessed by deflating the bronchial blocker cuff slowly under direct visualization with a bronchoscope. If there is improvement of bleeding, then the bronchial blocker may be left deflated. However, if the bleeding remains significant, then the bronchial blocker cuff should remain inflated until hemostasis can be achieved. Hemostasis is typically achieved within several hours after surgery. Coagulopathy should be corrected with administration of blood products. An institutional airway bleeding algorithm used is illustrated in Figure 20.2.

2. **Reperfusion pulmonary edema**

Pink frothy fluid return from the endotracheal tube suction indicates RPE. This is a result of pulmonary capillary—alveolar membrane dysfunction with increased capillary permeability.[13] RPE is typically noted within the first 24-48 hours post PTE surgery and can be a significant contributor to hypoxia and impaired gas exchange. Conservation management with institution of high PEEP with mechanical ventilation, diuretic treatment, and avoidance of hyperoxia usually allows for full lung recovery.[12,13] However, in refractory cases, veno-veno extracorporeal membrane oxygenation without systemic heparin use may be instituted while awaiting resolution of lung injury.[13]

III. Special Consideration

A. Sickle Cell Disease

PH in sickle cell disease is not uncommon, and a growing number of patients with sickle cell disease with CTEPH are presenting for PTE. Sickle cell disease presents a challenge for cardiac surgery as hypothermia, stagnation of blood, anemia from hemodilution, use of CPB, and potential acidosis increase the likelihood of red blood cell sickling. It is generally recommended that for patients with sickle cell disease, exchange transfusion be performed to reduce the fraction of hemoglobin S to <10% before surgery.[14] Intraoperative plasmapheresis technique can also be used to separate out platelet and plasma components from native red blood cells during CPB.[15] Maintenance of normothermia and avoidance of hypoxia and hypercarbia off CPB are critical in preventing sickling of red blood cells.

B. Cold Agglutinins

Cold agglutinin disease is a type of autoimmune hemolytic anemia in which autoantibodies against red blood cell antigen get activated below certain temperature thresholds, leading to destruction of red blood cells. This presents a challenge as cooling the patient's temperature to <20 °C is needed for PTE. Testing of thermal amplitude and titer levels should be performed before surgery. Rituximab, cyclophosphamide, glucocorticoids, and IV immunoglobulins can be administered preoperatively to reduce the cold agglutinin titers.[16] Intraoperatively, systemic perfusion temperature should be maintained above the thermal amplitude. Warm CPB priming solutions and warm cardioplegia solution should be used.[17] If circulatory arrest is needed, arrest temperature should be maintained above the thermal amplitude.

C. Heparin-Induced Thrombocytopenia

A unique anticoagulation strategy must be utilized for those patients with heparin-induced thrombocytopenia (HIT). Direct thrombin inhibitors may be used to achieve anticoagulation during the use of CPB; however, the lack of reversal agent and unpredictable clinical response makes the titration of these medications challenging. Cangrelor is a direct ultra-short-acting P2Y12 receptor antagonist that blocks the P2Y12 receptor site, which is responsible for platelet aggregation and thromboembolism formation that occurs in HIT. Before case start, a baseline P2Y12 reaction unit (PRU) assay is obtained, with normal values being >180. Once the surgeon is ready to cannulate the great vessels, then cangrelor dose of 30 μg/kg is bolused IV over 1 minute and an infusion is started at 4 μg/kg/min. A repeat PRU assay is obtained with a goal PRU <180, indicating adequate blockade of the P2Y12 receptor activity. Then a normal loading dose of heparin is given, and once adequate activated clotting time (ACT) is achieved, CPB can be initiated. The cangrelor is run as an infusion during the CPB to continuously inhibit the P2Y12 receptor site on platelets.[18] During circulatory arrest, the infusion is halted for the duration and then started again with resumption of bypass. About 10 minutes before termination of bypass, the cangrelor infusion is turned off. Once CPB is terminated, protamine can be given in a standard manner with observation of ACT levels. The cangrelor protocol used at UCSD is demonstrated in Figure 20.3.

D. Use of Extracorporeal Membrane Oxygenator Life Support

In cases of refractory hemodynamic instability or ventricular dysfunction, persistent oxygenation, or ventilation problems, the use of ECMO may be considered. Venoarterial ECMO should be considered in cases of biventricular dysfunction and persistent oxygenation/ventilation problems. Veno-veno ECMO can be considered if oxygenation and ventilation is the main problem with normal biventricular function. Systemic heparinization is not utilized in this case. RA inflow and PA outflow cannula ECMO can be considered if isolated RV dysfunction persists.

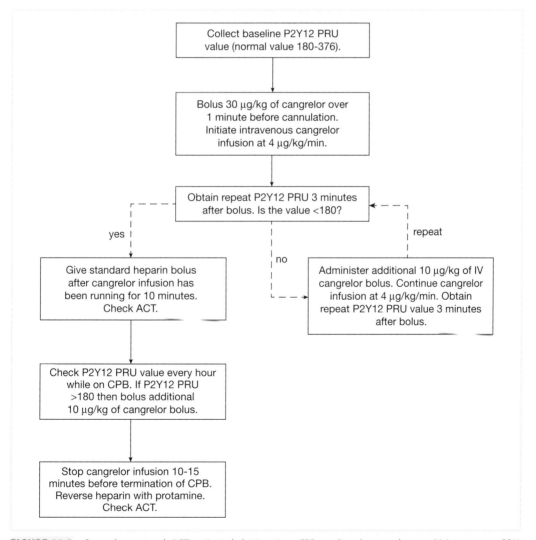

FIGURE 20.3   Cangrelor protocol. ACT, activated clotting time; CPB, cardiopulmonary bypass; IV, intravenous; PRU, P2Y12 reaction unit.

REFERENCES

1. Stuart RLR, Abenhaim L, Barst RJ, et al. Primary pulmonary hypertension. Paper presented at: Executive summary from the World Symposium; September 6-10, 1998; Evian, France.
2. Kim NH, Lang IM. Risk factors for chronic thromboembolic pulmonary hypertension. *Eur Respir Rev.* 2012;21:27-31.
3. Guth S, D'Armini AM, Delcroix M, et al. Current strategies for managing chronic thromboembolic pulmonary hypertension: results of the worldwide prospective CTEPH Registry. *ERJ Open Res.* 2021;7:1-11.
4. Auger WR, Fedullo PF, Moser KM, et al. Chronic major-vessel thromboembolic pulmonary artery obstruction: appearance at angiography. *Radiology.* 1992;182:393-398.
5. He J, Fang W, Lv B, et al. Diagnosis of chronic thromboembolic pulmonary hypertension: comparison of ventilation/perfusion scanning and multidetector computed tomography pulmonary angiography with pulmonary angiography. *Nucl Med Commun.* 2012;33:459-463.
6. Brookes JDL, Li C, Chung STW, et al. Pulmonary thromboendarterectomy for chronic thromboembolic pulmonary hypertension: a systematic review. *Ann Cardiothorac Surg.* 2022;11:68-81.
7. Jamieson SW. Historical perspective: surgery for chronic thromboembolic disease. *Semin Thorac Cardiovasc Surg.* 2006; 18:218-222.
8. Madani MM, Jamieson SW. Pulmonary endarterectomy for chronic thromboembolic disease. *Oper Tech Thorac Cardiovasc Surg.* 2006;11:264-274.
9. Thistlethwaite PA, Madani M, Jamieson SW. Pulmonary thromboendarterectomy surgery. *Cardiol Clin.* 2004;22:467-478.
10. Higgins J, Kim N, Kerr K, et al. A comparison of short term outcomes of minimally invasive versus sternotomy pulmonary thromboendarterectomy. *J Heart Lung Transplant.* 2018;37:S25-S26.
11. Jamieson SW, Kapelanski DP, Sakakibara N, et al. Pulmonary endarterectomy: experience and lessons learned in 1,500 cases. *Ann Thorac Surg.* 2003;76:1457-1462; discussion 1462-1454.
12. Banks DA, Pretorius GV, Kerr KM, et al. Pulmonary endarterectomy: part II. Operation, anesthetic management, and postoperative care. *Semin Cardiothorac Vasc Anesth.* 2014;18:331-340.
13. Thistlethwaite PA, Madani MM, Kemp AD, et al. Venovenous extracorporeal life support after pulmonary endarterectomy: indications, techniques, and outcomes. *Ann Thorac Surg.* 2006;82:2139-2145.
14. Firth PG, Head CA. Sickle cell disease and anesthesia. *Anesthesiology.* 2004;101:766-785.
15. Bocchieri KA, Scheinerman SJ, Graver LM. Exchange transfusion before cardiopulmonary bypass in sickle cell disease. *Ann Thorac Surg.* 2010;90:323-324.
16. Pecsi SA, Almassi GH, Langenstroer P. Deep hypothermic circulatory arrest for a patient with known cold agglutinins. *Ann Thorac Surg.* 2009;88:1326-1327.
17. Barbara DW, Mauermann WJ, Neal JR, et al. Cold agglutinins in patients undergoing cardiac surgery requiring cardiopulmonary bypass. *J Thorac Cardiovasc Surg.* 2013;146:668-680.
18. Gernhofer YK, Banks DA, Golts E, et al. Novel use of cangrelor with heparin during cardiopulmonary bypass in patients with heparin-induced thrombocytopenia who require cardiovascular surgery: a case series. *Semin Thorac Cardiovasc Surg.* 2020;32:763-769.

Heart Transplantation 21

John Hartnett, Joshua B. Cohen, and James M. Anton

KEY POINTS

1. Nonischemic cardiomyopathy (49%) is the most common pretransplant diagnosis worldwide.
2. Nearly 85% of recipients in the United States require some form of life support before cardiac transplantation. For example, the number of pretransplant patients with ventricular assist devices (VADs) has risen dramatically (29% in 2008 vs 45% in 2015).
3. Increased preoperative pulmonary vascular resistance (PVR) in the recipient predicts early graft dysfunction and an increased incidence of right heart dysfunction. Right ventricular (RV) failure accounts for nearly 20% of early mortality after transplantation.
4. During orthotopic cardiac transplantation, the cardiac autonomic plexus is transected, leaving the transplanted heart without autonomic innervation. The denervated heart responds to direct-acting agents, such as catecholamines, which are utilized frequently in the post-bypass period.
5. In contrast to the nontransplanted patient, where increases in cardiac output (CO) can be quickly achieved through a sympathetically mediated increase in heart rate (HR), the cardiac transplanted patient, whose sympathetic innervation to the heart will be interrupted, tends to require an increase in preload in order to increase CO.

ALTHOUGH "DESTINATION THERAPY" USING MECHANICAL CIRCULATORY SUPPORT (MCS) devices has increasingly become a viable option, and advances in MCS devices have resulted in a significant survival benefit, cardiac transplantation remains the gold standard for the treatment of heart failure (HF) refractory to medical therapy.[1] Since the first human cardiac transplant by Christiaan Barnard in 1967, over 118,000 cardiac transplants have been performed worldwide.[2] Currently, ~4,500 cardiac transplants are performed per year, with ~2,700 occurring in the United States.[2] Despite an increasingly high-risk patient population, survival rates continue to improve due to advances in immunosuppression, surgical technique, perioperative management, and the diagnosis and treatment of allograft rejection and allograft vasculopathy.[3] In the United States, cardiac transplantation is limited to member centers of the United Network for Organ Sharing (UNOS). The UNOS, in turn, administers the Organ Procurement and Transplantation Network (OPTN), which maintains the only national patient waiting list in the United States.

I. Heart Failure

About six million Americans >20 years of age have HF, with the prevalence projected to increase by 46% from 2012 to 2030, affecting >8 million people aged >18 years.[4] The American College of Cardiology (ACC) and the American Heart Association (AHA) define heart failure as a clinical syndrome that can result from any structural or functional cardiac disorder that impairs the ability of the ventricle to fill with or eject blood. The majority of patients with HF owe their symptoms to impairment of left ventricular (LV) myocardial function.[5] Because volume overload is not necessarily present, the term "heart failure" is now preferred to the older term "congestive HF."

The New York Heart Association (NYHA) scale is used to quantify the degree of functional limitation imposed by HF. Most patients with HF, however, do not show an uninterrupted and inexorable progression along the NYHA scale.[5] In 2005, the ACC/AHA created a staging scheme reflective of the fact that HF has established risk factors, a clear progression, and specific treatments at each stage that can reduce morbidity and mortality (Figure 21.1). Patients presenting for heart transplantation invariably present in stage D, refractory HF.

A. Etiology

Nonischemic cardiomyopathy (49%) is the most common pretransplant diagnosis worldwide.[2] Ischemic cardiomyopathy accounts for 35%, with valvular cardiomyopathy, restrictive cardiomyopathy, hypertrophic cardiomyopathy, viral cardiomyopathy, retransplantation, and congenital heart disease accounting for the remaining percentage of adult heart transplant recipients.

B. Pathophysiology

The neurohormonal model portrays HF as a progressive disorder initiated by an index event, which either damages the myocardium directly or disrupts the ability of the myocardium to

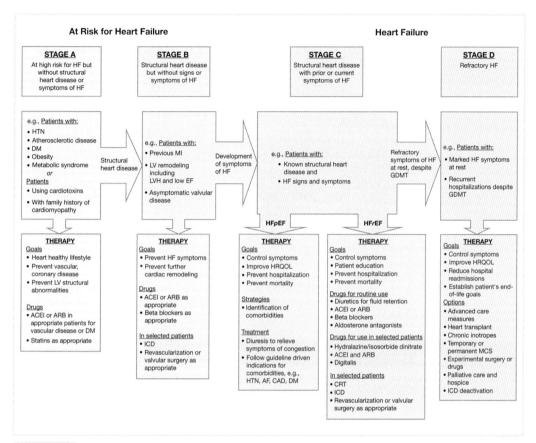

FIGURE 21.1   Stages in the development of heart failure and recommended therapy. ACEI, angiotensin-converting enzyme inhibitor; AF, atrial fibrillation; ARB, angiotensin receptor blocker; CAD, coronary artery disease; CRT, cardiac resynchronization therapy; DM, diabetes mellitus; EF, ejection fraction; GDMT, goal-directed medical therapy; HF, heart failure; HFpEF, heart failure with preserved ejection fraction; HFrEF, heart failure with reduced ejection fraction; HRQoL, health-related quality of life; HTN, hypertension; ICD, implantable cardioverter defibrillator; LV, left ventricle; LVH, left ventricular hypertrophy; MCS, mechanical circulatory support; MI, myocardial infarction. (Reprinted with permission from Yancy CW, Jessup M, Bozkurt B, et al. 2013 ACCF/AHA guideline for the management of heart failure: executive summary: a report of the American College of Cardiology Foundation/American Heart Association Task Force on practice guidelines. *Circulation.* 2013;128(16):1810-1852. © 2013 American Heart Association, Inc.)

generate force.[6] HF progression is characterized by declining ventricular function and activation of compensatory adrenergic and salt/water retention pathways. Ejection fraction (EF) is initially maintained by increases in LV end-diastolic volume, myocardial fiber length, and adrenergically mediated increases in myocardial contractility. LV remodeling takes place during this time and, while initially adaptive, may independently contribute to HF progression.[6] The chronic overexpression of molecular mediators of compensation (eg, norepinephrine, angiotensin II, endothelin, natriuretic peptides, aldosterone, and tumor necrosis factor) may lead to deleterious effects on cardiac myocytes and their extracellular matrix.[6,7] The result is progressive LV dilation, as well as decreasing EF and cardiac output (CO). Fatigue, dyspnea, and signs of fluid retention develop. Other organ systems such as the liver and kidneys become compromised by persistent decreases in CO and elevated venous pressures. With continued progression of HF, stroke volume (SV) becomes unresponsive to increases in preload, and increases in afterload are poorly tolerated (Figure 21.2). Chronic exposure to circulating catecholamines may result in downregulation of myocardial β1-adrenergic receptors, making the heart less responsive to inotropic therapy.

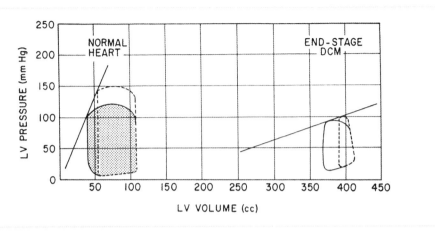

FIGURE 21.2   Pressure-volume (*P-V*) relationships in a normal heart and a heart with end-stage, dilated cardiomyopathy (DCM). Shown are the left ventricular (LV) *P-V* loops (dotted lines) obtained from a normal heart and a heart with end-stage DCM following an increase in afterload. The slope depicts the LV end-systolic *P-V* relationship. Note that the myopathic heart stroke volume (SV) is markedly decreased by increases in afterload. (Reprinted from Clark NJ, Martin RD. Anesthetic considerations for patients undergoing cardiac transplantation. *J Cardiothorac Anesth.* 1988;2(4):519-542. © 1988 Elsevier. With permission.)

CLINICAL PEARL

Patients with end-stage HF are chronically exposed to high circulating catecholamine levels and, as a result, are less responsive to inotropic therapy.

C. Medical Management of Heart Failure
  1. Therapeutic goals

The therapeutic goal for HF management is to slow or halt the progression from stages A to D. Lifestyle modifications and selected pharmacotherapy are the mainstays of the treatment for stages A and B. When stage C is reached, combination pharmacotherapy includes diuresis, interruption of the renin-angiotensin axis, and β-blockade. Selective use of direct vasodilators and inotropes is also indicated. Utilization of cardiac resynchronization therapy (CRT) and/or an implantable defibrillator may be recommended. Despite optimum medical management, some patients will progress to stage D, refractory HF. Chronic intravenous (IV) inotropes, MCS devices, and heart transplantation are the only measures available for palliation or treatment.

  a. Inotropes

Inotropic agents commonly used to treat cardiac failure include digitalis, catecholamines, and phosphodiesterase (PDE) III inhibitors. Digitalis, in combination with β-blockers, is effective in treating HF complicated by atrial fibrillation, but does not confer increased survival.[8] Similarly, recent evidence indicates that digitalis may have a role in the treatment of HF in patients with normal sinus rhythm, but this remains without documented mortality benefit.[9] Administered orally, digitalis exerts a positive inotropic effect by inhibiting the myocardial cell sodium pump and increasing cytosolic calcium concentrations. Digitalis also prolongs atrioventricular conduction time, leading to PR interval prolongation and possible heart block. Digitalis blood levels should be monitored as significant side effects, including atrial and ventricular arrhythmias, can occur particularly in the presence of hypokalemia.

Myocardial β1-adrenergic receptor stimulation by IV administration of catecholamines, such as epinephrine, norepinephrine, dobutamine, or dopamine, is often used to improve cardiac performance, diuresis, and clinical stability. PDE III inhibitors, such as milrinone and enoximone, may also be used. PDE inhibitors combine both positive inotropic and vasodilatory activity by inhibiting cyclic adenosine monophosphate (cAMP) metabolism. Occasionally, patients may not be weaned from IV inotropic support despite repeated attempts. At such times, an indwelling IV catheter may be placed to allow for the continuous infusion of an inotrope for patients awaiting transplantation, or to facilitate home palliation. However, chronic inotrope use has not been shown to increase survival.[10]

b. Diuretics

Diuretics provide symptomatic relief to patients with HF more quickly than any other class of drug and are the only class of drug used in HF that can adequately control fluid retention. Classes of diuretics used include the loop diuretics (eg, furosemide, bumetanide, torsemide), the thiazide diuretics (eg, hydrochlorothiazide), and the thiazide-like drug metolazone. Adverse diuretic effects include electrolyte disturbances (particularly of potassium and magnesium), hypotension, intravascular volume depletion, and azotemia.

c. Renin-angiotensin-aldosterone system inhibitors

Inhibition of the renin-angiotensin-aldosterone system may occur at the level of the angiotensin-converting enzyme inhibitors (ACEIs), the angiotensin receptor blockers (ARBs), or the aldosterone receptor. In combination with β1-antagonists, ACEIs have been shown to reduce HF progression by interfering with the neurohormonal pathways that modulate LV remodeling. ACEIs alleviate symptoms, enhance the overall sense of well-being, and reduce the risk of hospitalization and death in patients with HF.[11,12] Adverse effects of ACEIs include hypotension, worsening renal function, and hyperkalemia. If the adverse effects of ACEIs cannot be tolerated, ARBs may be considered an alternative. ARBs have been shown to reduce morbidity and mortality in patients with HF.[12] The propensity of ARBs to increase serum potassium levels limits their usage in patients with impaired renal function. A new class of medication, combined angiotensin receptor blocker neprilysin inhibitors (ARNIs), has been associated with significant reductions in hospital admissions and mortality as compared to ACEIs. Guidelines now recommend substituting ARNIs for ACEIs or ARBs in appropriate patients.[11,12] Aldosterone exerts an adverse effect on heart structure and function, independent of angiotensin II.[13] Spironolactone is the most widely used aldosterone antagonist in patients with HF, although eplerenone has been studied in HF after myocardial infarction.

d. Vasodilators

Vasodilators are used in the acute treatment of HF to reduce myocardial preload and afterload, thereby reducing myocardial work and oxygen demand. By preferentially reducing preload via venodilation, nitroglycerin may be useful for relieving the symptoms of pulmonary edema. β-Type natriuretic peptide (nesiritide) is used effectively for the medical management of decompensated HF.[10] Nesiritide, an arterial and venous dilator, acts by increasing cyclic guanosine monophosphate (cGMP).[10] In hospitalized patients, a dose-dependent reduction of pulmonary capillary wedge pressure (PCWP), right atrial pressure, and mean pulmonary artery (PA) pressure was demonstrated, along with improvements in cardiac index and clinical outcome.[14] A recent meta-analysis found reduced readmission rates and in-hospital mortality rates with nesiritide therapy as compared to dobutamine therapy for patients with acute decompensated HF.[14]

e. β-Adrenergic receptor blockade

In combination with interruption of the renin-angiotensin-aldosterone axis and diuresis, β-adrenergic receptor blockade is now standard treatment for HF. Carvedilol, bisoprolol, and sustained-release metoprolol have been demonstrated to be effective in reducing mortality in patients with chronic HF.[11] Chronic adrenergic stimulation initially supports the failing heart but may lead to progression of HF through neurohormonal-mediated LV remodeling. β-Blockers likely exert their benefit through attenuation of this influence. Adverse reactions to β-blockers in patients with HF include fluid retention, fatigue, bradycardia, heart block, and hypotension.

f. Anticoagulants

Patients with HF are at increased risk of thromboembolism as a result of low CO and a high incidence of coexistent atrial fibrillation. Long-term prophylactic anticoagulation with agents such as warfarin is common and may contribute to perioperative bleeding at the time of cardiac transplantation.

g. Cardiac implantable electronic devices

Cardiac implantable electronic devices (CIEDs) broadly consist of devices that seek to manage bradyarrhythmias (pacemakers), tachyarrhythmias (implantable cardiac defibrillators), and ventricular dyssynchrony (biventricular pacing/CRT). These devices are used to reduce the incidence of sudden cardiac death and to slow HF progression.[15] Their presence may complicate the placement of central venous catheters and require the involvement of the electrophysiology team for interrogation and reprogramming.[16]

D. Mechanical Circulatory Support Devices

Nearly 80% of recipients in the United States require some form of life support before heart transplantation.[17] These include IV medications, mechanical ventilation, intra-aortic balloon pump (IABP), extracorporeal life support (ELS), ventricular assist devices (VADs), and total artificial hearts (TAHs). IV medications, IABPs, ELS, and extracorporeal VADs are useful in temporizing a hospitalized patient with cardiogenic shock. Intracorporeal MCS devices offer the potential for discharge to home and may yield the greatest potential improvement in quality of life for patients with class D HF who are awaiting heart transplant surgery.

Extracorporeal membrane oxygenation (ECMO) used as a bridge to transplant (BTT) does not appear to affect survival following transplantation. Among those supported on ECMO as BTT, mortality was associated with an increasing number of risk factors, and those without risk factors had similar mortality to patients who were not on ECMO.[18]

The number of patients undergoing heart transplantation with a preexistent VAD has decreased from its peak in 2017, from 48% to 33%. Meanwhile, the percentage of patients with IABP has increased from 8% to 26%.[17] The increased use of VADs has contributed to a decline in the heart transplant waiting list mortality despite increased waiting times secondary to their use as a BTT.[17,19] One-year survival while being supported on a VAD has risen to 85%.[20] However, the influence of VADs on post–heart transplant survival remains controversial, with some studies suggesting an increased 6-month mortality after transplant, while others suggest no increase in mortality.[20,21]

The improved outcomes among patients with LVADs are now approaching the outcomes of transplantation, with similar 1- and 2-year mortality, albeit with a high risk of stroke.[22,23]

CLINICAL PEARL

The increased use of VADs has resulted in a decline in heart transplant waiting list mortality; however, the influence of VADs on post–heart transplant survival remains controversial.

II. Cardiac Transplant Recipient Characteristics

The number of active transplant candidates in the United States has increased from 5,506 in 2009 to 7,386 in 2020.[17] In 1999, the UNOS modified its listing system to be two-tiered (Table 21.1), and in 2006, the UNOS modified the allocation of donor hearts to expand organ sharing within geographic regions. In 2014-2015, the median time to transplantation was 12.4 months. Among adults, there was an increase in the number of candidates aged >65 years (12% in 2009 vs 16% in 2020).[17] Among all age groups, there was an increase in cardiomyopathy as a primary diagnosis, a decrease in coronary artery disease (CAD), and a stable number of those listed for other causes. Cardiomyopathy remains the most common diagnosis, comprising 60% in 2020, and this trend is not expected to change. The proportion of candidates listed for congenital heart disease has remained stable.[17]

The UNOS updated its listing system again in 2018. This update implemented a six-tier system designed to improve both the stratification of high-risk groups and the equitable geographic

TABLE 21.1 UNOS Adult Heart Allocation System

Status 1	ECMO Nondischargeable BiVAD MCS with VT
Status 2	IABP Percutaneous VADs Surgical nondischargeable LVAD Total artificial heart MCS with device failure VT/VF
Status 3	LVAD × 30 d (discretionary use) High dose or >1 inotrope Status 1 or 2 after 14 d MCS with other complication
Status 4	Stable LVAD Inotropes without monitoring Retransplant Complex congenital heart disease Hypertrophic CMP Restrictive CMP Ischemic CMP with refractory angina Amyloidosis
Status 5	Combined organs
Status 6	All others

BiVAD, biventricular assist device; CMP, cardiomyopathy; ECMO, extracorporeal membrane oxygenation; IABP, intra-aortic balloon pump; LVAD, left ventricular assist device; MCS, mechanical circulatory support; UNOS, United Network for Organ Sharing; VADs, ventricular assist devices; VF, ventricular fibrillation; VT, ventricular tachycardia.
Adapted from Estep JD, Soltesz E, Cogswell R. The new heart transplant allocation system: Early observations and mechanical circulatory support considerations. *J Thorac Cardiovasc Surg.* 2020:S0022-5223(20)32638-6. © 2020 by The American Association for Thoracic Surgery. With permission.

access to donor organs. This new allocation system has resulted in more transplants for patients on temporary MCS (41% vs 10%) and fewer patients with durable LVADs (23% vs 42%). Regional and national sharing increased, as did the ischemia time (3.4 vs 3 hours). Early data demonstrate no difference in patient and graft survival at 6 months, though continued follow-up is needed.[24]

A. Cardiac Transplantation Indications

Indications for heart transplantation are listed in Table 21.2.[25] Potential cardiac transplant candidates must have all reversible causes of HF excluded, and their medical management optimized.

B. Cardiac Transplantation Contraindications

There has been a gradual relaxation in the cardiac transplantation exclusion criteria as experience with increasingly complex cases has grown.[2] Absolute exclusion criteria have been simplified (Table 21.3).[25]

TABLE 21.2 Indications for Heart Transplantation

Refractory HF/cardiogenic shock requiring continuous IV inotropic support or MCS

Persistent NYHA class IV HF symptoms refractory to maximal medical therapy (LVEF <20%; peak Vo_2 <12 mL/kg/min with β-blockade, Vo_2 <14 mL/kg/min without β-blockade)

Intractable or severe anginal symptoms in patients with CAD not amenable to percutaneous or surgical revascularization

Intractable life-threatening arrhythmias unresponsive to medical therapy, catheter ablation, and/or implantation of a intracardiac defibrillator

CAD, coronary artery disease; HF, heart failure; IV, intravenous; LVEF, left ventricular ejection fraction; MCS, mechanical circulatory support; NYHA, New York Heart Association; Vo_2, oxygen consumption.
Reprinted with permission from Mancini D, Lietz K. Selection of cardiac transplantation candidates in 2010. *Circulation.* 2010;122(2):173-183.

TABLE 21.3   Contraindications to Heart Transplantation

Absolute contraindications

Systemic illness with a life expectancy <2 y despite transplant, including:
  Active or recent solid-organ or blood malignancy within 5 y
  AIDS with frequent opportunistic infections
  Systemic lupus erythematosus, sarcoidosis, or amyloidosis that has multisystem involvement and is still active
  Irreversible renal or hepatic dysfunction in patients considered only for heart transplant
  Significant obstructive pulmonary disease (FEV$_1$ <1 L/min)
Fixed pulmonary hypertension
  PA systolic pressure >60 mm Hg
  Mean transpulmonary gradient >15 mm Hg
  PVR >6 Wood units

Relative contraindications

Age >72 y
An active infection excepting device-related infection in patients with VAD
Severe peripheral vascular or cerebrovascular disease
  Symptomatic carotid stenosis
  Uncorrected abdominal aortic aneurysm >6 cm
  Severe diabetes mellitus with end-organ damage (neuropathy, nephropathy, or retinopathy)
  Peripheral vascular disease not amenable to percutaneous or surgical therapy
Morbid obesity (BMI >35 kg/m^2)
Recent pulmonary infarction (6-8 wk)
Irreversible neurologic or neuromuscular disorder
Drug, tobacco, or alcohol abuse within 6 mo
Active mental illness or psychosocial instability
Difficult-to-control hypertension
Active peptic ulcer disease
Heparin-induced thrombocytopenia within 100 d
Creatinine >2.5 mg/dL or creatinine clearance <25 mL/min
Bilirubin >2.5 mg/dL, serum transaminases >3× upper limit of normal, INR >1.5 off Coumadin

AIDS, acquired immune deficiency syndrome; BMI, body mass index; FEV$_1$, forced expiratory volume in 1 second; INR, international normalized ratio; PA, pulmonary artery; PVR, pulmonary vascular resistance; VAD, ventricular assist device.
Reprinted with permission from Mancini D, Lietz K. Selection of cardiac transplantation candidates in 2010. *Circulation.* 2010;122(2):173-183.

Increased preoperative pulmonary vascular resistance (PVR) predicts early graft dysfunction and increased mortality, due to an increased incidence of right heart dysfunction.[25-27] Methods used to quantify the severity of pulmonary hypertension (HTN) include calculation of PVR and the transpulmonary gradient (mean PA pressure—PCWP). At most centers, patients are not considered orthotopic cardiac transplant candidates if they demonstrate a PVR >5 Wood units or transpulmonary gradient >15 mm Hg without evidence of pharmacologic reversibility.[27] The reversibility of pulmonary HTN can be evaluated by vasodilator administration, including IV sodium nitroprusside, inhaled nitric oxide (iNO), inhaled epoprostenol (PGI2), and levosimendan.[28] In patients who receive VADs, "fixed" elevated PVR may be reduced and thus improve posttransplant outcome, or qualify a previously excluded patient for heart transplant.[25-27] The only transplant options for patients with severe irreversible pulmonary HTN include heterotopic cardiac or combined heart-lung transplantation (HLT).

III.   The Cardiac Transplant Donor

A.   Donor Selection

The primary factor limiting cardiac transplantation is a shortage of donors. Standard criteria for donors, first outlined in the 1980s, resulted in a paucity of donor organs relative to the number of patients who could benefit from heart transplantation. In an attempt to increase donor numbers, the criteria for cardiac organ donation have been relaxed. The so-called "marginal donor" hearts may be transplanted into borderline heart transplant candidates with good results when compared to their expected prognosis without transplantation.[29] Characteristics of marginal donors include older age (>55 years), the presence of CAD, donor/recipient size

TABLE 21.4 Contraindications to Heart Donation

Absolute contraindications
Positive serology for syphilis, HTLV-4, and HIV
Presence of malignancy with extracranial metastatic potential
LVEF <40%
Significant valvular abnormality
Significant CAD
Relative contraindications
Sepsis
Hepatitis B surface antigen positive
Hepatitis C antibody positive
Repeated need for cardiopulmonary resuscitation
High-dose inotropic support exceeding 24 h

CAD, coronary artery disease; HIV, human immunodeficiency virus; HTLV-4, human T-lymphotropic virus type 4; LVEF, left ventricular ejection fraction.

mismatch, history of donor drug abuse, and increased ischemic times.[29-31] Nonetheless, the risk of failed transplantation has been shown to increase with increased donor age, LV hypertrophy, and the presence of concomitant disease.[31] In an effort to further expand the donor pool, donation after circulatory death (DCD) for heart transplantation has been described recently using ex vivo perfusion. Early evidence suggests that with strict limitations and the use of ex vivo perfusion systems, DCD for heart transplantation may be feasible.[30,32] Contraindications to heart donation are listed in Table 21.4.

A trial of 93 extended criteria donor (ECD) hearts using the Organ Care System (OCS Heart System) for ex vivo perfusion resulted in a utilization rate of 81% with a mean ischemia time of 6.35 hours. A 90-day and 6-month survival was 94.7% and 88%, respectively.[33]

DCD transplantations have shown good promise, with one trial demonstrating a 4-year mortality rate of 4.4% and good clinical outcomes among the surviving patients.[34]

The success of antiviral therapy for hepatitis C virus (HCV) has allowed for the safe transplantation from donors who are seropositive, with documentation of safe and successful treatment of HCV viremia among recipients.[35]

Before a donor heart may be harvested, permission for donation must be obtained, the suitability of the heart for donation must be ascertained, and the diagnosis of brain death must be made. Initial functional and structural evaluation of the potential donor heart should be done with electrocardiography (ECG) and transthoracic echocardiography. Normal LV function predicts suitability for heart transplantation, and subsequent management of the donor may be guided by other invasive monitors, such as PA catheters or serial echocardiography.[29] Coronary angiography may be performed on patients ≥40 years of age.[29] Donor-recipient factors such as size, ABO compatibility, and antihuman leukocyte antigen (HLA)-antibody compatibility are also assessed. Logistic factors, including ischemic organ time, must be considered. Finally, the harvesting surgeon will directly inspect the donor heart.[29]

B. Determination of Brain Death

In the United States, The Uniform Determination of Death Act defines death as either (1) the irreversible cessation of circulatory and respiratory functions or (2) irreversible cessation of all functions of the entire brain, including the brainstem. A determination of death must be made in accordance with accepted medical standards. For the diagnosis of brain death to be made, the patient's core body temperature must be >32.5 °C, and no drug with the potential to alter neurologic or neuromuscular function must be present.

C. Pathophysiology of Brain Death

When brain death results from severe brain injury, increased intracranial pressure results in progressive herniation and ischemia of the brainstem. Subsequent hemodynamic instability and endocrine and metabolic disturbances disrupt homeostasis and may render organs unsuitable for transplantation (Table 21.5).

TABLE 21.5 Incidence of Pathophysiologic Changes After Brainstem Death

Hypotension	80%
Diabetes insipidus	46%-86%
Disseminated intravascular coagulation	28%-55%
Cardiac arrhythmias	25%-32%
Pulmonary edema	13%-18%
Systolic myocardial dysfunction	42%
Thrombocytopenia	56%

Reprinted by permission from Springer: Maciel CB, Greer DM. ICU Management of the potential organ donor: state of the art. *Curr Neurol Neurosci Rep.* 2016;16(9):86. © 2016 Springer Science Business Media New York.

1. **Cardiovascular function**

   In an attempt to maintain cerebral blood flow to the increasingly ischemic brain stem, blood pressure (BP) and HR rise. While usually transient, this adrenergically mediated "sympathetic storm" may precipitate ECG and echocardiographic findings, consistent with myocardial ischemia.[36,37] Occasionally, severe systemic HTN may persist and require management.[36,37] Hypotension will affect most brain-dead patients and may be refractory to pressors.[36,37] Hypotension may result from hypovolemia caused by traumatic blood loss, central diabetes insipidus (DI), or osmotic therapy for the management of elevated intracranial pressure. Loss of sympathetic tone resulting in blunted vasomotor reflexes, vasodilatation, and impaired myocardial contractility also contributes to hypotension.[36,37] Noxious stimuli may induce exaggerated hypertensive responses mediated by intact spinal sympathetic reflexes that are no longer inhibited by descending pathways. Despite optimal donor support, terminal cardiac arrhythmias may occur within 48-72 hours of brain death.

2. **Endocrine dysfunction**

   Dysfunction of the posterior pituitary gland occurs in a majority of brain-dead organ donors. The loss of antidiuretic hormone (ADH) results in DI, which is manifested by polyuria, hypovolemia, and hypernatremia.[36,37] Derangements in other electrolytes including potassium, magnesium, and calcium may also occur as a result of DI. Dysfunction of the anterior pituitary gland has been inconsistently described, with hemodynamic and electrolyte disturbances attributable in part to loss of thyroid-stimulating hormone (TSH), growth hormone (GH), and adrenocorticotropic hormone (ACTH).[36-38] Plasma concentrations of glucose may become variable (most often elevated), due to changes in serum cortisol levels, the use of catecholamine therapy, progressive insulin resistance, and the administration of glucose-containing fluids.[37]

3. **Pulmonary function**

   Hypoxemia resulting from lung trauma, infection, or pulmonary edema may occur following brain death. Pulmonary edema in this setting may be neurogenic, cardiogenic, or inflammatory in origin.[37]

4. **Temperature regulation**

   Thermoregulation by the hypothalamus is lost after brain death. Increased heat loss occurs because of an inability to vasoconstrict, along with a reduction in metabolic activity, which puts brain-dead organ donors at risk for hypothermia. Adverse consequences of hypothermia include cardiac dysfunction, arrhythmias, decreased tissue oxygen delivery, coagulopathy, and cold-induced diuresis.[36]

5. **Coagulation**

   Coagulopathy may result from hypothermia and from dilution of clotting factors following massive transfusion and fluid resuscitation. Disseminated intravascular coagulation occurs in 28%-55% of brain-dead organ donors due to the release of tissue thromboplastin and activation of the coagulation cascade by the ischemic brain.[37]

D. **Management of the Cardiac Transplant Donor**

   Posttransplant graft function is in part dependent on optimal donor management before organ harvesting. Strategies for the management of brain-dead organ donors seek to stabilize their physiology through active resuscitation so that the functional integrity of potentially transplantable organs is maintained.[36,37]

1. **Cardiovascular function**

   Donor systemic BP and central venous pressure (CVP) should be monitored continuously using arterial and central venous catheters.[31] Goals include a mean arterial pressure >60-70 mm Hg, a CVP of 6-10 mm Hg, urinary output >1 mL/kg/h, and a left ventricular ejection fraction (LVEF) of >45%.[36,37] The initial treatment step in maintaining hemodynamic stability is maintenance of euvolemia using aggressive replacement of intravascular volume with crystalloids, colloids, and packed red blood cells (pRBCs) if the hemoglobin (Hgb) concentration is <10 g/dL or the hematocrit is <30%.[31,36]

   If hemodynamic stability is not restored with fluid resuscitation, placement of a PA catheter, use of echocardiography, or continuous CO monitoring should be used to assess right- and left-sided intracardiac pressures, CO, and systemic vascular resistance (SVR).[36,37] The use of inotropes and vasopressors should be guided by these additional diagnostics. Dopamine and vasopressin are recommended as first-line agents, with epinephrine, norepinephrine, phenylephrine, and dobutamine utilized for severe shock.[37] However, prolonged use of catecholamines at high doses should be avoided due to potential downregulation of β-receptors on the donor heart and the negative impact this may have on graft function after cardiac transplant.[36] High-dose α-adrenergic receptor agonists should be used cautiously, as peripheral and splanchnic vasoconstriction may result in decreased perfusion of other potential donor organs and metabolic acidosis. Vasopressin has catecholamine-sparing effects without impairing graft function.[31,36]

   Hormonal replacement is indicated in brain-dead donors with hemodynamic instability refractory to fluids, catecholamines, and vasopressin; however, its efficacy has not been completely validated.[37] Regimens vary widely, but a combination of thyroid hormone, corticosteroid, ADH, and insulin seems to maximize organ yield.[37] All are part of the UNOS standard donor management protocol.

2. **Fluid and electrolytes**

   Hypernatremia (sodium >155 mEq/L) in the donor has been associated with higher rates of primary graft failure, particularly in liver transplantation.[36,37] Aggressive treatment of DI with 1-desamino-8-D-arginine vasopressin (ddAVP) is indicated. IV fluids should be given to replace urinary losses and to maintain urine output.[37] Normoglycemia (120-180 mg/dL) should be achieved through the use of dextrose-containing fluids and/or an insulin infusion.[37] Metabolic acidosis and respiratory alkalosis should be corrected, with a goal pH of 7.40-7.45.[37]

3. **Pulmonary function**

   If lung procurement is also being considered, a lung protective management protocol consisting of lower tidal volumes (6-8 mL/kg) and higher positive end-expiratory pressure (PEEP) of 8-10 cm H_2O and optimal positioning of the patient (head of bed >30°) should be initiated. Optimal volume management with goal CVP of 6-8 mm Hg and PCWP of 6-10 mm Hg has been shown to improve donor lung function without increasing other organ (heart/liver/kidney) dysfunction.[37]

   Efforts to prevent pulmonary aspiration, atelectasis, and infection are warranted. Neurogenic pulmonary edema should be managed with PEEP, careful diuresis, and iNO in appropriate donors.[37]

4. **Temperature**

   Monitoring of core temperature is mandatory, as hypothermia adversely affects coagulation, cardiac rhythm, and oxygen delivery. The use of warmed IV fluids, blankets, and humidifiers may prevent hypothermia.

5. **Coagulation**

   Different transplant centers have individual guidelines for blood component therapy for the management of coagulopathy. In general, component therapy should be guided by repeated donor platelet and clotting factor measurements. Generally accepted goals include an international normalized ratio (INR) of <1.5 and a platelet count of >100,000/mm³.[37] Antifibrinolytics to control donor bleeding are not recommended due to the risk of microvascular thrombosis.

E. **Anesthetic Management of the Donor**

Anesthetic management of the donor during organ harvesting is an extension of preoperative management. If the lungs are to be harvested, a lung protective ventilation strategy should be employed as well as judicious fluid management to keep the CVP <10 cm H_2O.[39] Vasopressors to maintain adequate BP, hormone replacement, and transfusion per institutional protocol to keep Hgb >8 g/dL and to manage coagulopathy should be continued through the intraoperative period.[39] Although intact spinal reflexes may result in HTN, tachycardia, and muscle movement, these signs do not indicate cerebral function or pain perception. Nondepolarizing muscle relaxants may be used to prevent spinal reflex–mediated muscle contraction.

F. **Organ Harvest Technique**

After initial dissection, the patient is fully heparinized. The perfusion-sensitive organs (ie, kidneys and liver) are removed before cardiectomy. The donor heart is excised en bloc via median sternotomy after dissection of the pericardial attachments. The superior (SVC) and inferior venae cavae (IVC) are ligated first, allowing exsanguination. The aorta is cross-clamped, and cold cardioplegia administered. The aorta and PAs are transected, leaving the native donor arterial segments as long as possible. Finally, the pulmonary veins are individually divided after lifting the donor organ out of the thoracic cavity. Most donor hearts are currently preserved with specialized cold colloid solutions (eg, University of Wisconsin [UW], histidine-tryptophan-ketoglutarate [HTK], or Celsior solution) and placed in cold storage at 4 °C.[32] When this technique is used, optimal myocardial function after transplantation is achieved when the donor heart ischemic time is <4 hours.[40]

Ex vivo machine perfusion (EVMP) has emerged in recent years as an opportunity to expand the donor pool and assess the viability of grafts between procurement and transplantation. In the United States, The TransMedics Organ Care System (OCS) is Food and Drug Administration (FDA) approved for lung transplantation, and its use is under evaluation for HLT. In the OCS model, the donor heart is arrested with warm cardioplegia solution, then cannulated onto the OCS. The system is primed with donor blood and a proprietary perfusate that includes steroids, antibiotics, and vitamins. This is circulated through the circuit and an oxygenator via a pulsatile pump. The OCS permits the evaluation of marginal grafts before transplantation, potentially increasing the supply of organs. It also has promise for patients whose operative time is prolonged due to re-entry sternotomy, the presence of a VAD, or complex anatomy, such as congenital heart disease. Initial trials have demonstrated similar recipient survival and rates of severe rejection, despite longer out-of-body times among the OCS grafts.[41]

IV. **Surgical Techniques for Cardiac Transplantation**

A. **Orthotopic Cardiac Transplantation**

Over 98% of cardiac transplants performed are orthotopic. The recipient is placed on standard cardiopulmonary bypass (CPB) and, if present, the PA catheter withdrawn into the SVC. The femoral vessels are often selected for arterial and venous CPB cannulation in patients undergoing repeat sternotomy. Otherwise, the distal ascending aorta is cannulated, as well as bicaval venous cannulas with snares placed around the SVC and IVC, so that the heart can be completely excluded from the native circulation. The aorta and PAs are then clamped and divided. Depending on the implantation technique (Figure 21.3), either both native atria or a single left atrial cuff containing the pulmonary veins is preserved. The native atrial appendages are discarded because of the risk of postoperative thrombus formation.

The donor heart is inspected for the presence of a patent foramen ovale. If patent, it is surgically closed, as right-to-left interatrial shunting and hypoxemia may occur in the presence of elevated right-sided pressures following transplantation. The donor and recipient left atria are anastomosed first, followed by the right atria, or both cavae when a bicaval anastomotic technique is chosen. The subsequent order of anastomoses varies depending on the donor heart ischemic time and the experience of the surgeon. The donor and recipient aortas are joined, and the aortic cross-clamp removed with the patient in Trendelenburg position to decrease air embolism. After completion of the PA anastomosis and placement of temporary epicardial pacing wires, the heart is de-aired and the patient separated from CPB.

1. **Biatrial implantation**

Biatrial implantation is the technique originally described by Barnard. It preserves portions of the recipient's native atria to create two atrial anastomoses. Biatrial orthotopic heart transplantation has been performed successfully for over four decades and has the advantage of being relatively simple and possibly faster to perform.[42] It is, however, falling out of favor. The biatrial technique puts the sinoatrial node at risk of injury, redundant atrial tissue

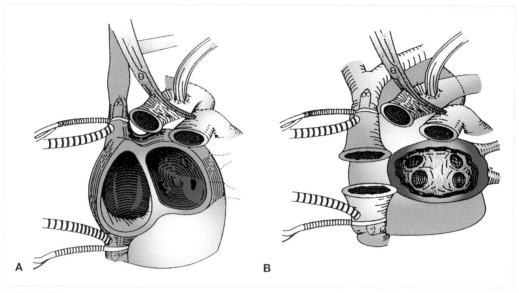

FIGURE 21.3 Surgical techniques for cardiac transplantation. **(A)** Biatrial technique. The donor heart is anastomosed to the main bulk of the recipient's native right and left atria. **(B)** Bicaval technique. The donor heart left atrium is anastomosed to a single left atrial cuff, including the pulmonary veins, in the recipient. (From Aziz TM, Burgess MI, El Gamel A, et al. Orthotopic cardiac transplantation technique: A survey of current practice. *Ann Thorac Surg.* 1999;68:1242–1246. Figure 1.)

may contribute to atrial dysrhythmias, and distortion of the right atrium may contribute to a higher risk for tricuspid regurgitation.[42] Although patients receiving biatrial transplant experience a higher incidence of permanent pacemakers (2.0% vs 9.1%) and tricuspid regurgitation, no definitive difference in long-term survival has been demonstrated.[42-44]

2. **Bicaval implantation**

The bicaval implantation technique is a modification of the biatrial technique. Only a single, small left atrial cuff containing the pulmonary veins is preserved in the recipient. Bicaval and left atrial anastomoses are performed (Figure 21.3B). The bicaval technique is growing in popularity, particularly at higher volume transplant centers.[42] Demonstrated advantages of the bicaval technique include a higher incidence of postoperative sinus rhythm, lower right atrial pressures, a reduced need for permanent pacemaker, and lower incidence of tricuspid regurgitation.[42-44] A decreased risk of perioperative mortality may exist.[42]

B. **Heterotopic Cardiac Transplantation**

Heterotopic transplantation accounts for <1% of cardiac transplantation procedures performed annually. In this technique, the recipient's heart is not excised. Instead, the donor heart is placed within the right anterior thorax and anastomosed to the recipient's native heart such that a parallel circulation is established. The recipient and donor atria are anastomosed, followed by the aortas. An artificial conduit usually joins the PAs, with the native and donor RVs ejecting into the native PA. Similarly, both the native and donor LVs eject into the native aorta. Thus, the recipient's RV, which is conditioned to eject against elevated PA pressures, will provide most of the right-sided ventricular output, whereas the healthy donor LV will make the major contribution to left-sided ventricular output. Situations in which heterotopic cardiac transplantation may be advantageous include recipients with severe pulmonary HTN, a small donor-to-recipient size ratio, and a marginal donor heart.[45] Disadvantages of heterotopic cardiac transplantation include relatively high operative mortality, a requirement for continued medical treatment of the failing native heart, the potential for the native heart to be a thromboembolism source, compromised pulmonary function due to placement of donor heart in the right chest, and possible increased incidence of tachyarrhythmias in both the native and heterotopic hearts.[45]

V. **Preoperative Management of the Cardiac Transplant Patient**

A. **Timing and Coordination**

When planning cardiac transplantation, important considerations include the time required for donor organ transport and potential for failure to complete recipient cannulation in a timely manner (eg, repeat sternotomy). Since the timing of heart transplants is dictated by donor availability, transplantation can take place at any hour of the day. Ideally, to minimize ischemic time, anesthetic induction of the recipient should be timed so that the recipient is already on CPB when the donor heart arrives. However, since the attendant risks of general anesthesia are magnified in the recipient, who, by definition, has advanced HF, induction of anesthesia ought to be delayed until a definitive "go" is received from the procurement team.

B. **Preoperative Evaluation**

The anesthesiologist usually has limited time for preoperative assessment of the cardiac transplant recipient. The presentation of this patient population varies widely, from a stable outpatient requiring no inotropic or mechanical support to a critically ill inpatient requiring cardiac support ranging from inotropes to IABP to ECMO.[46] These recipients will have been under the care of a medical team experienced in the management of HF, and their medical therapy is likely to have already been optimized. When the recipient is already admitted to the intensive care unit (ICU), all aspects of their ongoing care should be reviewed, including pulmonary status and ventilation settings, the presence of invasive monitors and existing venous access, the use of inotropes and/or pressors, and the use of MCS devices. In any case, the preoperative anesthetic evaluation should include a thorough history, physical examination, review of the patient's medical record, and assessment of the patient's functional status.[46] The ECG, echocardiogram, chest x-ray, and cardiac catheterization results should be noted, and all hematologic, renal, and liver function tests reviewed.

1. **Concomitant organ dysfunction**

Chronic systemic hypoperfusion and venous congestion in the recipient may produce reversible hepatic and renal dysfunction. Mild-to-moderate elevations of hepatic enzymes, bilirubin, and prolongation of prothrombin time are common. Preoperative hepatic dysfunction and anticoagulant medication may also contribute to the abnormal coagulation profile frequently observed in cardiac transplant recipients. Blood urea nitrogen is commonly elevated in patients with end-stage heart disease due to chronic hypoperfusion and the concomitant prerenal effects of high-dose diuretics.

2. **Preoperative medications**

Preoperative inotropic support should be continued throughout the pre-CPB period. Patients receiving digitalis and diuretics have an increased risk of dysrhythmias in the presence of hypokalemia. Anticoagulants such as warfarin, heparin, and aspirin may increase the need for perioperative blood product administration. Prothrombin complex concentrates (PCCs) can safely be used to reverse warfarin while reducing the transfusion of fresh-frozen plasma before transplantation.[47] Preoperative use of amiodarone is associated with an increased rate of primary graft dysfunction (PGD) and increased mortality.[48,49]

3. **Preoperative monitoring**

The position, function, and duration of invasive monitoring catheters should be noted. The function and settings of IABPs and VADs should be reviewed. If a CIED is present, it should be interrogated and the antitachyarrhythmia/rate responsiveness functions suspended in the operating room after external defibrillation pads have been applied.[46] Patients with invasive monitoring and/or MCS require extra personnel and vigilance to ensure safe transport from the ICU to the operating room.

4. **The combined heart-lung recipient**

The combined HLT recipient often requires special preoperative evaluation. Cystic fibrosis recipients should first have an otolaryngologic evaluation before being placed on a waiting list. Many of these patients will require endoscopic maxillary antrostomies for sinus access and monthly antibiotic irrigation. This measure has decreased the incidence of serious posttransplant bacterial infections in that patient population. Previous smokers must undergo screening to exclude malignancy. A negative sputum cytology, thoracic CT scan, bronchoscopy, and otolaryngologic evaluation are required. In addition, left heart catheterization, coronary angiography, and a carotid duplex scan may be performed in previous smokers.

VI. **Anesthetic Management of the Cardiac Transplant Recipient**

  A. **Premedication**

  The patient with HF has elevated levels of circulating catecholamines and is preload dependent. Even a small dose of sedative medication may result in vasodilatation and hemodynamic decompensation. Therefore, sedatives should be avoided or carefully titrated, along with supplemental oxygen.

  Patients presenting for cardiac transplantation should be considered "full stomach," as most present with short notice. If oral cyclosporine or azathioprine is started preoperatively, gastric emptying is slowed. Oral sodium citrate and/or IV metoclopramide may be useful in raising gastric pH and reducing gastric volumes.

  B. **Importance of Aseptic Technique**

  Perioperative immunosuppressive therapy places the cardiac transplant recipient at increased risk of infection. All invasive procedures should be done under aseptic or sterile conditions.

  Many patients will arrive to the operating room with central venous lines for the administration of inotropes. The removal of existing lines should be considered before the start of surgery, as they carry a known infectious risk.[50]

  C. **Monitoring**

  Noninvasive monitoring should include a standard 5-lead ECG, BP measurement, pulse oximetry, capnography, and nasopharyngeal temperature. If not already in situ, large-bore peripheral and central venous access should be obtained. Invasive monitoring should include systemic arterial as well as CVP and/or PA pressures and a urinary catheter. Intraoperative transesophageal echocardiography (TEE) is standard practice.[46] A PA catheter may be helpful in the post-CPB period, allowing monitoring of CO, ventricular filling pressures, and calculation of SVR and PVR. The PA catheter can be floated preoperatively, however will have to be pulled back into the SVC before cardiectomy and transplant, and then refloated afterward. Alternatively, the PA catheter can be placed initially into the SVC and placed into the PA with assistance of the surgeon during PA anastomosis or floated into the PA after separation from CPB. Additional monitors (eg, cerebral oximetry) may be indicated in selected patients.[46] Traditionally, catheterization of the right internal jugular vein has been avoided to preserve this route for endomyocardial biopsies (EMBs) that are routinely performed after transplant to screen for myocardial rejection. It can be noted, however, that difficulty with EMB by alternative routes has not been reported in circumstances where the right internal jugular vein was used for central venous access.

  D. **Considerations for Repeat Sternotomy**

  Many cardiac transplant recipients will have undergone previous cardiac surgery and are at increased risk of inadvertent trauma to the great vessels or preexisting coronary artery bypass grafts during sternotomy. Patients having repeat sternotomy should have external defibrillation pads placed before induction and cross-matched, irradiated pRBCs available in the operating room before sternotomy. The potential for a prolonged surgical dissection time in these patients may necessitate anesthetic induction earlier than usual in order to coordinate with donor heart arrival. Other considerations for repeat sternotomy include the potential for bleeding and the need for femoral or axillary CPB cannulation.

  E. **Anesthetic Induction**

   1. **Hemodynamic goals**

   Cardiac transplant recipients typically have hypokinetic, noncompliant ventricles sensitive to alterations in myocardial preload and afterload. Hemodynamic priorities for anesthetic induction are to maintain HR and contractility, avoid acute changes in preload and afterload, and prevent increases in PVR. Inotropic support is very often required during anesthetic induction and throughout the pre-CPB period. Owing to afterload sensitivity, epinephrine or norepinephrine infusions are probably preferable to phenylephrine or vasopressin infusions for BP support.

2. **Aspiration precautions**

Rapid sequence induction with maintenance of cricoid pressure should be considered when the patient is not appropriately fasted, as is often the case in these situations.

3. **Anesthetic agents**

Due to the slow circulation time in patients with end-stage HF, a delayed response to IV anesthetic agents is common. IV drugs commonly used for anesthetic induction of the cardiac transplant recipient include etomidate (0.1-0.3 mg/kg) in combination with fentanyl (2.5-10 μg/kg) or sufentanil (5-8 μg/kg). High-dose narcotic regimens (eg, fentanyl 25-50 μg/kg) have also been used successfully. Bradycardia occurring in response to high-dose narcotics should be treated promptly, as CO in patients with end-stage heart disease is HR dependent. Small doses of midazolam, ketamine, or scopolamine help ensure amnesia but should be used cautiously as they may synergistically lower SVR and induce hypotension.

4. **Muscle relaxants**

Muscle relaxants with minimal cardiovascular effects (eg, rocuronium, cisatracurium, or vecuronium) are most commonly utilized. As an added advantage, their relatively rapid onset facilitates rapid sequence induction in patients at risk for aspiration.[46]

F. **Anesthetic Maintenance**

During the pre-CPB period, anesthetic goals include maintenance of hemodynamic stability and end-organ perfusion. Anesthetic maintenance regimens have historically been narcotic based with supplemental inhalational agents and benzodiazepines. Although most inhalational agents have negative inotropic effects, low concentrations of these agents are usually well tolerated and decrease the risk of awareness. Anesthetic depth can be difficult to assess in this patient population, as the sympathetic response to light planes of anesthesia is often blunted. The use of narcotic-based anesthetic regimens may also increase the risk of awareness during anesthesia. Antifibrinolytics such as tranexamic acid or epsilon-aminocaproic acid should be administered following anesthetic induction to reduce bleeding, especially in the case of a repeat sternotomy.

In recent years, narcotic-based techniques seem to have fallen out of favor, and lower dose narcotic-based techniques have become popular to facilitate so-called "Fast-Track" anesthesia, with the goal of extubation in <6-8 hours. A 2016 Cochran review found that risks of mortality and postoperative complications were similar in fast-track patients compared to those receiving conventional techniques.[51] Whether this translates to heart transplant recipients remains to be seen.

G. **Cardiopulmonary Bypass**

CPB for cardiac transplantation is similar to that employed for routine cardiac surgical procedures. Femoral venous and arterial cannulation sites are frequently chosen in patients undergoing repeat sternotomy. Moderate hypothermia (28-30 °C) is commonly used during CPB to improve myocardial protection. Hemofiltration and/or mannitol administration are common during CPB, as patients with HF often have a large intravascular blood volume and coexistent renal impairment. Although immunosuppressive regimens vary among transplantation centers, high-dose IV glucocorticoids such as methylprednisolone are frequently administered before aortic cross-clamp release to reduce the likelihood of hyperacute rejection. Immunosuppressive induction therapy with an interleukin-2 receptor (IL2R) antagonist, or a polyclonal antilymphocyte antibody, has been employed in over 50% of patients between 2009 and 2014 in order to reduce the risk of T-cell rejection.[2] However, no consensus on the safety and efficacy of induction therapy exists.[46,52] The availability and timing of immunosuppressive medications should be discussed with the transplant team ahead of time.

VII. **Postcardiopulmonary Bypass**

Before CPB termination, the patient should be normothermic, and all electrolyte and acid-base abnormalities corrected. Complete de-airing of the heart before aortic cross-clamp removal is essential. TEE may be particularly useful for assessing the efficacy of cardiac de-airing maneuvers, as well as initial impressions of donor heart contractility and valvular function. Infusion of inotropic agents should be initiated before separation from CPB. An HR of 90-110 beats/min, a systemic mean arterial BP >65 mm Hg, and ventricular filling pressures of ~12-16 mm Hg (CVP) and 14-18 mm Hg (PCWP) are often required in the immediate post-CPB period. Although inotropic support is usually required for several days, patients are often extubated within 24 hours and discharged from the ICU by the third postoperative day. Clinical considerations in the immediate postoperative period include the following:

A. **Autonomic Denervation of the Transplanted Heart**

During orthotopic cardiac transplantation, the cardiac autonomic plexus is transected, leaving the transplanted heart without autonomic innervation. The transplanted heart thus does not respond to direct autonomic nervous system stimulation or to drugs that act indirectly through the autonomic nervous system (eg, atropine). The denervated, transplanted heart responds to direct-acting agents, such as catecholamines. Transient bradycardia and slow nodal rhythms are common following aortic cross-clamp release. An infusion of a direct-acting β-adrenergic receptor agonist such as isoproterenol or dobutamine is frequently initiated before termination of CPB and titrated to achieve an HR around 100 beats/min. Newly transplanted hearts unresponsive to pharmacologic stimulation may require temporary epicardial pacing. Although most initial dysrhythmias resolve, some cardiac transplant recipients require placement of a permanent pacemaker.

B. **Right Ventricular Dysfunction**

RV failure is a significant cause of early morbidity and mortality and is one of the most common causes of failure to separate from CPB.[46] Acute RV failure following cardiac transplantation may be due to prolonged donor heart ischemic time, mechanical obstruction at the level of the PA anastomosis, pulmonary HTN (both preexisting and protamine induced), donor-recipient size mismatch, and acute rejection.[46] RV distension and hypokinesis may be diagnosed by TEE or direct observation of the surgical field. Other findings suggesting RV failure include elevations in the CVP, PA pressure, or the transpulmonary gradient (>15 mm Hg).

Goals for managing RV dysfunction include maintaining systemic BP, lowering PVR, and minimizing RV dilation. Maintaining atrioventricular synchrony is especially important in optimizing RV preload. Correction of electrolyte and acid-base disturbances and the use of inotropic support may improve RV function. Optimizing ventilator settings and the use of inhaled pulmonary vasodilators may reduce RV afterload. Useful inotropes include epinephrine, dobutamine, isoproterenol, and milrinone; the latter three agents may also reduce PVR.[46] Inhaled pulmonary vasodilators include prostacyclin (PGI2), prostaglandin E1 (PGE1), and nitric oxide (NO).[46] NO selectively reduces PVR by activating guanylate cyclase in vascular smooth muscle cells, producing an increase in cGMP and smooth muscle relaxation. Little systemic effect is seen as it is inactivated by Hgb and thus has a very short half-life of only 6 seconds. NO administration results in the formation of the toxic metabolites nitrogen dioxide and methemoglobin. In the presence of severe LV dysfunction, selective dilation of the pulmonary vasculature by NO may lead to an increase in PCWP and pulmonary edema. PGI2 is an arachidonic acid derivative with a half-life of 3-6 minutes. It binds to a prostanoid receptor and causes an increase in intracellular cAMP, and consequently vasodilation. PGI2 has been shown to be efficacious for over 20 years in heart transplant patients.[46] Relative to NO, PGI2 is less costly, easier to administer, and does not create toxic metabolites. It may, however, cause a degree of systemic hypotension due to its longer half-life and may be implicated in increased bleeding due to inhibition of platelet function.[53] RV failure refractory to medical treatment may require insertion of a right-sided VAD or initiation of extracorporeal circulation (ie, ECMO).

C. **Left Ventricular Dysfunction**

Post-CPB LV dysfunction may result from prolonged donor heart ischemic time, inadequate myocardial perfusion, intracoronary embolization of intracavitary air, or surgical manipulation. The incidence of post-CPB LV dysfunction is greater in donors requiring prolonged, high-dose inotropic support before organ harvest. Continued postoperative inotropic support with dobutamine, epinephrine, or norepinephrine may be required. MCS, with IABP or even ECMO, might occasionally be required as well.

D. Coagulation

Coagulopathy following cardiac transplantation is common, and perioperative bleeding should be treated early and aggressively. Potential etiologies include hepatic dysfunction secondary to chronic hepatic venous congestion, preoperative anticoagulation, CPB-induced platelet dysfunction, hypothermia, and hemodilution of clotting factors. After ruling out surgical bleeding, blood product administration should be guided by repeated measurements of platelet count and plasma coagulation. Thromboelastography may also be helpful, especially if thromboelastograms can be viewed in real time as they develop, allowing treatment decisions to be made within minutes. Due to an increased risk of infection and graft-versus-host disease, all administered blood products should be cytomegalovirus (CMV) negative and irradiated or leukocyte depleted. RBCs and platelets should be administered through leukocyte filters. Desmopressin (ddAVP) has been shown to reduce postoperative blood loss in selected surgical patients but has not been shown to reliably decrease transfusion requirements post-CPB.[54]

E. Renal Dysfunction

Renal dysfunction, as evidenced by increased serum creatinine and oliguria, is common in the immediate postoperative period. Contributing factors include preexisting renal impairment, cyclosporine-associated renal toxicity, perioperative hypotension, and CPB. Treatment of renal dysfunction includes optimization of CO and systemic BP, as well as judicious use of diuretics to avoid volume overload.

F. Pulmonary Dysfunction

Postoperative pulmonary complications such as atelectasis, pleural effusion, and pneumonia are common and may be reduced by ventilation using PEEP, regular endobronchial suctioning, and chest physiotherapy. Bronchoscopy to clear pulmonary secretions is often useful. Pulmonary infection in the immunosuppressed recipient should be treated early and aggressively.

G. Hyperacute Allograft Rejection

Cardiac allograft hyperacute rejection is caused by preformed HLA antibodies present in the recipient. There are several explanations for the preexisting antibodies that initiate hyperacute rejection. First, prior recipients of blood transfusions may develop antibodies to major histocompatibility complex (MHC) antigens in the transfused blood. Multiple pregnancies may also expose females to fetal paternal antigens, resulting in antibody formation. Finally, prior transplant recipients may have already formed antibodies to other MHC antigens so that they may be present at the time of a second transplant. Collectively, these antibodies are formulated into a panel reactive antibody (PRA) score that represents the percentage of the population to which the recipient will likely react. Higher scores are thus associated with longer wait times as donors without these antibodies are more difficult to find. Although extremely rare, hyperacute rejection results in severe cardiac dysfunction and death within hours of transplantation. MCS until cardiac retransplantation is the only therapeutic option.

VIII. The Role of Intraoperative Transesophageal Echocardiography

Intraoperative TEE is a valuable tool for the evaluation and management of the cardiac transplant recipient. In addition to monitoring ventricular function, TEE in the pre-CPB period may be used to identify intracavitary thrombus, estimate recipient PA pressures in the absence of a PA catheter, and evaluate the aortic cannulation and cross-clamp sites for the presence of atherosclerotic disease. TEE is also used in the post-CPB period to evaluate the efficacy of cardiac de-airing, cardiac function, and surgical anastomoses. The caval and left atrial anastomoses should be evaluated for any evidence of obstruction or distortion.[55] Pulmonary venous flow should be assessed. Stenosis of the main PA should also be excluded by continuous-wave Doppler measurement of the pressure gradient across the anastomosis. After orthotopic cardiac transplantation, the long axis of the left atrium often appears larger than usual because of joining of the donor and recipient left atria. Occasionally, excess donor atrial tissue may obstruct the mitral valve orifice, resulting in pulmonary HTN and RV failure. TEE findings in the immediate post-CPB period frequently include impaired ventricular contractility, decreased diastolic compliance, septal dyskinesis, and acute mild-to-moderate tricuspid, pulmonic, and mitral valve regurgitation. Although LV size and function is typically normal on long-term echocardiographic follow-up of healthy cardiac transplant recipients, RV enlargement and tricuspid valve regurgitation persist in up to 33% of patients. Persistent tricuspid valve regurgitation may result from geometrical alterations of the right atrium or RV, asynchronous contraction of the donor and recipient atria, or valvular damage that might occur during EMB.

IX. Cardiac Transplantation Survival and Complications

Survival following cardiac transplantation in the United States in 2019 was 92.6% at 6 months and 90.6% at 12 months. Of those who underwent transplant in 2017, 3-year survival was 86%.[17] One-year survival among those aged ≥65 years was slightly lower than younger groups, though by year 5, survival was comparable among all age groups.[17] However, the cause of death varies by patient age, with younger patients being more susceptible to inadequate immunosuppression (acute rejection, cardiac allograft vasculopathy [CAV], and graft failure) and older patients being more susceptible to excessive immunosuppression (infection and renal failure).[56] Beyond the first-year posttransplant, lower survival was seen in recipients aged 18-35 years and African American recipients (5-year survival of 77.4% and 77.5%, respectively).[17] Adult death rates have declined since 2009, although they increased in the interval from 2015 to 2020 (Figure 21.4). Important causes of morbidity and mortality are infection, acute rejection, graft failure and CAV, renal insufficiency (RI), and malignancy. Other causes of long-term morbidity after transplantation include HTN, diabetes mellitus, and hyperlipidemia.

A. Infection

Infections in the early period (<30 days) are mainly nosocomial and bacterial in nature and account for 14% of deaths.[2] With the routine use of bacterial and viral prophylaxis, there has been a significant reduction in pneumocystis pneumonia infection and herpes viridae (including CMV).[57] Beyond 30 days, infection remains an important cause of mortality, reaching its peak as a primary cause of death (32%) from 31 days to 1 year posttransplant.[2]

B. Acute Rejection

Improvements in management have rendered acute rejection of the transplanted heart a less common cause of death (9%) between 2009 and 2015.[2] However, within the first year, acute rejection is seen in 28% of those aged 18-49 years and occurred less frequently among older patients (20.5% among those >65 years old).[17] Female recipients are at higher risk than males.[17] EMB remains the gold standard for confirming acute allograft rejection. Repeated EMB is associated with an increased incidence of tricuspid valve regurgitation.

C. Graft Failure and Cardiac Allograft Vasculopathy

Graft failure is the leading cause of death in the first 30 days after transplant (40%), presumably due to primary graft failure,[2] and the severity of PGD is correlated with increased mortality

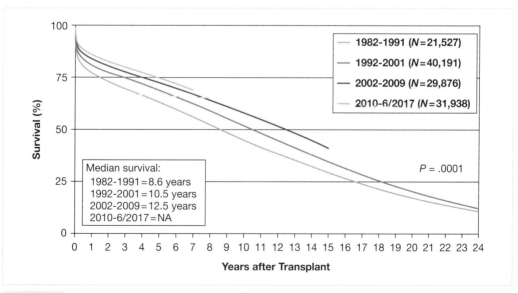

FIGURE 21.4 Survival for adult heart transplants performed between January 1982 and June 2017, stratified by era of transplant. (Reprinted from Khush KK, Cherikh WS, Chambers DC, et al. The International Thoracic Organ Transplant Registry of the International Society for Heart and Lung Transplantation: thirty-sixth adult heart transplantation report—2019; focus theme: donor and recipient size match. *J Heart Lung Transplant.* 2019;38(10):1056-1066. © 2019 Elsevier. With permission.)

risk.[58] After 30 days, chronic processes such as antibody-mediated rejection and CAV are more likely causes of graft failure. Graft failure continues to be a significant cause of death after 1 year, accounting for 17% of deaths.[2] Graft failure confirmed due to CAV becomes prominent between 1 and 3 years posttransplant and accounts for 26% of deaths.[2] The prevalence of CAV is 27% at 5 years and 47% at 10 years.[2] Significant CAV is defined angiographically by a stenosis of at least 50%. Unlike atherosclerotic CAD, CAV is characterized by a diffuse intimal hyperplasia.[57] Nonimmune risk factors for CAV include HTN, hyperlipidemia, diabetes mellitus, explosive etiology of donor brain death, hyperhomocysteinemia, and older donor age. Immune risk factors include HLA donor/recipient mismatch, recurrent cellular rejection, and antibody-mediated rejection (high PRA score). Aggressive management of risk factors is the primary strategy for preventing CAV. The diffuse nature of the vasculopathy defies percutaneous or surgical revascularization strategies.

D. **Renal Insufficiency**

RI is a strong predictor of reduced survival after transplant. Defined as a serum creatinine >2.5 mg/dL, or necessitating dialysis or kidney transplant, severe RI is identified as the primary cause of death in a significant number of patients.[59] Risks for early RI, developing within 1 year of transplant, are increased donor and recipient age, increased recipient serum creatinine at the time of transplant, the presence of a VAD, female recipient, rapamycin use at discharge, and IL2R antagonist induction.[59] Fortunately, the incidence of impaired renal function after heart transplant is decreasing, with 86% of patients transplanted between 1994 and 2005 being free of severe renal dysfunction at 5 years.[2]

E. **Malignancy**

Presumably as a consequence of long-term immunosuppression, solid-organ transplant recipients experience a higher risk for malignancy than the general population. Skin cancer is the most common malignancy in heart transplant recipients, with incidence at 1, 5, and 10 years of 1.7%, 9.3%, and 18.1%, respectively.[2] Lymphoproliferative malignancies occur less frequently than do malignancies of the skin, but their treatments are much less likely to be curative. Incidence at 1, 5, and 10 years is 0.5%, 1.1%, and 1.9%, respectively.[2] Mortality attributed to malignancy depends on the time after transplant and is as high as 21% after 10 years.[2]

F. **Immunosuppressive Drug Side Effects**

Cardiac transplant recipients require lifelong immunosuppression. Protocols vary among transplant centers; however, most regimens include triple therapy with corticosteroids, a calcineurin inhibitor, and an antiproliferative agent.[3] Immunosuppressants increase the risk of infection and are associated with numerous side effects (Table 21.6).[60] Furthermore, chronic immunosuppression increases the risk of malignancies, including skin cancers; lymphoproliferative malignancies; various adenocarcinomas; cancers of the lung, bladder, kidney, breast, and colon; and Kaposi sarcoma.

G. **Postoperative Vasoplegia Syndrome**

Postoperative vasoplegia syndrome has been described as persistent hypotension and reduced SVR immediately after cardiac surgery. It is associated with increased time on CPB and preoperative creatinine. In the cardiac transplant population, it is not associated with increased rates of PGD or mortality, though it is associated with prolonged intubation, greater blood product usage, and lengthened hospital stay.[61,62]

X. **Pediatric Cardiac Transplantation**

In the United States in 2015, children accounted for 13% of cardiac transplant recipients.[2] The primary indications for pediatric cardiac transplantation are complex congenital heart disease and idiopathic dilated cardiomyopathy (DCM).[17] At present, the majority of pediatric heart transplants take place in children >1 year of age at highly specialized pediatric centers.[17] Five-year survival rates for transplant recipients younger than 1 year, ages 1-5 years, ages 6-10 years, and ages 11-17 years are 71.2%, 78.4%, 87.5%, and 77.4%, respectively.[17] Like adult programs, pediatric cardiac transplant programs face a severe donor heart shortage. The use of implantable VADs for BTT is limited by the small body size of most pediatric transplant candidates, with only 21% of pediatric heart transplant recipients being supported by a VAD.[17]

TABLE 21.6   Immunosuppressive Agents

Agent	Mechanism of Action	Side Effects
Cyclosporine	Inhibits T-cell proliferation Inhibits interleukin-2 (IL-2) expression	Nephrotoxicity, hypertension, tremors, headache
Azathioprine	Inhibits DNA synthesis Inhibits lymphocyte proliferation	Leukopenia, thrombocytopenia, anemia, infection, hepatotoxicity, pancreatitis, nausea, vomiting, diarrhea
Corticosteroids	Decrease T-cell activation Inhibit cytokine production Inhibit leukocyte chemotaxis	Infection, hyperglycemia, hypertension, osteoporosis, adrenal suppression, myopathy, peptic ulcer disease, hyperlipidemia, psychological disturbances
Mycophenolate mofetil	Inhibits DNA synthesis Inhibits lymphocyte proliferation	Nausea, abdominal cramps, diarrhea, neutropenia, rarely hepatic and bone marrow toxicity
Tacrolimus (FK506)	Inhibits T-cell activation	Nephrotoxicity, anemia, hyperkalemia, hyperglycemia, hypertension, nausea, vomiting
OKT3	Opsonizes and lyses T cells	Fever, chills, hypotension, bronchospasm, pulmonary edema, aseptic meningitis, seizures, nausea, vomiting, diarrhea
Antilymphocyte globulin	Opsonizes and lyses T cells	Anaphylaxis, leukopenia, thrombocytopenia, hypotension, infection, fever, chills, hepatitis, serum sickness
Rapamycin	Promotes T-cell apoptosis	Abdominal pain; weakness; back pain; headache; upset stomach; swelling of the hands, feet, ankles, or lower legs; joint pain; insomnia; tremor; rash; fever
Basiliximab or daclizumab	Interleukin-2 receptor blocker inhibits IL-2 dependent T-cell activation	Anaphylaxis, abdominal pain, back pain, fever or chills, loss of energy or weakness, sore throat, vomiting, white patches in the mouth or throat, tremor

XI. **Combined Heart-Lung Transplantation**

Since 2014, an average of only 37 HLTs were done in the United States per year.[63] Donor procurement is of critical importance to the success of the operation, especially with respect to lung preservation. However, current techniques have led to safe procurement with ischemic times up to 6 hours.

The operation is performed using a double- or single-lumen endotracheal tube with the patient in the supine position. The surgical approach is generally through a median sternotomy, with particular emphasis on preservation of the phrenic, vagal, and recurrent laryngeal nerves.[64] After fully heparinizing the recipient, the ascending aorta is cannulated near the base of the innominate artery, and the venae cavae are individually cannulated laterally and snared. CPB with systemic cooling to 28-30 °C is instituted, and the heart is excised at the midatrial level. The aorta is divided just above the aortic valve, and the PA is divided at its bifurcation. The left atrial remnant is then divided vertically at a point halfway between the right and left pulmonary veins. Following division of the pulmonary ligament, the left lung is moved into the field, allowing full dissection of the posterior aspect of the left hilum, being careful to avoid the vagus nerve posteriorly. After this is completed, the left main PA is divided, and the left main bronchus is stapled and divided. The same technique of hilar dissection and division is repeated on the right side, and both lungs removed from the chest. Meticulous hemostasis of the bronchial vessels is necessary, as this area of dissection is obscured once graft implantation is completed. Once hemostasis is achieved, the trachea is divided at the carina.

The donor heart-lung block is removed from its transport container, prepared, and then lowered into the chest, passing the right lung beneath the right phrenic nerve pedicle. The left lung is then gently manipulated under the left phrenic nerve pedicle. The tracheal anastomosis is then performed, and the lungs ventilated with room air at half-normal tidal volumes to inflate the lungs and reduce atelectasis. The heart is then anastomosed as previously described. After separation from CPB, the patient is usually ventilated with an F_{IO_2} of 40% and PEEP at 3-5 cm H_2O, being very careful to avoid high inspiratory pressures that may disrupt the tracheal anastomosis.

III. Cardiac Anesthesia

XII. **Anesthesia for the Patient With History of Heart Transplant**

Many heart transplant recipients will undergo additional surgical procedures in their lifetime. Common surgical procedures following cardiac transplantation are listed in Table 21.7. Many of these subsequent surgical procedures are attributable to sequelae of the transplant surgery itself, atherosclerosis, and immunosuppression. Optimal anesthetic management of the previous transplant recipient requires full understanding of the patient's ongoing physiology and pharmacology.

A. **Physiology of the Previously Transplanted Patient**

During orthotopic cardiac transplantation, the cardiac autonomic plexus is transected, leaving the transplanted heart without autonomic innervation.[65] Due to the absence of parasympathetic innervation of the sinoatrial node, the transplanted heart will exhibit a resting HR of 90-110 beats/min. In addition, reflex bradycardia does not occur. Increases in HR and SV in response to stress are blunted, as they depend on circulating adrenal hormones. Although most transplanted hearts have near-normal contractility at rest, stress may reveal a reduction in functional reserve. The Starling volume-CO relationship, however, tends to remain intact.

A higher rate of dysrhythmia is seen due to the absence of parasympathetic tone coupled with conduction abnormalities. First-degree atrioventricular block is common, and 30% of patients will have right bundle branch block.[65]

B. **Pharmacology of the Previously Transplanted Patient**

Autonomic denervation of the transplanted heart alters the pharmacodynamic activity of many drugs (Table 21.8). Drugs that mediate their actions through the autonomic nervous system are ineffective in altering HR and contractility. In contrast, drugs that act directly on the heart are effective. The β-adrenergic response of the transplanted heart to direct-acting catecholamines such as epinephrine is often increased. Reflex bradycardia or tachycardia in response to changes in systemic arterial BP is absent. Narcotic-induced decreases in HR are frequently diminished in the transplanted heart. Drugs with mixed activity (eg, dopamine and ephedrine) will mediate an effect only through their direct actions. Vagolytic drugs such as atropine and glycopyrrolate will not alter HR, although their peripheral anticholinergic activity remains unaffected. Anticholinergic coadministration with reversal of neuromuscular blockade is still warranted to counteract the noncardiac muscarinic effects of neostigmine or edrophonium.

C. **Preoperative Evaluation**

A thorough medical history, physical examination, and review of the medical record should be undertaken. Current medications should be noted. Particular attention should be paid to determining cardiac allograft function, evidence of rejection or infection, complications of

---

TABLE 21.7 Common Surgical Procedures Following Cardiac Transplantation

Reexploration for mediastinal bleeding

Infectious complications

Laparotomy

Craniotomy

Thoracotomy

Abscess drainage

Bronchoscopy

Steroid-related complications

Hip arthroplasty or pinning

Laparotomy for perforated viscus

Cataract excision

Vitrectomy

Scleral buckle

Aortic or peripheral vascular surgery and amputation

Pancreatic and biliary tract surgery

Retransplantation

TABLE 21.8   Drug Effects on the Denervated Heart

Drug	Action	Heart Rate	Blood Pressure
Atropine	Indirect	–	–
Digoxin	Direct	–/↓	–
Dopamine	Indirect and direct	↑	↑
Ephedrine	Indirect and direct	–/↑	–/↑
Fentanyl	Indirect	–	–
Isoproterenol	Direct	↑	–/↓
Neostigmine	Indirect	–/↓	–
Norepinephrine	Direct	↑	↑
Pancuronium	Indirect	–	–
Phenylephrine	Direct	–	↑
Verapamil	Direct	↓	↓

↑, increased; ↓, decreased; –, no effect.

immunosuppression, and end-organ disease. Systemic HTN is common, and a significant proportion of patients will have CAV within 1 year of cardiac transplantation. The absence of angina pectoris does not exclude significant CAD because the transplanted heart is denervated. The patient's activity level and exercise tolerance are good indicators of allograft function. Symptoms of dyspnea and HF suggest significant CAD or myocardial rejection. The presentation of infection may be atypical in immunosuppressed patients, with fever and leukocytosis often absent. Soft-tissue changes in the patient's airway may occur due to lymphoproliferative disease and corticosteroid administration. Cyclosporine may cause gingival hyperplasia and friability. Hematocrit, coagulation profile, electrolytes, and creatinine should be checked because immunosuppressive therapy is commonly associated with anemia, thrombocytopenia, electrolyte disturbances, and renal dysfunction. Recent chest x-rays, ECGs, and coronary angiograms should be reviewed. More than one P wave may be seen on the ECG in patients in whom cardiac transplantation was performed using a biatrial technique (Figure 21.5). Although seen on the ECG, the P wave originating in the native atria does not conduct impulses across the anastomotic line.

D. **Anesthesia Management**
   1. **Clinical implications of immunosuppressive therapy**
      All cardiac transplant patients are immunosuppressed and consequently at higher risk of infection. All vascular access procedures should be carried out using aseptic or sterile technique. Antibiotic prophylaxis should be considered for any procedure with the potential to produce bacteremia. Oral immunosuppressive medication should be continued without interruption or given IV to maintain blood levels within the therapeutic range. IV and oral doses of azathioprine are approximately equivalent. Administration of large volumes of IV fluids will decrease blood levels of immunosuppressants, and therefore, levels should be checked daily. Immunosuppressant nephrotoxicity may be exacerbated by coadministration of other potentially renal toxic medications, such as nonsteroidal anti-inflammatory agents or gentamicin. Chronic corticosteroid therapy to prevent allograft rejection may result in adrenal suppression. Supplemental "stress" steroids should thus be administered to critically ill patients or patients undergoing major surgical procedures.

   2. **Monitoring**
      Standard anesthetic monitors should be used, including 5-lead ECG to detect ischemia and dysrhythmias. Cardiac transplant patients frequently have fragile skin and osteoporotic bones secondary to chronic corticosteroid administration. Care with tape, automated BP cuffs, and patient positioning is essential to avoid skin and musculoskeletal trauma. As in all patients undergoing anesthesia, invasive monitoring should only be considered for situations in which the benefits outweigh the risks. Importantly, cardiac transplant patients have an increased risk of developing catheter-related infections with a high associated morbidity

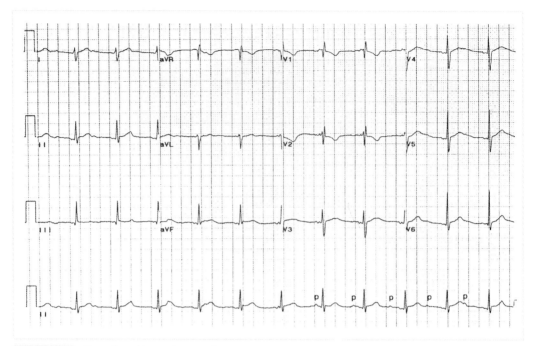

FIGURE 21.5 Transplanted heart electrocardiogram (ECG). The transplanted heart ECG is commonly characterized by two sets of P waves, right-axis deviation, and incomplete right bundle branch block (with biatrial technique). The donor heart P waves are small and precede the QRS complex, whereas P waves originating from the recipient's atria (labeled as *p*) are unrelated to the QRS complex. (Reprinted with permission from Fowler NO. *Clinical Electrocardiographic Diagnosis: A Problem-Based Approach.* Lippincott Williams & Wilkins; 2000:225.)

and mortality. Intraoperative TEE permits rapid evaluation of volume status, cardiac function, and ischemia and may be a useful substitute for invasive monitoring. Should central venous access be required, alternatives to the right internal jugular vein should be considered to preserve its use for EMB. Careful monitoring of neuromuscular blockade with a peripheral nerve stimulator is recommended in the previously transplanted patient, as cyclosporine may prolong neuromuscular blockade following administration of nondepolarizing neuromuscular blocking agents. In contrast, an attenuated response to nondepolarizing muscle relaxants may be seen in patients receiving azathioprine.

3. **Anesthesia techniques**

   Both general and regional anesthesia techniques have been used safely in cardiac transplant patients. In the absence of significant cardiorespiratory, renal, or hepatic dysfunction, there is no absolute contraindication to any anesthetic technique. For any selected anesthetic technique, maintenance of ventricular filling pressures is essential, as the transplanted heart increases CO primarily by increasing SV.

   a. General anesthesia

      General anesthesia is frequently preferred over regional anesthesia for cardiac transplant patients, as alterations in myocardial preload and afterload may be more predictable. Cyclosporine and tacrolimus decrease renal blood flow and glomerular filtration via thromboxane-mediated renal vasoconstriction. Thus, renally excreted anesthetics and muscle relaxants should be used with caution in patients receiving these medications. Cyclosporine and tacrolimus also lower the seizure threshold; hence, hyperventilation should be avoided. Elevations in the resting HR and a delayed sympathetic response to noxious stimuli in cardiac transplant recipients may make anesthetic depth difficult to assess.

b. Regional anesthesia

Many immunosuppressants cause thrombocytopenia and alter the coagulation profile. Both the platelet count and coagulation profile should be within normal limits if spinal or epidural regional anesthesia is planned. Ventricular filling pressures should be maintained following induction of central neural axis blockade to prevent hypotension caused by the delayed response of the denervated, transplanted heart to a rapid decrease in sympathetic tone. Volume loading, ventricular filling pressure monitoring, and careful titration of local anesthetic agents may avoid hemodynamic instability. Hypotension should be treated with vasopressors that directly stimulate their target receptors.

4. Blood transfusion

The cardiac transplant recipient is at increased risk for blood product transfusion complications. Adverse reactions include infection, graft-versus-host disease, and immunomodulation. The use of irradiated, leukocyte-depleted, CMV-negative blood products and white blood cell filters for blood product administration reduces the incidence of adverse transfusion reactions. The blood bank should receive early notification if the use of blood products is anticipated, because the presence of reactive antibodies delaying cross-match is not infrequent.

E. Pregnancy Following Cardiac Transplantation

Despite an increased incidence of preeclampsia and preterm labor, increasing numbers of cardiac transplant recipients are successfully carrying pregnancies to term. In general, the transplanted heart is able to adapt to the physiologic changes of pregnancy. Due to an increased sensitivity to the β-adrenergic effects of tocolytics such as terbutaline and ritodrine, the use of alternative drugs such as magnesium and nifedipine may be considered. Although pregnancy does not adversely affect cardiac allografts, the risk of acute cardiac allograft rejection may be increased postpartum. All immunosuppressive drugs used to prevent cardiac allograft rejection cross the placenta, though most are not thought to be teratogenic.

XIII. Future Directions

As medical management of HF continues to improve, a patient's need for definitive therapy with heart transplantation may become delayed or diminished. Based on trends over the previous decade, it is to be expected that patients who do present for heart transplant will have an increasing number and severity of comorbidities.[3] The continued role of MCS devices for destination therapy will also affect future developments in heart transplantation.[1] Intensive investigation into the use of stem cells and bioengineered organs may someday obviate the current organ shortage. Further understanding and widespread use of ex vivo perfusion systems could also greatly expand the pool of potential donor organs, resulting in greater numbers of transplants per year. Continuing advances in our understanding of mechanisms of rejection are likely to improve immunomodulation and delay graft failure. Improvements in surveillance, such as intravascular ultrasound, may eliminate the need for routine EMB. For the immediate future, however, heart transplantation continues to offer patients with advanced HF their best opportunity for a better quality and length of life.

REFERENCES

1. Mohamed A, Mehta N, Eisen HJ. New role of mechanical assist device as bridge to transplant: USA perspective. *Curr Opin Organ Transplant.* 2017;22(3):231-235.
2. Lund LH, Edwards LB, Dipchand AI, et al. International Society for Heart and Lung Transplantation. The Registry of the International Society for Heart and Lung Transplantation: thirty-third adult heart transplantation report-2016; Focus theme: primary diagnostic indications for transplant. *J Heart Lung Transplant.* 2016;35:1158-1169.
3. Andrew J, Macdonald P. Latest developments in heart transplantation: a review. *Curr Opin Organ Transplant.* 2017;22(3):231-235.
4. Benjamin EJ, Blaha MJ, Chiuve SE, et al. American Heart Association Statistics Committee and Stroke Statistics Subcommittee. Heart Disease and Stroke Statistics-2017 Update: a report from the American Heart Association. *Circulation.* 2017;135(10):e146-e603.
5. Yancy CW, Jessup M, Bozkurt B, et al. 2013 ACCF/AHA guideline for the management of heart failure: executive summary: a report of the American College of Cardiology Foundation/American Heart Association Task Force on practice guidelines. *Circulation.* 2013;128(16):1810-1852.

6. Mann DL, Bristow MR. Mechanisms and models in heart failure: the biomechanical model and beyond. *Circulation.* 2005;111:2837-2849.

7. Neubauer S. The failing heart—an engine out of fuel. *N Engl J Med.* 2007;356:1140-1151.

8. Ziff OJ, Kotecha D. Digoxin: the good and the bad. *Trends Cardiovasc Med.* 2016;26(7):585-595.

9. Hood WB Jr, Dans AL, Guyatt GH, et al. Digitalis for treatment of heart failure in patients in sinus rhythm. *Cochrane Database Syst Rev.* 2014;2014(4):CD002901.

10. Yandrapalli S, Tariq S, Aronow WS. Advances in chemical pharmacotherapy for managing acute decompensated heart failure. *Expert Opin Pharmacother.* 2017;18(5):471-485.

11. Metra M, Teerlink JR. Heart failure. *Lancet.* 2017;390(10106):1981-1995.

12. Yancy CW, Jessup M, Bozkurt B, et al. 2016 ACC/AHA/HFSA focused update on new pharmacological therapy for heart failure: an update of the 2013 ACCF/AHA guideline for the management of heart failure: a report of the American College of Cardiology/American Heart Association Task Force on Clinical Practice Guidelines and the Heart Failure Society of America. *Circulation.* 2016;134(13):e282-e293.

13. Murphy KM, Rosenthal JL. Progress in the presence of failure: updates in chronic systolic heart failure management. *Curr Treat Options Cardiovasc Med.* 2017;19(7):50.

14. Kong LG, Wang CL, Zhao D, et al. Nesiritide therapy is associated with better clinical outcomes than dobutamine therapy in heart failure. *Am J Ther.* 2017;24(2):e181-e188.

15. Choi AJ, Thomas SS, Singh JP. Cardiac resynchronization therapy and implantable cardioverter defibrillator therapy in advanced heart failure. *Heart Fail Clin.* 2016;12(3):423-436.

16. Epstein AE, DiMarco JP, Ellenbogen KA, et al. American College of Cardiology Foundation; American Heart Association Task Force on Practice Guidelines; Heart Rhythm Society. 2012 ACCF/AHA/HRS focused update incorporated into the ACCF/AHA/HRS 2008 guidelines for device-based therapy of cardiac rhythm abnormalities: a report of the American College of Cardiology Foundation/American Heart Association Task Force on Practice Guidelines and the Heart Rhythm Society. *Circulation.* 2013;127(3):e283-e352.

17. Colvin M, Smith JM, Ahn Y, et al. OPTN/SRTR 2020 annual data report: heart. *Am J Transplant.* 2022;22(Suppl. 2):350-437. doi:10.1111/ajt.16977

18. Ivey-Miranda JB, Maulion C, Farrero-Torres M, et al. Risk stratification of patients listed for heart transplantation while supported with extracorporeal membrane oxygenation. *J Thorac Cardiovasc Surg.* 2023;165(2):711-720. doi:10.1016/j.jtcvs.2021.05.032

19. Taghavi S, Jayarajan SN, Komaroff E, et al. Continuous flow left ventricular assist device technology has influenced wait times and affected donor allocation in cardiac transplantation. *J Thorac Cardiovasc Surg.* 2014;147(6):1966-1971.

20. Holley CT, Harvey L, John R. Left ventricular assist devices as a bridge to cardiac transplantation. *J Thorac Dis.* 2014; 6(8):1110-1119.

21. Kamdar F, John R, Eckman P, et al. Postcardiac transplant survival in the current era in patients receiving continuous-flow left ventricular assist devices. *J Thorac Cardiovasc Surg.* 2013;145:575-581.

22. Zhang B, Guo S, Ning J, Li Y, Liu Z. Continuous-flow left ventricular assist device versus orthotopic heart transplantation in adults with heart failure: a systematic review and meta-analysis. *Ann Cardiothorac Surg.* 2021;10(2):209-220. doi:10.21037/acs-2020-cfmcs-fs-197

23. Goldstein DJ, Naka Y, Horstmanshof D, et al. Association of clinical outcomes with left ventricular assist device use by bridge to transplant or destination therapy intent: the Multicenter Study of MagLev Technology in patients undergoing Mechanical Circulatory Support Therapy with HeartMate 3 (MOMENTUM 3) randomized clinical trial. *JAMA Cardiol.* 2020;5(4):411-419. doi:10.1001/jamacardio.2019.5323

24. Estep JD, Soltesz E, Cogswell R. The new heart transplant allocation system: early observations and mechanical circulatory support considerations. *J Thorac Cardiovasc Surg.* 2020;16:S0022-5223(20)32638-6. doi:10.1016/j.jtcvs.2020.08.113

25. Mancini D, Lietz K. Selection of cardiac transplantation candidates in 2010. *Circulation.* 2010;122:173-183.

26. Kanwar M, Raina A, Aponte MP, et al. Pulmonary hypertension in potential heart transplant recipients: current treatment strategies. *Curr Opin Organ Transplant.* 2015;20(5):570-576.

27. Fang JC, DeMarco T, Givertz MM, et al. World Health Organization Pulmonary Hypertension group 2: pulmonary hypertension due to left heart disease in the adult—a summary statement from the Pulmonary Hypertension Council of the International Society for Heart and Lung Transplantation. *J Heart Lung Transplant.* 2012;31(9):913-933.

28. Tavares-Silva M, Saraiva F, Pinto R, et al. Comparison of levosimendan, NO, and inhaled iloprost for pulmonary hypertension reversibility assessment in heart transplant candidates. *ESC Heart Fail.* 2021;8(2):908-917. doi:10.1002/ehf2.13168

29. Toyoda Y, Guy TS, Kashem A. Present status and future perspectives of heart transplantation. *Circ J.* 2013;77(5):1097-1110.

30. Andrew J, Macdonald P. Latest developments in heart transplantation: a review. *Clin Ther.* 2015;37(10):2234-2241.

31. DePasquale EC, Schweiger M, Ross HJ. A contemporary review of adult heart transplantation: 2012 to 2013. *J Heart Lung Transplant.* 2014;33(8):775-784.

32. Dhital KK, Iyer A, Connellan M, et al. Adult heart transplantation with distant procurement and ex-vivo preservation of donor hearts after circulatory death: a case series. *Lancet.* 2015;385:2585-2591.

33. Schroder JN, D'Alessandro D, Esmailian F, et al. Successful utilization of Extended Criteria Donor (ECD) hearts for transplantation—results of the OCS™ Heart EXPAND Trial to evaluate the effectiveness and safety of the OCS Heart System to preserve and assess ECD Hearts for transplantation. *J Heart Lung Transplant.* 2019;38(Suppl. 4):S42. doi:10.1016/j.healun.2019.01.088

34. Chew HC, Iyer A, Connellan M, et al. Outcomes of donation after circulatory death heart transplantation in Australia. *J Am Coll Cardiol.* 2019;73(12):1447-1459. doi:10.1016/j.jacc.2018.12.067

35. Schlendorf KH, Zalawadiya S, Shah AS, et al. Early outcomes using hepatitis C-positive donors for cardiac transplantation in the era of effective direct-acting anti-viral therapies. *J Heart Lung Transplant.* 2018;37(6):763-769. doi:10.1016/j.healun.2018.01.1293

36. Dictus C, Vienenkoetter B, Esmaeilzadeh M, et al. Critical care management of potential organ donors: our current standard. *Clin Transplant.* 2009;23(Suppl. 21):2-9.
37. Maciel CB, Greer DM. ICU management of the potential organ donor: state of the art. *Curr Neurol Neurosci Rep.* 2016;16:86.
38. Floerchinger B, Oberhuber R, Tullius SG. Effects of brain death on organ quality and transplant outcome. *Transplant Rev (Orlando).* 2012;26(2):54-59.
39. Anderson TA, Bekker P, Vagefi PA. Anesthetic considerations in organ procurement surgery: a narrative review. *Can J Anaesth.* 2015;62(5):529-539.
40. Minasian SM, Galagudza MM, Dmitriev YV, et al. Preservation of the donor heart: from basic science to clinical studies. *Interact Cardiovasc Thorac Surg.* 2015;20(4):510-519.
41. Pinnelas R, Kobashigawa JA. Ex vivo normothermic perfusion in heart transplantation: a review of the TransMedics® Organ Care System. *Future Cardiol.* 2022;18(1):5-15. doi:10.2217/fca-2021-0030
42. Davis RR, Russo MJ, Morgan JA, et al. Standard versus Bicaval techniques for orthotopic heart transplantation: an analysis of the United Network for Organ Sharing database. *J Thorac Cardiovasc Surg.* 2010;140:700-708.
43. Mallidi HR, Bates M. Pacemaker use following heart transplantation. *Ochsner J.* 2017;17(1):20-24.
44. Berger Y, Har Zahav Y, Kassif Y, et al. Tricuspid valve regurgitation after orthotopic heart transplantation: prevalence and etiology. *J Transplant.* 2012;2012:120702.
45. Flécher E, Fouquet O, Ruggieri VG, et al. Heterotopic heart transplantation: where do we stand? *Eur J Cardiothorac Surg.* 2013;44(2):201-206.
46. Ramakrishna H, Rehfeldt KH, Pajaro OE. Anesthetic pharmacology and perioperative considerations for heart transplantation. *Curr Clin Pharmacol.* 2015;10(1):3-21.
47. Wanek MR, Hodges K, Persaud RA, et al. Prothrombin complex concentrates for warfarin reversal before heart transplantation. *Ann Thorac Surg.* 2019;107(5):1409-1415. doi:10.1016/j.athoracsur.2018.10.032
48. Wright M, Takeda K, Mauro C, et al. Dose-dependent association between amiodarone and severe primary graft dysfunction in orthotopic heart transplantation. *J Heart Lung Transplant.* 2017;36(11):1226-1233. doi:10.1016/j.healun.2017.05.025
49. Cooper LB, Mentz RJ, Edwards LB, et al. Amiodarone use in patients listed for heart transplant is associated with increased 1-year post-transplant mortality. *J Heart Lung Transplant.* 2017;36(2):202-210. doi:10.1016/j.healun.2016.07.009
50. Haglund NA, Cox ZL, Lee JT, et al. Are peripherally inserted central catheters associated with increased risk of adverse events in Status 1B patients awaiting transplantation on continuous intravenous Milrinone? *J Card Fail.* 2014;20(9):630-637. doi:10.1016/j.cardfail.2014.06.004
51. Wong WT, Lai VK, Chee YE, Lee A. Fast-track cardiac care for adult cardiac surgical patients. *Cochrane Database Syst Rev.* 2016;9(9):CD003587. doi:10.1002/14651858.CD003587.pub3
52. Penninga L, Møller CH, Gustafsson F, et al. Immunosuppressive T-cell antibody induction for heart transplant recipients. *Cochrane Database Syst Rev.* 2013;12:CD008842.
53. Khan TA, Schnickel G, Ross D, et al. A prospective, randomized, crossover pilot study of inhaled nitric oxide versus inhaled prostacyclin in heart transplant and lung transplant recipients. *J Thorac Cardiovasc Surg.* 2009;138:1417-1424.
54. Wademan BH, Galvin SD. Desmopressin for reducing postoperative blood loss and transfusion requirements following cardiac surgery in adults. *Interact Cardiovasc Thorac Surg.* 2014;18(3):360-370.
55. Asante-Korang A. Echocardiographic evaluation before and after cardiac transplantation. *Cardiol Young.* 2004;14:88-92.
56. Wever-Pinzon O, Edwards LB, Taylor DO, et al. Association of recipient age and causes of heart transplant mortality: implications for personalization of post-transplant management-an analysis of the International Society for Heart and Lung Transplantation Registry. *J Heart Lung Transplant.* 2017;36(4):407-417. doi:10.1016/j.healun.2016.08.008
57. Costello JP, Mohanakumar T, Nath DS. Mechanisms of chronic allograft rejection. *Tex Heart Inst J.* 2013;40(4):395-399.
58. Buchan TA, Moayedi Y, Truby LK, et al. Incidence and impact of primary graft dysfunction in adult heart transplant recipients: a systematic review and meta-analysis. *J Heart Lung Transplant.* 2021;40(7):642-651. doi:10.1016/j.healun.2021.03.015
59. Lachance K, White M, de Denus S. Risk factors for chronic renal insufficiency following cardiac transplantation. *Ann Transplant.* 2015;20:576-587.
60. Page RL II, Miller GG, Lindenfeld J. Drug therapy in the heart transplant recipient: part IV: drug-drug interactions. *Circulation.* 2005;111:230-239.
61. Chan JL, Kobashigawa JA, Aintablian TL, et al. Characterizing predictors and severity of Vasoplegia syndrome after heart transplantation. *Ann Thorac Surg.* 2018;105(3):770-777. doi:10.1016/j.athoracsur.2017.09.039
62. Chan JL, Kobashigawa JA, Aintablian TL, et al. Vasoplegia after heart transplantation: outcomes at 1 year. *Interact Cardiovasc Thorac Surg.* 2017;25(2):212-217. doi:10.1093/icvts/ivx081
63. Organ Procurement and Transplantation Network. Selected data for heart/lung transplants by state. Accessed December 28, 2023. https://optn.transplant.hrsa.gov/data/view-data-reports/national-data
64. Roselli EE, Smedira NG. Surgical advances in heart and lung transplantation. *Anesthesiol Clin North Am.* 2004;22:789-807.
65. Blasco LM, Parameshwar J, Vuylsteke A. Anaesthesia for noncardiac surgery in the heart transplant recipient. *Curr Opin Anaesthesiol.* 2009;22:109-113.

Thoracic Anesthesia

22

Lung Transplantation

Ashley Jones, Daniel A. Tolpin, and James M. Anton

KEY POINTS

1. End-stage pulmonary disease (ESPD) is one of the five leading causes of mortality and morbidity in adults in the United States. ESPD results from destruction of the pulmonary parenchyma and vasculature. Lung transplantation is the definitive treatment for these patients.

2. Advances in organ allocation via the lung allocation score, lung preservation via ex vivo lung perfusion (EVLP), and bridging to transplantation via extracorporeal membrane oxygenation (ECMO) have allowed for an increased number of lung transplantations annually and a decrease in waiting list mortality.

3. In certain situations in which the patient is not expected to tolerate surgery "off-pump," mechanical circulatory support (MCS), such as cardiopulmonary bypass (CPB) or ECMO, may be utilized intraoperatively. CPB and ECMO allow for greater hemodynamic stability and improved oxygenation/ventilation during the procedure but can be linked to complications postoperatively.

4. Primary graft dysfunction (PGD) is the number one cause of early postoperative morbidity and mortality after lung transplant surgery. Factors such as increased fluid and blood administration intraoperatively have been linked to increases in PGD.

END-STAGE PULMONARY DISEASE (ESPD) is one of the five leading causes of mortality and morbidity in adults in the United States. ESPD results from destruction of the pulmonary parenchyma and vasculature. Lung transplantation is the definitive treatment for these patients. Depending on the patient's pathophysiology, there are several surgical options: single-lung transplantation (SLT), bilateral sequential lung transplantation (BSLT), or heart-lung transplantation (HLT). Before 1989, the most common type of lung transplant was combined HLT. Currently, BSLT has become the most common approach. Historically, a severe shortage of suitable donor organs led to many patients succumbing to their disease while awaiting transplantation. In the past few decades, advances in donor organ allocation, mechanical circulatory support (MCS) options for critically ill patients awaiting transplantation, and new technology in lung allograft preservation such as ex vivo lung perfusion (EVLP) have led to an increased number of lung transplantations annually and a decrease in waiting list mortality.[2] Similarly, several improvements in the management of a selected group of patients with emphysema via lung volume reduction surgery (LVRS), patients with cystic fibrosis (CF) via newer antibiotic agents, and patients with pulmonary hypertension via long-term prostacyclin therapy have been reported as viable options.

I. End-Stage Pulmonary Disease
    A. Epidemiology
        1. **Total candidates:** In the United States, there are in excess of one million potential lung transplant recipients among those suffering from ESPD.
        2. **Survival of candidates:** Because the number of lung transplant recipients far exceeds the number of suitable lung donors, up to one-third of recipients die while awaiting transplantation. Improvements to the method for allocation of lungs have decreased recipient waiting time for transplantation. In May 2005, the lung allocation score (LAS) was adopted in the United States.[1] This system is based on the severity of the recipient's disease coupled with medical urgency for transplantation. The LAS attempts to balance the risk of death while awaiting transplantation with posttransplant survival. In the years following the adoption of the LAS, the total number of recipients on the waiting list decreased by 50% and the total waiting time also decreased from a median of 792 days in 2004 to 200 days or less from 2005 to 2008.[2] According to the 2020 annual report from the U.S. Department of Health and Human Services, the average wait time on the waiting list for a lung transplant is 1.4 months.[3] Statistics from November 2022 indicate that there are 992 lung recipients and 36 heart-lung recipients awaiting transplantation[4] (see Table 22.1).
        3. **Total procedures:** According to the most recent data supplied by the International Society of Heart and Lung Transplant (ISHLT) Registry, a total of 69,200 lung transplants have been performed between January 1992 and June 2018. It is estimated that those centers reporting to the ISHLT represent only three-quarters of the world's transplant activity.
    B. Etiology and Pathophysiology of End-Stage Pulmonary Disease
        1. **Parenchymal end-stage pulmonary disease** is classified as obstructive, restrictive, or infectious.
            a. Obstructive diseases are characterized by elevation of airway resistance, diminished expiratory flow rates, severe ventilation/perfusion (V/Q) mismatching, and pronounced air trapping. The most common cause is smoking-induced emphysema; however, other causes include asthma and several comparatively rare congenital disorders. Among these, α1-antitrypsin deficiency is associated with severe bullous emphysema that manifests in the fourth or fifth decade of life.

TABLE 22.1	Factors for Calculating the Lung Allocation Score

Diagnosis
Age
Height
Weight
Cardiac index (at rest)
Bilirubin
Functional status
Pulmonary artery systolic pressure
O_2 required at rest
6-min walk distance
Continuous mechanical ventilation
P_{CO_2}
Increase in P_{CO_2} (%) over past 6 mo
Creatinine

Adapted from Organ Procurement and Transplantation Network, https://optn.transplant.hrsa.gov/data

(1) **Cystic fibrosis:** CF is a unique subset of obstructive lung disease. It is an autosomal recessive disorder with an incidence of 0.2% of live births in the United States. It is hallmarked by a mutation in the *CFTR* gene, which leads to disordered production of bodily secretions. Thickened respiratory secretions cause these patients to develop mucus plugging and frequent infections, which eventually lead to bronchiectasis, lung parenchymal destruction, and failure. These patients are much more likely to present young for lung transplantation and exhibit some unique challenges.

(a) Patients with CF are prone to be colonized by pan-resistant bacteria, such as *Pseudomonas* and *Burkholderia* species. Patients with pan-resistant bacteria, in particular, *Burkholderia cepacia*, are controversial.[5] Although the international guidelines do not regard the presence of *B. cepacia* as an absolute contraindication to transplantation, there are multiple transplant centers that limit organ allocation in these patients because previous data indicate a much higher incidence of preoperative and postoperative morbidity and mortality in this population. It has been reported that triple antimicrobial therapy can be bactericidal toward multiresistant *B. cepacia*.[6,7] Ultimately, the decision to transplant patients with CF with this microbe rests with each transplant center.

(b) Patients with CF are more likely to have had prior thoracic procedures, such as pleurodesis for pneumothorax, which may lead to increased pleural bleeding during the operation.

(c) Due to their underlying disease, patients with CF will have dysfunction of other organ systems as well. Gastrointestinal (GI) comorbidities include liver dysfunction from cholestasis, pancreatic exocrine deficiency, and malnutrition. Endocrine comorbidities include CF-related diabetes mellitus.[8]

b. Restrictive diseases are characterized by interstitial fibrosis that results in a loss of lung elasticity and compliance. Most fibrotic processes are idiopathic in nature (idiopathic interstitial pneumonia [IIP]), but they may also be caused by an immune mechanism or inhalation injury. Interstitial lung diseases may affect the pulmonary vasculature as well; therefore, pulmonary hypertension is frequently present. Functionally, diseases in this category are associated with diminished lung volumes and diffusion capacities, albeit with preserved airflow rates. Respiratory muscle strength is usually adequate because of the increased work of breathing experienced by this patient population.

2. **Pulmonary vascular diseases** are disorders that affect the blood vessels of the lungs. They are characterized by an elevation of pulmonary vascular resistance (PVR) secondary to hyperplasia of the muscular pulmonary arteries (PAs) combined with fibrosis and obliteration of the smallest arterioles. This disordered PVR can be a primary disorder of the pulmonary

vasculature itself (pulmonary arterial hypertension or PAH), or it can be secondary to heart and lung dysfunction, such as congenital heart disease with Eisenmenger syndrome. Primary PAH is rare and most frequently idiopathic. Due to long-standing elevation in PVR, these patients often develop secondary right heart dysfunction as well. If their disease progresses to the point of necessitating transplantation, these patients are often considered for combined HLT.

II. Lung Transplant Recipient Characteristics
A. Recipient Selection Criteria: Indications and Contraindications
   1. Recipient selection criteria and indications for lung transplantation are listed in Table 22.2.[9] Referral and listing of potential candidates are based on the progression of the patient's disease along with their risk of death on the waiting list balanced with the likelihood of survival

TABLE 22.2 Indications and Contraindications for Lung Transplantation

Indications	• High (>50%) risk of death from lung disease within 2 y • High (>80%) likelihood of surviving >90 d after lung transplantation • High (>80%) likelihood of 5-y posttransplant survival from a general medical perspective provided adequate graft function
Risk factors	• Age 65-70 • Mild-to-moderate CAD • Patients with prior CABG • LVEF 40%-50% • Moderate kidney dysfunction • Peripheral vascular disease • Connective tissue disease • Severe gastroesophageal reflux disease • Esophageal dysmotility • Thrombocytopenia, leukopenia, anemia • Osteoporosis • BMI 30-34.9 • BMI 16-17 • Frailty • Hypoalbuminemia • Poorly controlled diabetes • Edible marijuana use • HIV infection with undetectable viral load • Previous thoracic surgery or pleurodesis • Mechanical ventilation • Retransplant >1 y for obstructive CLAD
Risk factors with substantially increased risk	• Age >70 • Severe coronary artery disease that requires coronary artery bypass grafting at transplant • LVEF <40% • Significant cerebrovascular disease • Severe esophageal dysmotility • Untreatable hematologic conditions with risk of bleeding • BMI >35 or <16 • Limited functional status • Psychiatric conditions with potential to interfere with medical adherence • Unreliable support system • Lack of understanding of disease despite teaching • Multidrug-resistant infections (ie, *Mycobacterium abscessus, Lomentospora prolificans, Burkholderia cenocepacia,* or *Burkholderia gladioli*) • Hepatitis B or C with detectable viral load • Chest wall or spinal deformity • Extracorporeal life support • Retransplant <1 y following initial transplant • Retransplant for restrictive CLAD • Retransplant with AMR as etiology for CLAD

(continued)

TABLE 22.2	Indications and Contraindications for Lung Transplantation (*continued*)
Absolute contraindications	• Patient refusal • Malignancy with high risk of death • Advanced dysfunction of other organ system (heart, liver, kidney) • Acute coronary syndrome within 30 d • Stroke within 30 d • Septic shock • Active extrapulmonary or disseminated infection • Active tuberculosis • HIV with detectable viral load • Poor potential for posttransplant rehabilitation • Progressive cognitive impairment • Repeated medical nonadherence • Active substance abuse (tobacco, marijuana, IV drugs) • Other severe medical conditions expected to limit survival after transplant

AMR, antibody-mediated rejection; BMI, body mass index; CABG, coronary artery bypass grafting; CAD, coronary artery disease; CLAD, chronic lung allograft dysfunction; IV, intravenous; LVEF, left ventricular ejection fraction.
Derived from Chambers DC, Perch M, Zuckermann A, et al. The International Thoracic Organ Transplant Registry of the International Society for Heart and Lung Transplantation: thirty-eighth adult lung transplantation report—2021; Focus on recipient characteristics. *J Heart Lung Transplant.* 2021;40(10):1060-1072.

after transplantation; however, each patient must be considered on an individual basis and subjected to standardized selection criteria. According to the 2019 ISHLT report, the most common indication for lung transplant in recent years is restrictive lung disease, specifically IIP, found in 32.4% of transplants. This was followed by chronic obstructive pulmonary disease (COPD), at 26.1%.[10] Overall, there has been a trend toward increasing transplants for restrictive disease and decreasing for obstructive disease in recent years. This has been attributed to the introduction of the LAS and the allocation of organs to sicker patients on the waiting list.[11]

2. **Relative and absolute contraindications** to lung transplantation are listed in Table 22.2. Although candidates for organ transplantation frequently have abnormal physical or laboratory findings, such information must be distinguished from concurrent primary organ failure or a systemic disease that otherwise might disqualify candidacy. The relative contraindications to lung transplant have changed as improvements in the medical management of potential recipients have evolved. For example, coronary artery disease (CAD), previous coronary artery bypass grafting (CABG), and corticosteroid usage, once absolute contraindications, are now not prohibitive, particularly if left ventricular (LV) function is preserved and corticosteroid doses are moderate.[12,13] In situations of preexisting CAD, patients may even be considered for concomitant coronary revascularization at the time of lung transplant at certain transplant centers.

B. **Medical Evaluation of Lung Transplant Candidates**

All candidates are systematically evaluated by history, physical examination, and laboratory studies. In addition, pretransplant evaluation includes chest radiographs, computed tomography (CT) scans, arterial blood gas (ABG) values, spirometric and respiratory flow studies, V/Q scanning, 6-minute walk test, right heart catheterization, and echocardiography. On the basis of studies of the natural history of ESPD, specific laboratory criteria for referral to most lung transplantation programs that depend on the specific underlying disease have been developed (eg, cardiac index <2 L/min/m^2 in patients with PAH and FEV$_1$ $<30\%$ predicted in patients with COPD or CF). Most centers provide documentation of the evaluation results on a summary sheet that is readily available to the anesthesiology team on short notice (see Table 22.3).

C. **Impact of the COVID-19 Pandemic**

In the year 2020, the COVID-19 global pandemic introduced a new population of patients with ESPD to the realm of consideration for organ transplantation. Within the first year of the pandemic, millions of people worldwide tested positive for COVID-19. Of the patients who were admitted to the hospital, early reports from 2020 estimated that 33% progressed to acute respiratory distress syndrome (ARDS) and the mortality rate of COVID-associated ARDS was

TABLE 22.3 Standard Workup for Lung Transplantation

Pulmonary	• Chest imaging (radiographs and CT scans) • Arterial blood gas (room air) • Spirometry • Ventilation and perfusion scan • 6-min walk test
Cardiac	• Echocardiogram with bubble study • ECG • Right heart catheterization • Left heart catheterization for patients aged >40 y
Labs	• Complete blood count • Chemistry panel • Coagulation studies • Flow cytometry for HLA antibodies • Viral serologies (cytomegalovirus, herpes simplex, Epstein-Barr, hepatitis B and C, HIV, etc)
Other	• Barium swallow • Esophageal manometry • Possible liver ultrasound or liver CT

CT, computed tomography; ECG, electrocardiogram; HLA, human leukocyte antigen.
Data from Gray AL, Mulvihill MS, Hartwig MG. Lung transplantation at Duke. *J Thorac Dis.* 2016;8(3):E185-E196.

45%.[14] On October 28, 2020, COVID-19 diagnosis codes were added to the Organ Procurement and Transplantation Network (OPTN) system. At the end of 2020, 21 patients had been listed for transplant with a COVID-19 diagnosis code and 17 of those patients eventually received a lung transplantation.[3] Since that time, more centers have begun offering lung transplantation to patients with COVID-related lung failure refractory to medical therapy. Although data on these patients are still limited, a few reports have been published, detailing the outcomes of these transplants. One single-center, retrospective case series of patients with COVID-19 who underwent lung transplant found that patients with COVID-19 had higher LASs, were more likely to be on veno-veno extracorporeal membrane oxygenation (VV-ECMO), and had shorter waiting times on the transplant list, longer surgical times, and higher rates of intraoperative blood transfusion compared to the other lung transplants at that center.[15]

III. The Lung Transplant Donor

A. Selection Criteria for the Donor Lung

1. Suitable lung allografts are characterized by **ABO compatibility, no chest trauma or cardiopulmonary surgery, no aspiration sepsis, negative sputum Gram stain, no purulent secretions.**

2. The donor should **ideally be younger than 55 years**, although older donors have increasingly been accepted in recent years with minimal effect on outcomes.[16]

3. A possible donor lung will be evaluated on an FIO_2 of 1.0 with a positive end-expiratory pressure (PEEP) of 5 cm H_2O and the PaO_2 will be measured. Previously, it was believed that the PaO_2 should be >300 mm Hg, but this cutoff has not been associated with increased posttransplant survival. Currently, most centers will accept a PaO_2 >250 mm Hg, but practices vary.[16]

4. A donor should ideally have **no smoking history**, although ≤20 pack-years is often deemed acceptable.[17]

5. **Extended donor criteria:** Age >55 years, compatible nonidentical ABO group, chest x-ray with focal or unilateral abnormality, smoking history >20 pack-years, the absence of extensive chest trauma, prior cardiopulmonary surgery, secretions in upper airways, positive serology (eg, hepatitis B or C)[18]

6. The most common causes of donor death include cerebrovascular accident (CVA), anoxia, or head trauma, all of which lead to a diagnosis of brain death.

7. In an attempt to provide a larger pool of suitable lung donors, the lungs from **non–heart-beating donors** (donation after cardiac death) have been transplanted and reported to produce a successful recipient outcome.[19]

8. As experience in the field of genetic therapy continues to grow, **cytokine profiling** has become an important method to identify organs suitable for donation and transplantation. Fisher et al[20] reported that elevated levels of interleukin-8 in donor lungs were associated with early graft failure and decreased recipient survival. These data suggest that cytokine profiles could be an early indicator of recipient outcome.

B. Procurement Procedure

Because both the heart and the lungs are often harvested from the same donor for different recipients, a method has been developed to perform cardiectomy and reduce the risk of lung injury. During cardiectomy, a residual atrial cuff is left attached to the donor lungs. The trachea is stapled and divided at its midpoint, and the lungs are removed en bloc. Subsequently, the pulmonary vasculature is flushed and immersed in a hypothermic preservative (most commonly Euro-Collins or University of Wisconsin solution with or without prostaglandin E1 [PGE1]).

1. **Lung allograft preservation**

   a. There are several relevant issues surrounding donor lung preservation; however, all focus on methods to provide ready sources of energy and cryoprotection and to prevent vasospasm, cellular swelling, and accumulation of toxic metabolites. For example, free radical scavengers such as superoxide dismutase and catalase can be added to prevent oxygen-derived free radicals from damaging key intracellular constituents after reperfusion, and PGE1 can be added to promote uniform cooling and distribution of preservative solutions.

   b. Standard preservation techniques allow a reported maximum allograft ischemic time of 6-8 hours; however, ischemic times of 10-12 hours may be tolerated depending on the preservative solution.

2. **Normothermic ex vivo lung perfusion** is a newer preservation technique aimed at reconditioning and improving the function of marginal donor lungs. Donor lungs that may be considered for EVLP often have marginal Pao_2/Fio_2 ratios (<300 mm Hg), poor lung compliance, evidence of pulmonary edema on imaging, or some high-risk medical history, such as possible aspiration.[21] The harvested donor lung is perfused in an ex vivo circuit using a normothermic perfusate while they are ventilated at body temperature to mimic physiologic conditions. Perfusate solutions vary by protocol and can be cellular or acellular. They generally contain some combination of heparin, antimicrobial agents, and steroids. Cypel et al[22] demonstrated that transplantation of high-risk donor lungs that were physiologically stable during 4 hours of EVLP had a lower incidence of primary graft dysfunction (PGD) 72 hours posttransplant compared with controls. In addition, recent studies have shown that utilization of EVLP may expand the donor pool by including organs that would otherwise not be considered suitable for transplant. The EXPAND trial implemented EVLP for marginal donor lungs, and of the lungs selected for EVLP, 87% were eventually transplanted. The transplanted EVLP organs had similar clinical outcomes to that of the control, which implies that EVLP could be a safe and effective option for expanding lung transplantation into the future[23] (see Figure 22.1).

3. **Clinical immunology of organ matching:** ABO matching is essential before transplantation, because the donor-specific major blood group isoagglutinins have been implicated as a cause of allograft hyperacute rejection. Once procured, the practical matter of a 6- to 8-hour donor lung ischemic time limit severely restricts prospective matching of histocompatibility antigens, panel reactive antibody (PRA) screens, and the geography of organ donation. One study suggests that the total ischemic time alone does not predict a poor outcome after transplantation. Rather, the additive effect of increased donor age (>55 years) plus increased ischemic allograft time (>6-7 hours) is a more reliable indicator of poor posttransplant survival.[24]

IV. Choice of Lung Transplant Procedure

Choice of lung transplant procedure is based upon (a) the consequences of leaving a native lung in situ, (b) the procedure most likely to yield the best functional outcome for a given pathophysiologic process, and (c) the relative incidence of perioperative complications associated with a particular procedure. Currently, the vast majority of lung transplants are performed using the BSLT technique.

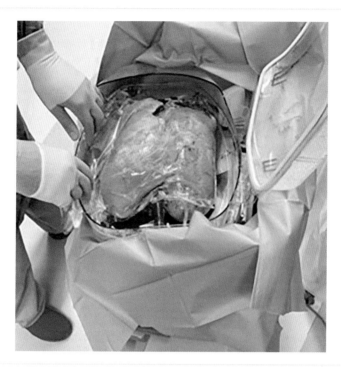

FIGURE 22.1 Image of donor lungs on ex vivo lung perfusion circuit.

A. **Single-Lung Transplantation**
1. SLT can be selected for transplant recipients with noninfectious lung pathophysiology. SLT is a frequent option for older patients with end-stage pulmonary fibrosis or emphysema, as it poses a lower perioperative risk[25]; however, in patients with severe bullous emphysema, SLT may exacerbate native lung hyperinflation and result in severe acute and/or chronic allograft compromise secondary to compression atelectasis. Preoperative measurement of the recipient static lung compliance has been suggested as a screening technique to determine whether SLT alone, SLT plus LVRS, or BSLT is most beneficial.
2. SLT offers several advantages.
   a. SLT may extend the limited supply of donor organs to more patients (but has less functional reserve as a buffer for complications). It is also associated with a worse outcome.[26]
   b. SLT is feasible in many patients without the use of cardiopulmonary bypass (CPB), so complications arising from coagulopathic states are less frequent.
3. The incision for SLT is a unilateral thoracotomy incision.
4. SLT involves pneumonectomy and implantation of the lung allograft. The choice of the native lung to be extracted is determined preoperatively. The lung with the poorest pulmonary function as delineated by V/Q scanning is generally chosen for replacement by the allograft. If the native lungs are equally impaired and pleural scarring is absent, the left lung is chosen for relative technical simplicity:
   a. The native left pulmonary veins are more accessible than those on the right.
   b. The left hemithorax can more easily accommodate an oversized donor lung.
   c. The recipient's left mainstem bronchus is longer.
B. **Bilateral Sequential Lung Transplantation**
1. Since 1996, there has been a proportional increase in adult BSLT for every major indication for lung transplantation, except for CF (which remains essentially a 100% indication for BSLT), and in 2017, it accounted for 81% of lung transplant procedures.[10]

2. In recent data, BSLT shows an increased long-term survival with a median survival of 7.8 years versus 4.8 years for SLT.[10]

3. While SLT is still performed frequently for end-stage idiopathic pulmonary fibrosis (IPF) and emphysema in older recipients (>65 years of age), BSLT is also increasingly utilized for these conditions.[9]

4. BSLT is the procedure of choice for septic lung disease (eg, generalized bronchiectasis), CF, young patients with COPD, and PAH.

5. Incision for BSLT will vary depending on the medical institution and surgeon preference but may include median sternotomy, clamshell incision, or bilateral anterior thoracotomies.

C. **Heart-Lung Transplantation**

1. The indications for HLT are diminishing as experience with isolated lung transplantation evolves. The latter operations will suffice in most cases when it is performed before irreversible heart failure (HF) occurs or in concert with intracardiac repair of simple congenital defects. The total number of centers performing HLT has increased from 37 in 2003 to 184 in 2019. Participating centers reported a total of 59 adult and pediatric HLTs for calendar year 2017. Most centers perform only one HLT on average per calendar year.[10]

2. HLT is **indicated** for patients with ESPD complicated by irreversible HF. PAH and congenital heart disease remain the main indications for adult HLT.[26]

D. **Living donor lobar lung transplantation (LDLLT)** is a surgical technique developed in the mid-1990s to circumvent the chronic shortage of available donor organs. Since introduction of the LAS in 2005, LDLLT has fallen out of favor as the waitlist mortality for lung transplantation has decreased and overall annual number of transplants has increased.[27] Although outcomes in adult recipients are similar to that of cadaveric transplantation,[28] there remain ethical and safety concerns for the donor.

V. **Preanesthetic Considerations**

A. Because of a chronic shortage of suitable lungs available for transplantation, many patients experience long waiting periods ranging from several months to several years. **Interval changes** may occur since completion of the initial medical evaluation. Specifically, reduction in exercise tolerance, new drug regimens or requirements for oxygen and steroids, appearance of purulent sputum, signs or symptoms indicative of right HF (eg, hepatomegaly, peripheral edema), and the presence of fever are among the most common occurrences that should be explored in the immediate preoperative period.

B. Evaluation of the patient on the day of operation is of the utmost importance and will provide clinical information that may affect the course of surgery. The **level of oxygenation and ventilatory support** should be ascertained. Asking the patient if they are **able to lay flat** may be predictive of respiratory compromise at the time of induction of anesthesia. The patient should be evaluated for any inotropic support, pulmonary vasodilator therapy, or even MCS, as these may affect the complexity of patient management.

C. Because of the relatively short safe ischemic time for allografts, there may be a short time interval between patient notification and operating room (OR) start time. As is customary for any emergent surgical procedure, the time of **last oral intake** should be ascertained before induction of general anesthesia.

D. Patients undergoing lung transplantation may exhibit anxiety. They usually have not received anxiolytic **premedication** before their arrival in the OR. One should be vigilant when administering anxiolytic agents to these patients so that their impaired respiratory drive is not further compromised, as hypercarbia secondary to sedation could lead to further increased PVR and possible catastrophic cardiovascular collapse.

CLINICAL PEARL

One should be vigilant when administering anxiolytic agents to lung transplant recipients so that their impaired respiratory drive is not further compromised.

E. **Regional Anesthesia**
1. Insertion of a **thoracic epidural catheter** for both intraoperative and postoperative analgesia may be performed before induction of general anesthesia. The catheter should be inserted at a spinal level that provides appropriate anesthesia and analgesia in concordance with the surgical incision site (eg, T-4 to T-5 or T-5 to T-6).[29] Alternatively, bilateral paravertebral catheters may be inserted. Placement of a thoracic epidural catheter or bilateral paravertebral catheters when anticoagulation is anticipated for CPB remains controversial. A newer alternative that may be safer with systemic anticoagulation is the erector spinae block. A catheter may be left in place (either unilateral or bilateral) for continued local anesthetic infusion postoperatively.
2. Another option for postoperative pain control is intercostal nerve blocks via **cryoanalgesia**. Studies have shown analgesic outcomes similar to that of thoracic epidural analgesia. Advantages of cryoablation include less hemodynamic instability compared to thoracic epidurals and less bleeding risk in the setting of possible anticoagulation.[30]

CLINICAL PEARL

Regional anesthesia is an option for perioperative analgesia. A thoracic epidural catheter, bilateral paravertebral catheters, or bilateral erector spinae catheters may be used for this purpose, but placement of these catheters remains controversial when anticoagulation is anticipated for the use of CPB in lung transplantation. Other techniques such as intercostal nerve blocks using cryoanalgesia may be preferred as they avoid some of the risks associated with anticoagulation and indwelling catheters.

F. Chronically cyanotic patients are frequently severely polycythemic (hematocrit >60%) and may manifest clotting abnormalities. In these instances, phlebotomy and hemodilution may be beneficial in minimizing the occurrence of end-organ infarction.
G. **Size matching** between donor and recipient is facilitated by comparing the vertical and transverse radiologic chest dimensions of the donor and recipient. Undersizing in regard to height and weight is associated with inferior posttransplant survival.[10] Organs are also matched on the basis of ABO compatibility, because the value of histocompatibility matching is still unknown and requires time in excess of the tolerable ischemic time for the lung allograft.
H. Close **coordination and effective communication** between the transplant team and the organ harvesting team is vital so that excess allograft ischemic time is avoided.
I. Arrangements should be made for intraoperative **availability of a multimodality ventilator** for patients with the most severe forms of lung disease. Useful ventilator settings include the ability to deliver minute volumes >15 L/min (especially helpful if airway leaks are present), adjustable inflation pressure "pop-offs" (to allow high inflation pressures to be delivered to noncompliant lungs), adjustable respiratory cycle waveforms, and availability of high levels of PEEP (eg, 15-20 cm H_2O during reperfusion pulmonary edema).
J. Before the initiation of surgery, the possible need for **inhaled vasodilators** should be considered, particularly in those patients with elevated PA pressures and right heart dysfunction at baseline. Inhaled nitric oxide (iNO) and inhaled nebulized prostacyclin (epoprostenol) have been proven effective for the treatment of pulmonary hypertension and early reperfusion injury in some patients. Recent studies show no difference in the rate of severe PGD between iNO and inhaled epoprostenol in the lung transplant population.[31]

CLINICAL PEARL

iNO and inhaled nebulized prostacyclin have been proven effective for the treatment of pulmonary hypertension and early reperfusion injury in some patients.

VI. **Anesthetic Management of the Lung Transplant Recipient**
  A. **Induction of Anesthesia**
  1. **Selection of induction agents:** Agents that promote hemodynamic homeostasis are preferred for induction of general anesthesia. One example is etomidate and a nondepolarizing neuromuscular blocking agent, such as rocuronium, which may be used during a modified rapid sequence induction technique. Modest amounts of fentanyl (5-10 µg/kg) administered intravenously (IV) may be used if indicated to control cardiovascular responses to endotracheal intubation.
  2. **Intraoperative monitoring**
      a. Both **systemic and PA pressure monitoring** are essential during lung transplant procedures. Dyspnea, arrhythmias, right ventricular (RV) dilation, and pulmonary hypertension may complicate PA catheter insertion before induction of general anesthesia. Oximetric PA catheters are useful in this setting to evaluate tissue oxygen delivery in patients who are subject to sudden cardiac instability. Some suggest that RV ejection fraction catheters may be useful for the diagnosis of right HF. Radial arterial cannulation with or without femoral artery cannulation is appropriate for monitoring of systemic arterial blood pressure. Femoral arterial catheters may interfere with groin cannulation for CPB; however, they can also serve as a means of quick access should venoarterial (VA)-ECMO be required.
      b. Pulse oximetry should be considered mandatory and is especially useful for continuous monitoring of SpO_2 during stressful intervals, such as the onset of one-lung ventilation (OLV) or cross-clamping of the PA.
      c. Near-infrared reflectance spectroscopy (NIRS) monitoring has proven very useful in monitoring the adequacy of cerebral oxygenation during both ECMO and CPB as well as in detecting lower limb ischemia related to femoral cannulation.
  3. **Transesophageal echocardiography:** Transesophageal echocardiography (TEE) is perhaps the most useful monitor available. TEE evaluation during lung transplantation should include:
      a. Evaluation of RV and LV wall motion and function as well as assessment of intracardiac valvular function
          (1) Special attention should be given to assessing RV size and function as well as tricuspid valve function. Impairments of the right heart may suggest a more tenuous course following lung reperfusion and may necessitate a bridge with MCS.
          (2) One should routinely evaluate the heart for intracardiac shunts, such as patent foramen ovale and atrial or ventricular septal defects, as these may require surgical closure.
      b. Assessment of PA and pulmonary vein anastomoses and blood flow
          (1) PA anastomoses should exhibit unobstructed, laminar flow with color-flow Doppler and no significant gradient on spectral Doppler.
          (2) Although there are no official guidelines regarding PA anastomosis diameter, it is commonly accepted that the minimal diameter should be at least 75% of the proximal PA diameter.[32]
          (3) The pulmonary vein anastomoses should have a diameter >0.5 cm and velocity of <1 m/s. Significant pulmonary vein stenosis has been associated with graft failure.[33]
          (4) The anesthesiologist should look for and rule out thrombi in the PAs and pulmonary veins.
      c. Assessment of the elimination of intracardiac air that occurs during pulmonary venous anastomosis
      d. Calculation of PA pressure as measured by Doppler flow velocity
      e. In addition, TEE will continuously assist in the assessment of hemodynamics during the case. Decisions regarding volume status, initiation of inotropic or vasopressor medications, and, possibly, the need for mechanical support with CPB or ECMO may be elucidated using TEE (see Figure 22.2).

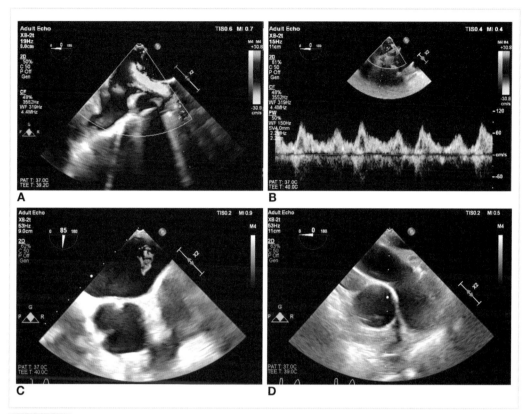

FIGURE 22.2 **(A)** Pulmonary vein color Doppler assessment for laminar flow. **(B)** Pulmonary vein pulsed-wave Doppler to assess velocity. **(C)** Left atrial clot translocated from pulmonary vein following allograft reperfusion. **(D)** Pulmonary artery anastomoses.

CLINICAL PEARL

TEE is perhaps the most useful monitor available. TEE allows for (a) direct visualization of RV and LV wall motion and function as well as assessment of intracardiac valvular function, (b) assessment of PA and pulmonary vein anastomoses and blood flow, (c) assessment of the elimination of intracardiac air that occurs during pulmonary venous anastomosis, and (d) calculation of PA pressure as measured by Doppler flow velocity.

4. **Intravenous access:** Large-caliber IV catheters are often inserted peripherally and centrally (eg, 14-G peripheral IV, 9-12F central venous introducer). In operations in which massive transfusion requirements are anticipated (eg, HLT for congenital heart disease with Eisenmenger syndrome, BSLT for CF with pleural scarring), a rapid infusion device should be available and primed. For patients with significant PAH and RV dysfunction, preinduction femoral vascular access for rapid cannulation for ECMO or CPB should be considered.

5. **Positioning:** Full lateral decubitus position is typically used during SLT, even when CPB is anticipated (eg, SLT for primary pulmonary hypertension [PPH]). One groin is usually prepped into the field to allow for the option of femoral cannula insertion for CPB. The supine position is used for BSLT, facilitating either median sternotomy, clamshell incision, or bilateral anterior thoracotomy incision.

6. **Securing the airway:** Lung isolation is required for optimal surgical exposure. Both double-lumen endobronchial tubes (EBTs) and bronchial blockers are useful for this purpose. A general discussion of these choices is provided in Chapter 15.

    a. Advantages of double-lumen EBTs in the setting of lung transplantation include the following:

        (1) Facilitation of lung isolation

        (2) Ability to suction the nonventilated lung

        (3) Ability to apply continuous positive airway pressure (CPAP) to the nonventilated lung

        (4) Provision for postoperative independent lung ventilation

    b. Left-sided EBTs (eg, Broncho-Cath) are recommended for both right and left SLTs as well as for BSLT (right-sided double lumen tube [DLTs] are still used for left SLT in some centers). There is a higher incidence of right upper lobe obstruction when right-sided double-lumen EBTs are used because the right upper lobe orifice is relatively close to the right mainstem bronchus.

    c. **Selecting the correct size of EBT:** In general, the largest-sized EBT that can be placed without causing airway trauma is preferred to facilitate therapeutic flexible bronchoscopy both intraoperatively and postoperatively. This is typically 39F for a male and 37F for a female recipient. Patients with CF are generally of lesser build and may require a 35F EBT.

    d. Many lung transplant recipients have limited pulmonary reserve, and desaturation during intubation may occur rapidly. Therefore, **initial EBT positioning** can be accomplished quickly and accurately with the aid of a flexible fiberoptic bronchoscopy (FOB).

CLINICAL PEARL

Many lung transplant recipients have limited pulmonary reserve, and desaturation during intubation may occur rapidly. Therefore, initial EBT positioning can be accomplished quickly and accurately with the aid of a flexible FOB.

B. **Maintenance of Anesthesia**

    1. **Volatile anesthetics versus** total intravenous anesthesia

        a. Volatile anesthetic agents (eg, isoflurane, sevoflurane) are frequently used during lung transplantation, but it is prudent to remember that ESPD and pneumonectomy may affect the uptake of inhaled agents. Depending on the severity of the patient's pathology, it may be advisable to administer a continuous IV agent, such as propofol infusion, for the maintenance of anesthesia.

        b. There are currently no data showing differences in outcomes between maintenance with volatile anesthetics versus total intravenous anesthesia (TIVA).

        c. Depth of anesthesia should be closely monitored, as these patients are at risk of awareness under anesthesia. Processed electroencephalogram (EEG) monitoring may be of particular benefit.

        d. While there had previously been some concern with volatile agents and inhibition of hypoxic pulmonary vasoconstriction, this was primarily seen with older inhaled anesthetics (eg, halothane). It has not been shown to occur with newer agents at <1 minimum alveolar concentration (MAC) equivalent.[34]

    2. **Opioids:** A balanced regimen of short-acting opioids, such as fentanyl, should be utilized to blunt the sympathetic response to surgery, thereby minimizing increases in PVR and worsening pulmonary hypertension. One must keep in mind that excessive opioid administration could worsen intraoperative hypotension and possibly delay time to extubation in certain patient populations.

    3. **Thoracic regional anesthesia**, in addition to providing excellent postoperative analgesia, may be used to enhance general anesthesia intraoperatively. Continuous infusion of a local anesthetic, such as 0.2%-0.5% ropivacaine, provides ideal surgical anesthesia and analgesia and allows for reduced doses of both IV opioids and inhaled agents.

4. **Nitrous oxide** is generally avoided for the following reasons: (a) 100% oxygen is almost always required to maintain an acceptable arterial saturation during OLV; (b) bullae may expand and compress the residual normal lung parenchyma, thus exacerbating V/Q mismatching; and (c) occult pneumothoraces may occur.

5. **Management of ventilation**

   a. Although there is a lack of strong data regarding optimal ventilation strategies in the lung transplant population, lung-protective ventilatory strategies as outlined by the ARDSNet Protocol is recommended: tidal volumes 6 mL/kg ideal body weight, plateau pressure <30 cm H_2O, and permissive hypercapnia to maintain pH >7.25.[35]

   b. PEEP should be tailored to the oxygenation needs of the patient but often initiated at 6-8 cm H_2O. PEEP may need to be increased for ventilation of the donor lungs.

   c. Independent or differential ventilation is often used during SLT for emphysema recipients, particularly those with gross V/Q mismatching. Independent lung ventilation allows PEEP to be selectively delivered to the allograft and avoid air trapping and over-inflation of the native lung.

   d. Alteration of the inspired-to-expired ratio during mechanical ventilation may be useful during SLT in patients with emphysema. Increasing the expiratory time during each respiratory cycle allows for adequate exhalation, thus reducing the possibility of overinflating of the native lung (breath stacking) and subsequent compromise of the allograft.

   e. Lateral decubitus positioning may be associated with significant alterations in oxygenation and ventilation, depending on the underlying pulmonary pathophysiology. Positional improvement or deterioration in blood gas values is sometimes predictable on the basis of the patient's preoperative V/Q scan.

   f. After allograft implantation, **the lowest possible FIO_2** should be used to maintain adequate oxygenation (PaO_2 of 60-80 mm Hg or SaO_2 of >91%). High FIO_2 at the time of reperfusion (>40%) has been linked to PGD.[36]

   g. In the setting of high inspiratory pressure, the transplanted bronchial circulation is susceptible to impaired perfusion. Impaired bronchial circulation can lead to anastomotic complications, including infection, poor healing, and dehiscence. Therefore, it is important to maintain peak inspiratory pressure (PIP) of <30 cm H_2O.[35]

   h. Frequent **suctioning and lavage** via **flexible FOB** is helpful to maintain airway patency during BSLT for CF or whenever airway bleeding and secretions are sufficient to cause obstruction and impair gas exchange.

   i. General strategies for supporting oxygenation during OLV (ie, during SLT and BSLT) are discussed in Chapter 15.

6. **Management of blood transfusion**

   a. Lung transplantation operations are high risk for necessitating blood transfusion. Packed red blood cells (pRBCs) and coagulation products should thus be readily available. In all cases, the benefits of blood transfusion must be weighed against the potential harms, and transfusion strategy should remain conservative and judicious.

   b. Large volume pRBC transfusion is an independent risk factor for PGD. In one study, >1 L pRBC transfusion was associated with a 2-fold increase in grade 3 PGD.[36]

   c. Platelet transfusion has been identified as an independent risk factor for increased short- and long-term mortality following lung transplantation[37] and, therefore, should only be given when clinically indicated.

   d. Intraoperative coagulation studies, thromboelastogram (TEG), and rotational thromboelastometry (ROTEM) should be employed to guide the management of coagulopathy.

   e. Cytomegalovirus (CMV)-seronegative blood products must be available for seronegative recipients if CMV sepsis is to be avoided. When transplantation of CMV-negative donors and recipients occurs, leukocyte filters are used to reduce exposure to CMV during transfusion of blood and blood products. Likewise, if human leukocyte antigen (HLA) alloimmunization is to be avoided, leukocyte-reduced blood is necessary for transplant candidates, particularly if they require transfusion before organ transplantation (see Table 22.4).

TABLE 22.4	Risk Factors for Increased Transfusion
Patient factors	Increased age
	Cystic fibrosis
	Extensive pleural adhesions
	Eisenmenger syndrome
	Preexisting anemia or coagulopathy
Surgical factors	BSLT
	Use of MCS
	Increased time on CPB
	Reoperation

BSLT, bilateral sequential lung transplantation; CPB, cardiopulmonary bypass; MCS, mechanical circulatory support.
Adapted from Pena JJ, Bottiger BA, Miltiades AN. Perioperative management of bleeding and transfusion for lung transplantation. *Semin Cardiothorac Vasc Anesth.* 2020;24(1):74-83.

7. **Fluid management**
   a. The transplanted lung is at high risk for developing postoperative pulmonary edema. In addition, increased fluid administration has been linked to PGD. Crystalloid should be administered sparingly.[38]
8. **Considerations for mechanical circulatory support**

   Over the past decade, much research regarding lung transplantation has revolved around the role of MCS and how it affects postoperative outcomes. In certain situations, in which the patient is not expected to tolerate surgery "off-pump," CPB or ECMO may be utilized. CPB and ECMO allow for greater hemodynamic stability and improved oxygenation/ventilation. Patients with very poor native lung function may develop hypoxia and hypercarbia during single-lung ventilation, which will worsen acidosis and pulmonary vasoconstriction and could further hinder right heart function. MCS alleviates some of these challenges but not without consequences. Although there is still much debate in this area, a few things should be noted:
   a. During all lung transplant operations, regardless of surgical plan, a perfusion team with a CPB machine should be on standby and ready to emergently initiate MCS at any time during the operation.
   b. It has been shown that cases emergently converted to CPB had worse outcomes than those with a planned CPB courses.[39]
   c. CPB has been associated with worse early postoperative outcomes, including PGD, increased duration of mechanical ventilation, and increased transfusion requirement.[40,41] This is secondary to the fact that CPB provokes a known inflammatory response in the patient. In addition, CPB requires full anticoagulation, leading to more bleeding, which can further lead to transfusion-related lung injury.[42]
   d. Increasing evidence shows that VA-ECMO may be preferable to CPB if MCS is required. It has been linked to fewer blood transfusions, fewer reoperations, less PGD, and decreased renal complications.[43,44] ECMO leads to less of an inflammatory response due to a smaller blood-air interface.[42]
   e. Hoetzenecker et al showed improved mortality and reduced PGD with routine use of VA-ECMO (as opposed to off-pump) during lung transplantation. This was thought to be secondary to attenuation of the ischemic-reperfusion injury due to controlled reperfusion via the ECMO circuit.[45]
   f. Many patients awaiting lung transplantation may be bridged to transplantation with VV-ECMO. In situations with severe PGD, VV-ECMO may be necessary postoperatively as well.
C. **Surgical Procedures and Anesthesia-Related Interventions**
   1. **Surgical dissection** may be complicated by extensive pleural adhesions, vascular anomalies, vascular collaterals, or previous cardiac or thoracic surgery.

2. **OLV** is almost always used during lung transplantation to facilitate dissection. In BSLT, the preoperative V/Q scan is used to determine which lung will be transplanted first and can also be predictive of how the patient will tolerate OLV. With the onset of OLV, acute deterioration in gas exchange and hemodynamics must be anticipated. Strategies for improving oxygenation under these circumstances include the following:
   a. PEEP applied to the nonoperative (ventilated) lung, provided that bullous disease or emphysema is absent
   b. CPAP or high-frequency jet ventilation in the operative (nonventilated) lung
   c. Ligation of the branch PA of the operative lung
   d. Initiation of MCS

3. **Clamping the branch PA** when PA pressures are low is usually well tolerated and improves V/Q matching and ABG values. If elevated PA pressures exacerbate right HF, vasodilators and inotropes may improve systemic hemodynamics; however, gas exchange may be further impaired, depending on the agents that are selected (eg, sodium nitroprusside may worsen V/Q mismatching). Should the patient's condition deteriorate despite pharmacologic intervention, implementation of CPB or ECMO should be considered.

4. Immediately before implantation of the donor lung, the donor hilar structures are trimmed to match the size of the recipient bronchus, branch PA, and atrial cuff containing the pulmonary venous orifices. While the allograft is kept scrupulously cold, the bronchial anastomoses, atrial cuff, and PA anastomoses are completed in sequence.

5. The **ischemic interval** ends with the removal of vascular clamps, but until ventilation is restored, systemic arterial saturation remains unchanged. Immediately before vascular unclamping, **methylprednisolone** (250-500 mg) is administered IV to minimize the potential for hyperacute allograft rejection.

6. **Reperfusion** of the allograft is a critical moment during the lung transplantation and may be associated with profound hemodynamic instability. Systemic hypotension may occur due to washout of vasoactive substances from the ischemic allograft, blood loss through vascular anastomoses, or entrainment of air into the coronaries. The anesthesiologist should be prepared to maximally support the patient through this period, and it may require preemptive adjustment of hemodynamic support.

7. **Reinflation of the allograft** follows, sometimes with the aid of a flexible FOB to clear airway secretions. This procedure allows for direct viewing of the airway anastomosis to ensure patency.

8. After SLT for emphysema, independent lung ventilation can be instituted if indicated using the anesthesia ventilator for the native lung (increased expiratory time, low-tidal volume, no PEEP) and an intensive care unit (ICU)-quality ventilator for the allograft (increased respiratory rates, low-tidal volumes of 5-7 mL/kg, 10 cm H_2O PEEP, and FIO_2 ≤0.3).

9. **Reperfusion injury**, characterized by increasing alveolar-arterial gradients, deteriorating compliance, and gross pulmonary edema, may follow allograft reperfusion within minutes to hours. The most effective treatments are PEEP and strict limitation of volume infusion, both crystalloid and colloid. Rarely, reperfusion injury may be accompanied by pulmonary hypertension. iNO (40-80 ppm) has been the agent of choice in this instance; however, inhaled prostacyclin has also been effective in decreasing PA pressure.[46] If evidence of right HF occurs, continuous IV infusion of vasopressin (0.01-0.04 units/min) or norepinephrine (0.01-0.2 μg/kg/min) plus inotropic support with epinephrine (0.01-0.2 μg/kg/min), dobutamine (2-20 μg/kg/min), or milrinone (0.375-0.5 μg/kg/min) may prove efficacious.

CLINICAL PEARL

The most effective treatments for reperfusion injury are PEEP and strict limitation of volume infusion, both crystalloid and colloid. Rarely, reperfusion injury may be accompanied by pulmonary hypertension. iNO (40-80 ppm) has been the agent of choice in this instance; however, inhaled prostacyclin has also been effective in decreasing PA pressure.

10. At the conclusion of surgery, the EBT can be exchanged for a standard single-lumen endotracheal tube (ETT) or retained for independent lung ventilation in the ICU. The anesthesia provider should proceed very cautiously with tube exchange, as fluid administration intraoperatively can lead to airway edema. In addition, caution is needed if a tube exchange catheter is utilized to avoid damaging fresh bronchial anastomoses.

VII. **Postoperative Management and Complications**

A. **Respiratory and Cardiovascular Support**

1. Early **respiratory insufficiency** is usually due to reperfusion injury, which is characterized by large alveolar-arterial O_2 gradients, poor pulmonary compliance, and parenchymal infiltrates despite low cardiac filling pressures. Mechanical ventilation with PEEP is essential, but inflation pressures are kept to a minimum in consideration of the new airway anastomoses.

   a. FIO_2 is maintained at the lowest levels compatible with an acceptable arterial oxygen saturation.

   b. Fifteen percent of lung transplant recipients may develop severe lung injury secondary to reperfusion injury and lymphatic disruption during the surgical procedure. This pattern of lung injury can be treated with ECMO, iNO, or selective lung ventilation if indicated.

   c. Acute allograft dysfunction can occur and is associated with a mortality rate of up to 60%.

   d. Cardiovascular deterioration may be secondary to hemorrhage, PA or pulmonary venous anastomotic obstruction, tension pneumothorax, or pneumopericardium. TEE may be a useful diagnostic tool in the setting of vascular obstructive lesions. Hemorrhage most frequently occurs in patients with pleural disease and Eisenmenger syndrome. Tension pneumothorax occurs more frequently in patients with concomitant end-stage emphysema.

B. **Primary graft dysfunction** is the number one cause of early postoperative morbidity and mortality after lung transplant surgery. It is characterized by a combination of hypoxia with evidence of radiographic infiltrates that occurs within the first 72 hours following transplants. It is graded on a scale of 0-3, with grade 3 PGD being the most severe. Although not fully understood, the etiology of PGD likely stems from a combination of medical and surgical factors in the perioperative period. Treatment is primarily supportive (see Table 22.5).

C. **Immunosuppressive drug regimens** have been developed to control the recipient's immune response and prevent allograft rejection.[47] Clinical immunosuppression for lung transplant can be considered in several different contexts: (1) induction therapy, (2) maintenance therapy, and (3) antirejection therapy. Most centers use a triple-drug maintenance regimen that includes

---

TABLE 22.5   PGD Grading According to 2016 ISHLT Consensus Statement

Grade	Oxygenation	Radiographic Infiltrates
0	Any Pao_2/FIO_2 Extubated, w/ or w/o supplemental O_2	Absent
1	Pao_2/FIO_2 >300 Extubated patient on supplemental oxygen with FIO_2 <30%	Present bilaterally SLT, absent in native lung
2	Pao_2/FIO_2 200-300	Present bilaterally SLT, absent in native lung
3	Pao_2/FIO_2 <200 Mechanical ventilation with FIO_2 >50% Hypoxemia requiring ECLS	Present bilaterally SLT, absent in native lung

ECLS, extracorporeal life support; SLT, single-lung transplantation.
Adapted from Snell GI, Yusen RD, Weill D, et al. Report of the ISHLT Working Group on Primary Lung Graft Dysfunction, part I: definition and grading-A 2016 Consensus Group statement of the International Society for Heart and Lung Transplantation. *J Heart Lung Transplant.* 2017;36(10):1097-1103. © 2017 International Society for the Heart and Lung Transplantation. With permission.

corticosteroids, a calcineurin inhibitor (eg, cyclosporine or tacrolimus), and an antiprolifera-tive agent (eg, azathioprine). Although these regimens may adequately control acute rejection, chronic rejection still accounts for a majority of long-term morbidity and mortality.

1. **Cyclosporine** is a cyclic polypeptide derived from a soil fungus. Its major actions are to inhibit macrophage and T-cell production of interleukins and to block activation of helper T cells.

2. **Azathioprine** blocks de novo purine biosynthesis, which is important to both DNA and RNA production, thus inhibiting both T- and B-cell proliferation.

3. **Prednisone** is an anti-inflammatory drug that suppresses helper T-cell proliferation and interleukin production by T cells. Tacrolimus is a macrolide antibiotic with immunosup-pressant properties that blocks interleukin production and proliferation of T lymphocytes. It is used as a substitute for cyclosporine in the setting of acute allograft rejection.

4. **Tacrolimus**, in comparison to cyclosporine, has been associated with a lower rate of rejec-tion, similar infection rates, and increased incidence of new-onset diabetes mellitus. It is effective in slowing progression of bronchiolitis obliterans. Some suggest using tacrolimus as a primary immunosuppressive agent for these reasons.

5. Approximately 50% of lung transplant centers also utilize induction therapy with polyclonal antibody (antithymocyte globulin), interleukin-2 receptor antagonists (daclizumab or basi-liximab), or alemtuzumab.

D. **Postoperative Complications**

1. The rate of **postoperative infectious complications** is higher in lung transplant patients compared with other solid organ transplant recipients. Therefore, one must be able to dif-ferentiate **infection versus allograft rejection**.

   a. **Several factors increase the susceptibility of transplanted lungs to infection:** (a) Exposure to the external environment, (b) pulmonary lymphatic disruption, (c) impair-ment of mucociliary function, (d) prolonged mechanical ventilation predisposing the patient to nosocomial infection and airway colonization, and (e) the presence of airway foreign bodies (eg, sutures).

   b. Proper diagnosis is crucial to successful outcome and is usually performed via a trans-bronchial biopsy using flexible FOB. Occasionally, open lung biopsy is necessary.

   c. During the initial 2 postoperative months, **nosocomial Gram-negative bacteria are the most frequent causes of pneumonia**. Thereafter, CMV pneumonitis becomes more common and is associated with progression to a state of chronic allograft rejection.

E. **The vagus, phrenic, and recurrent laryngeal nerves are jeopardized during lung trans-plantation.** Their injury complicates weaning from mechanical ventilation and can lead to long-term disability and vocal disorders.

F. **Postoperative airways complications** include bronchial anastomotic dehiscence, bronchial stenosis (most common), obstructive granulomas, bronchomalacia, and bronchial fistula formation.[48]

VIII. Outcomes

A. **Survival:** Recent reports from the ISHLT Registry indicate that the the 1- and 5-year survival fol-lowing lung transplantation is 85% and 59%, respectively, based on transplants between the years 2010 and 2018.[10] While survival following lung transplantation continues to improve, overall long-term survival still lags behind that of other solid organ transplants.

1. Categorical risk factors significantly associated with mortality during the first posttrans-plant year include recipient male gender, type of underlying lung disease (eg, COPD), pre-transplant long-term steroid use, retransplantation, earlier era of transplantation, increased severity of illness at the time of transplantation (mechanical ventilation or dialysis), donor cause of death other than anoxia, CVA or stroke or head trauma, higher mismatching of do-nor and recipient HLA type, CMV mismatch, and nonidentical donor and recipient blood groups.

2. Continuous risk factors significantly associated with mortality include older recipient and donor age at transplantation, lower transplant center volume, shorter donor height, ex-tremes of donor height minus recipient height difference, lower donor-recipient body mass

index (BMI) ratio, higher pretransplantation bilirubin, higher amount of supplemental O_2 at rest, lower percentage predicted value of forced vital capacity (FVC), and increased serum creatinine.

   3. Post–lung transplant morbidity factors include (a) hypertension, (b) renal dysfunction, (c) hyperlipidemia, (d) diabetes mellitus, (e) bronchiolitis obliterans, and (f) coronary artery vasculopathy.

B. Exercise tolerance has been shown to improve after lung transplantation, as have the quality-of-life factors for survivors.

C. Posttransplant lymphoproliferative disorders are more likely to develop in immunosuppressed patients. Posttransplant lymphoproliferative disorder is the third leading cause of death outside the perioperative period, with an incidence ranging from 1.8% to 20%. Other neoplasms have been associated with immunosuppression, including (a) non-Hodgkin lymphoma, (b) squamous cell carcinoma of the skin and lip, (c) Kaposi sarcoma, and (d) carcinoma of the vulva, perineum, kidney, and hepatobiliary tree.

IX. Special Considerations for Pediatric Lung Transplantation

A. Epidemiology

   1. Between 1992 and 2018, there have been 3,257 lung transplant procedures reported in children aged ≤17 years.[49]

   2. CF, idiopathic PAH, interstitial lung disease, and proliferative bronchiolitis obliterans account for almost all diagnoses in pediatric lung recipients. BSLT is the most frequent procedure.

B. Outcome: One-year survival is currently comparable with that reported for adults.[50]

C. Pathophysiology: In children with severe developmental anomalies of the lung (eg, congenital diaphragmatic hernia with pulmonary hypoplasia, cystadenomatous malformations), isolated lung transplantation may offer the only chance for survival. Rarely, HLT may be indicated during childhood for PPH, CF, or Eisenmenger syndrome.

D. Donor Lungs: Size considerations place additional limitations on organ matching for pediatric recipients and thereby exacerbate shortages. The scarcity of suitable donor organs has propagated living-related lung lobe donation; however, the success of this approach is somewhat uncertain. In addition, donor and recipient morbidity and mortality inherent to this operation have sparked considerable controversy.

E. Intubation: In smaller children, using DLTs is not feasible; instead, selective endobronchial intubation with a conventional cuffed single-lumen tube is the most frequent choice.

X. Anesthesia for the Post–Lung-Transplant Patient

In addition to certain specific considerations, several general principles apply to all patients who have undergone successful lung transplantation, including the toxicity of immunosuppressants, potential for infectious and malignant complications, and interactions between immunosuppressants and other pharmacologic agents (including anesthetics).

A. Airway anastomoses may be associated with chronic strictures and **inadequate clearance of secretions.**

B. Toxic Systemic Effects of Immunosuppressants

   1. Cyclosporine is a potent nephrotoxin. Blood urea nitrogen and creatinine levels increase, and most patients develop systemic hypertension. Cyclosporine can produce hepatocellular injury, hyperuricemia, gingival hypertrophy, hirsutism, and tremors or seizures (at high serum levels).

   2. Azathioprine suppresses all formed elements in the bone marrow. Anemia, thrombocytopenia, and, occasionally, aplastic anemia may result. Azathioprine is associated with hepatocellular and pancreatic impairment, alopecia, and GI distress. There may be an increased requirement in the dosage of nondepolarizing neuromuscular blocking agents in this patient population.

   3. Prednisone produces adrenal suppression, glucose intolerance, peptic ulceration, aseptic osteonecrosis, and integument fragility. Controversy surrounds the need to administer intraoperative "stress doses" of glucocorticoids to patients with chronic adrenal suppression.

4. **Tacrolimus** exhibits a spectrum of toxicities (including nephrotoxicity) similar to those for cyclosporine.

5. **Infections**

   a. Early posttransplant bacterial infections are typically related to **pneumonia** (*Streptococcus pneumoniae*; Gram-negative bacilli), **wound infection** (*Staphylococcus aureus*), and the use of **urinary catheters** (*Escherichia coli*). Because of the particular susceptibility of pneumonia, early extubation of the trachea after general anesthesia is highly recommended.

   b. CMV is the most frequent viral pathogen in lung transplant recipients and results from either primary infection (after contaminated allograft implantation or blood transfusion in seronegative recipients) or secondary to reactivated infection in a seropositive patient.

   c. After the first few months of immunosuppression, vulnerability to **opportunistic pathogens** increases (CMV, *Pneumocystis carinii*, herpes zoster). If diagnosis is rapid and treatment decisive, survival prevails. Prophylactic antibiotic regimens are available and have been successful in reducing the prevalence of some of these infections (eg, trimethoprim-sulfamethoxazole for *P. carinii*).

6. **Drug interactions**

   a. Both cyclosporine and prednisone are metabolized by the cytochrome P450 enzyme system in hepatocytes. Drugs that inhibit those enzymes (eg, calcium channel blockers) may increase their serum concentrations and promote toxic side effects.

   b. Other drugs (eg, barbiturates and phenytoin) may induce the P450 enzymes and decrease cyclosporine levels below therapeutic range.

XI. Future Directions

Lung transplantation is a viable therapeutic option for many patients with ESPD. Although advances in surgical techniques, organ preservation, and perioperative care have led to improved recipient survival and quality of life, a limited availability of suitable donor organs remains an obstacle. Efforts to enlarge the donor organ pool through expanded donor criteria, donation after cardiac death, and new allograft preservation technologies such as EVLP are continuing. These efforts, coupled with refinement of the organ allocation and prioritization criteria, should ideally expedite transplantation for the most critically ill patients. The COVID-19 global pandemic marked a turning point in lung transplantation with the introduction of a new cohort of patients with ESPD. In coming years, we will likely see a continual growth in lung transplants offered to patients with viral pulmonary disease. Development of perioperative optimization protocols and a more widespread use of mechanical life support such as ECMO have been instrumental in improving patient survival in both the pre- and posttransplantation periods. An increased understanding of perioperative factors that affect PGD will hopefully continue to decrease posttransplant morbidity and mortality. Ongoing research about mechanisms, prevention, and treatment of bronchiolitis obliterans offers hope that this devastating complication can be reduced or eliminated.

REFERENCES

1. Egan TM, Murray S, Bustami RT, et al. Development of the new lung allocation system in the United States. *Am J Transplant.* 2006;6:1212-1227.
2. Yusen RD, Shearon TH, Qian Y, et al. Lung transplantation in the United States 1999-2008. *Am J Transplant.* 2010;10:1047-1068.
3. Scientific Registry of Transplant Recipients. OPTN/SRTR 2020 annual data report: lung. U.S. Department of Health and Human Services. https://srtr.transplant.hrsa.gov/annual_reports/2020/Lung.aspx
4. Organ Procurement and Transplantation Network. Data Reports Open Database, Waiting List, Overall by Organ. https://optn.transplant.hrsa.gov/data
5. DeSoyza A, Corris PA. Lung transplantation and the *Burkholderia cepacia* complex. *J Heart Lung Transplant.* 2003;22:954-958.
6. Aris RM, Gilligan PH, Neuringer IP, et al. The effects of pan-resistant bacteria in cystic fibrosis patients on lung transplant outcome. *Am J Respir Crit Care Med.* 1997;155:1699-1704.
7. Meachery GJ, Archer L, DeSoyza A, et al. Survival outcomes following lung transplantation for cystic fibrosis patients infected with *Burkholderia cenocepacia*—a UK experience. *J Heart Lung Transplant.* 2007;26(25):S126-S127.
8. Moran A, Dunitz J, Nathan B, et al. Cystic fibrosis-related diabetes: current trends in prevalence, incidence, and mortality. *Diabetes Care.* 2009;32:1626-1631.
9. Weill D, Benden C, Corris PA, et al. A consensus document for the selection of lung transplant candidates: 2014-an update from the Pulmonary Transplantation Council of the International Society for Heart and Lung Transplantation. *J Heart Lung Transplant.* 2015;34:1-15.

10. Chambers DC, Cherickh WS, Harhay MO, et al. The international thoracic organ transplant registry of the international society for heart and lung transplantation: thirty-sixth adult lung and heart-lung transplantation report—2019; focus theme: donor and recipient size match. *J Heart Lung Transplant*. 2019;38:1042-1055.
11. Egan TM, Edwards LB. Effect of the lung allocation score on lung transplantation in the United States. *J Heart Lung Transplant*. 2016;35:433-439.
12. Snell GI, Richardson M, Griffiths AP, et al. Coronary artery disease in potential lung transplant recipients greater than 50 years old: the role of coronary intervention. *Chest*. 1999;116:874-879.
13. McKellar SH, Bowen ME, Baird BC, et al. Lung transplantation following coronary artery bypass surgery-improved outcomes following single-lung transplant. *J Heart Lung Transplant*. 2016;35:1289-1294.
14. Tzotzos SJ, Fischer B, Fischer H, Zeitlinger M. Incidence of ARDS and outcomes in hospitalized patients with COVID-19: a global literature survey. *Crit Care*. 2020;24(1):516. doi:10.1186/s13054-020-03240-7
15. Kurihara C, Manerikar A, Querrey M, et al. Clinical characteristics and outcomes of patients with COVID-19-associated acute respiratory distress syndrome who underwent lung transplant. *JAMA*. 2022;327(7):652-661. doi:10.1001/jama.2022.0204
16. Chambers DC, Zuckermann A, Cherikh WS, et al. The International Thoracic Organ Transplant Registry of the International Society for Heart and Lung Transplantation: 37th adult lung transplantation report—2020; focus on deceased donor characteristics. *J Heart Lung Transplant*. 2020;39(10):1016-1027. doi:10.1016/j.healun.2020.07.009
17. Reyes KG, Mason DP, Thuita L, et al. Guidelines for donor lung selection: time for revision? *Ann Thorac Surg*. 2010;89:1756-1764.
18. Bhorade SM, Vigneswaran W, McCabe MA, et al. Liberalization of donor criteria may expand the donor pool without adverse consequence in lung transplantation. *J Heart Lung Transplant*. 2000;19:1199-1204.
19. Snell GI, Levvy BJ, Oto T, et al. Early lung transplantation success utilizing controlled donation after cardiac death donors. *Am J Transplant*. 2008;8:1282-1289.
20. Fisher AJ, Donnelly SC, Hirani N, et al. Elevated levels of interleukin-8 in donor lungs is associated with early graft failure after lung transplantation. *Am J Respir Crit Care Med*. 2001;163:259-265.
21. Garijo JM, Roscoe A. Ex-vivo lung perfusion. *Curr Opin Anaesthesiol*. 2020;33(1):50-54. doi:10.1097/ACO.0000000000000804
22. Cypel M, Yeung JC, Liu M, et al. Normothermic ex vivo lung perfusion in clinical lung transplantation. *N Engl J Med*. 2011;364:1431-1440.
23. Loor G, Warnecke G, Villavicencio MA, et al. Portable normothermic ex-vivo lung perfusion, ventilation, and functional assessment with the Organ Care System on donor lung use for transplantation from extended-criteria donors (EXPAND): a single-arm, pivotal trial. *Lancet Respir Med*. 2019;7(11):975-984. doi:10.1016/S2213-2600(19)30200-0
24. Novick RJ, Bennett LE, Meyer DM, et al. Influence of graft ischemic time and donor age on survival after lung transplantation. *J Heart Lung Transplant*. 1999;18:425-431.
25. Low DE, Trulock EP, Kasier LR, et al. Morbidity, mortality and early results of single versus bilateral lung transplantation for emphysema. *J Thorac Cardiovasc Surg*. 1992;103:1119-1126.
26. Yusen RD, Edwards LB, Dipchand AI, et al. The Registry of the International Society for Heart and Lung Transplantation: thirty-third adult lung and heart-lung transplant report—2016; focus theme: primary diagnostic indications for transplant. *J Heart Lung Transplant*. 2016;35:1170-1184.
27. Rinewalt D, Wong M, Cruz SM, Fynn-Thompson F, Singh S. Donor directed lobar lung transplantation. *Ann Cardiothorac Surg*. 2019;9(1):56-57.
28. Starnes VA, Woo MS, MacLaughlin EF, et al. Comparison of outcomes between living donor and cadaveric lung transplantation in children. *Ann Thorac Surg*. 1999;68:2279-2283.
29. Feltracco P, Barbieri S, Milefoy M, et al. Thoracic epidural analgesia in lung transplantation. *Transplant Proc*. 2010;42:1265-1269.
30. Isaza E, Santos J, Haro GJ, et al. Intercostal nerve cryoanalgesia versus thoracic epidural analgesia in lung transplantation: a Retrospective Single-Center Study. *Pain Ther*. 2023;12(1):201-211. doi:10.1007/s40122-022-00448-z
31. Ghadimi K, Cappiello J, Cooter-Wright M, et al. Inhaled pulmonary vasodilator therapy in adult lung transplant: a randomized clinical trial. *JAMA Surg*. 2022;157(1):e215856. doi:10.1001/jamasurg.2021.5856
32. Hausmann D, Daniel WG, Mugge A, et al. Imaging of pulmonary artery and vein anastomoses by transesophageal echocardiography after lung transplantation. *Circulation*. 1992;86:II251-II258.
33. Evans A, Dwarakanath S, Hogue C, et al. Intraoperative echocardiography for patients undergoing lung transplantation. *Anesth Analg*. 2014;118(4):725-730.
34. Pruszkowski O, Dalibon N, Moutafis M, et al. Effects of propofol vs sevoflurane on arterial oxygenation during one-lung ventilation. *Br J Anaesth*. 2007;98:539-544.
35. Barnes L, Reed R, Parekh K, et al. Mechanical ventilation for the lung transplant recipient. *Curr Pulmonol Rep*. 2015;4:88-96.
36. Diamond J, Lee J, Kawut S, et al. Lung Transplant Outcomes Group: clinical risk factors for primary graft dysfunction after lung transplantation. *Am J Respir Crit Care Med*. 2013;187:527-534.
37. Ong, LP, Thompson E, Sachdeva A, et al. Allogeneic blood transfusion in bilateral lung transplantation: impact on early function and mortality. *Eur J Cardiothorac Surg*. 2016;49:668-674.
38. Geube MA, Perez-Protto SE, McGrath TL, et al. Increased intraoperative fluid administration is associated with severe primary graft dysfunction after lung transplantation. *Anesth Analg*. 2016;122:1081-1088.
39. Sabashnikov M, Garcia-Saez D, Zych B, et al. The role of cardiopulmonary bypass in lung transplantation. *Clin Transplant*. 2015;30:202-209.
40. Nagendran M, Maruthappu M, Sugand K. Should double lung transplant be performed with or without cardiopulmonary bypass? *Interact Cardiovasc Thorac Surg*. 2012;12:799-805.
41. Wang Y, Kurichi J, Blumenthal N, et al. Multiple variables affecting blood usage in lung transplantation. *J Heart Lung Transplant*. 2006;25:533-538.
42. Kukreja J, Venado A. *Lung Transplantation: An issue of Thoracic Surgery Clinics*. Elsevier; 2022.

43. Biscotti M, Yang J, Sonett J, et al. Comparison of extracorporeal membrane oxygenation versus cardiopulmonary bypass for lung transplantation. *J Thorac Cardiovasc Surg*. 2014;148(5):2410-2415.

44. Bermudez CA, Shiose A, Esper SA, et al. Outcomes of intraoperative venoarterial extracorporeal membrane oxygenation versus cardiopulmonary bypass during lung transplantation. *Ann Thorac Surg*. 2014;98(6):1936-1942 [discussion: 1942-1943].

45. Hoetzenecker K, Schwarz S, Muckenhuber M, et al. Intraoperative extracorporeal membrane oxygenation and the possibility of postoperative prolongation improve survival in bilateral lung transplantation. *J Thorac Cardiovasc Surg*. 2018;155:2193.e2193-2206.e2193.

46. Khan TA, Schnickel G, Ross D, et al. A prospective, randomized, crossover pilot study of inhaled nitric oxide versus inhaled prostacyclin in heart transplant and lung transplant recipients. *J Thorac Cardiovasc Surg*. 2009;138:1417-1424.

47. Scheffert JL, Raza K. Immunosuppression in lung transplantation. *J Thorac Dis*. 2014;6(8):1039-1053.

48. Dutau H, Vandermoortele T, Laroumagne S, et al. A new endoscopic grading system for macroscopic central airways complications following lung transplantation: the MDS classification. *Eur J Cardiothorac Surg*. 2014;45(2):e33-e38.

49. Hayes D Jr, Cherikh WS, Harhay MO, et al. The International Thoracic Organ Transplant Registry of the International Society for Heart and Lung Transplantation: twenty-fifth pediatric lung transplantation report—2022; focus on pulmonary vascular diseases. *J Heart Lung Transplant*. 2022;41(10):1348-1356. doi:10.1016/j.healun.2022.07.020

50. Goldfarb SB, Levvey BJ, Edwards LB, et al. The Registry of the International Society for Heart and Lung Transplantation: nineteenth pediatric lung and heart-lung transplantation report—2016; focus theme: primary diagnostic indications for transplant. *J Heart Lung Transplant*. 2016;35(10):1196-1205.

Anesthetic Management for Thoracic Aortic Aneurysm and Dissection

Ali Khalifa, Amanda A. Fox, John R. Cooper, Jr., and Sreekanth Cheruku

KEY POINTS

1. An aortic aneurysm is an area of dilation of the aorta of varying extent involving all three layers of the aortic wall.
2. The natural history of aortic aneurysms is for them to expand until they reach a critical threshold, after which they are likely to dissect or rupture.
3. An aortic dissection occurs when blood penetrates the aortic intima, forming either an expanding hematoma within the aortic wall or a false channel that propagates blood flow within the medial layer.
4. Medical management of acute aortic dissection includes the use of β-blockers and arterial vasodilators to reduce aortic wall stress and prevent further propagation of aortic dissection or aortic rupture.
5. Anesthetic goals during open surgical repair of the thoracic aorta include maintaining end-organ perfusion, preventing progression of aortic pathology, managing bleeding and coagulopathy, and preventing other complications.

6. Transesophageal echocardiography is helpful and often necessary for evaluating for progression of aortic pathology, monitoring cardiac function, determining the etiology of intraoperative hypotension, and evaluating valvular function after ascending aortic repair.

7. Because it is generally associated with better outcomes than open surgical repair of the descending thoracic aorta, thoracic endovascular aortic repair (TEVAR) is the preferred approach for most aortic pathologies involving the descending thoracic aorta, including aneurysms, dissections, and traumatic injuries.

8. TEVAR is associated with some unique complications, which can include endoleak, endograft migration, access site complications, retrograde aortic dissection, and unintentional coverage of the arch vessels or other critical arteries branching from the aorta.

ANESTHESIOLOGISTS CARING FOR THORACIC AORTIC SURGICAL PATIENTS encounter considerable variation among patients with regard to the cause and location of aortic disease. It is vital that anesthesiologists understand the implications of and the challenges related to these variations in order to provide optimal perioperative care. The 2022 American College of Cardiology/American Heart Association (ACC/AHA) guidelines for the diagnosis and management of patients with thoracic aortic disease were developed in collaboration with the Society of Cardiovascular Anesthesiologists and other professional societies.[1] These guidelines reflect decades of progress in thoracic aortic surgery. Thoracic endovascular aortic repairs (TEVARs) now have largely replaced open surgical repair for many descending thoracic or thoracoabdominal aortic pathologies, because TEVAR has been associated with improved perioperative outcomes.[2] The 2022 guidelines also emphasize the role of multidisciplinary team expertise in the management of patients with aortic disease. This chapter provides a concise overview of the pathophysiology of thoracic aortic disease and the key aspects of anesthetic management required to successfully treat thoracic aortic disease with open surgery and/or endovascular (EV) repair.

CLINICAL PEARL

Anesthetic management of patients with thoracic aortic aneurysm (TAA) requires knowledge of aortic anatomy, planned surgical and/or EV approaches and corresponding adjuncts needed, and excellent communication with the surgeon.

I. Classification and Natural History

A. Aneurysm

1. **Epidemiology:** The incidence of TAAs is 5.3 per 100,000 individuals-year, and the prevalence is 0.16%.[3] Patients with TAA were more frequently male (61%), with a mean age between 59 and 84 years at diagnosis, depending on the methodology of the study. Twenty percentage of patients with TAA had a first-degree relative with aneurysmal disease.[2]

2. **Pathophysiology:** The etiology and pathophysiology of aortic aneurysms are related to their anatomic location. Forty-five percentage of thoracic aneurysms involve the ascending aorta, 10% the aortic arch, 35% the descending aorta, and 10% the thoracoabdominal aorta.[4] Most commonly, ascending aortic aneurysms are due to cystic medial degeneration, whereas descending and thoracoabdominal aortic aneurysms result from intimal lesions and degenerative conditions associated with atherosclerosis.

3. **Natural history:** The natural history of aortic aneurysms is one of progressive dilation to a critical threshold diameter, after which it is likely to rupture. In general, TAAs enlarge at a rate of 0.42 cm/y, and aneurysms involving the aortic arch grow even faster at a rate of 0.56 cm/y.[5] Other complications of TAAs include mycotic infection, atheroembolism to peripheral vessels, and dissection.

B. Dissection

An aortic dissection usually occurs when blood penetrates the aortic intima, forming either an expanding hematoma within the aortic wall or simply a false channel for flow between the medial layers. Because the dissection does not necessarily involve the entire circumference of

TABLE 23.1 Conditions Predisposing to Aortic Dissection

History of hypertension	Present in ≈90% of patients
Advanced age	>60 y
Sex	Male preponderance age <60 y
Arachnodactyly	Connective tissue disorders (eg, Marfan syndrome)
Congenital heart disease	Coarctation of aorta, bicuspid aortic valve
Pregnancy	Uncommon
Other causes	Toxins and diet

the aorta, branching vessels may be unaffected, they may be occluded, or they may arise from the false lumen.

1. **Epidemiology**
   a. **Incidence:** The incidence of thoracic aortic dissection is 3-4 cases per 100,000 per year and is increasing because of improvements in screening and detection.[6]
   b. **Predisposing conditions:** The medical conditions predisposing to aortic dissection are listed in Table 23.1. Interestingly, atherosclerosis by itself may not contribute to the risk of subsequent aortic dissection. Genetic factors associated with thoracic aortic dissection include bicuspid aortic valve and Marfan syndrome.[7]
   c. **Inciting event:** The onset of aortic dissection has been associated with increased physical activity or emotional stress. Dissection also has been associated with blunt trauma to the chest. It also can occur during cannulation for cardiopulmonary bypass (CPB), either antegrade from the ascending aorta or retrograde from the femoral artery.
   d. **Mechanism of aortic tear:** An intimal tear is the initial event in aortic dissection. The tear usually occurs in a weakened portion of the aortic wall and typically also involves the middle and outer layers of the media. In this area of weakening, the aortic wall is more susceptible to shear forces produced by pulsatile blood flow through the aorta. Thus, intimal tears most frequently arise in the areas subject to the greatest mechanical shear forces: The ascending aorta and isthmic portion of the aorta just distal to the left subclavian artery takeoff are particularly vulnerable because they are relatively fixed.
2. **Classification of dissections:** The DeBakey classification consists of three different types based on the location of the intimal tear and the section of the aorta involved (Figure 23.1). The Stanford classification is simpler than DeBakey and consists of two types based on whether or not the dissection involves the ascending aorta (Figure 23.2).
3. **Natural history**
   a. **Mortality untreated:** The survival rate of patients with unrepaired Stanford type A dissection is poor, with 2-day mortality of up to 50% in some series and 3-month mortality approaching 90%.[8,9] The usual cause of death is rupture of the false lumen into the pleural space or pericardium.
   b. **Surgical mortality:** Overall mortality from open surgery ranges from 3% to 24% and varies with the section of aorta that is affected. Dissection involving the aortic arch carries the highest mortality.[10]

C. **Thoracic Aortic Rupture**
1. **Etiology:** Most thoracic aortic ruptures occur after trauma, most often as a result of a deceleration injury from a motor vehicle accident. Sudden deceleration places significant mechanical shear stress on points of the aortic wall that are relatively immobile.
2. **Location:** Most thoracic aortic ruptures occur just distal to the origin of the left subclavian artery (isthmus), because of the relative fixation of the aorta at this point by the ligamentum arteriosum. The second most common site of aortic rupture is in the ascending aorta, just distal to the aortic valve.

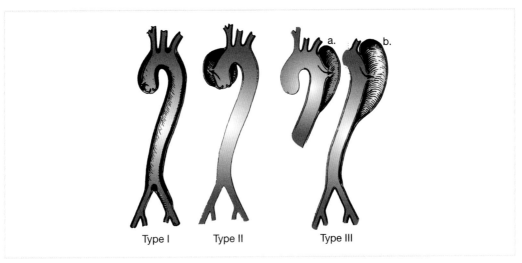

FIGURE 23.1   DeBakey classification of aortic dissections by location: type I, with intimal tear in the ascending portion and dissection extending to descending aorta; type II, ascending intimal tear and dissection limited to ascending aorta; type III, intimal tear distal to left subclavian, but dissection extending for a variable distance, either to the diaphragm (a) or to the iliac artery (b). (Reprinted from DeBakey ME, Henly WS, Cooley DA, Morris GC Jr, Crawford ES, Beall AC Jr. Surgical management of dissecting aneurysms of the aorta. *J Thorac Cardiovasc Surg.* 1965;49:130-149. © 1965 American Association for Thoracic Surgery. With permission.)

II. **Diagnosis**

    A. **Clinical Signs and Symptoms (Table 23.2)**

        1. Aneurysm: Aneurysms of the thoracic aorta are often asymptomatic until late in their course. In many circumstances, the aneurysm is not detected until medical evaluation is conducted for an unrelated problem or for a problem related to a complication of the aneurysm.

        2. Dissection: Aortic dissection usually presents with a dramatic onset and a fulminant course. Clinical presentations of Stanford types A and B are listed in Table 23.5.

        3. Traumatic rupture: Rupture most commonly occurs just distal to the left subclavian. If the patient survives the initial trauma, signs and symptoms are similar to those of aneurysms of the descending thoracic aorta.

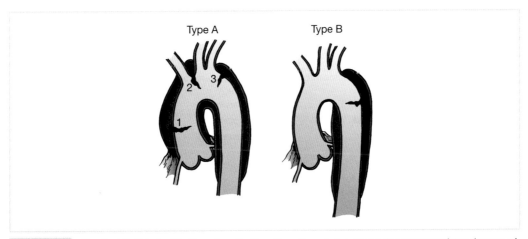

FIGURE 23.2   Stanford (Daily) classification of aortic dissections. Type A describes a dissection involving the ascending aorta regardless of site of intimal tear (1, ascending; 2, arch; 3, descending). In type B, both the intimal tear and the extension are distal to the left subclavian. (Reprinted from Miller DC, Stinson EB, Oyer PE, et al. Operative treatment of aortic dissections. Experience with 125 patients over a sixteen-year period. *J Thorac Cardiovasc Surg.* 1979;78(3):365-382. © 1979 American Association for Thoracic Surgery. With permission.)

TABLE 23.2 Presenting Clinical Signs and Symptoms by Location and Type of Aortic Pathology

	Aneurysm	Dissection	Aortic Tear
General presentation	Chronic symptoms, but leaking or ruptured aneurysm can lead to fulminant course (see Aortic Tear for symptoms and signs)	Dramatic onset and fulminant course; symptoms depend on location (type A or type B) Patient presents in shock, anxious, diaphoretic	History of deceleration injury; usually fulminant course (good chance of survival if patient gets to treatment center). Patient can present in hypovolemic shock
Symptoms and signs			
Ascending and arch		**Type A dissection**[a]	
Location of pain	Anterior chest pain secondary to compression of 1. Coronary arteries 2. Sensory mediastinal nerves	Anterior chest pain secondary to 1. Extension of dissection (ripping or tearing sensation) 2. Angina, from dissection of coronaries	Chest pain secondary to compression of structures by enlarging adventitia (the only structure maintaining aortic integrity)
Cardiovascular	CHF symptoms secondary to aortic annular enlargement 1. Widened pulse pressure 2. Diastolic murmur Facial and upper trunk venous congestion secondary to superior vena cava compression BP usually elevated chronically	CHF symptoms 1. Murmur of aortic valve insufficiency 2. Narrowing of true lumen (increased afterload), systolic ejection murmur BP 1. Hypotension secondary to rupture into the retroperitoneum, intra-abdominal, intrathoracic, or pericardial spaces 2. Hypertension secondary to pain, anxiety Asymmetry of pulses, or pulseless extremity	BP 1. Hypotension from hypovolemia 2. Hypertension from pain
Respiratory	Hoarseness secondary to compression of recurrent laryngeal nerve Dyspnea or stridor due to tracheal compression Hemoptysis due to erosion into trachea Rales secondary to CHF	Hoarseness secondary to compression of recurrent laryngeal nerve Dyspnea and stridor due to tracheal compression Hemoptysis due to erosion into trachea (chronic) Rales secondary to CHF	Lung contusion if chest trauma is significant
Gastrointestinal	Not usually affected	See under descending	Not usually affected
Renal	Not usually affected	See under descending	Decreased function secondary to hypotension
Neurologic	Possible because of emboli to carotid artery from aortic valve or aneurysmal segment (see Dissection, at right)	Hemiparesis or hemiplegia secondary to involvement of single carotid artery Reversible or progressive coma	Symptoms related to hypoperfusion
Descending		**Type B dissection**	
Location of pain	Chronic back pain may occur	Located in back, midscapular region	Located in midscapular region

TABLE 23.2   Presenting Clinical Signs and Symptoms by Location and Type of Aortic Pathology (*continued*)

	Aneurysm	Dissection	Aortic Tear
Cardiovascular	BP usually normal or elevated (chronic hypertension)	BP 1. Elevated secondary to pain (common) 2. Hypotension if rupture of dissection has occurred	BP 1. Elevated secondary to pain (especially with other injuries from trauma) 2. Hypotension if hypovolemic
Respiratory	Dyspnea from left mainstem bronchial obstruction Hemoptysis due to erosion into left bronchus Hemorrhagic pleural effusion	Dyspnea due to left mainstem bronchial obstruction Hemorrhagic pleural effusion	Sequelae of lung contusion or rib fracture
Gastrointestinal	Usually normal	Mimics an acute abdomen 1. Pain, rigid abdomen, nausea, and vomiting 2. Gastrointestinal bleeding Bowel ischemia secondary to compression or dissection of mesenteric or celiac artery	Usually normal
Renal	Renal insufficiency or renovascular hypertension if occlusive aortic disease develops	Ischemia due to involvement of renal arteries in dissection 1. Infarction and renal failure 2. Renal insufficiency	Renal hypofunction from hypoperfusion or hypovolemia
Neurologic	Usually not affected	Paraparesis or paraplegia possible secondary to occlusion of critical spinal cord blood flow	Paraplegia possible

BP, blood pressure; CHF, congestive heart failure.
[a]Type A dissections may involve the entire aorta; therefore, symptoms of both ascending and descending pathology may be present.

B. Diagnostic Tests

1. **Electrocardiogram:** Many patients with aortic disease will have evidence of left ventricular (LV) hypertrophy on electrocardiogram (ECG), secondary to the high incidence of hypertension in these patients. In patients with aortic dissection, the ECG may show ischemic changes caused by coronary artery involvement, or evidence of pericarditis from hemopericardium.

2. **Chest radiograph:** A widened mediastinum is a classic radiographic finding with thoracic aortic pathology. Widening of the aortic knob is often seen, with disparate ascending-to-descending aortic diameter. A double shadow has been described in patients with aortic dissection, secondary to visualization of the false lumen.

3. **Serum laboratory tests:** There are no laboratory findings specifically associated with asymptomatic aortic aneurysms. Aortic dissection or rupture lowers hemoglobin levels. Dissection may raise cardiac enzyme levels by causing coronary artery occlusion, increase creatinine levels due to kidney hypoperfusion, and lead to metabolic acidosis due to low cardiac output or ischemic bowel. D-Dimer, a fibrin degradation product, can be elevated in acute aortic dissection and has been proposed as a biomarker to rule out aortic dissection.[11]

4. **Computed tomography scans and magnetic resonance imaging:** Computed tomography (CT) using intravenous (IV) contrast is a useful tool for ascertaining aneurysm size and location and is the standard modality for diagnosing and planning the surgical repair of aortic dissections and aneurysms. It is also useful for following the progression of aortic disease. Magnetic resonance imaging is extremely sensitive and specific in identifying the entry tear location, presence of false lumen, aortic regurgitation, and pericardial effusion accompanying aortic dissection.[12]

5. **Transesophageal echocardiography:** Transesophageal echocardiography (TEE) has proved highly sensitive and specific for diagnosing aortic dissection. In many cases, pulsed-wave and color-flow Doppler imaging can aid in determining the presence, extent, and type of dissection. Identifying a mobile intimal flap constitutes a prompt bedside diagnosis that can be lifesaving.

C. **Indications for Endovascular and Open Surgical Repair**

1. **Ascending aorta**

   a. **Aneurysm:** Indications for surgical resection include the following:

      (1) Persistent pain despite a small aneurysm

      (2) Aortic valve involvement producing aortic insufficiency

      (3) Angina from LV strain secondary to aneurysmal involvement of the aortic valve or coronary arteries

      (4) Rapidly expanding aneurysm, or an aneurysm >5-5.5 cm in diameter[1] because the chance of aortic rupture increases with the size of the diameter

   b. **Dissection:** Acute type A dissection should be surgically corrected, given its virulent course and high associated mortality rate if not surgically treated.

2. **Aortic arch**

   a. **Aneurysm:** Isolated aneurysm of the aortic arch is rare. However, arch involvement is often seen together with ascending aneurysm (less so with descending aneurysm) and is thus dealt with at the time of surgical repair of the ascending aortic lesion. Indications to operate on the aortic arch include the following:

      (1) Persistent symptoms

      (2) Aneurysm >5.5 in transverse diameter

      (3) Progressive aneurysmal expansion

      (4) EV repair of the aortic arch is performed by specialized centers in patients with severe comorbidities and others who cannot tolerate open surgical repair. This approach is associated with lower mortality and risk of stroke but a higher reintervention rate.[13]

   b. **Dissection:** Acute dissection limited to the aortic arch is rare but is an indication for surgery.

3. **Descending aorta**

   a. **Multiple thoracic aortic segments diseased:** It is not uncommon for a surgeon to do an ascending and/or aortic arch replacement with open surgery and then coordinate a TEVAR of the descending thoracic aorta either at the end of the surgery or later as a staged procedure.

   b. **Aneurysm:** Indications for surgical or EV repair of descending thoracic aneurysm include the following:

      (1) Aneurysm >5.5 in diameter. In patients with known connective tissue disorders, the diameter threshold for repair may be lower.[1]

      (2) Aneurysm expanding

      (3) Aneurysm leaking

      (4) Chronic aneurysm causing persistent pain or symptoms

      (5) TEVAR using expandable stent grafts is the preferred approach for treating most aneurysms of the descending thoracic aorta, including ruptured aneurysms, because of lower morbidity and mortality when compared to open repair.[2] Open repair of descending TAAs is indicated for patients whose vascular anatomy is unsuitable for the EV approach, young patients with few comorbid conditions, and patients with genetic syndromes.[1]

   c. **Dissection:** Some controversy remains concerning the best treatment for an acute type B dissection. Because in-hospital mortality statistics are better for medical versus surgical interventions and similar for medical versus EV management, type B dissection is often treated medically in the acute phase, especially if the patient's comorbidities make the risk of surgical mortality prohibitively high.[1] However, patients with type

B dissection are treated surgically or with EV repair if they have any of the following complications:

(1) Failure to control hypertension medically
(2) Continued pain (indicating progression of dissection)
(3) Aneurysm enlargement on chest radiograph, CT scan, or angiogram
(4) Development of a neurologic deficit
(5) Evidence of renal or gastrointestinal ischemia
(6) Development of aortic insufficiency

III. Preoperative Management of Patients Requiring Surgery of the Thoracic Aorta
Key considerations in emergency preoperative management of acute aortic syndromes, including aortic dissection, aortic rupture, and contained rupture, are discussed later.

A. Blood Pressure Management
The initial management of patients with acute aortic syndromes is focused on reducing aortic wall stress by controlling blood pressure (BP), heart rate, and velocity of ventricular ejection velocity (dP/dt). The ideal drug to control BP is administered IV, is rapidly acting, has a short half-life, and causes few, if any, side effects.

B. β-Blockers
Both the 2022 AHA/ACC guidelines and the 2014 European Society of Cardiology (ESC) guidelines recommend treatment with IV β-blockers in acute aortic syndromes in order to decrease aortic wall stress.[1,14] β-Blockers can also attenuate the reflex tachycardia and increased ventricular contractility that can occur with the concurrent use of vasodilators, such as nicardipine, sodium nitroprusside, and clevidipine.

1. Labetalol is a combined α- and β-blocker and offers an alternative to the vasodilator-selective β1-antagonist combination. The disadvantage of labetalol is that it has a longer half-life, so it is not rapidly titratable if BP fluctuates.
2. Esmolol is a β1-selective adrenergic antagonist with a 9-minute half-life that can be useful in these cases when rapid titration is needed. Tachyphylaxis is commonly encountered with esmolol.
3. Metoprolol, another β1-selective agent, is longer acting than esmolol.

C. Vasodilators
Vasodilators are important adjunctive agents to achieve BP control in acute aortic syndromes.

1. Nicardipine is a calcium channel blocker that inhibits calcium influx into vascular smooth muscle and the myocardium.
2. Clevidipine is newer calcium channel blocker with a faster onset (2-4 vs 5-10 minutes) and shorter half-life than nicardipine (5-15 minutes vs 2-4 hours).
3. Nitroglycerin is a less potent vasodilator than sodium nitroprusside, and it causes more venous than arterial dilation. It can be useful in patients whose aortic pathology is coupled with myocardial ischemia because it can improve coronary blood flow by inducing coronary artery vasodilation.
4. Nitroprusside is a useful agent for controlling BP in patients with critical aortic lesions because its rapid onset and offset make it quickly effective and easily regulated. A vasodilator that relaxes both arterial and venous smooth muscles, it is given as an IV infusion, and although central administration is probably optimal, it can be administered through a peripheral vein with good effect. Higher doses (>8 μg/kg/min) have been associated with cyanide toxicity.
5. Desired endpoints: To decrease the chance of propagating aortic dissection or rupture, these pharmacologic agents should be titrated in most patients to achieve a heart rate <60 bpm and a systolic BP <100-120 mm Hg.[1,14]

D. Bleeding and Transfusion
1. Coagulopathy is frequently encountered in the thoracic aortic surgical patient. Patients who undergo open repair may require left heart bypass (LHB) or full CPB, both of which require heparinization. CPB may cause a consumptive coagulopathy and enhanced fibrinolysis, thus increasing blood loss. Patients requiring deep hypothermic circulatory arrest

(DHCA) for aortic arch surgery also may have substantial platelet dysfunction secondary to extreme hypothermia. In patients undergoing thoracoabdominal aortic aneurysm repairs, "back-bleeding" through intercostal vessels also contributes to blood loss.

2. Large-bore central venous access is required for open thoracic aortic surgical procedures. At least 8 units of packed red blood cells should be available before surgery, with an understanding that more packed red blood cells and other blood products may be needed.

3. Using blood-scavenging devices decreases the amount of banked blood transfused, but extensive bleeding and the logistics of effectively scavenging autologous blood during these operations frequently necessitate transfusing packed cells and other blood components. It is also important to recognize that reprocessed autologous blood is deficient in coagulation factors, so fresh-frozen plasma or other factor replacement treatment may likely be needed.

4. Antifibrinolytic agents, such as ε-aminocaproic acid and tranexamic acid, should be used prophylactically in patients who require CPB despite the lack of evidence supporting their use in thoracic aortic surgery patients. This is because of strong evidence that they reduce bleeding in patients undergoing other types of cardiac surgery with CPB. ε-Aminocaproic acid may be preferable to tranexamic acid because it is associated with a lower risk of postoperative seizures.[15] This is particularly important because thoracic aortic surgery with circulatory arrest is associated with a significant incidence of neurologic complications.

5. Thromboelastography (TEG), rotational thromboelastometry (ROTEM), or viscoelastic testing (VET) should be used to assess the coagulation system and guide the transfusion of blood components and adjuncts, such as desmopressin and prothrombin complex concentrates. Currently available prothrombin complex concentrates include three-factor (factors II, IX, and X) and four-factor (factors II, VII, IX, and X) concentrates, which can be used to rapidly increase the levels of vitamin K–dependent clotting factors.

E. **Assessment of Other Organ Systems**

1. **Neurologic:** Preoperatively, a thorough neurologic examination should be performed if time permits to establish the patient's baseline. The examination should include an evaluation of cognition, assessment of upper and lower extremity strength, and a determination of any focal neurologic deficits to allow better recognition of any postoperative deficits. The patient should also be monitored closely for acute changes in mental status and new focal neurologic deficits, as these may be indications for immediate surgical intervention.

CLINICAL PEARL

Involvement of the artery of Adamkiewicz can lead to lower extremity paralysis, whereas propagation of a dissection into a cerebral vessel can result change in mental status or cause stroke symptoms.

2. **Pulmonary:** Both physical examination and radiologic imaging should be used to evaluate any compression of airway structures by the aneurysm. Expiratory wheezing can indicate trachea-bronchial compression by a large thoracic aneurysm. Large TAAs can displace the left main bronchus and complicate double-lumen endotracheal tube placement.

3. **Gastrointestinal:** A preoperative abdominal examination should be performed, and arterial blood gases should be analyzed to assess changes in acid-base status. Ischemic bowel can cause significant metabolic acidosis and will require surgical intervention to try to reperfuse the intestine and to remove necrotic portions of the bowel.

F. **Pain Management**

Patients with aortic dissection may be anxious and in severe pain. Pain management is not only important for patient comfort but also beneficial in reducing sympathetic tone and optimizing hemodynamics. Oversedation should be avoided so that ongoing patient assessments can be made. Worsening of back pain may indicate aneurysm expansion or further aortic dissection and is regarded by many surgeons as an emergent situation.

IV. Surgical and Anesthetic Considerations

CLINICAL PEARL

The foremost goal in treating acute aortic syndromes is avoiding hemorrhage if possible and otherwise controlling and managing hemorrhage if it occurs. Once control is achieved, the objectives of managing both acute and chronic lesions are to repair the diseased aorta and to restore its relations with major arterial branches.

A. **Goal of Surgical Therapy (From Aortic Aneurysm, Dissection, Rupture, or Penetrating Ulcer)**

Surgical repair of TAAs involves replacing the entire diseased segment of the aorta with a synthetic graft and then reimplanting major arterial branches into the graft, if necessary. When repairing an aortic dissection, the goal is to resect the segment of the aorta that contains the intimal tear. When this segment is removed, it may be possible to obliterate the origin of the false lumen and interpose graft material.

CLINICAL PEARL

It is usually not possible or necessary to replace the entire dissected portion of the aorta because, if the origin of dissection is controlled, reexpansion of the true lumen usually compresses and obliterates the false lumen. With contained aortic rupture, the objective is to resect the area of the aorta that ruptured and either anastomose the natural aorta to itself in an end-to-end manner or interpose graft material for the repair.

B. **Overview of Intraoperative Anesthetic Management (for Aortic Aneurysm, Dissection, Rupture, or Penetrating Ulcer)**
1. **Key principles**
   a. **Managing hemodynamics:** BP and heart rate control should be monitored and managed to allow end-organ perfusion while preventing progression of a dissection, rupture, or hemorrhage.
   b. **Monitoring of organ ischemia:** If possible, the central nervous system, heart, and kidneys should be monitored for adequacy of perfusion. The liver and gut's metabolic functions can be checked periodically.
   c. **Treating coexisting disease:** Patients with aortic pathology often have associated cardiovascular and systemic diseases (Table 23.3).

TABLE 23.3 Incidence of Coexisting Diseases in Patients With Aortic Pathology Presenting for Surgery	
Coronary artery disease	66%
Hypertension	42%
Chronic obstructive pulmonary disease	23%
Peripheral vascular disease	22%
Cerebrovascular disease	14%
Diabetes mellitus	8%
Other aneurysms	4%
Chronic renal disease	3%

Reprinted with permission from Romagnoli A, Cooper JR Jr. Anesthesia for aortic operations. *Cleve Clinic Q*. 1981;48(1):147-152. © 1981 The Cleveland Clinic Foundation. All Rights Reserved.

   d. **Controlling bleeding:** Patients may have an inflammatory response to foreign graft material and the surfaces of the CPB circuit or the LHB circuits. This can interact with the coagulation cascade and lead to significant perioperative coagulopathy. Furthermore, patients with acute dissection and lower fibrinogen and platelet counts may already have a consumptive process from the clotting that often occurs in the false lumen. Coagulation abnormalities and their treatment are discussed in Chapter 28.

2. **Induction and anesthetic agents:** Many thoracic aortic operations are emergent procedures that require aspiration precautions while the airway is being secured. However, a typical rapid sequence induction and intubation is often not appropriate, as wide swings in hemodynamics can occur. A "modified" rapid sequence induction may be preferable, titration of anesthetic induction drugs to better control BP (ie, avoid hypertension) while laryngoscopy is being performed. The use of nonparticulate antacids, H_2-blockers, and metoclopramide should be considered. Other anesthetic considerations and agents are described more fully in Section IV.D. Despite precautions, marked changes in hemodynamics are common when the patient's airway is being secured, and vasoactive drugs should be available to treat an undesirable hemodynamic response to intubation.

3. **Importance of site of lesion (Table 23.4):** Knowing the location of the thoracic aortic lesion is important for intraoperative management because surgery on different segments of the aorta may require different perioperative monitoring and interventions.

TABLE 23.4 Anesthetic and Surgical Management for Thoracic Aortic Surgery

	Surgical Site		
	Ascending	**Arch**	**Descending**
Surgical approach	Median sternotomy	Median sternotomy	Left thoracotomy
Perfusion	CPB—aortic cannula distal to lesion, or in FA or right axillary artery	CPB—FA cannula or right axillary artery cannula	Simple cross-clamp Heparinized Gott shunt ECC with LHB or CPB (femoral-femoral)
Involvement of the following:			
Aortic valve	Sometimes	Sometimes	No
Coronary arteries	Sometimes	Sometimes	No
Pericardium	Sometimes	Sometimes	No
Invasive monitoring	Left radial or FA catheter PA catheter[b]	Arterial catheter—either arm or femoral[a] PA catheter[b]	Proximal arterial (right radial or brachial) Distal arterial (femoral)[b] PA catheter[b]
Special techniques	Renal preservation EEG	DHCA Cerebral protection (DHCA, DHCA with RCP, or anterograde cerebral perfusion) Renal preservation EEG	MEPs[b] One-lung ventilation Renal preservation CSF drainage[b]
Common complications	Bleeding Cardiac dysfunction	Bleeding Hypotension from cerebral protective doses of thiopental Neurologic deficits	Bleeding Paralysis Renal failure Cardiac dysfunction

CPB, cardiopulmonary bypass; CSF, cerebrospinal fluid; DHCA, deep hypothermic circulatory arrest; ECC, extracorporeal circulation; EEG, electroencephalogram; FA, femoral artery; LHB, left heart bypass; MEPs, motor-evoked potentials; PA, pulmonary artery; RCP, retrograde cerebral perfusion.
[a]Depends on whether the left subclavian or innominate arteries are involved in the pathologic process or if axillary arterial cannulation is used. If there is uncertainty preoperatively, use a FA catheter.
[b]Optional, depending on physician's preferences.

C. **Ascending Aortic Surgery**
1. **Surgical approach:** Ascending aortic surgery is conducted through a midline sternotomy.
2. **Cardiopulmonary bypass:** CPB is required because of proximal aortic involvement.
   a. If the aneurysm ends in the proximal or middle portion of the ascending aorta, the arterial cannula for CPB can be placed in the upper ascending aorta or proximal arch.

CLINICAL PEARL

Many ascending aneurysms extend into the proximal aortic arch. Such an extension may not be detected until the aorta is exposed, so further modification of management for the surgery may be needed.

   b. If the entire ascending aorta is involved, the femoral artery can be cannulated because an aortic cannula cannot be placed distal to the lesion without jeopardizing perfusion to the great vessels. Arterial flow on CPB in this case is retrograde from the femoral artery toward the great vessels. Often, a more advantageous approach is to cannulate the right axillary or innominate artery, allowing blood to flow retrograde into the innominate artery and then antegrade into the aorta. This allows for both CPB and selective antegrade cerebral perfusion (ACP) during DHCA.
   c. Venous cannulation is usually done through the right atrium; however, femoral venous cannulation may be necessary if the aneurysm is very large and obscures the atrium.
3. **Aortic valve involvement:** Aortic valve resuspension, valvuloplasty, or replacement is often needed with repair of ascending aortic dissection or aneurysm. Which procedure is used depends on the degree of involvement of the aortic root sinuses of Valsalva and the aortic annulus.
4. **Coronary artery involvement:** Ascending aortic dissection or aneurysm may involve the coronary arteries. Aortic dissection can cause coronary occlusion if an expanding false lumen compresses the coronary ostia; such occlusion necessitates surgical coronary artery bypass grafting to restore myocardial blood flow. In cases of proximal aortic aneurysm, displacement of the coronary arteries from their normal position distal to the aortic annulus usually requires coronary artery reimplantation into the reconstructed aortic tube graft, or coronary artery bypass grafting.
5. **Surgical techniques:** An example of the usual cross-clamp placement used in surgery of the ascending aorta is shown in Figure 23.3. The distal clamp is placed more distally than it is in coronary artery bypass surgery, and the surgeon needs to be sure that the clamped segments do not include part of the innominate artery. If aortic insufficiency is present, a large portion of the cardioplegia solution infused into the aortic root will flow through the incompetent aortic valve and into the LV instead of into the coronary arteries. This can cause distention of the LV with increased myocardial oxygen utilization and diminished myocardial protection from reduced distribution of cardioplegia. Thus, an aortotomy is often performed immediately after aortic cross-clamping, with direct infusion of cardioplegia into the individual ostia of the coronary arteries. Many centers also use retrograde coronary sinus perfusion for cardioplegia administration as an alternative or in addition to an antegrade technique. If the aortic valve and annulus are both normal size and unaffected by concurrent ascending aortic pathology, surgery is limited to replacing the diseased section of the aorta with graft material. If the annulus is normal size but the aortic valve is incompetent, the valve may be resuspended or replaced. If both aortic insufficiency and annular dilation are present, either a composite graft (ie, a tube graft with an integral artificial valve) or an aortic valve replacement with a graft sewn to the native annulus can be used. If the aortic root is replaced, the coronary arteries must be reimplanted into the wall of a composite graft. In contrast, if the sinuses of Valsalva are spared by doing a separate aortic valve replacement and then a supracoronary tube graft, the coronary arteries may not need to be reimplanted (Figure 23.4). The posterior wall of the native aneurysm can be wrapped around the graft material and sewn into place to help with hemostasis.

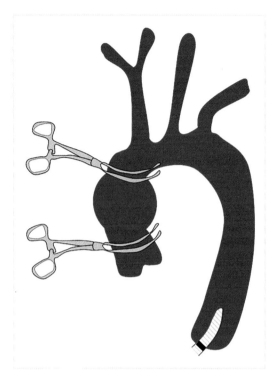

FIGURE 23.3 Circulatory support and clamp placement for surgery of the ascending aorta if femoral arterial cannulation is used; the distal clamp must be distal to the diseased segment. This may be the only clamp required. (Reprinted by permission from Springer: Cheruku S, Fox A. Anesthetic Management in Open Descending Thoracic Aorta Surgery. In: Cheng DCH, Martin J, David TE, eds. Evidence-Based Practice in Perioperative Cardiac Anesthesia and Surgery. Springer; 2021:111-122. Copyright © 2021 Springer Nature Switzerland AG.)

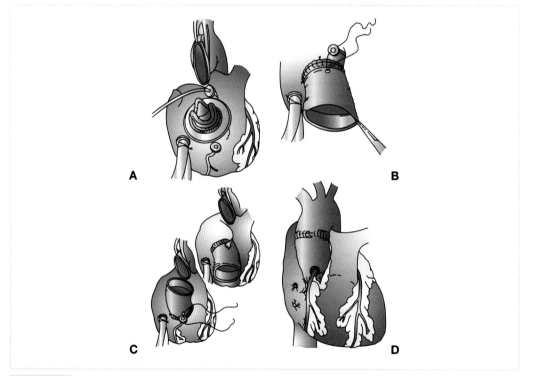

FIGURE 23.4 Surgical repair of ascending aortic aneurysm or dissection. **(A)** Aortic valve has been replaced and the aorta is transected at native annulus, leaving "buttons" of aortic wall around coronary ostia. **(B)** Graft material anastomosed to the annulus, with left coronary reimplantation. **(C)** Completion of left and beginning of right coronary reimplantation. **(D)** Completion of distal graft anastomosis. (Reprinted from Miller DC, Stinson EB, Oyer PE, et al. Concomitant resection of ascending aortic aneurysm and replacement of the aortic valve—operative results and long-term results with "conventional" techniques in ninety patients. *J Thorac Cardiovasc Surg.* 1980;79(3):394. Figure 5. © 1980 American Association for Thoracic Surgery. With permission.)

In patients with ascending aortic dissection, the aortic root is opened to expose the site of the intimal tear. The section of the aorta that includes the intimal tear is excised, and the edges of the true and false lumens are sewn together. Tube graft is used to replace the excised portion of the aorta.

D. Anesthetic Considerations for Ascending Aortic Surgery

1. **Monitoring**

   a. **Arterial line placement:** Since there may be involvement of the innominate artery, a left radial or femoral arterial line is inserted for direct BP monitoring. A right radial line could also be used as a surrogate for ACP pressure during DHCA if right axillary cannulation is performed. Right radial arterial pressure measurement will be falsely elevated when on CPB because of increased flow (see later).

   b. **Electrocardiogram:** Five-lead, calibrated ECG should be used to monitor both leads II and V_5 for ischemic changes.

   c. **Pulmonary artery catheter:** Because of the advanced age of many of these patients and the presence of severe systemic disease that may lead to pulmonary hypertension or low cardiac output, a pulmonary artery (PA) catheter may be useful in selected patients, particularly in the postoperative period.

   d. **Transesophageal echocardiography:** TEE is a useful and often necessary adjunct for the intraoperative management of these patients. Hypovolemia, hypocontractility, myocardial ischemia, intracardiac air, the location of an intimal tear, and the presence and extent of valvular dysfunction can all be detected and assessed with TEE. Caution should be exercised when placing this probe in patients with a large ascending aortic aneurysm because of the theoretical risk of rupture.

   e. **Neuromonitoring**

      (1) **Electroencephalogram:** Either raw or processed electroencephalographic (EEG) data may be helpful for judging the adequacy of cerebral perfusion during CPB. Monitoring the bispectral (BIS) or patient state index (PSI, SedLine) might help assess the depth of anesthesia during these procedures, but the benefits of such monitoring are unproven. Utilization of bilateral monitoring and displaying the compressed spectral array allow for easy detection of unilateral changes.

      (2) **Cerebral near-infrared spectroscopy or oximetry:** It may provide early warning of problematic cannulas or aortic clamp placement.[16] See the Aortic arch surgery section for further discussion.

      (3) **Temperature:** A nasopharyngeal or oropharyngeal temperature probe probably gives the anesthesiologist the best overall approximation of brain temperature. During CPB, the oxygenator's arterial outlet blood temperature can be used as a surrogate for cerebral temperature and can be used to guide the rewarming process.[17]

   f. **Renal monitoring:** As with all cases involving CPB, urine output should be monitored.

2. **Induction and anesthetic agents** (see Table 23.5)

3. **Cooling and rewarming:** Moderate hypothermic CPB is used in most ascending aortic aneurysm repairs. If femoral cannulation is to be used and the femoral artery is small, a smaller femoral arterial cannula may be needed. This may delay cooling and rewarming because blood flows on CPB will have to be lower to avoid excessive arterial line pressures between the pump and the arterial cannula.

E. Aortic Arch Surgery

1. **Surgical approach:** Repair of aortic arch lesions is typically done with an open surgical approach performed through a median sternotomy. A hybrid (open EV) approach to arch repair can be performed for aortic lesions that extend from the arch into the descending thoracic aorta. In this hybrid approach, either median sternotomy or a supraclavicular incision can be used to revascularize the affected arch vessels and create a proximal landing zone for subsequent TEVAR in the descending thoracic aorta.

2. **Cardiopulmonary bypass:** For open repair of the aortic arch, CPB with femoral or right axillary arterial cannulation and right atrial venous cannulation is required. This is often done with a Dacron graft. The hybrid and total EV approaches are designed to minimize or eliminate the need for CPB and DHCA.

TABLE 23.5   Anesthetic Considerations and Choice of Anesthetic Agent for Surgery of the Aorta

Patient Variables	Opioids[a]	Volatile Agent[b]	Other IV Agents
Full stomach	Rapid acting (especially sufentanil, alfentanil)	Prolonged induction	Rapid acting if tolerated
Hemodynamic instability	Minimal myocardial depression Potent analgesics useful for treating intraoperative hypertension	Dose-dependent myocardial depression Indicated if hypertensive with adequate cardiac output	T, P: Myocardial depression M, E: Minimal myocardial depression K: Worsens hypertension
Ventricular function (VF)	Indicated with poor VF	Use in patients with good VF	M, E, and K maintain VF Avoid T, P if VF is poor
Neurologic function	Decrease CMRo$_2$	Decrease CMRo$_2$, especially isoflurane; unclear in vivo protective effects	T, P decrease CMRo$_2$, probably protective, used with hypothermic arrest or open ventricle
Myocardial ischemia (coronary involvement)	Oxygen balance: Increases supply/demand ratio and, therefore, will have adverse effects in the presence of hypertension	Decrease supply/demand ratio but will have negative effect in the presence of hypotension	T, P: Adversely affect supply secondary to hypotension K: Increases oxygen demand, decreases supply (secondary to tachycardia)

CMRo$_2$, cerebral metabolic rate of oxygen consumption; E, etomidate; IV, intravenous; K, ketamine; M, midazolam; P, propofol; T, thiopental.
[a]Refers to fentanyl, sufentanil, and alfentanil.
[b]Halothane, sevoflurane, desflurane, and isoflurane.

3. **Technique:** Typical aortic clamp placement for this procedure is shown in Figure 23.5. Note that blood flow to the innominate, left carotid, and left subclavian artery will cease during resection of the aneurysmal or dissected section of the aortic arch, thus necessitating hypothermic circulatory arrest (HCA).

4. **Cerebral protection:** Open repair of the aortic arch requires interrupting or altering cerebral blood flow, which may contribute to postoperative stroke and neurocognitive dysfunction—both significant causes of morbidity and mortality in patients undergoing aortic arch surgery. Although various surgical approaches are used to reduce cerebral ischemia, all include lowering patient temperature with CPB to decrease the cerebral metabolic rate, the corresponding oxygen demand, and the production of toxic metabolites.

   a. Turning off CPB and partially draining the patient's blood volume into the venous reservoir provides a bloodless surgical field while protecting the brain and other organs. DHCA requires cooling the patient's core temperature to 15-22 °C, depending on the complexity and duration of the procedure and the adjunctive technique used (ACP or retrograde cerebral perfusion [RCP]). More recently, moderate HCA (21°-28°) with ACP has been employed to minimize the morbidities associated with DHCA.[18] Moderate hypothermia has been shown to decrease CPB and ischemic time, renal failure requiring dialysis, and blood transfusion requirements.[19] Multiple studies have identified prolonged DHCA time as an independent risk factor for temporary or permanent neurologic dysfunction and for stroke.[20,21] The accepted upper limit for DHCA duration without ACP is 40 minutes, after which stroke risk increases significantly. DHCA for >65 minutes is associated with significantly increased postoperative mortality.[22] DHCA has improved overall outcomes of aortic arch surgery but is associated with longer aortic cross-clamp and CPB times, which are needed to adequately cool and rewarm the patient.[23] Animal studies suggest that it is important to rewarm patients relatively slowly after DHCA and not to rewarm the brain above 37 °C, because this increases the risk of cerebral injury[24] (see illustration of surgical technique in Figure 23.6.).

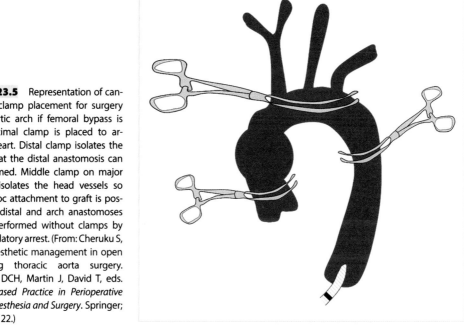

FIGURE 23.5 Representation of cannula and clamp placement for surgery of the aortic arch if femoral bypass is used. Proximal clamp is placed to arrest the heart. Distal clamp isolates the arch so that the distal anastomosis can be performed. Middle clamp on major branches isolates the head vessels so that en bloc attachment to graft is possible. The distal and arch anastomoses may be performed without clamps by using circulatory arrest. (From: Cheruku S, Fox A. Anesthetic management in open descending thoracic aorta surgery. In: Cheng DCH, Martin J, David T, eds. *Evidence-Based Practice in Perioperative Cardiac Anesthesia and Surgery*. Springer; 2021:111-122.)

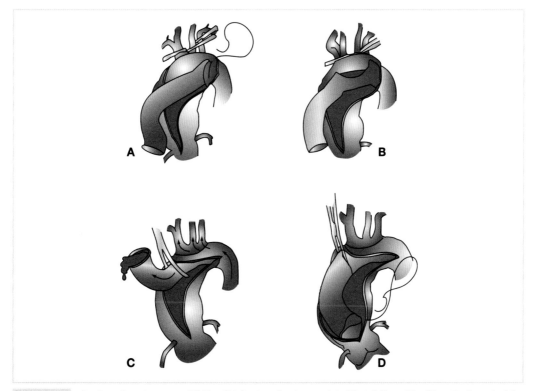

FIGURE 23.6 Aortic arch replacement. **(A)** The distal suture line is completed first, followed by **(B)** reattachment of the arch vessels. **(C)** Flow is reestablished to these vessels by moving the clamp more proximally. **(D)** The proximal suture line is completed. (Derived from Crawford ES, Saleh SA. Transverse aortic arch aneurysm: improved results of treatment employing new modifications of aortic reconstruction and hypothermic cerebral circulatory arrest. *Ann Surg.* 1981;194(2):180-188.)

    b. RCP necessitates individual cannulations of the superior and inferior venae cavae. After initiating DHCA, the arterial line of the CPB circuit is connected to the superior vena cava cannula and then low flows are directed through this cannula to maintain a central venous pressure (CVP) of ~20 mm Hg. This CVP is not necessarily associated with better outcomes. Advantages of RCP include relative simplicity, uniform cerebral cooling, efficient de-airing of the cerebral vessels (thus reducing the risk of embolism), and provision of oxygen and energy substrates. Outcome studies have identified three risk factors for mortality and morbidity in patients undergoing RCP during DHCA, including CPB time, urgency of surgery, and patient age.[25] Controversy exists as to how much RCP flow is actually directed to the brain and how much flow courses through the extracranial vessels. Clinical outcomes have been shown to be comparable between patients undergoing RCP versus ACP. In addition, RCP combined with HCA provides better neuroprotection than HCA alone. However, animal studies have shown that RCP can result in impaired cerebral perfusion and neurologic recovery.[26]

    c. Antegrade cerebral perfusion: The brain is selectively perfused via the innominate or carotid arteries. One method of administering ACP is to take blood from the CPB circuit's oxygenator and deliver it via arterial access to the brain by using a roller pump separate from the one used for CPB (Figure 23.7). Many centers use this same technique to deliver antegrade or retrograde cardioplegia.

    Figure 23.7 depicts direct cannulation of both carotid arteries for ACP, but this technique has been simplified in many practices by cannulating the right axillary artery or other arteries, as discussed earlier, instead of the femoral artery for placement of the arterial line from the CPB circuit. After CPB is initiated, the patient is cooled, circulatory arrest is initiated, the surgeon clamps the base of the innominate artery, and ACP is delivered at lower flow rates (eg, 10 mL/kg/min) through the axillary arterial cannula and thus up the right carotid artery (Figure 23.8). This allows bilateral cerebral perfusion, assuming that the circle of Willis is intact. The left common carotid artery also can be cannulated directly in the surgical field, as shown. There is mixed evidence concerning the use of bilateral (ie, left carotid artery) versus unilateral ACP. Some studies report decreased CPB time, milder hypothermia, and lower incidence of neurologic dysfunction when bilateral ACP is utilized, but adequately powered prospective randomized trials are needed to validate this assertion.

    Some centers use near-infrared spectroscopy to try to detect unilateral cerebral perfusion during ACP via the right carotid. Results of a small study suggest that this may be effective.[27] Cannulating the right axillary artery instead of the femoral artery to provide CPB before and after circulatory arrest reduces the risk for atheroembolic events. This is because right axillary artery cannulation provides antegrade aortic flow whereas femoral arterial cannulation produces retrograde flow through an atherosclerotic descending aorta.[28]

    In addition, HCA is required only for the completion of the distal and arch anastomoses. Then the aortic graft can be clamped proximally and full CPB perfusion reinitiated to the rest of the body while the proximal anastomosis and any concomitant aortic valve procedure are performed.

  5. Complications: Cerebral ischemia resulting in permanent brain damage is a distinct possibility. Hemostatic difficulties may be increased secondary to the multiple suture lines, long CPB times, and prolonged periods of intraoperative hypothermia.

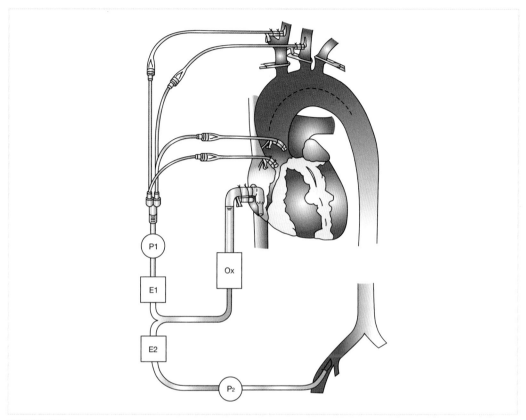

FIGURE 23.7 Perfusion circuit for anterograde cerebral perfusion for aortic arch surgery. Venous blood from the right atrium drains to the oxygenator (*Ox*) and is cooled to 28 °C by heat exchange (*E2*) before passing via the main roller pump (*P2*) to a femoral artery. A second circuit derived from the oxygenator with a separate heat exchanger (*E1*) and roller pump (*P1*) provides blood at 6-12 °C to the brachiocephalic and coronary arteries. (Reprinted from Bachet J, Guilmet D, Goudot B, et al. Antegrade cerebral perfusion with cold blood: a 13-year experience. *Ann Thorac Surg.* 1999;67(6):1874-1894. © 1999 The Society of Thoracic Surgeons. With permission.)

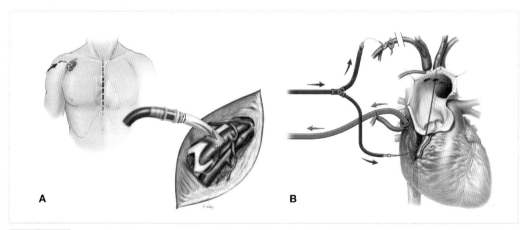

FIGURE 23.8 Antegrade cerebral perfusion (ACP) by right axillary artery cannulation. **(A)** Detail of surgical cutdown and graft anastomosis to the right axillary artery, showing relationship to the sternal incision. **(B)** Direction of blood flow when the right axillary artery is used for ACP. The brain is perfused via the right carotid artery and (optionally) via the left carotid artery from a balloon-tipped catheter inserted through the surgical field into the base of the artery. Venous return to the pump is via the right atrium. Note occlusion of the base of the innominate artery, allowing opening of the ascending aorta and aortic arch. (Printed with permission from Baylor College of Medicine.)

F. Anesthetic Considerations for Aortic Arch Surgery

1. Monitoring

a. Arterial blood pressure: An intra-arterial catheter can be placed in either the right or left radial artery, depending on which of the head and neck arteries that extend from the aortic arch are involved. If both the right- and left-sided arteries are involved, the femoral artery may need to be catheterized. Some have advocated monitoring right radial or brachial pressures to assess flow during ACP via the right axillary artery or the innominate artery. There is no consensus on this point. Also, with profound hypothermia, many have found that the radial artery does not provide accurate pressures for a period during rewarming, and they electively and preemptively also insert a femoral arterial catheter.[29]

b. Neurologic monitors

(1) Electroencephalography: It is often used to ensure that the patient has been cooled such that the EEG is isoelectric before HCA. Propofol or barbiturates are given by some anesthesiologists to achieve or extend this isoelectric state.

(2) Near-infrared regional spectroscopy: This technology measures frontal cerebral oxygenation through light transmittance. It can be particularly useful when ACP is used. Significant reductions in left-sided sensor values compared with right-sided ones may indicate an incomplete circle of Willis, and left-sided sensor values are usually restored when separate left carotid perfusion is initiated. Longer periods of lower cerebral oxygenation during HCA, as indicated by near-infrared regional spectroscopy (NIRS), have been associated with longer postoperative hospital stays.[30]

c. Transesophageal echocardiography: As in ascending aortic surgery (see Section IV.D.1), TEE can be used to assess ventricular function (VF), volume status, etc. TEE imaging of the arch is limited by the location of the trachea.

2. Choice of anesthetic agents (see Table 23.5)

3. Management of hypothermic circulatory arrest: The technique involves core cooling to a temperature as low as 15-20 °C. Some large centers use a target temperature of 24 °C (moderate hypothermia), pack the head in ice, use pharmacologic adjuncts to aid in cerebral protection, avoid glucose-containing solutions, and use appropriate monitoring for selective cerebral perfusion.

4. Management of acid-base disturbances: The primary philosophies involved are pH-stat versus alpha-stat for arterial blood gas assessment. pH-stat management is temperature corrected, aiming for a pH of 7.40 and $Paco_2$ of 40 mm Hg at the patient's actual temperature. During hypothermia, CO_2 is usually added to maintain a $Paco_2$ of 40 mm Hg. This typically causes an increased $Paco_2$ and subsequently increased cerebral blood flow and cerebral vasodilation.[31] pH-stat management is, therefore, often used in pediatric cardiac surgery. In adult cardiac surgeries, the alpha-stat approach is more typically used, meaning blood cases are not temperature corrected. A $Paco_2$ of 40 mm Hg and pH of 7.40 are maintained at a temperature of 37 °C. The patient's blood sample is warmed to 37 °C, and values are reported at this temperature. This allows for better preservation of cerebral autoregulation and cerebral flow-metabolism coupling.[32] The expected decrease in $Paco_2$ results in cerebral vasoconstriction. There are no randomized controlled trials in adults undergoing HCA that definitively establish superiority of one strategy to the other.

5. Complications: Complications related directly to anesthesia for aortic arch surgery are uncommon.

G. Descending Thoracic and Thoracoabdominal Aortic Surgery

1. Surgical approach: Aneurysms of the descending thoracic aorta frequently extend into the abdominal cavity and involve the entire aorta. They are often grouped according to Crawford classification (Figure 23.9). The affected segment of aorta can be exposed through a left thoracotomy incision alone or a thoracoabdominal incision. Extent IV aneurysms involve the supraceliac abdominal aorta but still require low thoracic aortic clamping. For aneurysms of any extent, the patient is placed in a full right lateral decubitus position with

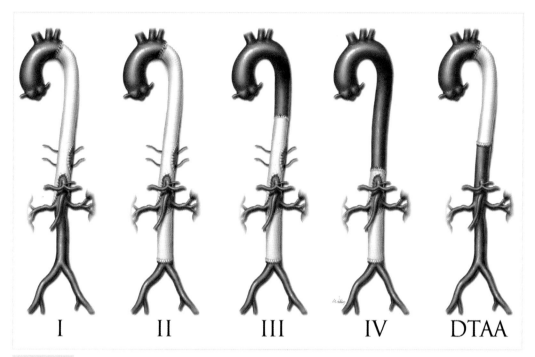

I   II   III   IV   DTAA

FIGURE 23.9 The Crawford classification of repair for thoracoabdominal aortic aneurysm surgery, with a descending thoracic aortic repair for comparison. The descending aortic repair does not extend beyond the diaphragm, whereas all the others do. Extent I aneurysms involve an area that begins just distal to the left subclavian artery and extends to most or all of the abdominal visceral vessels, but not the infrarenal aorta. Extent II aneurysms also begin distal to the left subclavian and involve most of the aorta above the abdominal bifurcation. Extent III lesions begin in the midthoracic aorta and involve various lengths of the abdominal aorta. Finally, Extent IV lesions originate above the celiac axis and end below the renal arteries; these aneurysms necessitate a thoracoabdominal approach for proximal aortic cross-clamping. DTAA, descending thoracic aortic aneurysm. (Printed with permission from Baylor College of Medicine.)

the hips rolled slightly to the left so that the femoral vessels can be cannulated for LHB or CPB if necessary. When positioning the patient, it is important to protect pressure points by measures such as using an axillary roll, placing pillows between the knees, and padding the head and elbows. It is also important to maintain the occiput in line with the thoracic spine to prevent traction on the brachial plexus. Various methods can be used to position the left arm.

2. **Surgical techniques:** Regardless of whether a patient has a descending TAA, a thoracoabdominal aneurysm, a dissection, or aortic rupture, surgical repair usually involves placing aortic cross-clamps both above and below the affected region of the aorta and then opening the aorta and replacing the diseased segment with a graft.

a. **Simple cross-clamping:** Some groups report success with cross-clamping the aorta above and below the lesion without using additional measures to provide perfusion distal to the aortic lesion. This technique has the advantage of simplifying the operation and reducing the amount of heparin needed (Figure 23.10) because more heparin is required when bypass circuits are used. An obvious disadvantage is potentially compromising flow to the distal aorta and its perfused organs when the simple cross-clamp technique is used. This approach is more often used with aneurysms confined to descending thoracic aorta and Extent III and IV thoracoabdominal aneurysms. Clamping the descending thoracic aorta generally causes profound *hypertension* in the proximal aorta and *hypotension* distal to the cross-clamp. The increase in afterload can cause acutely elevated LV filling pressures and a corresponding progressive decline in cardiac

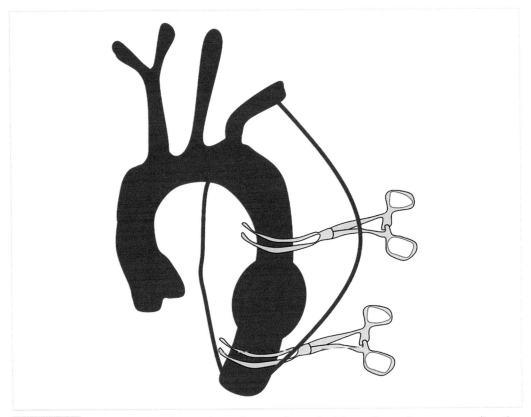

FIGURE 23.10 Illustration of simple cross-clamp placement for repair of descending aortic aneurysm or dissection. Distal clamp placement dictates that flow to the spinal cord and major organs proceeds through collateral vessels. (Reprinted by permission from Springer: Cheruku S, Fox A. Anesthetic Management in Open Descending Thoracic Aorta Surgery. In: Cheng DCH, Martin J, David TE, eds. *Evidence-Based Practice in Perioperative Cardiac Anesthesia and Surgery.* Springer; 2021:111-122. Copyright © 2021 Springer Nature Switzerland AG.)

output and, possibly, LV failure. Furthermore, hypertension in the proximal aorta could precipitate a catastrophic cerebral event, particularly in patients with unidentified cerebral aneurysm. Mean arterial pressure (MAP) distal to the aortic cross-clamp may decrease to <10%-20% of the patient's baseline BP, causing an obvious decline in renal perfusion and, perhaps, spinal cord perfusion. The physiology of aortic cross-clamping can change depending on the actual site of the clamp and is influenced by many factors, a discussion of which is beyond the scope of this chapter. Gelman's review of the subject remains an excellent reference.[33]

Aortic coarctation repair is another procedure in which simple cross-clamping is often used. Chronic obstruction of distal aortic blood flow, such as that which occurs with aortic coarctation, generally results in well-developed collateral flow and lessens the hemodynamic changes usually encountered when a cross-clamp is placed on the descending thoracic aorta. This is illustrated by BP measurements taken proximal and distal to the aortic cross-clamp in a series of patients with aortic coarctation versus descending TAA (Table 23.6).[34]

Another simple method of aortic cross-clamping is an "open" technique, in which no cross-clamp is placed distal to the aortic pathology. This technique allows direct inspection of the distal aorta for debris, such as thrombus and atheroma, and graft material can be anastomosed in an oblique manner that reincorporates the maximal number of intercostal arteries.

TABLE 23.6 Proximal Versus Distal Blood Pressure (BP) in Simple Aortic Clamp

	Proximal Systolic/ Diastolic; Mean (mm Hg)	Distal Mean (mm Hg)
Coarctation	160/85; 110	23
	145/80; 102	54
	150/85; 107	18
	155/80; 105	36
Average	152/82; 106	33
Thoracic aneurysm	260/160; 194	12
	240/135; 170	8
	245/150; 182	24
	235/140; 172	4
	240/155; 184	10
	255/160; 192	6
Average	245/150; 182	10

Reprinted with permission from Romagnoli A, Cooper JR Jr. Anesthesia for aortic operations. *Cleve Clinic Q.* 1981;48(1):147-152. © 1981 The Cleveland Clinic Foundation. All Rights Reserved.

  b. **Shunts:** Placing a heparin-bonded (Gott) extracorporeal shunt from the LV, aortic arch, or left subclavian artery to the femoral artery (Figure 23.11) provides decompression of the proximal aorta and perfusion to the distal aorta. Systemic heparinization is usually not required. However, there may be technical difficulties with placement and kinking of the shunt, which can result in inadequate distal flows. Also, relatively small shunt diameters can limit blood flow and thereby limit how much proximal LV decompression and augmentation of distal aortic perfusion can be accomplished.

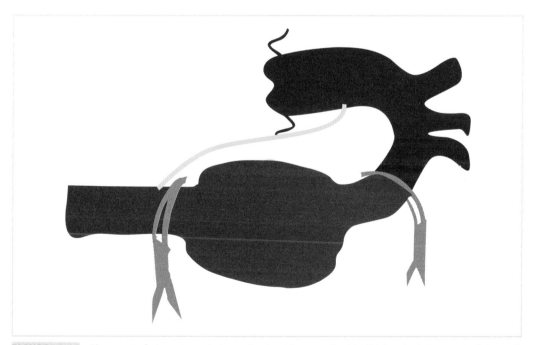

FIGURE 23.11 Placement of a heparin-coated vascular shunt from proximal to distal aorta during repair of descending aneurysm or dissection. (Reprinted by permission from Springer: Cheruku S, Fox A. Anesthetic management in open descending thoracic aorta surgery. In: Cheng DCH, Martin J, David TE, eds. *Evidence-Based Practice in Perioperative Cardiac Anesthesia and Surgery.* Springer; 2021:111-122. © 2021 Springer Nature Switzerland AG.)

c. **Extracorporeal circulation:** There are several ways to perform ECC, but all involve removal of blood from the patient, passage into an extracorporeal pump, and reinfusion into the femoral artery or another site to provide perfusion distal to the aortic cross-clamp (Figure 23.12). An alternative technique is perfusing the body of the aneurysm with extracorporeal circulation (ECC) while the proximal anastomosis is being performed and then opening the aneurysm and perfusing the major visceral vessels individually until they can be incorporated into the anastomosis.

Blood can be drained from the patient into the extracorporeal pump via the femoral vein. However, this necessitates placing an oxygenator in the ECC circuit to provide oxygenated blood for reinfusion. This form of CPB in conjunction with HCA may be necessary to repair descending TAAs that involve the distal aortic arch.

Alternatively, LHB can be used. A pulmonary vein or the left atrium, LV apex, or left axillary artery can be cannulated to carry oxygenated patient blood to the ECC pump; this blood is then returned via the distal aorta, the body of the aneurysm, or the femoral artery. This technique does not require an oxygenator in the LHB circuit (Figure 23.13).

Both ECC techniques have disadvantages. Using an oxygenator requires complete systemic heparinization, which is associated with increased risk of hemorrhage, especially into the left lung. Left atrial or LV cannulation for LHB without an oxygenator may allow the use of less heparin, but this approach increases the risk of systemic air embolism. Also, in the venous-to-arterial circulation CPB technique, a heat exchanger is included in the ECC circuit, which helps to avoid significant perioperative hypothermia and corresponding coagulopathy, although some degree of hypothermia is probably advantageous for spinal cord protection. When LHB is used, a heat exchanger is often not added to the ECC circuit. Table 23.7 summarizes the possible cannulation sites and the major differences between heparinized shunts and ECC for perfusion distal to the aortic cross-clamp.

3. **Complications of descending thoracic aortic repairs**

a. **Cardiac:** The rate of major cardiac morbidity and mortality was ~12% in one large series of thoracoabdominal aneurysm repairs.[35] Cardiac complications including arrhythmias, heart failure, myocardial infarction, need for pacemaker, or pericardial effusion have been reported in up to 30% of patients.[36]

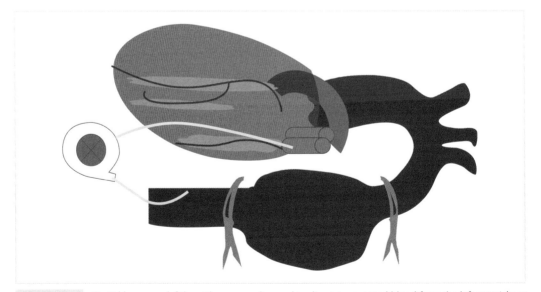

FIGURE 23.12 Partial bypass or left heart bypass can be used to direct oxygenated blood from the left ventricle or atrium and pump it using an extracorporeal pump into the femoral artery. Use of an oxygenator dictates the use of a full heparinizing dose. (Reprinted by permission from Springer: Cheruku S, Fox A. Anesthetic management in open descending thoracic aorta surgery. In: Cheng DCH, Martin J, David TE, eds. *Evidence-Based Practice in Perioperative Cardiac Anesthesia and Surgery.* Springer; 2021:111-122. © 2021 Springer Nature Switzerland AG.)

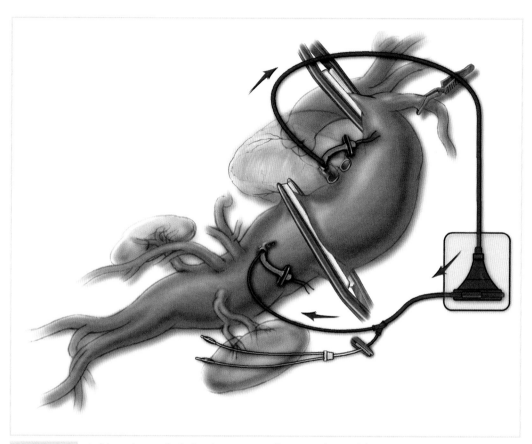

FIGURE 23.13 Left heart bypass. Perfusing the aneurysm allows completion of the proximal anastomosis while distal perfusion is maintained. After the aneurysm is opened, perfusion of the celiac, superior mesenteric, and renal arteries may be performed by individual cannulation before these arteries are attached to the graft. (Reprinted from Coselli JS, LeMaire SA. Tips for successful outcomes for descending thoracic and thoracoabdominal aortic aneurysm procedures. *Semin Vasc Surg.* 2008;21(1):13-20. © 2008 Elsevier. With permission.)

TABLE 23.7 Options for Increasing Distal Perfusion in Descending Aortic Surgery

Blood Removed From	Blood Infused Into	Heparinized Shunt	Perfusion Apparatus		Extracorporeal Bypass	
			Roller	Centrifugal	Oxygenator	Heparin (ACT)[a]
LV, AoA, LSA	FA, DAo	Yes	No	No	No	None (nl)
FV	FA, DAo	No	Either		Yes	Full (>480)
LA, AoA, LSA, LV	FA, DAo	No	No	Yes	No	Minimum (nl–250)[b]

ACT, activated clotting time; AoA, aortic arch; DAo, descending aorta; FA, femoral artery; FV, femoral vein; LA, left atrium; LSA, left subclavian artery; LV, left ventricle; nl, normal.
[a]Refers to the activated clotting time (in seconds); if used, optimum ACT is controversial.
[b]Some groups will not use heparin when using a centrifugal pump.

b. **Hemorrhage:** Significant perioperative bleeding is a common complication.

c. **Renal failure:** The incidence of acute kidney injury (AKI) in large case series ranges from 13% to 18%, depending on the extent of aortic pathology, preoperative comorbidities, and definition of AKI used.[35,37-39] The mortality rate is substantially higher in patients who develop postoperative renal failure.[35] The etiology of postoperative AKI is thought to be related to decreased renal blood flow during aortic cross-clamping, hemodynamic instability, bleeding, blood transfusion, atheroembolism, or a combination of these factors. Preexisting renal dysfunction increases a patient's risk of postoperative renal failure.

d. **Paraplegia:** The reported incidence of paraplegia after open surgical repair of the descending thoracic or thoracoabdominal aortic aneurysms ranges from 0.5% to 38%.[35,39,40] The largest risk factor associated with spinal cord injury is the extent of aortic coverage. The cause is either complete interruption of blood supply or prolonged hypoperfusion (>30 minutes) of the spinal cord via the anterior spinal artery (ASA). It receives collateral blood supply from radicular branches of the intercostal arteries (Figure 23.14).

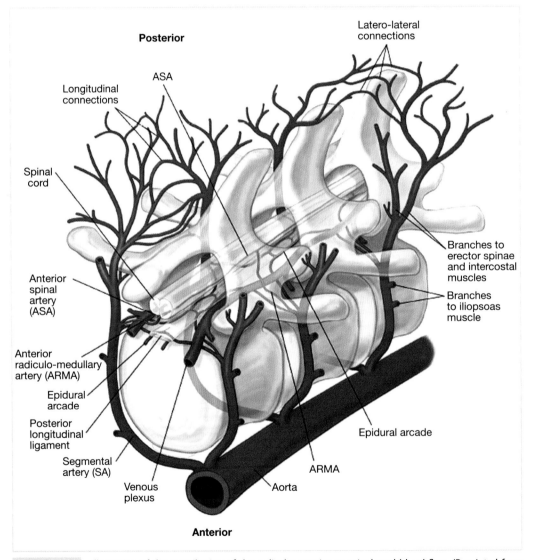

FIGURE 23.14 Illustration of the contribution of the radicular arteries to spinal cord blood flow. (Reprinted from Etz CD, Kari FA, Mueller CS, et al. The collateral network concept: a reassessment of the anatomy of spinal cord perfusion. *J Thorac Cardiovasc Surg.* 2011;141(4):1020-1028. © 2011 The American Association for Thoracic Surgery. With permission.)

In most patients, the **great radicular artery (of Adamkiewicz)** provides a major portion of the blood supply to the midportion of the spinal cord. This vessel is difficult to identify by angiography or by inspection during surgery. Interruption of flow can lead to paraplegia, depending on the contribution of other collateral arteries to spinal cord perfusion. With ASA hypoperfusion, an **anterior spinal syndrome** can result, in which motor function is usually completely lost (anterior horns) but some sensation may remain intact (posterior columns).

　　e. **Miscellaneous:** Patients who undergo thoracoabdominal aortic repair may develop postoperative diaphragmatic dysfunction. Cerebrovascular accidents are seen in a small number of these patients. Also, left vocal cord paralysis due to recurrent laryngeal nerve damage commonly occurs during descending thoracic aortic surgery because of the proximity of the nerve to the site of the aneurysm. Table 23.8 provides the incidence rates of various complications.

CLINICAL PEARL

All descending thoracic and thoracoabdominal aneurysms can be associated with major complications, but Crawford Extent II lesions involve more potential hazards because more of the aorta is affected.

　H. **Anesthetic Considerations in Descending Thoracic Aortic Surgery**
　　1. **General considerations:** Providing anesthesia for open descending thoracic aortic surgery can be extremely demanding because of profound hemodynamic changes and compromised perfusion of organs distal to the aortic cross-clamp. Anesthesia for descending thoracic aortic surgery is summarized in several good reviews.[41,42]

TABLE 23.8　Early Outcomes After Open Thoracoabdominal Aortic Aneurysm Repair (n = 3,309)

Adverse outcome	478 (14.4%)
Operative mortality	249 (7.5%)
In-hospital death	237 (7.2%)
30-Day death	159 (4.9%)
Permanent spinal cord deficits	178 (5.4%)
Paraplegia	97 (2.9%)
Paraparesis	81 (2.4%)
Immediate	79 (2.4%)
Delayed	99 (3.0%)
Stroke	98 (3.0%)
Acute renal dysfunction	406 (12.3%)
Renal failure necessitating dialysis	250 (7.6%)
Permanent	189 (5.7%)
Transient	61 (1.8%)
Cardiac complication	860 (26.0%)
Pulmonary complication	1,185 (35.8%)
Bleeding necessitating reoperation	110 (3.3%)
Left vocal cord paralysis	502 (15.2%)
Postoperative ICU length of stay, days; median [interquartile range]	4 [3-6]
Postoperative hospital length of stay, days; median [interquartile range]	12 [9-17]

ICU, intensive care unit.
Adapted from Coselli JS, LeMaire SA, Preventza O, et al. Outcomes of 3309 thoracoabdominal aortic aneurysm repairs. *J Thorac Cardiovasc Surg.* 2016;151(5):1323-1337.

2. **Monitoring**
   a. **Arterial blood pressure:** A right radial or brachial arterial catheter is needed to monitor pressures above the proximal clamp because aortic cross-clamping may occlude the left subclavian artery. To assess perfusion distal to the lower aortic cross-clamp, many centers place a femoral arterial catheter. If the LHB technique of ECC is used, the left femoral artery is typically cannulated for distal perfusion of the aorta and the right femoral artery can be used for monitoring BP.
   b. **Ventricular function:** The TEE probe in the esophagus can interfere with surgical placement of retractors or clamps. In those cases, TEE cannot be used. A PA catheter allows indirect assessment of LV filling and cardiac output. However, a PA catheter is not as helpful as TEE for intraoperative real-time patient monitoring.
   c. **Other monitors:** ECG lead V_5 cannot be used because of the surgical approach, which limits the assessment of anterior myocardial ischemia. However, TEE may allow good assessment of LV wall motion.
3. **One-lung anesthesia:** Double-lumen endobronchial tubes not only improve surgical exposure but also protect the left lung from trauma associated with surgical manipulation, particularly in heparinized patients. Furthermore, the double-lumen tube can protect the right lung from blood spillage. A left-sided double-lumen endotracheal tube is generally easier to place; however, in some patients, the aortic aneurysm distorts the trachea or left mainstem bronchus to the degree that placing a left-sided double-lumen tube is impossible. Patients with aortic rupture may also have a distorted left mainstem bronchus. Right-sided double-lumen endobronchial tubes may be used, but proper alignment with the right upper lobe bronchus should be checked with a fiberoptic bronchoscope. Alternatively, a single-lumen endotracheal tube with an endobronchial blocker can be used. For a detailed description of double-lumen and endobronchial blocker tube placement and single-lung ventilation, see Chapter 25.
4. **Anesthetic management before and during aortic cross-clamping:** Before the aorta is cross-clamped, mannitol (0.5 g/kg) is sometimes administered for its perceived reno-protective antioxidant properties. The evidence for using mannitol remains ambiguous.

   If simple aortic cross-clamping without shunting or ECC is used, proximal hypertension should be controlled, again with awareness that distal organ flow may be diminished. In treating proximal hypertension, regional blood flow studies have shown that infusing nitroprusside may decrease renal and spinal cord blood flow in a dose-related manner. Ideally, aortic cross-clamp time (regardless of technique) should be <30 minutes because the incidence of complications, especially paraplegia, starts to increase substantially beyond this time.

   If a heparinized shunt is used and proximal **hypertension** cannot be treated without producing subsequent distal **hypotension** (<60 mm Hg), the surgeon should be made aware that there could be a technical problem with the shunt's placement. If LHB is used, pump speed can be increased to reduce proximal hypertension by moving blood volume from the proximal to the distal aorta. This also increases lower body perfusion. Usually, little or no pharmacologic intervention is needed during LHB because changing the pump speed allows rapid control of proximal and distal aortic pressures. Table 23.9 lists the treatment options for several clinical scenarios when using ECC.

   Before the surgeon removes the aortic cross-clamp, the patient should be adequately volume resuscitated and a vasopressor should be available in case substantial hypotension occurs after the aorta is unclamped.

CLINICAL PEARL

The anesthesiologist must be constantly aware of the stage of the operation so that major events such as clamping and unclamping of the aorta are anticipated.

TABLE 23.9 Management of Extracorporeal Circulation for Surgery of the Descending Aorta

Proximal Arterial Pressure	Distal Arterial Pressure	Pulmonary Wedge Pressure	Treatment
↑	↓	↓	Volume; increase pump flow
↑	↓	↑	Increase pump flow
↑	↑	↓	Volume; vasodilator
↑	↑	↑	Vasodilator; diuretic; maintain pump flow, hold volume in pump reservoir (if in use)
↓	↓	↓	Volume; look for partial occlusion of arterial outflow cannula (if reservoir in use)
↓	↓	↑	Increase pump flow; inotrope
↓	↑	↑	Decrease pump flow; inotrope; diuretic
↓	↑	↓	Decrease pump flow; may need volume

↑, increase; ↓, decrease.

5. **Declamping shock:** When **simple cross-clamping** of the aorta is used, subsequent unclamping can have serious and even life-threatening consequences, usually from severe hypotension or myocardial depression. Declamping shock has several theoretical causes, including washout of acid metabolites, vasodilator substances, sequestration of blood in the gut or lower extremities, and reactive hyperemia.

CLINICAL PEARL

The usual cause of declamping shock, however, is relative or absolute hypovolemia.

To attenuate the effects of clamp removal, the patient's volume should be optimized, particularly in the 10-15 minutes before unclamping the aorta. This includes elevating filling pressures by infusing blood products, colloids, or crystalloids. Some advocate prophylactic bicarbonate administration just before clamp removal to minimize myocardial depression from "washout acidosis." It is advisable for the surgeon to release the cross-clamp slowly over a period of 1-2 minutes to allow enough time for compensatory hemodynamic changes to occur and for the anesthesiologist to determine whether further volume resuscitation is indicated. With a volume-resuscitated patient and a slow cross-clamp release, significant postclamp hypotension is usually short lived and well tolerated. If hypotension is severe, the easiest intervention is for the surgeon to reapply the aortic clamp and for the anesthesiologist to give the patient additional volume.

If shunts or ECC are used, declamping hypotension is usually mild, as the vascular bed below the clamp is less "empty," and there will be less proximal to distal aortic volume shifting after the aortic cross-clamp is released. If a volume reservoir is used in the bypass circuit, ECC also provides a means for rapid volume infusion after the aortic cross-clamp is removed. Some type of rapid infusion device is most useful in these cases.

6. **Fluid therapy and transfusion:** Blood loss can be considerable in these cases because of back-bleeding from the intercostal arteries, which are often ligated when the aorta is opened. The use of intraoperative cell–scavenging devices has become common and has reduced the need for banked blood transfusions. Hemorrhage can result in estimated blood loss exceeding the patient's blood volume and has been cited as the cause of death in 12%-39% of deaths in patients that do not survive thoracic aneurysm repairs.[43,44] After heparinization, shed whole blood harvested from the field via suction can be returned to a cardiotomy reservoir and propelled to a rapid infusion device. The rapid infuser can then be managed by the anesthesiologist to return autologous whole blood back to the patient (Figure 23.15). Of note, acid-citrate-dextrose solution is added to the cardiotomy blood to prevent clot formation, and calcium supplementation may be necessary.

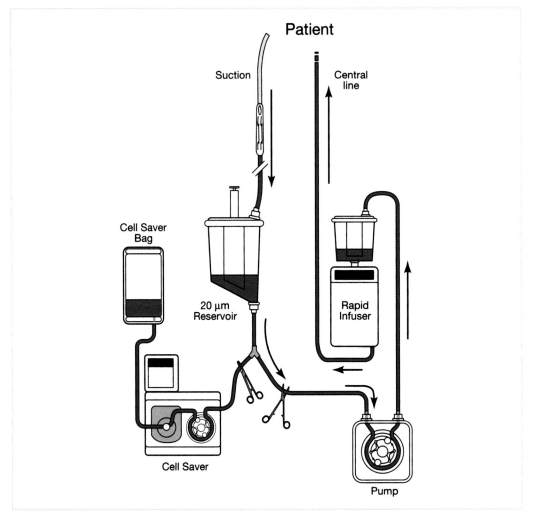

FIGURE 23.15 Schematic of reinfusion system where shed whole blood is filtered and directly returned to the patient through a rapid infusion device for patients undergoing thoracoabdominal aortic aneurysm repair. (Printed with permission from Baylor College of Medicine.)

CLINICAL PEARL

Thoracic aneurysm repair, particularly with simple clamping, presents a unique situation because hepatic arterial blood flow to the liver may be compromised, perhaps for an extended period. In this circumstance, transfusing banked blood may rapidly produce citrate toxicity, resulting in myocardial depression that requires vigilant calcium chloride infusion. One should never wait for an ionized calcium level if citrate toxicity is suspected.

7. **Spinal cord protection:** In addition to the use of ECC, shunts, and expeditious surgery, several other methods have been promoted to protect the spinal cord during aortic cross-clamping.

   a. **Maintaining perfusion pressure:** Some groups prefer to maintain the perfusion pressure of the distal aorta in the range of 40-60 mm Hg to increase blood flow to the middle and lower spinal cord. **No method used to maintain blood flow to the distal aorta (ie, shunt or partial bypass [PB]) guarantees that spinal cord blood flow, and therefore function, will be preserved.** Sequential clamping of the aorta may reduce ischemic periods for individual segments of the spinal cord and allow for faster reperfusion of reimplanted segmental arteries; however, no large trials have evaluated the efficacy. Distal perfusion may be hindered by atherosclerotic disease in the abdominal aorta, which can also compromise blood flow to the kidneys and spinal cord. Crucial arterial vessels may be disrupted in gaining surgical exposure.

b. **Somatosensory-evoked potentials:** Although it has been used intraoperatively to help identify intercostal arteries that should be reimplanted to preserve spinal cord perfusion, somatosensory-evoked potential (SEP) monitoring has not been shown to decrease the incidence of postoperative paraplegia.

c. **Motor-evoked potentials:** Because of the noted deficiencies in SEPs monitoring, using motor-evoked potentials (MEPs) has been advocated as a potentially superior method of monitoring for spinal cord ischemia, because MEP monitoring can accurately assess the integrity of the anterior horn of the spinal cord. Some groups have successfully used MEPs, particularly as an adjunct to SEPs, to detect spinal cord injury in patients undergoing thoracic and thoracoabdominal aortic aneurysm repair. Although studies have shown these neuromonitoring techniques to be helpful for predicting spinal cord injury, they cannot definitively rule out intraoperative spinal cord injury that will result in paraplegia.

d. **Hypothermia:** Allowing the core body temperature to passively drift down to 32-34 °C may provide some protection from reduced or interrupted blood flow. At temperatures below 32 °C, the myocardium may become more prone to ventricular arrhythmias, and hypothermia increases the risk of coagulopathy. Despite these potential problems, using vigorous methods to rewarm the patient is ill advised because of the risk of rapidly warming neural tissue that may be ischemic.

e. **Cerebrospinal fluid drainage:** Spinal cord damage may also be mediated by the increases in cerebrospinal fluid pressure (CSFP) that often accompanies aortic cross-clamping. CSFP can increase to levels as high as the mean distal **aortic** pressure. Placing a lumbar spinal drain not only allows measurement of the CSFP but also, by removal of CSF, reduces CSFP and increases spinal cord perfusion pressure (SCPP), which apparently reduces the risk of paraplegia.[45] In a randomized controlled trial, CSF drainage significantly decreased postoperative paraplegia and paraparesis rates in 145 patients who underwent surgical repair of Extent I or II thoracoabdominal aneurysm: 13% and 2.6% of patients experienced postoperative paraplegia or paraparesis in the control group versus the spinal drain group.[40]

   (1) **Potential complications of spinal drain placement:** Draining CSF in patients with elevated intraspinal pressure can provide a gradient for herniation of cerebral structures. Also, rapid drainage can cause intracranial bleeding from traction of the brain on the meninges, torn bridging veins, and the formation of subdural hematomas.[46,47] Risk of intracranial bleeding can be decreased by maintaining CSFP above at least 10 cm H_2O (7.4 mm Hg) during CSF drainage.[47] CSF drainage is now targeted to less aggressive minimum CSFP thresholds, such as 10-15 mm Hg, and the rate of drainage is not to exceed 15 mL/h even if CSFP is above the minimum. If the patients develop paraplegia postoperatively, CSF drainage is then liberalized to try to provoke resolution of the paralysis. If a subdural hematoma develops and CSF is still leaking from the insertion site after drain removal, an epidural blood patch may be warranted at the site.[47] In addition, spinal drain placement followed by systemic heparinization could lead to the formation of an epidural hematoma at the insertion site.[46] This is of more concern in patients who are undergoing concurrent aortic arch and descending thoracic aortic repairs that involve CPB with full heparinization and HCA and who are thus at increased risk of bleeding. Another risk associated with drain placement is catheter fracture in the subarachnoid space.

   (2) **Technique for inserting and monitoring spinal drains:** A variety of spinal drain catheters are commercially available, but the insertion technique is similar for all. Spinal drain catheters are generally placed according to anatomic landmarks through a 14-G (or smaller) Touhy needle that has been inserted into the

subarachnoid space at a lumbar interspace (usually L_3 to L_4 or L_4 to L_5). Once the catheter is threaded into the subarachnoid space and the needle is removed, the drain is attached to a stopcock that allows toggling between CSFP measurement and drainage collection (Figure 23.16).

CLINICAL PEARL

Although many try maintaining CSFP at 8-10 mm Hg to balance benefit of increasing SCPP against the risk of supratentorial bleeding with a lower CSFP, there is no consensus in the literature regarding what the optimal target CSFP is or how much CSF should be drained over a set time period.

---

(3) **Spinal drain pressure transducer management:** Another point of controversy concerning the use of spinal drains is at what level relative to the patient should the pressure be measured, that is, where is the transducer placed? Some anesthesiologists when faced with this simply chose to place the transducer at the approximate midlevel of the cord, and others estimate the distance between the two points and allow for it in their estimation of pressure. As far as we know, this question has not received adequate research. It is also possible that one specific level does not matter significantly for the time that the patient is in the operating room.

(4) **Postoperative spinal drain management:** There is no consensus regarding when spinal drains should be removed. This is of concern because ≥30% of all neurologic deficits have delayed onset.[48] Spinal drains are commonly left in for 48-72 hours postoperatively[40] and are replaced if neurologic deficits occur after the drain is removed. If delayed-onset paraparesis or paraplegia evolves, systemic hypotension should be treated and CSF drained. This combination of measures can result in some recovery of neurologic function. As with any patient with a dural puncture, headaches related to residual CSF leaks may be expected, and some will require therapy with epidural blood patches. The incidence of postdural puncture headaches and need for an epidural blood patch is elevated in patients with connective tissue diseases, such as Marfan syndrome.[49]

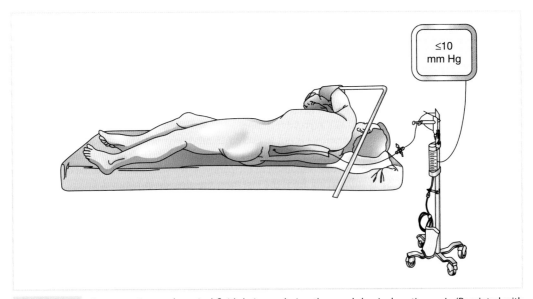

FIGURE 23.16 Intraoperative cerebrospinal fluid drainage during thoracoabdominal aortic repair. (Reprinted with permission from Safi HJ, Miller CC III, Huynh TT, et al. Distal aortic perfusion and cerebrospinal fluid drainage for thoracoabdominal and descending thoracic aortic repair: ten years of organ protection. *Ann Surg.* 2003;238(3):372-381.)

8. **Pain relief:** Thoracic and thoracoabdominal aortic surgical patients can be given IV opioid and oral analgesics to relieve postoperative pain. Anesthesiologists may also consider using a thoracic epidural anesthesia as an adjunctive perioperative pain control measure, although analgesic coverage may not be complete. In a patient who will undergo partial or even full heparinization and who may have significant intraoperative and early postoperative coagulopathy, instrumenting the epidural space can increase the risk of epidural hematoma (just as placing a spinal drain does). This possibility is particularly worrisome because these patients already have a primary risk of significant neurologic complications. In addition, using a thoracic epidural may mask neurologic complications related to the removal of a CSF drainage catheter.[50]

9. **Preventing renal failure:** Acute renal failure is a strong postoperative determinant of mortality after open thoracoabdominal aortic repair.[51] Renal failure is thought to be caused by ischemia from interruption of blood flow during clamping, although embolism remains another possibility. Using CPB or a shunt may be protective, but definitive outcome data are lacking. Adequate volume loading is probably important for renal protection. In some centers, cold crystalloid or cold blood renal perfusion is administered during thoracoabdominal aneurysm repair. If the renal arteries can be surgically exposed during periods of the operation when renal arterial blood flow is interrupted, perfusate can be administered with a roller-head pump into perfusion catheters that are inserted into the renal arteries.[34]

I. **Endovascular Graft Repair of the Thoracic Aorta**

EV graft design has improved to allow reliable deployment in the higher pulse pressure zones of the thoracic aorta. There has also been a progressive increase in "hybrid" procedures combining EV intervention with an adjunctive surgical procedure that is less extensive than a purely surgical operation would be (eg, use of an EV graft to treat a thoracic aneurysm plus a carotid-to-subclavian bypass because the EV graft occludes the origin of the left subclavian artery).

1. **Surgical approach:** Placing EV grafts in the thoracic aorta generally requires femoral arterial access through which fluoroscopically guided wires and catheters can be passed to allow optimal EV graft positioning. The femoral artery can be accessed percutaneously, or it can be exposed and isolated via a small groin incision. If the artery is too small or stenotic to accommodate the relatively large thoracic EV graft delivery system, retroperitoneal dissection may be required to attain access to the iliac artery. The delivery system is positioned fluoroscopically at the desired implantation site, and when the delivery device is withdrawn, the endograft expands at this final aortic position. After EV graft deployment, fluoroscopy and TEE are generally used to reassess for blood leakage around the graft. Patients are positioned supine on the fluoroscopy table throughout the procedure.

2. **Surgical techniques**
   a. Patients must be systemically anticoagulated, usually with heparin, during the procedure.
   b. It is important that patients do not move during angiography, particularly during EV graft deployment. Sometimes, the interventionalist will ask the anesthesiologist to hold ventilation during the procedure so that the portion of the aorta in which the EV graft will be deployed can be more closely assessed. This is one reason why EV graft placement in the descending thoracic aorta is usually performed with general anesthesia.
   c. Advances have led to the development of self-expanding stents that reliably adhere to the aortic wall after deployment and do not require temporarily occlusive balloon inflation in the aorta. This removes the risks of proximal hypertension associated with occluding the thoracic aorta.
   d. The patient's aortic pathology must ideally have a proximal "landing zone" at least 10-15 mm in length and a diameter no greater than that of the largest available EV graft. Many descending thoracic aneurysms and dissections involve the distal aortic arch, including the takeoff of the left subclavian artery. EV stent grafts are now placed that cover the ostia, but prophylactic preprocedural left subclavian artery transposition or left subclavian-to-left common carotid artery bypass is frequently performed, as noted earlier, to prevent post–EV graft complications, including left arm ischemia, stroke, and spinal cord ischemia.[52,53] Myocardial ischemia in patients who have a patent

left internal mammary arterial bypass graft is also possible when the subclavian artery takeoff is covered by an EV graft.[52] It is important to note that stroke can also occur as a complication of transposition or left subclavian-to-left common carotid artery bypass, so patients' cerebral blood flow anatomy and institutional comfort with the procedure should be considered before subclavian artery revascularization is performed.[52] The distal site for EV graft attachment needs to be nonaneurysmal and also of sufficient length. Furthermore, fenestrated stents can be used to accommodate aortic side branches,[54] but the location of these side branches still must be carefully evaluated and considered when one is selecting and placing EV grafts.

3. **Complications of endovascular repair**
   a. Emergency conversion to open repair may be necessary if the aorta is ruptured or dissected during manipulations to place the EV graft, or if the EV graft becomes malpositioned such that it poses a substantial risk of visceral ischemia.
   b. **Bleeding:** Although blood loss during EV repair of the thoracic aorta is markedly less (by ~500 mL)[55] than during open surgery, bleeding does occur from the femoral artery introducer when it is traversed by wires and catheters during EV repair. Large-volume blood loss can also occur if the internal iliac artery is damaged during removal of a large-diameter graft-deployment device.
   c. **Endoleak:** Endoleak occurs when blood continues to flow into the aneurysmal sac after EV graft placement. It confers continued risk of aortic rupture and thus requires early identification and intervention. The degree of intervention depends on the type of leak identified (Figure 23.17). Type I endoleak occurs with an inadequate seal between the EV graft and the wall of the aorta at either the proximal or distal attachment sites, such that there is persistent flow into the native aneurysm. Type II endoleak occurs when the portion of the aorta that was to be excluded by the graft fills in a retrograde manner from back-bleeding collateral vessels, such as the lumbar or inferior mesenteric arteries. No definitive approach exists for addressing type II endoleak: Both observation and side branch embolization are used. Type III endoleak results from EV graft failure and requires conversion to open repair so that the EV graft does not dislodge. Type IV endoleak is rare and occurs secondary to increased graft porosity. It is typically seen in the immediate postoperative period and usually resolves with correction of coagulopathy. Improvements in graft fabric have significantly decreased the incidence as well. Type V endoleak consists of a continued expansion of an aneurysmal sac without signs of a leak on imaging. This is also referred to as *endotension*.

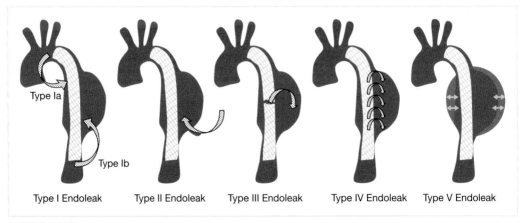

Type Ia
Type Ib

Type I Endoleak   Type II Endoleak   Type III Endoleak   Type IV Endoleak   Type V Endoleak

FIGURE 23.17 Classification of endoleaks. (Reprinted from Cheruku S, Huang N, Meinhardt K, Aguirre M. Anesthetic management for endovascular repair of the thoracic aorta. *Anesthesiol Clin.* 2019;37(4):593-607. © 2019 Elsevier. With permission.)

d. **Stroke:** The incidence of periprocedural stroke is ~5%[56] and appears to be highest in patients whose EV graft is placed in the region of the distal arch that includes the takeoff of the left subclavian. The risk of stroke may be lower in those who undergo a staged carotid-to-subclavian artery bypass procedure first, as this may prevent vertebrobasilar arterial insufficiency and potential ensuing posterior cerebral infarction.[52] Stroke risk is elevated in patients who have a history of stroke, whose CT scans reveal severe atheromatous disease of the aortic arch, or in whom EV grafting involves the distal aortic arch.[57]

CLINICAL PEARL

Although some data suggest that risk of lower extremity paraparesis or paralysis is lower in patients undergoing EV graft versus open thoracic aortic repair, its incidence is still 3%-4%.[55,56,58]

e. **Paraplegia:** Many surgeons and interventional radiologists, therefore, prefer that a lumbar spinal drain be placed before the procedure and that CSF drainage be conducted in the same manner described in Section IV.H.7.e for open thoracoabdominal operations.

f. **Contrast nephropathy:** Patients with preexisting renal insufficiency, especially those with diabetic nephropathy, are particularly susceptible to contrast nephropathy (CN).[59] Older age, hypertension, repeat contrast exposure within a short time, use of high osmolality contrast, and preprocedural medications such as nonsteroidal anti-inflammatory drugs and angiotensin-converting enzyme (ACE) inhibitors also increase patients' risk of CN.[59] Although the pathogenesis of CN is not completely understood, it appears to be related to decreased renal medullary perfusion and associated ischemia, as well as a direct toxic effect of contrast on the renal epithelial cells. We refer the reader to two excellent reviews of CN for a more detailed discussion.[59,60]

J. **Anesthetic Considerations for Patients Undergoing Endovascular Stent Graft Repair of the Thoracic Aorta**

1. **General considerations**

a. The possibility of aortic rupture, dissection, or malposition of the EV graft should be considered when the location for the procedure is selected and the anesthetic approach is chosen. If a cardiac or vascular surgeon is not performing the EV graft procedure, one should be immediately available if conversion to open surgery is necessary. Table 23.10 summarizes the perioperative management of TEVAR.

b. Although there are reports of placing thoracic aortic EV grafts under regional anesthesia, this approach has several disadvantages in comparison to general anesthesia.

(1) Should emergency conversion to open aortic repair be necessary, this conversion will be slowed by the need to establish airway control before positioning the patient for the operation.

(2) If the patient is intubated at the start of the procedure and the surgeon believes that the patient is at substantial risk for open conversion, the anesthesiologist can place a bronchial blocker in the left mainstem bronchus without inflating it. The bronchial blocker could then be quickly inflated during emergency conversion to provide single-lung ventilation.

(3) Many thoracic aortic EV graft procedures are too lengthy for regional anesthesia.

(4) General anesthesia with endotracheal intubation allows the anesthesiologist or cardiologist to conduct TEE evaluation throughout the procedure. This is particularly useful in assessing for endoleaks and for differentiating slow leakage associated with the porosity of the EV stent graft from true high-velocity persistent endoleak.[61,62] In patients undergoing EV stent graft placement for complicated type B dissection, TEE can also be helpful for repositioning the guidewire from the false to the true lumen and for detecting new intimal tears in the thoracic aorta after EV stent placement.[61] Such new distal aortic tears might require additional EV stents to be placed.

TABLE 23.10 Perioperative Management for Thoracic Endovascular Aortic Repair

Preoperative evaluation	1. Common comorbidities: CAD, COPD, CKD
	2. Optimize renal function due to contrast use
Monitors	1. Standard monitors and arterial line in all patients
	2. Consider central venous monitor depending on patient comorbidities extent of aortic disease and complexity of procedure
	3. Consider TEE depending on patient comorbidities and procedures involving the aortic arch
	4. Neuromonitoring with motor- and sensory-evoked potentials can be used to monitor spinal cord function
Intraoperative considerations	1. General anesthesia is most often used to immobilize the patient and maintain a secure airway during procedures, which can be long and hemodynamically turbulent.
	2. Anesthesia can be maintained with a combination or volatile anesthetics and opioids or using a total intravenous anesthetic technique if necessary to enable evoked potential monitoring.
	3. Anticoagulation with heparin is necessary to facilitate insertion of the endovascular device and graft.
	4. A lower BP may be necessary to stabilize the graft during deployment.
	5. Patients should be extubated at the end of the procedure to facilitate neurologic examination.
Complications	1. Hematoma and pseudoaneurysm at access site
	2. Dissection of the aorta and branch vessels
	3. Endoleak and endograft migration
	4. End-organ injury (AKI, mesenteric ischemia)
	5. Spinal cord injury
Postoperative care	1. Serial neurologic evaluations
	2. Lay flat for up to 6 h to facilitate access site hemostasis
	3. Pain management and anxiolysis to prevent excessive movement during the lay flat period

AKI, acute kidney injury; BP, blood pressure; CAD, coronary artery disease; COPD, chronic obstructive pulmonary disease; CKD, chronic kidney disease; TEE, transesophageal echocardiography.

2. **Monitoring:** All patients should have standard ASA monitors and a radial arterial line for BP monitoring to help maintain hemodynamic stability. Furthermore, surgeons may request transient, mild hypotension during stent deployment to help prevent graft migration. In the event that emergent conversion to open surgery is needed, an arterial line will be extremely useful in guiding volume resuscitation and possible cardiopulmonary resuscitation. Typically, a right radial arterial line is ideal for hemodynamic monitoring because it allows monitoring of arterial pressure proximal to the distal aortic arch. Some centers monitor SEPs and/or MEPs, as well as CSF pressure, during placement of thoracic aortic EV grafts. Urine output should be monitored to help assess adequacy of fluid administration during what can often be long procedures. A fluid warmer and warming blanket should be used to help prevent hypothermia, and oropharyngeal temperature should be monitored.
3. **Fluid therapy and transfusion**
   a. Large-bore IV access should be established in case rapid volume resuscitation is needed.
   b. Cross-matched, packed red blood cells should be available.
   c. A system for rapidly infusing blood products and other fluids should be immediately available in cases in which volume resuscitation is needed.
4. **Cerebrospinal fluid drainage:** As with patients who undergo open surgical repair of the descending thoracic aorta, delayed-onset paraparesis or paraplegia can occur in patients who receive EV stent grafts,[63,64] so patients should undergo frequent postprocedural neurologic examination; if signs of spinal cord ischemia/injury are detected, aggressive efforts should be made to increase MAP and to drain more CSF.

5. **Contrast nephropathy:** While the ability of a single dose of IV contrast to cause nephropathy is controversial,[65] because EV grafting of the thoracic aorta is often a long procedure that involves a substantial volume of IV contrast, the anesthesiologist should consider strategies to attenuate the risk of CN, particularly in patients with renal insufficiency.
   a. **Hydration:** There is no consensus regarding duration of IV 0.9% normal saline infusion before or after the procedure, but avoiding hypovolemia in these patients during the procedure is advisable.[60]
   b. **N-Acetylcysteine:** N-Acetylcysteine (NAC) has antioxidant and vasodilatory effects. Some studies have shown the benefit of pretreating patients with NAC for 24 hours before procedures requiring IV contrast, while other studies have shown no such benefit.[59,60]
   c. **Diuretics:** Diuretic use does not seem to prevent CN. Some advocate that, if possible, diuretics be withdrawn for 24 hours before procedures requiring contrast[59] because of concern that they may increase the risk of CN.
   d. **Dopamine and fenoldopam:** Neither of these drugs has been found to prevent CN in human studies.[59]

REFERENCES

1. Isselbacher EM, Preventza O, Black JH, et al. 2022 ACC/AHA guideline for the diagnosis and management of aortic disease. *J Am Coll Cardiol.* 2022;80(24):e223-e393. doi:10.1016/j.jacc.2022.08.004
2. Upchurch GR Jr, Escobar GA, Azizzadeh A, et al. Society for Vascular Surgery clinical practice guidelines of thoracic endovascular aortic repair for descending thoracic aortic aneurysms. *J Vasc Surg.* 2021;73(1):55S-83S.
3. Melo RG, Duarte GS, Lopes A, et al. *Incidence and Prevalence of Thoracic Aortic Aneurysms: A Systematic Review and Meta-Analysis of Population-Based Studies.* Elsevier; 2021.
4. Bickerstaff LK, Pairolero PC, Hollier LH, et al. Thoracic aortic aneurysms: a population-based study. *Surgery.* 1982;92(6):1103-1108.
5. Hirose Y, Hamada S, Takamiya M, Imakita S, Naito H, Nishimura T. Aortic aneurysms: growth rates measured with CT. *Radiology.* 1992;185(1):249-252.
6. LeMaire SA, Russell L. Epidemiology of thoracic aortic dissection. *Nat Rev Cardiol.* 2011;8(2):103-113.
7. Januzzi JL, Isselbacher EM, Fattori R, et al. Characterizing the young patient with aortic dissection: results from the International Registry of Aortic Dissection (IRAD). *J Am Coll Cardiol.* 2004;43(4):665-669.
8. Hirst AE Jr, Johns VJ Jr, Kime SW Jr. Dissecting aneurysm of the aorta: a review of 505 cases. *Medicine.* 1958;37(3):217.
9. Hagan PG, Nienaber CA, Isselbacher EM, et al. The International Registry of Acute Aortic Dissection (IRAD): new insights into an old disease. *JAMA.* 2000;283(7):897-903.
10. Kouchoukos NT, Dougenis D. Surgery of the thoracic aorta. *N Engl J Med.* 1997;336(26):1876-1889.
11. Shimony A, Filion KB, Mottillo S, Dourian T, Eisenberg MJ. Meta-analysis of usefulness of d-dimer to diagnose acute aortic dissection. *Am J Cardiol.* 2011;107(8):1227-1234.
12. Hartnell GG. Imaging of aortic aneurysms and dissection: CT and MRI. *J Thorac Imaging.* 2001;16(1):35-46.
13. Verscheure D, Haulon S, Tsilimparis N, et al. Endovascular treatment of post type A chronic aortic arch dissection with a branched endograft: early results from a multicenter international multicenter study. *Ann Surg.* 2021;273(5):997-1003.
14. Erbel R, Aboyans V, Boileau C, et al. 2014 ESC guidelines on the diagnosis and treatment of aortic diseases. *Russ J Cardiol.* 2015;123(7):7-72.
15. Martin K, Knorr J, Breuer T, et al. Seizures after open heart surgery: comparison of ε-aminocaproic acid and tranexamic acid. *J Cardiothorac Vasc Anesth.* 2011;25(1):20-25.
16. Thiele RH, Shaw AD, Bartels K, et al. American Society for Enhanced Recovery and Perioperative Quality Initiative Joint Consensus Statement on the role of neuromonitoring in perioperative outcomes: cerebral near-infrared spectroscopy. *Anesth Analg.* 2020;131(5):1444-1455.
17. Engelman R, Baker RA, Likosky DS, et al. The Society of Thoracic Surgeons, The Society of Cardiovascular Anesthesiologists, and The American Society of ExtraCorporeal Technology: clinical practice guidelines for cardiopulmonary bypass—temperature management during cardiopulmonary bypass. *Ann Thorac Surg.* 2015;100(2):748-757.
18. Liu Z, Wang C, Zhang X, Wu S, Fang C, Pang X. Effect of different types of cerebral perfusion for acute type A aortic dissection undergoing aortic arch procedure, unilateral versus bilateral. *BMC Surg.* 2020;20(1):286.
19. Abdelgawad A, Arafat H. Moderate versus deep hypothermic circulatory arrest for ascending aorta and aortic arch surgeries using open distal anastomosis technique. *J Egypt Soc Cardiothorac Surg.* 2017;25(4):323-330.
20. Damberg A, Carino D, Charilaou P, et al. Favorable late survival after aortic surgery under straight deep hypothermic circulatory arrest. *J Thorac Cardiovasc Surg.* 2017;154(6):1831.e1-1839.e1.
21. Goldstein LJ, Davies RR, Rizzo JA, et al. Stroke in surgery of the thoracic aorta: incidence, impact, etiology, and prevention. *J Thorac Cardiovasc Surg.* 2001;122(5):935-945.
22. Ziganshin BA, Elefteriades JA. Deep hypothermic circulatory arrest. *Ann Cardiothorac Surg.* 2013;2(3):303.
23. Vallabhajosyula P, Jassar AS, Menon RS, et al. Moderate versus deep hypothermic circulatory arrest for elective aortic transverse hemiarch reconstruction. *Ann Thorac Surg.* 2015;99(5):1511-1517.
24. Shum-Tim D, Nagashima M, Shinoka T, et al. Postischemic hyperthermia exacerbates neurologic injury after deep hypothermic circulatory arrest. *J Thorac Cardiovasc Surg.* 1998;116(5):780-792.

25. Ueda Y, Okita Y, Aomi S, Koyanagi H, Takamoto S. Retrograde cerebral perfusion for aortic arch surgery: analysis of risk factors. *Ann Thorac Surg.* 1999;67(6):1879-1882.
26. Ueda Y. A reappraisal of retrograde cerebral perfusion. *Ann Cardiothorac Surg.* 2013;2(3):316.
27. Urbanski PP, Lenos A, Kolowca M, et al. Near-infrared spectroscopy for neuromonitoring of unilateral cerebral perfusion. *Eur J Cardiothorac Surg.* 2013;43(6):1140-1144.
28. Strauch JT, Spielvogel D, Lauten A, et al. Axillary artery cannulation: routine use in ascending aorta and aortic arch replacement. *Ann Thorac Surg.* 2004;78(1):103-108.
29. Rich GF, Lubanski RE Jr, McLoughlin TM. Differences between aortic and radial artery pressure associated with cardiopulmonary bypass. *Anesthesiology.* 1992;77(1):63-66. PMID: 1610010
30. Fischer GW, Lin H-M, Krol M, et al. Noninvasive cerebral oxygenation may predict outcome in patients undergoing aortic arch surgery. *J Thorac Cardiovasc Surg.* 2011;141(3):815-821.
31. du Plessis AJ, Jonas RA, Wypij D, et al. Perioperative effects of alpha-stat versus pH-stat strategies for deep hypothermic cardiopulmonary bypass in infants. *J Thorac Cardiovasc Surg.* 1997;114(6):991-1001.
32. Henriksen L. Brain luxury perfusion during cardiopulmonary bypass in humans: a study of the cerebral blood flow response to changes in CO_2, O_2, and blood pressure. *J Cereb Blood Flow Metab.* 1986;6(3):366-378.
33. Gelman S. The pathophysiology of aortic cross-clamping and unclamping. *J Am Soc Anesth.* 1995;82(4):1026-1057.
34. Coselli JS. Strategies for renal and visceral protection in thoracoabdominal aortic surgery. *J Thorac Cardiovasc Surg.* 2010;140(6):S147-S149.
35. Cambria RP, Clouse WD, Davison JK, Dunn PF, Corey M, Dorer D. Thoracoabdominal aneurysm repair: results with 337 operations performed over a 15-year interval. *Ann Surg.* 2002;236(4):471-479.
36. LeMaire SA, Price MD, Green SY, Zarda S, Coselli JS. Results of open thoracoabdominal aortic aneurysm repair. *Ann Cardiothorac Surg.* 2012;1(3):286.
37. Wynn MM, Acher C, Marks E, Engelbert T, Acher C. Postoperative renal failure in thoracoabdominal aortic aneurysm repair with simple cross-clamp technique and 4 C renal perfusion. *J Vasc Surg.* 2015;61(3):611-622.
38. Safi HJ, Harlin SA, Miller CC, et al. Predictive factors for acute renal failure in thoracic and thoracoabdominal aortic aneurysm surgery. *J Vasc Surg.* 1996;24(3):338-345.
39. Svensson LG, Crawford ES, Hess KR, Coselli JS, Safi HJ. Experience with 1509 patients undergoing thoracoabdominal aortic operations. *J Vasc Surg.* 1993;17(2):357-370.
40. Coselli JS, LeMaire SA, Köksoy C, Schmittling ZC, Curling PE. Cerebrospinal fluid drainage reduces paraplegia after thoracoabdominal aortic aneurysm repair: results of a randomized clinical trial. *J Vasc Surg.* 2002;35(4):631-639.
41. O'Connor CJ, Rothenberg DM. Anesthetic considerations for descending thoracic aortic surgery: part 1. *J Cardiothorac Vasc Anesth.* 1995;9(5):581-588.
42. O'Connor CJ, Rothenberg DM. Anesthetic considerations for descending thoracic aortic surgery: part II. *J Cardiothorac Vasc Anesth.* 1995;9(6):734-747.
43. Gilling-Smith G, Worswick L, Knight P, Wolfe J, Mansfield A. Surgical repair of thoracoabdominal aortic aneurysm: 10 years' experience. *J Br Surg.* 1995;82(5):624-629.
44. Janusz MT. Experience with thoracoabdominal aortic aneurysm resection. *Am J Surg.* 1994;167(5):501-504.
45. Ling E, Arellano R, Fisher DM. Systematic overview of the evidence supporting the use of cerebrospinal fluid drainage in thoracoabdominal aneurysm surgery for prevention of paraplegia. *J Am Soc Anesth.* 2000;93(4):1115-1122.
46. Murakami H, Yoshida K, Hino Y, Matsuda H, Tsukube T, Okita Y. Complications of cerebrospinal fluid drainage in thoracoabdominal aortic aneurysm repair. *J Vasc Surg.* 2004;39(1):243-245.
47. Dardik A, Perler BA, Roseborough GS, Williams GM. Subdural hematoma after thoracoabdominal aortic aneurysm repair: an underreported complication of spinal fluid drainage? *J Vasc Surg.* 2002;36(1):47-50.
48. Wong DR, Coselli JS, Amerman K, et al. Delayed spinal cord deficits after thoracoabdominal aortic aneurysm repair. *Ann Thorac Surg.* 2007;83(4):1345-1355.
49. Youngblood SC, Tolpin DA, LeMaire SA, Coselli JS, Lee V-V, Cooper JR Jr. Complications of cerebrospinal fluid drainage after thoracic aortic surgery: a review of 504 patients over 5 years. *J Thorac Cardiovasc Surg.* 2013;146(1):166-171.
50. Heller LB, Chaney MA. Paraplegia immediately following removal of a cerebrospinal fluid drainage catheter in a patient after thoracoabdominal aortic aneurysm surgery. *J Am Soc Anesth.* 2001;95(5):1285-1287.
51. Nathan DP, Brinster CJ, Woo EY, Carpenter JP, Fairman RM, Jackson BM. Predictors of early and late mortality following open extent IV thoracoabdominal aortic aneurysm repair in a large contemporary single-center experience. *J Vasc Surg.* 2011;53(2):299-306.
52. Rehman SM, Vecht JA, Perera R, et al. How to manage the left subclavian artery during endovascular stenting of the thoracic aorta. *Eur J Cardiothorac Surg.* 2011;39(4):507-518.
53. Weigang E, Parker JA, Czerny M, et al. Should intentional endovascular stent-graft coverage of the left subclavian artery be preceded by prophylactic revascularisation? *Eur J Cardiothorac Surg.* 2011;40(4):858-868.
54. Eagleton MJ, Follansbee M, Wolski K, Mastracci T, Kuramochi Y. Fenestrated and branched endovascular aneurysm repair outcomes for type II and III thoracoabdominal aortic aneurysms. *J Vasc Surg.* 2016;63(4):930-942.
55. Makaroun MS, Dillavou ED, Kee ST, et al. Endovascular treatment of thoracic aortic aneurysms: results of the phase II multicenter trial of the GORE TAG thoracic endoprosthesis. *J Vasc Surg.* 2005;41(1):1-9.
56. Cheng D, Martin J, Shennib H, et al. Endovascular aortic repair versus open surgical repair for descending thoracic aortic disease: a systematic review and meta-analysis of comparative studies. *J Am Coll Cardiol.* 2010;55(10):986-1001.
57. Gutsche JT, Cheung AT, McGarvey ML, et al. Risk factors for perioperative stroke after thoracic endovascular aortic repair. *Ann Thorac Surg.* 2007;84(4):1195-1200.

58. Leurs LJ, Bell R, Degrieck Y, Thomas S, Hobo R, Lundbom J. Endovascular treatment of thoracic aortic diseases: combined experience from the EUROSTAR and United Kingdom Thoracic Endograft registries. *J Vasc Surg.* 2004;40(4):670-679.
59. Maeder M, Klein M, Fehr T, Rickli H. Contrast nephropathy: review focusing on prevention. *J Am Coll Cardiol.* 2004;44(9):1763-1771.
60. Barrett BJ, Parfrey PS. Preventing nephropathy induced by contrast medium. *N Engl J Med.* 2006;354(4):379-386.
61. Rocchi G, Lofiego C, Biagini E, et al. Transesophageal echocardiography–guided algorithm for stent-graft implantation in aortic dissection. *J Vasc Surg.* 2004;40(5):880-885.
62. Swaminathan M, Lineberger CK, McCann RL, Mathew JP. The importance of intraoperative transesophageal echocardiography in endovascular repair of thoracic aortic aneurysms. *Anesth Analg.* 2003;97(6):1566-1572.
63. Baril DT, Carroccio A, Ellozy SH, et al. Endovascular thoracic aortic repair and previous or concomitant abdominal aortic repair: is the increased risk of spinal cord ischemia real? *Ann Vasc Surg.* 2006;20(2):188-194.
64. Gravereaux EC, Faries PL, Burks JA, et al. Risk of spinal cord ischemia after endograft repair of thoracic aortic aneurysms. *J Vasc Surg.* 2001;34(6):997-1003.
65. Goulden R, Rowe BH, Abrahamowicz M, Strumpf E, Tamblyn R. Association of intravenous radiocontrast with kidney function: a regression discontinuity analysis. *JAMA Intern Med.* 2021;181(6):767-774. doi: 10.1001/jamainternmed.2021.0916

24

Anesthesia for Esophageal Surgery

Bruno Maranhao, Jaclyn Yeung, Furqaan Sadiq, and Thomas Graetz

KEY POINTS

1. Patients undergoing esophageal procedures are at elevated risk for aspiration.
2. Procedural management depends heavily on the procedure being performed—from sequential major thoracic and abdominal procedures to transluminal endoscopy—the positioning, monitoring, and anesthetic techniques will depend on the procedural plan. General endotracheal anesthesia is almost always required, and esophageal surgery may necessitate one-lung ventilation.
3. Operative therapies for gastroesophageal reflux disease (GERD) include various wrappings of the stomach around the esophagus; these are generally performed laparoscopically with general endotracheal anesthesia and do not require lung isolation.
4. Paraesophageal hernia is typically repaired with a laparoscopic technique and requires general endotracheal anesthesia with peripheral intravenous access.
5. Achalasia can result in massive esophageal dilation and significant amounts of esophageal contents despite several days of a liquid diet followed by multiple days of nil per os (NPO) status.
6. Post–esophagectomy anastomotic leaks are associated with significant morbidity and the need for reoperation.
7. Decompressive nasogastric tubes and jejunal feeding tubes are both placed at the conclusion of esophagectomy, and durably securing any tubes is essential.
8. Esophageal perforations are associated with high morbidity and mortality.
9. Endotracheal tube position in patients with tracheoesophageal fistulas is ideally verified beyond the fistula, or the fistula is excluded from positive pressure ventilation by a lung isolation technique.

I. Introduction

Esophageal surgery encompasses a broad range of operations and procedures, including open and endoscopic approaches, involving both the chest and abdominal cavities. A clinical concern that is relevant to all esophageal procedures is the risk of pulmonary aspiration. The priority of other issues, particularly lung isolation with one-lung ventilation and postoperative pain control, can vary depending on the operation or procedure.

II. Preoperative Assessment

A. Overview and Patient Factors

The preoperative assessment of a patient presenting for esophageal surgery is similar to assessments for other surgery, with additional attention to distinct areas. The nature of the underlying disease process of patients undergoing esophageal procedures is such that the patient should be treated as high risk for pulmonary aspiration, regardless of their nil per os (NPO) duration. A patient's history, frequency, and severity of any reflux symptoms, as well as their ability to tolerate lying flat, are important to elicit. One particularly concerning group of patients is those with achalasia, which many times have significant contents in their esophagus, even if they have been NPO for >8 hours (Figure 24.1). In an effort to minimize aspiration risk, it is appropriate to plan for rapid sequence induction and intubation. Consequently, special attention to the airway examination should be undertaken, and plans made to address any concerns of an anticipated or known difficult airway. Patients typically continue their home gastric acid suppression medications, histamine type 2 receptor blocker, or proton-pump inhibitor (PPI), up to the time of their operation; some clinicians also advocate for the administration of a nonparticulate oral antacid before induction of anesthesia to mitigate the consequences of pulmonary aspiration, should it occur.

In the setting of severe reflux or esophageal outlet obstruction, mass, stricture, or achalasia, a preoperative decompressive nasoenteric tube can be considered in an effort to decrease the volume of contents in the esophagus and stomach. Difficulty tolerating oral intake either secondary to obstruction or reflux symptoms can lead to malnourishment in this patient

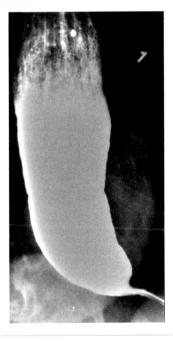

FIGURE 24.1 Idiopathic (primary) achalasia. (Reprinted from Farrokhi F, Vaezi MF. Idiopathic (primary) achalasia. *Orphanet J Rare Dis.* 2007;2:38. http://creativecommons.org/licenses/by/2.0)

population. If malnourishment is suspected, and the operation can be delayed, the patient may benefit from preoperative nutritional assessment and dietary supplementation—typically a high protein, simple carbohydrate supplement diet, possibly via an enteric feeding tube.[1]

Patients presenting for esophagectomy may have undergone neoadjuvant chemoradiation therapy. Some chemotherapeutic agents have been implicated in the development of cardiomyopathy; patients' exercise tolerance should be assessed, and if their history is concerning, the appropriate diagnostic studies, potentially including a preoperative transthoracic echocardiogram, be performed. It is important to consider individual patient factors when making decisions about preoperative testing or interventions and ensure clarity on how tests could impact management, particularly for procedures being performed because of a cancer diagnosis; risks, benefits, and alternatives should be carefully considered. Patients should be included in the decision-making noted previously; delaying an operation for esophageal cancer comes at the risk of tumor progression and should only be considered after carefully weighing the risks and benefits of a delay.

B. Procedural and Operation Factors

[2]

When anesthetic plans are being made, it is important to consider the details of the planned procedure, including whether the procedure is planned to be open thoracic, open abdominal, thoracoscopic, laparoscopic, or endoscopic. It is appropriate to determine if lung isolation is necessary, and if so, plan for an appropriate technique, including the placement of a double-lumen tube or a bronchial blocker. If lung isolation is appropriate for the planned operation, the approach can be impacted by the anticipated ease of intubation, because a difficult airway can make a double-lumen endotracheal tube (ETT) technically more difficult to place than a single-lumen tube with a bronchial blocker. If the planned operation requires one-lung ventilation, a history of pulmonary disease that could make one-lung ventilation or oxygenation challenging should be elicited.[2] Patients presenting with esophageal cancer often have a history of smoking and its sequela. Patients should be counseled to abstain from smoking in preparation for surgery; if present, chronic obstructive pulmonary disease therapy should be optimized.

CLINICAL PEARL

If intraoperative administration of inhaled bronchodilators is likely, preemptive administration in the awake spontaneously breathing patient offers a superior drug delivery profile compared to intraoperative delivery via an ETT.

If the planned surgery involves a thoracotomy or thoracoscopic approach, a discussion should take place regarding postoperative analgesia and the potential for regional anesthetic techniques (epidural, paravertebral, erector spinae, or other block) to reduce postoperative pain. Timing of cessation of some anticoagulants may affect patients' ability to receive certain regional anesthetic techniques. A review of anticoagulation therapy and ensuring appropriate timing of discontinuation should occur before performing any regional anesthetic technique based on the planned operation.

III. Intraoperative Management

A. Positioning

Patients undergoing limited endoscopic procedures can often be positioned supine on a standard patient stretcher rather than an operating room (OR) table; patients undergoing operative procedures, however, must be moved to an OR table that permits bed adjustments and better patient access. After intubation and appropriate access is obtained, positioning will take place based on the operative plan. Positioning approaches can include supine, lithotomy, as well as lateral position. In addition, for some esophagectomies, the operation involves an abdominal and thoracic portion, which requires a change in position during the procedure. As with any anesthetic, the anesthesia team must remain vigilant regarding adequate access to the patient, intravascular access, and ensuring there is sufficient padding to minimize the risk of nerve and other soft-tissue injuries. Furthermore, after repositioning, it is prudent to verify the continued adequacy of lung isolation, because of the potential for ETT and airway movement.

CLINICAL PEARL

The left lateral decubitus position is often utilized for thoracoscopic and thoracotomy approaches in esophageal surgery. Patients in this position are stabilized with the use of a bean bag, rolled blankets, or devices attached to the OR table. Care should be taken to maintain the left axilla free of direct pressure and the neck in a midline neutral position. Padding, often a pillow, should be placed between the knees, and the knees flexed to prevent the ankles from lying directly on top of each other.

More recently, the prone position has been utilized for a minimally invasive thoracoscopic approach to esophageal surgery. The perceived benefit of this positioning and approach is that lung isolation may not be required and that the lung and any bleeding fall away from the esophagus by gravity.[3] The tradeoff with this approach is all the risks inherent to the prone position, for example, ophthalmic complications resulting in vision loss, decreased stroke volume resulting in decreased cardiac output, anterior pressure injuries resulting in neuropathy and/or ulcers, dependent edema of the tongue and sclera, and difficulty with airway manipulation, including lung isolation, if necessary.

B. **Monitoring and Access**

Standard American Society of Anesthesiologists (ASA) monitors must be utilized and are often sufficient for endoscopic procedures. For patients undergoing larger operations, particularly those requiring one-lung ventilation, an arterial line for continuous blood pressure monitoring and intermittent arterial blood gas monitoring may be appropriate, depending on the extent of the specific operation and patient comorbidities. Central venous catheters (CVCs) are not routinely necessary in all circumstances, though they may be helpful for administering vasoactive infusions. Central venous pressure may also be monitored, though its use as a predictor of a particular patient's intravascular volume status or preload responsiveness is no longer considered best practice.[4] For nonendoscopic procedures, adequate intravenous (IV) access is necessary for rapid volume administration since injury to nearby great vessels is always a possibility when operating on the esophagus; depending on patient positioning, obtaining this venous access during the procedure may be challenging, if not prohibitive. Quantitative neuromuscular monitoring to ensure adequate reversal of neuromuscular blocking drugs is universally recommended and is especially important in a patient population at high risk for postoperative pulmonary complications.

C. **Anesthetic Technique**

If one-lung ventilation is necessary for the operative approach, the advantages and disadvantages of lung isolation techniques must be considered carefully. A double-lumen tube has the benefit of permitting one-lung ventilation, selective lung suctioning, passive oxygenation including the application of continuous positive airway pressure (CPAP) to the nonventilated lung, and, though not typically necessary during esophageal surgery, the rapid switching between which lung is ventilated and which is not. One major disadvantage of double-lumen tubes is that they are larger than the single-lumen tubes, potentially making double-lumen tube placement more challenging and increasing the risk of airway trauma. If the patient is to remain intubated after the surgical procedure, a double-lumen tube is typically exchanged for a single-lumen tube, requiring additional instrumentation of the patient's airway. This added procedure comes with risk of airway loss during the exchange, as well as leading to potential trauma and swelling from multiple instrumentations. A bronchial blocker is another option for lung isolation and is placed via a single-lumen tube. A single-lumen tube intubation is typically considered easier, but the use of a bronchial blocker limits the ability for suctioning or application of CPAP to the nonventilated lung. Intentional intubation of a mainstem bronchus with a single-lumen ETT likewise does not permit interventions to the nonventilated lung, but it can be used in the setting of unplanned need for lung isolation, in addition to the use of a bronchial blocker; specific endobronchial tubes, which are longer than the standard ETT and have a modified cuff design to facilitate intentional intubation of a mainstem bronchus, may not be readily available. Generally, size 8.0 ETTs, or larger, are used when planning to utilize a bronchial blocker.

In addition, while not well studied in one-lung ventilation, based on evidence in standard two-lung mechanical ventilation, it follows that a lung-protective ventilation strategy is also important. Typically, recommended parameters for one-lung ventilation include targeting 5 mL/kg of predicted body weight, plateau pressures to ≤30 cm H_2O, permissive hypercapnia, and minimizing the fraction of inspired oxygen while maintaining blood oxygen saturation >90%.[5] Intraoperative management of patients undergoing esophageal surgery should be tailored to the individual patient's comorbidities as well as the specific operation being performed. Intraoperative anesthetic management of patients is an important component of a multidisciplinary continuum of care that begins with preoperative assessment and concludes with postoperative rehabilitation and surgical wound care. Several evidence-based Enhanced Recovery after Surgery (ERAS) protocols have been developed to improve short-term outcomes associated with a variety of surgeries. Adherence to ERAS protocols has been shown to reduce hospital length of stay and cost, and to reduce the incidence and severity of postoperative complications. Esophagectomy was the first intrathoracic surgery for which the ERAS society developed a protocol.[6] Though this protocol is specific to esophagectomy, some aspects of the anesthetic care of the protocol are generalizable to other esophageal surgeries.

Another important consideration for esophageal surgery is muscle relaxation. Depolarizing neuromuscular blockers are commonly used to facilitate rapid sequence tracheal intubation. Based on the specific needs of the procedure being performed, muscle relaxation may be helpful to facilitate operative exposure or prevent movement of structures adjacent to the operative field, for example, diaphragm during an esophageal fundoplication. While avoiding patient movement is helpful during endoscopic procedures, muscle relaxation is not generally necessary. While muscle relaxation may be helpful during esophageal procedures, residual neuromuscular blockade has the potential to predispose patients to significant patient morbidity. Quantitative monitoring at the adductor pollicis is currently recommended; achieving a train-of-four ratio of >0.9 ensures adequate recovery from neuromuscular blockade. Sugammadex can be used successfully from deeper levels of neuromuscular blockade, while antagonism from less intense levels of blockade may be achieved with neostigmine.[7]

IV. Operations for Gastroesophageal Reflux Disease

A. Disease Overview

Gastroesophageal reflux disease (GERD) is common worldwide with an estimated prevalence of 20% in the United States. Typical GERD symptoms include heartburn and regurgitation, while nontypical symptoms can include chronic cough, hoarseness, laryngitis, and wheezing. GERD involves loss of lower esophageal sphincter (LES) competence. LES incompetence leads to acidic gastric contents refluxing into the esophagus. Surgical management may be offered to control severe GERD symptoms if refractory to optimal medical therapy and lifestyle modifications. GERD can lead to complications including esophagitis, strictures, ulcers, and Barrett metaplasia with its associated risk of adenocarcinoma.

B. Traditional Operative Approaches

Laparoscopic Nissen fundoplication, circumferential wrapping of the esophagus by the proximal stomach, is frequently used as the benchmark when comparing other operations for GERD; improvement in symptoms occurs in up to 90% of patients. Fundoplication, however, is associated with the potential for adverse effects, including dysphagia, difficulty vomiting, bloating, and dumping syndrome, as well as the potential for procedural complications. While surgical variations of the fundoplication exist (robotic vs laparoscopic approach and partial vs complete fundoplication), the procedure is designed to create an antireflux barrier. A partial 270° posterior wrap (Toupet) and an anterior 180° wrap (Dor) are variations of the 360° Nissen fundoplication. The benefits of a minimally invasive surgical technique involving robotic or laparoscopic fundoplication (vs open procedure) include reduced pain, shorter hospital stay, smaller incisions, and decreased risk of wound infections and hernias.

C. Newer Therapies

Newer approaches include transoral incisionless fundoplication (TIF) performed with an endoscope inserted through the mouth into the stomach to plicate tissue at the gastroesophageal (GE) junction, creating a functionally longer LES. In addition, a magnetic sphincter augmentation, the LINX Reflux Management system, involves implantation of a small flexible band of magnetic titanium beads around the LES, which is designed to allow food to pass but minimize reflux of gastric contents. The LINX is typically inserted via laparoscopic approach. General endotracheal anesthesia is appropriate for these procedures, and one-lung ventilation is not routinely needed.

V. **Operations for Paraesophageal Hernia Repair**

A. **Hernia Types**

The distal end of the esophagus is tethered at the diaphragm by the phrenoesophageal membrane. The degree to which the GE junction and portions of the stomach herniate through this membrane determines the classification and informs management approach. Of the four types of hiatal hernias, the most common is Type I, or sliding hernia, where the GE junction herniates above the diaphragm, with the fundus of the stomach remaining below. This type of herniation is commonly associated with pathologies of the GE junction's mucosa, such as in GERD. Type II, III, and IV hiatal hernias are typically referred to as *paraesophageal hernias*; defects in the phrenoesophageal membrane result in varying degrees of herniation. Type II paraesophageal hernia involves the GE junction remaining below the diaphragm with the gastric fundus herniating adjacent to the esophagus. A Type III hiatal hernia involves both a portion of the stomach and the GE junction herniating through the hiatus. Rarely, a large enough defect can result in herniation of the stomach and other abdominal organs, including small bowel and/or colon, resulting in a Type IV paraesophageal hernia.

B. **Operative Approaches**

Typically, operations for asymptomatic Type I hiatal hernias are not offered. For symptomatic hernias, management of GERD with oral medications is often sufficient, though if medical therapies fail, an operation may be offered. The likelihood that a patient with a Type II or Type III paraesophageal hernia will develop acute symptoms, necessitating emergency repair is estimated to be near 1%. However, when repair is required in emergent situations, including volvulus, strangulation, or perforation, the risk of mortality can be as high as 7%. Patients who suffer from chronic, persistent symptoms may report GERD, dysphagia, postprandial chest or abdominal pain, and frequent emesis. Elective surgical repair for these patients is associated with an improved quality of life. A thorough history and physical examination can help mitigate potential perioperative complications, including cardiac and pulmonary issues. Most pertinent to the hernia repair are upper endoscopy findings and biopsy reports as well as results from barium swallow studies. Regarding the surgical approach for paraesophageal hernia repair, laparoscopy may be preferred over open transabdominal or open thoracotomy approaches, even in emergent indications, but there are instances when an open approach may be preferential, for example, prior abdominal surgeries and need for significant adhesiolysis. Potential complications include injury to the pericardium, pneumothorax, and bleeding.

General endotracheal anesthesia is appropriate for paraesophageal hernia repairs with consideration for lung isolation, depending on the operative plan. Adequate prophylaxis for postoperative nausea and vomiting cannot be overstated as excessive increases in intra-abdominal pressure from retching can lead to early reoccurrence of the hernia.

VI. **Operations for Achalasia**

Achalasia results from progressive degeneration of ganglion cells of the esophageal wall, leading to unopposed cholinergic stimulation, reduced peristalsis, and subsequent esophageal dilation with impaired esophageal emptying into the stomach. The etiology of primary idiopathic achalasia is unknown. Secondary achalasia is due to diseases that cause esophageal motor abnormalities. In addition, disorders such as Chagas disease, amyloidosis, sarcoidosis, neurofibromatosis, eosinophilic esophagitis, multiple endocrine neoplasia, Sjögren syndrome, and Fabry disease may lead to achalasia-like esophageal dysmotility.

Symptoms of achalasia include dysphagia with both liquids and solids, regurgitation of undigested food, heartburn, and chest pain; pulmonary aspiration is common. Patients may induce vomiting to relieve a sensation of retrosternal fullness, and some patients have difficulty belching, due to a defect in relaxation of the upper esophageal sphincter. Achalasia is associated with increased risk of esophageal cancer. Pseudoachalasia due to cancer at the GE junction should be excluded by endoscopic evaluation. Diagnosis of achalasia via barium esophagram demonstrates a classic "bird's-beak" appearance (Figure 24.1). Esophageal manometry is the standard for definitive diagnosis and is used to classify achalasia into one of three distinctive subtypes. Type I involves minimal esophageal pressurization with swallowing. Type II involves pressurization of the entire esophagus with swallowing. Type III involves esophageal spasm with premature contractions during swallowing.

All treatments for achalasia are palliative and aimed at decreasing the resting pressure in the LES to facilitate passage of consumed material. Obstruction caused by the LES can be relieved; however, the normal peristaltic motility of the esophagus is not restored. Medical therapy includes nitrates and calcium channel blockers targeted at improving LES relaxation, while endoscopic botulinum toxin therapy may be considered in patients who are poor candidates for more invasive therapies. Botulinum toxin injected into the LES inhibits the excitatory neurons; their inhibition leads to a decrease in LES muscle tone, with a subsequent decrease in LES pressure and improved emptying of the esophagus. More invasive approaches include pneumatic dilation, laparoscopic Heller myotomy, and per oral endoscopic myotomy (POEM). Patients with achalasia are at high risk of perioperative aspiration, regardless of NPO duration, and must be treated using full stomach (full esophagus) precautions. The dilated, hypomotile esophagus may retain food for many days after ingestion; thus, it is not uncommon to prescribe a liquid diet for a period followed by fasting for 24-48 hours before anesthesia. A nasoenteric tube can be inserted to decompress and attempt to empty the esophagus before rapid sequence induction and intubation.

Multiple endoscopies are frequently used for graded pneumatic dilation, involving endoscopic balloon dilation, which stretches and tears muscle fibers circumferentially. Ideally, patients undergoing pneumatic dilation are good surgical candidates because perforations can occur which may require surgical repair. Serial pneumatic dilations may be necessary due to relapse.

Surgical myotomy, in which the LES is weakened by cutting its muscle fibers, is an alternative to pneumatic balloon dilation for achalasia. One particular approach is the Heller myotomy; this is usually performed laparoscopically and often combined with a fundoplication to minimize postoperative reflux. Both Dor and Toupet partial fundoplications may be used; the circumferential Nissen fundoplication is typically not performed. Symptom relief is achieved in 90% of patients after surgical myotomy; however, symptom relapse may occur with need for reintervention. The POEM procedure endoscopically divides the muscular layer of the LES. Unlike surgical myotomy, which is often combined with a fundoplication to prevent reflux, POEM does not include an antireflux procedure and may result in severe GERD. Without treatment, patients may develop progressive dilation of the esophagus, leading to megaesophagus (diameter >6 cm). Patients with advanced disease may require esophagectomy. These procedures for achalasia require a general anesthetic with ETT placement.

VII. Operations for Esophageal Diverticula

Esophageal diverticula are outpouchings of the esophageal wall that can be one or more tissue layers thick. They can be located near the upper esophageal sphincter (Zenker diverticulum), at the mid-esophagus (commonly a traction diverticulum), or immediately above the LES (epiphrenic diverticulum). Zenker diverticula emerge from an area of muscular wall weakness. While small diverticula may be asymptomatic, larger Zenker diverticula may be aligned with the pharynx and allow food to preferentially pass into the diverticulum. Retained food contents may result in halitosis, regurgitation, or appearance of a neck mass. In severe cases, the Zenker diverticulum may enlarge significantly and compress the true esophageal lumen, obstructing the esophagus.

Complications of esophageal diverticula include aspiration pneumonia, ulceration, retained food and medication, and fistula formation between the diverticulum and tracheal lumen. Diagnosis is made with barium swallow and upper endoscopy, revealing what appears to be a separate esophageal lumen.

Asymptomatic patients with small diverticula (<1 cm) are typically not offered intervention; patients may be managed expectantly until symptoms occur or the diverticulum size increases. Treatment of patients with symptomatic or large diverticula (>1 cm) may be considered, with treatment of symptomatic Zenker diverticula often being surgical. Decision-making on open versus transoral approach is made on the basis of visualization, body habitus, and anatomic features. Patients with short necks, decreased hyomental distance, and high body mass index (BMI) are most often associated with difficult exposure and may require an open approach. Diverticula <2 cm long are usually treated with endoscopic methods. Open repairs of more proximal diverticula are typically performed through a neck incision in which case a general anesthetic with single-lumen tube is appropriate; lung isolation is not necessary unless a thoracotomy is required for a more distal diverticulum.

Transoral endoscopic techniques are less invasive than open surgery and are generally associated with shorter procedural times, decreased duration of hospital admissions, earlier oral intake, and decreased rates of complications. Endoscopic approaches, however, may be associated with less durable repairs with recurrence of symptoms. For patients who are poor operative candidates, a flexible endoscopic approach for diverticulotomy may be the procedure of choice. Endoscopic approaches may be performed under monitored anesthesia care (MAC) or general anesthesia (GA). Complications include microperforations or esophageal leak, which patients may experience as chest or back pain along with subcutaneous emphysema. Symptoms typically subside after several days with conservative management to heal the leak, including tube feeding, antibiotics, and pain control.

Rigid endoscopy is usually performed under GA. An endoscope is used to expose the common wall between the diverticulum and the esophagus, and various techniques are used to divide the septum. Complications of the rigid endoscopic technique include dental injuries, perforations, and recurrent laryngeal nerve injury.

Complications of open transcervical approach for Zenker diverticula include mediastinitis, vocal cord paralysis, esophageal stenosis, and pharyngocutaneous fistula. Open approaches to Zenker diverticulum typically do not require one-lung ventilation because of extrathoracic approaches, but for more distal diverticula, thoracoscopy or thoracotomy could be utilized with the use of one-lung ventilation.

CLINICAL PEARL

The presence of esophageal disease should be carefully assessed in patients presenting for any surgical procedures requiring transesophageal echocardiography (TEE). Esophageal pathologies including diverticulum, stricture, tumor, perforation or laceration, perforated viscus, and an active upper gastrointestinal bleed represent *absolute* contraindications to TEE. Other esophageal pathologies may represent relative contraindications to TEE.

VIII. Other Endoscopic Esophageal Procedures/Surgeries

A. Foreign Body

Ingestion of foreign bodies often requires general endotracheal anesthesia to allow for endoscopic retrieval and typically requires no more than a single IV. A carefully taken social history may uncover recreational activities that impact the appropriate dose of anesthetic drugs to administer. Foreign bodies that have potential to lacerate or puncture the esophagus when removed, for example, razor blades or bones, may require the placement of an esophageal overtube to minimize such damage, though the overtube use itself carries a risk of mucosal abrasions/tears and esophageal perforation among other complications.

B. Esophageal Stricture

Esophageal strictures impeding ingestion may be due to various causes, including, but not limited to, prior esophageal surgery, GERD, esophagitis, or ingestion of caustic material. A common therapy for esophageal strictures is serial dilations. This procedure involves an initial endoscopic examination for diagnosis of the stricture, dilation of the stricture itself, and a postdilation endoscopy to assess the adequacy of dilation and any complications. Dilation is frequently performed with bougie or balloon dilators, which may be passed through the stricture directly or over a guidewire with the assistance of fluoroscopy. These procedures are typically relatively short, do not require more than a single IV and single-lumen ETT, and should not require any prolonged muscle relaxant. These are not typically very painful procedures, and care should be taken to avoid administering more opioids than necessary.

C. Esophageal Varices

Venous drainage of the cephalad two-thirds of the esophagus is via the azygous vein into the superior vena cava, while the distal third of the esophagus is drained via the gastric veins into the portal vein. Esophageal varices develop at the collateral venous communications between the portal and systemic circulations in the distal esophagus usually due to portal hypertension from cirrhosis, though there are other causes, including splenic vein thrombosis. The collateral flow can lead to an increase in the diameter of the esophageal veins with an increase in vessel wall stress and higher risk of overlying mucosal ulceration and bleeding.

Acute management of bleeding esophageal varices should focus on stabilizing hemodynamics, including assessment of intravascular volume status, as well as ensuring adequate oxygenation and airway protection since bleeding varices can lead to significant bleeding with the risk of pulmonary aspiration. Early endoscopy is typically the initial therapy after stabilization. Endoscopic approaches commonly utilize variceal ligation and endoscopic sclerotherapy. Patients are at risk for rebleeding, particularly if they have not previously received a transjugular intrahepatic portosystemic shunt (TIPS). TIPS is a catheter-based technique used to create a portosystemic shunt within the liver. Historically, operative shunts were created between the portal and systemic venous circulation, but these had significant morbidity because of the major abdominal surgery that was required. Pharmacologic therapy for acute variceal bleeding includes octreotide and somatostatin to decrease portal blood flow.

For patients on anticoagulation therapy, it is appropriate to clarify indication and appropriateness of reversal of anticoagulants. Oral intubation is generally used in the setting of significant variceal bleeding to minimize aspiration risk during endoscopic therapy. Active hemorrhage and hematemesis may significantly complicate airway management. An awake intubation of patients not in extremis may be ideal, but even small amounts of hematemesis can render video laryngoscopy and fiberoptic intubation techniques impossible. Airway devices like the light-wand or lighted stylet may be helpful when there is significant airway bleeding, since direct glottic visualization is not necessary for successful intubation. In the case of active hematemesis, the anesthesiologist should have a plan in place to obtain an emergency front-of-neck airway (eFONA). As with any airway, it is important to have backup plans in place for airway management.

IX. Esophagectomy

Esophagectomies are most often performed for either squamous cell carcinoma or adenocarcinoma of the esophagus, though they may also be performed for esophageal atresia, achalasia, or a nonhealing injury to the esophagus. Most often, the excised portion of the esophagus is replaced with a gastric conduit, though jejunal and colonic interpositions may also be performed.[8] The three main types of esophagectomy are categorized by their surgical approaches. Subsequently, the introduction of laparoscopic and thoracoscopic surgical techniques with or without robotic assistance has resulted in minimally invasive variants of the esophagectomies described earlier.

A. Transhiatal

The oldest form of esophagectomy is the transhiatal esophagectomy. Originally performed by two surgical teams operating simultaneously, now more commonly performed by a single team operating sequentially. Via a laparotomy and left neck dissection, the stomach is mobilized, and the esophagus is digitally dissected from both ends; the stomach is then pulled into the mediastinum as the mediastinal esophagus is delivered via the left neck incision. The esophagus is then excised, and the cervical esophagus anastomosed to the stomach before closure.

B. Ivor Lewis

The Ivor Lewis esophagectomy is named after the Welsh surgeon and was introduced to address concerns that the transhiatal esophagectomy did not permit adequate sampling of mediastinal lymph nodes and to reduce injuries to neighboring mediastinal structures that resulted from digital dissection. The Ivor Lewis esophagectomy involves a laparotomy for the formation of the gastric conduit, and a right thoracotomy for dissection of the mediastinal esophagus and associated lymph nodes. A partial esophagectomy is performed, and a GE anastomosis is made in the mediastinum. The benefits of the Ivor Lewis esophagectomy come at the expense of a thoracic anastomosis site. The thoracic anastomosis results in a less extensive proximal resection margin, anastomosis of esophagus likely within a prior radiation field, and a greater frequency of reflux symptoms. While a thoracic anastomosis as compared to a cervical anastomosis is associated with a lower failure rate if an anastomotic leak does occur, mediastinitis and a more complicated surgical repair are necessary.

6

CLINICAL PEARL

In case series, the mortality associated with a thoracic anastomotic leak ranges from 35% to 60%, whereas that of a cervical anastomotic leak is comparatively low at ≤5%.[9]

C. **McKeown**
This esophagectomy approach, also known as a three-field or three-hole esophagectomy, is a hybrid of the transhiatal and Ivor Lewis esophagectomies. Like the Ivor Lewis esophagectomy, the McKeown esophagectomy involves a laparotomy to form a gastric conduit and a right thoracotomy to dissect the mediastinal esophagus and associated lymph nodes, but these steps are then followed by a left neck dissection and cervical anastomosis of the stomach to the esophagus.

D. **Anesthetic Management**
The anesthetic management of the patient undergoing esophagectomy will depend upon the planned surgical approach. Irrespective of the specific operative plan, patients should undergo rapid sequence intubation to minimize the risk of aspiration. Due to the intrathoracic approaches of the Ivor Lewis and McKeown esophagectomies, these approaches require one-lung ventilation. A multimodal, opioid-sparing approach to analgesia consisting of acetaminophen, nonsteroidal anti-inflammatory drugs (NSAIDs), gabapentinoids, ketamine, and regional anesthetic techniques is a key part of most esophagectomy ERAS protocols. When the procedure involves open laparotomy and/or thoracotomy incision, patients generally benefit from having a preoperative thoracic epidural for intraoperative and postoperative analgesia, though paravertebral[10] and erector spinae plane catheters[11] are gaining favor as they are shown to be equally efficacious from an analgesic perspective with an added benefit of less vasodilation and hypotension as compared to thoracic epidurals.

The use of vasopressors during and after esophagectomies is an area of debate and practice patterns vary, with much of the variation due to institutionally dependent approaches. The concern of those who advocate against vasopressor use is that they function by shunting blood flow from the viscera to the more vital organs, that is, the heart and brain, and vasopressor use could compromise perfusion to the region of the esophageal anastomosis.[12] Historically, this has led to the liberal administration of fluids to patients both intraoperatively and postoperatively. More recently, liberal fluid resuscitation has been implicated in increased tissue edema, poor wound healing, delayed return of bowel function, as well as increased rates of pulmonary edema, respiratory failure, and pneumonia in the major abdominal surgery literature. Current recommendations target judicious fluid administration and a neutral fluid balance with an upper limit on daily weight gain <2 kg.[6] Colloids have not been shown to be superior to crystalloids for fluid administration; given the higher costs of colloids, it is appropriate to administer crystalloids. Balanced electrolyte solutions may be helpful to avoid electrolyte disturbances, but there is no clear benefit over normal saline.[13] It is appropriate to avoid long-acting neuromuscular blockade in an effort to facilitate early extubation, a key aspect of ERAS. It is possible to use electroencephalographic phenotypes to monitor the depth of anesthesia, in addition to the use of proprietary processing algorithms such as the Bispectral Index (BIS).[14] These monitoring tools may also lead to less anesthetic-mediated vasodilation and thus less fluid administration intraoperatively.

7

At the conclusion of an esophagectomy, a decompressive nasoenteric tube is positioned across the anastomosis to ensure it is adequately decompressed. Typically, a postanastomotic enteral access site is established either via a nasojejunal tube or through percutaneous jejunal tube to allow for enteral nutrition as the esophageal anastomosis heals. The durable securement of these tubes cannot be understated as their placement is under endoscopic and/or surgical visualization and replacement may require another anesthetic to replace.

X. Repair of Esophageal Perforation or Rupture

8

Esophageal perforations and ruptures are surgical emergencies with high mortality. While associated with sustained bouts of emesis, Boerhaave syndrome, esophageal perforations, can also be iatrogenic. Indeed, probe placement during TEE, gastrointestinal endoscopies, electrophysiology ablation procedures, and other intrathoracic procedures including mediastinoscopies and thoracoscopies all carry a risk of esophageal injury.

CLINICAL PEARL

Esophageal perforation has a mortality rate of almost 10% if treated within 24 hours but is nearly 20% if treatment started after 24 hours.[15]

In addition, patients can also ingest substances that inadvertently lead to esophageal perforation. At initial presentation, a patient's hemodynamics may be reassuring, but as foregut contents leak into the mediastinum and potentially the chest, inflammation and shock will eventually develop. Surgical approaches may include stenting or primary repair, depending on the time course of the presentation and the underlying comorbidities of the patient.

Obtaining IV access for fluid and vasoactive agents is paramount for the initial resuscitation before taking the patient to the OR for definitive management. Typically, two large-bore IV lines are adequate, though a central line would provide added utility if able to be placed. GA with endotracheal intubation is required; lung isolation may be necessary depending on the surgical approach. Proper preoxygenation (denitrogenation) is essential since mask ventilation with positive pressure could increase esophageal wall strain and further exacerbate a patient's esophageal perforation or rupture. It is not advisable for anesthesiologists to independently place a decompressive gastric tube before induction of anesthesia when there is a known esophageal injury. Perioperative pain management should take into consideration regional blockade of the thoracic wall, as untreated pain may result in delay of extubation and/or worsening respiratory insufficiency due to splinting. Thoracic epidural catheters are proven methods for relieving pleuritic chest pain, but there is increasing evidence for the utilization of erector spinae and paravertebral regional blocks as well.[10,11]

XI. Repair of Tracheoesophageal Fistula

While tracheoesophageal fistula (TEF) typically presents as a congenital anomaly of the esophagus in the pediatric population, the focus of this section is on the surgical repair and anesthetic management of TEF and bronchoesophageal fistula in adults. Although uncommon, they are a significant source of morbidity and mortality for patients with esophageal or lung cancer.[16] While malignancy accounts for the majority of TEFs, prolonged endotracheal intubation and surgical or endoscopic interventions may also lead to a pathologic connection between the esophagus and the trachea or major bronchi; diagnosis may be difficult due to nonspecific symptoms. TEF should be suspected in patients with known risk factors and frequent coughing following solid and liquid intake, recurrent purulent pneumonia, recurrent aspiration, or unexplained malnutrition. Patients on mechanical ventilation can develop TEF from prolonged endotracheal intubation and may present with respiratory distress, worsening gas exchange, loss of returned tidal volume during ventilation, and gastric distention. Presentation may develop over days to weeks, in the context of malignancy, or may present more acutely over hours to days in the context of intubation and mechanical ventilation; large proximal TEFs may present earlier than smaller more distal TEFs.[17]

Spontaneous closure of TEFs is rare, and efforts should be made to identify and treat as promptly as possible; left untreated, patients typically progress to respiratory failure and death. Both esophagram and endoscopy can be used for diagnostic evaluation in patients with concern for TEF. Diagnosis of TEF can be made based on a combination of clinical, radiographic, and endoscopic findings. A barium esophagram will show passage of contrast into the lung. In patients who cannot swallow, e.g. patients on mechanical ventilation, chest computed tomography (CT) with oral or IV contrast may be used to help localize the fistula, but bronchoscopy and endoscopy are then frequently performed to confirm imaging findings and localize the fistula.

In general, curative surgery is performed for noncancerous TEF, whereas palliative management is reserved for malignancy-associated TEF. Conservative management is targeted at minimizing the risk of aspiration by making the patient NPO, elevating the head of bed, suppressing acid production with a PPI, a decompressive gastric tube, and frequent oral suctioning; any present or suspected pneumonia should be appropriately treated, and nutrition should be provided by either small bowel enteral tube feeds or total parenteral nutrition (TPN).

[9]   In patients receiving mechanical ventilation, extubation is preferable, but not always appropriate. It can be helpful to decrease the tidal volume and positive end-expiratory pressure in an attempt to minimize air leak through the fistula, until ETT adjustment. For those who cannot be extubated, advancing the ETT distal to the site of the TEF and ensuring that the inflated cuff is below the fistula should be performed. Some surgeons may prefer to delay surgical repair until patients are weaned off mechanical ventilation to optimize their preoperative state and potentially minimize the incidence of anastomotic dehiscence and restenosis associated with positive pressure ventilation.

Patients with malignant TEF >5 mm are commonly treated with palliative stenting of the esophagus and/or airway. Smaller lesions (those <5 mm) have been treated with bronchoscopic clipping or fibrin glue. In many cases, palliative stenting allows patients to survive weeks or months longer with improved quality of life. Double stenting (concurrent esophageal and airway stents) is also an option advocated by some, though there is not broad consensus on the best management approach (double vs single stenting) for a stent-based approach in TEF.

Distal esophageal fistulas are less common than mid- or proximal TEFs and are more likely to communicate with major bronchi (bronchoesophageal fistula) than with the trachea. Management may be with esophageal stent or possibly double stenting utilizing a bronchial and esophageal stent.

For patients who are suitable surgical candidates with noncancerous TEFs, curative surgery is appropriate. Surgical repair is a technically difficult surgery involving a cervicotomy, cervicosternotomy, or thoracotomy approach. For small lesions, the fistula can be divided and repaired using omental or muscle flaps. Large TEFs may require major operations for repair, including esophageal diversion, esophageal reconstruction, and/or tracheal or laryngotracheal reconstruction. Prompt extubation after surgery should be facilitated to minimize complications associated with prolonged mechanical ventilation, including wound dehiscence and fistula recurrence. Perioperative morbidity and mortality are high, with major complications including wound dehiscence, pneumonia, recurrent TEF, vocal cord dysfunction, and tracheal stenosis.

Anesthetic management of patients with TEF includes maintaining a patent airway and preventing aspiration of secretions. Patients should remain NPO, be started on IV fluids, and be placed in a head-up position to minimize regurgitation of gastric secretions through the fistula. Awake, fiberoptic, or rapid sequence induction and intubation should be considered. Proper placement of the ETT is critical, as it should be above the carina but below the TEF to avoid worsening of the lesion. If the TEF is below the carina, then a double-lumen tube could be used to isolate the TEF and allow positive pressure ventilation to the airway.

REFERENCES

1. Gillis C, Buhler K, Bresee L, et al. Effects of nutritional prehabilitation, with and without exercise, on outcomes of patients who undergo colorectal surgery: a systematic review and meta-analysis. *Gastroenterology.* 2018;155(2):391-410.
2. Campos J, Feider A. Hypoxia during one-lung ventilation—a review and update. *J Cardiothorac Vasc Anesth.* 2018; 32(5):2330-2338.
3. Schizas D, Papaconstantinou D, Krompa A, et al. Minimally invasive oesophagectomy in the prone versus lateral decubitus position: a systematic review and meta-analysis. *Dis Esophagus.* 2022;35(4):doab042.
4. Marik PE, Cavallazzi R. Does the central venous pressure predict fluid responsiveness? An updated meta-analysis and a plea for some common sense. *Crit Care Med.* 2013;41(7):1774-1781.
5. Lohser J. Evidence-based management of one-lung ventilation. *Anesthesiol Clin.* 2008;26(2):241-272.
6. Low DE, Allum W, De Manzoni G, et al. Guidelines for perioperative care in esophagectomy: enhanced recovery after surgery (ERAS®) society recommendations. *World J Surg.* 2019;43(2):299-330.
7. Thilen SR, Weigel WA, Todd MM, et al. 2023 American Society of Anesthesiologists Practice Guidelines for monitoring and antagonism of neuromuscular blockade: a report by the American Society of Anesthesiologists Task Force on Neuromuscular Blockade. *Anesthesiology.* 2023;138(1):13-41.
8. Bartels K, Fiegel M, Stevens Q, et al. Approaches to perioperative care for esophagectomy. *J Cardiothorac Vasc Anesth.* 2015;29(2):472-480.
9. Whooley BP, Law S, Alexandrou A, Murthy SC, Wong J. Critical appraisal of the significance of intrathoracic anastomotic leakage after esophagectomy for cancer. *Am J Surg.* 2001;181(3):198-203.

10. Davies RG, Myles PS, Graham JM. A comparison of the analgesic efficacy and side-effects of paravertebral vs epidural blockade for thoracotomy—a systematic review and meta-analysis of randomized trials. *Br J Anaesth.* 2006;96(4):418-426.

11. Elsabeeny WY, Ibrahim MA, Shehab NN, Mohamed A, Wadod MA. Serratus anterior plane block and erector spinae plane block versus thoracic epidural analgesia for perioperative thoracotomy pain control: a randomized controlled study. *J Cardiothorac Vasc Anesth.* 2021;35(10):2928-2936.

12. Walsh KJ, Zhang H, Tan KS, et al. Use of vasopressors during esophagectomy is not associated with increased risk of anastomotic leak. *Dis Esophagus.* 34(4):doaa090.

13. Tyagi A, Maitra S, Bhattacharjee S. Comparison of colloid and crystalloid using goal-directed fluid therapy protocol in non-cardiac surgery: a meta-analysis of randomized controlled trials. *J Anesth.* 2020;34(6):865-875.

14. Wildes TS, Mickle AM, Abdallah AB, et al. Effect of electroencephalography-guided anesthetic administration on postoperative delirium among older adults undergoing major surgery—the ENGAGES randomized clinical trial. *JAMA.* 2019;321(5):473-483.

15. Biancari F, D'Andrea V, Rosalba P, et al. Current treatment and outcome of esophageal perforations in adults: systematic review and meta-analysis of 75 studies. *World J Surg.* 2013;37(5):1051-1059.

16. Cerfolio RJ, Laliberte A-S, Blackmon S, et al. Minimally invasive esophagectomy: a consensus statement. *Ann Thorac Surg.* 2022;110(4):1417-1426.

17. Diddee R, Shaw IH. Acquired tracheo-oesophageal fistula in adults. *BJA Educ.* 2006;6(3):105-108.

Anesthetic Management for Surgery of the Lungs and Mediastinum

Alexander Huang, Peter Slinger, and Erin A. Sullivan

KEY POINTS

1. Preoperatively, respiratory function should be assessed in three related but independent areas: respiratory mechanics, gas exchange, and cardiopulmonary interaction.
2. The most useful preoperative predictor of difficult endobronchial intubation is the chest film.
3. The most important predictor of Pao_2 during one-lung ventilation (OLV) is the Pao_2 during two-lung ventilation in the lateral position before OLV.
4. Absolute indications for lung isolation include purulent secretions, massive pulmonary hemorrhage, bronchopleural fistula, blebs, and bullae (blood, pus, and air).
5. Iatrogenic injury has been estimated to occur in 0.5-2 per 1,000 cases using double-lumen tubes (DLTs).
6. The rapidity of the fall in Pao_2 after the onset of OLV is an indicator of the risk of subsequent desaturation.
7. Because of the risk of increased shunt and pulmonary edema in the dependent lung, no volume should be given for theoretical third-space losses during thoracotomy.
8. Desaturation during bilateral lung procedures is particularly a problem during the second period of OLV.
9. The postoperative mortality following pneumonectomy is 17% in patients who develop arrhythmias versus 2% in those without this complication.
10. During induction of general anesthesia in patients with an anterior mediastinal mass, airway obstruction is the most common and feared complication.
11. Hemoptysis in a patient with a pulmonary artery (PA) catheter must be assumed to be caused by perforation of a pulmonary vessel by the catheter until proven otherwise. The mortality rate may exceed 50%.
12. Lung volume reduction surgery (LVRS) is a viable option for a select group of patients with emphysema. Goals of treatment include improvements in dyspnea, exercise tolerance, quality of life, and prolonged patient survival.

I. Preoperative Assessment

A. Overview

Advances in anesthetic management, surgical techniques, and perioperative care have expanded the envelope of patients now considered to be operable. The principles described apply to all types of pulmonary resections and other chest surgery. In patients with malignancy, the risk/benefit ratio of canceling or delaying surgery pending other investigation/therapy is always complicated by the risk of further spread of cancer during any interval before resection.

1. **Risk assessment:** It is the anesthesiologist's responsibility to use the preoperative assessment to identify patients at elevated risk and then to use that risk assessment to stratify perioperative management and focus resources on the high-risk patients to improve their outcomes. This is the primary function of the preanesthetic assessment.

2. **Initial and final assessments:** Commonly, the patient is initially assessed in a clinic and often not by the member of the anesthesia staff who will administer the anesthesia. The actual contact with the responsible anesthesiologist may be only 10-15 minutes before induction. It is necessary to organize and standardize the approach to preoperative evaluation for these patients into two temporally disconnected phases: the initial (clinic) assessment and the final (day-of-admission) assessment.

3. **"Lung-sparing" surgery:** Postoperative preservation of respiratory function has been shown to be proportional to the amount of functioning lung parenchyma preserved. To assess patients with limited pulmonary function, the anesthesiologist must understand these surgical options in addition to conventional lobectomy and pneumonectomy.

   Prethoracotomy assessment involves all aspects of a complete anesthetic assessment: past history, allergies, medications, and upper airway. Respiratory complications comprise the major cause of perioperative morbidity and mortality in thoracic surgery. Atelectasis, pneumonia, and respiratory failure occur in 15%-20% of patients, and cardiac complications (eg, arrhythmia and ischemia) occur in 10%-15% of them.

B. Risk Stratification

1. **Assessment of respiratory function:** The best assessment of respiratory function comes from a history of the patient's quality of life. An asymptomatic American Society of Anesthesiologists (ASA) class I or II patient with full exercise capacity does not need screening cardiorespiratory testing. Assess respiratory function in three related but independent areas (see Figure 25.1).

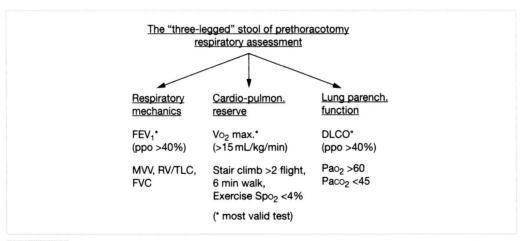

FIGURE 25.1 "Three-legged" stool of prethoracotomy respiratory assessment. DLCO, diffusing capacity for carbon monoxide; FEV$_1$, forced expiratory volume in 1 second; FVC, forced vital capacity; MVV, maximum voluntary ventilation; Paco$_2$, arterial partial pressure of carbon dioxide; Pao$_2$, arterial partial pressure of oxygen; parench., parenchymal; ppo, predicted postoperative; pulmon., pulmonary; RV/TLC, residual volume/total lung capacity; Spo$_2$, oxygen saturation by pulse oximetry; Vo$_2$ max, maximum oxygen consumption.

a. **Lung mechanics:** The most valid single test[1] for post-thoracotomy respiratory complications is the predicted postoperative forced expiratory volume in 1 second (ppoFEV$_1$%), which is calculated as follows:

$$ppoFEV_1\% = \text{pre-op } FEV_1\% \times (1 - \%\text{functional lung tissue removed}/100)$$

Consider the right upper and middle lobes combined as approximately equivalent to each of the other three lobes and the right lung as 10% larger than the left lung.

Low risk = ppoFEV$_1$ >40% of preoperative predicted FEV$_1$

Moderate risk = ppoFEV$_1$ 30%-40% of preoperative predicted FEV$_1$

High risk = ppoFEV$_1$ <30% of preoperative predicted FEV$_1$

b. **Pulmonary parenchymal function:** Traditionally, arterial blood gas (ABG) data such as preoperative Pao$_2$ <60 mm Hg or Paco$_2$ >45 mm Hg have been used as cutoff values for pulmonary resection. Cancer resections now have been successfully done or even combined with volume reduction in patients who do not meet these criteria, although they remain useful as warning indicators of increased risk. The most useful test of the gas exchange capacity of the lungs is the diffusing capacity for carbon monoxide (DLCO). DLCO correlates with the total functioning surface area of the alveolar-capillary interface. A ppoDLCO <40% correlates with both increased respiratory and cardiac complications.[2]

c. **Cardiopulmonary interaction:** The traditional test in ambulatory patients is stair climbing. The ability to climb three flights of stairs or more is associated with decreased mortality. Formal laboratory exercise testing is currently the "gold standard" for the assessment of cardiopulmonary function. The maximal oxygen consumption (Vo$_2$ max) is the most valid exercise predictor of post-thoracotomy outcome. An estimate of Vo$_2$ max can be made by dividing the distance walked in meters in 6 minutes (6MWT) by 30 (ie, 450 m/30 = 15 mL/kg/min):

Low risk = Vo$_2$ max >20 mL/kg/min

Moderate risk = Vo$_2$ max of 15-20 mL/kg/min

High risk = Vo$_2$ max <15 mL/kg/min

CLINICAL PEARL

Patients who can climb at least three flights of stairs without stopping or who can walk at least 600 m in 6 minutes most often have a low risk of perioperative mortality following pulmonary resection.

d. Ventilation-perfusion (V/Q) scintigraphy is particularly useful in pneumonectomy patients and should be considered for any patient who has ppoFEV$_1$ <40%. Assessments of ppoFEV$_1$, DLCO, and Vo$_2$ max can be upgraded if the lung region to be resected is nonfunctioning.

e. **Split-lung function studies:** These tests have not shown sufficient predictive validity for universal adoption in potential lung resection patients.

f. **Combination of tests (Figure 25.2):** If a patient has ppoFEV$_1$ >40%, it should be possible for the patient to be extubated in the operating room at the conclusion of surgery, assuming the patient is alert, warm, and comfortable ("AWaC"). If ppoFEV$_1$ is >30% and exercise tolerance and lung parenchymal function exceed the increased risk thresholds, then extubation in the operating room should be possible depending on the status of associated diseases. Patients with ppoFEV$_1$ 20%-30% and favorable predicted cardiorespiratory and parenchymal function can be considered for early extubation if thoracic epidural analgesia (TEA) is used.

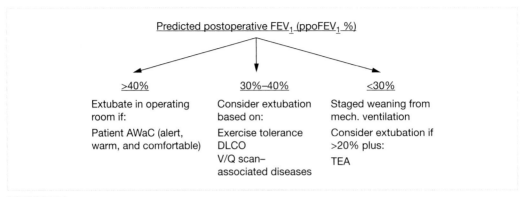

FIGURE 25.2 Post-thoracotomy anesthetic management. DLCO, diffusing capacity for carbon monoxide; FEV_1, forced expiratory volume in 1 second; mech., mechanical; ppo, predicted postoperative; TEA, thoracic epidural analgesia; V/Q, ventilation/perfusion.

2. **Intercurrent medical conditions**
   a. **Age:** For patients older than 80 years, the rate of respiratory complications (40%) is double that expected in a younger population and the rate of cardiac complications (40%), particularly arrhythmias, nearly triples. The mortality from pneumonectomy (22% in patients older than 70 years), particularly right pneumonectomy, is excessive.

CLINICAL PEARL

As compared to that for middle-aged patients, the risk of pulmonary complications in patients over 80 years of age doubles and the risk of cardiac complications almost triples.

   b. **Cardiac disease**
      (1) **Ischemia:** Pulmonary resection is generally regarded as an intermediate-risk procedure for perioperative ischemia. Beyond the standard history, physical examination, and electrocardiogram, routine screening for cardiac disease does not appear to be cost-effective for prethoracotomy patients. Noninvasive testing is indicated in patients with active cardiac conditions (unstable ischemia, recent infarction, decompensated heart failure, severe valvular disease, significant arrhythmia), multiple clinical predictors of cardiac risk (stable angina, remote infarction, previous congestive failure, diabetes, renal insufficiency, or cerebrovascular disease), or in the older patients. Lung resection surgery should ideally be delayed 4-6 weeks after placement of a bare-metal coronary artery stent and 6-12 months after a drug-eluting stent. After a myocardial infarction, limiting the delay to 4-6 weeks in a medically stable and fully investigated and optimized patient seems acceptable.
      (2) **Arrhythmia:** Atrial fibrillation is a common complication (10%-15%) of pulmonary resection surgery. Factors correlating with an increased incidence of arrhythmia are the amount of lung tissue resected, age, intraoperative blood loss, esophagectomy, and intrapericardial dissection. The American Association of Thoracic Surgery guidelines recommend the continuation of β-blockers in patients already receiving them and the replacement of magnesium in any patient with low magnesium stores.[3]
   c. **Chronic obstructive pulmonary disease:** Assessment of the severity of chronic obstructive pulmonary disease (COPD) is based on FEV_1% predicted, as follows—stage I: >50%, stage II: 35%-50%, and stage III: <35%. The following factors in COPD need to be considered:
      (1) **Respiratory drive:** Many patients with stage II or III COPD have an elevated $Paco_2$ at rest. It is not possible to differentiate "CO_2 retainers" from nonretainers

on the basis of history, physical examination, or spirometry. These patients need an ABG preoperatively. Supplemental oxygen causes the $Paco_2$ to increase in CO_2 retainers by a combination of decreased respiratory drive and increased dead space.

CLINICAL PEARL

In patients with advanced COPD, neither history, physical examination, nor FEV_1 predicts chronic CO_2 retention.

    (2) **Nocturnal hypoxemia:** Patients with COPD desaturate more frequently and severely than normal patients during sleep. This results from the rapid/shallow breathing pattern that occurs during rapid eye movement sleep.

    (3) **Right ventricular dysfunction:** Cor pulmonale occurs in 40% of adult patients with COPD with FEV_1 <1 L and in 70% with FEV_1 <0.6 L. Pneumonectomy candidates with ppoFEV_1 <40% should have transthoracic echocardiography to assess right heart function.

3. **Preoperative therapy of chronic obstructive pulmonary disease:** The four complications of COPD that must be actively sought and treated at the initial prethoracotomy assessment are atelectasis, bronchospasm, chest infection, and pulmonary edema (PE). Patients with COPD have fewer postoperative pulmonary complications when a perioperative program of chest physiotherapy is initiated preoperatively. Pulmonary complications decrease in thoracic surgical patients who are not smoking versus those who continue to smoke up until the time of surgery.

4. **Lung cancer considerations:** At the time of initial assessment, patients with cancer should be assessed for the "4 Ms" associated with malignancy: **M**ass effects, **M**etabolic abnormalities, **M**etastases, and **M**edications. Prior use of medications that can exacerbate oxygen-induced pulmonary toxicity, such as bleomycin, should be considered (Table 25.1).

5. **Postoperative analgesia:** The risks and benefits of the various forms of post-thoracotomy analgesia should be explained to the patient at the time of initial preanesthetic assessment. Potential contraindications to specific methods of analgesia should be determined, such as coagulation problems, sepsis, and neurologic disorders. If the patient will receive prophylactic anticoagulants and epidural analgesia is elected, appropriate timing of anticoagulant administration and neuraxial catheter placement must be arranged.

6. **Premedication:** Avoid inadvertent withdrawal of drugs that are being taken for concurrent medical conditions (bronchodilators, antihypertensives, β-blockers). For esophageal reflux surgery, oral antacids and H_2-blockers are routinely ordered preoperatively. In patients with copious secretions, an antisialagogue (eg, glycopyrrolate 0.2 mg intravenous [IV]) is useful to facilitate fiberoptic bronchoscopy (FOB) for positioning of a double-lumen tube (DLT) or bronchial blocker (BB).

TABLE 25.1   Anesthetic Considerations in Patients With Lung Cancer (the "4 Ms")

   I. **Mass effects:** Obstructive pneumonia, superior vena cava syndrome, tracheobronchial distortion, Pancoast syndrome, recurrent laryngeal nerve, or phrenic nerve paresis
  II. **Metabolic effects:** Lambert-Eaton syndrome, hypercalcemia, hyponatremia, Cushing syndrome
 III. **Metastases:** Particularly to brain, bone, liver, and adrenal gland
 IV. **Medications:** Chemotherapy agents, pulmonary toxicity (bleomycin, mitomycin), cardiac toxicity (doxorubicin), renal toxicity (*cis*-platinum)

TABLE 25.2   Summary of Preanesthetic Assessment

Initial Preanesthetic Assessment for Pulmonary Resection

   I.   All patients: Exercise tolerance, ppoFEV$_1$%, discuss postoperative analgesia, D/C smoking
   II. Patients with ppoFEV$_1$ <40%: DLCO, V/Q scan, Vo$_2$ max
   III. Patients with cancer: The "4 Ms": Mass effects, metabolic effects, metastases, medications
   IV. Patients with COPD: ABG, physiotherapy, bronchodilators

Final Preanesthetic Assessment for Pulmonary Resection

   I.   Review initial assessment and test results
   II. Assess difficulty of lung isolation: Chest x-ray film, CT scan
   III. Assess risk of hypoxemia during OLV

ABG, arterial blood gas; COPD, chronic obstructive pulmonary disease; CT, computed tomography; D/C, discontinue; DLCO, diffusing capacity for carbon monoxide; OLV, one-lung ventilation; ppoFEV$_1$, predicted postoperative forced expiratory volume in 1 second; Vo$_2$ max, maximum oxygen consumption; V/Q, ventilation/perfusion.

CLINICAL PEARL

In patients with copious secretions, prophylactic glycopyrrolate often facilitates visualization for FOB-assisted DLT positioning.

   7. **Final preoperative assessment:** The final preoperative anesthetic assessment is made immediately before the patient is brought to the operating room. Review the data from the initial prethoracotomy assessment (Table 25.2) and the results of tests ordered at that time. Two other concerns for thoracic anesthesia need to be assessed: (i) the potential for difficult lung isolation and (ii) the risk of desaturation during one-lung ventilation (OLV).

   2
   a. **Assessment of difficult endobronchial intubation:** The most useful predictor of difficult endobronchial intubation is the chest imaging. Clinically important tracheal or bronchial distortions or compression from tumors or previous surgery can usually be detected on plain chest radiographs (CXRs). Distal airway (including distal trachea and proximal bronchi) problems not detectable on the plain x-ray film may be visualized on chest computed tomographic (CT) scans. These abnormalities often will not be mentioned in a written or verbal report from the radiologist or surgeon. The anesthesiologist must examine the chest image before placing a DLT or BB.

   b. **Prediction of desaturation during one-lung ventilation:** It is possible to determine patients at high risk for desaturation during OLV for thoracic surgery. Factors that correlate with desaturation during OLV are listed in Table 25.3. The most important predictor of Pao$_2$ during OLV is the Pao$_2$ during two-lung ventilation in the lateral position
   3
   before OLV. The proportion of perfusion or ventilation to the nonoperated lung on preoperative V/Q scans also correlates with the Pao$_2$ during OLV. The side of the thoracotomy has an effect on Pao$_2$ during OLV. With the left lung being 10% smaller than the right lung, there is less shunt when the left lung is collapsed. The degree of obstructive lung disease correlates inversely with Pao$_2$ during OLV. Patients tend to desaturate more in the supine position during OLV than in the more usual lateral position.

TABLE 25.3   Factors That Correlate With an Increased Risk of Desaturation During OLV

   I.   High percentage of ventilation (V) or perfusion (Q) to the operative lung on preoperative V/Q scan
   II. Poor Pao$_2$ during two-lung ventilation, particularly in the lateral position intraoperatively
   III. Right-sided surgery
   IV. Supine position

OLV, one-lung ventilation; Pao$_2$, arterial oxygen pressure; V/Q, ventilation/perfusion.

Stratifying the perioperative risks allows the anesthesiologist to develop a systematic approach to these patients that can be used to guide anesthetic management (Figure 25.2).

II. Intraoperative Management

A. Lung Separation

There are three basic options for lung separation: single-lumen endobronchial tubes (EBTs), double-lumen endotracheal tubes (DLTs) (left- or right-sided) (see Figures 25.3 and 25.4), and BBs. The second half of the 20th century saw refinements of the DLT from that of Carlens to a tube specifically designed for intraoperative use (Robertshaw) with larger, D-shaped lumens and without a carinal hook. Current disposable polyvinyl chloride DLTs have incorporated high-volume/low-pressure tracheal and bronchial cuffs. Recently, there has been a revival of interest in BBs due to several factors: new blocker designs (see Figures 25.5 and 25.6)[4] and greater familiarity of anesthesiologists with fiberoptic placement of BBs (see Figure 25.7).

4

1. **Indications for lung separation:** Absolute indications for lung isolation include purulent secretions, massive pulmonary hemorrhage, and bronchopleural fistula, blebs, and bullae (blood, pus, and air). More commonly, lung separation is provided intraoperatively to facilitate surgical exposure.

2. **Techniques of lung separation:** The optimal methods for lung isolation are listed in Table 25.4. Because it is impossible to describe one technique as best in all indications for OLV, the various indications are considered separately.

   a. **Elective pulmonary resection, right-sided:** The first choice is a left DLT. The widest margin of safety in positioning is with left DLTs. During OLV, this technique maintains

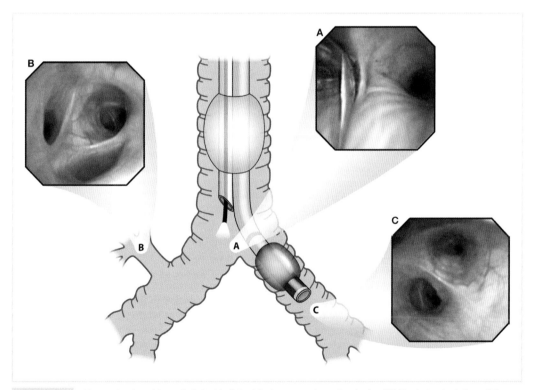

FIGURE 25.3 The optimal position of a left-sided double-lumen endotracheal tube. **(A)** Unobstructed view of the entrance of the right mainstem bronchus as seen from the tracheal lumen. **(B)** Takeoff of the right upper lobe bronchus with the three segments. **(C)** Unobstructed view of the left upper and left lower bronchus as seen from the bronchial lumen. (Reprinted by permission from Springer: Campos J. Lung isolation. In: Slinger P, ed. *Principles and Practice of Anesthesia for Thoracic Surgery*. Springer; 2011:227-246. © 2011 Springer Science+Business Media, LLC.)

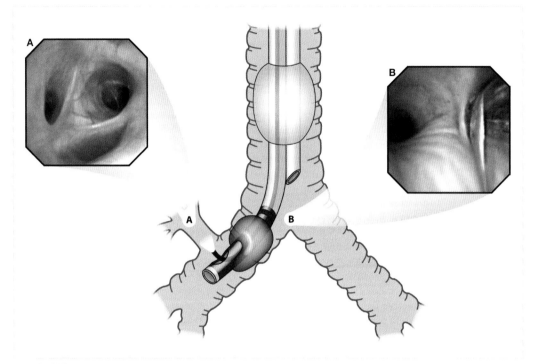

FIGURE 25.4 Optimal position of a right-sided double-lumen endotracheal tube as seen with a fiberoptic broncho-scope. **(A)** View of the right upper lobe bronchus seen through the ventilating side slot of the bronchial lumen. **(B)** View of the carina showing the left mainstem bronchus and the bronchial lumen in the right mainstem bronchus seen from the tracheal lumen. (Reprinted by permission from Springer: Campos J. Lung isolation. In: Slinger P, ed. *Principles and Practice of Anesthesia for Thoracic Surgery.* Springer; 2011:227-246. © 2011 Springer Science+Business Media, LLC.)

continuous access to the nonventilated lung for suctioning, fiberoptic monitoring of position, and continuous positive airway pressure (CPAP). There are two possible alternatives: (i) single-lumen EBT: a standard 7.5-mm diameter, 32-cm long endotracheal tube (ETT) can be advanced over an FOB into the left mainstem bronchus. (ii) A BB can be placed external to or intraluminally with an ETT.

b. **Elective pulmonary resection, left-sided**
  (1) **Not pneumonectomy:** There is no obvious best choice between a BB and a left DLT. The use of a left DLT for a left thoracotomy can be associated with obstruction of the tracheal lumen by the lateral tracheal wall and subsequent problems with gas exchange in the ventilated lung. A right DLT is a good alternate choice.
  (2) **Left pneumonectomy:** When a pneumonectomy is foreseen, a right DLT is the best choice. A right DLT will permit the surgeon to palpate the left hilum during OLV without interference from a tube or blocker in the left mainstem bronchus. The disposable right DLTs currently available in North America vary greatly in design, depending on the manufacturer (Mallinckrodt, Rusch, Kendall). All three designs include a ventilating side slot (fenestration) in the distal bronchial lumen for right upper lobe ventilation. The optimal positioning technique includes bronchoscopically confirming that this fenestration aligns with the right upper lobe orifice as shown in Figure 25.4. If left lung isolation is impossible despite extremely high pressures in the right DLT bronchial cuff, a Fogarty catheter can be passed into the left main bronchus as a BB. As an alternative, there is no clear preference between a left DLT and BB. These all require repositioning before clamping the left mainstem bronchus.

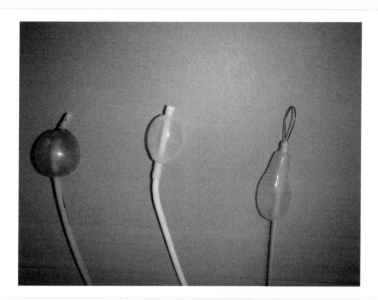

FIGURE 25.5 Three of the endobronchial blockers currently available in North America. **(Left)** The Cohen tip-deflecting endobronchial blocker (Cook Critical Care), which allows anesthesiologists to establish one-lung ventilation by directing its flexible tip left or right into the desired bronchus using a control wheel device on the proximal end of the blocker in combination with fiberoptic bronchoscopic (FOB) guidance. **(Middle)** The Fuji Uniblocker (Fuji Corp). It has a fixed distal curve that allows it to be rotated for manipulation into position with FOB guidance. Unlike its predecessor, the Univent blocker, the Uniblocker is used with a standard endotracheal tube. **(Right)** The wire-guided endobronchial blocker (Arndt bronchial blocker; Cook Critical Care) introduced in 1999. It contains a wire loop in the inner lumen; when used as a snare with a fiberoptic bronchoscope, it allows directed placement. The snare is then removed, and the 1.4-mm lumen may be used as a suction channel or for oxygen insufflation. (Reprinted by permission from Springer: Campos J. Lung isolation. In: Slinger P, ed. *Principles and Practice of Anesthesia for Thoracic Surgery*. Springer; 2011:227-246. © 2011 Springer Science+Business Media, LLC.)

    c. **Thoracoscopy:** Lung biopsies, wedge resection, bleb/bullae resections, and some lobectomies can be done using video-assisted thoracoscopic surgery (VATS). During open thoracotomy, the lung can be compressed by the surgeon to facilitate collapse before the inflation of a BB. A left DLT is generally preferred for thoracoscopy.

    d. **Pulmonary hemorrhage:** Life-threatening pulmonary hemorrhage can result from a wide variety of causes, such as aspergillosis, tuberculosis, and pulmonary artery (PA) catheter trauma. The primary risk for these patients is asphyxiation, and the first-line treatment is lung isolation and suctioning the lower airways. Lung isolation can be with a DLT, BB, or single-lumen EBT, depending on availability and the clinical circumstances. Tracheobronchial hemorrhage from blunt chest trauma usually resolves with suctioning; only rarely is lung isolation necessary.

    e. **Bronchopleural fistula:** The anesthesiologist is faced with the triple problem of avoiding tension pneumothorax, ensuring adequate ventilation, and protecting the healthy lung from any fluid collection in the involved hemithorax. Management depends on the site of the fistula and the urgency of the clinical situation. For a peripheral bronchopleural fistula in a stable patient, a BB may be acceptable. For a large central fistula and in urgent situations, the most rapid and reliable method of securing one-lung isolation and ventilation is a DLT. In life-threatening situations, a DLT can be placed in awake patients with direct FOB guidance.

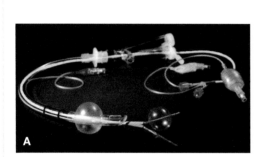
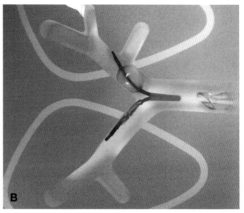

FIGURE 25.6 **(A, B)** The recently introduced EZ Blocker (Teleflex). This bronchial blocker has two blockers and is placed at the carina with fiberoptic guidance and the corresponding cuff to the operative lung is inflated when required.

CLINICAL PEARL

Because positive-pressure ventilation risks tension pneumothorax in patients with bronchopleural fistula (and massive air leak in the presence of a chest tube), either preservation of spontaneous ventilation until lung isolation is achieved or rapid attainment of lung isolation is highly recommended.

    f. Purulent secretions (lung abscess, hydatid cysts): Lobar or segmental blockade is ideal. Loss of lung isolation in these cases is not merely a surgical inconvenience but may be life threatening. A left DLT is usually preferred.

    g. Nonpulmonary thoracic surgery: Thoracic aortic and esophageal surgeries require OLV. Because there is no risk of ventilated lung contamination, a left DLT and a BB are equivalent choices.

    h. Bronchial surgery: An intrabronchial tumor, bronchial trauma, or bronchial sleeve resection during a lobectomy requires that the surgeon have intraluminal access to the ipsilateral mainstem bronchus. Either a single-lumen EBT or a DLT in the ventilated lung is preferred.

    i. Unilateral lung lavage, independent lung ventilation, and lung transplantation are all best accomplished with a left DLT.

  3. Upper airway abnormalities: It is occasionally necessary to provide OLV in patients who have abnormal upper airways due to previous surgery or trauma or in patients who are known for difficult intubations. There are four basic options for these patients: (i) fiberoptic-guided intubation with a DLT, (ii) secure the airway with an ETT and then use a "tube exchanger" to place a DLT, (iii) use a BB, and (iv) use an uncut single-lumen tube as an EBT.

    The optimal choice will depend on the patient and the operation. At all times, it is best to maintain spontaneous ventilation and to do nothing blindly in the presence of blood or pus. Awake FOB intubation with a DLT requires thorough topical anesthesia of the airway. It is important when using a tube exchanger to have a second person perform a direct laryngoscopy to expose as much of the glottis as possible during the tube change. Direct laryngoscopy decreases the angles between the oropharynx and the trachea and reduces the chance of trauma to the airway from the DLT. Video-laryngoscopes are very useful for this.

    BBs are often the best choice for these patients. If the ETT is too narrow to easily accommodate both a bronchoscope and a BB, the BB can be introduced through the glottis

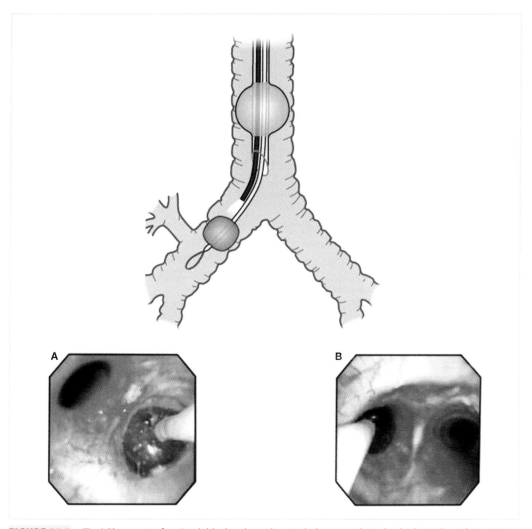

FIGURE 25.7 **(Top)** Placement of an Arndt blocker through a single-lumen endotracheal tube in the right mainstem bronchus with the fiberoptic bronchoscope. **(Bottom)** Optimal position of an endobronchial blocker in the right **(A)** or left **(B)** mainstem bronchus as seen through a fiberoptic bronchoscope. Note that the right-sided placement is deliberately closer to the carina in an effort to avoid overlapping the origin of the right upper lobe bronchus. (Reprinted by permission from Springer: Campos J. Lung isolation. In: Slinger P, ed. *Principles and Practice of Anesthesia for Thoracic Surgery.* 2nd ed. Springer; 2019:283-309. © 2019 Springer Science+Business Media, LLC.)

independently external to the ETT with fiberoptic guidance. Bilateral BBs can be used for bilateral resections, or the same blocker can be manipulated from side to side. Bilateral single-lumen EBTs or BBs can be used for lung isolation in patients with tracheal fistulas, trauma, or other abnormalities in the region of the carina. Smaller DLTs (32, 28, and 26F) are available, but they will not permit passage of an FOB of the diameter commonly available to monitor positioning (3.5-4.0 mm). An ETT designed for microlaryngoscopy (5- to 6-mm inner diameter [ID] and >30 cm long) can be used as an EBT, with FOB positioning, but beware of right upper lobe obstruction if placed in the right mainstem bronchus. If the patient's trachea can accept a 7-mm ETT, a Fogarty catheter (8F venous thrombectomy catheter with a 10-mL balloon) can be passed through the ETT via an FOB adapter for use as a BB.

TABLE 25.4 Selection of Airway Device for Lung Isolation

Surgery	Primary Choice[a]	Secondary Options (in Order of Preference)
Pulmonary resection, right-sided	Left DLT	BB, EBT
Pulmonary resection, left-sided, not pneumonectomy	Left DLT	BB, right DLT
Pulmonary resection, left-sided pneumonectomy/left main bronchial surgery	Right DLT	BB, left DLT
Thoracoscopy	Left DLT	Right DLT, BB, EBT
Pulmonary hemorrhage	DLT/BB/EBT	
Bronchopleural fistula/abscess	Left DLT	Right DLT, BB, EBT
Esophageal, thoracic aortic, transthoracic vertebral surgery	Left DLT/BB	Right DLT, EBT
Lung transplantation, bilateral/right single	Left DLT	EBT, BB
Lung transplantation, left single	Right DLT	BB, left DLT
Abnormal upper airway, left thoracotomy	BB	Right DLT/left DLT, EBT
Abnormal upper airway, right thoracotomy	EBT/BB	Left DLT/right DLT

BB, bronchial blocker ipsilateral to side of surgery; EBT, single-lumen tube placed endobronchially contralateral to surgery; left DLT, left-sided double-lumen tube; right DLT, right-sided double-lumen tube.
[a]Options separated by a slash (/) are equivalent choices.

4. **Chest trauma:** It is common in both open and closed chest trauma to have some hemoptysis from alveolar hemorrhage. The majority of these cases can be managed without lung isolation after bronchoscopy and suction. The majority of the deaths in these patients are due to their other injuries and not from airway hemorrhage or air embolus.

5. **Avoiding iatrogenic airway injury:** Iatrogenic injury has been estimated to occur in 0.5-2 per 1,000 cases with DLTs.[5]
   a. Examine the CXR film or CT scan, which can help predict the majority of difficult endobronchial intubations.
   b. Use an appropriate size tube. Too small a tube will make lung isolation difficult. Too large a tube is more likely to cause trauma. Useful guidelines for DLT sizes in adults are as follows:
      (1) Females' height <1.6 m (63 inch): 35F (possibly 32F if <1.5 m)
      (2) Females >1.6 m: 37F
      (3) Males <1.7 m (67 inch): 39F (possibly 37F if <1.6 m)
      (4) Males >1.7 m: 41F

CLINICAL PEARL

Avoid the natural tendency to place a DLT that is too small because this often complicates tube positioning, successful lung isolation, and suctioning.

   c. **Depth of insertion of DLT:** Tracheobronchial dimensions correlate with height. The average depth at insertion, from the teeth, for a left DLT is 29 cm in an adult and varies ±1 cm for each 10 cm of patient height ±170 cm.
   d. **Avoid nitrous oxide:** Nitrous oxide 70% can increase the bronchial cuff volume by 5-16 mL intraoperatively.
   e. Inflate the bronchial cuff/blocker only to the minimal volume required for lung isolation and for the minimal time. This volume is usually <3 mL for a DLT bronchial cuff and <7 mL for a BB. Inflating the bronchial cuff does not stabilize the DLT position when the patient is turned to the lateral position.
      (1) Endobronchial intubation must be done gently and with fiberoptic guidance if resistance is met. A significant number of case reports of airway injury are from

cases of esophageal surgery, where the elastic-supporting tissue may be weakened (eg, by preoperative radiation treatments) and predisposed to rupture from DLT placement.

6. **Other complications of lung separation**
   a. **Malpositioning:** Initial malpositioning of DLTs with blind placement can occur in >30% of cases. Verification and adjustment with FOB immediately before initiating OLV is mandatory because these tubes will migrate during patient positioning.
   b. **Airway resistance:** The resistance from a 37F DLT during two-lung ventilation is less than that of an 8-mm ID ETT but exceeds that of a 9-mm ETT. For short periods of postoperative ventilation and weaning, airflow resistance is not a problem with a DLT.

7. **The ABCs of lung separation will always apply**
   a. Know the tracheobronchial **a**natomy.[6]
   b. Use the fiberoptic **b**ronchoscope (see Figure 25.8).[7]
   c. Look at the **c**hest x-ray film and CT scan in advance.

B. **Positioning**

The majority of thoracic procedures are performed with the patient in the lateral position, but, depending on the surgical technique, a semi-supine or semi-prone lateral position may be used. It is awkward to induce anesthesia in the lateral position; thus, monitors will be placed and anesthesia will be usually induced in the supine position, and the anesthetized patient will then be repositioned for surgery. Due to the loss of venous vascular tone in the anesthetized

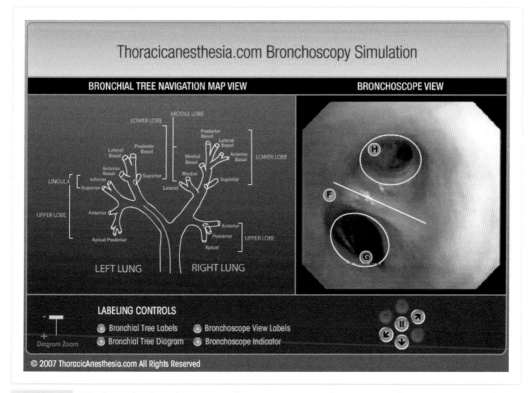

FIGURE 25.8 The free online bronchoscopy simulator at **www.pie.med.utoronto.ca.** The user can navigate the tracheobronchial tree using real-time video by clicking on the *lighted directional arrows* under the "bronchoscopic view" **(right)**. Clicking on the labels on the "bronchoscopic view" gives details of the anatomy seen. The process is aided by the "Bronchial Tree Navigational Map" **(left)**, which shows the simultaneous location of the bronchoscope as the orange line in the airway. The free online **Ruffle Flash Emulator** must be downloaded to run the simulator. (Reprinted by permission from Springer: Campos J. Lung isolation. In: Slinger P, ed. *Principles and Practice of Anesthesia for Thoracic Surgery*. 2nd ed. Springer; 2019:283-309. © 2019 Springer Science+Business Media, LLC.)

patient, it is not uncommon to see hypotension from redistribution of systemic venous blood when the patient is turned to or from the lateral position.

All lines and monitors will have to be secured during position change and their function reassessed after repositioning. The anesthesiologist should take responsibility for the head, neck, and airway during position change and must be in charge of the operating team to direct repositioning. It is useful to make an initial "head-to-toe" survey of the patient after induction and intubation, checking oxygenation, ventilation, hemodynamics, lines, monitors, and potential nerve injuries. This survey must be repeated after repositioning. The patient's head, neck, and EBT should be turned en bloc with the patient's thoracolumbar spine. The margin of error in positioning EBTs or blockers is often so narrow that even small movements can have significant clinical implications. EBT/blocker position and adequacy of ventilation must be rechecked by auscultation and FOB after patient repositioning.

1. **Neurovascular complications:** The brachial plexus is the site of the majority of intraoperative nerve injuries related to the lateral position. The brachial plexus is fixed at two points: proximally by the transverse process of the cervical vertebrae and distally by the axillary fascia. This two-point fixation plus the extreme mobility of neighboring skeletal and muscular structures make the brachial plexus extremely liable to injury. The patient should be positioned with padding under the dependent thorax to keep the weight of the upper body off the dependent arm brachial plexus. This padding will exacerbate the pressure on the brachial plexus if it migrates superiorly into the axilla. It is useful to survey the patient from the side of the table immediately after the patient is turned to ensure that the entire vertebral column is aligned properly.

   The dependent leg should be slightly flexed with padding under the knee to protect the peroneal nerve lateral to the proximal head of the fibula. The nondependent leg is placed in a neutral straight position and padding placed between it and the dependent leg. The dependent leg must be observed for vascular compression. Excessively tight strapping at the hip level can compress the sciatic nerve of the nondependent leg. A "head-to-toe" protocol to monitor for possible neurovascular injuries related to the lateral decubitus position is given in Table 25.5.

2. **Physiologic changes in the lateral position**
   a. **Ventilation:** Significant changes in ventilation develop between the lungs when the patient is placed in the lateral position. The compliance curves of the two lungs are different because of their difference in size. The lateral position, anesthesia, paralysis, and opening the thorax all combine to magnify these differences between the lungs.

   In a spontaneously breathing patient, ventilation of the dependent lung will increase by ~10% when the patient is turned to the lateral position. Once the patient is anesthetized and paralyzed, ventilation of the dependent lung will decrease by 15%. The compliance of the entire respiratory system will increase once the nondependent hemithorax is open, yet will decrease from interpleural insufflation in a VATS.

TABLE 25.5 Avoiding Neurovascular Injuries Specific to the Lateral Position

Routine "Head-to-Toe" Survey

I. Dependent eye
II. Dependent ear pinna
III. Cervical spine alignment
IV. Dependent arm: (i) brachial plexus, (ii) circulation
V. Nondependent arm[a]: (i) brachial plexus, (ii) circulation
VI. Nondependent leg sciatic nerve
VII. Dependent leg: (i) peroneal nerve, (ii) circulation

[a]Neurovascular injuries of the nondependent arm are more likely to occur if the arm is suspended or held in an independently positioned armrest.

Applying positive end-expiratory pressure (PEEP) to both the lungs in the lateral position, PEEP preferentially goes to the most compliant lung regions and hyperinflates the nondependent lung without causing any improvement in gas exchange. In the lateral position, atelectasis will develop in a mean of 5% of total lung volume, all in the dependent lung.

b. **Perfusion:** Turning the patient to the lateral position decreases the blood flow of the nondependent lung due to gravity by ~10% of the total pulmonary blood flow.

The matching of ventilation and perfusion will usually decrease in the lateral position compared to the supine position.

C. **Intraoperative Monitoring**

1. **General to all pulmonary resections:** The majority are major operative procedures of moderate duration (2-4 hours) and performed in the lateral position with either induced pneumothorax (VATS) or open. Consideration for monitoring and maintenance of body temperature and fluid volume should be given to all of these cases. All cases should have standard ASA monitoring. Additional monitoring is guided by a knowledge of which complications are likely to occur (Table 25.6).

2. **Specific to certain types of resection:** There are complications that are more prone to occur with certain resections, such as hemorrhage from an extrapleural pneumonectomy, contralateral lung soiling with resection of a cyst or bronchiectasis, air leak hypoventilation, or tension pneumothorax with a bronchopleural fistula.

3. **Oxygenation:** Significant arterial oxygen desaturation (<90%) during OLV occurs in ~1% of the surgical population with a high inspired oxygen concentration (FIO_2) of 1. Pulse oximetry (SpO_2) has not negated the need for direct measurement of arterial PaO_2 via intermittent blood gases in the majority of thoracotomy patients. The rapidity of the fall in PaO_2 after the onset of OLV is an indicator of the risk of subsequent desaturation. Consequently, we recommend measuring PaO_2 by ABG before OLV and 20 minutes after the start of OLV.

4. **Capnometry:** End-tidal CO_2 ($P_{et}CO_2$) is a less reliable indicator of the $PaCO_2$ during OLV than during two-lung ventilation, and the $P_{a-et}CO_2$ gradient increases during OLV. As the patient is turned to the lateral position, the $P_{et}CO_2$ of the nondependent lung falls relative to the dependent lung because of increased perfusion of the dependent lung and increased dead space of the nondependent lung. At the onset of OLV, the $P_{et}CO_2$ of the dependent lung usually falls transiently, as all the minute ventilation is transferred to this lung. The $P_{et}CO_2$ then rises as the fractional perfusion is increased to this dependent lung by collapse and pulmonary vasoconstriction of the nonventilated lung. If there is no correction of minute ventilation, the net result will be increased baseline $PaCO_2$ and $P_{et}CO_2$, with an increased gradient. Severe (>5 mm Hg) or prolonged falls in $P_{et}CO_2$ indicate a maldistribution of perfusion between ventilated and nonventilated lungs and may be an early warning of a patient who will desaturate during OLV.

TABLE 25.6   Intraoperative Complications That Occur With Increased Frequency During Thoracotomy

Complication	Etiology
I. Hypoxemia	Intrapulmonary shunt during one-lung ventilation
II. Sudden severe hypotension	Surgical compression of the heart or great vessels
III. Sudden changes in ventilating pressure or volume	Movement of endobronchial tube/blocker, air leak
	Direct mechanical irritation of the heart
IV. Arrhythmias	Direct airway stimulation, increased frequency of reactive airways disease
V. Bronchospasm	Surgical blood loss from great vessels or inflamed pleura
VI. Massive hemorrhage	Heat loss from the open hemithorax
VII. Hypothermia	

5. **Invasive hemodynamic monitoring**
   a. **Arterial catheter:** There is a significant incidence of transient severe hypotension from surgical compression of the heart or great vessels during intrathoracic procedures. For this reason, plus the utility of intermittent ABG sampling, it is useful to have beat-to-beat assessment of systemic blood pressure during many thoracic surgery cases. Exceptions are limited procedures, such as "wedge" segmental resections and/or thoracoscopic resections in younger/healthier patients.
   b. **Central venous pressures:** Central venous pressure (CVP) readings obtained intraoperatively with the chest open are not reliable indicators of right atrial pressure or right ventricle (RV) preload. It is often practice to routinely place CVP lines in pneumonectomy patients, but not for lesser resections unless there is significant other concurrent illness or risk of bleeding.
   c. **Pulmonary artery catheters:** The risk/benefit ratio for the routine use of PA catheters for pulmonary resection surgery favors their infrequent use, such as patients with life-threatening coexisting cardiac disease or possibly active septicemia. Several recently developed systems of noninvasive cardiac output monitoring may prove equally useful for this purpose (eg, FloTrac, Edwards Lifesciences).
6. **Fiberoptic bronchoscopy:** Significant malpositions of left-sided or right-sided DLTs that can lead to desaturation during OLV are often not detected by auscultation or other traditional methods of confirming placement. Positioning of DLTs or BBs should be confirmed after placing the patient in the surgical position because a substantial percentage of tubes/blockers migrate during repositioning of the patient.

CLINICAL PEARL

Head and neck extension or rotation during patient repositioning risks displacement of a previously perfectly positioned DLT.

7. **Continuous spirometry:** The adequacy of lung isolation can be monitored by breath-to-breath comparison of inspiratory and expiratory tidal volumes. This also gives a sense of the magnitude of air leaks from the ventilated lung. Changes in the position of a DLT can be detected by changes in the pressure-volume loops.
D. **Anesthetic Technique**
   Any anesthetic technique that provides safe and stable general anesthesia for major surgery can and has been used for lung resection. Many centers use combined regional (eg, TEA or paravertebral blocks) and general anesthesia for thoracic surgery. Commonly, neuromuscular blockers are used, but they are not essential to the safe conduct of thoracotomies or to DLT management.
1. **Intravenous fluids:** Because of hydrostatic effects, excessive administration of IV fluids can cause increased shunt and lead to PE of the dependent lung. Because the dependent lung is the lung that must carry on gas exchange during OLV, it is best to be as judicious as possible with fluid administration (Table 25.7).
2. **Nitrous oxide:** Nitrous oxide/oxygen mixtures are more prone to cause atelectasis in poorly ventilated lung regions than oxygen by itself.

TABLE 25.7 Fluid Management for Pulmonary Resection Surgery

I. Total positive fluid balance in the first 24 h perioperatively should not exceed 20 mL/kg.
II. For an average adult patient, crystalloid administration should be limited to <3 L in the first 24 h.
III. No fluid administration for "third-space" fluid losses during pulmonary resection.
IV. Urine output >0.5 mL/kg/h is unnecessary.
V. If increased tissue perfusion is needed postoperatively, it is preferable to use invasive monitoring and inotropes rather than to cause fluid overload.

3. **Temperature:** Maintenance of body temperature can be a problem during thoracic surgery because of heat loss from the open hemithorax. This is particularly a problem at the extremes of the age spectrum. Most of the body's physiologic functions, including hypoxic pulmonary vasoconstriction (HPV), are inhibited during hypothermia. Increasing the ambient room temperature and using lower and upper body forced-air patient warmers are the best methods to prevent inadvertent intraoperative hypothermia.

4. **Prevention of bronchospasm:** Due to the high incidence of coexisting reactive airways disease in the thoracic surgical population, it is generally advisable to use an anesthetic technique that decreases bronchial irritability. This is particularly important because the added airway manipulation caused by the placement of a DLT or BB potently triggers bronchoconstriction. Avoid manipulation of the airway in a lightly anesthetized patient, use bronchodilating anesthetics, and avoid drugs that release histamine.

   For IV induction of anesthesia, either propofol or ketamine diminishes bronchospasm. For maintenance of anesthesia, propofol and/or any of the volatile anesthetics will diminish bronchial reactivity.

E. **Management of One-Lung Ventilation**
   1. **Hypoxemia:** There is an incidence of <4% of hypoxemia (arterial saturation <90%) during OLV for thoracic surgery. Hypoxemia is more likely to occur when OLV is in the supine position.
   2. **Hypoxic pulmonary vasoconstriction:** HPV is thought to decrease the blood flow to the nonventilated lung by 50%. The stimulus for HPV is primarily the alveolar oxygen tension (PAO_2), which stimulates precapillary vasoconstriction to redistribute pulmonary blood flow away from hypoxemic lung regions via a pathway involving nitric oxide (NO) and/or cyclooxygenase synthesis inhibition. All of the volatile anesthetics inhibit HPV. This inhibition is dose-dependent.[8] No clinical benefit has been shown for total IV anesthesia beyond that seen with isoflurane ≤1 MAC (minimum alveolar concentration). HPV is decreased by all vasodilators, such as nitroglycerin and nitroprusside.
   3. **Cardiac output:** The net effects of an increase in cardiac output during OLV tend to favor an increase in Pao_2. However, the elevation of cardiac output beyond physiologic needs tends to oppose HPV and may cause Pao_2 to fall.
   4. **Ventilation during one-lung anesthesia:** It is possible to improve gas exchange for selected individual patients by altering the ventilatory variables that are under the control of the anesthesiologist: tidal volume, rate, inspiratory/expiratory ratio, $Paco_2$, peak and plateau airway pressures, and PEEP (Table 25.8).

TABLE 25.8   Recommended Ventilation Parameters for OLV

Parameter	Suggested	Note
Tidal volume	5-6 mL/kg (ideal body weight)	Maintain Peak airway pressure <35 cm H_2O Plateau airway pressure <25 cm H_2O
PEEP	5 cm H_2O (recruitment maneuver at start of OLV and as needed), increase prn	Avoid added PEEP in patients with moderate-severe COPD who have auto-PEEP
Respiratory rate	12/min, adjust based on $Paco_2$	$P_{a-et}CO_2$ gradient usually will increase 1-3 mm Hg during OLV. Mild hypercapnia ($Paco_2$ 50-55 mm Hg) is OK
Mode	Volume or pressure control	Patients at risk for lung injury (pneumonectomy, lung transplantation, bullae): pressure-control ventilation preferred
FiO_2	0.8-1.0 initially	Add air to decrease FiO_2 guided by oxygen saturation after 20 min of stable OLV

COPD, chronic obstructive pulmonary disease; FiO_2, inspired oxygen concentration; OLV, one-lung ventilation; $Paco_2$, arterial partial pressure of CO_2; $P_{a-et}CO_2$, arterial end-tidal CO_2 partial pressure; PEEP, positive end-expiratory pressure.

a. **Respiratory acid-base status:** The overall efficacy of HPV is optimal with normal pH and $Paco_2$.

b. **Tidal volume:** A 5-6 mL/kg ideal body weight for OLV is a reasonable starting point. The tidal volume should be adjusted during OLV to keep the airway peak pressure <35 cm H_2O and the plateau airway pressure <25 cm H_2O.

c. **Positive end-expiratory pressure:** Most patients with either normal or supranormal (restrictive lung disease) lung elastic recoil will benefit from low levels (5 cm H_2O) of PEEP during OLV. A recruitment maneuver (eg, static inflation to 20 cm H_2O for 20 seconds, observing for hypotension) to the ventilated lung is useful at the start of OLV. Auto-PEEP is prone to occur in patients with decreased lung elastic recoil, such as those with emphysema.

d. **Volume control versus pressure control:** Pressure-control OLV is useful in patients with severe obstructive disease and to limit airway pressure in patients with blebs, bullae, or fresh resections in the lung, and also in patients at risk of acute lung injury (pneumonectomies, lung transplantation).

e. **Inspired oxygen concentration:** The Fio_2 should be increased at the start of OLV to 0.8-1.0 and then can be decreased as tolerated over the next 20 minutes.

5. **Treatment of hypoxemia during one-lung ventilation (see Table 25.9):** In cases of severe and/or acute desaturation, resume two-lung ventilation immediately, deflate the bronchial cuff or blocker, and then check the position of the DLT or BB with FOB. In cases of desaturation that have not become life threatening:

a. **Increase inspired oxygen concentration:** The first-line therapy is to increase the Fio_2, which is an option in essentially all patients, except those who received bleomycin or similar therapy that potentiates pulmonary oxygen toxicity.

b. **Positive end-expiratory pressure:** PEEP to the ventilated dependent lung will improve oxygenation in patients with normal lung mechanics and those with increased elastic recoil due to restrictive lung diseases. Apply a recruitment maneuver to the ventilated lung before application of PEEP.

c. **Pharmacologic manipulations:** Increasing cardiac output will result in a small but clinically useful increase in both Pvo_2 and Pao_2 if cardiac output has decreased. Selective inhaled pulmonary vasodilators such as iloprost or prostacyclin administered by a nebulizer to the ventilated lung may also be useful.

TABLE 25.9 Treatment Options for Hypoxemia During OLV

Severe/acute: Resume two-lung ventilation

Gradual desaturation:

  I. Assure $Fio_2 = 1$
  II. Check position of DLT/BB with FOB
  III. Optimize cardiac output
  IV. Recruitment maneuver of ventilated lung
  V. Apply PEEP 5 cm H_2O to ventilated lung (except COPD)
  VI. Apply CPAP 1-2 cm H_2O to nonventilated lung (recruitment maneuver first, avoid during VATS)
  VII. Intermittent reinflation of nonventilated lung
  VIII. Partial ventilation of nonventilated lung:
    A. Segmental oxygen insufflation via FOB
    B. Lobar reinflation
    C. Lobar collapse
    D. Oxygen insufflation
    E. High-frequency ventilation
  IX. Mechanical restriction of nonventilated lung pulmonary blood flow

BB, bronchial blocker; COPD, chronic obstructive pulmonary disease; CPAP, continuous positive airway pressure; DLT, double-lumen tube; Fio_2, inspired oxygen concentration; FOB, fiberoptic bronchoscopy; OLV, one-lung ventilation; PEEP, positive end-expiratory pressure; VATS, video-assisted thoracoscopic surgery.

d. **Continuous positive airway pressure:** This must be applied to a fully inflated or re-inflated lung for optimal effect. When CPAP is applied to a fully inflated lung, as little as 2-3 cm H_2O can be used. When the bronchus of the operative lung is obstructed or open to atmosphere, CPAP will not improve oxygenation. During thoracoscopic surgery, CPAP can significantly interfere with surgery.

CLINICAL PEARL

When CPAP is applied to the nondependent, surgical lung to treat hypoxemia, the lung must first be reinflated.

---

e. **Alternative ventilation methods:** Several alternative methods of OLV, all of which involve partial ventilation of the nonventilated lung, have been described. All improve oxygenation during OLV.
   (1) Oxygen insufflation (5 L/min) for brief periods via the suction channel of an FOB to partially recruit a segment of the nonventilated lung remote from the site of surgery (eg, a basilar segment of the lower lobe for upper lobe surgery). This is particularly useful in VATS.[9] Surgeon's direct observation is useful to prevent over-reinflation.
   (2) Selective lobar collapse of only the operative lobe in the open hemithorax by placement of a blocker in the appropriate lobar bronchus of the ipsilateral operative lung
   (3) Differential lung ventilation by only partially occluding the lumen of the DLT to the operative lung
   (4) Intermittent reinflation of the nonventilated lung by regular reexpansion of the operative lung via an attached CPAP circuit
   (5) Conventional OLV of the nonoperative lung and high-frequency jet ventilation of the operative lung
f. **Mechanical restriction of pulmonary blood flow:** It is possible for the surgeon to directly compress or clamp the blood flow to the nonventilated lung. This can be done temporarily in emergency desaturation situations or definitively in cases of pneumonectomy or lung transplantation.

6. **Prevention of hypoxemia:** The treatments outlined as therapy for hypoxemia can be used prophylactically to prevent hypoxemia in patients who are at high risk for desaturation during OLV. Desaturation during bilateral lung procedures is particularly a problem during a second period of OLV (eg, bilateral thoracotomy). It is advisable to operate first on the lung that has better gas exchange.

III. **Specific Procedures**
   A. **Thoracotomy**
      1. **Operations**
         a. **Lobectomy:** Lobectomy is the most common pulmonary resection for lung cancer. Early functional loss exceeds the amount of lung tissue resected, but function recovers over a period of 6 weeks so that the final net loss of respiratory function is equivalent to the amount of functioning lung tissue excised. The recovery of pulmonary function after thoracotomy is unique because it shows a plateau with no early recovery during the first 72 hours postoperatively. This period coincides with the occurrence of the majority of post-thoracotomy respiratory complications (atelectasis, pneumonia), which are the major causes of mortality after pulmonary resection.
         b. **Sleeve lobectomy:** A sleeve lobectomy is the excision of a lobe plus the adjacent segment of mainstem bronchus with bronchoplastic repair of the bronchus by end-to-end anastomosis to preserve the distal functioning pulmonary parenchyma. It is done to preserve functioning lung tissue when the tumor encroaches to <2 cm from the lobar bronchial orifices, precluding simple lobectomy. This procedure is usually done for right upper lobe tumors but can be used for other lobes. The anesthetic implications of this procedure are that, most often, no airway catheter (single lumen or DLT) or BB can be

placed in the ipsilateral mainstem bronchus, although some surgeons prefer to use a carefully positioned left-sided DLT during left upper lobe sleeve lobectomies. Mucus clearance across the bronchial anastomosis may be impaired after sleeve resection, and local tumor recurrence is a problem.

c. **Bilobectomy:** In the right lung, a bilobectomy may be used to conserve either a functioning upper or lower lobe when the tumor extends across the lobar fissure or for malignancies involving the bronchus intermedius (the portion of the right mainstem bronchus distal to the right upper lobe orifice). The complication rate is slightly higher than for a simple lobectomy but is less than for a pneumonectomy. The residual lobe cannot completely fill the hemithorax, and all patients will have a degree of pneumothorax that can be expected to resolve gradually.

d. **Pneumonectomy:** Complete removal of the lung is required when a lobectomy or its modifications are not adequate to remove the local disease and/or ipsilateral lymph node metastases. The mortality rate after pneumonectomy exceeds that for lobectomy because of complications that are more likely with pneumonectomy.

   (1) **Post-pneumonectomy pulmonary edema:** This syndrome presents clinically with dyspnea and an increased alveolar-arterial oxygen gradient on the second or third postoperative day[10] and has a high fatality rate. Radiologic changes precede clinical symptoms by ~24 hours. The factors that are known about this syndrome are listed in Table 25.10.

   (2) **Atrial fibrillation:** Up to 50% of post-pneumonectomy patients will develop supraventricular arrhythmias in the first week postoperatively, the majority of which are atrial fibrillation. The perioperative mortality is 17% in patients who develop arrhythmias versus 2% in those without them. Prophylactic digoxin is not effective in preventing them.[11]

   (3) **Mechanical effects:** A variety of potentially lethal intrathoracic mechanical derangements of cardiorespiratory function can occur after pneumonectomy. The most important of these is cardiac herniation through an incompletely closed pericardium. This is particularly a risk after right pneumonectomy and presents with acute severe hypotension in the immediate postoperative period. The only useful therapy is immediate reoperation to return the heart into the pericardium. A subacute form of cardiac herniation can occur after a left pneumonectomy and presents with a picture of myocardial ischemia as the apex of the heart herniates through the pericardial defect and compresses the coronary arteries.

CLINICAL PEARL

If sudden, severe hypotension occurs in the early postoperative period after pneumonectomy, a diagnosis of cardiac herniation should be assumed unless proven otherwise.

TABLE 25.10 Post-Pneumonectomy Pulmonary Edema

Incidence 2%-4% of pneumonectomies
Case fatality >50%
Incidence right > left pneumonectomy (3-4:1)
Clinical onset 2-3 d postoperatively
Associated with increased pulmonary capillary permeability
Not associated with increased PA pressures
Exacerbation by fluid overload

PA, pulmonary artery.

e. **Sleeve pneumonectomy:** Tumors involving the most proximal portions of the main-stem bronchus and the carina may require a sleeve pneumonectomy. These are per-formed most commonly for right-sided tumors and usually can be performed without cardiopulmonary bypass (CPB) via a right thoracotomy. A long single-lumen EBT can be advanced into the left mainstem bronchus during the period of anastomosis, or the lung can be ventilated via a separate sterile ETT and circuit that is passed into the operating field and used for temporary intubation of the open distal bronchus. High-frequency positive-pressure ventilation (HFPPV) also has been used for this procedure.

Because the carina is surgically more accessible from the right side, left sleeve pneu-monectomies are commonly performed as a two-stage operation, first a left thoracot-omy and pneumonectomy and then a right thoracotomy for the carinal excision.

f. **Lesser resections (segmentectomy, wedge):** These procedures are commonly per-formed in older patients or in those with limited cardiopulmonary reserves to preserve functioning pulmonary parenchyma. These lesser resections are associated with a lower 5-year survival rate compared to lobectomy due to locoregional recurrence of cancer. The decrease in pulmonary function (FEV_1) for lesser resections is in proportion to the amount of lung tissue removed.

g. **Extended resections:** Portions of the chest wall, diaphragm, pericardium, left atrium, vena cava, brachial plexus, or vertebral body may be excised with an adjacent lung tumor. Resection of any of these structures has important anesthetic implications for the choice and placement of intraoperative monitors and lines and for postoperative management.

h. **Subsequent pulmonary resections:** Lung resection surgery after previous lung re-section is increasingly frequent. These operations can be performed for either benign or malignant diseases. Prediction of postoperative lung function for these patients is accurate based on the assessment of preoperative function (lung mechanics, gas ex-change, and cardiopulmonary reserve) and estimation of the amount of functional lung tissue removed at surgery (Figure 25.1). Intraoperative hemorrhage is the specific anesthetic concern with this procedure, as >50% of patients experience blood loss of >1,000 mL. Hemorrhage is particularly a problem in completion pneumonectomy for nonmalignant lung disease (lung abscess, bronchiectasis, tuberculosis). Inflammatory lung disease tends to destroy the tissue planes around the hilum and makes the surgical dissection more difficult, with an attendant increase in perioperative mortality.

i. **Incomplete resections:** In general, prognosis of a patient with lung cancer is not im-proved from an incomplete resection. There are several exceptions. Incompletely re-sected tumors with direct mediastinal invasion or tumors of the superior sulcus may benefit if the resection is combined with adjuvant brachytherapy or external irradiation. Also, if the residual tumor is limited to microscopic involvement of the cut mucosal margin of the bronchus, 5-year survival is increased beyond that seen without surgery. Incomplete resections may be indicated for palliation in cases of airway obstruction or hemoptysis if these are not amenable to endoscopic or radiologic procedures.

2. **Surgical approaches:** Any given pulmonary resection can be accomplished by a variety of surgi-cal approaches. The approach used in an individual case depends on the interaction of several factors, which include the site and pathology of the lesion(s) and the training and experience of the surgical team. Each approach has specific anesthetic implications. Common thoracic surgical approaches and their generally accepted advantages and disadvantages are listed in Table 25.11.

a. **Posterolateral thoracotomy:** For decades, this was the traditional incision in thoracic surgery. The patient is placed in the lateral decubitus position. Chest access is usually via the fifth or sixth intercostal space. The left seventh or eighth space may be used for access to the esophageal hiatus. Exposure to all ipsilateral intrathoracic structures is excellent.

b. **Muscle-sparing lateral thoracotomy:** The lateral muscle-sparing thoracotomy has been advocated to reduce the pain and disability associated with a standard posterolat-eral thoracotomy. The skin incision may or may not be smaller, but an extensive subcu-taneous dissection is required to mobilize the latissimus and serratus muscles.

TABLE 25.11 Surgical Approaches for Pulmonary Resections

Incision	Pro	Con
Posterolateral thoracotomy	Excellent exposure to entire operative hemithorax	Postoperative pain; with or without respiration dysfunction (short and long term)
Lateral muscle-sparing thoracotomy	Decreased postoperative pain	Increased incidence of wound seromas
Anterolateral thoracotomy	Better access for laparotomy, resuscitation, or contralateral thoracotomy, especially in trauma	Limited access to posterior thorax
Axillary thoracotomy	Decreased pain; adequate access for first rib resection, sympathectomy, apical blebs, or bullae	Limited exposure
Sternotomy	Decreased pain, bilateral access	Decreased exposure of posterior structures
Trans-sternal bilateral ("clamshell")	Good exposure for bilateral lung transplantation	Postoperative pain and chest wall dysfunction
Video-assisted thoracoscopic/robotic surgery	Less postoperative pain and respiratory dysfunction	Technically difficult with lung adhesions

    c. **Anterolateral thoracotomy:** This is a particularly useful incision in trauma because it allows complete access to the patient for ongoing resuscitation and does not require repositioning for laparotomy or exploration of the contralateral chest. Exposure to the posterior hemithorax is limited in comparison to a posterolateral incision.

    d. **Axillary thoracotomy:** The transaxillary approach provides access only to the apical areas of the hemithorax. The ipsilateral arm must be draped free or suspended, and access to this arm will be limited intraoperatively. Thus, it is preferable for vascular access and monitoring to use the contralateral arm. This is an adequate incision for the first rib resection, resection of apical bullae/blebs, or thoracic sympathectomy.

    e. **Median sternotomy:** This incision, which is the standard for cardiac surgery, has potential benefits for certain thoracic procedures. Bilateral excisions for metastases and bullae are best performed via this incision. It has been demonstrated that postoperative spirometry is superior and pain is less after median sternotomy than thoracotomy. Most pulmonary resections can be performed via a median sternotomy, which obviates the need for a separate incision in cases of combined cardiac and thoracic surgery. Certain procedures are more difficult via a median sternotomy, including procedures performed for superior sulcus tumors, tumors with posterior chest wall extension, and left lower lobe tumors. OLV is more of a necessity for surgical exposure than for lateral thoracotomies because of the limited surgical access, and oxygen desaturation is more common with OLV in the supine than the lateral position.

    f. **Trans-sternal bilateral thoracotomy (the "clamshell" incision):** This is the common incision for bilateral lung transplantation. Because of increased pain and postoperative chest wall dysfunction, it is not commonly used for other intrathoracic procedures. It has been used for resection of bilateral metastases, pericardiectomy, resection of a posterior ventricular aneurysm, and cardiac surgery in a patient with a tracheotomy.

  B. **Video-Assisted Thoracoscopic Surgery**

    Essentially, any surgical procedure that is performed via thoracotomy has been attempted by VATS. VATS has been advocated for pulmonary resection of lung cancer in patients with limited respiratory reserves because of decreased postoperative pain and loss of early postoperative spirometric respiratory function that is only approximately half of that seen when the same operation is performed by thoracotomy. VATS is the procedure of choice for resection of nonmalignant pulmonary lesions (blebs, bullae, granulomas). Bilateral VATS can be performed in the supine position for apical lesions, but for most operations, bilateral VATS requires change from one lateral position to the other intraoperatively. Robotic thoracic surgery is being used increasingly for minimally invasive procedures due to better visualization.

Some procedures are attempted by VATS initially with conversion to thoracotomy if the surgery proves impractical. OLV with complete collapse of the operative lung is more of a priority than for open thoracotomy, and application of CPAP to the nonventilated lung is more detrimental to surgery than to open thoracotomy. To aid collapse of the lung, particularly in patients with COPD and poor lung elastic recoil, it is best to ventilate with oxygen instead of air/oxygen mixtures during the period of two-lung ventilation before lung collapse and to apply suction (-20 cm H_2O) to the nonventilated lung after the start of OLV until collapse is complete. Postoperative management is essentially the same as for thoracotomy, and most patients initially will have chest drains. The amount of postoperative pain after VATS varies greatly depending on the surgical procedure performed.

CLINICAL PEARL

Complete collapse of the operative lung is more critical to VATS than to open thoracotomies, and the application of CPAP to that lung is relatively contraindicated because it severely compromises surgical exposure.

C. Bronchopleural Fistula

A persistent communication between the airway and the interpleural space can develop after medical conditions, such as rupture of a bleb or bulla, infection, or malignancy. Bronchopleural fistula can develop as a postoperative complication after lung surgery. The large majority of persistent lung air leaks will heal with drainage and conservative management.

Surgical intervention is indicated when conservative therapy is unable to permit adequate gas exchange (this is more likely to occur in the immediate postoperative period, particularly after pneumonectomy) or when conventional chest tube drainage and suction are unable to reexpand the ipsilateral lung, or for a second ipsilateral or first contralateral pneumothorax.

There are three specific **anesthetic goals** in all patients with a bronchopleural fistula:

1. Healthy lung regions must be protected from soiling by extrapleural fluid from the affected hemithorax (eg, coexisting empyema).
2. The ventilation technique must avoid development of a tension pneumothorax in the affected hemithorax.
3. The anesthetic technique must ensure adequate alveolar gas exchange in the presence of a low-resistance air leak.

   To achieve these goals, there are two **management principles** that should be used in essentially all cases:

1. A functioning chest drain should be placed before the induction of anesthesia and connected to an underwater seal without suction.
2. A method of lung separation should be placed so that the fistula can be isolated as necessary intraoperatively.

   After placement of a chest drain, there are three **options for induction** of anesthesia[12]:

1. A single-lumen or double-lumen EBT or blocker can be placed in an awake patient with topical anesthesia and its position checked fiberoptically before induction. This is often not the best choice in a patient with severely compromised gas exchange because maintaining adequate oxygenation in an already hypoxemic patient can be a problem during awake intubation.
2. Induction of anesthesia while maintaining spontaneous ventilation until lung isolation is secured. A spontaneous ventilation induction may not be desirable if there is a risk of aspiration and in patients with compromised hemodynamics.
3. IV induction of general anesthesia and muscle relaxation after meticulous preoxygenation and manual ventilation using small tidal volumes and low airway pressures until the lung isolation is confirmed. The efficiency of this technique can be improved by using a bronchoscope to guide DLT placement during intubation.

The air leak through a bronchopleural fistula is dependent on the pressure gradient between the mean airway pressure at the site of the fistula and the interpleural space. High-frequency ventilation, with and without lung or lobar blockade, has been used in certain cases. High-frequency techniques may permit relatively lower proximal mean airway pressures than conventional mechanical ventilation and may be more useful in large central air leaks.

D. **Bullae and Blebs**
Whenever positive-pressure ventilation is applied to the airway of a patient with a bulla or bleb, there is the risk of lesion rupture and development of a tension pneumothorax that will require drainage and may progress to a bronchopleural fistula. The anesthetic considerations are similar to those for a patient with a bronchopleural fistula, except that it is best not to place a chest drain prophylactically because the chest tube may enter the bulla and create a fistula and there is not the risk of soiling healthy lung regions from extrapleural fluid that exists with fistulas. For induction of anesthesia, it is usually optimal to maintain spontaneous ventilation until the lung or lobe with the bulla or bleb is isolated. When there is a risk of aspiration or it is believed that the patient's gas exchange or hemodynamics may not permit spontaneous ventilation for induction, the anesthesiologist will need to use small tidal volumes and low airway pressures during positive-pressure ventilation until the airway is isolated. Nitrous oxide will diffuse into a bleb or bulla, causing it to enlarge, and must be avoided.

E. **Abscesses, Bronchiectasis, Cysts, and Empyema**
As with bronchopleural fistulas, there is the risk of soiling healthy lung regions by uncontrolled spillage from these lesions. Lung isolation is a primary requirement for anesthesia, and the anesthetic principles and management are similar to those described for fistulas. When an intrathoracic space–occupying lesion is removed, there is the potential for reexpansion PE to develop after reinflation of the ipsilateral lung. A slow and gradual reinflation may decrease the severity of this complication.

F. **Mediastinoscopy**
Cervical mediastinoscopy is a diagnostic sampling of the mediastinal nodes to assess if a pulmonary resection will improve outcome. Mediastinoscopy can be done during a separate anesthetic before pulmonary resection, often as an outpatient, or after induction of anesthesia preceding pulmonary resection. Apart from the specific anesthetic considerations of mediastinoscopy itself, the anesthetic implication of starting the case with these diagnostic procedures is that the resection may be aborted based on the initial mediastinoscopy findings. The likelihood of not proceeding to thoracotomy must enter into each individual assessment of risk/benefit when considering placing an epidural catheter before induction.

Mediastinoscopy is most commonly done via a cervical approach with an incision in the suprasternal notch. Any structure in the upper chest can be injured during the procedure, including great vessels, pleura (pneumothorax), nerves (recurrent laryngeal), and airways. Hemorrhage is the most frequent major complication, particularly due to inadvertent PA biopsy, and this must always be considered with respect to vascular access, monitoring, and the availability of means for resuscitation. Fortunately, significant hemorrhage during mediastinoscopy can usually be tamponaded temporarily by the surgeon when resuscitation is required. In only a minority of mediastinoscopy hemorrhages, it is necessary to proceed to thoracotomy for surgical control of bleeding.

A frequent complication of cervical mediastinoscopy is transient compression of the brachiocephalic (innominate) artery by the mediastinoscope. The surgeon is usually unaware that this is occurring, so it is essential to incorporate continuous pulse monitoring in the right arm (pulse oximetry, arterial line, or palpation) into the anesthetic plan. The surgeon can then be immediately notified and avoid the risk of cerebral ischemia in patients who may not have good collateral cerebral circulation.

CLINICAL PEARL

During mediastinoscopy, continuous pulse monitoring in the right arm is essential to early recognition of innominate artery compression.

Because of the different pattern of lymphatic drainage of the left upper lobe, patients with left upper lobe tumors often will have an anterior left parasternal mediastinoscopy or median sternotomy instead of or in addition to a cervical mediastinoscopy. The serious complications associated with cervical mediastinoscopy are not as frequent with parasternal mediastinoscopy.

Endobronchial ultrasound (EBUS)-guided mediastinal nodal biopsies via an FOB are increasingly used as an alternative to traditional mediastinoscopy as a lung cancer staging procedure. These can be performed awake with topical anesthesia of the airway or under general anesthesia.

G. **Anterior Mediastinal Mass**

Patients with anterior mediastinal masses present unique problems to the anesthesiologist. A large number of such patients require anesthesia for biopsy of these masses by mediastinoscopy or VATS, or they may require definitive resection via sternotomy or thoracotomy. Tumors of the anterior mediastinum include thymoma, teratoma, lymphoma, cystic hygroma, bronchogenic cyst, and thyroid tumors. Anterior mediastinal masses may cause obstruction of major airways, main PAs, atria, and the superior vena cava. Any one of these complications can be life threatening. During induction of general anesthesia in patients with an anterior mediastinal mass, airway obstruction is the most common and feared complication.

It is important to note that the point of tracheal compression usually occurs distal to the ETT. A history of supine dyspnea or cough should alert the clinician to the possibility of airway obstruction upon induction of anesthesia. Life-threatening complications may occur in the absence of symptoms. The other major complication is cardiovascular collapse secondary to compression of the heart or major vessels. Symptoms of supine syncope suggest vascular compression. Death upon induction of general anesthesia in patients with an anterior mediastinal mass is always a risk. Anesthetic deaths have mainly been reported in children. These deaths may be the result of the more compressible cartilaginous structure of the airway in children or because of the difficulty in obtaining a history of positional symptoms in children.

The most important diagnostic test in the patient with an anterior mediastinal mass is the CT scan of the trachea and chest.[13] Flow-volume loops, specifically exacerbation of a variable intrathoracic obstruction pattern (expiratory plateau) when supine, are unreliable for predicting which patients will have intraoperative airway complications. Echocardiography is indicated for patients with vascular compressive symptoms.

Management: General anesthesia will exacerbate extrinsic intrathoracic airway compression in at least three ways. First, reduced lung volume occurs during general anesthesia; second, bronchial smooth muscle relaxes during general anesthesia, allowing greater compressibility of large airways; and third, paralysis eliminates the caudal movement of the diaphragm seen during spontaneous ventilation. This reduces or eliminates the normal transpleural pressure gradient that dilates the airways during inspiration and minimizes the effects of extrinsic intrathoracic airway compression.

Management of these patients is guided by their symptoms (Tables 25.12-25.14) and the CT scan. All of these patients need a step-by-step induction of anesthesia with continuous monitoring of gas exchange and hemodynamics. This **"NPIC" (Noli Pontes Ignii Consumere, ie, don't burn your bridges)** anesthetic induction can be an inhalation induction with a volatile agent such as sevoflurane or IV titration of propofol with or without ketamine, which maintains spontaneous ventilation until either the airway is definitively secured or the procedure is completed.[14] Awake intubation of the trachea before induction is a possibility in some adult patients if the CT scan shows an area of noncompressed distal trachea to which the ETT can be

TABLE 25.12 Grading Scale for Symptoms in Patients With an Anterior Mediastinal Mass

Asymptomatic

Mild: Can lie supine with some cough/pressure sensation
Moderate: Can lie supine for short periods but not indefinitely
Severe: Cannot tolerate supine position

TABLE 25.13	Anterior Mediastinal Mass Patient Safety Stratification for "NPIC" General Anesthesia
A. Safe	**I.** Asymptomatic adult **II.** CT minimum tracheal/bronchial diameter >50% of normal
B. Unsafe	**I.** Severely symptomatic adult or child **II.** Children with CT tracheal/bronchial diameter <50% of normal
C. Uncertain	**I.** Mild/moderate symptomatic adult **II.** Asymptomatic adult with CT tracheal/bronchial diameter <50% of normal **III.** Mild/moderate symptomatic child with CT tracheal/bronchial diameter >50% of normal **IV.** Adult or child unable to give history

CT, computed tomography; NPIC, Noli Pontes Ignii Consumere (ie, Don't burn your bridges).

advanced before induction. If muscle relaxants are required, ventilation should first be gradually taken over manually to assure that positive-pressure ventilation is possible and only then can a muscle relaxant be administered. Development of airway or vascular compression requires that the patient be awakened as rapidly as possible and then other options for the surgery to be explored. Intraoperative life-threatening airway compression has usually responded to one of two therapies: either **repositioning** of the patient (which should be determined before induction if there is one side or position that causes less compression) or **rigid bronchoscopy** and ventilation distal to the obstruction. This means that an experienced bronchoscopist and equipment must always be immediately available in the operating room in these cases.

CLINICAL PEARL

Loss of airway during induction of a patient with an anterior mediastinal mass requires rapid rescue by repositioning the patient or by rigid bronchoscopy.

Femoro-femoral CPB before induction of anesthesia is a possibility for some patients who are considered "unsafe" for "NPIC" general anesthesia.[15] Other options for "unsafe" patients include local anesthetic biopsy of the mediastinal mass or biopsy of another node (eg, supraclavicular), preoperative radiotherapy with a nonradiated "window" for subsequent biopsy, preoperative chemotherapy or short course steroids, and CT-guided biopsy of mass or drainage of a cyst.

H. Tracheal and Bronchial Stenting

Regional narrowing of the trachea or bronchi can be treated temporarily or definitively by placement of tracheal or bronchial stents.[16] Anesthetic management for tracheal stenting is similar to management of patients with mediastinal masses. General anesthesia with muscle relaxation is optimal, but in patients with severe symptoms of airway obstruction, induction of anesthesia should follow a step-by-step "NPIC" protocol as discussed earlier. Further details on airway stent placement can be found in Chapter 26.

TABLE 25.14	Anterior Mediastinal Mass Management for All "Uncertain" Patients for "NPIC" General Anesthesia

I. Secure airway beyond stenosis awake if feasible
II. Rigid bronchoscope and surgeon available at induction
III. Laryngeal mask airway available
IV. Determine optimal positioning of patient
V. Preserve spontaneous respiration capability until tolerance for positive-pressure ventilation is proven
VI. Monitor for airway compromise postoperatively "NPIC"

NPIC, Noli Pontes Ignii Consumere (ie, Don't burn your bridges).

I. **Tracheal Resection**

Anatomically, the trachea has a necessary structural rigidity and a segmental blood supply that complicate its resection and repair. Endotracheal intubation and resulting strictures were once the primary cause of the need for tracheal resection, but using less irritating ETT materials and limiting the duration of prolonged endotracheal intubation have decreased this complication. Benign and malignant tumors (eg, adenocarcinomas and cylindromas) constitute the remaining indications for tracheal resection.

For a controlled and methodical operation on the trachea, full control of the airway must be maintained at all times. Cooperation between the surgeon and the anesthesiologist is of utmost importance. Both should visualize the lesion preoperatively (CT and bronchoscopy). With preoperative planning and discussions, they can avoid unnecessary hasty procedures that might compromise the end result or worse. Benign lesions can be dilated preoperatively to allow the passage of a small ETT through the lesion. Operatively, the area below the lesion is addressed first. If the degree of obstruction increases, a sterile ETT can be placed directly from the surgical field. The patient should be spontaneously ventilating at the end of the case to allow for extubation. Some surgeons will temporarily place a Montgomery "T" tube distal to the anastomosis with the side arm of the "T" brought out anteriorly through the neck incision to ensure gas exchange in case of proximal trachea-glottic obstruction or edema. Some surgeons will leave a temporary "chin retention" suture for several days postoperatively. This heavy suture between the chin and the sternum restricts head extension and limits traction on the fresh tracheal anastomosis.

J. **Pulmonary Hemorrhage**

Massive hemoptysis is defined as expectoration of >200 mL of blood in 24-48 hours. The commonest causes are carcinoma, bronchiectasis, and trauma (blunt, penetrating, or secondary to a PA catheter). Death can occur quickly due to asphyxia. Management requires four sequential steps: lung isolation, resuscitation, diagnosis, and definitive treatment. The anesthesiologist is often called to deal with these cases outside the operating room. There is no consensus on the best method of lung isolation. The initial method for lung isolation will depend on the availability of appropriate equipment and an assessment of the patient's airway. FOB is usually not helpful in positioning EBTs or blockers in the presence of torrential pulmonary hemorrhage, and lung isolation must be guided by clinical signs (primarily auscultation). DLTs will achieve rapid and secure lung isolation. Even if a left-sided tube enters the right mainstem bronchus, only the right upper lobe will be obstructed. However, suctioning large amounts of blood or clots is difficult through the narrow lumens of a DLT. An option is the initial placement of a single-lumen tube for oxygenation and suctioning and then replacement with a DLT either by laryngoscopy or with an appropriate tube exchanger. An uncut single-lumen ETT can be advanced directly into the right mainstem bronchus or rotated 90° counterclockwise for advancement into the left mainstem bronchus (less reliable than right mainstem intubation). A BB will normally pass easily into the right mainstem bronchus and is useful for right-sided hemorrhage (90% of PA catheter–induced hemorrhages are right-sided). After lung isolation and resuscitation have been achieved, both diagnosis and definitive therapy are now most commonly performed by radiologists[17] (except for blunt and penetrating trauma).

11

1. **Pulmonary artery catheter–induced hemorrhage:** Hemoptysis in a patient with a PA catheter must be assumed to be caused by the perforation of a pulmonary vessel by the catheter until proven otherwise. The mortality rate may exceed 50%. Therapy for PA catheter–induced hemorrhage should follow an organized protocol with some variation depending on the severity of the hemorrhage (see Table 25.15).

2. **During weaning from cardiopulmonary bypass:** Weaning from CPB is one of the times when PA catheter–induced hemorrhage is most likely to occur. Management of the PA catheter during CPB by routinely withdrawing the catheter 2-3 cm to avoid wedging during CPB may decrease the risk of this complication. When hemoptysis does occur in this situation, there are several management options available (see Figure 25.9). The anesthesiologist should resist the temptation to rapidly reverse the anticoagulation in order to quickly get off CPB since this can lead to disaster. Resumption of full CPB ensures oxygenation while

TABLE 25.15	Management of the Patient With a PA Catheter–Induced Pulmonary Hemorrhage

I. Initially position the patient with the bleeding lung dependent.
II. Endotracheal intubation, oxygenation, airway toilet
III. Lung isolation. Endobronchial DLT or single-lumen tube or BB
IV. Withdraw the PA catheter several centimeters, leaving it in the main PA. Do not inflate the balloon (except with fluoroscopic guidance).
V. Position the patient with the isolated bleeding lung nondependent. PEEP to the bleeding lung if possible.
VI. Transport to medical imaging for diagnosis and embolization if feasible.

BB, bronchial blocker; DLT, double-lumen tube; PA, pulmonary artery; PEEP, positive end-expiratory pressure.

the tracheobronchial tree is suctioned and then visualized with FOB. The use of a PA vent or full-flow CPB may be required to decrease the pulmonary blood flow sufficiently to define the bleeding site (usually the right lower lobe). The pleural cavity should be opened to assess the lung parenchymal damage. When possible, conservative management with lung isolation constitutes optimal therapy. In patients with persistent hemorrhage who are not candidates for lung resection, temporary lobar PA occlusion with a vascular loop may be an option.

K. **Post-Tracheostomy Hemorrhage**

Hemorrhage in the immediate postoperative period following a tracheostomy is usually from local vessels, such as the anterior jugular or inferior thyroid veins. Massive hemorrhage 1-6 weeks postoperatively is most commonly due to tracheo-innominate artery fistula.[18] A small sentinel bleed occurs in most patients before a massive bleed. The management protocol for tracheo-innominate artery fistula is outlined in Table 25.16.

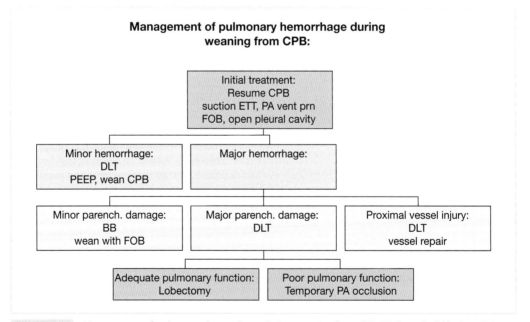

FIGURE 25.9 Management of pulmonary hemorrhage during weaning from CPB. BB, bronchial blocker; CPB, cardiopulmonary bypass; DLT, double-lumen tube; ETT, endotracheal tube; FOB, fiberoptic bronchoscopy; PA, pulmonary artery; parench., lung parenchyma; PEEP, positive end-expiratory pressure; prn (pro re nata), as needed.

TABLE 25.16	Management of Tracheo-Innominate Artery Fistula Hemorrhage

1. Overinflate the tracheostomy cuff to tamponade the hemorrhage. If this fails:
2. Replace the tracheostomy tube with an oral ETT. Position the cuff with FOB guidance just above the carina.
3. Digital compression of the innominate artery against the posterior sternum using a finger passed through the tracheostomy stoma. If this fails:
4. Slow withdrawal of the ETT and overinflation of the cuff to tamponade.
5. Then proceed with definitive therapy: sternotomy and ligation of the innominate artery.

ETT, endotracheal tube; FOB, fiberoptic bronchoscopy.

IV. Lung Volume Reduction Surgery

According to the National Heart, Blood, and Lung Institute, ~13.5 million persons in the United States are afflicted with COPD, and 3.1 million of these patients have emphysema (Cure Researchtm.com, http://www.cureresearch.com) as the primary manifestation. Airflow obstruction associated with chronic bronchitis or emphysema occurs due to a loss of the elastic recoil properties of the lung and chest wall. As the disease progresses, patients become increasingly debilitated. They exhibit symptoms of severe dyspnea, require supplemental oxygen, and display poor exercise tolerance. Lung volume reduction surgery (LVRS) offers a select group of patients the possibility of improved exercise tolerance, reduction in dyspnea, improved quality of life, and extended life span. It has been suggested that LVRS may provide these patients with a benefit that otherwise cannot be achieved by any means other than lung transplantation.

A. Anesthetic Management for Lung Volume Reduction Surgery

Anesthesiology expertise is essential to successful outcomes for patients undergoing LVRS. Our expertise in cardiopulmonary physiology, pharmacology, and pain management allows us to minimize postoperative complications.

1. **Preoperative assessment:** All patients scheduled for LVRS receive the following preoperative physiologic studies: (a) standard pulmonary function studies, (b) plethysmographic measurement of lung volumes, (c) standardized 6MWT, (d) ABG values, (e) quantitative nuclear lung perfusion scans, and (f) radionuclide cardiac ventriculogram and/or dobutamine stress echocardiogram.

2. **Preoperative pulmonary rehabilitation program:** After the initial preoperative evaluation, all patients are enrolled in a pulmonary rehabilitation program for a minimum of 6 weeks before surgical intervention.

3. **Monitors:** In addition to the standard monitors, large-bore IV access and an arterial catheter are recommended. The use of central venous catheters and PA catheters should be considered on an individual patient basis.

4. The judicious use of **TEA**, both intraoperatively and postoperatively, affords advantages as follows: (a) preserved ability to cough and clear secretions, thus decreasing atelectasis and possibly reducing pulmonary infection; (b) decreased airway resistance; (c) improved phrenic nerve function; (d) stabilization of coronary endothelial function; (e) improved myocardial perfusion; (f) earlier return of bowel function; (g) preservation of immunocompetence; and (h) decreased cost of perioperative care through reduction of perioperative complications. Best results are obtained with catheters placed in the T4-T5 or T5-T6 spinal interspaces.

   a. **Intraoperative thoracic epidural analgesia:** TEA can be used as an adjunct to general anesthesia. Local anesthetics, such as 2% lidocaine, 0.5% ropivacaine, or 0.25% bupivacaine, provide optimal surgical conditions. The local anesthetics can be delivered via intermittent bolus or as a continuous infusion.

      (1) Because persistent air leaks may be a problem in the postoperative period and may be exacerbated by positive-pressure ventilation, it is optimal to extubate the patients either at the conclusion of surgery or as soon as possible thereafter.

      (2) Caution must be exercised if opioids are added to the infusate because they have the potential to severely depress the patient's respiratory efforts.

  b. Postoperative thoracic epidural analgesia: TEA provides superior postoperative analgesia for both median sternotomy and bilateral thoracoscopic surgical procedures. A reduced concentration of local anesthetic plus a small dose of opioids delivered by continuous infusion is suggested (eg, 0.2% ropivacaine plus 0.01 mg/mL hydromorphone).

  c. Paravertebral nerve blocks (PVNBs) may be used as an alternative to TEA. They may be performed either by multiple injections or by inserting a catheter into the paravertebral space for use with a continuous infusion of local anesthetic. This technique requires the use of a multimodal analgesic regimen, including IV opioids and nonsteroidal anti-inflammatory agents. The effect of PVNB on morbidity and mortality following thoracic surgery, in particular LVRS, has yet to be determined.

 5. A left-sided double-lumen EBT should be used to secure the patient's airway.

 6. General anesthesia: Induction of general anesthesia can be conducted with agents that promote hemodynamic homeostasis. The anesthetic plan for each patient should be individualized appropriately.

 7. Postoperative management: Problems that should be anticipated in the postoperative period include (a) oversedation, (b) accumulation of airway secretions, (c) pneumothorax, (d) bronchospasm, (e) PE, (f) pneumonia, (g) persistent air leaks, (h) arrhythmias, and (i) myocardial infarction. Reintubation and mechanical ventilation are associated with high morbidity and mortality. Several measures can be taken to minimize these adverse side effects:

  a. Judicious pulmonary toilet

  b. Bronchodilators

  c. Effective analgesia with TEA or PVNB/multimodal analgesia

  d. Avoidance of systemic corticosteroids

B. Endobronchial Valves and Blockers for Lung Volume Reduction

Although LVRS has been shown to benefit patients with a heterogeneous pattern of emphysema, this constitutes only about 20% of patients who are eligible candidates for this treatment. Currently available bronchoscopic techniques include endobronchial blockers/valves, biologic glues, and airway bypass. Further details on this can be found in Chapter 26.

C. Conclusions

LVRS is a viable option for a select group of patients with emphysema. Regardless of the selection of treatment modality, the goals remain the same: improvements in dyspnea, exercise tolerance, quality of life, and prolonged survival. The anesthesiologist must be actively engaged in the perioperative management of these patients. Patient history and preoperative status as well as the results obtained from the evaluation of CXRs, high-resolution CT scans, and right heart catheterizations should be carefully weighed when planning these procedures.

REFERENCES

1. Hanley C, Donahoe L, Slinger P. Fit for surgery? What's new in preoperative assessment of the high-risk patient undergoing pulmonary resection. *J Cardiothorac Vasc Anesth.* 2021;35(12):3760-3773.
2. Brunelli A, Kim AW, Berger KI, et al. Physiologic evaluation of the patient with lung cancer being considered for resectional surgery. Diagnosis and management of lung cancer, 3rd ed: American College of Chest Physicians evidence-based clinical practice guidelines. *Chest.* 2013;143(Suppl. 5):e166S-e190S.
3. Frendl G, Sodickson AC, Chung MK, et al. 2014 AATS guidelines for the prevention and management of perioperative atrial fibrillation and flutter for thoracic surgical procedures. *J Thorac Cardiovasc Surg.* 2014;148(3):772-791.
4. Campos JH. An update on bronchial blockers during lung separation techniques in adults. *Anesth Analg.* 2003;97(5):1266-1274.
5. Knoll H, Ziegeler S, Schreiber JU, et al. Airway injuries after one-lung ventilation: a comparison between double-lumen tube and endobronchial blocker: a randomized, prospective, controlled trial. *Anesthesiology.* 2006;105(3):471-477.
6. Campos JH, Hallam E, Van Natta T, et al. Devices for lung isolation used by anesthesiologists with limited thoracic experience: comparison of double-lumen endotracheal tube, Univent torque control blocker, and Arndt wire-guided endobronchial blocker. *Anesthesiology.* 2006;104:261-266.
7. Slinger P. Fiberoptic bronchoscopic positioning of double-lumen tubes. *J Cardiothorac Anesth.* 1989;3:486-496. For photographs see "Bronchoscopic positioning of Double-Lumen Tubes" in the Living Library section at the website www.thoracicanesthesia.com.
8. Karzai W, Schwarzkopf K. Hypoxemia during one-lung ventilation. *Anesthesiology.* 2009;110(6):1402-1411.

9. Ku CM, Slinger P, Waddell TK. A novel method of treating hypoxemia during one-lung ventilation for thoracoscopic surgery. *J Cardiothorac Vasc Anesth*. 2009;23(6):850-852.

10. Slinger P. Postpneumonectomy pulmonary edema: good news, bad news. *Anesthesiology*. 2006;105(1):2-5.

11. Amar D, Roistacher N, Burt ME, et al. Effects of diltiazem versus digoxin on dysrhythmias and cardiac function after pneumonectomy. *Ann Thorac Surg*. 1997;63(5):1374-1381.

12. Riley RH, Wood BM. Induction of anaesthesia in a patient with a bronchopleural fistula. *Anaesth Intensive Care*. 1994;22(5):625-626.

13. Shamberger RC, Hozman RS, Griscom NT, et al. Prospective evaluation by computed tomography and pulmonary function tests of children with mediastinal masses. *Surgery*. 1995;118(3):468-471.

14. Frawley G, Low J, Brown TC. Anaesthesia for an anterior mediastinal mass with ketamine and midazolam infusion. *Anaesth Intensive Care*. 1995;23(5):610-612.

15. Turkoz A, Gulcan O, Tercan F, et al. Hemodynamic collapse caused by a large unruptured aneurysm of the ascending aorta in an 18 year old. *Anesth Analg*. 2006;102(4):1040-1042.

16. Licker M, Schweizer A, Nicolet G, et al. Anesthesia of a patient with an obstructing tracheal mass: a new way to manage the airway. *Acta Anaesthesiol Scand*. 1997;41:84-86.

17. Fortin M, Turcotte R, Gleeton O, et al. Catheter-induced pulmonary artery rupture: using occlusion balloon to avoid lung isolation. *J Cardiothorac Vasc Anesth*. 2006;20(3):376-378.

18. Grant CA, Dempsey G, Harrison J, et al. Tracheo-innominate artery fistula after percutaneous tracheostomy: three case reports and a clinical review. *Br J Anaesth*. 2006;96(1):127-131.

Anesthetic Management for Interventional Pulmonology Procedures

Julia Scarpa and Alessia Pedoto

KEY POINTS

1. Interventional pulmonology (IP) techniques are rapidly and increasingly being used to diagnose, stage, and treat a large variety of lung and airway diseases.
2. These procedures are commonly done in an IP lab that may be some distance from the operating rooms. In addition to the acuity of the pulmonary patients cared for in the IP suite, the distance to the operating room and other surgical and interventional collaborators further necessitates good planning and communication among all the IP team members. Fortunately, serious complications in the IP suite are not frequent, but when they do occur, they can be life-threatening. It is imperative that rescue protocols are in place in case of major complications.
3. Most of the IP cases where an anesthesiologist is involved are done under general anesthesia, with an endotracheal tube or a supraglottic airway device in place.
4. Interventional procedures may require the use of jet ventilation and total intravenous anesthesia (TIVA). Airway bleeding, airway obstruction, bronchospasm, and pneumothorax are the most common perioperative complications requiring immediate management.
5. Many of these procedures are done as outpatients; therefore, the anesthetic should be tailored to expedite discharge.
6. Good regional anesthesia is essential for the success of pleural procedures done with sedation. Neuraxial and peripheral nerve blocks have been successfully used.

I. **Introduction**

Interventional pulmonology (IP) is a subspecialty of pulmonary medicine focused on using minimally invasive diagnostic and therapeutic techniques in patients with lung, mediastinal, pleural, and complex airway diseases.

A. **Indications:** Referral to an IP specialist is prioritized for the diagnosis and treatment of a variety of chest-related disorders. In recent years, as the minimally invasive techniques of IP procedures have advanced, patients who would have previously required more invasive thoracic surgical or interventional radiology (IR) approaches are now increasingly referred to undergo IP procedures instead. Due to the endoscopic nature of the procedures, patients can recover and be discharged faster than if they had undergone an open diagnostic or therapeutic intervention.

B. **Alternatives:** Not all pulmonary disease processes are amenable to IP therapies or accessible with IP diagnostic technologies. Alternatives to IP procedures include computed tomography (CT)-guided percutaneous biopsy, as would be performed by IR specialists, or video-assisted thoracic surgery (VATS) biopsy, performed by a thoracic surgeon. Both CT-guided and VATS biopsies have a high diagnostic yield but are limited to one side at a time. In addition, CT-guided procedures for mediastinal lymphadenopathy staging are associated with a higher risk of complications. The higher yield of CT-guided percutaneous biopsy, as compared to IP advanced bronchoscopy, is related to the quality of the preprocedural CT, navigational ability, and real-time confirmation.[1]

II. **Anesthetic Approaches**

A. **Local: Airway Topicalization**

1. **Anatomy:** Key structures requiring topicalization include the nasopharynx, posterior oropharynx including tonsillar pillars, vocal cords, and the trachea. Topical anesthesia to these areas will cover sensory innervation, including the pharyngeal branch of the maxillary nerve (nasopharynx), the glossopharyngeal nerve (oropharynx), the internal laryngeal branch of the superior laryngeal nerve (larynx above the vocal cords), and the recurrent laryngeal nerve (trachea below the vocal cords). Inadequate topicalization increases the risk of cough and laryngospasm during instrumentation of the pharynx and larynx.

2. **Methods for topicalizing:** Commonly used techniques include nebulization of 4% lidocaine; spraying of 4% lidocaine with the McKenzie technique or a mucosal atomizer; application of 4% lidocaine ointment or solution on cotton swabs, gauze, or nasal trumpets; and nerve blocks of the glossopharyngeal, superior laryngeal, and recurrent laryngeal nerves. Relevant anatomy is shown in Figure 26.1. The use of one technique does not preclude the others, and frequently more than one method of topicalization is employed. Lidocaine spray has been shown to be more effective than nebulized lidocaine.[2] Cricothyroid lidocaine administration has been shown to result in less cough and superior operator-rated procedural satisfaction, at a lower cumulative lidocaine dose, when compared to spray-as-you-go lidocaine administration.[3]

3. **Toxicity:** While systemic absorption of topically administered local anesthetic is lower than expected, there is always the possibility of toxicity with excessive administration. Methemoglobinemia can develop with benzocaine, although other local anesthetics have also been described as causal; this is characterized by hypoxemia and cyanosis, which can be fatal if untreated. Treatment is with intravenous methylene blue. In addition, local anesthetic systemic toxicity (LAST) has been reported and is characterized first by tinnitus or perioral tingling, escalating to seizure and ultimately cardiac arrest. Treatment is with intravenous lipid emulsion therapy and supportive care.

CLINICAL PEARL

Lidocaine nebulization is the most common modality for airway topicalization.

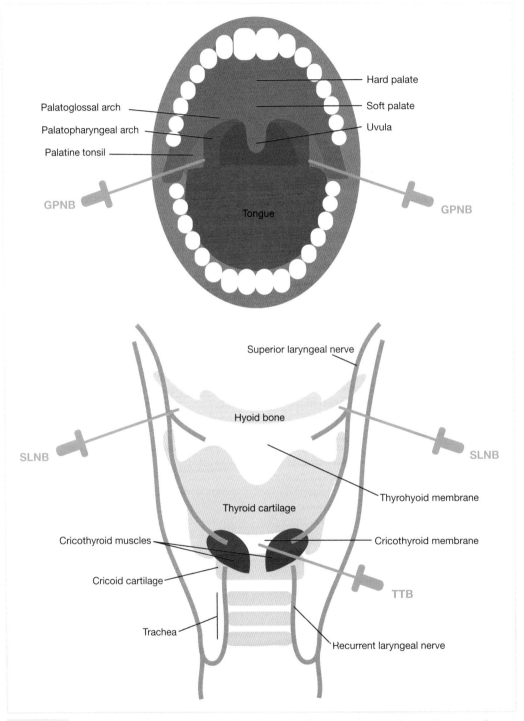

FIGURE 26.1   Topicalization of the oropharynx and upper airway. The glossopharyngeal nerve innervates the oropharynx, including the tongue and upper epiglottis; it mediates the afferent limb of the gag reflex. It can be blocked transorally by injecting just medial to the palatine tonsils bilaterally (GPNB). The superior laryngeal nerve can be blocked (SLNB) at the thyrohyoid membrane bilaterally; the internal branch provides sensation above vocal cords, and the external branch provides motor function to the cricothyroid muscle. The recurrent laryngeal nerve can be blocked by transcricothyroid (transtracheal) injection (TTB [transtracheal block]); it provides sensation to the trachea and motor function to all intrinsic laryngeal muscles, except the cricothyroid muscle. The superior and the recurrent laryngeal nerves are branches of the vagus nerve. (Courtesy of Julia Scarpa.)

B. **Sedation: Monitored Anesthesia Care**

1. **To facilitate topicalization:** Except in rare circumstances with exceptional concern for airway compromise, airway topicalization to facilitate awake fiberoptic intubation is typically performed with some degree of light sedation for patient comfort. Intravenous medications routinely used for this purpose include benzodiazepines such as midazolam; short-acting opioids such as remifentanil infusion; and low-dose nonbenzodiazepine sedative-hypnotics such as ketamine, dexmedetomidine, and propofol. Many of these agents are satisfactory but have different clinical profiles. For example, ketamine-propofol and dexmedetomidine-propofol combinations are both adequate for awake intubation, but the former has a faster onset of sedation, a shorter time to successful intubation, and greater hemodynamic stability.[4]

2. **As the primary anesthetic:** In IP procedures that do not require intubation, such as awake diagnostic bronchoscopy, intravenous sedation is employed to facilitate patient comfort and proceduralist satisfaction. Many of the same agents are used as earlier, with the goal of maintaining not only spontaneous ventilation but also tolerance of the procedure. However, combinations are often used; for example, dexmedetomidine bolus and infusion alone were demonstrated to be insufficient for sedation without the need for rescue sedation with midazolam or propofol in many patients.[5]

3. **Adjuvant regional anesthetic techniques:** Regional blocks can be performed in addition to the provision of sedation for medical thoracoscopy. They provide excellent intraoperative and postoperative analgesia, minimizing pleuritic chest pain and opioid requirements, therefore facilitating respiratory recovery. Epidural or paravertebral anesthesia is the most invasive regional technique. Fascial plane blocks are typically preferred due to their increased safety profile. Chest wall coverage can be achieved with epidural, paravertebral, midpoint transverse process to pleura,[6] erector spinae, serratus plane, intercostal nerve blocks, or transversus thoracis muscle plane blocks, depending on the procedural or injury site (Figure 26.2).

C. **General Anesthesia:** The use of general anesthesia for IP procedures is increasing, due to advances in bronchoscopy that allow for deeper endobronchial tree access and, therefore, require complete immobility of the patient. The incidence of atelectasis under general anesthesia during bronchoscopy is extraordinarily high, close to 90%, and correlates with body mass index (BMI) and duration of anesthesia.[7] Given the detrimental effects of atelectasis on patient ventilatory status and recovery, as well as on peripheral bronchoscopy efficacy, vigilance for and prevention of atelectasis during bronchoscopy is key. In a multicenter randomized controlled trial, when compared to usual care, endotracheal intubation with a recruitment maneuver, titrated FIO_2, and a positive end-expiratory pressure (PEEP) of 8-10 cm H_2O demonstrated a clinically significant decrease in the incidence and extent of atelectasis in patients undergoing bronchoscopy under general anesthesia.[8] These interventions were well tolerated and highly effective, and they should be considered for all patients undergoing bronchoscopy under general anesthesia.

CLINICAL PEARL

- Prevention of atelectasis is instrumental in avoiding CT-patient divergence.
- Most IP cases are done under general anesthesia as outpatient procedures.

III. **Procedural Approaches**

A. **Flexible Bronchoscopy**

1. **Procedure:** Visualization of the tracheobronchial tree with a flexible white light bronchoscope that allows access to the lower airways including the third order of bronchi. Typically performed in conjunction with one or more other procedures

4 5

2. **Anesthesia:** Airway topicalization with or without sedation, or general anesthesia (volatile or total intravenous anesthesia, TIVA) with an endotracheal tube (ETT) or a supraglottic airway (SGA), with or without paralysis, depending on additional procedures or interventions

3. **Complications:** Bronchospasm, laryngospasm, hypercarbia, hypoxemia, pneumothorax, vocal cord trauma or edema, and airway trauma[9]

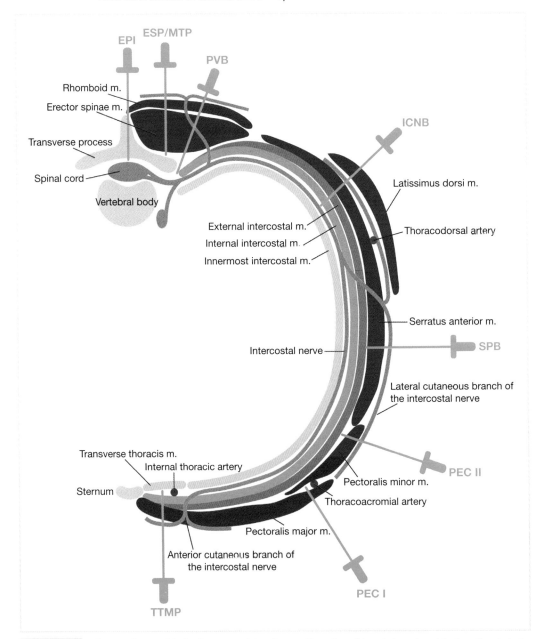

FIGURE 26.2 Chest wall nerve blocks. Coverage of the chest wall can be achieved via various blocks, either in isolation or in combination, depending on the location of injury, surgery, or pain. Epidural block (EPI), midtransverse process to pleura block (MTP), erector spinae block (ESP), paravertebral block (PVB), serratus plane block (SPB), intercostal nerve block (ICNB), pectoralis nerve block (PEC I and PEC II), and transversus thoracis muscle plane (TTMP) block can all be performed and block progressively more distal nerves. (Courtesy of Julia Scarpa.)

B. **Endobronchial Ultrasound Bronchoscopy**
   1. **Procedure:** Flexible bronchoscopy is performed via a bronchoscope with an ultrasound probe that is used to visualize central structures within the tracheobronchial walls, mediastinum, and lungs.
   2. **Anesthesia:** General anesthesia with an ETT or SGA, with or without paralysis. TIVA is usually preferred, given the presence of air leak around the bronchoscopy adapter. If the patient cannot accommodate an 8.0 or larger ETT, a smaller (7.0) ETT is sufficient for flexible bronchoscopy with a subsequent switch to SGA for the endobronchial ultrasound (EBUS) portion of the procedure.
   3. **Additional considerations:** Typically performed with transbronchial needle aspiration to access mediastinal lymph nodes for sampling. Higher paratracheal nodes can only be accessed with an SGA in place, while lower nodes remain accessible with an ETT.
   4. **Complications:** Same as flexible bronchoscopy, plus airway bleeding and tension pneumothorax from the biopsy needle

CLINICAL PEARL

Vocal cord trauma is more common with EBUS due to the 45° location of the light source.

C. **Navigational Bronchoscopy**
   1. **Procedure:** Electromagnetic navigation with real-time CT images is used to create a three-dimensional (3D) map of the lungs. Following high-resolution CT acquisition, a 3D image of the patient's chest is generated, and lesion targets are identified. A virtual pathway through the endobronchial tree is planned. Flexible bronchoscopy is performed, and a navigational catheter is introduced through the working channel to the target area; real-time location is shown on intraprocedural CT, and the catheter is adjusted by the physician. Once it is locked in place, a standard endoscopic tool is introduced to obtain a sample.
   2. **Anesthesia:** General with an ETT with paralysis
   3. **Additional considerations:** The locator board and sensors must be correctly placed, and nothing with metal in close proximity. Accuracy is limited by lack of visualization during sample acquisition. Cough or patient motion must be avoided to prevent losing the target area.
   4. **Complications:** Same as EBUS

CLINICAL PEARL

General anesthesia with endotracheal intubation and paralysis is most commonly used to avoid motion, which interferes with the mapping and finally the accuracy of tissue sampling.

D. **Robotic-Assisted Bronchoscopy**
   1. **Procedure**
      a. **Electromagnetic navigation:** The Monarch system relies on electromagnetic guidance, requiring reference sensors around the patient to triangulate the lesion location and thus requires registration. This allows for continuous visualization, which is required to extend a telescopic "mother-daughter" catheter controlled by a joystick.[1]
      b. **Shape sensing:** The ION system is based on shape-sensing technology. Once the target lesion is identified, the camera is removed and a uniform catheter controlled by a trackball and scroll wheel is used. A 3D reconstruction from a dedicated detailed CT also requires registration before the start.[1,10]
   2. **Indications and advantages:** This technique allows for endobronchial navigation into lung periphery (Figure 26.3) with catheter stabilization to maximize precision and diagnostic yield.

3. **Anesthesia:** General anesthesia (volatile or TIVA) with an 8.5 ETT and paralysis. Positive-pressure ventilation is maintained, with a tidal volume of 8-10 mL/kg of ideal body weight, PEEP of 8-10 cm H_2O, the lowest possible FIO_2, and intermittent breath holding with the adjustable pressure-limiting (APL) valve at 20-40 cm H_2O for recruitment.[11] Due to the elevated intrathoracic pressures, continuous invasive or noninvasive blood pressure monitoring may be required.

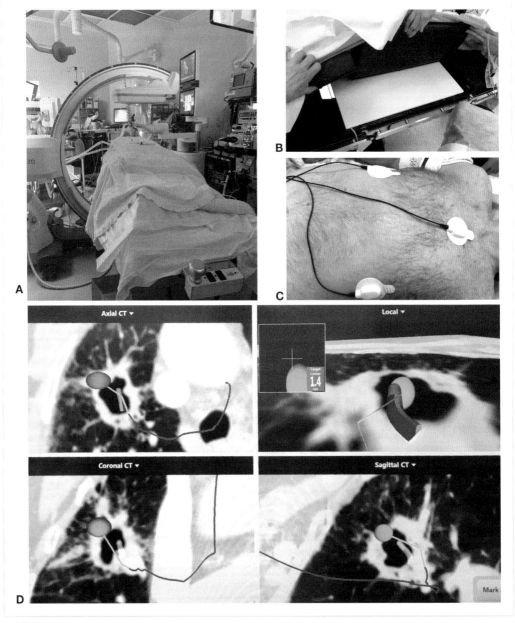

FIGURE 26.3 Navigational bronchoscopy. **(A)** The patient is under general endotracheal anesthesia with neuromuscular blockade. Patient positioning requires placement of a location board under the thorax **(B)** and three sensors on the chest **(C)**. This allows for registration of the patient with a previously acquired computed tomography scan, so that path navigation to the periphery can be calculated **(D)**. (Images courtesy of Dr Alessia Pedoto.)

4. **Additional considerations:** CT-to-body divergence is a mismatch in lung volumes between the high-resolution CT acquired at maximal inspiration in the preoperative period and at the end of expiration while mechanically ventilated. This is minimized by using the proposed ventilatory settings. Lateral positioning has been suggested to decrease atelectasis and obviate the high-pressure high-volume ventilatory need;[12] however, this is not clinically feasible.

5. **Complications:** Similar to EBUS. In particular, due to elevated intrathoracic pressures, hypotension, and pneumothorax

---

CLINICAL PEARL

CT-to-body divergence is the limiting factor to good sampling with the least associated complications, especially bleeding.

E. **Rigid Bronchoscopy**
1. **Procedure:** A rigid bronchoscope is introduced through the vocal cords and above the carina, to visualize the trachea and proximal bronchi.
2. **Indications:** Hemoptysis, large airway obstruction, foreign body, respiratory papillomatosis, airway dilation, or stent placement or removal
3. **Anesthesia:** General anesthesia with TIVA, with or without paralysis. While spontaneous ventilation is possible, jet ventilation is frequently used[13] with paralysis.
4. **Additional considerations:** The rigid bronchoscope effectively acts as an airway device while in place; upon its removal, it is sometimes necessary to place a temporary airway, such as an ETT or SGA, during emergence from anesthesia, depending on patient anatomy and level of sedation. Mask ventilation is also a possibility.
5. **Complications:** Barotrauma, airway obstruction, pneumothorax, pneumomediastinum, dental injury, tongue injury, tracheal injury, esophageal injury, hypoxia, hypercapnia, inability to ventilate

---

CLINICAL PEARL

General anesthesia with paralysis is commonly used for this procedure to facilitate the placement of the rigid bronchoscope and jet ventilation.

F. **Pleuroscopy**
1. **Procedure:** Also known as medical thoracoscopy, this procedure involves placing a camera through the chest wall and into the pleural space for diagnostic and therapeutic purposes.
2. **Indications:** Pleurodesis, pleural biopsy, pleural fluid drainage
3. **Anesthesia:** Typically, general anesthesia is used, with or without selective lung ventilation; however, deep sedation with regional analgesia is also a good option in certain candidates.[6]
4. **Complications:** Air leak, subcutaneous emphysema, pneumothorax, hemorrhage, air embolism, reexpansion pulmonary edema

---

6 **CLINICAL PEARL**

Regional analgesia and proper patient selection are instrumental in the success of sedation for these procedures. Paravertebral, erector spinae, and midtransverse process to pleura (MTP) block are good analgesic options.

IV. Diagnostic Techniques

    A. Bronchoalveolar Lavage

        1. Compatible with flexible bronchoscopy

        2. Technique: Once the bronchoscope is wedged into the subsegmental bronchus of choice, sterile saline is instilled and then gently suctioned into a separate canister and sent to cytology.

        3. Indications: Specimen acquisition for the diagnosis of various infectious, inflammatory, immunologic, and cancerous disorders

        4. Complications: Rarely: bronchospasm, hypoxia, pneumothorax

    B. Transbronchial Needle Aspiration

        1. Compatible with flexible bronchoscopy, EBUS, and robotic bronchoscopy

        2. Technique: A needle is introduced through the bronchial wall and aspirates samples.

        3. Advantages: Less invasive alternative to mediastinoscopy or mediastinotomy for sampling of mediastinal lymph nodes or masses; also with a higher diagnostic yield than mediastinoscopy[14] and high specificity for mediastinal lymph node staging.[15] Less invasive alternative to cervical mediastinoscopy, thoracoscopy, or thoracotomy for peripheral lung nodule sampling

        4. Indications: Lung carcinoma, sarcoidosis, lymphoma, mediastinal and hilar node sampling

        5. Complications: Hypoxia, hypercapnia, pneumothorax, airway bleeding, airway irritation, conversion to mediastinoscopy requiring a thoracic surgeon[16]

    C. Spray Cryotherapy

        1. Compatible with flexible, navigational, robotic, and rigid bronchoscopy

        2. Technique: Insufflation of liquid nitrogen through a flexible catheter via a bronchoscope to rapidly freeze tissue and induce cellular death and hemostasis

        3. Indications: Treatment of obstructing endobronchial tumors and hemoptysis

        4. Advantages: Compared to heat-producing methods (eg, laser therapy, electrocautery, argon plasma coagulation, photodynamic therapy), there is no airway fire risk and there is rapid hemostasis.

        5. Complications: Hypotension, bradycardia, hemodynamic instability, cardiopulmonary arrest, death[17]

CLINICAL PEARL

Due to high complication rates, spray cryotherapy (SCT) has lost popularity. Be aware of bradycardia, atrioventricular block (AVB), conduction pauses, pneumothorax, and bronchospasm. Invasive hemodynamic monitoring and intraoperative transthoracic echocardiography may be required.

    D. Transbronchial Lung Cryobiopsy

        1. Compatible with flexible, navigational, robotic, and rigid bronchoscopy

        2. Procedure: Cryobiopsy has 1 second of contact time followed by 1 minute of tamponade via bronchial blocker of the sampled area before the next biopsy. Typically, two biopsies at two sites are performed, with significantly greater sample yield compared to traditional forceps biopsy.[18]

        3. Indications: Lung biopsy

        4. Additional anesthetic considerations: General anesthesia with paralysis is required. A bronchial blocker is placed before the biopsy to tamponade the source of bleeding. If an ETT is used, the blocker is inserted via direct laryngoscopy before the intubation. The cuff of the ETT is used to keep the device in place.

        5. Complications: Hemorrhage, pneumothorax, hypoxemia, bradycardia (from cold transmission to myocardium and/or cardiac conduction system)

CLINICAL PEARL

Bleeding can be significant at the site of biopsy and is usually tamponaded via bronchial blocker.

V. **Therapeutic Techniques**
    A. **Airway Dilation**
        1. **Compatible with** flexible and rigid bronchoscopy
        2. **Procedure:** Serial dilatations may occur either with a balloon passed distally to the obstruction and inflated to dilate the stenosed airway or via rigid bronchoscopes of increasing size. It can be performed in combination with debulking techniques to maximize airway recanalization, depending on the etiology of disease. Due to the short-lived results, this procedure is usually combined with stent placement.
        3. **Indications:** Benign or malignant airway stenosis
        4. **Complications:** Airway injury, pneumothorax, pneumomediastinum, hemorrhage[19]
    B. **Airway Stent Placement (and Removal)**
        1. **Compatible with** rigid bronchoscopy. Some stents can also be placed using flexible bronchoscopy with fluoroscopy confirmation.[20]
        2. **Procedure:** Various types and shapes of stents are available, depending on the location and etiology of the diseased airway. Retrievability and repositioning of the stent depend on the stent material.[21]
        3. **Indications:** Benign and malignant central airway stenosis, obstructions, and fistulae
        4. **Additional anesthetic considerations:** The more central the diseased conducting airway, the more complex the anesthetic management. For very severe tracheal obstruction, standby veno-venous extracorporeal membrane oxygenation (ECMO) should be available. Jet ventilation is commonly used with rigid bronchoscopy. Stent removal may be complicated by bleeding and difficulty with ventilation if performed for stents placed months or years prior.
        5. **Complications:** Acute airway obstruction, hypoxia, hypercarbia, stent migration or erosion into surrounding structures, in-stent stenosis or plugging, airway or vascular injury

CLINICAL PEARL

Carinal stents are difficult to place and tend to dislodge, impairing ventilation. Ventilation may also be difficult during placement and can be facilitated via Jet.

    C. **Endobronchial Valves**
        1. **Compatible with** flexible bronchoscopy
        2. **Procedure:** Bronchoscopic lung volume reduction can be achieved by the placement of one-way valves in bronchi, leading to the most emphysematous portions of the lung to limit air entry and allow air expulsion. Unidirectional endobronchial valves can be used to treat air leaks after lung surgery (Figure 26.4).
        3. **Indications:** Severe chronic obstructive pulmonary disease (COPD) with hyperinflation, persistent postoperative air leak
        4. **Complications:** Pneumothorax, pneumonia, respiratory failure, COPD exacerbation, valve migration, and erosion into surrounding structures

CLINICAL PEARL

Pneumothorax can occur on induction in patients with severe COPD and should be in the differential diagnosis of refractory hypotension. Tension pneumothorax may occur with positive-pressure ventilation in the presence of an air leak.

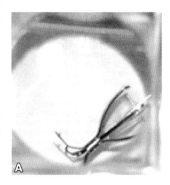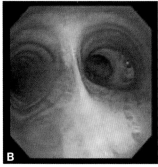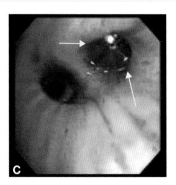

FIGURE 26.4 Endobronchial valves. **(A)** Deployed endobronchial valve. **(B)** Rigid bronchoscopy view of bronchi before endobronchial valve deployment. **(C)** Rigid bronchoscopy view of bronchi following endobronchial valve deployment, as indicated by the arrows. (Images courtesy of Dr Alessia Pedoto.)

    D. Bronchial Thermoplasty
        1. **Compatible with** flexible bronchoscopy
        2. **Procedure:** Radiofrequency energy is applied directly to large airway mucosa, to decrease airway smooth muscle mass and contractility, as well as neuroendocrine cells and autonomic fibers.[22]
        3. **Indications:** Nonpharmacologic treatment of severe, refractory asthma
        4. **Complications:** Worsening of respiratory symptoms
    E. Laser Debulking
        1. **Compatible with** flexible and rigid bronchoscopy
        2. **Procedure:** Lasers of various wavelengths (eg, CO_2, Nd-YAG, argon plasma) are used to burn away tissue. CO_2 lasers have limited tissue penetration and are useful for superficial airway lesions; Nd-YAG lasers are higher energy and are useful for tumor ablation.[25] All lasers require the use of very low FIO_2 (typically <30%) to reduce the risk of airway fire.
        3. **Indications:** Debulking of malignant and benign endobronchial, carinal, or tracheal airway tumors; treatment of various upper airway stenoses[23]
        4. **Complications:** Hemorrhage, tracheobronchial perforation, gas embolism, airway fire, hypoxemia, hypercarbia, pneumothorax, pneumomediastinum, tracheoesophageal fistula, eye injury[24]

CLINICAL PEARL

Low FIO_2 is necessary to prevent airway fire during laser use.

    F. Cryoablation
        1. **Compatible with** flexible, navigational, robotic, and rigid bronchoscopy
        2. **Procedure:** Argon gas expansion rapidly cools the probe tip to <−140 °C to freeze the target. Cycles of freezing and thawing cause cell necrosis.
        3. **Indications/advantages:** Indicated for tumor ablation and nerve ablation (pain therapy). Compared to other ablative techniques, such as microwave ablation and radiofrequency ablation, cryoablation is less painful and preserves tissue architecture, making it preferred for sensitive areas such as the pleura or areas where structural integrity is critical, such as the large airways and diaphragm. It has the lowest complication rate of currently available ablative techniques.[25] Since there are no FIO_2 limitations, this technique is indicated for patients on O_2.
        4. **Complications:** Hemoptysis, hemorrhage, pleural effusions, pneumothorax, prolonged air leak, bronchopleural fistula, arrhythmias, bronchospasm

CLINICAL PEARL

Bradyarrhythmias may be prolonged and profound during cryoablation, requiring continuous hemodynamic monitoring and possible pacing.

    G. **Whole Lung Bronchopulmonary Lavage**
       1. **Compatible with** fiberoptic bronchoscopy and double-lumen ETT
       2. **Procedure:** 15-20 L of warmed normal saline is instilled in multiple, serial aliquots of about 1 L each. Following each instillation, chest percussion is performed, followed by fluid drainage (Figure 26.5). Typically, one lung is lavaged in each session with a separation of days to allow for recovery; bilateral sequential lung lavage in a single session is also possible, but not common.
       3. **Indications:** Pulmonary alveolar proteinosis, refractory asthma, cystic fibrosis, bronchiectasis, lipoid pneumonitis, silicosis
       4. **Complications:** Hypoxemia, hypercarbia, hydrothorax, pneumothorax, aspiration of lavage fluid, atelectasis (due to removal of surfactant), severe bronchospasm, airway reactivity
       5. **Additional anesthetic considerations:** General anesthesia with volatile or TIVA, paralysis, and one-lung ventilation via a double-lumen ETT. If the patient cannot tolerate one-lung ventilation, partial venoarterial or venovenous cardiopulmonary bypass or ECMO can be used.[26]

CLINICAL PEARL

Bronchodilation via nebulizers may be required during and after whole lung bronchopulmonary lavage due to airway reactivity.

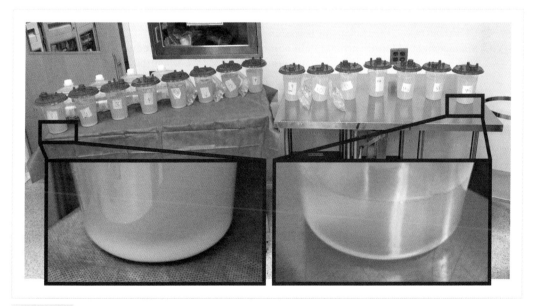

FIGURE 26.5   Whole lung lavage. Endobronchial washings collected by whole lung lavage in a patient with pulmonary alveolar proteinosis. Suction canisters of lavage washings were collected sequentially to demonstrate the volume and clearance of the lavage fluid, starting with the first lavage on the left through the last lavage on the right. Cropped images are close-ups of the first and last lavage washings. (Images courtesy of Dr Alessia Pedoto.)

H. Foreign Body Removal
   1. **Compatible with** flexible bronchoscopy (with basket forceps) or rigid bronchoscopy
   2. **Indications:** Endotracheal or proximal bronchial foreign body
   3. **Complications:** Tracheal injury, esophageal injury, airway bleeding, aspiration
   4. **Additional anesthetic considerations:** Maintenance of spontaneous ventilation until foreign body is retrieved, to avoid distal dislocation with positive pressure.

VI. Preoperative Assessment for Interventional Pulmonology Procedures
   A. Most IP procedures are done on an outpatient basis, and patients are seen by the anesthesiologist on the same day, in the presurgical area, unless severe comorbidities are present and the patient needs to be optimized. Therefore, a thorough preoperative evaluation that is tailored to the needs of the IP procedure and the most relevant patient-related factors is necessary to plan a safe anesthetic.
      1. Patients with **reactive airway disease** should continue their inhalers and steroids on the day of surgery. Additional bronchodilators may be needed throughout the perioperative period.
      2. Patients with **cardiac disease** should be optimized before elective procedures. For patients with a pacemaker or automatic implantable cardioverter defibrillator (AICD), basic information about the device (eg, indication for placement, last battery check, dependency, and underlying rhythm) should be available on the day of the procedure.
      3. **Additional comorbidities and medications** should be reviewed, and the plan customized accordingly.
   B. The need for transfusion is fairly rare during IP procedures. However, in the presence of anemia or known antibodies, a type and screen should be available on the day of the procedure.
   C. **Hemodynamic Instability** may occur in patients with severe COPD (due to high intrathoracic pressure secondary to increased lung volumes, causing a decrease in venous return and cardiac output), or as a consequence of the ventilator settings or pneumothorax, requiring continuous blood pressure monitoring either via arterial line or noninvasive devices.
   D. A detailed conversation with the interventional pulmonologist should take place before the start of the case about the specific procedure and the possible complications, including the potential for loss of the airway. A plan for airway rescue should be developed that is tailored to patient and procedural factors. Any additional equipment that may be needed for rescue should be collected before the procedure starts.

VII. Management of Interventional Pulmonology–Specific Intraprocedural Complications
   While complications are uncommon during IP procedures, when they do occur, they may be life-threatening, since the airway is being manipulated and patients undergoing these procedures may have limited reserve.
   A. **Airway Irritability:** Cough, bronchospasm, and laryngospasm are the most common complications. Nebulized lidocaine is usually effective in suppressing cough. Bronchospasm responds well to nebulized β-agonists (albuterol), anticholinergics (ipratropium), and racemic epinephrine. Laryngospasm can be managed by deepening the anesthetic, positive pressure, and/or administration of paralytics.
   B. **Airway Loss:** IP procedures involve sharing the airway, and loss of airway control can result in respiratory arrest and death. Communication with the interventional pulmonologist and detailed planning are instrumental in preventing this potentially fatal complication. Specifically, different ETT and SGA sizes, an airway exchange catheter, jet ventilation, or ECMO may be needed and should be set up ahead of time, if necessary.
   C. **Airway Bleeding:** Certain procedures (eg, cryobiopsy, stent placement) can cause significant airway bleeding, and this risk is exacerbated by certain patient-specific factors (eg, history of chest irradiation, renal cell, or sarcoma metastasis to the airway). Bronchial blockers can be used to tamponade the source of bleeding and are placed at the hemorrhagic source until bleeding stops, which may take only minutes or may take longer to abate. Ongoing airway bleeding may require arterial embolization by an interventional radiologist, postprocedural mechanical ventilation, and intensive care unit (ICU) care. When transferring patients on

mechanical ventilated with a bronchial blocker in place, providers should monitor for the potential dislodgment of the blocker, resulting in a tracheal conclusion and causing an inability to deliver tidal volumes.

D. Airway Fire: The use of lasers or any other heat source in the presence of high FIO_2 can result in airway fire. Prevention is paramount and can be achieved by lowering the FIO_2 before using the laser. In case of airway fire, the patient should be disconnected from the circuit, the fresh gas flow stopped, and the ETT removed. Saline should be used to extinguish the fire. After the fire is quenched, the patient should be reintubated and bronchoscopy should be done to assess the extent of damage. Maintenance FIO_2 should be minimized, and administration of steroids should be considered to decrease airway edema.

E. Pneumothorax: This can occur as a result of needle biopsy, especially in at-risk patients, such as those with severe COPD or emphysema. If real-time CT is used during the procedure, the diagnosis can be made before leaving the IP suite. The diagnosis can also be made via physical examination, ultrasound, or chest x-ray in the postanesthesia care unit (PACU); this may be done routinely after high-risk procedures, or it may be prompted by hypoxemia and/or dyspnea. If the patient is asymptomatic, the pneumothorax can be observed. Oxygen delivered via nasal cannula can expedite the reabsorption of air and decrease the size of the pneumothorax. If the patient is symptomatic, a pigtail catheter should be placed to decompress the chest cavity.

F. Failure to Extubate: At the end of the procedure, patients need to meet extubation criteria before extubation; the patient must be awake, fully reversed from residual muscle paralysis, normothermic, and have adequate vital signs and minute ventilation. Extra vigilance and caution should be exerted when extubating patients following an IP procedure, due to their underlying compromised pulmonary status and the additional irritation caused by the procedure. Patients may need short-term mechanical ventilation if they are unable to meet extubation criteria or have excessive airway irritability. Patients must remain stable following extubation before being transferred out of the IP suite. The sitting position improves respiratory compliance and is recommended after extubation; noninvasive positive-pressure ventilation may be considered for postextubation respiratory support, especially in patients with COPD. Reintubation may be necessary in the presence of severe bronchospasm, unrecognized airway edema, or inadequate ventilation.

REFERENCES

1. Folch E, Mittal A, Oberg C. Robotic bronchoscopy and future directions of interventional pulmonology. *Curr Opin Pulm Med.* 2022;28(1):37-44.
2. Dhooria S, Chaudhary S, Ram B, et al. A randomized trial of nebulized lignocaine, lignocaine spray, or their combination for topical anesthesia during diagnostic flexible bronchoscopy. *Chest.* 2020;157(1):198-204.
3. Madan K, Mittal S, Gupta N, et al. The cricothyroid versus spray-as-you-go method for topical anesthesia during bronchoscopy: the CRISP randomized clinical trial. *Respiration.* 2019;98(5):440-446.
4. El Mourad MB, Elghamry MR, Mansour RF, et al. Comparison of intravenous dexmedetomidine-propofol versus ketofol for sedation during awake fibeoptic intubation: a prospective, randomized study. *Anesth Pain Med.* 2019;9(1):e86442.
5. Lee K, Orme R, Williams D, et al. Prospective pilot trial of dexmedetomidine sedation for awake diagnostic flexible bronchoscopy. *J Bronchology Interv Pulmonol.* 2010;17(1):323-328.
6. Pedoto A, Kalchiem-Dekel O, Baselice S, et al. Ultrasound-guided midpoint transverse process to pleura nerve block for medical thoracoscopy: a case report. *A A Pract.* 2020;14(8):e01240.
7. Sagar AS. Sabath BF, Eapen GA, et al. Incidence and location of atelectasis developed during bronchoscopy under general anesthesia: the I-LOCATE trial. *Chest.* 2020;158(6):2658-2666.
8. Salahuddin M, Sarkiss M, Sagar AS, et al. Ventilatory strategy to prevent atelectasis during bronchoscopy under general anesthesia: a multicenter randomized controlled trial (VESPA trial). *Chest.* 2022;162(6):1393-1401.
9. Goudra BG, Singh PM, Borle A, et al. Anesthesia for advanced bronchoscopic procedures: state-of-the-art review. *Lung.* 2015;193(4):453-465.
10. Klachiem-Dekel O, Connolly JG, Lin IH, et al. Shape-sensing robotic-assisted bronchoscopy in the diagnosis of pulmonary parenchymal lesions. *Chest.* 2022;161(2):572-582.
11. Bhadra K, Setser RM, Condra W, et al. Lung navigation ventilation protocol to optimize biopsy of peripheral lung lesions. *J Bronchology Interv Pulmonol.* 2022;29(1):7-17.
12. Lin J, Sabath BF, Sarkiss M, et al. Lateral decubitus positioning for mobile CT-guided robotic bronchoscopy: a novel technique to prevent atelectasis. *J Bronchology Interv Pulmonol.* 2022;29(3):220-223.
13. Putz L, Mayné A, Dincq AS. Jet ventilation during rigid bronchoscopy in adults: a focused review. *Biomed Res Int.* 2016;2016:4234861.

14. Ernst A, Anantham D, Eberhardt R, et al. Diagnosis of mediastinal adenopathy-real-time endobronchial ultrasound guided needle aspiration versus mediastinoscopy. *J Thorac Oncol.* 2008;3(6):577-582.
15. Adams K, Shah PL, Edmonds L, et al. Test performance of endobronchial ultrasound and transbronchial needle aspiration biopsy for mediastinal staging in patients with lung cancer: systematic review and meta-analysis. *Thorax.* 2009;64(9):757-762.
16. Vaidya PJ, Munavvar M, Leuppi JD, et al. Endobronchial ultrasound-guided transbronchial needle aspiration: safe as it sounds. *Respirology.* 2017;22(6):1093-1101.
17. Pedoto A, Desiderio DP, Amar D, et al. Hemodynamic instability following airway spray cryotherapy. *Anesth Analg.* 2016;123(5):1302-1306.
18. Dhillon, SS, Harryanto H, Randhawa S, et al. Transbronchial lung cryobiopsy: a meticulous technique. *J Bronchology Interv Pulmonol.* 2020;27(2):e19-e22.
19. Ratwani AP, Davis A, Maldonado F. Current practices in the management of central airway obstruction. *Curr Opin Pulm Med.* 2022;28:45-51.
20. Pertzov B, Gershman E, Izhakian S, et al. Placement of self-expanding metallic tracheobronchial Y stent with laryngeal mask airway using conscious sedation under fluoroscopic guidance. *Thorac Cancer.* 2021;12(4):484-490.
21. Barnwell N, Lenihan M. Anaesthesia for airway stenting. *BJA Educ.* 2022;22(4):160-166.
22. Hashmi MD, Khan A, Shafiq M. Bronchial thermoplasty: state of the art. *Respirology.* 2022;27(9):720-729.
23. Bolliger CT, Sutedja TG, Strausz J, et al. Therapeutic bronchoscopy with immediate effect: laser, electrocautery, argon plasma coagulation and stents. *Eur Respir J.* 2006;27(6):1258-1271.
24. Sullivan EA. Anesthetic considerations for special thoracic procedures. *Thorac Surg Clin.* 2005;15(1):131-142.
25. Murphy MC, Wrobel MM, Fisher DA, et al. Update on image-guided thermal lung ablation: society guidelines, therapeutic alternatives, and postablation imaging findings. *AJR Am J Roentgenol.* 2022;219(3):471-485.
26. Tan Z, Tan KT, Poopalalingam R. Anesthetic management for whole lung lavage in patients with pulmonary alveolar proteinosis. *A A Case Rep.* 2016;6(8):234-237.

V Perioperative Medicine

27

Perioperative Evaluation

Kenneth Cheung and Stefan Dieleman

KEY POINTS

1. Investigations can be divided into cardiac and noncardiac categories.
2. Specific tests should be guided by a patient's pathology and medical history.
3. Investigations should not be repeated and performed only when necessary.

I. Introduction

Patients undergoing cardiothoracic surgery generally have an established diagnosis. The purpose of preoperative investigations is to identify the severity and stability of their disease, to aid surgical planning, and to guide perioperative medical management, including preoperative optimization. Investigations can be divided into cardiac and noncardiac-specific tests. Additional testing is guided by the patient's comorbidities and symptoms. These range from serologic testing to specific imaging and physiologic testing. It is important for the anesthesiologist to be able to review, interpret, and understand the implications of the results.

It is important to practice responsibly and be able to justify the need for a given test. Tests not only carry a financial cost, but invasive tests may also carry inherent risk or lead to unnecessary treatments or procedures. Therefore, it is essential that investigations are performed only when necessary.

II. Noncardiac Evaluation

A. Laboratory Tests

Blood tests such as a complete blood count, a metabolic panel (electrolytes, glucose, renal function), a coagulation profile, and blood group testing are routinely performed.

1. **Complete blood count:** Specifically identifying anemia, low platelet count, infection
   a. In the case of preoperative anemia and/or thrombocytopenia, causes should be identified, investigated, and treated as able.
   b. Preoperative infection may be associated with altered white blood cell counts and significantly increases perioperative morbidity. Prompt investigation, treatment, and, possibly, a delay in surgery are warranted.
2. **Metabolic panel**
   a. **Renal function:** Identifying renal dysfunction and associated electrolyte imbalance, such as hyperkalemia, hypermagnesemia, or hyponatremia
      (1) Preexisting renal dysfunction may put a patient at a high risk of postoperative acute kidney injury, potentially requiring renal replacement therapy.
      (2) Electrolyte imbalances place a patient at high risk of arrhythmias.

3. **Hemoglobin A1c:** Detects diabetes mellitus and adequacy of blood sugar control
   a. Optimal hemoglobin A1c (HbA1c) is <6.5%. Higher levels represent suboptimal glycemic control, which is associated with increased morbidity, sternal wound infection/breakdown, and perioperative ischemic events.[1]
   b. Patients with untreated diabetes before elective cardiac surgery will require specialist input and optimization before their surgery, provided that the acuity of their surgical condition allows for a delay.
4. **Coagulation profile:** This includes prothrombin time (PT), activated partial thromboplastin clotting time (aPTT), and international normalized ratio (INR). Dynamic tests such as thromboelastography (TEG) or rotational thromboelastometry (ROTEM) can also be utilized to better characterize coagulation status.
   a. In the absence of anticoagulation therapy, abnormal PT/aPTT could identify patients with bleeding diathesis, who may need a hematology consult and possibly preoperative correction.
   b. TEG or ROTEM, with or without platelet mapping, could be utilized in patients in an emergency setting with perioperative bleeding or those with ongoing antiplatelet therapy. This will help guide early preparation to manage bleeding, such as the use of cell salvage, blood products, or adjuncts, such as DDAVP.

CLINICAL PEARL

In patients who have been on prolonged heparin infusion and/or who have a borderline aPTT despite seemingly adequate rates of heparin infusion preoperatively, the assessment of antithrombin III levels should be considered. A relative lack of antithrombin III can make heparin less effective and may, therefore, need to be corrected, for example, by administration of fresh-frozen plasma or antithrombin III concentrate (where locally available) before heparinization.

5. **Blood type and screen, and crossmatching:** Cardiac surgery is major surgery with high risk of perioperative bleeding.
   a. Preoperative type and screen should always be performed in patients scheduled for cardiac surgery. Testing defines the ABO group and Rhesus (Rh) factor type. Screening detects atypical antibodies. Crossmatching packed red blood cells is recommended before most open cardiac surgical procedures.
   b. Some patients may have additional antibodies that require specific blood products. Anesthesiologists should be aware of this and ensure the availability of such products to minimize delay in treatment in case blood product transfusion is warranted.
B. **Noncardiac-Specific Imagining**
   1. **Chest x-ray:** A preoperative x-ray can provide important information regarding lung fields, cardiac silhouette, and, on a lateral view, proximity of the right ventricular (RV) free wall to the sternum.
      a. Lung-field abnormalities, such as pleural effusion or pulmonary edema, may indicate congestive cardiac failure, which can then be optimized before surgery.
      b. Coarse lung markings, bullae, or hyperexpanded lung fields suggestive of respiratory disease may prompt further pulmonary function testing (PFT).
      c. Baseline chest x-ray (CXR) may provide subsequent comparisons for CXRs made postoperatively.
      d. Lateral CXR could help assess the risk of unintentional right atrial/RV/aortic injury in patients undergoing repeat cardiac surgery. However, computed tomography (CT) scanning is more commonly used for such an assessment.
   2. **Computed tomographic angiography:** CT angiography provides reliable assessment of mediastinal structures, especially their relationship between chest wall and cardiovascular structures, coronary artery grafts, and the RV.
      a. Close proximity to the sternum of an adherent coronary artery graft (Figure 27.1) or the RV-free wall (Figure 27.2). Modification to a different surgical technique and/or peripheral cannulation for cardiopulmonary bypass may need to occur before sternotomy.

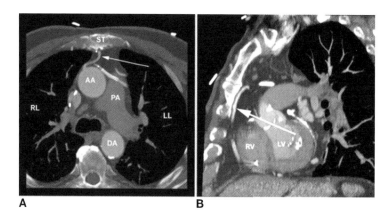

FIGURE 27.1 **(A)** Axial views of a contrast-enhanced multidetector computed tomographic angiography (MDCTA) of the chest demonstrating an adherent aortocoronary graft (arrow) to the underside of the ST. **(B)** Sagittal views of a contrast-enhanced MDCTA of the chest demonstrating an adherent aortocoronary graft (arrow) to the underside of the ST. AA, ascending aorta; DA, descending aorta; LL, left lung; LV, left ventricle; PA, pulmonary artery; RL, right lung; RV, right ventricle; ST, sternum. (Reprinted from Kamdar AR, Meadows TA, Roselli EE, et al. Multidetector computed tomographic angiography in planning of reoperative cardiothoracic surgery. *Ann Thorac Surg.* 2008;85(4):1239-1245. © 2008 The Society of Thoracic Surgeons. With permission.)

3. **Carotid duplex ultrasound:** The incidence of cerebrovascular complications after coronary artery bypass grafting (CABG) is estimated to be between 1.6% and 3%.[2] According to the American Heart Association, preoperative carotid duplex ultrasound should be performed in patients who are >65 years and have left main coronary disease, peripheral vascular disease, a history of tobacco use, a history of prior cerebral vascular disease, or a carotid bruit.

   a. Patients with significant carotid stenosis may benefit from precardiac surgery carotid intervention to minimize perioperative stroke risk. However, there are conflicting data regarding the benefit of preoperative carotid interventions.

   b. Consider higher cerebral perfusion pressure when the patient is on cardiopulmonary bypass if there is significant carotid stenosis.

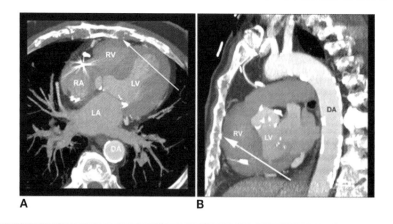

FIGURE 27.2 **(A)** Axial views of a contrast-enhanced multidetector computed tomographic angiography (MDCTA) of the chest demonstrating an adherent RV-free wall (arrow) to the underside of the sternum. **(B)** Sagittal views of a contrast-enhanced MDCTA of the chest demonstrating an adherent RV-free wall (arrow) to the underside of the sternum. DA, descending aorta; LA, left atrium; LV, left ventricle; RA, right atrium; RV, right ventricle. (Reprinted from Kamdar AR, Meadows TA, Roselli EE, et al. Multidetector computed tomographic angiography in planning of reoperative cardiothoracic surgery. *Ann Thorac Surg.* 2008;85(4):1239-1245. © 2008 The Society of Thoracic Surgeons. With permission.)

4. **Pulmonary function test:** PFTs are only indicated if a patient's history, examination, and smoking history are suggestive of significant lung disease. It can be used for identification of obstructive or restrictive lung disease and assessment of its severity.

   a. A poor preoperative lung function is associated with a much higher risk of morbidity and mortality in patients undergoing cardiac surgery.

   b. Reversible obstruction found on a PFT can be treated with bronchodilators.

III. **Cardiac-Specific Evaluation**

A. **Resting Electrocardiogram**

Although, in most patients presenting for cardiac surgery, a resting electrocardiogram (ECG) will have been done at some point, it is good to make sure that a recent preoperative ECG is available. This can be used to determine a baseline for rate, rhythm, infarct location, and other preexisting abnormalities.

B. **Echocardiography**

Transthoracic echocardiography (TTE) is an integral component of preoperative evaluation. It provides an essential qualitative and quantitative assessment of valvular pathologies, regional wall abnormalities, chamber size and function, pericardial disease, and septal defects. This can guide surgical planning and anesthesia management and can also provide a good indication of any potential issues in the postoperative period.

Transesophageal echocardiogram (TEE) is not routinely performed preoperatively; however, certain pathology identified by TTE may need further evaluation before surgery. TEE may be indicated in patients with intracardiac mass or for patients with congenital cardiac abnormalities to evaluate previous repairs/shunts and valvular/subvalvular pathology. In particular, the mitral valve is in an ideal position to examine with TEE, given its close proximity to the probe, allowing closer two-dimensional (2D) and 3D inspection (Figure 27.3A,B) of any valvular pathology and aiding in surgical planning. For a detailed overview of perioperative echocardiography, refer to Chapter 4.

C. **Diagnostic Cardiac Catheterization**

1. **Overview**

All patients for CABG and most other open-heart surgery would have had cardiac catheterization performed. Left heart catheterization is the gold standard investigation to definitively assess coronary anatomy, as well as the location and severity of coronary lesions. Ventricular and valvular function can also be assessed if indicated. Right heart catheterization (RHC) is only indicated to assess the severity of pulmonary hypertension, right-sided pressures, or pulmonary and systemic vascular resistance.

Cardiac catheterization is an invasive procedure and carries risk. There is a 0.1% incidence of stroke, death, or myocardial infarction. Other issues relating to access site complications occur in ~0.5% of patients.

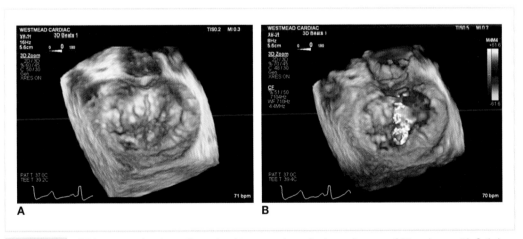

FIGURE 27.3 **(A)** Intraoperative three-dimensional transesophageal echocardiogram of P2 prolapse with flail chordae. **(B)** Corresponding anteriorly directed mitral regurgitant jet. (Courtesy of Echo Library, Westmead Hospital.)

2. Left heart catheterization

Arterial access for left heart catheterization is gained via femoral or radial approach. Specific catheters are placed at the coronary ostia, and radioopaque contrast is injected to visualize and assess the coronary anatomy and degree of stenosis.

a. Anatomy

Coronary arterial dominance is defined by the vessel that gives rise to the posterior descending artery (PDA) that supplies the inferior septum. Right coronary artery (RCA) dominance is most common (80%-85% of patients). Left dominance (15%-25% of patients) is where the PDA is supplied by the left circumflex (LCx) artery. Codominance implies that the supply of the inferior septum is shared by both RCA and LCx artery. Knowledge of coronary anatomy (Figure 27.4) as well as the location and severity of stenotic lesions is important for the cardiac anesthesiologist. It allows for correlation of intraoperative ischemic changes on ECG as well as regional wall motion abnormalities detected on TEE.

b. Assessment of coronary arteries

Lesion severity can be characterized visually, physiologically, or via intravascular ultrasound.

(1) Visual assessment: Upon visual assessment, significant stenosis is diagnosed when there is ≥70% stenosis of the coronary lumen in all branches, except the main left coronary artery, where the cutoff for significant stenosis is ≥50%. Length of lesion should also be considered; however, there is no consensus to classify a severe stenosis. More objective assessment could be performed using quantitative coronary

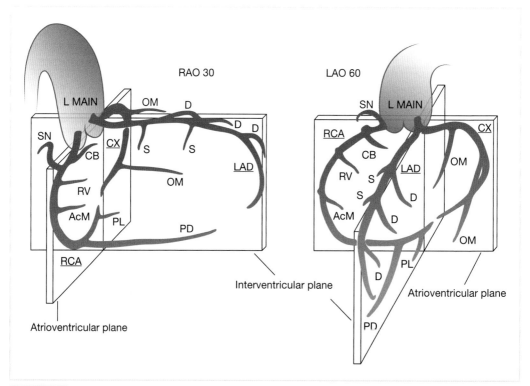

FIGURE 27.4 Representation of coronary anatomy relative to the interventricular and atrioventricular valve planes. AcM, acute marginal; CB, conus branch; CX, circumflex; D, diagonal; LAD, left anterior descending; LAO 60, left anterior oblique 60° view; L MAIN, left main; PD, posterior descending; PL, posterolateral left ventricular; OM, obtuse marginal; RAO 30, right anterior oblique 30° view; RCA, right coronary artery; RV, right ventricle; S, septal; SN, sinus node. (Reprinted with permission from Moscucci M. Coronary angiography. In: Moscucci M, ed. *Grossman & Baim's Cardiac Catheterization, Angiography, and Intervention.* 9th ed. Wolters Kluwer; 2021:303-342. Figure 15.17.)

angiography (QCA) (Figure 27.5). QCA uses computer-generated edge-detection systems and 3D reconstruction from various orthogonal views to objectively assess luminal diameter. The difference in mean diameter of the lumen between these two methods varies between 10% and 20%. Therefore, assessment of a lesion, especially when it concerns an intermediate-grade stenosis, requires multiple projections as well as other modalities described later.

(2) **Physiologic assessment:** Fractional flow reserve (FFR) is one of the most common physiologic methods of further assessing lesion significance, especially when there is an intermediate stenosis (40%-69%) on visual assessment. FFR is defined as the ratio of maximum flow in the presence of a stenosis to normal maximum flow. For example, an FFR of 0.70 means that the stenosis causes a 30% drop in flow. An FFR <0.8 may warrant intervention.[3]

c. Intravascular ultrasound

Intravascular ultrasound (IVUS) is performed using a specialized catheter with ultrasound crystals at the distal end (Figure 27.6). This allows in vivo examination of atherosclerotic lesions with visualization of plaque burden and characteristics within the vascular wall. IVUS allows precise tomographic measurement of lumen area, plaque size, distribution, and composition.[4] In contrast, angiography only visualizes the 2D silhouette of the lumen.

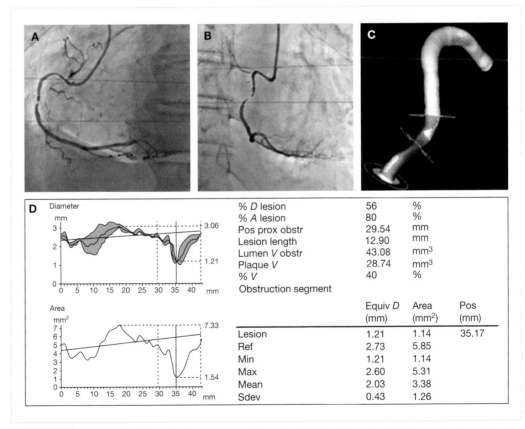

FIGURE 27.5 An example of quantitative coronary angiography with three-dimensional (3D) reconstruction of the right coronary artery **(Panel C)** of two selected 2D views **(Panel A:** Left anterior, **Panel B:** Right anterior oblique). Parameters such as lesion length and percentage luminal obstruction can be obtained via 3D contour detection and reconstruction of the artery in question **(Panel D).** A, area; D, diameter; V, volume. (Reprinted from Nishi T, Kitahara H, Fujimoto Y, et al. Comparison of 3-dimensional and 2-dimensional quantitative coronary angiography and intravascular ultrasound for functional assessment of coronary lesions. *J Cardiol.* 2017;69(1):280-286. © 2016 Japanese College of Cardiology. With permission.)

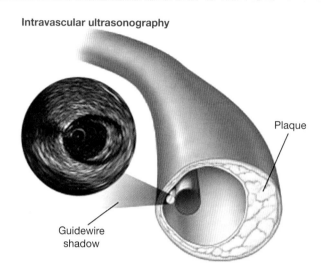

FIGURE 27.6   Intravascular ultrasonography. (Reprinted with permission from Schoenhagen P, White RD, Nissen SE, Tuzcu EM. Coronary imaging: angiography shows the stenosis, but IVUS, CT, and MRI show the plaque. *Cleve Clin J Med.* 2003;70(8):713-719. © 2003 The Cleveland Clinic Foundation. All Rights Reserved.)

CLINICAL PEARL

Particular attention must be paid to patients with severe left main coronary artery disease as it is responsible for supplying 75% of the left ventricle in right dominant type or 100% in the left dominant type. Significant reduction in blood flow will lead to cardiac failure and arrhythmias.[5] During the induction of anesthesia, this requires meticulous attention to preserve blood flow by maintaining adequate systemic blood pressure as well as the ability to perform immediate cardioversion.

3. **Right heart catheterization**

There is a vast amount of information that could be gained from RHC. Measurements could be either direct or indirect (Table 27.1).

In the preoperative setting, the most common reason to perform RHC is to confirm the diagnosis of pulmonary hypertension, guide treatment options, as well as to assess the contribution of left-sided heart disease. Other uses include assessing patients with complex congenital heart disease, left-to-right shunts, or severe valvular disease.

D. **Computed Tomographic Coronary Angiography:** CT with radioopaque contrast can be used as an initial, noninvasive test to screen for the presence of coronary artery disease. This test has a high sensitivity but lower specificity, meaning that a negative computed tomographic coronary angiography (CTCA) predominantly rules out coronary artery disease. Similar to IVUS, CTCA also allows for visualization of vessel walls and identifies high-risk plaques that are associated with acute coronary syndrome.

Calculating a so-called calcium score from a CTCA can also be used to risk stratify coronary artery disease. High-calcium deposit is an independent marker for risk of major adverse cardiac events. It should be noted that this is a screening test, and a positive test will warrant cardiac catheterization as outlined earlier.

E. **Aortic Assessment With Computed Tomography:** CT angiography of the aorta is performed in patients with suspected aortic dissection or aortic aneurysm. This allows assessment of the extent of the dissection/aneurysm and involvement of any other vessels, particularly the three branches of the aortic arch, which may have a significant impact on intraoperative/surgical planning.

TABLE 27.1   Possible Direct and Indirect Measurements From Right Heart Catheterization

Direct	Indirect
Central venous pressure	Systemic vascular resistance
Right-sided cardiac pressures	Pulmonary vascular resistance
Pulmonary artery pressure	Cardiac index
Pulmonary capillary occlusion pressure	Stroke volume index
Cardiac output	Oxygen delivery and uptake
Mixed venous oxyhemoglobin saturation	Left and right ventricle stroke work index

F. **Cardiac Magnetic Resonance Imaging:** In recent years, cardiac magnetic resonance (CMR) imaging has emerged as a highly specialized option for noninvasive evaluation of the heart. Although the clinical utility of CMR is extremely broad, it is particularly useful in the assessment of myocardial/pericardial/valvular heart disease, chamber anatomy, motion and function, myocardial morphology or mass, and complex congenital cardiac disease. Despite the breadth of CMR's clinical application, more simple, accessible, and cost-effective investigations such as echocardiography should be used as the first line.

1. **Myocardial disease**

   CMR can assess diseases ranging from ischemic, inflammatory, infiltrative, and other causes of cardiomyopathy. With the use of gadolinium contrast, viability and reversibility of myocardial damage can be quantified, and it, therefore, is an excellent prognostication tool.

   Due to CMR's high-spatial resolution, it is also excellent in assessing hypertrophic cardiomyopathy or infiltrative diseases, such as cardiac sarcoidosis, amyloidosis, or hemochromatosis.

2. **Valvular heart disease**

   For the evaluation of valvular heart disease, echocardiography is still the first-line modality due to its high temporal resolution. However, valve pathology can be better assessed by CMR, especially in patients with suboptimal or indeterminate echocardiography images. Similar to echocardiography, quantitative analysis of regurgitant/stenotic lesions could also be performed.

3. **Intracardiac mass**

   High-spatial resolution allows for the evaluation of intracardiac masses with the use of different magnetic resonance imaging (MRI) sequences. CMR could be used to differentiate between an actual intracardiac mass and normal variants. Examples include differentiation between a possible thrombus and a coumadin ridge or a Chiari network (a thrombus will have a low T2 and postcontrast sequence signal), between lipomatous hypertrophy of interatrial septum and a lipoma, or between benign cardiac lesions and potential metastatic lesions.

4. **Congenital cardiac disease**

   CMR is particularly useful in congenital cardiac disease. It helps not only to better evaluate the type of previous repairs performed but also to evaluate scarring/fibrosis, delineate anatomy, as well as quantify any shunts that may be present. Furthermore, the absence of radiation is ideal for the ongoing follow-up that usually occurs in this patient group.

G. **Provocative Testing**

1. **Overview**

   Cardiac exercise stress testing (EST) is a diagnostic and prognostic tool to evaluate patients with suspected ischemic heart disease. Although all patients undergoing cardiac surgery will have a coronary angiogram, provocative testing is usually the first step in the process of risk assessment and diagnosing ischemic heart disease due to its low-cost and noninvasive nature.

   In order to perform an EST, a baseline resting state is initially recorded. Stress is usually in the form of physical exertion, such as a treadmill or an exercise bike. Pharmacologic

TABLE 27.2 Absolute Contraindications for Exercise Stress Testing

Absolute Contraindication

- Acute myocardial infarction, within 2 d
- Ongoing unstable angina
- Uncontrolled cardiac arrhythmia with hemodynamic compromise
- Active endocarditis
- Symptomatic severe aortic stenosis
- Decompensated heart failure
- Acute pulmonary embolism, pulmonary infarction, or deep vein thrombosis
- Acute myocarditis or pericarditis
- Acute aortic dissection
- Physical disability that precludes safe and adequate testing

stress, such as dobutamine to increase myocardial workload, is usually reserved for patients who are unable to exercise.

Assessment of myocardial ischemia during an EST can be done in several ways. The most commonly used modalities include continuous ECG, stress echocardiography, and radionuclide myocardial perfusion imaging (rMPI). Each assessment has its own advantages and disadvantages as well as different performance compared to invasive coronary angiography as the reference standard (Table 27.3). There are a number of contraindications for EST[6] (Table 27.2), and the potential risks should always be weighed against the perceived benefits.

2. **Exercise electrocardiographic test**
This is the most common form of stress test, due to its simplicity, relatively cost efficiency, and results being well validated. Continuous ECG monitoring during protocolized exercise allows indirect detection of myocardial ischemia, which manifests as ST-segment depression or elevation.

3. **Stress echocardiography**
A resting echocardiography is usually obtained for baseline comparison as patients may have preexisting regional wall abnormalities. Stress echocardiography helps to detect hemodynamically significant coronary artery disease and localized regions of ischemia. New or worsened regional wall abnormalities, a decrease in left ventricular ejection fraction, or an increased left ventricular end-systolic volume may indicate obstructive coronary artery disease.

TABLE 27.3 Sensitivity and Specificity of Noninvasive Tests to Diagnose the Presence of Coronary Heart Disease

	Diagnosis of Coronary Artery Disease	
	Sensitivity (%)	Specificity (%)
Exercise ECG	45-61	70-90
Exercise stress echocardiography	70-85	77-89
Exercise stress SPECT	73-92	63-88
Pharmacologic stress echocardiography	72-90	79-95
Pharmacologic stress SPECT	88-91	75-90
CT coronary angiogram	93-99	64-90

CT, computed tomography; ECG, electrocardiography; SPECT, single-photon emission computed tomography.

Garber AM, Hlatky MA, Chareonthaitawee P. Stress testing for the diagnosis of obstructive coronary heart disease. *UpToDate*. Accessed November 21, 2022. http://www.uptodate.com

4. **Radionuclide myocardial perfusion imaging**

This modality involves the administration of radioactive perfusion tracer, a specialized camera system, and equipment to detect γ photons. Resting and stress series images are taken. The distribution of the tracer in myocardium is proportional to coronary blood flow, thus allowing comparison of relative blood flow to different regions of the heart. Furthermore, myocytes with intact membrane transport mechanisms facilitate tracer uptake and retention, therefore indicating viable myocytes. Resting images convey the presence or absence of viable myocardium, while stress images relay information regarding stress-induced ischemia. Viability testing is particularly important for surgical planning as grafting to nonviable myocardium is not beneficial.

CLINICAL PEARL

Emergency cardiac surgery carries a higher risk of morbidity and mortality. These patients often have limited investigations performed before surgery due to the time-sensitive nature of their disease. Minimum requirements would include blood work, blood group, ECG, coronary angiogram, CXR, and, where feasible, an echocardiogram. TEG with platelet mapping and coagulation profile should also be considered in a patient requiring emergency bypass surgery if they have had recent loading of dual-antiplatelet drugs.

REFERENCES

1. Engelman DT, Ali WB, Williams JB, et al. Guidelines for perioperative care in cardiac surgery: enhanced recovery after surgery society recommendations. *JAMA Surg.* 2019;154(8):755-766.
2. Nah HW, Lee JW, Chung CH, et al. New brain infarcts on magnetic resonance imaging after coronary artery bypass graft surgery: lesion patterns, mechanism, and predictors. *Ann Neurol.* 2014;76:347.
3. Lawton JS, Tamis-Holland JE, Bangalore S, et al. 2021 ACC/AHA/SCAI guideline for coronary artery revascularization: a report of the American College of Cardiology/American Heart Association Joint Committee on Clinical Practice Guidelines. *Circulation.* 2022;145(3):e18-e114.
4. Nissen SE, Yock P. Intravascular ultrasound: novel pathophysiological insights and current clinical applications. *Circulation.* 2001;103(4):604-616.
5. Kalbfleisch H, Hort W. Quantitative study on the size of coronary artery supplying areas postmortem. *Am Heart J.* 1977;94:183-188.
6. Fletcher GF, Ades PA, Kligfield P, et al. Exercise standards for testing and training: a scientific statement from the American Heart Association. *Circulation.* 2013;128(8):873-934.

28

Patient Blood Management

Nadia B. Hensley, Megan P. Kostibas, Colleen G. Koch, and Steven M. Frank

KEY POINTS

1. Blood transfusion is the most common procedure performed in U.S. hospitals and has been named one of the top five overused procedures by The Joint Commission.
2. Both anemia and transfusion carry significant risks. Balancing these risks is the key to appropriate blood transfusion decisions.
3. Despite published guidelines, clinical transfusion practice still varies substantially among clinicians and centers and often falls outside recommended guidelines.
4. Transfusion-associated circulatory overload (TACO) is the most frequent cause of mortality from blood transfusion. The second most frequent cause of mortality is transfusion-related acute lung injury (TRALI).
5. Three large hemoglobin (Hb) trigger trials in cardiac surgery support the use of a restrictive transfusion strategy with Hb triggers of 7.5-8 g/dL; no improvement in primary outcomes was attained with higher triggers (9-10 g/dL).
6. Treating preoperative anemia and intraoperative antifibrinolytic therapy represent important opportunities to reduce unnecessary transfusions in cardiac surgery.
7. Viscoelastic testing assesses whole-blood clotting characteristics, which allows targeted transfusion therapy.

"**BLOOD TRANSFUSION IS LIKE MARRIAGE:** *it should not be entered upon lightly, unadvisedly or wantonly or more often than is absolutely necessary.*"

—*R. Beale*[1]

I. **Introduction**

Blood transfusion is the most common procedure performed in U.S. hospitals and has been named one of the top five overused procedures by The Joint Commission. Competing risks form the core of perioperative transfusion. Patients face tangible risk if hemoglobin (Hb) values fall too low, and different but equally real risk when exposed to allogeneic blood transfusion. The risks of both anemia and transfusion vary depending on the patient's comorbidities, degree of and ability to tolerate anemia, and surgical procedure. In the dynamic milieu of the operating rooms, clinicians caring for cardiovascular surgical patients encounter challenging transfusion decisions daily. No measures can definitively direct transfusion decisions; rather, clinical judgment based on the balance of perceived risks and benefits must guide individual transfusion decisions. Given this background, the substantial variability of transfusion even within a single institution becomes understandable.[2,3]

A. **Practice Patterns Vary Widely for Transfusion of All Three Major Blood Components in Cardiac Surgery**

   1. **The wide variation in transfusion practice patterns was highlighted in a nationwide study in 2010. More than 100,000 patients undergoing isolated coronary artery bypass graft surgery were included from almost 800 hospitals.**[3] Such variability often serves as the impetus for evidence-based guidelines that are intended to reconcile disparate evidence.

   2. The most widely cited guideline for transfusion practice in cardiac surgery is the guideline for patient blood management (PBM) in cardiac surgery published jointly by the Society of Thoracic Surgeons (STS) and Society of Cardiovascular Anesthesiologists, which was last updated in 2021.[4]

B. **Patient Blood Management Programs**

   1. **PBM programs are somewhat new but are being implemented in many hospitals with the goal of reducing risks, improving outcomes, and lowering costs.**[5]

   2. The Society for Advancement of Blood Management defines patient blood management as "Patient blood management is a patient-centered, systematic, evidence-based approach to improve patient outcomes by managing and preserving a patient's own blood, while promoting patient safety and empowerment."

   3. The primary goal of PBM is to reduce unnecessary transfusions. Several methods of blood conservation discussed in this chapter are being effectively utilized in PBM programs.

   4. The Joint Commission, along with Association for the Advancement of Blood and Biotherapies (AABB), introduced a certification for PBM in 2016. Certification enables hospitals to be recognized for successfully implementing these valuable methods of care that are considered advancements in patient safety and quality.

CLINICAL PEARL

Anemia, bleeding, and transfusion are all associated with adverse outcomes. It is, therefore, important to treat and prevent anemia, minimize bleeding, and transfuse blood and blood components according to evidence-based indications.

C. **Complications of Transfusion**

   1. Complications of transfusion have always been a major concern, highlighted by the threat of transfusion-transmitted viral infections, such as human immunodeficiency virus (HIV).[6] Now, with nucleic acid testing for HIV and hepatitis C, the risk for transmission of these viruses is similar to that of dying from an airline crash or lightning strike.[7]

   2. The decrease in infection risk has led some to assume that blood is incredibly safe; however, transfusion poses much more common and potentially life-threatening events that should be recognized.

4

3. **The Food and Drug Administration's (FDA) summary of fatalities related to transfusion for fiscal years 2018-2020 listed transfusion-associated circulatory overload (TACO) and transfusion-related acute lung injury (TRALI) as the first and second most frequent causes of mortality from transfusion, respectively (Figure 28.1).**[8] Between 2018 and 2020, 32% of deaths were from TACO, and 22% were from TRALI. Hemolytic transfusion reactions caused by non-ABO (17%) and ABO (8%) incompatibilities were also the causes for mortality. Microbial contamination and allergic/anaphylactic reactions each accounted for 10% of transfusion-related mortalities.

   a. TACO presents as pulmonary edema and is thought to occur in ~1 in 100 transfusions, but it may also be underreported. The Mayo group has reported a frequency as high as 5 in 100 transfusions.[9] TACO can be difficult to differentiate from heart failure or generalized intravascular volume overload, which can present with the same clinical picture.

   b. TRALI also presents as pulmonary edema. The diagnosis is primarily clinical and can vary from mild to severe with evidence of hypoxemia and pulmonary edema on chest x-ray within 6 hours of transfusion. The purported mechanism for TRALI likely involves human leukocyte antigen (HLA) incompatibility, which triggers a cytokine-mediated inflammatory response in the lungs.[10,11] The incidence has been reported as about 1 in 5,000 transfusions; however, recent data from the Mayo Clinic suggest that TRALI or possible TRALI may occur in as many as 1 in 100 transfusions.[12]

4. **A recent investigation noted that TRALI, a diagnosis of exclusion, can be difficult to diagnose in patients undergoing cardiac surgery.** The authors reported greater pulmonary morbidity in the postoperative period for patients transfused with red blood cells (RBCs) and fresh-frozen plasma (FFP); this pulmonary morbidity may have been related to TRALI, TACO, both, or neither. Nevertheless, transfusion of either RBCs or FFP was independently associated with pulmonary morbidity in the postoperative period.[13]

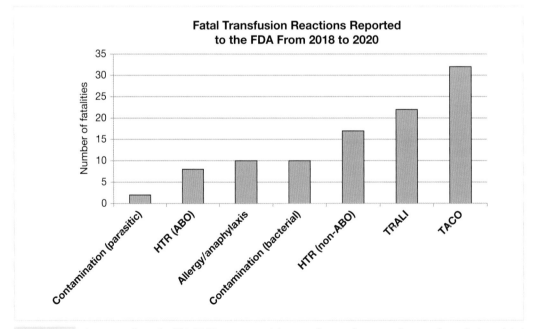

FIGURE 28.1 In a report from the FDA, TACO represented the most frequently reported cause of transfusion-related mortality, and TRALI was the second most common cause.[8] FDA, Food and Drug Administration; HTR (ABO), hemolytic transfusion reactions related to ABO incompatibility; HTR (non-ABO), hemolytic transfusion reactions unrelated to ABO incompatibility; TACO, transfusion-associated circulatory overload; TRALI, transfusion-related acute lung injury.

5. Stokes and colleagues[14] recently examined the effect of bleeding-related complications, blood product use, and costs on a population of inpatient surgical patients. They documented that inadequate surgical hemostasis leads to bleeding complications as well as transfusion. The authors were able to rank incremental cost per hospitalization associated with bleeding-related complications and adjust for covariates. For example, in cardiac surgery, a bleeding complications added $10,279 of incremental cost on average. These findings support the need for further implementation of blood conservation strategies.

6. **Bleeding complications and the associated need for reoperation correlate with increased morbidity in cardiac surgical patients.** Recent work attempted to delineate whether increased morbidity risk was related to the reoperation, blood transfusion, or both. The patients who underwent reoperation for bleeding had greater subsequent morbidity (1% vs 8.5%), prolonged ventilation, increased rates of renal failure, prolonged postoperative length of stay, and increased resource utilization even after risk adjustment (Figure 28.2).[15]

7. A recent investigation in patients undergoing noncardiac thoracic surgery showed that postoperative outcomes were worse in patients transfused with 1-2 units of RBCs than in those who received no transfusion. The negative effect of transfusion was dose dependent and was associated with increased morbidity and resource utilization. The authors urged clinicians to be cautious in transfusing patients for mild degrees of anemia.[16]

CLINICAL PEARL

TACO and TRALI are the current number one and two causes of transfusion-related death, respectively. Hemolytic transfusion reactions are the next most common cause.

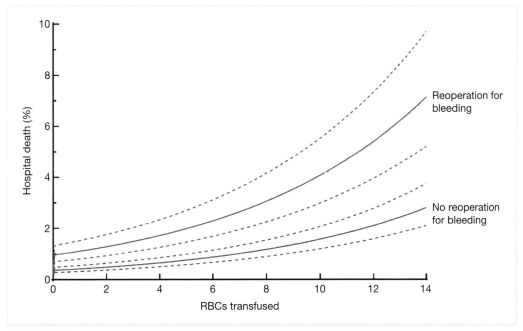

FIGURE 28.2 Predicted probability of operative mortality stratified by reoperation for bleeding and RBC transfusion. RBC transfusion and reoperation for bleeding were independently associated with increased mortality. RBCs, red blood cells. (Reprinted from Vivacqua A, Koch CG, Yousuf AM, et al. Morbidity of bleeding after cardiac surgery: is it blood transfusion, reoperation for bleeding, or both? *Ann Thorac Surg.* 2011;91(6):1780-1790. © 2011 The Society of Thoracic Surgeons. With permission.)

II. Red Blood Cell Transfusion and Clinical Outcomes

RBC units contain red cells that have been separated from whole blood by centrifugation or apheresis (Table 28.1).[17] Isbister and colleagues reported on the abundance of data supporting morbidity risk associated with transfusion, yet noted that transfusion remains "ingrained" in current medical practice almost as a "default" position.[18] Recently, several large studies have examined clinical outcomes related to transfusion to determine the ideal Hb thresholds for transfusion in postoperative cardiac surgery patients. In addition, the AABB's most recent red cell transfusion guidelines advocate a restrictive transfusion strategy for cardiac surgery patients.[19]

A. Hemoglobin Transfusion Trigger Trials

1. **In the past decade, practice has moved toward transfusing less blood to patients, including those undergoing cardiac surgery.** This change in practice is supported by large randomized trials showing noninferiority when a restrictive transfusion strategy is compared to a liberal strategy. The three large studies carried out in cardiac surgical patients were the Transfusion Requirements after Cardiac Surgery (TRACS) trial in 2010,[20] the Transfusion Indication Threshold Reduction (TITRe2) trial in 2015,[21] and the Transfusion Requirements in Cardiac Surgery (TRICS-III) trial in 2017.[22] None of these trials demonstrated a difference in the primary outcome (mortality) between a liberal and a restrictive transfusion strategy, which means that giving extra blood to cardiac surgery patients above a threshold of 7.5-8.0 g/dL only adds risks and costs without benefit.[7]

   a. TRACS trial ($n = 502$)
      (1) Compared hematocrit of 24% (restrictive) to hematocrit of 30% (liberal)
      (2) Primary outcome was a composite of morbidity and mortality.
      (3) The primary outcome occurred with similar frequency in the liberal (10%) and restrictive (11%) groups ($P = .85$). The various event rates in the two groups are shown in Figure 28.3.

   b. TITRe2 trial ($n = 2,003$)
      (1) Compared Hb triggers of 7.5 (restrictive) and 9.0 g/dL (liberal)
      (2) Primary outcome was a serious infection or ischemic event.
      (3) The primary outcome occurred with similar frequency in the liberal (33.0%) and restrictive (35.1%) groups ($P = .30$). The primary event rates after 90 days are shown in Figure 28.3.
      (4) Although the restrictive group had a higher mortality at 90 days postoperatively in the TITRe2 trial (4.2% vs 2.6%, $P = .045$), this was a secondary outcome with no statistical adjustment for multiple comparisons, making the significance questionable.

TABLE 28.1 Fast Facts: Red Blood Cells From American Red Cross Compendium[17]

Fast facts: RBC units	
Concentrated from whole blood	By centrifugation or collected by apheresis
Hematocrit	55%-65% or 65%-80%
Plasma content	20-100 mL
Typical volume	300-400 mL
Volume of hemoglobin	50-80 g
Iron content	**~250 mg**
1 unit RBC transfusion	Increases hematocrit by 3%
Perioperative/periprocedural/critically ill indications for RBC transfusion	**When hemoglobin is <6 g/dL in a young healthy patient; when hemoglobin is <7 g/dL in critically ill patients; 7-8 g/dL in patients with cardiovascular disease**
Indication intermediate hemoglobin 6-10 g/dL	Based on patient symptoms, comorbidities, ongoing bleeding, or end-organ ischemia

RBC, red blood cell.

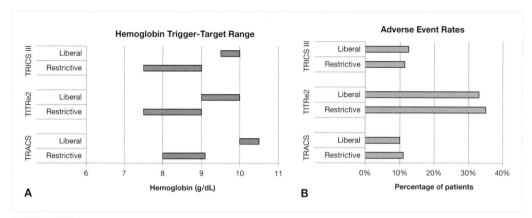

FIGURE 28.3 Hemoglobin and primary outcome data are shown for the liberal and restrictive transfusion groups in the TRACS, TITRe2, and TRICS III trials.[20-22] In postoperative cardiac surgery patients, adverse event rates for the primary outcome (as defined by these trials) were similar in the groups assigned to a lower (restrictive) or a higher (liberal) hemoglobin transfusion threshold **(panel B)**. In **panel A**, the left edge of the red bars represents the hemoglobin trigger (before transfusion), and the right edge of the red bars represents the hemoglobin target (after transfusion). TRACS, Transfusion Requirements after Cardiac Surgery; TITRe2, Transfusion Indication Threshold Reduction; TRICS III, Transfusion Requirements in Cardiac Surgery.

    c. TRICS-III trial ($n = 4,860$)

        (1) In moderate- to high-risk cardiac surgery patients, this trial compared Hb triggers of 7.5 (restrictive) and 9.5 g/dL (liberal) during the intraoperative and postoperative (intensive care unit [ICU]) time periods, however, the 9.5 g/dL group was transfused at a trigger of 8.5 g/dL after leaving the ICU.

        (2) The primary outcome was death, myocardial infarction, stroke, or new-onset renal failure with dialysis, which occurred with similar frequency in the restrictive (11.4%) and liberal (12.5%) groups (odds ratio 0.90; 95% CI, 0.76-1.07; $P < .001$ for noninferiority). Red cell transfusion occurred in 52.3% versus 72.6% in the restrictive and liberal groups, respectively (odds ratio 0.41; 95% CI, 0.37-0.47).

        (3) Interestingly, for the subgroup of patients aged ≥75 years, which was half of all patients enrolled, the primary outcome occurred less frequently in the restrictive transfusion group (10.2%) than in the liberal group (14.1%; $P = .004$).

        (4) This is the first trial to show that older patients may actually do worse when transfused liberally. It is hard to say this definitively with findings from a subgroup of the trial; however, this subgroup was larger than the sample size in any previous Hb trigger trial.

CLINICAL PEARL

Three large randomized trials, comparing restrictive transfusion triggers (Hb 7.5-8 g/dL) to liberal transfusion triggers (Hb 9-10 g/dL) in postoperative cardiac surgery patients, showed no difference in the primary outcome that was measured. This supports giving less blood, since we only add risk and cost when giving more blood than is necessary.

    B. Intraoperative Transfusion Triggers

        1. In contrast to the postoperative setting, the ideal intraoperative Hb transfusion trigger for cardiac surgical patients has not been rigorously studied.

2. In the 2011 STS and Society of Cardiovascular Anesthesiologists Blood Conservation Clinical Practice Guidelines,[23] the authors suggest a lower limit of 6 g/dL for patients on cardiopulmonary bypass (CPB) with moderate hypothermia, although they recognize that high-risk patients may need higher Hb levels and that this recommendation is supported by relatively weak evidence.

3. Some centers have begun monitoring cerebral tissue oxygen content with near-infrared spectroscopy technology; however, no conclusive evidence shows that this type of monitoring can reliably guide transfusion therapy.

4. An analysis of the French Society of Intensive Care Medicine recommendations for transfusion in critically ill patients (which are context sensitive) found that in patients with SvO_2 <70%, $ScvO_2$ increased by over 10% following transfusion; however, in those with $ScvO_2$ >70%, blood transfusion had no impact on SvO_2.[24]

5. By lowering the metabolic rate, hypothermic bypass reduces oxygen demands for all vital organs, meaning that lower Hb levels will be tolerated. However, some groups now use either very mild or no systemic hypothermia. Instead, they use selective regional cooling of the chest cavity, leaving the brain and kidneys at normal temperature.

C. **Red Blood Cell Storage Duration**
   1. **As storage duration increases, RBCs undergo alterations in both structural shape and biochemical properties.** Implications of these time-dependent changes may contribute to adverse clinical outcomes associated with RBC transfusion. However, findings from clinical and experimental animal studies have been inconsistent.[25-27]
   2. In a 2008 retrospective investigation that included over 6,000 cardiac surgical patients at a single center, patients who received exclusively older blood exhibited greater mortality.[27] This pivotal study was the impetus for the large randomized controlled trials (RCTs) carried out in a variety of settings, including adult cardiac surgical patients (the RECESS trial),[28] critically ill adult ICU patients (the ABLE study),[29] and the largest study to date, which enrolled all types of hospitalized patients (the INFORM study with over 20,000 patients).[30] Each of these trials found no difference in any major clinical outcomes. A follow-up secondary analysis from the INFORM study showed that even blood stored for the longest duration (35-42 days) was not associated with a worse outcome compared to the freshest blood (stored for ≤7 days).[31]

CLINICAL PEARL

Randomized trials over the past decade have shown no difference in outcomes between blood stored for shorter versus longer durations.

III. **Component Therapy**
   A. **Restrictive Red Blood Cell Transfusion Practices** have become a standard of care; yet, evidence-based indications for the use of blood component therapy, such as FFP and platelet concentrate transfusion, have been more limited.[32] Though RBCs can be stored for up to 42 days at 1-6 °C, platelets are stored at room temperature for a much shorter storage duration of 5 days. Plasma and cryoprecipitate can be stored frozen for 1 year.
      1. The use of predetermined ratios of component therapy to RBCs has gained increased attention as a result of recent research into military and civilian trauma resuscitation. These investigations focus on earlier and increased use of component therapy.
      2. Though retrospective evidence supports the premise that survival increases with more aggressive use of plasma and platelets in massive transfusion, it was not until 2015 when the PROPPR trial[33] was published that we had good evidence to support a balanced ratio of FFP and platelets to RBCs. The results of this study are described in Section E3, under massive transfusion.

B. **Platelet Therapy (Table 28.2)**

1. General recommendations for platelet therapy stress that platelet transfusion cannot be based simply on platelet count. In the cardiac surgery population, platelets can be dysfunctional or impaired due to CPB, mechanical circulatory support, valve disease, end-stage renal disease, or in those on antiplatelet drugs.[34] In general, for major surgical procedures or during massive transfusion (eg, replacement of one or more blood volumes), a platelet count of at least 50,000/μL is recommended.[35] However, many cardiac programs target platelet counts of 100,000/μL when patients are actively bleeding, especially with abnormal findings on viscoelastic testing. A standard dose of platelets for adults is approximately one unit per 10 kg body weight. Transfusing six units of platelets harvested from whole blood (or one "apheresis" single donor unit containing an equivalent number of platelets) increases the platelet count by ~30,000/μL (Table 28.2).[17]

2. When patients do not show the expected increase in platelet counts, they may need HLA-matched units, as HLA antibodies in the recipient are associated with platelet refractoriness.

3. Historically, of all the major blood components, platelets are associated with the highest risk and cost. The foremost major adverse outcome with platelet transfusion is bacterial sepsis. One in 3,000 platelet concentrates may have bacterial contamination, with an estimated mortality from sepsis occurring in between 1 in 17,000 and 1 in 61,000 transfusions.[36] In 2021, however, new FDA requirements were introduced across the United States for risk mitigation, leading to the widespread use of pathogen-reduced platelets. Amotosalen and ultraviolet light (INTERCEPT Blood System, Cerus) is now the most widely used method for pathogen reduction, which works by interrupting DNA and RNA replication. This reduces risk for virtually all viral, bacterial, and other pathogens (eg, babesiosis, Zika virus), but has resulted in increased platelet cost (by ~30%).

   a. Room temperature storage is the primary reason that platelets are more likely to have bacterial growth than other blood components. Therefore, platelets are routinely cultured before transfusion is allowed.

   b. TRALI has been associated with platelet transfusion more than with other blood components. TRALI reduction strategies have excluded women from donating plasma. However, women are not excluded from donating platelets, and they have a higher rate of HLA antigens owing to fetal blood exposure during childbirth.

CLINICAL PEARL

Platelets are the highest risk and cost of all the blood components. The primary risk is bacterial sepsis, since platelets are stored at room temperature. The new requirements for pathogen-reduced platelets result in risk reduction, along with increased cost.

TABLE 28.2 Fast Facts: Platelets From American Red Cross Compendium[17]

Fast Facts: Platelets	
Derived from whole blood	5.5×10^{10} platelets per bag
Plasma content (whole blood derived)	40-70 mL
Apheresis platelets	3.0×10^{11} platelets per bag
Plasma content (apheresis derived)	100-500 mL
Average platelet count increase in (70 kg) adult per each random donor platelet transfusion	5,000-10,000/μL
In general, appropriate indication for transfusion	Platelet count <50,000/μL with active bleeding or invasive procedures/surgery
In cardiac surgery, appropriate indication for transfusion	Platelet count <100,000/μL and microvascular bleeding, or impaired platelet function

Data from American Red Cross Compendium of Transfusion Practice Guidelines. 2021.

C. **Plasma Therapy (Table 28.3)**[17]

1. FFP refers to human donor plasma that is separated and frozen at -18 °C within 8 hours of collection; frozen plasma-24 (FP-24) refers to plasma separated and frozen at -18 °C within 24 hours of collection. FFP from a collection of whole blood has a volume of ~300 mL. Both products contain necessary plasma coagulation factors that are maintained after thawing and storage at 1-6 °C for up to 5 days. In general, the dose of FFP is 10-20 mL/kg.[37] FFP should be ABO compatible but does not require crossmatching.

2. **Excessive blood loss, coagulation factor consumption, and specific deficiencies in coagulation factors are among a number of factors that can lead to inadequate hemostasis and the need for an FFP transfusion**. In patients who require massive transfusion, it is well recognized that the use of crystalloids, colloids, and RBCs can lead to a dilutional coagulopathy. A number of publications address limited adherence to published guidelines and rational use of FFP transfusion.[38]

3. Interestingly, Holland and Brooks[39] reported that FFP transfusion failed to change the international normalized ratio (INR) in patients with a minimally prolonged INR (<1.6); INR decreased only with treatment of the disease causing the elevated INR.

4. Prophylactic use of FFP is not supported by evidence from good-quality RCTs. **Evidence indicates that prophylactic plasma for transfusion is not effective across a range of clinical settings**.[38]

5. Although the INR test is routinely used to determine when FFP is given, the INR was designed to follow anticoagulant dosing with vitamin K antagonist drugs and is likely too sensitive and inadequately specific to guide FFP dosing accurately. For example, in our experience, until the INR is ≥ 2.0, the thromboelastogram (TEG) will usually be normal, suggesting that coagulation is unimpaired.[40]

6. Four-factor prothrombin complex concentrate (4-PCC) can be considered in replacing coagulation factors as demonstrated by viscoelastic testing. Clinically, 4-PCC is used especially when the patient is at risk for right ventricular volume overload, such as during left ventricular assist device implant, heart transplant, or in moderate to massive bleeding. One recent randomized trial comparing 4-PCC (15 IU/kg) to plasma (10-15 mL/kg) showed less intraoperative red cells transfused in those treated with 4-PCC (13.7% vs 30.6%), improved prothrombin time (PT) and INR correction, and a higher incidence of allogeneic transfusion avoidance.[41]

TABLE 28.3   Fast Facts: Fresh Plasma From American Red Cross Compendium[17]

Fast Facts: FFP	
Noncellular portion of blood	From whole blood or apheresis
Volume of 1 unit (approximate)	250 mL
Frozen at -18 °C	Within 6-8 h of collection
Contains all coagulation factors	At usual plasma concentration (1 unit of activity/mL of plasma)
Thawed and used or stored at 1-6 °C for 24 h	
Transfusion should be guided by coagulation testing	Prothrombin time $>1.5\times$ normal, activated partial thromboplastin time $>1.5\times$ normal, or factor assay $<25\%$
Dose	10-20 mL/kg
Selected indications	Massive transfusion with coagulopathic bleeding, active bleeding due to coagulation multiple factor deficiency, severe bleeding due to warfarin therapy

FFP, fresh-frozen plasma.

D. **Cryoprecipitate (Table 28.4)**[17]

   1. When FFP is thawed for 24 hours at 1-6 °C, high-molecular-weight proteins separate out from the plasma; this cryoprecipitate can be frozen at -18 °C for up to 1 year.
   2. One bag of cryoprecipitate contains 10-15 mL of insoluble protein.
   3. Cryoprecipitate contains Factors I (fibrinogen), VIII, and XIII, von Willebrand factor, fibronectin, and platelet microparticles.
   4. **Cryoprecipitate is most commonly used as a concentrated source of fibrinogen,** except in some European countries and Canada where fibrinogen concentrate is approved (and preferred) to treat acquired fibrinogen deficiency.[42] In the United States, fibrinogen concentrate is approved by the FDA only for congenital, not acquired, deficiency. This product is more expensive than cryoprecipitate and has been shown to be noninferior in efficacy but faster to prepare and deliver.[43]
   5. Hypofibrinogenemia occurs in patients undergoing cardiac surgery, most often in those with hemorrhage. In such patients, even a balanced ratio of RBCs, FFP, and platelets will eventually result in fibrinogen deficiency, as FFP has some fibrinogen, but not enough to maintain normal levels during massive transfusions. Depending upon the weight of the recipient, 10 pooled units of cryoprecipitate will increase plasma fibrinogen by 70-100 mg/dL.[37,42]
   6. Recent guidelines for treating hemorrhage suggest that fibrinogen levels be maintained >150-200 mg/dL. Ideally, viscoelastic point-of-care testing is used to guide such therapy, focusing on clot strength (α-angle and maximum amplitude).

E. **Massive Transfusion and Component Ratios**

   1. The formal definition of massive transfusion is one entire blood volume replacement in a 24-hour time period. When a patient undergoes massive transfusion or experiences any other large, rapid blood loss, it is important to administer an optimal ratio of blood components to avoid dilutional coagulopathy.
   2. Given the complexity of cardiac surgery and extracorporeal support, the incidence of massive transfusion is substantial, especially in tertiary referral centers that perform revision cardiac surgeries, transplants, and extracorporeal life support (ECMO).
   3. Most studies in this area have been retrospective and focused on trauma patients with active hemorrhage. These studies support using a high ratio of plasma and platelets to RBCs in order to reconstitute a mixture similar to that of whole blood. **As a large RCT, the PROPPR study showed that in actively bleeding trauma patients, the primary outcomes of 24-hour and 30-day mortality were similar in the 1:1:1 and 1:1:2 groups (platelet:plasma:RBC ratios).**[33] However, early exsanguination, which was the

TABLE 28.4   Fast Facts: Cryoprecipitate From American Red Cross Compendium[17]

Fast Facts: Cryoprecipitate	
Unit is prepared from 1 unit of FFP at 1-6 °C	Recovering cold insoluble precipitate
Refrozen within 1 h	
Contains concentrated levels of	Fibrinogen, Factor VIII:C, Factor VIII:vWF, Factor XIII, and fibronectin
Factor VIII:C in 1 unit	At least 80 IU
Fibrinogen in 1 unit	Minimum of 150 mg
Plasma volume of 1 unit	5-20 mL
Dose and response from 1 pool or "bag" (5 units)	Fibrinogen increases by ~50 mg/dL for average adult
Selected indications	Bleeding associated with fibrinogen deficiencies; massive transfusion when fibrinogen <150-200 mg/dL

FFP, fresh-frozen plasma; vWF, von Willebrand factor.

predominant cause of death, occurred less frequently in the 1:1:1 group. This secondary outcome suggests that a balanced ratio of components, similar to whole blood, was efficacious in improving outcomes. Whether this finding applies to massive hemorrhage in cardiac surgical patients is unclear, as trauma patients may have unique characteristics. Ideally, the ratio can be tailored based on laboratory testing, including viscoelastic (TEG, rotational thromboelastometry [ROTEM], or the new Quantra)[44,45] testing, to avoid coagulopathy.

IV. Blood Conservation Measures

A. Preoperative Anemia Management

1. **Best practices for PBM include the diagnosis and treatment of preoperative anemia with the goal of reducing the need for allogeneic transfusion.**[46] This type of care applies primarily to elective surgical patients because there is insufficient time for medical treatment in urgent or emergent cases, which are not infrequent in cardiac surgery.

2. For patients undergoing elective surgery, effective and specific treatments, such as iron replacement for iron deficiency (either oral or intravenous), can make a difference.[47]

3. Erythropoietic-stimulating agents (eg, erythropoietin or darbepoetin) can also be used to increase Hb levels preoperatively,[48] although the FDA warnings for thrombotic events and promotion of tumor growth should be considered when weighing the risks and benefits of such therapy.

4. A comprehensive review on preoperative anemia management in cardiac surgery advocates for targeted therapy with intravenous iron and erythropoietic-stimulating agents as the most promising therapies.[49]

5. Since perioperative anemia has been linked to long-term survival after cardiac surgery—even out to 7 years[50]—attention to prevention and treatment of anemia is prudent.

B. Antifibrinolytics

The use of lysine analogs, ε-aminocaproic acid (EACA) and tranexamic acid (TXA), suppresses pathologic hyperfibrinolysis associated with CPB.[51] **In a 2011 Cochrane review, Henry et al[52] conducted a meta-analysis on antifibrinolytic use that included 34 studies of TXA, 11 studies of EACA, and 6 trials comparing the two. The findings showed that TXA use was associated with a 32% reduction in the need for allogeneic blood transfusion. Those who received EACA had a 30% reduction.** On average, patients who received either TXA or EACA saw reductions in both intraoperative and postoperative blood loss. Neither drug has been shown to increase thrombotic events; however, TXA in high doses is associated with increased risk for seizures.[53] These drugs have now replaced aprotinin as the drugs of choice because aprotinin was removed from the U.S. marketplace in 2008 for safety concerns (increased mortality) after the BART trial.[54]

CLINICAL PEARL

6 | Antifibrinolytic drugs are commonly used intraoperatively, to reduce bleeding and transfusion requirements in cardiac surgery patients. There is no evidence that they are associated with increased venous thromboembolic events.

C. Acute Normovolemic Hemodilution

1. For acute normovolemic hemodilution (ANH), a certain amount of blood is withdrawn from a patient before heparinization and CPB, and the intravascular volume is replaced to maintain isovolemia. The autologous whole blood is then readministered, usually after CPB. The use of ANH reduces requirements for allogeneic transfusion by preserving RBCs, coagulation factors, and platelets and improving perfusion during CPB by decreasing blood viscosity.[55]

2. Barile et al[56] conducted a meta-analysis of 29 RCTs that included 2,439 patients to compare the use of ANH with standard intraoperative care. They assessed the number of allogeneic RBC units transfused, rate of perioperative transfusion, and estimated total blood loss. They found that ANH reduced the number of allogeneic RBC units used, the incidence of transfusion, and the amount of bleeding.

3. **ANH is associated with reduced allogeneic transfusion, most notably when a large volume of ANH phlebotomy is accomplished.**[57] Three recent studies on ANH for complex cardiac or thoracic aortic surgery reported an average of 826,[58] 1,200,[59] and 960 mL[60] of whole-blood phlebotomy. These studies also showed reduced allogeneic blood requirements (both red and yellow products) and improved hemostatic profiles by laboratory and viscoelastic testing results. In a multicenter, observational study of over 13,000 patients,[61] researchers found that at all volumes of ANH, the number of allogeneic transfusions was reduced. Perhaps unsurprisingly, this reduction became more pronounced with increased ANH volume removal. They also noted a lower rate of plasma and platelet transfusion in those who had ANH, as well as less acute kidney injury and lower rates of prolonged length of stay.

4. Other studies have not demonstrated a reduction in transfusion requirements with ANH.[62] It is also important to note potential confounding variables. For example, patients who undergo ANH tend to be younger and male, have a larger body surface area, have less preoperative anemia, and have lower STS mortality scores.

5. In the 2021 STS guidelines on PBM in cardiac surgery,[4] the evidence supporting ANH was considered Class IIa and it was recognized as underutilized. Accordingly, the guidelines indicated that ANH could be considered as part of a multipronged approach to blood conservation.

D. **Methods Used by Perfusionists**
   1. **Cell salvage**
      a. Cell salvage is a technique in which whole blood from a patient is centrifuged to collect platelets and other clotting factors into the cell-washing supernatant.
      b. Cell salvage has become a standard of care in cardiac surgery owing to the recent emphasis on blood conservation. In addition, salvaged RBCs may be higher in quality than stored (banked) RBCs. Compared with banked RBCs, salvaged blood has normal levels of 2,3-DPG, no left shift in the Hb-oxygen saturation curve, and better cell membrane deformability.[63,64]
   2. **Modified ultrafiltration**
      a. Membrane oxygenators activate the coagulation cascade, dilute platelets and clotting factors, and induce fibrinolysis and systemic inflammatory response syndrome. Various studies have attempted to mitigate these risks with a technique known as modified ultrafiltration (MUF), which has been shown to reduce postoperative blood loss and blood product utilization.
      b. MUF involves the use of a hydrostatic pressure gradient to remove water and some low-molecular-weight substances from plasma at the termination of CPB, producing protein-rich whole blood to be returned to the patient. When this technique is used during CPB, it is considered conventional ultrafiltration, or zero-balance ultrafiltration (Z-BUF).
      c. **In a meta-analysis that compared MUF to no ultrafiltration, Boodhwani et al[65] demonstrated that MUF significantly reduced transfusion requirements.** In a prospective randomized trial of 573 patients, Luciani et al[66] found not only that the mean volume of RBCs transfused for each patient was lower but also that the proportion of patients who did not receive any blood products was higher with MUF (51.8% vs 38.1%, $P = .001$). In a recent meta-analysis that included 13 RCTs, MUF was shown to increase postoperative hematocrit, while reducing postoperative chest tube drainage, transfusion requirements, and duration of ICU stay.[67]
      d. MUF is a blood conservation strategy that is likely underutilized in adults and has become the standard of care for pediatric cardiac surgical patients. MUF is considered to be supported at the evidence level Class II-B in the 2021 STS guidelines.[4]
   3. **Zero-balance ultrafiltration**
      a. For Z-BUF, or conventional ultrafiltration, ultrafiltration occurs during CPB, and the ultrafiltrate is replaced with an equal volume of balanced electrolyte solution. The Z-BUF

filter unit is connected to the CPB pump, takes blood from a premembrane port, and runs in parallel to the main cardiopulmonary circuit. To prevent patient blood flow from dropping, the arterial pump rate is increased to compensate for the blood flow through the hemofilter.

b. The main theoretical advantage is that Z-BUF can be used to reduce the inflammatory mediators that are activated when blood contacts a foreign surface. A recent meta-analysis of RCTs, however, showed no significant difference in clinical outcomes.[68]

4. **Low-volume cardiopulmonary bypass circuits**
   a. Smaller diameter and shorter length tubing as well as low-volume oxygenators can reduce the hemodilution that occurs when patients are placed on CPB, which may reduce transfusion requirements.[69]

5. **Retrograde autologous prime**
   a. By using the patient's own venous blood to prime the CPB circuit by retrograde flow, a reduction in hemodilution can be achieved, resulting in less anemia and transfusion requirements. A recent meta-analysis including 11 RCTs and 10 observational studies found a decrease in both intraoperative and whole hospital RBC requirements, but no increase in adverse events (acute kidney injury or stroke).[70]
   b. Both low-volume "minicircuits" and retrograde autologous prime are supported at evidence level Class I in the 2021 STS guidelines.[4]

CLINICAL PEARL

Perfusionists play a prominent role in achieving blood conservation in cardiac surgery patients. There are several methods they can employ to reduce the incidence of anemia and transfusion.

E. **Viscoelastic Testing**
   1. TEG, ROTEM, and the newer Quantra hemostasis analyzer system are viscoelastic hemostatic assays that are used to assess whole-blood clot formation: initiation, propagation, strength, and dissolution.[44,45] The diagnosis of a specific cause of coagulopathic bleeding allows for targeted hemostatic correction and potentially prevents the use of unwarranted blood products. Early utilization of viscoelastic testing (while the patient is still on CPB) allows for prompt decision-making about FFP, platelets, and cryoprecipitate transfusions when the patients are coming off of CPB. Basic interpretation of viscoelastic test results is illustrated in Figure 28.4.
   2. **Transfusion algorithms that use viscoelastic parameters have been shown to reduce transfusion requirements in cardiac surgery by allowing targeted transfusion therapy.**[71,72] Viscoelastic-guided therapy has been shown to reduce bleeding (by ~30%), along with mortality for patients requiring long duration of CPB (>115 minutes).[73]
   3. More recent studies have continued to show that viscoelastic testing not only reduces the need for transfusion but also potentially correlates with a reduced mortality.[74] Conventional kaolin-activated viscoelastic testing methods are unable to detect the effect of antiplatelet medications (P2Y12 inhibitors or aspirin) on platelet function; however, the use of point-of-care platelet function tests or platelet mapping TEG has been suggested as an additional modality to assess platelet dysfunction caused by antiplatelet agents and CPB.[75,76] Corredor et al[77] found that platelet function testing within a blood transfusion algorithm resulted in a significant reduction in bleeding at longest follow-up and reduced transfusion of RBCs and FFP.
   4. Platelet mapping TEG was recently shown to reduce cardiac surgery waiting time to at least 3 days earlier than STS recommendations without increased bleeding.[78]

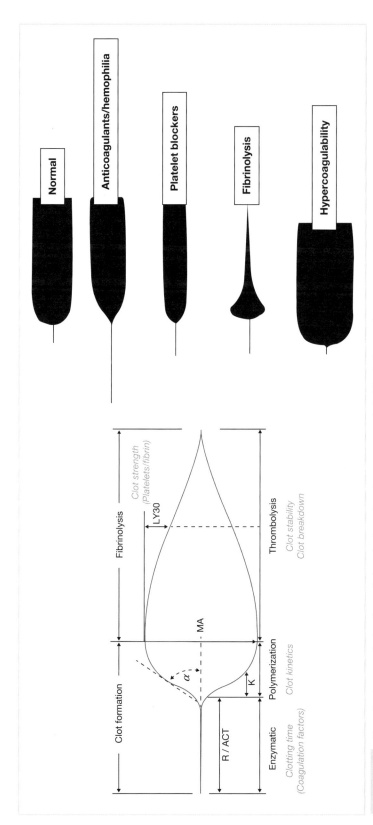

FIGURE 28.4 Thromboelastography is a form of viscoelastic testing that measures whole-blood clotting characteristics. The tracings can be interpreted by both shape and numeric attributes derived from the images. Such testing allows targeted transfusion therapy. α; ACT, activated clotting time; R, K, MA, LY30.
α - Alpha angle: Angle between the baseline at initial clot formation, and a tangent line that intersects the tracing curve; **R - R time:** Time to initial clot formation; **K - K time:** Time from initial clot formation until reaching 20 mm in amplitude; **MA - Maximum amplitude:** Maximum clot strength; **LY30 – Lysis30:** Percentage of clot lysis at 30 minutes time.

V. Conclusion

Although transfusion is a necessary treatment strategy for selected patients, it is associated with a number of morbidity risks, as is anemia. Recent work suggests moving from the current blood banking, "supply-centric" perspective to a "patient-centric" PBM approach. Implementation of institutional PBM protocols enhances practitioners' knowledge base and the consistency of transfusion practices while encouraging a more restrictive approach to blood utilization.

REFERENCES

1. Beal RW. The rational use of blood. *Aust N Z J Surg*. 1976;46(4):309-313.
2. Frank SM, Savage WJ, Rothschild JA, et al. Variability in blood and blood component utilization as assessed by an anesthesia information management system. *Anesthesiology*. 2012;117(1):99-106. doi:10.1097/ALN.0b013e318255e550
3. Bennett-Guerrero E, Zhao Y, O'Brien SM, et al. Variation in use of blood transfusion in coronary artery bypass graft surgery. *JAMA*. 2010;304(14):1568-1575.
4. Tibi P, McClure RS, Huang J, et al. STS/SCA/AmSECT/SABM update to the clinical practice guidelines on patient blood management. *Ann Thorac Surg*. 2021;112(3):981-1004. doi:10.1016/j.athoracsur.2021.03.033
5. Shander A, Hardy JF, Ozawa S, et al. A global definition of patient blood management. *Anesth Analg*. 2022;135(3):476-488. doi: 10.1213/ANE.0000000000005873
6. Vamvakas EC, Blajchman MA. Transfusion-related mortality: the ongoing risks of allogeneic blood transfusion and the available strategies for their prevention. *Blood*. 2009;113(15):3406-3417. doi:10.1182/blood-2008-10-167643
7. Carson JL, Stanworth SJ, Guyatt G, et al. Blood, Bleeding, and Transfusion. *JAMA*, 2023 Nov 21;330(19):1892-1902. doi: 10.1001/jama.2023.12914
8. Fatalities reported to the FDA following blood collection and transfusion. 2021. Accessed January 19, 2024. https://www.fda.gov/media/172382/download?attachment.
9. Clifford L, Jia Q, Yadav H, et al. Characterizing the epidemiology of perioperative transfusion-associated circulatory overload. *Anesthesiology*. 2015;122(1):21-28. doi:10.1097/ALN.0000000000000513
10. Toy P, Lowell C. TRALI definition, mechanisms, incidence and clinical relevance. *Best Pract Res Clin Anaesthesiol*. 2007;21(2):183-193.
11. Popovsky MA. Pulmonary consequences of transfusion: TRALI and TACO. *Transfus Apher Sci*. 2006;34(3):243-244. doi:10.1016/j.transci.2006.01.005
12. Clifford L, Jia Q, Subramanian A, et al. Characterizing the epidemiology of postoperative transfusion-related acute lung injury. *Anesthesiology*. 2015;122(1):12-20. doi:10.1097/ALN.0000000000000514
13. Koch C, Li L, Figueroa P, Mihaljevic T, Svensson L, Blackstone EH. Transfusion and pulmonary morbidity after cardiac surgery. *Ann Thorac Surg*. 2009;88(5):1410-1418. doi:10.1016/j.athoracsur.2009.07.020
14. Stokes ME, Ye X, Shah M, et al. Impact of bleeding-related complications and/or blood product transfusions on hospital costs in inpatient surgical patients. *BMC Health Serv Res*. 2011;11:135. doi:10.1186/1472-6963-11-135
15. Vivacqua A, Koch CG, Yousuf AM, et al. Morbidity of bleeding after cardiac surgery: is it blood transfusion, reoperation for bleeding, or both? *Ann Thorac Surg*. 2011;91(6):1780-1790. doi:10.1016/j.athoracsur.2011.03.105
16. Ferraris VA, Davenport DL, Saha SP, Bernard A, Austin PC, Zwischenberger JB. Intraoperative transfusion of small amounts of blood heralds worse postoperative outcome in patients having noncardiac thoracic operations. *Ann Thorac Surg*. 2011;91(6):1674-1680; discussion 1680. doi:10.1016/j.athoracsur.2011.01.025
17. American Red Cross Compendium of Transfusion Practice Guidelines. 2021. Accessed January 19, 2024. https://www.redcross.org/content/dam/redcrossblood/hospital-page-documents/334401_compendium_v04jan2021_bookmarkedworking_rwv01.pdf
18. Isbister JP, Shander A, Spahn DR, Erhard J, Farmer SL, Hofmann A. Adverse blood transfusion outcomes: establishing causation. *Transfus Med Rev*. 2011;25(2):89-101. doi:10.1016/j.tmrv.2010.11.001
19. Carson JL, Guyatt G, Heddle NM, et al. Clinical practice guidelines from the AABB: red blood cell transfusion thresholds and storage. *JAMA*. 2016;316(19):2025-2035. doi:10.1001/jama.2016.9185
20. Hajjar LA, Vincent JL, Galas FR, et al. Transfusion requirements after cardiac surgery: the TRACS randomized controlled trial. *JAMA*. 2010;304(14):1559-1567. doi:10.1001/jama.2010.1446
21. Murphy GJ, Pike K, Rogers CA, et al. Liberal or restrictive transfusion after cardiac surgery. *N Engl J Med*. 2015;372(11):997-1008. doi:10.1056/NEJMoa1403612
22. Mazer CD, Whitlock RP, Fergusson DA, et al. Restrictive or liberal red-cell transfusion for cardiac surgery. *N Engl J Med*. 2017;377(22):2133-2144. doi:10.1056/NEJMoa1711818
23. Ferraris VA, Brown JR, Despotis GJ, et al. 2011 Update to the Society of Thoracic Surgeons and the Society of cardiovascular anesthesiologists blood conservation clinical practice guidelines. *Ann Thorac Surg*. 2011;91(3):944-982.
24. Adamczyk S, Robin E, Barreau O, et al. Contribution of central venous oxygen saturation in postoperative blood transfusion decision. *Ann Fr Anesth Reanim*. 2009;28(6):522-530. Apport de la saturation veineuse centrale en oxygene dans la decision transfusionnelle postoperatoire. doi:10.1016/j.annfar.2009.03.013
25. Raat NJ, Verhoeven AJ, Mik EG, et al. The effect of storage time of human red cells on intestinal microcirculatory oxygenation in a rat isovolemic exchange model. *Crit Care Med*. 2005;33(1):39-45; discussion 238-239. doi:10.1097/01.CCM.0000150655.75519.02
26. Yap CH, Lau L, Krishnaswamy M, Gaskell M, Yii M. Age of transfused red cells and early outcomes after cardiac surgery. *Ann Thorac Surg*. 2008;86(2):554-559. doi:10.1016/j.athoracsur.2008.04.040
27. Koch CG, Li L, Sessler DI, et al. Duration of red-cell storage and complications after cardiac surgery. *N Engl J Med*. 2008;358(12):1229-1239. doi:10.1056/NEJMoa070403

28. Steiner ME, Ness PM, Assmann SF, et al. Effects of red-cell storage duration on patients undergoing cardiac surgery. *N Engl J Med.* 2015;372(15):1419-1429. doi:10.1056/NEJMoa1414219

29. Lacroix J, Hebert PC, Fergusson DA, et al. Age of transfused blood in critically ill adults. *N Engl J Med.* 2015;372(15):1410-1418. doi:10.1056/NEJMoa1500704

30. Heddle NM, Cook RJ, Arnold DM, et al. Effect of short-term vs. long-term blood storage on mortality after transfusion. *N Engl J Med.* 2016;375(20):1937-1945. doi:10.1056/NEJMoa1609014

31. Cook RJ, Heddle NM, Lee KA, et al. Red blood cell storage and in-hospital mortality: a secondary analysis of the INFORM randomised controlled trial. *Lancet Haematol.* 2017;4(11):e544-e552. doi:10.1016/S2352-3026(17)30169-2

32. Gajic O, Dzik WH, Toy P. Fresh frozen plasma and platelet transfusion for nonbleeding patients in the intensive care unit: benefit or harm? *Crit Care Med.* 2006;34(Suppl. 5):S170-S173. doi:10.1097/01.CCM.0000214288.88308.26

33. Holcomb JB, Tilley BC, Baraniuk S, et al. Transfusion of plasma, platelets, and red blood cells in a 1:1:1 vs a 1:1:2 ratio and mortality in patients with severe trauma: the PROPPR randomized clinical trial. *JAMA.* 2015;313(5):471-482. doi:10.1001/jama.2015.12

34. Squiccimarro E, Jiritano F, Serraino GF, Ten Cate H, Paparella D, Lorusso R. Quantitative and qualitative platelet derangements in cardiac surgery and extracorporeal life support. *J Clin Med.* 2021;10(4):615. doi:10.3390/jcm10040615

35. Kaufman RM, Djulbegovic B, Gernsheimer T, et al. Platelet transfusion: a clinical practice guideline from the AABB. *Ann Intern Med.* 2015;162(3):205-213. doi:10.7326/M14-1589

36. Stroncek DF, Rebulla P. Platelet transfusions. *Lancet.* 2007;370(9585):427-438. doi:10.1016/S0140-6736(07)61198-2

37. Stanworth SJ. The evidence-based use of FFP and cryoprecipitate for abnormalities of coagulation tests and clinical coagulopathy. *Hematology Am Soc Hematol Educ Program.* 2007;2007:179-186. doi:10.1182/asheducation-2007.1.179

38. Roback JD, Caldwell S, Carson J, et al. Evidence-based practice guidelines for plasma transfusion. *Transfusion.* 2010;50(6):1227-1239. doi:10.1111/j.1537-2995.2010.02632.x

39. Holland LL, Brooks JP. Toward rational fresh frozen plasma transfusion: the effect of plasma transfusion on coagulation test results. *Am J Clin Pathol.* 2006;126(1):133-139. doi:10.1309/NQXH-UG7H-ND78-LFFK

40. Patel IJ, Rahim S, Davidson JC, et al. Society of Interventional Radiology Consensus Guidelines for the periprocedural management of thrombotic and bleeding risk in patients undergoing percutaneous image-guided interventions-part II: recommendations: endorsed by the Canadian Association for Interventional Radiology and the Cardiovascular and Interventional Radiological Society of Europe. *J Vasc Interv Radiol.* 2019;30(8):1168.e1-1184.e1. doi:10.1016/j.jvir.2019.04.017

41. Smith MM, Schroeder DR, Nelson JA, et al. Prothrombin complex concentrate vs plasma for post-cardiopulmonary bypass coagulopathy and bleeding: a randomized clinical trial. *JAMA Surg.* 2022;157(9):757-764. doi:10.1001/jamasurg.2022.2235

42. Callum JL, Karkouti K, Lin Y. Cryoprecipitate: the current state of knowledge. *Transfus Med Rev.* 2009;23(3):177-188. doi:10.1016/j.tmrv.2009.03.001

43. Callum J, Farkouh ME, Scales DC, et al. Effect of Fibrinogen concentrate vs cryoprecipitate on blood component transfusion after cardiac surgery: the FIBRES randomized clinical trial. *JAMA.* 2019;322(20):1966-1976. doi:10.1001/jama.2019.17312

44. DeAnda A, Levy G, Kinsky M, et al. Comparison of the Quantra QPlus system with thromboelastography in cardiac surgery. *J Cardiothorac Vasc Anesth.* 2021;35(4):1030-1036. doi:10.1053/j.jvca.2020.11.058

45. Zghaibe W, Scheuermann S, Munting K, et al. Clinical utility of the Quantra((R)) point-of-care haemostasis analyser during urgent cardiac surgery. *Anaesthesia.* 2020;75(3):366-373. doi:10.1111/anae.14942

46. Guinn NR, Guercio JR, Hopkins TJ, et al. How do we develop and implement a preoperative anemia clinic designed to improve perioperative outcomes and reduce cost? *Transfusion.* 2016;56(2):297-303. doi:10.1111/trf.13426

47. Liu HM, Tang XS, Yu H, Yu H. The efficacy of intravenous iron for treatment of anemia before cardiac surgery: an updated systematic review and meta-analysis with trial sequential analysis. *J Cardiothorac Surg.* 2023;18(1):16. doi:10.1186/s13019-023-02119-2

48. Yoo YC, Shim JK, Kim JC, Jo YY, Lee JH, Kwak YL. Effect of single recombinant human erythropoietin injection on transfusion requirements in preoperatively anemic patients undergoing valvular heart surgery. *Anesthesiology.* 2011;115(5):929-937. doi:10.1097/ALN.0b013e318232004b

49. Klueser R, Buser A, Bolliger D. Treatment strategies in anemic patients before cardiac surgery. *J Cardiothorac Vasc Anesth.* 2022;37:266-275. doi:10.1053/j.jvca.2022.09.085

50. Schwann TA, Vekstein AM, Engoren M, et al. Perioperative anemia and transfusions and late mortality in coronary artery bypass patients. *Ann Thorac Surg.* 2023;115:759-769.

51. Pustavoitau A, Faraday N. Pro: antifibrinolytics should be used in routine cardiac cases using cardiopulmonary bypass (unless contraindicated). *J Cardiothorac Vasc Anesth.* 2016;30(1):245-247. doi:10.1053/j.jvca.2015.08.014

52. Henry DA, Carless PA, Moxey AJ, et al. Anti-fibrinolytic use for minimising perioperative allogeneic blood transfusion. *Cochrane Database Syst Rev.* 2011;11(3):CD001886. doi:10.1002/14651858.CD001886.pub4

53. Myles PS, Smith JA, Forbes A, et al. Tranexamic acid in patients undergoing coronary-artery surgery. *N Engl J Med.* 2017;376(2):136-148. doi:10.1056/NEJMoa1606424

54. Mangano DT, Tudor IC, Dietzel C, Multicenter Study of Perioperative Ischemia Research Group, Ischemia Research and Education Foundation. The risk associated with aprotinin in cardiac surgery. *N Engl J Med.* 2006;354(4):353-365. doi:10.1056/NEJMoa051379

55. Grant MC, Resar LM, Frank SM. The efficacy and utility of acute normovolemic hemodilution. *Anesth Analg.* 2015;121(6):1412-1414. doi:10.1213/ANE.0000000000000935

56. Barile L, Fominskiy E, Di Tomasso N, et al. Acute normovolemic hemodilution reduces allogeneic red blood cell transfusion in cardiac surgery: a systematic review and meta-analysis of randomized trials. *Anesth Analg.* 2017;124(3):743-752. doi:10.1213/ANE.0000000000001609

57. Henderson RA, Mazzeffi MA, Strauss ER, et al. Impact of intraoperative high-volume autologous blood collection on allogeneic transfusion during and after cardiac surgery: a propensity score matched analysis. *Transfusion.* 2019;59(6):2023-2029. doi:10.1111/trf.15253

58. Geube M, Sale S, Bakdash S, et al. Prepump autologous blood collection is associated with reduced intraoperative transfusions in aortic surgery with circulatory arrest: a propensity score-matched analysis. *J Thorac Cardiovasc Surg.* 2022;164(5):1572.e5-1580e5. doi:10.1016/j.jtcvs.2021.01.029

59. Henderson RA, Judd M, Strauss ER, et al. Hematologic evaluation of intraoperative autologous blood collection and allogeneic transfusion in cardiac surgery. *Transfusion.* 2021;61(3):788-798. doi:10.1111/trf.16259

60. Mladinov D, Eudailey KW, Padilla LA, et al. Effects of acute normovolemic hemodilution on post-cardiopulmonary bypass coagulation tests and allogeneic blood transfusion in thoracic aortic repair surgery: an observational cohort study. *J Card Surg.* 2021;36(11):4075-4082. doi:10.1111/jocs.15943

61. Goldberg J, Paugh TA, Dickinson TA, et al. Greater volume of acute normovolemic hemodilution may aid in reducing blood transfusions after cardiac surgery. *Ann Thorac Surg.* 2015;100(5):1581-1587; discussion 1587. doi:10.1016/j.athoracsur.2015.04.135

62. Hohn L, Schweizer A, Licker M, Morel DR. Absence of beneficial effect of acute normovolemic hemodilution combined with aprotinin on allogeneic blood transfusion requirements in cardiac surgery. *Anesthesiology.* 2002;96(2):276-282. doi:10.1097/00000542-200202000-00009

63. Frank SM, Abazyan B, Ono M, et al. Decreased erythrocyte deformability after transfusion and the effects of erythrocyte storage duration. *Anesth Analg.* 2013;116(5):975-981. doi:10.1213/ANE.0b013e31828843e6

64. Salaria ON, Barodka VM, Hogue CW, et al. Impaired red blood cell deformability after transfusion of stored allogeneic blood but not autologous salvaged blood in cardiac surgery patients. *Anesth Analg.* 2014;118(6):1179-1187. doi:10.1213/ANE.0000000000000227

65. Boodhwani M, Williams K, Babaev A, Gill S, Saleem N, Rubens FD. Ultrafiltration reduces blood transfusions following cardiac surgery: a meta-analysis. *Eur J Cardiothorac Surg.* 2006;30(6):892-897. doi:10.1016/j.ejcts.2006.09.014

66. Luciani GB, Menon T, Vecchi B, Auriemma S, Mazzucco A. Modified ultrafiltration reduces morbidity after adult cardiac operations: a prospective, randomized clinical trial. *Circulation.* 2001;104(12 Suppl. 1):I253-I259.

67. Low ZK, Gao F, Sin KYK, Yap KH. Modified ultrafiltration reduces postoperative blood loss and transfusions in adult cardiac surgery: a meta-analysis of randomized controlled trials. *Interact Cardiovasc Thorac Surg.* 2021;32(5):671-682. doi:10.1093/icvts/ivaa330

68. Zhu X, Ji B, Wang G, Liu J, Long C. The effects of zero-balance ultrafiltration on postoperative recovery after cardiopulmonary bypass: a meta-analysis of randomized controlled trials. *Perfusion.* 2012;27(5):386-392. doi:10.1177/0267659112450182

69. Yang K, Huang H, Dai R, et al. Modified cardiopulmonary bypass with low priming volume for blood conservation in cardiac valve replacement surgery. *J Cardiothorac Surg.* 2023;18(1):56. doi:10.1186/s13019-023-02175-8

70. Hensley NB, Gyi R, Zorrilla-Vaca A, et al. Retrograde autologous priming in cardiac surgery: results from a systematic review and meta-analysis. *Anesth Analg.* 2021;132(1):100-107. doi:10.1213/ANE.0000000000005151

71. Shore-Lesserson L, Manspeizer HE, DePerio M, Francis S, Vela-Cantos F, Ergin MA. Thromboelastography-guided transfusion algorithm reduces transfusions in complex cardiac surgery. *Anesth Analg.* 1999;88(2):312-319.

72. Wasowicz M, McCluskey SA, Wijeysundera DN, et al. The incremental value of thrombelastography for prediction of excessive blood loss after cardiac surgery: an observational study. *Anesth Analg.* 2010;111(2):331-338. doi:10.1213/ANE.0b013e3181e456c1

73. Haensig M, Kempfert J, Kempfert PM, Girdauskas E, Borger MA, Lehmann S. Thrombelastometry guided blood-component therapy after cardiac surgery: a randomized study. *BMC Anesthesiol.* 2019;19(1):201. doi:10.1186/s12871-019-0875-7

74. Wikkelso A, Wetterslev J, Moller AM, Afshari A. Thromboelastography (TEG) or rotational thromboelastometry (ROTEM) to monitor haemostatic treatment in bleeding patients: a systematic review with meta-analysis and trial sequential analysis. *Anaesthesia.* 2017;72(4):519-531. doi:10.1111/anae.13765

75. Kwak YL, Kim JC, Choi YS, Yoo KJ, Song Y, Shim JK. Clopidogrel responsiveness regardless of the discontinuation date predicts increased blood loss and transfusion requirement after off-pump coronary artery bypass graft surgery. *J Am Coll Cardiol.* 2010;56(24):1994-2002. doi:10.1016/j.jacc.2010.03.108

76. Preisman S, Kogan A, Itzkovsky K, Leikin G, Raanani E. Modified thromboelastography evaluation of platelet dysfunction in patients undergoing coronary artery surgery. *Eur J Cardiothorac Surg.* 2010;37(6):1367-1374. doi:10.1016/j.ejcts.2009.12.044

77. Corredor C, Wasowicz M, Karkouti K, Sharma V. The role of point-of-care platelet function testing in predicting postoperative bleeding following cardiac surgery: a systematic review and meta-analysis. *Anaesthesia.* 2015;70(6):715-731. doi:10.1111/anae.13083

78. Rogers AL, Allman RD, Fang X, et al. Thromboelastography-platelet mapping allows safe and earlier urgent coronary artery bypass grafting. *Ann Thorac Surg.* 2022;113(4):1119-1125. doi:10.1016/j.athoracsur.2021.07.068

Preservation of End-Organ Function

Christina Massoth and Alexander Zarbock

KEY POINTS

1. Preservation of kidney function requires early detection and targeted implementation of supportive measures.
2. Postoperative cognitive impairment is frequent and demands the routine use of screening tools.
3. Low cardiac output syndrome and vasoplegia are both contributors to postoperative hemodynamic compromise and require differentiated vasopressor and catecholamine regimens.
4. Protocols for lung-protective ventilation and timely extubation decrease pulmonary complications.
5. Impairment of abdominal and gastrointestinal organs occurs infrequently but is usually secondary to other organ system dysfunctions.

I. Introduction

Cardiac surgery is the intersection of a multimorbid population with high-risk procedures characterized by several nonphysiologic features. The result is a significantly increased hazard for intraoperative and postoperative functional decline in end-organ function.

The use of cardiopulmonary bypass (CPB) is considered a key factor in various mechanisms of organ damage. Characteristics of organ perfusion are altered by nonpulsatile instead of pulsatile flow and hemodilution caused by the priming fluids of the extracorporeal circuit.

Contact activation between blood and the artificial surfaces of the bypass circuits results in a systemic inflammatory response syndrome by inducing numerous inflammatory pathways, including the complement system, kallikrein-kinin and fibrinolytic cascades, and endothelial and leukocyte activation. Due to bypass circulation and red blood cell transfusion, hemolysis creates radical heme and iron species as further promotors of oxidative stress. Ischemia following aortic cross-clamping and cardioplegia causes first-hit damage, while the reestablishment of perfusion triggers a subsequent inflammatory mediator release.

The omission of CPB for off-pump coronary artery bypass grafting (CABG) seemed to be a promising approach to avoid the detrimental effects associated with extracorporeal circulation. However, two large randomized controlled trials (RCTs) with a total of 3,014 randomized patients failed to prove any difference in primary outcomes but reported higher revascularization rates, calling the specific role of CPB in causing end-organ dysfunction into question.[1,2]

Several pharmacologic strategies have targeted the systemic inflammatory response associated with CPB. However, an appropriate drug has yet to be identified: Glucocorticoids were ineffective in reducing mortality after cardiac surgery.[3] A perioperatively implemented statin therapy did not reduce myocardial complications but was associated with increased rates of acute kidney injury (AKI).[4,5] Hemadsorption during extracorporeal circulation failed to decrease postoperative organ dysfunction.[6] Remote ischemic preconditioning (RIPC) reduced AKI, but as with anesthetic-induced preconditioning, it was not associated with decreased mortality, myocardial infarction, or stroke.[7,8]

This chapter highlights the most common end-organ complications associated with cardiac surgery and discusses current preventive strategies. Although the organ systems are analyzed separately, it is of note that prophylactic and supportive measures usually provide multiplier effects with an impact on all systems.

II. Kidneys

AKI is among the most frequent organ dysfunction in cardiac surgery patients. It is associated with higher in-hospital mortality and decreased long-term survival and is an important contributor to overall rising healthcare expenditures, as indicated by increased lengths of hospital stay and adverse long-term outcomes, such as chronic kidney disease (CKD). Still, no pharmacologic therapy is available, but AKI is preventable in many cases and can be attenuated by the timely initiation of bundled interventions. This is especially important since the overall outcome worsens with increasing AKI severity. Although the need for renal replacement therapy (RRT) is not frequent in cardiac surgery–associated AKI (CS-AKI) and affects <5%, it is associated with a 50% mortality.[9] Consequently, the management of renal protection in cardiac surgery is focused on prevention, timely recognition, and goal-directed supportive measures.

A. **Diagnosis and Epidemiology**

1. Nowadays, the Kidney Disease Improving Global Outcome (KDIGO) criteria are used to diagnose and stage an AKI. These criteria are based on a rise in serum creatinine of at least 0.3 mg/dL within 48 hours or by 1.5 times baseline within 7 days or as a decline in diuresis to <0.5 mL/kg/h for at least 6 hours or by compliance with both criteria (Table 29.1).[10] AKI is differentiated by severity as mild, moderate, and severe and by duration as transient or when lasting >48 hours as persistent. In the broader spectrum of disease, AKI defines the intermediate stage between subclinical damage and acute kidney disease (AKD) after 7 days of persistence, which transforms into CKD after 90 days.[11]

2. The incidence of CS-AKI ranges between 20% and 40%, depending on the population, the type of procedure, and the application of diagnostic criteria. It is of note that the use of the oliguria criterion to determine AKI is still underrepresented in clinical practice and trial reporting. Recent data implied that up to 40% of patients undergoing cardiac surgery present with isolated postoperative oliguria, a finding that was associated with a doubled odds of persistent renal dysfunction after 6 years compared to patients with normal postoperative

TABLE 29.1 KDIGO AKI Stages

Stage	Serum Creatinine	Urine Output
1	1.5-1.9 times baseline OR ≥0.3 mg/dL increase	<0.5 mL/kg/h for 6-12 h
2	2.0-2.9 times baseline	<0.5 mL/kg/h for ≥12 h
3	3.0 times baseline OR Increase in serum creatinine to ≥4.0 mg/dL OR Initiation of renal replacement therapy	<0.3 mL/kg/h for ≥24 h OR Anuria for ≥12 h

AKI, acute kidney injury; KDIGO, Kidney Disease Improving Global Outcome.

kidney function.[12] However, a temporary decline in urine output may occur as a physiologic response to hypovolemia (or surgical stress) and is not necessarily related to kidney damage. While oliguria lacks specificity, serum creatinine has a low sensitivity and is influenced by several factors, including muscle mass, age, sex, or diet. Given these limitations, new biomarkers have been identified to detect renal damage before a loss of function becomes apparent. The translation of biomarkers into clinical practice for better risk stratification and guidance of therapy to reduce AKI was recommended by the 2019 enhanced recovery after surgery guidelines for perioperative care in cardiac surgery.[13] A consensus statement by the Acute Disease Quality Initiative Consensus Conference (ADQI) proposed enhancing the conventional AKI stages by biomarkers to better display the subclinical damage stage, which is not reflected by the traditional criteria so far.[14]

B. Biomarkers

In recent years, a large number of biomarkers of CS-AKI were proposed and assessed for their predictive abilities. Biomarkers were identified and categorized in terms of risk assessment and prediction of AKI, such as Dickkopf-3 and interleukin-18; biomarkers to diagnose and predict the severity of AKI, including cystatin C, liver-type fatty acid–binding protein (L-FABP), kidney injury molecule 1 (KIM-1), N-acetyl-β-D-glucosaminidase, and renin; and novel candidates such as C-C motif chemokine ligand 14 to predict renal recovery after AKI.

Among these, neutrophil gelatinase–associated lipocalin (NGAL) as a marker of proximal tubular damage and the product of two molecules that are involved in the G_1-cell cycle arrest, tissue metalloproteinase-2 (TIMP2), and insulin-like growth factor–binding protein-7 (IGFBP7) have been investigated most extensively.[14] However, [TIMP2]*[IGFBP7] provides a superior sensitivity of 0.79 (95% confidence interval [CI], 0.71-0.86) and a specificity of 0.76 (95% CI, 0.72-0.80) to predict AKI and shows a favorable kinetic by reaching its peak levels at 4 hours after CPB.[15] A point-of-care test is commercially available to measure urinary levels at the bedside. To date, biomarkers are not yet routinely applied in perioperative care, and further research is warranted to clarify their significance in clinical practice.

CLINICAL PEARL

Already 4 hours after CPB, biomarkers of early damage detect cell stress that proceeds in AKI.

C. Implementation of the Kidney Disease Improving Global Outcome Care Bundle

Measuring stress/damage biomarkers of CS-AKI can be a complementary measure in addition to the application of risk scores and offers the opportunity to identify patients at high risk for developing AKI. The 2012 KDIGO Clinical Practice Guideline for Acute Kidney Injury proposed a stage-based management to begin with a certain care bundle implementation already in patients at high risk for AKI (Figure 29.1). The following care bundle measures were recommended:

1. Discontinue all nephrotoxic agents when possible

The development of CS-AKI is considered a result of multiple insults, to which the perioperative application of nephrotoxic drugs poses an additional risk by providing tubular damage, decreased renal blood flow, and altered intraglomerular hemodynamics. Apart from single-drug effects, adverse effects may occur by drug-drug interactions. Triple therapy with renin-angiotensin system inhibitors (angiotensin-converting enzyme inhibitor [ACEi]), diuretics, and nonsteroidal anti-inflammatory drugs was identified to be associated with even a greater risk of AKI.[16]

Although the role of angiotensin blockers in cardiac surgery is somewhat controversial, ACEi and angiotensin receptor blockers are usually withheld on the day of surgery and the early postoperative period. Perioperative blockade of the renin-angiotensin-aldosterone system (RAAS) potentially contributes to the development of AKI by increasing the risk for intraoperative and postoperative vasoplegic syndrome with systemic hypotension and efferent arteriolar vasodilation. At least in patients who are critically ill, they should be stopped temporarily but reintroduced as early as possible.[17]

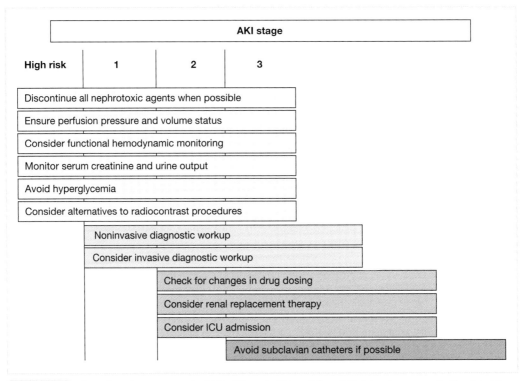

FIGURE 29.1 Stage-based management of AKI. AKI, acute kidney injury; ICU, intensive care unit. (Reprinted from Kidney Disease: Improving Global Outcomes (KDIGO) Acute Kidney Injury Work Group. KDIGO clinical practice guideline for acute kidney injury. *Kidney Int Suppl.* 2012;2:1-138. © 2012 KDIGO. With permission.)

2. **Optimize volume status and perfusion pressure**
   a. Ensuring an adequate perfusion pressure and avoiding postoperative hypovolemia or hypervolemia are crucial factors for the prevention and treatment of AKI. Fluid management should be guided by repeated assessments of fluid status and volume responsiveness since a higher positive fluid balance is associated with AKI and the requirement of RRT after cardiac surgery.[18] Although chloride-rich solutions can be used safely,[19,20] balanced crystalloid solutions are the first choice for fluid replacement and are preferred over chloride-rich solutions and synthetic colloids. However, the administration of higher volumes of chloride-rich solutions results in a worse outcome.[21-23]
   b. Given the potentially harmful effects of synthetic colloids, the use of albumin was discussed as a potentially preferable alternative. Albumin raises the colloid oncotic pressure, traps reactive oxygen species, stabilizes the endothelial glycocalyx function, and has essential binding and transporting properties, affecting almost all drug pharmacokinetics.
      However, a recent large single-center trial failed to prove beneficial effects on postoperative outcomes in cardiac surgery. The albumin infusion and acute kidney injury following cardiac surgery (ALBICS) trial randomized 1,386 patients to receive either albumin 4% or Ringer acetate solution for pump priming and perioperative volume therapy up to a total volume of 3,200 mL. Patients in the albumin group had a cumulative lower fluid intake, but no differences in regard to major adverse events, including AKI, were detectable between both groups. These findings do not support a routine use of albumin in cardiac surgery; nevertheless, the study did not include high-risk patients undergoing emergency procedures.[24]
   c. Although the optimum hemodynamic targets are yet to be defined and need to be developed on a case-by-case decision, a mean arterial blood pressure of >65 mm Hg is usually considered sufficient to maintain organ perfusion and was found to be a key driver

of AKI reversal. An individualized blood pressure management might provide further advantage regarding the altered autoregulation in patients with known hypertension. Venous congestion was lately identified to play a pivotal role in the development of CS-AKI, being even more important than arterial hypotension.[25] An elevated central venous pressure (CVP) increases renal venous pressure and subsequently decreases renal blood flow and glomerular filtration rate (GFR). At a threshold of >12 mm Hg, the odds for AKI increase by 6% and >16 mm Hg by 12%, and a CVP > 20 mm Hg is independently associated with a 30% increase in odds for AKI.[25]

3. **Consider functional hemodynamic monitoring**

   A comprehensive hemodynamic workup is completed by measurements of preload and cardiac output since a low cardiac output state with decreased systemic oxygen delivery is strongly associated with the development of organ dysfunctions. Optimization of stroke volume and preservation of cardiac index >3 L/min/m^2 were identified to be among the most important measures to prevent AKI.[26]

   Depending on the clinical context and local availability, either noninvasive methods, including transthoracic echocardiography (TTE), bioimpedance, or bioreactance devices, or invasive methods, such as pulse index continuous cardiac output (PiCCO) or Swan-Ganz catheters, are appropriate.

4. **Monitor serum creatinine and urine output**

   Close postoperative monitoring of renal function based on serum creatinine and diuresis is essential to establish an early diagnosis, classify the severity, and predict the outcome of AKI.

   Intensive urine output monitoring is associated with increased detection of AKI and decreased mortality at day 30 (hazard ratio, 0.85; 95% CI, 0.77-0.94; $P = .001$) due to improved fluid management and less cumulative volume overload.[27]

5. **Avoid hyperglycemia**

   High blood glucose levels induce inflammation, apoptosis, and fibrosis pathways; cause oxidative stress and volume depletion by osmotic diuresis; and are generally well recognized for their contribution to kidney disease. While a history of diabetes mellitus is common in patients undergoing cardiac procedures, CPB, surgical stress, and inotropic agents contribute additionally to the high incidence of intraoperative and postoperative hyperglycemia. The potential benefits of tight glycemic control have to be balanced against the risk of hypoglycemia. The 2012 KDIGO recommends an intermediate corridor between tight and conventional glycemic control, targeting plasma glucose of 110-149 mg/dL (6.1-8.3 mmol/L).

   However, it seems reasonable to differentiate between patients without diabetes and patients with diabetes since hyperglycemia is especially linked in patients without diabetes with increased AKI and mortality rates. Still, this association indicates the chicken-egg problem of stress hyperglycemia: It remains controversial whether high glucose needs to be treated more aggressively in these patients or occurs as a consequence of the critical condition.[28]

6. **Consider alternatives to radiocontrast procedures**

   A comparable dilemma applies to the application of iodinated radiocontrast agents and the subsequent development of AKI: Critically ill patients who already have an inherently increased risk for AKI are more likely to undergo contrast-enhanced diagnostic procedures involving radiocontrast agents. Given the potential nephrotoxic effects of iodinated contrast agents, the 2012 KDIGO guideline recommended avoiding these whenever possible and considering alternative approaches when available to minimize the overall exposure to nephrotoxic agents. However, more recent evidence suggests that this effect may have been overestimated, finding only a slightly increased risk in patients with mildly to moderately reduced kidney function.[29] A recent cohort study including 156,028 emergency patients with radiocontrast exposure found no association with a change in estimated GFR (−0.4 mL/min/1.73 m^2; 95% CI, −4.9 to 4.0), AKI, or the need for RRT.[30] Consequently, delaying urgent contrast-enhanced diagnosis with therapeutic implications is not legitimate regarding AKI prevention.

7. Increasing evidence supports the implementation of this six-measure care bundle in cardiac surgery patients. A prospective observational study reported less progression to more severe AKI stages and less mortality associated with the early implementation of the bundle.[31]

In a quality improvement initiative, the biomarker-guided use of the KDIGO recommendations was associated with a reduced incidence of moderate and severe AKI.[32]

The PrevAKI Single-Center trial used a biomarker-guided approach as well. It measured the urinary levels of [TIMP2]*[IGFBP7] 4 hours after CPB to identify patients at high risk for AKI. A total of 276 patients were randomized to receive either the standard of care or a strict implementation of the KDIGO bundle. This intervention significantly reduced the incidence of AKI within 72 hours after surgery (55.1% vs 71.7%; $P = .004$; odds ratio [OR], 0.483 [95% CI, 0.293-0.796]) and the occurrence of higher AKI severity stages.[33] The PrevAKI multicenter trial investigated the same intervention at 12 participating sites with 27 randomized patients and found the incidence of moderate and severe AKI to be significantly reduced (absolute risk reduction [ARR], 10.0% [95% CI, 0.9-19.1]; $P = .034$).[34]

In a secondary analysis of the combined data of both PrevAKI studies, the individual elements were tested for their impact on AKI prevention. The avoidance of nephrotoxic agents and hemodynamic optimization, defined as the avoidance of hypotension and low cardiac output, were identified as the most important measures for the effectiveness of the bundle.[26]

CLINICAL PEARL

The implementation of a care bundle consisting of six supportive and preventive measures in patients at high risk for AKI reduces the incidence of moderate and severe AKI stages (Figure 29.1).

D. Pharmacologic Strategies

The rationale for most pharmacologic interventions for AKI prevention is to attenuate the systemic inflammation in response to extracorporeal circulation.

1. For this purpose, the effects of different intraoperative corticosteroid treatment regimens were investigated in large RCTs. The steroids in cardiac surgery (SIRS) trial randomized 7,507 patients to receive 500-mg methylprednisolone or placebo and found no difference in the secondary outcome, "acute renal failure." However, the application of methylprednisolone was associated with elevated CK-MB enzyme levels, which might reflect a more extended myocardial injury.[3] In the dexamethasone for cardiac surgery (DECS) trial, 4,494 patients underwent randomization to receive an intraoperative dose of dexamethasone 1 mg/kg. However, AKI rate was not a prespecified outcome, and only in a post hoc analysis, steroid administration slightly reduced the incidence of acute renal failure with the need for RRT (0.4% vs 1.0%, $P = .04$).[35]

2. Statins are a class of drugs with antioxidant and anti-inflammatory effects and have been proposed to preserve renal function in cardiac surgery. The statin therapy in cardiac surgery (STICS) trial assessed the impact of a new-onset therapy with rosuvastatin on the rates of postoperative complications in 192 randomized patients compared to placebo. The new initiation of statin therapy or the change of class from any previously described statin to rosuvastatin was not associated with any beneficial effects but increased the incidence of AKI by 5.4% ± 1.9% (AKI 24.7% vs 19.3%, $P = .005$). Although the authors speculated that this finding might be a class effect, linked to the potential of rosuvastatin to cause proteinuria, meta-analyses including other statins failed to prove any benefit from a newly started statin therapy before cardiac surgery.[4,5]

3. The α2-adrenergic agonist dexmedetomidine provides, besides its sedative and analgesic properties, sympatholytic and anti-inflammatory effects by inhibiting apoptosis and reducing plasma levels of pro-inflammatory cytokines. Perioperative administration in cardiac surgery within a dose range between 0.1 and 0.8 mg/kg/h was reported to be safe in terms of bradycardia and hypotension, while the incidence of CS-AKI was significantly reduced (relative risk [RR], 0.60; 95% CI, 0.41-0.87, $P = .008$, $I^2 = 30\%$). A meta-analysis suggests that preoperative and/or intraoperative application with or without postoperative continuation seemed to provide beneficial effects compared to a postoperative administration alone.[36]

4. In experimental research, volatile anesthetics were found to provide cell-protective effects in conditions of ischemia-reperfusion injury. Despite these properties of anesthetic-induced preconditioning, meta-analyses came to conflicting results in terms of AKI reduction.[37,38] The large multicenter MYRIAD RCT compared an anesthetic regimen of intravenous induction and inhalational maintenance with total intravenous anesthesia for elective CABG. The trial was stopped for futility at 540 randomized patients since no difference in any of the prespecified outcomes, including AKI, became apparent.[7]

E. **Remote Ischemic Preconditioning**

RIPC is a procedure to provide organ protection from a subsequent injury by inducing repetitively short episodes of ischemia and reperfusion of a limb, usually, the forearm, by inflating and deflating a cuff. This intervention induces multiple anti-inflammatory and humoral signaling pathways, attenuating the systemic inflammatory response to cardiovascular surgery. While data from animal studies and some RCTs reported renal and cardioprotective effects, others, such as the 2015 landmark RIPHeart study (1,403 randomized patients) and the effect of remote ischaemic preconditioning on clinical outcomes in patients undergoing coronary artery bypass graft surgery (ERICCA) trial (1,612 randomized patients), failed to provide a proof of concept.[39,40] However, factors such as the inclusion of a low-risk population or the choice of anesthetic agents may have masked the potential effects of RIPC. In contrast, the multicenter RenalRIPC trial including 240 patients at high risk for AKI found RIPC to be associated with a significant reduction of AKI and RRT.[8] A recent meta-analysis including 79 RCTs with 10,814 patients indicated a reduction of postoperative AKI with RIPC (22% vs 24.4%; RR, 0.86; 95% CI, 0.77-0.97, $P = .01$, $I^2 = 34\%$). Subgroup analysis identified an association between the use of volatile anesthetics and the application in non–high-risk patients.[41] It has been shown that propofol attenuated the protective effects of RIPC. This may explain why the RIPHeart and ERICCA trials were negative, since >95% of patients in the RIPC groups were treated with propofol.

III. **Brain**

A. **Neurocognitive Disorders**

Cognitive changes are a common finding after cardiac surgery, affecting more than half of all patients. Even in the absence of symptoms, a decline in cognitive function can still be apparent after months up to years after the procedure.[42] In this continuum of several overlapping conditions, the latest nomenclature on perioperative cognitive disorders by the American Society of Anesthesiologists defines the terms *neurocognitive disorders* (NCDs) and *delayed postoperative recovery* (Table 29.2).

TABLE 29.2 Summary of Perioperative Cognitive Disorder Nomenclature

Time Period	Mild NCD		Major NCD	
Emergence from anesthesia	Emergence excitation or delirium			
Immediately postoperative to 30 d	Delirium OR delayed neurocognitive recovery	Delayed neurocognitive recovery	Delayed neurocognitive recovery	The time for expected resolution is based on perioperative conditions (complications, infections, etc)
30 d until 12 mo		Mild NCD postoperative (POCD)	Major NCD postoperative (POCD)	POCD is an indicator of the temporal association with anesthesia/surgery
Beyond 12 mo		Mild NCD	Major NCD	As in community if a new diagnosis after this time

NCD, neurocognitive disorder; POCD, postoperative cognitive dysfunction.
Reprinted with permission from Evered L, Silbert B, Knopman DS, et al. Recommendations for the nomenclature of cognitive change associated with anaesthesia and surgery—2018. Anesthesiology. 2018;129(5):872-879. © 2018 American Society of Anesthesiologists.

1. The generic concept of NCDs includes postoperative delirium and delayed neurocognitive recovery as short-term events up to 30 days from the initial procedures. After 30 days until 12 months, the term *postoperative cognitive dysfunction*, specified as mild or major NCD, applies. Diagnostic features are the subjective complaint by the patient, clinician, or an informant; the objective impairment, defined as mild at 1-2 standard deviations below controls or major ≥2 standard deviations below norms; and a decline in the activities of daily living.[42]

2. Postoperative delirium is a form of early NCD and usually occurs within 1 week after the procedure. Although it is associated with increased mortality and severe short- and long-term adverse outcomes, such as persistent cognitive decline and loss of independence, it is still an underrecognized condition.[43] Delirium can be differentiated by motoric phenotype as hyperactive with agitation and combativeness or hypoactive characterized by apathy and impaired awareness.

   According to the *Diagnostic and Statistical Manual of Mental Disorders* (*DSM-5*), it is defined as a disturbance in attention and awareness characterized by the reduced ability to focus and orient to the environment (a) compared to baseline cognitive function, usually with a fluctuation in severity (b). It is accompanied by additional cognitive dysfunctions in features of memory, language, orientation, visuospatial ability, or perception (c) and cannot be explained by a preexisting condition of NCD (d) with additional evidence to be a direct consequence of another medical condition or exposure.

3. The risk for postoperative delirium increases with age, preexisting neuropsychiatric conditions, cognitive impairment, and congestive heart failure. The constellation of the inherent baseline risk, the procedural stress of cardiac surgery, and additional postoperative stressors add up to the pathophysiology of delirium, which is still poorly understood so far.

   Precipitating factors to be aware of include the transfusion of blood products, silent cerebral ischemia, the length of surgery, and duration of mechanical ventilation and conscious sedation afterward.[44] Identifying the delirium risk at baseline provides the opportunity for individual preoperative optimization of conditions of frailty or malnutrition and increases postoperative vigilance.[43] Cardiac surgery patients should be monitored routinely for delirium by using validated tools, such as the Intensive Care Delirium Screening Checklist (ICDSC) or the Confusion Assessment Methods for the Intensive Care Unit (CAM-ICU). Both tests have high accuracy in detecting delirium—the ICDSC shows good performances with a pooled area under the summary receiver operating characteristic curve (area under curve [AUC]) of 0.89 and pooled sensitivity of 74% and specificity of 81.9%, and the CAM-ICU provides even superior features with a pooled AUC of 0.97 and a pooled sensitivity of 80% and specificity of 95.9%. However, both tools are less sensitive when it comes to the screening of the more prevalent hypodynamic subtype of delirium.[45]

4. Traditional management of delirium was usually based on the use of antipsychotic drugs, but recent society recommendations such as the 2018 Pain, Agitation/Sedation, Delirium, Immobility, and Sleep Disruption in Adult Patients in the ICU (PADIS) guidelines depart from this long-standing dogma and turn to a more comprehensive approach favoring nonpharmacologic interventions. First-line measures for delirium management include routine screening, restrictive postoperative use of opioids and sedatives, avoidance of sleep disruption, and early mobilization. The prophylactic or routine application of benzodiazepines or antipsychotics is not supported by current evidence and should be limited to the management of hyperactive states and attenuating-associated symptoms, such as hallucinations and delusion.[43] The prophylactic haloperidol use for delirium in icu patients at high risk for delirium (REDUCE) randomized clinical trial assessed the effects of a prophylactic haloperidol therapy in 178 randomized patients but found no differences in delirium rates or length of ICU and hospital stay compared to placebo.[46] The large MIND-USA trial with a total of 1,183 included patients failed to prove any effect of the therapeutic use of haloperidol or ziprasidone compared to placebo on the duration of delirium.[47] A small single-center RCT indicated a reduced incidence of delirium after cardiac surgery with risperidone.[48] The results of a systematic review and meta-analysis suggested protective effects for the perioperative administration of dexmedetomidine compared to saline (RR = 0.54 [0.32-0.90],

$P = .02)$.[36] However, patient selection, dosage, timing, and length of administration have yet to be defined, especially in the light of the latest findings of a secondary analysis of the SPICE III trial, which reported increased mortality associated with dexmedetomidine sedation in critically ill patients <65 years.[49]

CLINICAL PEARL

While the prevention of postoperative delirium relies on nonpharmacologic interventions, the prophylactic administration of dexmedetomidine might provide additional benefits.

B. **Perioperative Stroke**

Perioperative ischemic stroke is among the most feared complications of cardiac surgery and a significant contributor to postoperative mortality and long-term disability. While the clinical stroke risk is about 6%, the risk of brain ischemia on magnetic resonance imaging (MRI) approximates 36% for all comers, 27% for CABG, and about 50% for open valve surgery.[50,51]

Stroke can occur as an intraoperative event, becoming apparent at emergence from anesthesia, or as a postoperative complication with a clear onset after extubation.

1. Postoperative stroke is usually associated with atrial fibrillation or other arrhythmias.[52] Etiologies of intraoperative stroke include hypoperfusion and embolism of air or thrombotic material. Atheromatosis of the ascending aorta is accountable for the majority of intraoperative events due to plaque dislodgements during arterial cannulation, aortic cross-clamping, and the jet effect of the aortic cannula. Epiaortic ultrasound may help guide the insertion of the arterial cannula in patients at risk and thereby improve neurologic outcomes.[53]

CLINICAL PEARL

The use of epiaortic ultrasound in patients with atheromatosis may decrease the incidence of intraoperative stroke.

---

2. Intraoperative cerebral perfusion can be monitored and guided by techniques of electroencephalogram (EEG), evoked potentials, transcranial Doppler, or measurements of oxygenation. The most widely adopted method is near-infrared spectroscopy (NIRS), a noninvasive real-time monitor, which uses near-infrared light (700-1,000 nm) to transverse biologic tissues, including the skull, to measure the light absorption of oxyhemoglobin and deoxyhemoglobin. Unlike transmissive pulse oximetry, NIRS is independent of pulsatility and measures predominantly venous and capillary blood to determine regional cerebral oxygen saturation ($rScO_2$). This implies an important limitation to this technique, as the amounts of arterial versus capillary and venous blood are highly variable and changes in cerebral blood flow are not sufficiently reflected by the venous and capillary components.[54]

Although there is some uncertainty in defining the lower threshold at 60%, 55%, or 50%, a fall of >20% is generally considered indicative of cerebral hypoperfusion. While NIRS can successfully detect cannula malposition for cerebral perfusion in aortic surgery, data on the effects of NIRS-based algorithms on postoperative NCDs or stroke are conflicting, and high-quality studies are still lacking.[55]

3. Temperature management during CPB targeting mild (32-35 °C), moderate (28-32 °C), or deep (<28 °C) hypothermia is used for neuroprotection depending on length, complexity, and the need for circulatory arrest. Hypothermia lowers the cerebral metabolic rate of oxygen consumption, decreases reactive oxygen species, and downregulates excitatory neurotransmitter activity. To date, it remains inconclusive whether hypothermic CPB actually improves neurocognitive outcomes and if further insights on the effects during different stages of temperature management are needed. Hypothermia might as well induce

neuronal apoptosis and comes with the potential risks of hyperthermic states during the re-warming period. Most recent data from a meta-analysis including 58 studies on neurologic outcomes and mortality after normothermic or hypothermic CPB failed to demonstrate a relationship between temperature and postoperative NCD, stroke, or mortality.[56]

4. **Management of stroke**

Opioid reduction and the use of short-acting anesthetic agents accelerate the time to ex-tubation after surgery, but the evaluation of neurologic function during emergence from anesthesia for cardiac surgery can be challenging. Newly developed focal neurologic defi-cits suspicious of stroke should be addressed by the immediate initiation of diagnostic im-aging.[57] A noncontrast computed tomography (CT) scan identifies cerebral hemorrhage and may reveal early signs of ischemic lesions. CT angiography and CT perfusion detect large vessel occlusions and allow for differentiation between the penumbra and already infarcted brain tissue. Stroke patients should be cared for by interdisciplinary stroke teams. Intravenous thrombolytic therapy is usually not a therapeutic option due to the high risk of postoperative hemorrhage. Endovascular thrombectomy can be performed in patients with large vessel occlusions and is associated with significantly improved functional outcomes and reduced mortality.[58]

C. **Seizures**

Seizures emerging during weaning of sedation or in the early postoperative phase in patients without a history of epilepsy may occur in up to 1% of cardiac surgery cases.[59] Acute symp-tomatic seizures can occur not only as an early sign of intraoperative ischemic or hemorrhagic stroke but also as a result of a variety of triggers, such as metabolic disturbances, anesthetic drugs, or other pharmacologic interventions. After the introduction of tranexamic acid for in-traoperative antifibrinolytic therapy, the incidence of postoperative seizures increased, depend-ing on the dose administration and renal clearance. Given the variable etiology of postoperative seizures, there are no general treatment recommendations. Whether or not a temporary or permanent anticonvulsive therapy is required must be decided on a case-by-case basis.

IV. **Heart and Circulatory System**

A. **Low Cardiac Output Syndrome**

Postoperative low cardiac output syndrome (LCOS) is a severe complication of cardiac surgery associated with a high risk of mortality. It occurs in up to 15% of patients and is especially prevalent in those who present preoperatively with severely reduced left ventricular function. LCOS is not clearly defined but usually refers to a condition with a reduced cardiac index below a range between 1.8 and 2.2 L/min/m^2, hypotension, decreased mixed venous oxygen saturation (SvO_2), and impaired microcirculation with elevated lactate levels >2.0 mmol/L and signs of end-organ hypoperfusion.[60] Although LCOS and cardiogenic shock are more of a con-tinuum than two separate entities, the term *cardiogenic shock* is sometimes used to describe a life-threatening condition with insufficient oxygen supply and multiorgan dysfunction.

Management of LCOS usually relies on inotropes to increase myocardial contractility and reduce right and left ventricular afterload but at the cost of higher cardiac oxygen consumption and incidence of arrhythmias.

The choice of inotropic agents and general management of LCOS relies primarily on center-level preference and expert opinion. So far, there is insufficient evidence to clearly rec-ommend a certain inotrope for the prevention of LCOS.

1. Like enoximone and amrinone, milrinone is a phosphodiesterase-3 inhibitor in vascular smooth muscles and the cardiac sarcoplasmic reticulum. Phosphorylation of calcium chan-nels promotes calcium reuptake and increases inotropy, chronotropy, and lusitropy. Besides these effects on systolic and diastolic function, it is a potent vasodilator in the pulmonary vasculature with superior efficacy compared to β1-agonists, such as dobutamine. It offers theoretical benefits, especially in patients with impaired right ventricular function and pul-monary hypertension. However, while there is a large body of literature and widely spread use in pediatric cardiac surgery for preventing and treating LCOS, the role in adult surgical patients is less clear.

The dobutamine compared to milrinone (DOREMI) trial randomized 192 patients with cardiogenic shock but not specifically after cardiac surgery to receive treatment with either dobutamine or milrinone for inotropic support. In this population, no difference became apparent concerning primary end points, including in-hospital mortality, need for mechanical circulatory support, myocardial infarction, stroke, or RRT.[61]

Retrospective data and the results of a meta-analysis of RCTs implied that intraoperative use of milrinone might be associated with increased perioperative mortality. This effect became only apparent in studies comparing milrinone with other drugs such as levosimendan, but not in studies comparing milrinone with placebo, suggesting a superior protective effect of the other agents.[62,63]

2. Levosimendan improves inotropy without raising intracellular calcium levels and myocardial oxygen consumption by upregulating the affinity of troponin c for calcium.

   It also opens adenosine triphosphate (ATP)-sensitive potassium channels of mitochondria and vascular smooth muscle cells, causing vasodilation of the coronary arteries and resulting in improved myocardial oxygen supply. Due to this mechanism of action, it is considered especially beneficial in patients with ischemic cardiomyopathy undergoing CABG.[60]

   A meta-analysis and systematic review of six RCTs comparing levosimendan with placebo in high-risk patients implied a reduced mortality (OR, 0.51 [0.32, 0.82], $P = .005$, $I^2 = 0\%$) and decreased need for RRT (OR, 0.55 [0.31, 0.97], $P = .04$, $I^2 = 0\%$) in patients with left ventricular ejection fraction <35%. However, these findings are limited by the fact that the included trials were underpowered and had an increased risk of bias.[60] In contrast, three large multicenter RCTs published in 2017 challenged the effectiveness of levosimendan and found no differences in their primary composite end points compared to placebo. The LEVO-CTS trial as the most extensive of these studies indicated, however, a decreased incidence of LCOS, less need for other inotropic agents, and higher cardiac indices.[64]

   These findings indicate that a prophylactic infusion of levosimendan may be reasonable in certain subgroups, but further evidence is warranted to clarify patient selection.

CLINICAL PEARL

The prophylactic administration of levosimendan in patients with severe ischemic cardiomyopathy might reduce the risk of LCOS.

B. Postoperative Arrhythmias

Postoperative arrhythmias are a regular complication after cardiac surgery, with atrial fibrillation and atrial flutter being by far the most common types, affecting up to 30% of patients after CABG, 40% after valve replacement, and up to 50% after combined procedures.

Supraventricular tachyarrhythmias develop most frequently on the second and third postoperative day and are often self-limited within 2-24 hours.[65]

Nevertheless, these episodes are associated with increased morbidity, length of stay, and death. Loss of the atrial kick, impaired diastolic filling, and increased myocardial oxygen consumption promote or worsen hemodynamic compromise.[65] Irregular atrial contractions with blood stasis are a well-known risk factor for intra-atrial clot formation and stroke. Especially older patients with a history of atrial fibrillation and comorbidities such as renal failure, mitral valve pathologies, heart failure, or chronic obstructive pulmonary disease have an elevated risk of developing postoperative atrial fibrillation (POAF). Exposure to perioperative inflammation, structural remodeling, metabolic disturbances, catecholamine therapy, and pericardial effusion contributes to its pathophysiology.[66]

1. Both patients at normal and elevated risk should receive perioperative continuation and postoperative administration of β-receptor antagonists based on a Class I recommendation. In patients with normal sinus rhythm but at high risk of developing POAF, a Class II recommendation suggests considering a perioperative prophylactic administration of amiodarone.[65] Other pharmacologic strategies, including sotalol or colchicine, and non-pharmacologic measures, such as prophylactic atrial or biatrial pacing, were only graded as a Class IIb recommendation (Figure 29.2).[65] Implementing a posterior left pericardiotomy

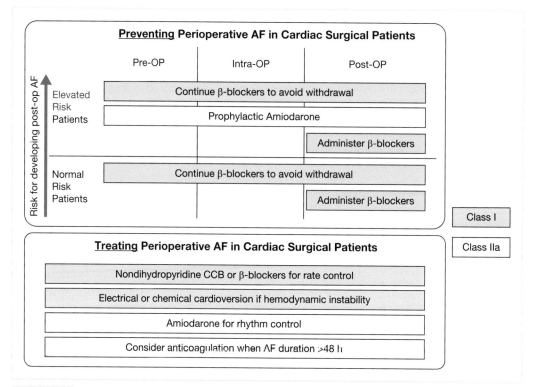

FIGURE 29.2 Practice advisory for the prevention and treatment of perioperative AF in patients undergoing cardiac surgery. AF, atrial fibrillation; CCB, calcium channel blocker. (Reprinted with permission from Muehlschlegel JD, Burrage PS, Ngai JY, et al. Society of Cardiovascular Anesthesiologists/European Association of Cardiothoracic Anaesthetists practice advisory for the management of perioperative atrial fibrillation in patients undergoing cardiac surgery. *Anesth Analg.* 2019;128(1):33-42. © 2018 International Anesthesia Research Society.)

was recently supported as an effective measure by the results of the large posterior left pericardiotomy for the prevention of atrial fibrillation after cardiac surgery (PALACS) trial. A total of 420 patients undergoing mixed cardiac procedures were randomly assigned whether or not to receive this intervention. Draining pericardial fluids into the left pleural cavity significantly reduced the incidence of POAF (17% vs 32%, P = .0007, OR, 0.44 [95% CI, 0.27-0.7], P = .0005) without increasing any potentially attributable complications.[67]

CLINICAL PEARL

Besides the perioperative continuation of β-receptor antagonists, posterior left pericardiotomy appears to be an effective measure to prevent POAF.

2. Electrolyte imbalances play a vital role in the development of cardiac arrhythmias, and conditions of hypokalemia and hypomagnesemia are common findings after cardiac surgery. However, despite it being common practice to maintain postoperative serum potassium levels at a high-normal range between 4.5 and 5.5 mmol/L, the evidence for a reductive effect of the incidence of POAF has yet to be provided.[68] Data on repletion of magnesium levels come to contradictory conclusions: While meta-analyses of studies with small sample sizes with different dosing regimens suggested beneficial effects, a large RCT with 389 randomized patients, testing a high intraoperative dose of 100 mg/kg versus placebo, found no reduction in the postoperative incidence of atrial fibrillation (Mg: 42.5% [95% CI, 35%-50%] vs placebo: 37.9% [95% CI, 31%-45%], P = .40).[66,69]

3. Therapeutic strategies distinguish between patients with stable and unstable hemodynamic conditions. POAF with hemodynamic compromise should be treated with electrical or chemical cardioversion. At the same time, rate control with β-blockers or calcium channel blockers is recommended as first-line therapy in POAF with hemodynamic stability.

   There is only a moderate quality of evidence and Class IIA recommendations supporting the initiation of a therapeutic anticoagulation.[65] While anticoagulation therapy significantly decreases the risk for thromboembolic events in patients with POAF, these benefits come at the cost of higher bleeding risk. The administration of anticoagulants can be considered if POAF lasts beyond 48 hours.[65]

C. **Vasodilatory Shock**

Despite adequate fluid resuscitation and preserved cardiac output, up to 20% of patients after cardiac surgery develop hemodynamic compromise due to reduced systemic vascular resistance (SVR). Although a consensual definition of vasodilatory shock is lacking, it is often described by a mean arterial pressure of <60-65 mm Hg, a cardiac index of >2.2 L/min/m², and an SVR of <800 dynes/s/cm⁵ at a vasopressor therapy of 0.2-0.5 μg/kg/min norepinephrine equivalent.[70]

1. Norepinephrine is the first-line vasopressor to restore SVR, but its administration can be limited by a refractory response and a dose-dependent increase in adverse events. In patients requiring high doses of >0.2 μg/kg/min norepinephrine equivalent, combined vasopressor therapy exerts synergistic effects to achieve perfusion goals while allowing a dose reduction of individual vasopressor compared to monotherapy.

2. Prolonged exposure to CPB is associated with depleted plasma levels of the hypopituitary hormone vasopressin, resulting in a decreased vasopressin-mediated reduction of nitric oxide (NO) release.[71] Unlike catecholamines, the administration of arginine vasopressin provides peripheral vasoconstriction by its agonism at the AVPR1a, AVPR1b, and AVPR2 receptors. The VANCS RCT found it to be associated with decreased mortality and severe complications compared to noradrenaline (hazard ratio, 0.55; 95% CI, 0.38-0.80; $P = .0014$), advocating its use as a first-line vasopressor.[72] However, the advantage in patients with preoperatively reduced left ventricular ejection fraction is less clear, as retrospective analyses indicated increased rates of atrial fibrillation and ventricular arrhythmias, but at comparable survival rates in this population.[73]

3. Recent data found the RAAS to be substantially involved in the pathophysiology of postoperative vasoplegia. Hypotension, decreased sodium levels, or activation of the sympathetic nervous system can each stimulate the release of renin from the extraglomerular apparatus. Renin converts angiotensinogen to angiotensin I (AT-I), the precursor of the active form AT-II, a potent vasoconstrictor, which inhibits further renin release in a feedback loop. Increased renin levels after cardiac surgery are indicative of hemodynamic instability and AKI.[74] Using renin as a biomarker to guide postoperative administration of AT-II was found to spare norepinephrine in patients with hypotension and decrease renin plasma levels compared to norepinephrine therapy alone.[75]

   A pilot study comparing AT-II to noradrenaline in cardiac surgery reported significantly decreased AKI rates in the AT-II group, but further research is warranted to clarify the target population and the risk-benefit-cost ratio of this substance.[70]

CLINICAL PEARL

AT-II appears as a promising novel candidate for the treatment of post-CPB vasodilatory shock, but more research is warranted.

4. There are several other drugs that have been discussed as a rescue treatment for vasodilatory shock. Methylene blue increases smooth vascular muscle tone by inhibiting NO but has been noted for its side effects and increased odds of morbidity and in-hospital mortality.[76] Hydroxocobalamin was described as another inhibitor of NO activity in case reports

and small case series. As mentioned earlier, glucocorticoid administration in cardiac surgery was assessed in different regimens, but vasoplegia was not among the prespecified outcomes.

V. Lung

Postoperative pulmonary complications occur in ~11% of patients undergoing cardiac surgery. About 6% require prolonged postoperative ventilation exceeding 24 hours, 4% present with impaired oxygenation at a PaO_2/FIO_2 ratio <100, about 3% undergo unplanned reintubation, and another 3% develop pneumonia.[77]

Patients in need of unplanned reintubation have a 7.5-fold increase in mortality and are at increased risk of weaning failure (OR, 30.81, 95% CI, 24.65-38.52) and infectious and thromboembolic complications.[78]

1. A poor functional status, pulmonary and renal or cardiac comorbidities along with systemic inflammation, and pulmonary collapse with low bronchial arterial perfusion during CPB are considered the key factors promoting acute respiratory failure after cardiac surgery.[77]

2. Enhanced recovery after surgery guidelines recommend early extubation within 6 hours after surgery to reduce ventilator-associated morbidity.[13]

   Adherence to a lung-protective ventilation regimen with basic measures, including a V_T <8 mL/kg predicted body weight, a driving pressure <16 cm H_2O, and a positive end-expiratory pressure (PEEP) of ≥5 cm H_2O, is associated with fewer pulmonary complications in cardiac surgery cohorts.[77]

CLINICAL PEARL

The use of an early extubation strategy minimizes pulmonary complications.

3. Maintenance of ventilation during CPB was discussed as a strategy to improve postoperative pulmonary function, but two larger trials failed to prove any effect of this approach. The perioperative open lung protective ventilation during cardiac surgery with cardiopulmonary bypass (PROVECS) trial assessed 493 cardiac surgical patients randomized to receive either a conventional ventilation strategy with a paused ventilation during CPB and the perioperative application of a low PEEP level at 2 cm H_2O or an open-long approach with the continuation of ventilation during CPB regular recruitment maneuvers and PEEP levels at 8 cm H_2O. Both groups had comparable incidences of postoperative pulmonary complications within 7 days.[79]

   The MECANO (Mechanical Ventilation Against No Ventilation During Cardiopulmonary Bypass in Heart Surgery) trial followed a similar approach in 75 randomized patients, comparing a treatment assignment with no ventilation during CPB with a ventilation strategy with 5 breaths per minute, a tidal volume of 3 mL/kg at a PEEP of 5 cm H_2O during CPB, and recruitment maneuvers at the end of surgery. As well, this trial was unable to report any differences in primary end points, including death, pneumonia, PaO_2/FIO_2 <200 during the first day at the ICU, and prolonged respiratory support on the second postoperative day.[80]

4. Noninvasive ventilation is frequently used in the ICU to treat hypoxemia and improve outcomes by avoiding reintubation, prolonged invasive ventilation, and reduced ICU length of stay. However, this technique is often limited by patient discomfort, skin erosions, and personnel resources. In recent years, high-flow nasal oxygen therapy with a continuous application of up to 60 L/min has become increasingly popular. Recent data support its use as a viable alternative to treat cardiac surgery–associated pulmonary failure.[81]

VI. Gastrointestinal Organs

Abdominal complications rarely occur following cardiac surgery but are often associated with devastating outcomes despite early recognition and treatment.[82]

Less than 2.5% of patients develop gastrointestinal complications, with about 0.5% needing surgical consultation.[82,83] Infections with *Clostridium difficile* occur most frequently, accounting for about one-third of gastrointestinal complications, followed by hepatic failure and gastrointestinal bleeding requiring blood transfusion in 22% and 20%, respectively. Gastrointestinal ischemia accounts for about 12% of cases. Increased age, comorbidities such as chronic obstructive pulmonary disease, congestive heart failure, serum creatinine levels, and surgical factors, including aortic cross-clamp time and preoperative use of intra-aortic balloon pump, are the most important predictors of gastrointestinal adverse events.[82]

5

Gastrointestinal complications frequently occur in a cluster effect subsequent to nongastrointestinal complications. This association implies that the prevention of other organ dysfunctions may help reduce their incidence.[82]

VII. Summary

Transient or permanent end-organ dysfunctions are a common finding within the perioperative course of cardiac surgery and are regularly associated with worse short- and long-term outcomes and increased mortality. Among these, AKI, NCDs, stroke, LCOS, arrhythmias, vasoplegia, and respiratory failure account for the greater part of postoperative complications. Since no single pharmacologic therapy has been identified so far to treat these sequelae of cardiac procedures driven mostly by the systemic inflammatory response, a variety of preventive and supportive measures need to be implemented to preserve end-organ function.

REFERENCES

1. Lamy A, Devereaux PJ, Prabhakaran D, et al. Off-pump or on-pump coronary-artery bypass grafting at 30 days. *N Engl J Med.* [Internet]. 2012 [cited 2019 Nov 10];366:1489-1497. http://www.ncbi.nlm.nih.gov/pubmed/22449296
2. Diegeler A, Börgermann J, Kappert U, et al. Off-pump versus on-pump coronary-artery bypass grafting in elderly patients. *N Engl J Med.* [Internet]. 2013 [cited 2019 Nov 27];368:1189-1198. http://www.ncbi.nlm.nih.gov/pubmed/23477657
3. Whitlock RP, Devereaux PJ, Teoh KH, et al. Methylprednisolone in patients undergoing cardiopulmonary bypass (SIRS): a randomised, double-blind, placebo-controlled trial. *Lancet.* [Internet]. 2015 [cited 2022 Aug 7];386:1243-1253. http://www.ncbi.nlm.nih.gov/pubmed/26460660
4. Zheng Z, Jayaram R, Jiang L, et al. Perioperative rosuvastatin in cardiac surgery. *N Engl J Med.* [Internet]. 2016 [cited 2019 Dec 27];374:1744-1753. http://www.ncbi.nlm.nih.gov/pubmed/27144849
5. Zhao B-C, Shen P, Liu K-X. Perioperative statins do not prevent acute kidney injury after cardiac surgery: a meta-analysis of randomized controlled trials. *J Cardiothorac Vasc Anesth.* [Internet]. 2017 [cited 2022 Aug 14];31:2086-2092. http://www.ncbi.nlm.nih.gov/pubmed/28803772
6. Poli EC, Alberio L, Bauer-Doerries A, et al. Cytokine clearance with CytoSorb® during cardiac surgery: a pilot randomized controlled trial. *Crit Care.* [Internet]. 2019 [cited 2022 Nov 5];23:108. http://www.ncbi.nlm.nih.gov/pubmed/30944029
7. Landoni G, Lomivorotov V, Neto CN, et al. Volatile anesthetics versus total intravenous anesthesia for cardiac surgery. *N Engl J Med.* [Internet]. 2019 [cited 2022 Aug 15];380:1214-1225. http://www.ncbi.nlm.nih.gov/pubmed/30888743
8. Zarbock A, Schmidt C, van Aken H, et al. Effect of remote ischemic preconditioning on kidney injury among high-risk patients undergoing cardiac surgery: a randomized clinical trial. *JAMA.* [Internet]. 2015 [cited 2022 Dec 6];313:2133-2141. http://www.ncbi.nlm.nih.gov/pubmed/26024502
9. O'Neal JB, Shaw AD, Billings FT IV. Acute kidney injury following cardiac surgery: current understanding and future directions. *Crit Care.* [Internet]. 2016 [cited 2021 May 24];20:187. http://www.ncbi.nlm.nih.gov/pubmed/27373799
10. Kellum JA, Lameire N, Aspelin P, et al. KDIGO clinical Practice guideline for acute kidney injury 2012. *Kidney Int Suppl.* [Internet]. 2012;2:1-138. http://www.kidney-international.org/
11. Chawla LS, Bellomo R, Bihorac A, et al. Acute kidney disease and renal recovery: consensus report of the acute disease quality initiative (ADQI) 16 workgroup. *Nat Rev Nephrol.* [Internet]. 2017;13:241-257. http://www.ncbi.nlm.nih.gov/pubmed/28239173
12. Priyanka P, Zarbock A, Izawa J, Gleason TG, Renfurm RW, Kellum JA. The impact of acute kidney injury by serum creatinine or urine output criteria on major adverse kidney events in cardiac surgery patients. *J Thorac Cardiovasc Surg.* [Internet]. 2021 [cited 2021 Jun 17];162:143-151.e7. http://www.ncbi.nlm.nih.gov/pubmed/32033818
13. Engelman DT, Ben Ali W, Williams JB, et al. Guidelines for perioperative care in cardiac surgery: enhanced recovery after surgery society recommendations. *JAMA Surg.* [Internet]. 2019 [cited 2019 Jun 12];154:755-766. http://www.ncbi.nlm.nih.gov/pubmed/31054241
14. Ostermann M, Zarbock A, Goldstein S, et al. Recommendations on acute kidney injury biomarkers from the acute disease quality initiative consensus conference: a consensus statement. *JAMA Netw Open.* [Internet]. 2020 [cited 2021 May 21];3:e2019209. http://www.ncbi.nlm.nih.gov/pubmed/33021646
15. Cummings JJ, Shaw AD, Shi J, Lopez MG, O'Neal JB, Billings FT. Intraoperative prediction of cardiac surgery-associated acute kidney injury using urinary biomarkers of cell cycle arrest. *J Thorac Cardiovasc Surg.* [Internet]. 2019 [cited 2021 Jun 18];157:1545.e5-1553.e5. http://www.ncbi.nlm.nih.gov/pubmed/30389130
16. Lapi F, Azoulay L, Yin H, Nessim SJ, Suissa S. Concurrent use of diuretics, angiotensin converting enzyme inhibitors, and angiotensin receptor blockers with non-steroidal anti-inflammatory drugs and risk of acute kidney injury: nested case-control study. *BMJ.* [Internet]. 2013 [cited 2022 Aug 20];346:e8525. http://www.ncbi.nlm.nih.gov/pubmed/23299844
17. Mangieri A. Renin-angiotensin system blockers in cardiac surgery. *J Crit Care.* [Internet]. 2015 [cited 2022 Aug 21];30:613-618. http://www.ncbi.nlm.nih.gov/pubmed/25813547

18. Haase-Fielitz A, Haase M, Bellomo R, et al. Perioperative hemodynamic instability and fluid overload are associated with increasing acute kidney injury severity and worse outcome after cardiac surgery. *Blood Purif.* [Internet]. 2017 [cited 2022 Aug 21];43:298-308. http://www.ncbi.nlm.nih.gov/pubmed/28142133

19. Finfer, S., Micallef, S., Hammond, N., et al. Balanced Multielectrolyte Solution versus Saline in Critically Ill Adults. *The New England Journal of Medicine.* 2022;386(9): 815–826. https://doi.org/10.1056/NEJMoa2114464

20. Hammond, D. A., Lam, S. W., Rech, M. A., et al. Balanced Crystalloids Versus Saline in Critically Ill Adults: A Systematic Review and Meta-analysis. *The Annals of Pharmacotherapy.* 2020;54(1):5–13. https://doi.org/10.1177/1060028019866420

21. Self WH, Semler MW, Wanderer JP, et al. Balanced crystalloids versus saline in noncritically ill adults. *N Engl J Med.* 2018;378(9):819-828.

22. Semler MW, Self WH, Wanderer JP, et al. Balanced crystalloids versus saline in critically ill adults. *N Engl J Med.* 2018;378(9):829-839.

23. Semler MW, Wanderer JP, Ehrenfeld JM, et al. Balanced crystalloids versus saline in the intensive care unit. The SALT randomized trial. *Am J Respir Crit Care Med.* 2017;195(10):1362-1372.

24. Pesonen E, Vlasov H, Suojaranta R, et al. Effect of 4% albumin solution vs ringer acetate on major adverse events in patients undergoing cardiac surgery with cardiopulmonary bypass: a randomized clinical trial. *JAMA.* [Internet]. 2022 [cited 2022 Aug 22];328:251-258. http://www.ncbi.nlm.nih.gov/pubmed/35852528

25. Lopez MG, Shotwell MS, Morse J, et al. Intraoperative venous congestion and acute kidney injury in cardiac surgery: an observational cohort study. *Br J Anaesth.* [Internet]. 2021 [cited 2022 Aug 22];126:599-607. http://www.ncbi.nlm.nih.gov/pubmed/33549321

26. von Groote TC, Ostermann M, Forni LG, Meersch-Dini M, Zarbock A, PrevAKI Investigators. The AKI care bundle: all bundle components are created equal-are they? *Intensive Care Med.* [Internet]. 2022 [cited 2022 Apr 6];48:242-245. http://www.ncbi.nlm.nih.gov/pubmed/34921624

27. Jin K, Murugan R, Sileanu FE, et al. Intensive monitoring of urine output is associated with increased detection of acute kidney injury and improved outcomes. *Chest.* [Internet]. 2017 [cited 2021 Jun 1];152:972-979. http://www.ncbi.nlm.nih.gov/pubmed/28527880

28. Gorelik Y, Bloch-Isenberg N, Hashoul S, Heyman SN, Khamaisi M. Hyperglycemia on admission predicts acute kidney failure and renal functional recovery among inpatients. *J Clin Med.* [Internet]. 2021 [cited 2022 Mar 26];11:54. http://www.ncbi.nlm.nih.gov/pubmed/35011805

29. McDonald JS, McDonald RJ, Williamson EE, Kallmes DF, Kashani K. Post-contrast acute kidney injury in intensive care unit patients: a propensity score-adjusted study. *Intensive Care Med.* [Internet]. 2017 [cited 2022 Aug 27];43:774-784. http://www.ncbi.nlm.nih.gov/pubmed/28213620

30. Goulden R, Rowe BH, Abrahamowicz M, Strumpf E, Tamblyn R. Association of intravenous radiocontrast with kidney function: a regression discontinuity analysis. *JAMA Intern Med.* [Internet]. 2021 [cited 2023 Feb 25];181:767-774. http://www.ncbi.nlm.nih.gov/pubmed/33818606

31. Kolhe NV, Staples D, Reilly T, et al. Impact of compliance with a care bundle on acute kidney injury outcomes: a prospective observational study. *PLoS One.* [Internet]. 2015 [cited 2018 Dec 2];10:e0132279. http://www.ncbi.nlm.nih.gov/pubmed/26161979

32. Engelman DT, Crisafi C, Germain M, et al. Using urinary biomarkers to reduce acute kidney injury following cardiac surgery. *J Thorac Cardiovasc Surg.* [Internet]. 2020 [cited 2020 Mar 2];160:1235.e2-1246.e2. http://www.ncbi.nlm.nih.gov/pubmed/31757451

33. Meersch M, Schmidt C, Hoffmeier A, et al. Prevention of cardiac surgery-associated AKI by implementing the KDIGO guidelines in high risk patients identified by biomarkers: the PrevAKI randomized controlled trial. *Intensive Care Med.* [Internet]. 2017 [cited 2018 Nov 30];43:1551-1561. http://www.ncbi.nlm.nih.gov/pubmed/28110412

34. Zarbock A, Küllmar M, Ostermann M, et al. Prevention of cardiac surgery–associated acute kidney injury by implementing the KDIGO guidelines in high-risk patients identified by biomarkers: the PrevAKI-multicenter randomized controlled trial. *Anesth Analg.* [Internet]. 2021 [cited 2021 Jun 18]; http://www.ncbi.nlm.nih.gov/pubmed/33684086

35. Jacob KA, Leaf DE, Dieleman JM, et al. Intraoperative high-dose dexamethasone and severe AKI after cardiac surgery. *J Am Soc Nephrol.* [Internet]. 2015 [cited 2022 Aug 8];26:2947-2951. http://www.ncbi.nlm.nih.gov/pubmed/25952257

36. Peng K, Li D, Applegate RL, Lubarsky DA, Ji F, Liu H. Effect of dexmedetomidine on cardiac surgery-associated acute kidney injury: a meta-analysis with trial sequential analysis of randomized controlled trials. *J Cardiothorac Vasc Anesth.* [Internet]. 2019 [cited 2019 Nov 5];34:603-613. http://www.ncbi.nlm.nih.gov/pubmed/31587928

37. Bonanni A, Signori A, Alicino C, et al. Volatile anesthetics versus propofol for cardiac surgery with cardiopulmonary bypass: meta-analysis of randomized trials. *Anesthesiology.* [Internet]. 2020 [cited 2022 Aug 14];132:1429-1446. http://www.ncbi.nlm.nih.gov/pubmed/32205551

38. Cai J, Xu R, Yu X, Fang Y, Ding X. Volatile anesthetics in preventing acute kidney injury after cardiac surgery: a systematic review and meta-analysis. *J Thorac Cardiovasc Surg.* [Internet]. 2014 [cited 2022 Aug 15];148:3127-3136. http://www.ncbi.nlm.nih.gov/pubmed/25218542

39. Meybohm P, Bein B, Brosteanu O, et al. A multicenter trial of remote ischemic preconditioning for heart surgery. *N Engl J Med.* [Internet]. 2015 [cited 2022 Aug 19];373:1397-1407. http://www.ncbi.nlm.nih.gov/pubmed/26436208

40. Hausenloy DJ, Candilio L, Evans R, et al. Remote ischemic preconditioning and outcomes of cardiac surgery. *N Engl J Med.* [Internet]. 2015 [cited 2022 Dec 6];373:1408-1417. http://www.nejm.org/doi/10.1056/NEJMoa1413534

41. Long Y-Q, Feng X-M, Shan X-S, et al. Remote ischemic preconditioning reduces acute kidney injury after cardiac surgery: a systematic review and meta-analysis of randomized controlled trials. *Anesth Analg.* [Internet]. 2022 [cited 2022 Aug 19];134:592-605. http://www.ncbi.nlm.nih.gov/pubmed/34748518

42. Evered L, Silbert B, Knopman DS, et al. Recommendations for the nomenclature of cognitive change associated with anaesthesia and surgery-2018. *Anesthesiology.* [Internet]. 2018 [cited 2022 Aug 29];129:872-879. http://www.ncbi.nlm.nih.gov/pubmed/30325806

43. Shaw AD, Guinn NR, Brown JK, et al. Controversies in enhanced recovery after cardiac surgery. *Perioper Med (Lond)*. [Internet]. 2022 [cited 2022 Sep 3];11:19. http://www.ncbi.nlm.nih.gov/pubmed/35477446

44. Russell MD, Pinkerton C, Sherman KA, Ebert TJ, Pagel PS. Predisposing and precipitating factors associated with postoperative delirium in patients undergoing cardiac surgery at a veterans affairs medical center: a pilot retrospective analysis. *J Cardiothorac Vasc Anesth*. [Internet]. 2020 [cited 2022 Sep 3];34:2103-2110. http://www.ncbi.nlm.nih.gov/pubmed/32127274

45. Gusmao-Flores D, Salluh JIF, Chalhub RÁ, Quarantini LC. The confusion assessment method for the intensive care unit (CAM-ICU) and intensive care delirium screening checklist (ICDSC) for the diagnosis of delirium: a systematic review and meta-analysis of clinical studies. *Crit Care*. [Internet]. 2012 [cited 2022 Aug 30];16:R115. http://www.ncbi.nlm.nih.gov/pubmed/22759376

46. van den Boogaard M, Slooter AJC, Brüggemann RJM, et al. Effect of haloperidol on survival among critically ill adults with a high risk of delirium: the REDUCE randomized clinical trial. *JAMA*. [Internet]. 2018 [cited 2022 Sep 5];319:680-690. http://www.ncbi.nlm.nih.gov/pubmed/29466591

47. Girard TD, Exline MC, Carson SS, et al. Haloperidol and ziprasidone for treatment of delirium in critical illness. *N Engl J Med*. [Internet]. 2018 [cited 2022 Sep 5];379:2506-2516. http://www.ncbi.nlm.nih.gov/pubmed/30346242

48. Prakanrattana U, Prapaitrakool S. Efficacy of risperidone for prevention of postoperative delirium in cardiac surgery. *Anaesth Intensive Care*. [Internet]. 2007 [cited 2022 Sep 5];35:714-719. http://www.ncbi.nlm.nih.gov/pubmed/17933157

49. Shehabi Y, Serpa Neto A, Howe BD, et al. Early sedation with dexmedetomidine in ventilated critically ill patients and heterogeneity of treatment effect in the SPICE III randomised controlled trial. *Intensive Care Med*. [Internet]. 2021 [cited 2022 Sep 5];47:455-466. http://www.ncbi.nlm.nih.gov/pubmed/33686482

50. Browne A, Spence J, Power P, et al. Perioperative covert stroke in patients undergoing coronary artery bypass graft surgery. *JTCVS Open*. [Internet]. 2020 [cited 2023 Feb 26];4:1-11. http://www.ncbi.nlm.nih.gov/pubmed/36004290

51. Indja B, Woldendorp K, Vallely MP, Grieve SM. Silent brain infarcts following cardiac procedures: a systematic review and meta-analysis. *J Am Heart Assoc*. [Internet]. 2019 [cited 2023 Feb 26];8:e010920. http://www.ncbi.nlm.nih.gov/pubmed/31017035

52. Wahba A, Milojevic M, Boer C, et al. 2019 EACTS/EACTA/EBCP guidelines on cardiopulmonary bypass in adult cardiac surgery. *Eur J Cardiothorac Surg*. [Internet]. 2020 [cited 2022 Sep 5];57:210-251. http://www.ncbi.nlm.nih.gov/pubmed/31576396

53. Rosenberger P, Shernan SK, Löffler M, et al. The influence of epiaortic ultrasonography on intraoperative surgical management in 6051 cardiac surgical patients. *Ann Thorac Surg*. [Internet]. 2008 [cited 2022 Sep 5];85:548-553. http://www.ncbi.nlm.nih.gov/pubmed/18222262

54. Ito H, Ibaraki M, Kanno I, Fukuda H, Miura S. Changes in the arterial fraction of human cerebral blood volume during hypercapnia and hypocapnia measured by positron emission tomography. *J Cereb Blood Flow Metab*. [Internet]. 2005 [cited 2023 Mar 3];25:852-857. http://www.ncbi.nlm.nih.gov/pubmed/15716851

55. Zheng F, Sheinberg R, Yee M-S, Ono M, Zheng Y, Hogue CW. Cerebral near-infrared spectroscopy monitoring and neurologic outcomes in adult cardiac surgery patients: a systematic review. *Anesth Analg*. [Internet]. 2013 [cited 2022 Sep 12];116:663-676. http://www.ncbi.nlm.nih.gov/pubmed/23267000

56. Linassi F, Maran E, de Laurenzis A, et al. Targeted temperature management in cardiac surgery: a systematic review and meta-analysis on postoperative cognitive outcomes. *Br J Anaesth*. [Internet]. 2022 [cited 2022 Aug 29];128:11-25. http://www.ncbi.nlm.nih.gov/pubmed/34862000

57. Beaty CA, Arnaoutakis GJ, Grega MA, et al. The role of head computed tomography imaging in the evaluation of postoperative neurologic deficits in cardiac surgery patients. *Ann Thorac Surg*. [Internet]. 2013 [cited 2023 Mar 3];95:548-554. http://www.ncbi.nlm.nih.gov/pubmed/23218967

58. Berkhemer OA, Fransen PSS, Beumer D, et al. A randomized trial of intraarterial treatment for acute ischemic stroke. *N Engl J Med*. [Internet]. 2015 [cited 2022 Sep 12];372:11-20. http://www.ncbi.nlm.nih.gov/pubmed/25517348

59. Shi J, Zhou C, Pan W, et al. Effect of high- vs low-dose tranexamic acid infusion on need for red blood cell transfusion and adverse events in patients undergoing cardiac surgery. *JAMA*. [Internet]. 2022 [cited 2022 Dec 7];328:336. https://jamanetwork.com/journals/jama/fullarticle/2794565

60. Sanfilippo F, Knight JB, Scolletta S, et al. Levosimendan for patients with severely reduced left ventricular systolic function and/or low cardiac output syndrome undergoing cardiac surgery: a systematic review and meta-analysis. *Crit Care*. [Internet]. 2017 [cited 2022 Sep 23];21:252. http://www.ncbi.nlm.nih.gov/pubmed/29047417

61. Mathew R, di Santo P, Jung RG, et al. Milrinone as compared with dobutamine in the treatment of cardiogenic shock. *N Engl J Med*. [Internet]. 2021 [cited 2022 Oct 6];385:516-525. http://www.nejm.org/doi/10.1056/NEJMoa2026845

62. Nielsen DV, Torp-Pedersen C, Skals RK, Gerds TA, Karaliunaite Z, Jakobsen C-J. Intraoperative milrinone versus dobutamine in cardiac surgery patients: a retrospective cohort study on mortality. *Crit Care*. [Internet]. 2018 [cited 2022 Sep 27];22:51. http://www.ncbi.nlm.nih.gov/pubmed/29482650

63. Zangrillo A, Biondi-Zoccai G, Ponschab M, et al. Milrinone and mortality in adult cardiac surgery: a meta-analysis. *J Cardiothorac Vasc Anesth*. [Internet]. 2012 [cited 2022 Oct 6];26:70-77. http://www.ncbi.nlm.nih.gov/pubmed/21943792

64. Mehta RH, Leimberger JD, van Diepen S, et al. Levosimendan in patients with left ventricular dysfunction undergoing cardiac surgery. *N Engl J Med*. [Internet]. 2017 [cited 2019 Dec 29];376:2032-2042. http://www.ncbi.nlm.nih.gov/pubmed/28316276

65. Muehlschlegel JD, Burrage PS, Ngai JY, et al. Society of Cardiovascular Anesthesiologists/European Association of Cardiothoracic Anaesthetists practice advisory for the management of perioperative atrial fibrillation in patients undergoing cardiac su.3rgery. *Anesth Analg*. [Internet]. 2019 [cited 2022 Oct 8];128:33-42. http://journals.lww.com/00000539-201901000-00011

66. Arsenault KA, Yusuf AM, Crystal E, et al. Interventions for preventing post-operative atrial fibrillation in patients undergoing heart surgery. *Cochrane Database Syst Rev*. [Internet]. 2013 [cited 2022 Oct 8];2013:CD003611. http://www.ncbi.nlm.nih.gov/pubmed/23440790

67. Gaudino M, Sanna T, Ballman KV, et al. Posterior left pericardiotomy for the prevention of atrial fibrillation after cardiac surgery: an adaptive, single-centre, single-blind, randomised, controlled trial. *Lancet*. [Internet]. 2021 [cited 2022 Oct 6];398: 2075-2083. http://www.ncbi.nlm.nih.gov/pubmed/34788640

68. Campbell NG, Allen E, Sanders J, et al. The impact of maintaining serum potassium ≥3.6 mEq/L vs ≥4.5 mEq/L on the incidence of new-onset atrial fibrillation in the first 120 hours after isolated elective coronary artery bypass grafting—study protocol for a randomised feasibility trial for the proposed Tight K randomized non-inferiority trial. *Trials*. [Internet]. 2017 [cited 2022 Oct 10];18:618. http://www.ncbi.nlm.nih.gov/pubmed/29282098

69. Klinger RY, Thunberg CA, White WD, et al. Intraoperative magnesium administration does not reduce postoperative atrial fibrillation after cardiac surgery. *Anesth Analg*. [Internet]. 2015 [cited 2022 Oct 10];121:861-867. http://www.ncbi.nlm.nih.gov/pubmed/26237622

70. Coulson TG, Miles LF, Serpa Neto A, et al. A double-blind randomised feasibility trial of angiotensin-2 in cardiac surgery. *Anaesthesia*. [Internet]. 2022 [cited 2022 Oct 18];77:999-1009. http://www.ncbi.nlm.nih.gov/pubmed/35915923

71. Ortoleva J, Shapeton A, Vanneman M, Dalia AA. Vasoplegia during cardiopulmonary bypass: current literature and rescue therapy options. *J Cardiothorac Vasc Anesth*. [Internet]. 2020 [cited 2022 Oct 23];34:2766-2775. https://www.sciencedirect.com/science/article/abs/pii/S1053077019312674?via%3Dihub

72. Hajjar LA, Vincent JL, Barbosa Gomes Galas FR, et al. Vasopressin versus norepinephrine in patients with vasoplegic shock after cardiac surgery: the VANCS randomized controlled trial. *Anesthesiology*. [Internet]. 2017 [cited 2022 Oct 24];126:85-93. http://www.ncbi.nlm.nih.gov/pubmed/27841822

73. Cheng Y, Pan T, Ge M, et al. Evaluation of vasopressin for vasoplegic shock in patients with preoperative left ventricular dysfunction after cardiac surgery: a propensity-score analysis. *Shock*. [Internet]. 2018 [cited 2022 Oct 24];50:519-524. http://www.ncbi.nlm.nih.gov/pubmed/29424795

74. Küllmar M, Saadat-Gilani K, Weiss R, et al. Kinetic changes of plasma renin concentrations predict acute kidney injury in cardiac surgery patients. *Am J Respir Crit Care Med*. [Internet]. 2021 [cited 2021 May 9];203:1119-1126. http://www.ncbi.nlm.nih.gov/pubmed/33320784

75. Meersch M, Weiss R, Massoth C, et al. The association between angiotensin II and renin kinetics in patients after cardiac surgery. *Anesth Analg*. [Internet]. 2022 [cited 2022 Oct 18];134:1002-1009. http://www.ncbi.nlm.nih.gov/pubmed/35171852

76. Weiner MM, Lin H-M, Danforth D, Rao S, Hosseinian L, Fischer GW. Methylene blue is associated with poor outcomes in vasoplegic shock. *J Cardiothorac Vasc Anesth*. [Internet]. 2013 [cited 2022 Oct 18];27:1233-1238. https://www.sciencedirect.com/science/article/pii/S1053077013001298

77. Mathis MR, Duggal NM, Likosky DS, et al. Intraoperative mechanical ventilation and postoperative pulmonary complications after cardiac surgery. *Anesthesiology*. [Internet]. 2019 [cited 2022 Oct 10];131:1046-1062. http://www.ncbi.nlm.nih.gov/pubmed/31403976

78. Beverly A, Brovman EY, Malapero RJ, Lekowski RW, Urman RD. Unplanned reintubation following cardiac surgery: incidence, timing, risk factors, and outcomes. *J Cardiothorac Vasc Anesth*. [Internet]. 2016 [cited 2022 Oct 12];30:1523-1529. http://www.ncbi.nlm.nih.gov/pubmed/27595531

79. Lagier D, Fischer F, Fornier W, et al. Effect of open-lung vs conventional perioperative ventilation strategies on postoperative pulmonary complications after on-pump cardiac surgery: the PROVECS randomized clinical trial. *Intensive Care Med*. [Internet]. 2019 [cited 2022 Oct 11];45:1401-1412. http://www.ncbi.nlm.nih.gov/pubmed/31576435

80. Nguyen LS, Estagnasie P, Merzoug M, et al. Low tidal volume mechanical ventilation against no ventilation during cardiopulmonary bypass in heart surgery (MECANO): a randomized controlled trial. *Chest*. [Internet]. 2021 [cited 2022 Oct 11];159:1843-1853. http://www.ncbi.nlm.nih.gov/pubmed/33217416

81. Stéphan F, Barrucand B, Petit P, et al. High-flow nasal oxygen vs noninvasive positive airway pressure in hypoxemic patients after cardiothoracic surgery: a randomized clinical trial. *JAMA*. [Internet]. 2015 [cited 2022 Oct 11];313:2331-2339. http://www.ncbi.nlm.nih.gov/pubmed/25980660

82. Hess NR, Seese LM, Hong Y, et al. Gastrointestinal complications after cardiac surgery: incidence, predictors, and impact on outcomes. *J Card Surg*. [Internet]. 2021 [cited 2022 Oct 13];36:894-901. http://www.ncbi.nlm.nih.gov/pubmed/33428223

83. Mangi AA, Christison-Lagay ER, Torchiana DF, Warshaw AL, Berger DL. Gastrointestinal complications in patients undergoing heart operation: an analysis of 8709 consecutive cardiac surgical patients. *Ann Surg*. [Internet]. 2005 [cited 2022 Oct 12];241:895-901; discussion 901-904. http://www.ncbi.nlm.nih.gov/pubmed/15912039

Regional Anesthesia Techniques for the Cardiac Surgery Population

Jessica Brodt and Ban Tsui

KEY POINTS

1. Unattenuated pain after cardiac surgery increases postoperative morbidity, impedes optimal patient recovery, and may increase the risk of chronic pain and persistent opioid use.

2. Regional anesthesia, including neuraxial techniques, fascial plane blocks, and isolated nerve blocks, can play a role in managing acute pain during and after cardiac surgery in adult and pediatric patients.

3. Neuraxial techniques, including epidural and intrathecal options, are considered the most effective analgesia. Broad adoption of these techniques in cardiac surgery patients is limited due to the risk of rare but potentially devastating neuraxial hematoma in patients receiving systemic anticoagulation and sympathectomy associated with neuraxial local anesthetics.

4. There is accumulating evidence on the role of chest wall fascial plane blocks, including parasternal intercostal (superficial and deep), interpectoral and pectoserratus (previously pectoralis I and II), serratus anterior, and erector spinae plane techniques in cardiac surgery patients. Benefits may include reduced opioid requirements, lower pain scores, and other improvements in recovery parameters.

5. There is currently insufficient evidence to recommend one single regional anesthesia technique, with choice driven by surgical incisions (sternotomy vs thoracotomy vs thoracoscopy), workflows (placement preoperatively vs intraoperatively vs postoperatively), infrastructure for postoperative management (single shot vs catheter), and provider preference.

6. High thoracic epidural anesthesia techniques and stellate ganglion blocks moderate sympathetic tone and may be considered in patients with ventricular storm.

7. Selection of a regional anesthetic technique must consider the risk profile of the technique, surgical incisions and postoperative pain profile, perioperative anticoagulation requirements, density and duration of technique, and local expertise.

8. Regional anesthesia techniques are ideally combined with systemic nonopioid pharmacotherapies as part of opioid-sparing–enhanced recovery pathways.

I. Introduction

Analgesia for the cardiac surgery population has traditionally relied on moderate- to high-dose systemic opioids and sedation and intubation in the immediate postoperative period.[1] The primary benefits of adequate analgesia are patient satisfaction and an improved recovery profile, including faster liberation from mechanical ventilation, improved postoperative respiratory mechanics, earlier mobilization and return of bowel function, shorter length of stay, enhanced immune function and wound healing, and reduced costs.[2] In addition to avoiding the unpleasant emotional aspects of pain, adequate analgesia may also reduce perioperative activation of the surgical stress response via reduced activation of neuroendocrine pathways, mitigating the release of humoral substances (eg, cortisol, vasopressin, renin, angiotensin), improving vagal tone, and avoiding increased sympathetic activation and oxygen consumption,[3] though any morbidity or mortality benefit of this reduction remain challenging to prove.

Regional anesthesia can provide potent analgesia, but there are risks associated with its use for cardiac anesthesia. Conventional regional techniques for the chest wall and trunk analgesia, such as neuraxial techniques, including epidural block, spinal block, and paravertebral block (PVB), not only still pose a risk of hematoma in cardiac patients who are not receiving cardiopulmonary bypass (CPB), but also create other concerns including hemodynamic instability and complexity around post-operative anticoagulation needs. Side effects, such as decreased peripheral vascular resistance from sympathectomy and local anesthetic cardiac toxicity, are of concern to cardiac anesthesiologists attempting to maintain stable physiology and manage the risk of placing blocks in anticoagulated patients.

Recent advanced ultrasound-guided techniques for regional anesthesia, such as interfascial plane blocks, may be associated with a reduced risk of hematoma and sympathetic effect. With the emergence and increasingly routine application of enhanced recovery pathways for cardiac surgery,[4] regional anesthesia techniques, particularly with the mostly superficial and somatic interfascial plane blocks, have regained interest and popularity to become a central component of efforts to refine perioperative opioid-sparing analgesic techniques further.[5,6]

This chapter focuses on the physiologic features, selection, timing, and practical application of individual blocks within the context of cardiac surgery and only briefly describes technical aspects, in order to provide a careful, balanced, evidence-based view on the risks and benefits of neuraxial blocks, targeted nerve blocks, and interfascial plane blocks (Table 30.1). The reader is directed to other specialized regional anesthesia literature for further information on the technical performance of the blocks.

II. Regional Anesthesia Techniques

A. Neuraxial Blocks

Epidural

1. **Anatomic consideration**
   a. Surgical incision dictates the selection of a specific interspace, aiming for an interspace in the middle of the desired range of coverage. Thoracic epidural analgesia (TEA) for cardiac surgery patients is generally placed between T4 and T10.
2. **Physiologic effect**
   a. Potent sympathetic and somatic blockade
   b. Depending on spread, may cause systemic hypotension
   c. Depending on level, some motor blockade
3. **Technique**
   a. Epidural catheters are placed in adult patients when awake to monitor for paresthesia. This may not be feasible or safe in pediatric patients.
   b. Prescanning with ultrasound can confirm midline and estimate the depth of epidural space before performing a classic blind tactile paramedian or midline approach with loss of resistance.
   c. Catheter should be threaded 4-6 cm into the epidural space, with at least 60 minutes delay from neuraxial instrumentation before any systemic anticoagulation is administered. Surgery should be postponed for 24 hours in the event of a traumatic tap.[7]
   d. Epidural stimulation test may be used to confirm the location of catheter tip before the administration of local anesthetic (Table 30.2).[8,9]

TABLE 30.1   Regional Techniques, Advantages, Disadvantages, Physiologic Effect, and Suitability of Catheter Use

Regional Technique	Advantages	Disadvantages	Physiologic Effects	Catheter
Neuraxial blocks				
Epidural	• Well studied • Reduced risk of myocardial infarction, respiratory depression, atrial arrhythmia • Reduced mortality	• Risk of hematoma • Risk of hypotension	Somatic and sympathetic blockade	Suitable
Spinal	• Well studied • Proven efficacy • Decreased stress response to surgery	• Risk of hematoma • Risk of postdural puncture headache	Somatic and sympathetic blockade	Suitable if desired
Posterior approach				
Paravertebral	• Equivalent analgesia to unilateral neuraxial anesthesia • Lower incidence of complications compared to neuraxial techniques	• Risk of hematoma • Risk of pneumothorax • Risk of epidural migration	Somatic and sympathetic blockade	Suitable
Erector spinae plane/retrolaminar	• Potentially opioid sparing • Less invasive compared to neuraxial and paravertebral techniques • Theoretically lower risk of hematoma and other major complications	• Effectiveness not well studied • Higher risk of back muscle spasm • Large studies are lacking	Somatic blockade Possible sympathetic blockade	Suitable
Anterior approach				
Serratus anterior plane	• Potentially opioid sparing • Theoretically lower risk of hematoma and other major complications	• Effectiveness not well studied • Large doses of anesthetic needed for analgesic effect	Somatic blockade only	Suitable if desired
Interpectoral/pectoserratus plane (previously PECS I/II)	• Opioid sparing • Theoretically lower risk of hematoma and other major complications	• Effectiveness not well studied • Large doses of anesthetic needed for analgesic effect	Somatic blockade only	Not suitable
Parasternal intercostal (previously PIF and TTMP)	• Opioid sparing • May facilitate early extubation • Theoretically lower risk of hematoma and other major complications	• Effectiveness not well studied • Risk of pneumothorax • Risk of injury to IMA	Somatic blockade only	Not suitable
Special situations				
Rectus sheath	• Opioid sparing • Theoretically lower risk of hematoma and other major complications	• Effectiveness not well studied • Risk of bowel puncture	Somatic blockade only	Not suitable
Ilioinguinal and iliohypogastric nerve	• Theoretically lower risk of hematoma and other major complications	• Risk of bowel puncture	Somatic blockade only	Not suitable
Stellate ganglion block	• Rescue therapy for ventricular tachycardia • Well studied for sympathetically maintained pain in the head, neck chest, and arm • Proven efficacy for complex pain syndrome	• Risk of hematoma • Risk of vascular injection • Horner syndrome • Hoarse voice • Phrenic nerve blockade	Sympathetic blockade	Suitable

IMA, internal mammary artery; PECs, pectoralis; PIF, pectointercostal fascial; TTMP, transversus thoracis muscle plane.

TABLE 30.2 Motor Responses and Threshold Currents With Different Catheter Locations During Epidural Stimulation Test

Catheter Location	Threshold Current	Motor Responses
Epidural space	1-10 mA (up to 17 mA for thoracic level)	Unilateral or bilateral
Subcutaneous	NA	No motor response
Subdural	<1 mA	Bilateral (many segments)
Subarachnoid	<1 mA	Unilateral or bilateral
Against nerve root	<1 mA	Unilateral
Nonintravascular	Threshold current increase upon local anesthetic injection	Unilateral or bilateral
Intravascular	No change in threshold current upon local anesthetic injection	Unilateral or bilateral

4. **Dosing**
   a. In order to detect inadvertent intravascular placement, a "test dose" is recommended before catheter use (in adult patients, lidocaine 1.5% 3 mL, 45 mg, with epinephrine 15 μg) after negative aspiration for blood or cerebrospinal fluid. A rise in heart rate in response to the epinephrine suggests the catheter may need replacing.
   b. Postoperative dosing generally includes a local anesthetic (eg, bupivacaine 0.05%-0.125%) and an opioid with intermediate lipid solubility (eg, hydromorphone, 10-20 μg/mL) administered by continuous infusion, starting dose 4-7 mL/h, with or without a patient-controlled epidural analgesia (PCEA) dose in extubated patients.
   c. Opioid-only dosing may be used in patients unable to tolerate TEA-induced sympathectomy.

5. **Risks and precautions**
   a. The true incidence of neuraxial hematoma in cardiac surgery patients is unclear. From the available literature, it appears to be anywhere from 1:1,528 to 1:3,500, compared to 1:5,000 to 1:10,000 in the general surgical population.[7,10]
   b. Epidural analgesia adds complexity in managing anticoagulation in cardiac surgery patients. Careful catheter manipulation and timing of removal are necessary for patients with residual coagulopathy or those receiving postoperative anticoagulation.
   c. Dose-dependent sympathetic blockade poses a hypotension risk.

6. **Clinical evidence**
   a. Of all published techniques, only TEA has the potential to provide complete pain relief for sternotomy and thoracotomy incisions.
   b. A 2015 meta-analysis reported improved pain scores, reduced tracheal intubation duration, and reduced supraventricular arrhythmias. Shorter hospital and intensive care unit (ICU) stays are also seen in patients receiving TEA with general anesthesia compared with general anesthesia alone.[11]
   c. A separate systematic review of 57 trials with 6,383 patients reported reduced mortality with TEA, and a number needed to treat of 70.[12]
   d. TEA reduces opioids and duration of mechanical ventilation in patients undergoing lung transplantation via clamshell or traditional thoracotomy.[13] Some centers utilize TEA in patients undergoing sternotomy, though evidence of benefit is more limited.[14]
   e. Not all literature is favorable, and the benefit on the duration of intubation is more evident in older trials,[10] before the current focus on enhanced recovery, multimodal analgesia, and protocolized extubation pathways.

CLINICAL PEARL

Modulation of the sympathetic nervous system with TEA has been used as a rescue therapy in patients with refractory ventricular arrhythmias. A high thoracic technique (T1-T3) reduces sympathetic tone, providing antiarrhythmic effects by decreased ventricular excitability. Dosing is local anesthetic only, titrated to abatement of arrhythmia, for example, bupivacaine 0.25% 1 mL bolus followed by an infusion starting at 2 mL/h. Some authors advocate for documented rhythm control with deep sedation as a positive predictor for success before TEA insertion.[15]

Spinal

1. **Anatomic consideration**
   a. Intrathecal analgesia for cardiac surgery patients is typically limited to single-shot techniques administered at the lumbar region before induction of general anesthesia.
2. **Physiologic effect**
   a. Potent sympathetic and somatic blockade
   b. May produce sympathectomy with systemic hypotension
   c. If local anesthetic is used, may have a profound motor blockade
3. **Technique**
   a. Utilize small-gauge noncutting spinal needles at the L3 or L4 level.
   b. Generally landmark-based technique. Ultrasound can identify the midline and confirm the level of injection.
4. **Dosing**
   a. Preservative-free morphine (4-10 μg/kg in adults), with or without clonidine (1 μg/kg)
   b. Onset in 1-2 hours, duration up to 24 hours
   c. Trendelenburg position immediately after intrathecal injection will raise the block level and increase sympathectomy and corresponding hypotension.
5. **Risks and precautions**
   a. Delayed respiratory depression can occur. Hourly respiratory rate and somnolence assessments with or without capnography are advised for 18-24 hours.
6. **Clinical evidence**
   a. Investigations of intrathecal morphine in cardiac surgery patients have been reported for nearly 30 years.[16]
   b. Generally, the literature supports that intrathecal morphine, with or without clonidine, reduces postoperative pain scores, opioid requirements, extubation times, pulmonary complications, and pain interference with activities.[17-19]
   c. Intrathecal morphine is considered an "opioid-sparing opioid" and may be considered in selected cases as part of a dedicated multimodal analgesic–enhanced recovery pathway.[6]

CLINICAL PEARL

Older patients are more susceptible to side effects of neuraxial techniques, especially delayed respiratory depression, so the total dose should be reduced. Intrathecal techniques including opioids are typically avoided in patients >85 years.

B. **Paravertebral Blocks**
1. **Anatomic consideration**
   a. This technique blocks nerve roots as they emerge from the intervertebral foramen, with anatomic connections to the intercostal space (laterally) and epidural space (medially).
   b. The paravertebral space is bordered anterolaterally by parietal pleura; medially by vertebral bodies, intervertebral discs, and intervertebral foramina; and posteriorly by the costotransverse ligament, transverse process (TP), and ribs. This close anatomic arrangement means injection in the paravertebral space can spread to epidural and intercostal spaces.

2. **Physiologic effect**
   a. Potent somatic blockade
   b. Can cause sympathetic block with systemic hypotension
3. **Technique**
   a. Ultrasound guidance has mostly replaced the traditional landmark technique.
   b. Sagittal or transverse approach
4. **Dosing**
   a. **Single-level injections:** May consider ropivacaine 0.25% 5-7 mL per injection
   b. **Catheters:** May consider lidocaine 0.25% or bupivacaine 0.0625%, 7-10 mL/h, with or without patient or nurse-controlled demand bolus of 3-5 mL
5. **Risks and precautions**
   a. PVB is considered a deep block—identical considerations should be taken around systemic heparinization and coagulopathy as neuraxial techniques.[7]
   b. Compared to epidural techniques, PVB offers comparable analgesia and fewer complications, including less risk of sympathectomy, particularly when unilateral techniques are used. However, patients should still be monitored for sympathectomy.
6. **Clinical evidence**
   a. Comparable efficacy to TEA regarding pain scores and opioid requirements[20-22]
   b. May have reduced side effects compared to TEA, including hypotension, urinary retention, nausea, and vomiting[23,24]
   c. Literature generally supports reduced pain scores, opioid requirements, and the time to extubation in cardiac surgery patients. One study reports no difference in efficacy compared to subcutaneous lidocaine infusion.[25]

CLINICAL PEARL

Paravertebral (PVB) spread from a single-level injection is generally no more than two levels, and analgesia is limited to the ipsilateral side. For extensive chest wall coverage, multiple injections or catheter insertion are necessary. For sternotomy or bilateral chest wall coverage, bilateral PVB techniques are required.

C. **Chest Wall Fascial Plane Blocks**

Fascial plane blocks are regional anesthesia techniques where local anesthetic is deposited in the space between two discrete fascial layers, usually between muscles or between a muscle and a bony landmark. Local anesthetic administered in this space blocks the nerve or nerves crossing through the plane or compartment by combining bulk flow and diffusion, with or without additional effects from systemic absorption.[26] Understanding the spread, mechanism, and ideal application of fascial plane blocks is still evolving, and readers are encouraged to seek additional literature as the field develops. Despite this, many blocks have already been applied in cardiac surgery patients.

For cardiac surgery, the most discussed and relevant fascial plane blocks are those that cover the chest wall (Figure 30.1), including the superficial and deep serratus anterior plane (SAP), the superficial and deep parasternal intercostal plane (PIP), the interpectoral plane (IPP, previously termed the *pectoralis I*) and pectoserratus plane (PSP, previously termed the *pectoralis II*), and the erector spinae plane (ESP).[27] Selection of a specific technique for chest wall coverage is discussed in Section II. Individual techniques are grouped into posterior and anterior approaches.

Posterior approach
Erector Spinae and Retrolaminar
1. **Anatomic consideration**
   a. The ESP block and retrolaminar block are two novel interfascial plane blocks that offer an alternative to the more invasive paravertebral nerve block and neuraxial techniques.
   b. Using the TP or laminae as an osseous backstop, and positioning away from neuraxial structures, blood vessels, and pleura reduce the risk of complications.
   c. Efficient spread from a single injection and ease of catheter placement have contributed to widespread application.

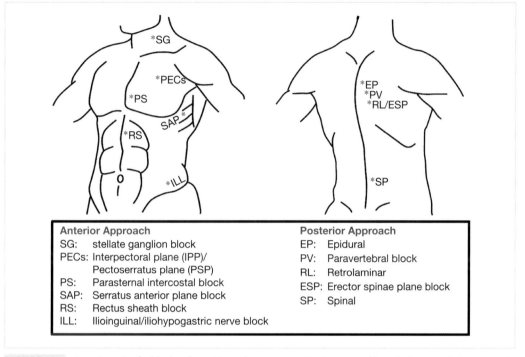

FIGURE 30.1 Insertion sites for blocks relevant to cardiac surgery patients, grouped by anterior or posterior approach. (Courtesy of Jessica Brodt and Ban C.H. Tsui.)

2. **Physiologic effect**
   a. The precise mechanism of analgesia is unknown, but it is thought to involve the injection of local anesthetic diffusing and spreading to the dorsal and ventral rami of the spinal and sympathetic nerve fibers, as well as the epidural space, where it blocks pain signals from both the somatic and visceral nervous systems.[28]
3. **Technique:** ESP
   a. Under ultrasound guidance, the erector spinae muscle is visualized laterally to the spine with the patient in a sitting, lateral, or prone position.
   b. The ultrasound probe is moved from side to side (while maintaining a sagittal orientation) until the TPs (seen as a rectangular structure) corresponding to the targeted ESP area are identified.
   c. Next, the needle is guided toward the TP, and hydrodissection of the erector spinae interfascial plane is performed, with injectate spreading cranially and caudally along the continuous plane of the vertebral column.
   d. Depending on the depth of the TP under the skin, a 50- or 100-mm needle (21-22 G for a single injection, 18 G for catheter placement) is typically used.
4. **Technique:** Retrolaminar
   a. The retrolaminar block is administered in the same manner as the ESP block, with the patient in a sitting, lateral, or prone position.
   b. After identifying the erector spinae muscle and TP, the probe is scanned medially to reveal the vertebral laminae, which appeared as sawtooth structures on the ultrasound. When the needle contacts the vertebral lamina, it is inserted cephalad to caudad or caudad to cephalad and in plane.
   c. The plane is then opened by hydrodissected between the lamina and the erector spinae muscle using local anesthetic or saline.

5. **Dosing**
    a. For a single shot, ropivacaine 0.2% 0.5 mL/kg (up to 20 mL) may be given via the needle while ultrasound imaging is performed in real time.
    b. **Catheter:** Ropivacaine 0.2% 0.3 mL/kg (up to 20 mL) per side (every 4 hours) or lidocaine 0.5% 0.5 mg/kg (up to 20 mL) per side (every 2 hours) with alternating side programmed intermittent boluses (Figure 30.2)[29]

6. **Risks and precautions**
    a. Due to their more superficial targets, ESP and the retrolaminar blocks have fewer risks and concerns than the deeper and more invasive PVB and epidural blocks.
    b. When ultrasound visualization is impeded, retrolaminar blocks may be used instead of ESP.[30]
    c. Any retrolaminar and ESP block should be cautiously administered to patients with a history of anticoagulation, even if administered in a compressible area.

7. **Clinical evidence**
    a. Postoperative analgesia and low risk for complications after cardiac and thoracic surgeries have been reported with the ESP[31,32] and retrolaminar[33] blocks, at least in the early postoperative period.
    b. However, large-scale randomized control trials demonstrating significant improvement in clinical outcomes comparing the ESP and retrolaminar blocks to others, like the neuraxial block and PVB, still need to be published.

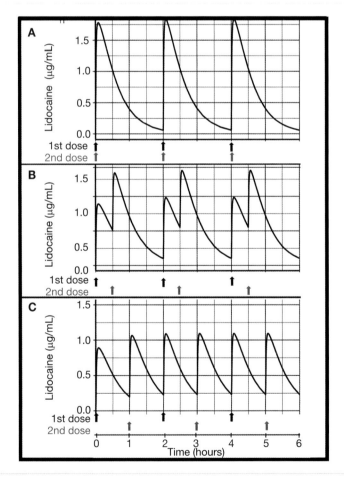

FIGURE 30.2 Effect of timing variation during intermittent bolus of local anesthetics. When modeled on intravenous administration of lidocaine every 2 hours, a lower and more stable serum level is achieved with alternating side programmed intermittent boluses that are optimally time staggered (eg, 1 hour apart) boluses **(C)**, compared to simultaneous bilateral boluses with no stagger **(A)** or a short stagger (eg, 1/2 hour) boluses **(B)**. (Courtesy of Jessica Brodt and Ban C.H. Tsui.)

CLINICAL PEARL

Inserting an ESP or retrolaminar catheter is a simple and uncomplicated process once the space has been opened with local anesthetic or saline. If resistance is felt during catheter insertion, the catheter should be removed from the needle, and the needle tip location verified with ultrasound. Do not attempt to manipulate the needle while the catheter is threaded through the needle's tip; doing so can result in shearing and compromise the catheter's integrity.

Anterior Approach

Serratus Anterior Plane

1. **Anatomic consideration**
   a. The serratus anterior plane (SAP) block is an ultrasound-guided interfascial plane block administered to anesthetize the axilla and anterior chest wall.[34]
   b. To perform a superficial SAP block, local anesthetic is injected between the serratus anterior and latissimus dorsi muscles.
   c. To perform a deep SAP block, local anesthetic is injected between the anterior serratus muscle and the fifth or sixth rib.

2. **Physiologic effect**
   a. Somatic block with no sympathectomy
   b. Ipsilateral coverage for intercostobrachial, lateral cutaneous, long thoracic, and thoracodorsal nerves, covering axilla and anterior chest wall
   c. Deep SAP block is as effective as a superficial SAP block.[35]

3. **Technique**
   a. At the midaxillary line, perpendicular to the fifth and sixth ribs, a linear (13-6 MHz) probe is positioned.
   b. The latissimus dorsi is superficial to the serratus anterior, with thoracodorsal artery running between them.
   c. Pleura can be visualized between the costal cartilage margins.
   d. Needle is inserted deep into the serratus anterior muscle under continuous in-plane ultrasound guidance, with the rib serving as a backstop.
   e. After the needle has touched the rib, the local anesthetic is injected beneath the serratus anterior muscle. A catheter may be inserted into the plane created by injection and subsequent lifting of the serratus anterior muscle.

4. **Dosing**
   a. **Single shot:** Ropivacaine 0.2% 0.5 mL/kg per injection can be utilized up to 3 mg/kg.[36]
   b. **Catheter:** Ropivacaine 0.2% 0.3 mL/kg (up to 20 mL) per side (every 4 hours) or lidocaine 0.5% 0.5 mg/kg (up to 20 mL) per side (every 2 hours) with alternating side programmed intermittent boluses (Figure 30.2)[29]

5. **Risks and precautions**
   a. Pneumothorax, infection, and bleeding are all possible complications.

6. **Clinical evidence**
   a. There is evidence that the SAP block is an effective analgesic block for major cardiac and thoracic procedures[37,38].
   b. Although PVB or ESP blocks may be considered first-line options for thoracoscopic surgery, SAP techniques should be considered a second-line alternative[39] and have been suggested as just as effective as PVB,[40] though with limited high-level evidence.

CLINICAL PEARL

Catheter placement with continuous or intermittent bolus can help mitigate the short duration of single-shot SAP. Although success is feasible with preoperative SAP catheter placement,[41] catheter dislodgement during surgery is a frequent concern, and post-surgical placement is feasible either in the operating room or in post-operative unit.

Parasternal Intercostal Plane
1. **Anatomic consideration**
   a. The superficial PIP was previously termed the pectointercostal fascial (PIF) block. The deep PIP was previously termed the *transversus thoracis muscle plane* (TTMP) block.[27]
   b. The internal mammary artery (IMA) runs in plane targeted by deep PIP block.
2. **Physiologic effect**
   a. Somatic block with no sympathectomy
   b. T2-T6 anterior cutaneous nerves
   c. Ipsilateral sternal and parasternal analgesia
3. **Technique**
   a. **Ultrasound guided, in plane:** Parasagittal or transverse approach depending on user preference; generally easier to visualize the IMA using a transverse approach
   b. **Superficial PIP:** Local anesthetic deposited between the pectoralis muscle and either the external or internal intercostal muscle
   c. **Deep PIP:** Local anesthetic deposited between the internal intercostal muscle and the transversus thoracis muscle
4. **Dosing**
   a. **Single shot:** 4-7 mL of local anesthetic (ropivacaine 0.2%, lidocaine 0.5%) at each space, up to 20 mL per side. One level injection may spread to multiple levels and, although unpredictable, can be visualized on ultrasound.
   b. **Catheter:** 8-15 mL/h of local anesthetic (ropivacaine 0.2%, lidocaine 0.5%) per side
5. **Risks and precautions**
   a. Injury to IMA during deep PIP techniques
   b. **Pneumothorax due to proximity of pleura:** Continuous visualization of needle tip is essential
6. **Clinical evidence**
   a. Multilevel single-shot bilateral superficial PIP blocks reduced intraoperative opioid use and improved spirometry in cardiac patients with median sternotomy.[42]
   b. Superficial PIP reduced pain and opioid use after median sternotomy for mediastinal mass resection.[43]
   c. Deep PIP reduced pain scores, postoperative analgesic doses, extubation times, and ICU length of stay in cardiac patients with median sternotomy.[44]

CLINICAL PEARL

In-plane transverse sonography with clear visualization of tip and trajectory of needle is essential, particularly for the deep PIP, due to proximity of the IMA and pleura. Maintaining preoperatively placed parasternal catheters near surgical sites is challenging and requires strict sterile techniques to reduce infection risk.

Interpectoral Plane and Pectoserratus Plane
1. **Anatomic consideration**
   a. IPP was previously termed the *pectoralis I*; PSP was previously termed the *pectoralis II*.[27,45]
   b. They are anterior interfascial chest wall blocks done with the patient supine.
   c. Due to their superficial anatomy and the presence of an osseous rib to reduce the risk of pleural penetration, these blocks are simple and safe to perform.
2. **Physiologic effect**
   a. Somatic blockade with no sympathectomy
   b. IPP blocks medial and lateral pectoral nerves. PSP blocks the long thoracic nerve, the intercostobrachial nerve, and the third to sixth intercostal nerves.
   c. IPP and PSP do not cover the anterior branches of the intercostal nerves, so no parasternal coverage is expected.
3. **Technique**
   a. Identify subclavian vessels and second rib using a linear probe caudal to the clavicle.

   b. Move the probe caudally to the lateral third and fourth ribs.

   c. The serratus anterior muscle is the narrow band of muscle on top of the ribs and beneath the pectoralis minor. The thoracoacromial artery may be visualized in the plane between the pectoralis major and pectoralis minor muscles.

   d. Use a 50- or 100-mm 22-G short bevel needle inserted in cephalad to caudad direction.

   e. For a PSP block, the target plane is between the pectoralis minor and serratus anterior muscles.

   f. For an IPP block, slowly withdraw the needle from the position used for PSP, then inject between the pectoralis major and pectoralis minor.

4. **Dosing**

   a. **Single shot:** Ropivacaine 0.2% 0.5 mL/kg per side (up to 3 mg/kg). In most cases, if two blocks are performed, each block will receive half the total recommended dose.

   b. **Catheter:** Not common

5. **Risk and precautions**

   a. Pneumothorax, hematoma, and scapular winging due to thoracic nerve compression are all possible complications.

   b. For patients undergoing pacemaker or defibrillator placement/revision, a strict sterile technique is essential to minimize the risk of infection.

6. **Clinical evidence**

   a. Surgical analgesia for procedures including pacemaker and defibrillator placement/revision,[46] and port insertion and removal,[47] have been reported using IPP and PSP blocks.

   b. The combination of PSP block with SAP block has been reported in the literature for use on awake patients undergoing video-assisted thoracoscopic surgery (VATS).[48]

   c. While there are no extensive randomized controlled studies directly comparing neuraxial and chest wall blocks to IPP and PSP blocks, a recent meta-analysis suggests that opioid requirements and pain scores are compared between PSP block and PVB.[49]

CLINICAL PEARL

It is feasible in adult patients to administer both IPP and PSP blocks in a single needle pass without needing needle repositioning. The deeper PSP block should be performed first to prevent the accidental deposition of air, which would impair visualization for IPP injection.

D. **Special Situations**

1. Regional anesthesia may also be used for nonsurgical patients in locations including the ICU and cardiac catheterization laboratory.

2. In the ICU, regional anesthesia may provide excellent analgesia, including epidural or chest wall blocks for improved postoperative lung transplantation recovery,[13,14] continuous ilioinguinal nerve block for pain from peripheral extracorporeal membrane oxygenation (ECMO) cannulation in awake patients,[50] or rectus sheath (RS) blocks for patients with intolerable pain at chest tube insertion sites.

3. In the cardiac catheterization laboratory, there are many opportunities to utilize regional anesthesia to enhance perioperative pain management, including traditional pacemaker or defibrillator generator placement/revision (IPP, PSP blocks) to subcutaneous defibrillators implantation (combination of serratus anterior, external oblique, IPP, and PSP) to provide complete analgesia.[51,52]

4. Regional techniques may serve as treatment or rescue therapy for refractory ventricular tachycardia in the form of stellate ganglion blocks (SGBs)[53] or high TEA.

Stellate Ganglion Block

1. **Anatomic consideration**

   a. The stellate ganglion is a bilateral nerve bundle originating at C6-C7 from fusion of the inferior cervical and first thoracic ganglions.

   b. The sympathetic chain is most prominent in the fascia between the longus colli muscle and the carotid artery.

2. **Physiologic effect**
   a. Right stellate ganglion is thought to be responsible for innervating the anterior left ventricular (LV) wall, while the left is responsible for posterior and inferior LV walls.[54]
   b. Reducing sympathetic outflow by modulating the cervical sympathetic (stellate) ganglion and the upper thoracic sympathetic ganglion has been demonstrated as an effective therapeutic in managing drug-resisted refractory tachycardia.
3. **Technique**
   a. At the C6-C7 level, relevant structures are first identified by ultrasound imaging, including the carotid artery, left internal jugular vein, longus coli muscle, vertebral artery, anterior scalene muscle, and brachial plexus.
   b. Use 1% (1-2 mL) of lidocaine to anesthetize the skin and superficial tissues.
   c. To avoid inadvertent puncture of vascular structures, ultrasound-guided in-plane, lateral-to-medial approach is used with a 22-G, 5-cm needle.
   d. Local anesthetic is injected anterior to the longus colli.
   e. Injections should be strictly incremental confirming negative aspiration each time.
4. **Dosing**
   a. **Single shot:** Lidocaine 0.5% 5-10 mL, ropivacaine 0.5% 5-10 mL, or bupivacaine 0.5% 6-12 mL
   b. **Catheter:** Infusions are more effective at sustained arrhythmia management.[53] Example doses are lidocaine 0.5% 5-10 mL bolus then 2-10 mL/h infusion, ropivacaine 0.5% 5-10 mL bolus then 0.2% 6-10 mL/h, or bupivacaine 0.5% 6-12 mL bolus then 0.05% 6-10 mL/h.
5. **Risks and precautions**
   a. The inferior thyroid artery crosses the longus colli muscle from lateral to medial. Avoid intravascular arterial injection checking for negative aspiration before each injection.
   b. The phrenic nerve passes over the anterior scalene muscle's anterior surface as it travels from lateral to medial.
   c. Stellate block performed caudal to C6, with needle directed laterally to medially reduces the risk of phrenic nerve block. The superficial cervical artery (transverse cervical artery), located directly over the anterior scalene muscle, can be similarly avoided.
6. **Clinical evidence**
   a. SGB has very specific indications.
   b. Percutaneous stellate has shown promise in stabilizing ventricular rhythm in patients where conventional therapies have failed, including in pediatric patients.[55,56]
   c. After single-shot SGB, over half of the patients in one study experienced electrical storm attenuation; no complications were reported from the procedure.[53,57]

CLINICAL PEARL

The key anatomic landmark for SGBs is the longus colli muscle, which is a hypoechoic structure. Horner syndrome is a useful clinical verification of block success. Finally, the thoracic sympathetic ganglion at T2-T4 provides sympathetic innervation to the heart, so a high TEA may be an acceptable alternative to SGB unless contraindicated by coagulopathy or anticoagulation, systemic infection, or hemodynamic instability.

E. **Rectus Sheath Blocks**
   1. **Anatomic consideration**
      a. The rectus sheath (RS) block is commonly described for postoperative pain relief following umbilical and midline surgery. It was originally used for abdominal wall relaxation for laparotomy before the introduction of muscle relaxants.
      b. Typical chest wall blocks like parasternal blocks have limited coverage over structures in the subxiphoid region, due to the anterior branches of the inferior six intercostal nerves passing through the posterior aspect of the RS compartment. RS blocks may provide analgesia for subxiphoid pain related to extended sternotomy or chest tubes.

   c. The oval-shaped rectus abdominis muscles run vertically on each side of the anterior abdominal wall, enclosed by the RS formed by the external, internal, and transversus abdominis aponeuroses.

   d. The linea alba joins the left and right RSs in the midline.

   e. The posterior RS, derived from the internal oblique and transversus abdominis aponeurosis, supports the rectus muscles above the arcuate line. The posterior RS ends below the arcuate line, and all three aponeuroses pass superficial to the rectus muscles, which sit directly on the fascia transversalis.

2. **Physiologic effect**

   a. Somatic block only. No sympathetic or viscus pain coverage

   b. RS blocks cover the lower seven intercostal nerves (T6-T12) and the L1 dermatome innervating the anterior abdominal wall. The nerves enter the posterior RS at the posterolateral edge, pass through the muscle, and exit anteriorly to supply the skin.

3. **Technique**

   a. Place a high-frequency (13-6 MHz) linear probe in a transverse plane above the umbilicus on one side of the anterior abdominal wall to scan the three muscle layers: external oblique, internal oblique, and transversus abdominis.

   b. Find the oval-shaped rectus abdominis medial to the internal oblique on the same plane.

   c. The posterior RS appears as a hyperechoic double line posterior to the rectus muscle above the arcuate line.

   d. The needle is inserted lateral to medial into the rectus muscle posterior RS plane. To avoid entering the muscle belly with epigastric vessels, slide the needle down from the lateral side of the rectus muscle.

   e. The anterior RS pops as the needle is advanced. After aspiration, the needle is advanced until the posterior RS resists, and local anesthetic is deposited.

   f. Superior and inferior epigastric vessels can be visualized (and avoided) with color Doppler in the rectus muscle. The nerve is usually invisible.

4. **Dosing**

   a. **A single shot:** Local anesthetic (such as 0.5% ropivacaine) is injected into both sides in a volume of 10 mL (0.2 mL/kg for children).

   b. **Catheter:** Alternating side programmed intermittent boluses of ropivacaine 0.2% 0.3 mL/kg (up to 10 mL) each side every 4 hours, or lidocaine 0.5% 0.5 mg/kg (up to 20 mL) each side every 2 hours

5. **Risks and precautions**

   a. Hematoma and bleeding risk from inadvertent puncture of the inferior epigastric vessels

   b. Peritoneal or abdominal viscus injury from inadvertent peritoneal puncture

6. **Clinical evidence**

   a. There is some anecdotal evidence that RS blocks can improve clinical outcomes by reducing the need for opioids during extended sternotomies[58] and chest tube pain following aortic valve replacement,[59] but not enough evidence to draw firm conclusions.

   b. While a catheter can be placed to prolong the analgesic effect, an RS block is unique in that a single injection can provide long-lasting pain relief.[60]

   c. Due to its frequent use with other chest wall blocks during cardiac surgery, a conservative dosing strategy is recommended. For example, single shot or intermittent catheter bolus of a local anesthetic for RS blocks instead of a continuous infusion, with careful calculation of total administered local anesthetic dose.

   d. The inferior epigastric vessels that travel through the rectus muscle can be located and avoided with the help of color Doppler imaging.

   e. The nerve is usually invisible, and local anesthetic targets the rectus muscle posterior RS plane.

III. **Selection of Technique**

Deciding on a particular regional anesthesia technique relies on understanding the distribution of pain associated with the procedure, feasible timing and workflow around performing the block, the anticipated duration of local anesthetics used, and available technical expertise.

A. **Distribution of Pain**
1. Complete understanding of the surgical incisions, chest tube sites, vein or arterial graft harvest sites, and any referred pain or preexisting pain patterns is essential.
2. It is not routinely feasible to cover all incisions and painful regions with a single regional anesthetic technique, and it is recommended that any technique be incorporated with multimodal systemic analgesia for comprehensive pain management (Figure 30.3).[6]
3. Any dermatomal level is likely innervated by two or more nerve roots, accounting for variability in dermatomal distribution.[61] Dermatomal maps are a valuable tool to plan for technique choice and level of insertion. Insertion, remembering that any midline structure, such as the sternum, receives innervation from each side, necessitating either neuraxial or bilateral peripheral regional anesthesia techniques.
4. The majority of chest wall innervation is via thoracic intercostal nerves (subcostal at the level of T12) originating from T1-T12 nerve roots, which branch to ventral rami, then run anteriorly as intercostal nerves with lateral cutaneous branches (at mid axillary line), then terminate as anterior cutaneous branches.
5. Branches of the brachial plexus innervate the superior chest wall, shoulders, and radial artery harvest sites.
6. The parietal pleura is innervated by intercostal nerves, likely in a similar distribution to the chest wall, with the phrenic nerve innervating the diaphragmatic portion of parietal pleura and the parietal pericardium. Visceral pleura and pericardium are insensate.
7. Literature is heterogeneous regarding specific chest wall blocks for specific procedures.

CLINICAL PEARL

Selection of an appropriate regional anesthesia technique must consider surgical incisions and other sites of pain, local expertise, infrastructure, and case mix. There is currently wide practice and literature variability, and no single technique can be recommended.

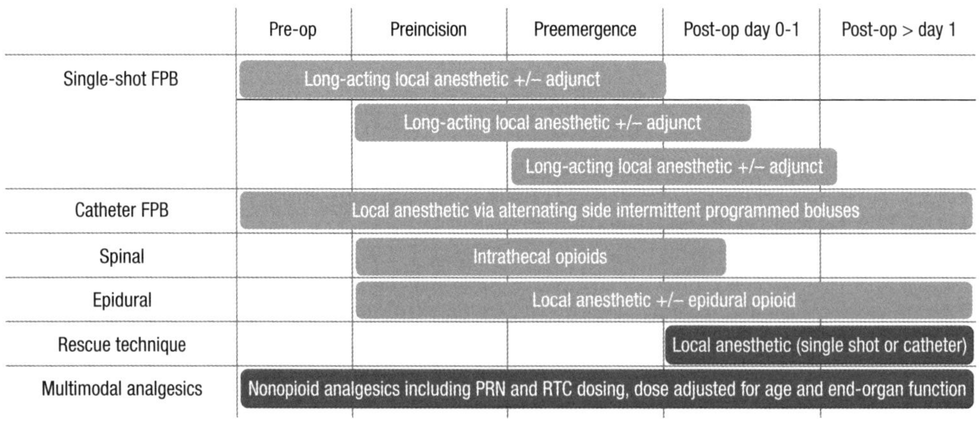

	Pre-op	Preincision	Preemergence	Post-op day 0-1	Post-op > day 1
Single-shot FPB	Long-acting local anesthetic +/− adjunct				
		Long-acting local anesthetic +/− adjunct			
			Long-acting local anesthetic +/− adjunct		
Catheter FPB	Local anesthetic via alternating side intermittent programmed boluses				
Spinal		Intrathecal opioids			
Epidural		Local anesthetic +/− epidural opioid			
Rescue technique				Local anesthetic (single shot or catheter)	
Multimodal analgesics	Nonopioid analgesics including PRN and RTC dosing, dose adjusted for age and end-organ function				

FPB, fascial plane block; PRN, pro re nata; RTC, round the clock.

FIGURE 30.3 Timing and potential duration of analgesia for different regional anesthesia techniques and nonopioid analgesics. Multimodal analgesics should supplement any regional anesthesia technique. (Courtesy of Jessica Brodt and Ban C.H. Tsui.)

B. **Timing of Technique**
   1. Table 30.3 shows the advantages and disadvantages of different timing paradigms for regional anesthesia, including placing before surgery, before emergence, or postoperatively. Figure 30.3 summarizes the anticipated duration of any technique, though this will vary based on medications and dosages used.
   2. The specific timing of blocks in any regional anesthesia pathway will vary based on provider preference, local workflow and practice patterns (including tolerance of delays or additional operating room [OR] time), and staff availability outside the OR.

IV. **Dosing and Safety Considerations**
   1. Safe local anesthetic dosing is essential. Do not dose more than the published maximum recommended doses (Table 30.4).
   2. Cardiac surgery patients are often older adults with altered end-organ function, including renal and hepatic metabolism. This necessitates reduced total local anesthetic dosing (as well as reducing dosing of other medications including multimodal analgesics).
   3. Systemic lidocaine (eg, del Nido cardioplegia, or systemic administration for ventricular arrhythmia management) further reduces the maximum amount of local anesthetic available for any concurrent regional anesthetic technique.
   4. **Single-shot dosing:** Total calculated dose should be divided among all sites and levels. Dosing varies by block, see individual block sections.

TABLE 30.3   Advantages and Disadvantages of Different Timing Options for Regional Anesthesia Techniques

Timing	Advantages	Disadvantages
Preoperative	Positioning may be easier with cooperative patient. Does not consume OR time. May provide intraoperative analgesia.	Duration of postoperative pain relief limited if using single-shot techniques. Resources (staff, space) needed in pre-op holding area.
Preinduction	Positioning may be easier with cooperative patient. May provide intraoperative analgesia.	Duration of postoperative pain relief limited if using single-shot techniques. Requires additional OR time before starting surgery (albeit minimal with experienced provider).
Preemergence	Minimal risk of regional anesthesia-related surgical delay for current case. Most positioning is achievable with intubated patient (sitting not recommended). Potentially longer postoperative pain relief than preoperative single-shot techniques.	Duration of postoperative pain relief may be limited if using single-shot techniques and patient is not rapidly weaned from mechanical ventilation. No intraoperative analgesia. Will require additional OR time at completion of surgery (minimal with experienced provider).
Postoperative	No risk of regional anesthesia-related surgical delay. No additional resources or time in pre-op. Does not consume OR time.	Positioning in ICU can be challenging. Resources (staff, equipment) need to travel to ICU/PACU/floor. No intraoperative analgesia.
Rescue	Provides regional anesthesia on as-needed basis for patients with intolerable pain. No risk of delays. Does not consume OR time.	Resources (staff, equipment) needed to go to ICU/PACU/floor. No intraoperative analgesia. Patients may require significant amounts of systemic analgesics before receiving blocks.

ICU, intensive care unit; OR, operation room; PACU, postoperative care unit.

TABLE 30.4   Maximum Recommended Doses and Pharmacokinetics for Common Local Anesthetics

Anesthetic	Usual Concentration (%)	Maximum Dose (No Epinephrine) (mg/kg)	Maximum Dose (With Epinephrine) (mg/kg)	Maximum Dose in 70 kg Patient (No Epinephrine) (mg)	Maximum Dose in 70 kg Patient (With Epinephrine) (mg)	Onset (min)	Duration of Analgesia (h)
Lidocaine	1-2	3	7	200	500	10-20	3-8
Ropivacaine	0.2-0.5	3	4[a]	225	225[a]	15-30	5-24
Bupivacaine	0.25-0.5	2	2.5[a]	150	175[a]	15-30	5-24
Mepivacaine	2-3	5	7	400	500	10-20	3-10

Maximum doses specific to infusions or repeated boluses have not been established.
Doses listed are for a healthy patient with no end-organ dysfunction.
[a]Epinephrine not routinely added to these anesthetics and may not reliably increase the maximum recommended dose. The addition of epinephrine may still prolong the duration of block.

     5. Catheter-based dosing: There is significant heterogeneity in the literature, and recommended dosing has not been established. For patients with more than one catheter, staggered dosing is recommended to reduce peak serum concentrations of local anesthetic (Figure 30.2).[29]

     6. Addition of adjuncts to local anesthetic doses in fascial plane blocks is an emerging technique. Addition of dexamethasone, dexmedetomidine, epinephrine, or other medications depends on local experience and provider preference.

V. Limitations of Regional Anesthesia Techniques

     1. Cardiac surgery may illicit pain at sites not amenable to regional anesthesia coverage, including pericarditis, referred pain, and muscle spasms. Multimodal analgesia including judicious opioid utilization is required to manage these pain sites.

     2. Evidence is currently lacking for the benefit of preemptive analgesia or reduction in chronic pain in patients receiving regional anesthesia.

VI. Summary

Regional anesthesia techniques have emerged as a promising addition to the analgesic toolkit for cardiothoracic anesthesiologists. Several techniques are available for chest wall analgesia, including neuraxial (epidural and spinal), anterior approach (IPP and PSP, parasternal intercostal, SAP), and posterior approach (ESP, retrolaminar, paravertebral), as well as techniques for special situations, including stellate ganglion, RS, and ilioinguinal/iliohypogastric blocks. Selection of a specific technique should be based on surgical incision/indication, local expertise, and workflow. All of these techniques are best utilized as part of a multimodal patient-specific analgesic strategy. The literature continues to evolve, and readers are encouraged to engage with specialty societies for ongoing education, follow the literature, and learn from colleagues already using these techniques in their practice.

REFERENCES

1. Wong WT, Lai VK, Chee YE, et al. Fast-track cardiac care for adult cardiac surgical patients. *Cochrane Database Syst Rev.* 2016;9:CD003587.
2. Gan TJ. Poorly controlled postoperative pain: prevalence, consequences, and prevention. *J Pain Res.* 2017;10:2287-2298.
3. Zubrzycki M, Liebold A, Skrabal C, et al. Assessment and pathophysiology of pain in cardiac surgery. *J Pain Res.* 2018;11:1599-1611.
4. Engelman DT, Ali WB, Williams, JB, et al. Guidelines for perioperative care in cardiac surgery: enhanced recovery after surgery society recommendations. *JAMA Surg.* 2019;154(8):755-766.
5. Mittnacht AJC, Shariat A, Weiner MM, et al. Regional techniques for cardiac and cardiac-related procedures. *J Cardiothorac Vasc Anesth.* 2019;33(2):532-546.
6. Grant MC, Chappell D, Gan TJ, et al. Pain management and opioid stewardship in adult cardiac surgery: joint consensus report of the PeriOperative quality initiative and the enhanced recovery after surgery cardiac society. *J Thorac Cardiovasc Surg.* 2023;166:1695.e2-1706.e2.

7. Horlocker TT, Vandermeuelen E, Kopp SL, et al. Regional anesthesia in the patient receiving antithrombotic or thrombolytic therapy: American Society of Regional Anesthesia and pain medicine evidence-based guidelines (fourth edition). *Reg Anesth Pain Med.* 2018;43(3):263-309.

8. Balki M, Malavade A, Ye XY, et al. Epidural electrical stimulation test versus local anesthetic test dose for thoracic epidural catheter placement: a prospective observational study. *Can J Anaesth.* 2019;66(4):380-387.

9. Tsui B. Epidural stimulation test vs epidural ECG test for checking epidural catheter placement. *Br J Anaesth.* 2005;95(6):836.

10. Guay J, Kopp S. Epidural analgesia for adults undergoing cardiac surgery with or without cardiopulmonary bypass. *Cochrane Database Syst Rev.* 2019;3:CD006715.

11. Zhang S, Wu X, Guo H, et al. Thoracic epidural anesthesia improves outcomes in patients undergoing cardiac surgery: meta-analysis of randomized controlled trials. *Eur J Med Res.* 2015;20:25.

12. Landoni G, Isella F, Greco M, et al. Benefits and risks of epidural analgesia in cardiac surgery. *Br J Anaesth.* 2015;115(1):25-32.

13. McLean SR, von Homeyer P, Cheng A, et al. Assessing the benefits of preoperative thoracic epidural placement for lung transplantation. *J Cardiothorac Vasc Anesth.* 2018;32(6):2654-2661.

14. Bowles C, Keeyapaj W, Brodt J, et al. Thoracic epidural analgesia improves outcomes after lung transplant. *J Heart Lung Transplant.* 2021;40(4):S355.

15. Do DH, Bradfield J, Ajijola OA, et al. Thoracic epidural anesthesia can be effective for the short-term management of ventricular tachycardia storm. *J Am Heart Assoc.* 2017;6(11):e007080.

16. Chaney MA, Barclay J, Aasen MK, et al. High dose intrathecal morphine for cardiac surgery. *Anesth Analg.* 1995;80:SCA91.

17. Chen IW, Sun CK, Ko CC, et al. Analgesic efficacy and risk of low-to-medium dose intrathecal morphine in patients undergoing cardiac surgery: an updated meta-analysis. *Front Med (Lausanne).* 2022;9:1017676.

18. Dhawan R, Daubenspeck D, Wroblewski KE, et al. Intrathecal morphine for analgesia in minimally invasive cardiac surgery: a randomized, placebo-controlled, double-blinded clinical trial. *Anesthesiology.* 2021;135(5):864-876.

19. dos Santos LM, Santos VC, Santos SR, et al. Intrathecal morphine plus general anesthesia in cardiac surgery: effects on pulmonary function, postoperative analgesia, and plasma morphine concentration. *Clinics (Sao Paulo).* 2009;64(4):279-285.

20. Mehta Y, Arora D, Sharma KK, et al. Comparison of continuous thoracic epidural and paravertebral block for postoperative analgesia after robotic-assisted coronary artery bypass surgery. *Ann Card Anaesth.* 2008;11(2):91-96.

21. Dhole S, Mehta Y, Saxena H, et al. Comparison of continuous thoracic epidural and paravertebral blocks for postoperative analgesia after minimally invasive direct coronary artery bypass surgery. *J Cardiothorac Vasc Anesth.* 2001;15(3):288-292.

22. El Shora HA, El Beleehy AA, Abdelwahab AA, et al. Bilateral paravertebral block versus thoracic epidural analgesia for pain control post-cardiac surgery: a randomized controlled trial. *Thorac Cardiovasc Surg.* 2018;68:410-416.

23. Xu M, Hu J, Yan J, et al. Paravertebral block versus thoracic epidural analgesia for postthoracotomy pain relief: a meta-analysis of randomized trials. *Thorac Cardiovasc Surg.* 2022;70(5):413-421.

24. Scarfe AJ, Schuhmann-Hingel S, Duncan JK, et al. Continuous paravertebral block for post-cardiothoracic surgery analgesia: a systematic review and meta-analysis. *Eur J Cardiothorac Surg.* 2016;50(6):1010-1018.

25. Lockwood GG, Cabreros L, Banach D, et al. Continuous bilateral thoracic paravertebral blockade for analgesia after cardiac surgery: a randomised, controlled trial. *Perfusion.* 2017;32(7):591-597.

26. Chin KJ, Lirk P, Hollmann MW, et al. Mechanisms of action of fascial plane blocks: a narrative review. *Reg Anesth Pain Med.* 2021;46(7):618-628.

27. El-Boghdadly K, Wolmarans M, Stengel AD, et al. Standardizing nomenclature in regional anesthesia: an ASRA-ESRA delphi consensus study of abdominal wall, paraspinal, and chest wall blocks. *Reg Anesth Pain Med.* 2021;46(7):571-580.

28. Chin KJ, El-Boghdadly K. Mechanisms of action of the erector spinae plane (ESP) block: a narrative review. *Can J Anaesth.* 2021;68(3):387-408.

29. Tsui BCH, Brodt J, Pan S, et al. Alternating side programmed intermittent repeated (ASPIRe) bolus regimen for delivering local anesthetic via bilateral interfascial plane catheters. *J Cardiothorac Vasc Anesth.* 2021;35(10):3143-3145.

30. Seol A, Tsui BCH. Retrolaminar continuous nerve block catheter for multiple rib fractures: a case report. *A A Pract.* 2022;16(8):e01614.

31. Wong J, Navaratnam M, Boltz G, et al. Bilateral continuous erector spinae plane blocks for sternotomy in a pediatric cardiac patient. *J Clin Anesth.* 2018;47:82-83.

32. Munoz-Leyva F, Chin KJ, Mendiola WE, et al. Bilateral continuous erector spinae plane (ESP) blockade for perioperative opioid-sparing in median sternotomy. *J Cardiothorac Vasc Anesth.* 2019;33(6):1698-1703.

33. Abdelbaser I, Mageed NA, Elfayoumy SI, et al. The effect of ultrasound-guided bilateral thoracic retrolaminar block on analgesia after pediatric open cardiac surgery: a randomized controlled double-blind study. *Korean J Anesthesiol.* 2022;75(3):276-282.

34. Biswas A, Castanov V, Li Z, et al. Serratus plane block: a cadaveric study to evaluate optimal injectate spread. *Reg Anesth Pain Med.* 2018;43(8):854-858.

35. Moon S, Lee J, Kim H, et al. Comparison of the intraoperative analgesic efficacy between ultrasound-guided deep and superficial serratus anterior plane block during video-assisted thoracoscopic lobectomy: a prospective randomized clinical trial. *Medicine (Baltimore).* 2020;99(47):e23214.

36. Kunigo T, Murouchi T, Yamamoto S, et al. Injection volume and anesthetic effect in serratus plane block. *Reg Anesth Pain Med.* 2017;42(6):737-740.

37. Gado AA, Abdalwahab A, Ali H, et al. Serratus anterior plane block in pediatric patients undergoing thoracic surgeries: a randomized controlled trial. *J Cardiothorac Vasc Anesth.* 2021;36:2271-2277.

38. Toscano A, Capuano P, Costamagna A, et al. The serratus anterior plane study: continuous deep serratus anterior plane block for mitral valve surgery performed in right minithoracotomy. *J Cardiothorac Vasc Anesth.* 2020;34(11):2975-2982.

39. Feray S, Lubach J, Joshi GP, et al. PROSPECT guidelines for video-assisted thoracoscopic surgery: a systematic review and procedure-specific postoperative pain management recommendations. *Anaesthesia.* 2022;77(3):311-325.

40. Zhang X, Zhang C, Zhou X, et al. Analgesic effectiveness of perioperative ultrasound-guided serratus anterior plane block combined with general anesthesia in patients undergoing video-assisted thoracoscopic surgery: a systematic review and meta-analysis. *Pain Med.* 2020;21(10):2412-2422.

41. Kim RK, Brodt J, MacArthur JW, et al. Continuous serratus anterior plane block: a team approach. *J Cardiothorac Vasc Anesth.* 2022;36(4):1217-1218.

42. Pascarella G, Costa F, Nonnis G, et al. Ultrasound guided parasternal block for perioperative analgesia in cardiac surgery: a prospective study. *J Clin Med.* 2023;12(5):2060.

43. Chen H, Song W, Wang W, et al. Ultrasound-guided parasternal intercostal nerve block for postoperative analgesia in mediastinal mass resection by median sternotomy: a randomized, double-blind, placebo-controlled trial. *BMC Anesthesiol.* 2021;21(1):98.

44. Shokri H, Ali I, Kasem AA. Evaluation of the analgesic efficacy of bilateral ultrasound-guided transversus thoracic muscle plane block on post-sternotomy pain: a randomized controlled trial. *Local Reg Anesth.* 2021;14:145-152.

45. Blanco R. The "pecs block": a novel technique for providing analgesia after breast surgery. *Anaesthesia.* 2011;66(9):847-848.

46. Yang JK, Char DS, Motonaga KS, et al. Pectoral nerve blocks decrease postoperative pain and opioid use after pacemaker or implantable cardioverter-defibrillator placement in children. *Heart Rhythm.* 2020;17(8):1346-1353.

47. Munshey F, Ramamurthi RJ, Tsui B. Early experience with PECS 1 block for Port-a-Cath insertion or removal in children at a single institution. *J Clin Anesth.* 2018;49:63-64.

48. Corso RM, Maitan S, Russotto V, et al. Type I and II pectoral nerve blocks with serratus plane block for awake video-assisted thoracic surgery. *Anaesth Intensive Care.* 2016;44(5):643-644.

49. Versyck B, van Geffen GJ, Chin KJ. Analgesic efficacy of the Pecs II block: a systematic review and meta-analysis. *Anaesthesia.* 2019;74(5):663-673.

50. Graber TJ, Meineke M, Said ET, et al. Continuous ilioinguinal nerve block for treatment of femoral extracorporeal membrane oxygenation cannula site pain. *J Cardiothorac Vasc Anesth.* 2021;35(8):2458-2461.

51. Miller MA, Bhatt HV, Weiner M, et al. Implantation of the subcutaneous implantable cardioverter-defibrillator with truncal plane blocks. *Heart Rhythm.* 2018;15(7):1108-1111.

52. Braver O, Semyonov M, Reina Y, et al. Novel strategy of subcutaneous implantable cardioverter defibrillator implantation under regional anesthesia. *J Cardiothorac Vasc Anesth.* 2019;33(9):2513-2516.

53. Sanghai S, Abbott NJ, Dewland TA, et al. Stellate ganglion blockade with continuous infusion versus single injection for treatment of ventricular arrhythmia storm. *JACC Clin Electrophysiol.* 2021;7(4):452-460.

54. Lobato E, Kern K, Paige G, et al. Differential effects of right versus left stellate ganglion block on left ventricular function in humans: an echocardiographic analysis. *J Clin Anesth.* 2000;12:315-318.

55. Franklin AD, Llobet JR, Sobey CM, et al. Stellate ganglion catheter effective for treatment of ventricular tachycardia storm in a pediatric patient on extracorporeal membrane oxygenation: a case report. *A A Pract.* 2019;13(7):245-249.

56. Parris W, Reddy B, White H, et al. Stellate ganglion blocks in pediatric patients. *Anesth Analg.* 1991;72:552-556.

57. Tian Y, Wittwer ED, Kapa S, et al. Effective use of percutaneous stellate ganglion blockade in patients with electrical storm. *Circ Arrhythm Electrophysiol.* 2019;12(9):e007118.

58. Jones J, Murin PJ, Tsui JH. Combined pectoral-intercostal fascial plane and rectus sheath blocks for opioid-sparing pain control after extended sternotomy for traumatic nail gun injury. *J Cardiothorac Vasc Anesth.* 2021;35(5):1551-1553.

59. Everett L, Davis TA, Deshpande SP, et al. Implementation of bilateral rectus sheath blocks in conjunction with transversus thoracis plane and pectointercostal fascial blocks for immediate postoperative analgesia after cardiac surgery. *Cureus.* 2022;14(7):e26592.

60. Primrose M, Al Nebaihi H, Brocks DR, et al. Rectus sheath single-injection blocks: a study to quantify local anaesthetic absorption using serial ultrasound measurements and lidocaine serum concentrations. *J Pharm Pharmacol.* 2019;71(8):1282-1290.

61. Lee MW, McPhee RW, Stringer MD. An evidence-based approach to human dermatomes. *Clin Anat.* 2008;21(5):363-373.

Postoperative Care of the Cardiac Surgical Patient

Anna Budde, Steven Insler, Daniel Lotz, and Michael H. Wall

KEY POINTS

1. Transport from the operating room (OR) to the intensive care unit (ICU) is a critical period for patient monitoring and vigilance. Emergency drugs and airway equipment should be present, and adequate transportation personnel (typically three people) should accompany the patient.
2. Patient "handoff" to the ICU should be consistent, careful, and structured and should not distract caregivers from continuous assessment of hemodynamics, oxygenation, and ventilation.
3. Early postoperative respiratory support ranges from full mechanical ventilation to immediate extubation in the OR. There is no "best" ventilation mode for cardiac surgery patients.
4. Weaning from mechanical ventilation involves assessment of oxygenation adequacy, hemodynamic stability, patient responsiveness to commands, and measured ventilatory parameters, such as vital capacity and the rapid shallow breathing index (RSBI).
5. Fast-tracking protocols designed to extubate cardiac surgery patients within several hours of completion of surgery are common. Early postoperative continuous infusions of propofol or dexmedetomidine may be helpful.
6. Enhanced recovery after cardiac surgery involves a multidisciplinary approach with physical therapists, occupational therapists, dieticians, and pharmacists, with the combined goal of shortening the convalescent time after cardiac surgery.
7. Early postoperative differential diagnosis of hypotension is often challenging and includes hypovolemia, heart valve dysfunction, left ventricular (LV) and/or right ventricular (RV) dysfunction, cardiac tamponade, cardiac dysrhythmia, and vasodilation. Once a diagnosis has been made, optimal therapy usually becomes clear.
8. Hypertension is not uncommon and must be acutely and effectively managed to minimize bleeding and other complications, such as LV failure and aortic dissection. The differential diagnoses include pain, hypothermia, hypercarbia, hypoxemia, intravascular volume excess, anxiety, and preexisting essential hypertension, among others.
9. Acute poststernotomy pain most often is managed by administering intravenous (IV) opioids, but other potentially helpful modalities include nonsteroidal anti-inflammatory drugs (NSAIDs), intrathecal opioids, and central neuraxial or peripheral nerve blocks.
10. Early postoperative acid-base, electrolyte, and glucose disturbances are common. They should be diagnosed and treated promptly.
11. Postoperative bleeding may be surgical, coagulopathic, or both. Aggressive diagnosis and treatment of coagulation disturbances facilitates early diagnosis and treatment of surgical bleeding (ie, return to OR for reexploration) and avoidance of cardiac tamponade.
12. Discharge from the ICU typically occurs in 1-2 days. Criteria vary with cardiac surgical procedures and with institutional capabilities for post-ICU patient care (eg, stepdown ICU beds vs traditional floor nursing care).
13. Adequate communication with patients' family members and adequate family visitation and support greatly facilitate postoperative recovery.

INTRODUCTION

The purpose of this chapter is to discuss the postoperative care of the cardiac surgery patient and common problems that occur in the first 24 hours in the intensive care unit (ICU).

I. Transition From Operating Room to Intensive Care Unit

A. General Principles

1. Interhospital or intrahospital transport of critically ill patients is associated with increased morbidity and mortality.
2. The American College of Critical Care Medicine (ACCM) guidelines state that "during transport, there is no hiatus in the monitoring or maintenance of a patient's vital signs."[1]
3. There are four major areas to optimize efficiency and safety of patient transport: communication (or handoffs), personnel, equipment, and monitoring.

B. The Transport Process
   1. **Before movement of the patient from operating room table to intensive care unit bed**
      a. **Airway/breathing:** The endotracheal tube should be checked for position and patency and securely attached to the patient. All chest tubes and drains should be checked for ongoing bleeding and for proper functioning.
      b. **Circulation:** The patient should be hemodynamically stable before transport. Proper settings and functioning of the pacemaker should be confirmed.
      c. **Coagulation:** Bleeding should be controlled.
      d. **Metabolic:** Metabolic abnormalities should be identified and corrected as much as possible before the transport.
      e. **Brief telephone report:** A brief verbal report to the ICU team should be provided before transport.
      f. **Special bed:** Patients at high risk for the development of pressure ulcers (preexisting pressure ulcers, poor nutritional status, older adult, poor ventricular function, etc) should be placed on special beds/mattresses in the operating room (OR).
      g. **Intravenous access:** Easy access to an intravenous (IV) is required.
   2. **Patient movement from the operating room table to the transport bed:** Movement can cause hemodynamic instability, fluid shifts, arrhythmias, loss of airway, loss of vascular access, and interruption of IV infusions. Transfer may also induce movement of residual intracardiac air or the pulmonary artery catheter. Ready access to a large-bore IV infusion port is required.

CLINICAL PEARL

If hemodynamic deterioration occurs in the OR even after transfer from the OR table to the ICU bed, it is always better to stop, reassess, and stabilize the patient in the OR.

   3. **Transport from the operating room to the intensive care unit**
      a. Personnel
         (1) **Minimum:** Anesthesia team, surgical team nurse, or tech
         (2) **Additional if needed:** Surgical team member, perfusion, respiratory therapy
      b. Equipment
         (1) Emergency airway management
         (2) Ambu bag
         (3) Backup batteries for mechanical support devices
         (4) Transport ventilator (if needed)
         (5) Adequate oxygen supply
         (6) Defibrillator and emergency drugs
      c. Monitoring
         (1) Should be the same as in the OR
      d. **Intravenous access:** One large-bore IV identified for rapid administration of fluids or drugs
II. **Transfer of Care to the Intensive Care Unit Team**
   A. **Importance of Handoffs**
      The handoff of care from the OR team to the ICU team is a potentially dangerous event. Numerous studies have shown that the best handoffs occur when they are structured, standardized, and use checklists.
   B. **Logistics**
      Each member of the OR and ICU teams should have specific tasks, and the handoff should occur in a standardized sequence. One simple sequence would be the transition from transport to ICU monitor, then initial ventilator settings, and then a formal structured handoff.

C. Transition to Intensive Care Unit Monitors

Based on local monitors, each parameter should be transferred from the transport monitor to the ICU monitor in series, or the monitors can be switched over as a group.

D. Initial Ventilator Settings

Intubated patients must have their endotracheal tube evaluated for patency, security, and position. Ventilator parameters and ventilator mode must be selected.

E. The Actual Handoff

Once the monitors have been transferred to the ICU bedside monitor and oxygenation and ventilation have been confirmed, a structured handoff should occur.

1. **Initial review**
   a. The patient's history, age, height, weight, preexisting medical conditions, any allergies, a list of preoperative medications, and a review of the most current laboratory findings
   b. Review of cardiac status, ventricular dysfunction, valvular disease, coronary anatomy, and details of the surgical procedure, including any events that were unexpected and might lead to postoperative problems (eg, unintended breach of a major vessel)
2. **Anesthetic review** should be presented, which includes:
   a. Types and location of IV catheters and invasive monitors, along with any complications that occurred during their placement
   b. Brief description of the anesthetic technique, including airway assessment at laryngoscopy
   c. Airway management and the need for continuing patient's home continuous positive airway pressure (CPAP) or bilevel positive airway pressure (BiPAP) should be addressed.
   d. A post-cardiopulmonary bypass (CPB) use of vasoactive, inotropic, and antiarrhythmic drugs, as well as any untoward events such as arrhythmias and presumed drug reactions
   e. The presence or absence of bleeding before chest closure
3. **Heart rate, rhythm, and blood pressure**
   a. Temporary pacemaker (epicardial wires)
      (1) Review mode, settings, and electrodes
   b. Permanent pacemaker or defibrillator
      (1) Settings should be reviewed.
      (2) Should be interrogated in the ICU and antitachycardia treatment reactivated
   c. Ventricular assist device
      (1) The monitor should be attached to a wall-based energy supply, and the output of the device should be attached to the display module.
      (2) The settings of the device and the position and location of the cannula should be reviewed.
   d. Extracorporeal membrane oxygenation
      (1) The O_2 and air supplies should be attached to the wall outlet supplies.
      (2) Backup tanks should be available.

F. Laboratory Tests/Electrocardiogram/Chest Radiograph

After the handoff is complete and questions are answered, baseline electrocardiogram (ECG), chest x-ray (CXR), and laboratory tests should be obtained.

III. Mechanical Ventilation After Cardiac Surgery

A. Hemodynamic Response to Positive-Pressure Ventilation and Predictable Pulmonary Changes After Sternotomy and Thoracotomy

In patients with normal left ventricular (LV) function, positive-pressure ventilation (PPV) increases intrathoracic pressure (ITP), reducing venous return, afterload, and stroke volume (SV) and cardiac output (CO). Positive end-expiratory pressure (PEEP) further increases ITP and decreases venous return. Following cardiac surgery, there is a significant reduction in all lung volumes compared to preoperative values that may persist up to ≥ 2 months. These findings suggest a marked tendency toward postoperative atelectasis and the possibility of hypoxemia from increased physiologic shunting. These changes in chest wall function can increase physiologic shunt to as much as 13% (compared to a baseline normal value of 5%).

B. Choosing Modes of Ventilation
1. Intubated patient
   a. Upon arrival from the OR, patients are immediately connected to mechanical ventilation if transported on manual bag/valve—ventilation. The ventilator prescription is typically the pressure-control ventilation (PCV) mode, with a low-dose PEEP of 5-8 cm of water, an F_{IO_2} of $\leq$40%-60% (depending on the respiratory history and intraoperative trends), and tidal volumes of 6-8 mL/kg (see Figure 31.1. Definition: cardiothoracic anesthesia [CTA] ICU staff).
   b. Careful attention is given to maintaining plateau pressure $\leq$30 cm of water while maintaining pH 7.35-7.45. An arterial blood gas (ABG) should be obtained upon admission as a baseline for comparative progress and ventilator weaning. Serum lactate levels should be followed as they may be suggestive of impaired oxygen delivery/hypoperfusion, but there are conflicting data regarding utility immediately following cardiac surgery, and trends need to be followed.[2] A chest radiograph is obtained on admission to evaluate endotracheal, nasogastric/orogastric tube, and central venous or pulmonary artery catheter placement as well as rule out pneumothorax and/or hemothorax, atelectasis, and pleural effusion(s).
C. Weaning From Mechanical Ventilation Is Multifactorial: This is best accomplished using an algorithm in order that weaning can proceed methodically and without interruption. Figure 31.1 shows an example of an algorithm that might facilitate efficient weaning. Before attempts at weaning, the following parameters must be met:
   1. Normothermia $\geq$ 36 °C
   2. Hemodynamically stable
   3. Normal acid-base and metabolic rate
      a. Lactate <3 and down trending
   4. Not bleeding excessively (criteria vary, but generally <150 mL/h chest tube drainage)
D. Liberation From Mechanical Ventilation
   1. The first step is to assess the following to determine "readiness to wean":
      a. Pao_2/F_{IO_2} >200 mm Hg with PEEP $\leq$5 cm H_2O
      b. Hemodynamically stable that is low dose vasopressor and/or inotropic support
      c. Awake, alert, and following commands, without excessive pain
      d. Able to cough effectively
      e. Adequate reversal of neuromuscular blockade
   2. If the patient passes the readiness to wean screen, a trial of spontaneous ventilation with low levels of pressure-support ventilation (PSV) (5-7 cm H_2O) and PEEP ($\leq$5 cm H_2O) for 30-45 minutes is done. At the end of the trial, if the rapid shallow breathing index (RSBI) is <80-100, the patient should be considered for extubation if they meet the following criteria. The RSBI is defined as respiratory rate (RR) divided by tidal volume in liters after a spontaneous breathing trial (SBT).
      a. Extubation criteria
         (1) Awake and alert, neurologically intact or at baseline
         (2) Able to cough and clear secretions
         (3) No airway edema (as judged crudely by edema of the tongue and the presence of both inspiratory and expiratory leak when endotracheal tube cuff is fully deflated)
         (4) Hemodynamically stable
         (5) Normal oxygenation and ventilation during SBT, minimal PEEP, pressure-support (PS) settings, and F_{IO_2} 40%
      b. Incentive spirometry, positive airway pressure systems, deep breathing, and coughing maneuvers
         (1) Patients must be encouraged to do deep breathing, coughing maneuvers, and spirometry after extubation in order to reduce atelectasis. Positive expiratory pressure therapies should be done at least 4 times a day for the first 48 hours post-op to mobilize secretions, reduce air trapping, and prevent atelectasis.

CVICU Mechanical Ventilation Protocol

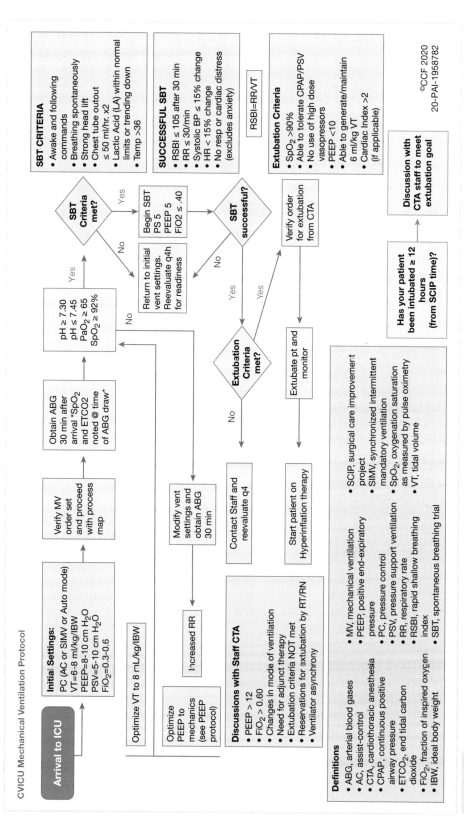

FIGURE 31.1 Weaning from mechanical ventilation following cardiac surgery. (Reprinted with permission, Cleveland Clinic Foundation ©2023. All Rights Reserved.)

E. **Rapid Mechanical Ventilation Weaning for Fast-Track Patients (<6 Hours)**

 1. While many patients should be extubated within 6 hours, some patients who have been deemed eligible for fast-track (FT) status can be safely and effectively liberated from the ventilator earlier than this utilizing the rapid weaning process described in Figure 31.1.

IV. **Principals of Fast-Tracking**

 A. **Goals of Fast-Tracking**

 FT cardiac surgery was introduced to speed recovery and increase the efficiency of a finite resource (ICUs). Key goals of an FT program include early extubation, ambulation, early rehabilitation to decrease the time in the ICU, and, ultimately, time to discharge. Time and time again, randomized controlled trials have shown that FT cardiac surgery programs are safe and less expensive than traditional cardiac anesthesia.

V. **Enhanced Recovery After Cardiac Surgery**

 A. **Goals of Enhanced Recovery After Cardiac Surgery**

 The goal of enhanced recovery after surgery (ERAS) program is to decrease the surgical stress response and thus reduce the length of stay (ICU and hospital) through standardization in order to improve patient outcomes. The ERAS-Cardiac Society released its first set of recommendations in 2019.[3]

VI. **Hemodynamic Management in the Postoperative Period**

 A. **Monitoring for Ischemia**

 In the postoperative period, ischemia is often detected utilizing a continuous ECG with ST-segment analysis. In continuous ST-segment analysis mode, leads II and V4 or V5 should be monitored, which improves sensitivity to around 90% when all three leads are used. Segmental wall motion abnormalities represent one of the most sensitive early detectors of myocardial ischemia and can be detected by either transesophageal (TEE) or transthoracic echocardiography. When in doubt, cardiac catheterization can be both diagnostic and therapeutic.

 B. **Ventricular Dysfunction After Cardiac Surgery**

 1. **Causes:** In addition to preexisting ventricular dysfunction, postoperative causes of ventricular dysfunction include inadequate myocardial protection, myocardial stunning, incomplete revascularization, and reperfusion injury. Preoperative predictors include cardiac enlargement, advanced age, diabetes mellitus, female gender, high LV end-diastolic pressures, small coronary arteries, and LV ejection fraction (EF) of <40%. Intraoperative predictors are prolonged (>120 minutes) CPB/aortic cross-clamp time.

 2. **Treatment**

 a. Catecholamines

 The inotropic response to β1/β2-adrenergic receptor stimulation occurs via activation of the G-protein and adenylyl cyclase, leading to increased intracellular cyclic adenosine monophosphate (cAMP). Lusitropy (myocardial relaxation) is an active energy-consuming process, and impaired relaxation can lead to both systolic and diastolic heart failure. Until recently, there have been no head-to-head clinical trials comparing the clinical outcomes of inotropes and vasopressors. Levy et al reported a study in which patients either received epinephrine or dobutamine in combination with norepinephrine. Both groups experienced an increased CO and a decrease in plasma creatinine concentrations. In this trial, the epinephrine group experienced more arrhythmias, transient lactic acidosis, and decreased splanchnic perfusion.[4]

 b. Phosphodiesterase type III inhibitors

 Phosphodiesterase type III inhibitors augment β-adrenergic–mediated stimulation via the inhibition of the breakdown of cAMP. Phosphodiesterase inhibitors (PDEIs) act synergistically with β-adrenergic agonists. PDEIs appear to have anti-ischemic effects and may favorably alter myocardial oxygen consumption.[4]

 C. **Fluid Management**

 Managing postoperative fluids after cardiac surgery can be challenging. The vasoconstricting effects of hypothermia combined with the vasodilating effects as the patient rewarms commonly complicate the delicate balance of fluid management during the first few hours after cardiac surgery. One approach is to ask whether a hypotensive patient may benefit from additional fluid boluses. Volume responsiveness can be defined as an increase in CO by >15% in response to a fluid challenge.

Cases that involve CPB typically result in fluid sequestration in the interstitial compartments, and when coupled with changes in circulating blood volume from blood loss, these can cause large-volume fluid shifts. Most patients will reach the postoperative period with an excess total-body fluid that will eventually need to be mobilized.

D. Managing Hypotension

The cardiovascular system depends on preload, afterload, and contractility to function properly, and a systematic evaluation of each must be performed on a postoperative patient who is hypotensive.

1. Vasodilatory shock

Approximately 8% of cardiac surgery patients will experience refractory vasodilatory shock after CPB. This shock is associated with an increased mortality estimated as high as 25%. While the exact cause is not well understood, it is usually multifactorial: long CPB times, preoperative angiotensin-converting-enzyme inhibitor (ACEi), calcium channel blockers, heart transplantation, ventricular assist device (VAD) placement, and preoperative myocardial dysfunction.

2. Cardiac tamponade

Any postcardiac surgery patient with hypotension may be developing cardiac tamponade, and this diagnosis should always be considered. Postcardiac surgery patients often do not present with classic diagnostic signs, such as equalized filling pressures, increased jugular venous pressure, and pulsus paradoxus. More importantly, these patients may not even present with large-volume collections, but rather focal posterior collections, which may be difficult to diagnose via echocardiography. Echocardiography can aid in diagnosis, but ultimately, cardiac tamponade is a clinical diagnosis.

E. Dysrhythmia Management

Managing postoperative dysrhythmias is an important part of ICU management in the cardiac surgery population, with a variety of atrial or ventricular dysrhythmias that can occur. Atrial fibrillation remains the most common (up to 30%) arrhythmia after heart surgery and can be a troublesome problem to manage, especially in patients with reduced systolic function.

F. Pulmonary Hypertension

1. Acute postoperative pulmonary hypertension

This should be identified early and managed aggressively in order to prevent RV failure. The main factors that can cause acute pulmonary hypertension (PHTN) in the cardiac surgery patient population are mitral stenosis, mitral regurgitation, clot/thrombus around the prosthetic mitral valve, perivalvular leak, acidosis, hypercarbia, hypoxia, increased mean airway pressure, and excessive sympathetic stimulation.

a. Volume status of the right ventricle

Echocardiography will be the primary tool in assessing volume and/or pressure overload in cases of RV dysfunction after heart surgery. This can be deciphered by close inspection of the shape of the interventricular septum in both systole and diastole.

b. Right ventricular function

This can be augmented by the addition of inotropic agents, such as dobutamine, PDEIs, and epinephrine. Before these drugs are commenced, however, optimization of both heart rate and rhythm is important to achieve.

c. Decrease pulmonary vascular resistance

By decreasing the pulmonary vascular resistance (PVR), we reduce the afterload the RV must work against. This can be as simple as correcting an underlying acidosis, hypercarbia, or hypoxemia. Also pulmonary artery vasodilators (inhaled nitric oxide, prostacyclin, PDEI, and IV nitroglycerin). Lastly, optimization of the ventilator with steps to minimize PEEP, mean airway pressure, and peak airway pressures will all help reduce RV afterload.

d. Maintaining adequate right coronary perfusion pressure

Increased systemic afterload by the addition of vasopressors or augmenting diastolic pressure with the support of an intra-aortic balloon pump (IABP) may enhance right coronary artery perfusion. In particular, the use of vasopressin may be helpful as it raises systemic blood pressure without a concomitant rise in pulmonary artery pressure.

VII. Postoperative Bleeding

Postoperative bleeding after cardiac surgery leads to increased morbidity and mortality and is a relatively common complication.[5]

A. Risk Factors

Multiple studies have found several risk factors that increase the likelihood of postoperative bleeding, including older age, smaller body mass index, nonelective cases and five or more distal anastomoses, length of bypass time, plasma fibrinogen levels, thrombocytopenia, and avoidance of antifibrinolytics.

B. Monitoring

Standard lab tests for coagulation complete blood count (CBC), partial thromboplastin time (PTT), prothrombin time (PT), international normalized ratio (INR), and fibrinogen all should be followed, but only capture small portions of the coagulation cascade. Newer tests such as thromboelastography (TEG) or viscoelastic testing are increasingly being used to evaluate the entire process of coagulation, especially in the cardiac surgery population.[6]

C. Treatment

For all postsurgical bleeding, the first decision must be whether this is surgical bleeding or microvascular bleeding. Surgical bleeding can be identified as probable when the chest tube output is > 200 mL in the first hour or 2 mL/kg/h for 2 consecutive hours. Surgical bleeding requires a return to the OR to secure hemostasis. For microvascular bleeding, the Society of Cardiovascular Anesthesiologists has published a targeted algorithm.[7]

VIII. Postoperative Pain Management Following Cardiac Surgery

A. Appropriate Pain Management following cardiac surgery has a close association with early extubation and maintenance of respiratory function, early ambulation, and reduced incidence of delirium.[3]

1. **Postoperative pain strategies begin in the preoperative period if possible**

   a. Patient- and family-centered assessment and tailored education have been associated with reduced opioid consumption, anxiety, anxiolysis, and reduced hospital length of stay.[8]

2. Evolving pain management strategies have been focused upon the use of the **multimodal analgesia regimens.**

   a. Multimodal strategies include the use of nonnarcotic agents such as nonsteroidal anti-inflammatory drugs (NSAIDs), acetaminophen, gabapentinoids, local and regional analgesia/neuraxial blockade, NMDA (N-methyl-D-aspartate) antagonists (eg, ketamine), and nonmedication techniques, such as music therapy.

B. Immediately Postoperative, short-acting parenteral opioids are recommended, given the rapid ability to titrate doses according to patient clinical need.

1. Assessing pain in the sedated, mechanically ventilated, or nonverbal patient is difficult. Validated tools should be used for nonverbal cues that are associated with pain estimates and may guide treatment.

2. Following surgery and in the neurologically intact, one may initiate intravenous patient-controlled analgesia (IVPCA). IVPCA may begin before extubation, without a basal infusion, but with a clinician set dose and dosing intervals (typically 6-10 doses per hour) and lockout periods set up on a patient-activated pump.

3. IVPCA may be associated with decreased opioid consumption, earlier extubation, and ambulation and greater patient satisfaction. **Fentanyl, hydromorphone, and morphine** are the most common parenteral opioids.

   a. Fentanyl is a synthetic derivative of morphine, but 100 times more potent and more lipid soluble.

   (1) **Rapid onset (within 2 minutes) and time-to-peak effect (4 minutes):** Given in titrated IV doses of 12.5-25 µg every 5 minutes until moderate-to-severe pain is relieved. The elimination half-life is 2-4 hours.

   (2) Frequently used as first-line IV and IVPCA medication, often used to provide analgesia because it is easily titratable

   b. Hydromorphone is a commonly used alternative if the pain is refractory to fentanyl and is 4-6 times more potent than morphine.

        (1) It has a rapid onset of action and achieves peak effect occurring within 10 minutes with a half-life of 2.4 hours.

        (2) May be administered in doses of 0.2-0.5 mg every 5 minutes until pain is relieved. May be used in IVPCA regimen

    c. Morphine is the prototypical opioid, commonly used for postoperative pain relief.

        (1) Rapid onset with peak effect within 20 minutes IV. Elimination half-time of 2-3 hours, duration of action of 3-4 hours. Causes histamine release and associated hypotension and bronchospasm

        (2) In acute pain, morphine can be administered in doses of 1-3 mg every 5 minutes until pain is relieved or respiratory depression and/or hemodynamic instability are evident.

    d. The NMDA antagonist, ketamine, can be used in low-dose IV infusions to manage refractory pain.[9,10]

        (1) Subanesthetic infusions can be used in mechanically ventilated or extubated patients with dosing range from 0.1 to 0.6 mg/kg/h. It is currently recommended that patients be monitored in the ICU setting.

C. **Following Extubation,** when neurologically intact, begin introducing oral analgesics and increasing ambulation.

    1. All patients receive scheduled oral acetaminophen (500-1,000 mg orally) every 6 hours unless contraindicated.

    2. Minimize opioids postoperatively, and introduce oral opioids such as oxycodone or hydrocodone as needed postextubation to supplement nonnarcotic therapies.

    3. Have discussion with the patient and home support network regarding the importance of limiting opioids by using pain treatment alternatives.

IX. **Metabolic Abnormalities**

A. **Electrolyte Abnormalities:** All electrolytes should be replaced until they are in normal range.

B. **Shivering:** Shivering can result in a 300%-600% increase in oxygen demand. Effective first-line treatments include active rewarming and prevention of further temperature loss. Pharmacologic interventions include IV meperidine (12.5-25 mg) or dexmedetomidine.

C. **Acidosis**[11]

    1. **Respiratory acidosis** results from hypoventilation or increased CO_2 production. Treatment consists of support of ventilation while treating the underlying cause.

    2. **Metabolic acidosis,** when present, is associated frequently with inadequate systemic perfusion because of compromised cardiac function. Treatment is directed at correcting the underlying cause of the acidosis. Metabolic acidosis in a cardiac surgery patient may require the administration of sodium bicarbonate as a temporizing measure, especially in patients who are hemodynamically unstable.

    3. **Lactic acidosis** needs to be managed by assuring adequate CO and avoidance of shivering. Epinephrine can produce a transient lactic acidosis that does not appear to reflect inadequate perfusion. For this reason, it is important to follow lactate-level trends rather than isolated results.

D. **Glucose Management:** Control of blood glucose levels should be between 140 and 180 mg/dL.[12]

X. **Complications in the First 24 Hours**

A. **Pulmonary Complications**

Postoperative pulmonary complications including postoperative respiratory failure, acute respiratory distress syndrome, pulmonary edema, pneumothorax, hypoxia, atelectasis, and pleural effusion occur at a rate of 5%-25% after cardiac surgery.[13] An intraoperative lung-protective ventilatory bundle including low-tidal volume ventilation and application of PEEP has been associated with reduced postoperative pulmonary complications.[14] Lung ultrasound may facilitate timely diagnosis of these complications, especially pneumothorax.

B. **Bleeding**
Postoperative bleeding requiring reoperation occurs at a rate of 2%-6% in the cardiac surgical population.[15] To differentiate between surgical and nonsurgical bleeding, measurement of coagulation parameters is essential, and utilization of point-of-care testing may reduce time to diagnosis. A restrictive transfusion strategy of red blood cells to a goal hematocrit of 24% has been shown to be noninferior to a more liberal strategy to a goal hematocrit of 30%.[16] Hemorrhage into the chest cavity can be life-threatening and may result in profound hypotension, which may require emergency resternotomy.

C. **Cardiac Tamponade**
Untreated cardiac tamponade can result in circulatory collapse and cardiac arrest. Despite the absence of an intact pericardium, cardiac surgical patients can develop regional tamponade due to compression by loculated effusions or localized adhesions. Clinical presentation of cardiac tamponade includes dyspnea, tachycardia, hypotension, and cardiogenic shock, and treatment consists of emergency surgical drainage.

D. **Hemothorax**
Hemothorax can complicate cardiac surgery, especially for those patients who have undergone internal mammary artery dissection. These patients often require return to the OR for hemostasis.

E. **Acute Graft Closure**
Acute coronary graft closure after cardiac surgery can result in myocardial ischemia, hemodynamic instability, and ventricular arrhythmias. Echocardiography can be utilized to identify myocardial wall motion abnormalities; however, cardiac catheterization is required to definitively diagnose acute bypass graft occlusion.

F. **Prosthetic Valve Failure**
Acute prosthetic valve failure typically presents with sudden hemodynamic changes and usually requires immediate surgical correction. TEE is the diagnostic modality of choice to evaluate prosthetic valve function.

G. **Neurologic Dysfunction**
Perioperative neurologic dysfunction including stroke, peripheral nerve injury, and cognitive dysfunction can occur postoperatively in the cardiac surgical patient. Common mechanisms for stroke in this patient population include emboli, hypoperfusion, and atrial fibrillation. Cognitive dysfunction and delirium are common and can lead to long-term cognitive decline and poor functional status. Assessment of delirium and prediction tools to identify high-risk patients may help clinicians prevent this complication. Peripheral nerve injury can occur due to sternal retractors, and this primarily affects the lower trunk of the brachial plexus.

H. **Acute Kidney Injury**
Acute kidney injury commonly complicates cardiac surgery; furthermore, patients with acute kidney injury in the postoperative period have an increased short-term and 10-year mortality, even if they have recovery of renal function.[17]

XI. Discharge From the Intensive Care Unit
Patients can be discharged from the ICU once they meet standard discharge criteria. Preoperative and postoperative risk factors for longer ICU length of stay include increasing age, impaired LV function, emergency surgery, more complex surgery, and the presence of pulmonary disease.[18]

XII. The Transplant Patient
Heart transplant recipients are at risk for graft dysfunction, rejection, and infection. Hyperacute rejection occurs immediately upon reperfusion of the allograft and can be treated with high-dose immunosuppression, plasmapheresis, and potentially retransplantation. Primary graft dysfunction occurs within the first 24 hours after transplantation and presents with ventricular dysfunction. Cardiac transplant patients should be monitored for arrhythmias, which can indicate rejection in this patient population. When compared with other solid organ transplant patients, lung transplant recipients continue to have higher mortality. The leading causes of mortality in the first 30 days include graft dysfunction and infection. Primary graft dysfunction thought to be caused by reperfusion injury occurs in the early postoperative period with management consisting of supportive care. Other common complications include bacterial and fungal pneumonias, atrial arrhythmias, and stroke. All transplant patients require careful attention to immunosuppression therapy.

XIII. **Patients With Mechanical Assist Devices**

   A. **Intra-Aortic Balloon Pump**

   IABPs are the most frequently used mechanical circulatory support devices and support cardiac function by inflating during diastole resulting in an increase in blood and oxygen delivery to the coronary arteries and by deflating during systole resulting in lower LV afterload. Appropriate function depends on correct anatomic location as well as coordination of inflation and deflation timing with diastole and systole. Placement is typically via the femoral artery and can be assessed via CXR and/or TEE. Complications include balloon rupture, aortic or iliac artery dissection, thromboembolism, distal ischemia, and thrombocytopenia.

   B. **Ventricular Assist Device**

   Left ventricular assist devices (LVADs) are increasingly placed to support patients with end-stage heart failure. Pump speed should be titrated to maintain adequate CO while ensuring sufficient LV cavity volume to sustain pump flow. Complications include RV failure, bleeding, stroke, thrombosis, hemolysis, or infection, particularly at the driveline site. All patients require anticoagulation to maintain LVAD patency and are, therefore, at high risk of bleeding postoperatively.

   C. **Extracorporeal Membrane Oxygenation**

   Some cardiac surgical patients require venoarterial extracorporeal membrane oxygenation (ECMO) support postoperatively, especially in the setting of inability to wean from CPB. Venoarterial ECMO can support both hemodynamics and oxygenation and ventilation in patients with cardiac dysfunction or combined cardiac and respiratory failure. Systemic anticoagulation is required to maintain circuit patency in patients requiring venoarterial ECMO.

XIV. **Family Issues in the Postoperative Period**

   Interaction with families is important in communicating any patient's status and in giving appropriate expectations about recovery.[19]

   A. **Family Visitation**

   Family visitation provides reassurance about the patient's clinical course progression as well as encouragement toward subsequent postoperative care. Family members can be very important in encouraging adequate pulmonary toilet, coughing, deep breathing, and early ambulation to improve postoperative outcomes.

   B. **The Role of Family Support**

   Family support is a vital link toward the early success of an FT program. Family members need adequate education by surgical and anesthesia staff, who can outline the expected early postoperative events. The role of family support is heightened when patients spend very short periods in postoperative areas, such as the recovery room or ICU. Family members who are educated about the expected postoperative course can facilitate postoperative care and smooth the transition from the ICU to a regular nursing floor and finally to the patient's home.

CLINICAL PEARL

Throughout the perioperative period, close communication with family members enhances patient outcomes.

ACKNOWLEDGMENTS

The authors would like to thank Breandon L. Sullivan, MD, and Lindsey Kreishner, MHA, RRT-ACCS, for their contributions to this chapter.

REFERENCES

1. Warren J, Fromm RE Jr, Orr RA, et al. Guidelines for the inter- and intrahospital transport of critically ill patients. *Crit Care Med.* 2004;32(1):256-262.
2. Anderson LW. Lactate elevation during and after major cardiac surgery in adults: a review of etiology, prognostic value, and management. *Anesth Analg.* 2017;125(3):743-752.
3. Engelman DT, Ben Ali W, Williams JB, et al. Guidelines for perioperative care in cardiac surgery: enhanced recovery after surgery society recommendations. *JAMA Surg.* 2019;154(8):755-766.

4. Levy B, Perez P, Perny J, et al. Comparison of norepinephrine–dobutamine to epinephrine for hemodynamics, lactate metabolism, and organ function variables in cardiogenic shock. A prospective, randomized pilot study. *Crit Care Med.* 2011;39(3):450-455.

5. Murphy GJ, Reeves BC, Rogers CA, et al. Increased mortality, post-operative morbidity and cost after red blood cell transfusion in patients having cardiac surgery. *Circulation.* 2007;116:254.

6. Meco M, Montisci A, Giustiniano E, et al. Viscoelastic blood tests use in adult cardiac surgery: meta-analysis, meta-regression and trial sequential analysis. *J Cardiothorac Vasc Anesth.* 2020;34:119-127.

7. Raphael J, Mazer CD, Subramani S, et al. Society of cardiovascular anesthesiologists clinical practice improvement advisory for management of perioperative bleeding and hemostasis in cardiac surgery patients. *Anesth Analg.* 2019;129(5):1209-1221.

8. Klein DG, Dumpe M, Katz E, Bena J. Pain assessment in the intensive care unit: development and psychometric testing of the nonverbal pain assessment tool. *Heart Lung.* 2010;39(6):521-528.

9. Maher DP, Chen L, Mao J. Intravenous ketamine infusions for neuropathic pain management: a promising therapy in need of optimization. *Anesth Analg.* 2017;124(2):661-674.

10. Buchheit JL, Yeh DD, Eikermann M, Lin H. Impact of low-dose ketamine on the usage of continuous opioid infusion for the treatment of pain in adult mechanically ventilated patients in surgical intensive care units. *J Intensive Care Med.* 2019;34(8):646-651.

11. Berend K, de Vries A, Gan R. Physiological approach to assessment of acid-base disturbances. *N Engl J Med.* 2014;371(15):1434-1445.

12. Jacobi J, Bircher N, Krinsley J, et al. Guidelines for the use of an insulin infusion for the management of hyperglycemia in critically ill patients. *Crit Care Med.* 2012;40(12):3251-3276. doi:10.1097/CCM.0b013e3182653269

13. Ball L, Costantino F, Pelosi P. Postoperative complications of patients undergoing cardiac surgery. *Curr Opin Crit Care.* 2016;22(4):386-392.

14. Mathis MR, Duggal NM, Likosky DS, et al. Intraoperative mechanical ventilation and postoperative pulmonary complications after cardiac surgery. *Anesthesiology.* 2019;131(5):1046-1062.

15. Whitlock R, Crowther MA, Ng HJ. Bleeding in cardiac surgery: its prevention and treatment—an evidence-based review. *Crit Care Clin.* 2005;21(3):589-610.

16. Hajjar LA, Vincent J-L, Galas FR, et al. Transfusion requirements after cardiac surgery: the TRACS randomized controlled trial. *JAMA.* 2010;304(14):1559-1567.

17. Hobson CE, Yavas S, Segal MS, et al. Acute kidney injury is associated with increased long-term mortality after cardiothoracic surgery. *Circulation.* 2009;119(18):2444-2453.

18. Bardell T, Legare J, Buth K, Hirsch G, Ali I. ICU readmission after cardiac surgery. *Eur J Cardiothorac Surg.* 2003;23(3):354-359.

19. Xyrichia A, Fletcher S, Philippou J, et al. Interventions to promote family member involvement in adult critical care settings: a systematic review. *BMJ Open.* 2021;11:e042556. doi:10.1136/bmjopen-2020-042556

Practice Management, Quality Assurance and Improvement, and Ethical and Legal Issues in Cardiothoracic Anesthesiology

Mariya Geube, Michael O'Connor, and Christopher A. Troianos

KEY POINTS

1. A well-managed practice, no matter which type of setting, ultimately drives quality patient care and continuous improvement.
2. Billing and coding within a cardiothoracic anesthesia service consists of several unique aspects of anesthesia care, including procedure-based services, transesophageal echocardiography, and staffing ratios.
3. The cardiac operating room is a highly complex environment, which relies on highly skilled multidisciplinary teams, process standardization, and redundancy to promote patient safety.
4. The main principles of "just culture" are to develop a local culture of safety in which speaking up is enabled, to create a blameless reporting system to capture and analyze errors, and to communicate back the lessons learned. This process leads to transparency and accountability, as well as a commitment from the entire team to generate a culture of safety.
5. Providing informed consent is an ethical obligation predicated on the foundational principle of respect for personal autonomy in Western medical practice. This principle grants the right of competent adults to make decisions about their own healthcare.
6. Conflict of interest occurs when clinician self-interest or other secondary interests assume priority over patient care with the potential to harm patients, impair clinician judgment, and undermine trust in the healthcare system.
7. The ethical principles supporting professionalism in patient-centered care include respect for patient autonomy, acting in the patient's best interests (beneficence), weighing the balance between benefit and harm for an intervention (nonmaleficence), equitable distribution of resources and benefits (distributive justice), and honoring the duties of confidentiality, veracity, and fidelity.

I. Introduction

This chapter addresses practice management, quality and safety, and the ethical and legal issues important in the practice of cardiothoracic anesthesia (CTA). The authors practice in the United States, and so many of the details are U.S. centric. Nevertheless, the principles discussed in this chapter are relevant wherever patients are receiving anesthesia care for cardiac surgery. Although practice management and legal considerations address the nonmedical aspects of providing care, and conversely quality, safety, and ethics are focused more on the clinical aspects of care, they are all interrelated. For example, a well-run practice is more likely to lead to a safer environment in which to provide care and which leads to higher quality clinical outcomes. The structure of the practice itself depends on a number of factors that include the hospital setting (tertiary, community, teaching hospital, nonteaching hospital), availability of physician anesthesiologist extenders (fellows, residents, certified registered nurse anesthetists [CRNAs], anesthesiology assistants [AAs]), practice type (employed, contracted, locum tenens), and service requirements beyond anesthesia care (intraoperative or perioperative transesophageal echocardiography [TEE], critical care, acute pain management). A well-managed practice, no matter which setting, ultimately drives quality patient care and continuous improvement of that care. Ethical dilemmas and legal issues are common to all practice settings and conclude the discussion within this chapter.

II. Practice Management

A. Staffing a Cardiac Operating Room

1. **Practice setting:** The practice setting is a key determinant for structuring a CTA service. Tertiary or quaternary care facilities generally require a more intense model or higher level of coverage, regardless of whether or not the facility is also a teaching hospital, as most (but not all) tend to be. From the perspective of providing and staffing for anesthesia services, this may require a lower concurrency coverage model (1:1 or 1:2) depending on the intensity of the work, or type of case. For example, an open repair of a descending thoracic aortic aneurysm that requires a spinal drain, one-lung ventilation, invasive monitoring, TEE, often requires 1:1 staffing with either a trainee or experienced provider, because of the magnitude of work, ongoing patient hemodynamic and cardiorespiratory management, and careful attention to spinal cord perfusion. Similarly, patients with severe cardiorespiratory failure receiving extracorporeal membrane oxygenation (ECMO), and patients undergoing lung transplantation, are best managed with a 1:1 staffing model, regardless of whether or not these are teaching cases, because of the severity of their comorbidities. Some practice settings where the availability of qualified physician extenders is limited may require 1:0 staffing, where the physician anesthesiologist is the only clinician providing anesthesia care.

2. **Concurrency:** Community hospitals that are not quaternary or tertiary care settings *may* be amenable to higher concurrency with experienced physician extenders who allow for staffing ratios of 1:2, 1:3, or 1:4 depending on the type and assignment of cases overall. However, the nature of work within a CTA practice is that case management and complexity can change very quickly to require a higher intensity of care. Staffing models should optimally allow for those unexpected occurrences as they often occur without warning or prediction. The additional variable that determines staffing is the experience of the physician extender. Trainees who are earlier in their training or CRNAs/AAs who lack extensive experience with providing anesthesia care to cardiothoracic surgical patients may also require medical direction at a lower concurrency. Physician trainees require a maximum of 1:2 concurrency as per the Accreditation Council for Graduate Medical Education (ACGME) regulations and for billing considerations.

3. **Academic mission:** An additional aspect within teaching hospitals that have an academic mission is to advance the subspecialty through research, education, and scholarship. All of these endeavors take time, effort, and experience to develop. The time for these activities is typically provided through a combination of the institution and the individual. Teaching programs are required to provide protected nonclinical time to the program director for the execution of the ACGME program requirements. But many other individuals, particularly those early in their careers, often utilize their own "off" time as they invest in themselves, before the institution or department invests in them, by providing protected time.

2

B. **Billing and Coding for Anesthesia Services**
   1. **Coding for anesthesia services:** Various practice parameters dictate how anesthesia services are billed. Coding for an anesthesia service follows a system that is distinct from other medical services that utilize the resource-based relative value system (RBRVS) for procedural-based care. Anesthesia services are based upon a combination of base units and time units, collectively termed "ASA units." Base units are valued according to the complexity, risk, and skill involved to provide each anesthetic specific to a particular surgical procedure. Preoperative evaluation, administration of blood and fluids, data interpretation, and post-op assessment are included with payment of the base unit value. The base unit values of the most common cardiac surgical procedures are available from the American Medical Association (AMA) Current Procedural Terminology (CPT) codes (https://www .ama-assn.org/topics/cpt-codes). If two distinct surgical procedures are performed with a single anesthetic encounter, the base unit associated with the surgical procedure that carries the highest base unit values is the one used for billing. For example, if coronary artery bypass grafting (CABG—18 base units) is performed within the same anesthetic as an aortic valve replacement (AVR—20 base units), the base units charged would be 20 ASA units. Time units are billed for each 15-minute interval, or proportion thereof. For example, 5 hours of anesthetic care during the AVR/CABG would generate 20 time units, for a total of 40 units (base plus time). Additional ASA units are billed for modifiers and qualifying circumstances, such as the physical status of the patient, extremes of age, and qualifying circumstances, such as emergencies and induced hypotension and hypothermia as listed in Table 32.1. Although the Centers for Medicare & Medicaid Services (CMS) does not provide payment for modifiers and qualifying circumstances, commercial payers vary in their payment of these modifiers. All payers recognize the payment modifiers associated with who is providing the anesthesia service for a particular patient as is indicated in Table 32.2.
   2. **Care team modifiers:** Anesthesia care can be provided through a variety of practice models, each with their own practice and billing implications. Cases personally performed by an anesthesiologist are indicated by payment modifier AA, while the medical direction of one or two residents is indicated by payment modifier AA-GC. The medical direction of one CRNA or AA is indicated by payment modifier QY for the physician component and QX for the CRNA or AA component, while the medical direction of two, three, or four CRNAs/AAs is indicated by payment modifier QK for the physician component and QX for the CRNA or AA component. When a physician is responsible for more than four simultaneous anesthetizing locations, the physician utilizes payment modifier AD, while the CRNA/AA component is indicated by payment modifier QX. A CRNA service without physician oversight is indicated by payment modifier QZ.

TABLE 32.1   Modifiers and Qualifying Services to Billing and Coding for an Anesthesia Service

Modifiers and Qualifying Circumstances	Unit Value
Physical status modifiers	
1 or 2	0
3	1
4	2
5	3
Age modifiers	
<1 or >70 y of age	1
Qualifying circumstances	
Emergency (threat to life or limb with delay in care)	2
Total-body hypothermia	5
Induced hypotension	5

TABLE 32.2 Modifiers to Billing Anesthesia Services According to Billing Category

Billing Category	Physician Modifier	Physician Payment	CRNA/CAA Modifier	CRNA/CAA Payment
Personally performed	AA	100%	NA	NA
Teaching case (medical direction of 1-2 residents and no >2 rooms total, including CRNA/AA)	AA-GC	100%	NA	NA
Medical direction of 1 CRNA/AA	QY	50%	QX	50%
Medical direction of 2-4 CRNAs/AAs	QK	50%	QX	50%
Medical supervision >4 sites	AD	3 base units + 1 time unit if present at induction	QX	50%

AA, anesthesiologist's assistant; CRNA, certified registered nurse anesthetist.

3. **Concurrency implications to billing:** Concurrency is the number of anesthetizing locations at which an anesthesiologist is providing anesthesia care at any one time during the course of the anesthetic. There is a negative impact on anesthesia billing under three distinct scenarios. It behooves the practice or the person responsible for clinical scheduling to be cognizant of these implications when assigning or relieving various anesthesiology professionals in the course of providing care. The first scenario is exceeding four simultaneous anesthetizing locations by a physician anesthesiologist under a medical direction model. The implication of exceeding four locations is that instead of using the billing base and time units as described earlier, the anesthesiologist can only bill three base units and no time units, unless present for induction, which would allow for billing one time unit. The second scenario is when an anesthesiologist is medically directing more than two locations and one of those locations involves a resident. Instead of billing as AA-GC, the anesthesiologist bills for medical direction (QX) at 50% of the rate of the teaching category for the resident room(s). The third scenario is when a teaching case (AA-GC) or personally performed case (AA) becomes medical direction. In this scenario, the entire case is billed as medical direction (QX) with payment at 50% *for the entire case*. Potential revenue is unrealized when "like-for-like" relief does not occur either intentionally (eg, fatigue of the primary anesthesia professional) or unintentionally (inattention to like-for-like relief).

CLINICAL PEARL

Potential anesthesia revenue is unrealized under specific circumstances related to how cases are assigned or how the handover of care is managed.

C. **Ancillary Services**
1. **Billing for procedural services:** Ancillary services associated with a CTA practice are billed according to the RBRVS payment system or work relative value units (wRVUs). Commonly performed procedures in a CTA service include invasive catheters, such as arterial and central venous catheters, postoperative pain management blocks, and intraoperative TEE. It is important to note that anesthesia time units cannot be billed during the time when these procedures are performed, unless the patient is under general anesthesia. It is also important to understand that although *interpretation* of these various monitors is included within the value of the base units, the *placement* of these lines and catheters is not and hence the allowance for billing the placement of these catheters separately. The wRVU value for the most common intravascular catheterization procedures used in a CTA practice is available from the American Society of Anesthesiologists (ASA) Relative Value Guide,[1] as developed by the ASA Committee on Economics and derived from the AMA's CPT codes (https://www.ama-assn.org/topics/cpt-codes).

D. **Echocardiography Services**

1. **Indication for transesophageal echocardiography:** Providing an intraoperative TEE service is an important aspect of the practice of CTA. TEE procedures require documentation of the medical necessity for performing the service. Two examples that could describe the medical necessity of providing a perioperative TEE service include an explanation or indication as to (1) how the surgical technique will be affected by the intraoperative echocardiographic findings, thus assisting in surgical management decisions, and (2) an evaluation of the thoracic and/or cardiac function that were not evaluated preoperatively and indicating why the information is necessary for the safe conduct of anesthesia and surgery.

2. **Transesophageal echocardiography billing codes:** The most common intraoperative TEE billing codes are available from the ASA Statement on Transesophageal Echocardiography,[2] as developed by the ASA Committee on Economics and amended on October 26, 2022 (www.asahq.org) and derived from the AMA's CPT codes (https://www.ama-assn.org/topics/cpt-codes). If a diagnostic TEE service is performed by the same anesthesiologist who is providing anesthesia services, modifier 59 should be appended to the TEE code to indicate that the diagnostic TEE is a separate and distinct service from the anesthesia service. When TEE is used solely for monitoring purposes during an anesthetic, TEE billing code 93318 is used to describe the work, but since monitoring is included within the base unit value of an anesthetic, no additional payment is made for the TEE when used solely for monitoring. When TEE is used during catheter-based interventional procedures, the best code that describes the work is 93315.

III. **Patient Safety and Quality Improvement**

A. **Call for Patient Safety and Improvement**

1. **Complex environment:** The cardiac operating room (OR) is a high-risk, high-complexity environment, which relies on highly skilled multidisciplinary teams, process standardization, and redundancy to promote patient safety. The incidence of adverse events in the cardiac ORs is 12%, compared with 3% in noncardiac surgery, and one-third to one-half of these are considered preventable.[3] Efforts to improve safety in the cardiac OR have been ongoing for more than two decades, in order to provide evidence-based guidance for a safer clinical environment and better outcomes for the patients.

2. **Patient safety:** The first call to work for improving patient safety was made with the publication of the National Academy of Medicine (previously Institute of Medicine) report "To Err is Human." The report provided an overview of the literature regarding errors and improved the understanding of the magnitude of this problem, and it identified barriers to the implementation of safety initiatives. This report highlighted that preventable adverse events are a leading cause of death in the United States. Before the year 2000, the number of deaths attributed to medical errors exceeded the number of deaths due to motor vehicle accidents.[4] In addition to the unfortunate consequences suffered by patients, there are direct and indirect costs borne by society from increased hospital expenses, lost productivity, and quality of life.

B. **Comprehensive Approach to Quality**

1. **Healthcare goals:** According to the Institute of Healthcare Improvement, the main goals of healthcare are improving the population health, improving the experience of care, and reducing the costs associated with healthcare services. In the National Academy of Medicine 2001 report, quality in healthcare was identified by six main domains—*safety* (prevent harm), *effectiveness* (science-based care to those who benefit from it), *efficiency* (avoid waste and promote cost-effectiveness), *timeliness* (reduce harmful delay), *equitability* (equal care and treatment for everyone), and *patient-centeredness* (care individualized to patient's needs and values). Given that the primary focus is on safe and efficient hospital-based care, anesthesiologists are in a unique position to lead efforts to improve clinical outcomes, efficiency, and patient experience.

C. **National Quality Organizations**

1. **The Joint Commission:** Founded in 1951, *The Joint Commission on Accreditation of Healthcare Organizations* (aka The Joint Commission) is an independent, not-for-profit, and the nation's largest regulatory and accrediting agency in healthcare. The standards

monitored by The Joint Commission address a broad spectrum of healthcare, from patient rights and education, infection control, medication compounding, preventing medical errors, physician and nursing credentials, emergency preparedness plans, and electronic quality data collection. The Joint Commission awards hospitals with *Disease-Specific Care Certification Programs*, which aim to provide consistency and standardized care, and to improve outcomes in certain disease entities, such as the Heart Failure and Ventricular Assist Device Advanced certification programs and the Stroke and Heart Attack Ready certification programs. Although hospital accreditation by The Joint Commission is pursued on a voluntary basis, it is an objective verification of the organization's commitment to the highest standards of patient care and continuous improvement of healthcare services. Apart from strengthening the community confidence in the quality and safety of care services, the hospital accreditation may increase the competitive value within the healthcare marketplace and provide needed recognition from medical insurance companies.

2. **Centers of Medicare & Medicaid Services:** The CMS is an organization responsible for certification of hospitals meeting eligibility standards, in order to receive reimbursement from the federally funded programs. The CMS has approved The Joint Commission as an accrediting body; thus, any healthcare organization accredited by The Joint Commission is deemed CMS compliant and eligible to receive Medicare and Medicaid incentives. Inversely, not all CMS compliant centers are accredited by The Joint Commission, if they have not applied for accreditation.

CLINICAL PEARL

Both The Joint Commission and CMS adhere to established standards that aim to continuously improve the public's healthcare, by assuring organizations are providing care of the highest quality, safety, and value. Achieving accreditation status from The Joint Commission ensures the organization meets CMS standards for reimbursement from federally funded programs; however, compliance with CMS does not mandate accreditation by The Joint Commission.

3. **National Quality Forum:** The *National Quality Forum* (NQF) is an independent national quality organization, which serves to promote and ensure patient protection and healthcare quality. The NQF has endorsed a portfolio of performance measures incorporated into federally funded incentive programs, evaluated by expert committees, composed of patients, providers, and payers. The federal government and many private-sector entities use NQF-endorsed measures above all others, because of the rigor and consensus process behind them.

4. **Anesthesia Quality Institute:** The ASA created the *Anesthesia Quality Institute* (AQI) in 2008, whose mission is to improve patient outcomes and decrease untoward events through quality feedback and education. The AQI has created the *National Anesthesia Clinical Outcome Registry* to serve as the exclusive source of information and guidance for anesthesia-related quality indicators and practice management and to consolidate efforts for society-driven quality initiatives. Although these external organizations function independently, there is significant overlap in the indicators they have endorsed. Table 32.3 lists the specific measures relevant to cardiothoracic anesthesiology and surgery, as endorsed by national quality organizations.

5. **Society of Thoracic Surgeons:** Public reporting of performance is the cornerstone of any effort to achieve better quality of healthcare at a lower cost. Public reporting increases transparency, affects market value, and helps patients and insurers make informed choices. The *Society of Thoracic Surgeons (STS) National Database* is the largest quality improvement and outcomes registry with voluntary public reporting in cardiothoracic surgery. The STS database has evolved as the major source for benchmark performance measures, risk adjustment models, development of guidelines and best practices, and outcomes research in cardiothoracic surgery. Since 2010, the STS publicly reports clinical outcomes for the

TABLE 32.3 The 2023 Performance Measures Relevant to Cardiothoracic Anesthesiology and Surgery, Endorsed by the National Regulatory Quality Organizations

Anesthesia Quality Institute Measures	Centers for Medicare & Medicaid MIPS Measures	National Quality Forum Measures
AQI 18: CABG prolonged intubation beyond 24 h for isolated CABG	Prolonged intubation beyond 24 h for isolated CABG	Prolonged intubation beyond 24 h for isolated CABG
AQI 41: Postoperative stroke	QID 076: Prevention of central venous catheter–related bloodstream infections	Postoperative stroke
AQI 42: Postoperative renal failure	QID 130: Documentation of current medications	Postoperative renal failure
AQI 49: Adherence to blood conservation guidelines for cardiac operations (excludes emergencies and non-CPB procedures)	QID 424: Perioperative temperature measurement	Operative mortality
AQI 65: Avoidance of cerebral hyperthermia for procedures involving CPB	QID 430: Prevention of postoperative nausea and vomiting combination therapy	30-d mortality
AQI 68: Obstructive sleep apnea mitigation strategies	QID 477: Multimodal Pain Management and pain assessment	Coronary artery disease bundle care
AQI 71: Intraoperative antibiotic redosing	QID 76: Prevention of central venous catheters–associated bloodstream infections	Preoperative β-blocker administration
AQI 72: Perioperative anemia management	QID 44: Preoperative β-blocker administration for CABG surgery	
AQI 73: Prevention of arterial line–related bloodstream infections		

CABG, coronary artery bypass grafting; CPB, cardiopulmonary bypass; MIPS, Merit-Based Incentive Payment System.
Derived from 2023 MIPS Measures from the Anesthesia Quality Institute.

following cardiac procedures—isolated CABG, mitral valve repair or replacement, AVR, and combined coronary artery bypass surgery with either mitral or aortic valve surgery: These data are based on voluntary participation in the database from cardiac surgery practices in the United States and Canada. Every year, the STS assigns a *star rating* to each cardiac practice group. The star-rating calculation determines statistically the probability that the cardiac group performance is lower than average (designates one star) or higher than average (designates three stars). Every year, reports of the star rating are published and show that most of the programs receive two stars, and about 10%-15% of the participants receive one or three stars.

D. **Performance Assessment and Shared Accountability**

1. **Quality reporting:** Healthcare organizations are required to demonstrate the capability to capture, analyze, and report clinical data, based on national quality organizations–endorsed quality indicators and outcomes. Quality reporting helps institutions identify improvement opportunities, provide objective comparisons between similar practices, and show value to patients and payers.

2. **Quality measures:** Quality measures in anesthesiology are categorized according to the Donabedian principles of structure metrics, process metrics, and outcomes metrics.[5] *Structure metrics* refer to the anesthesia care team model and concurrency and are viewed as administrative metrics. *The process metrics* are based on societal management guidelines and assume that compliance with these metrics will eventually result in improved clinical outcomes, without directly measuring the outcomes themselves. Examples are antibiotic

administration within 60 minutes before incision, management of hyperglycemia or hypoglycemia, administration of neuromuscular reversal agent or antiemetic agent before emergence, and avoidance of hypothermia.

3. **Outcome measures:** Cardiac surgery is a "team sport," and the ultimate clinical outcome is determined by the performance of all specialties involved and not just the surgeon. While some of the clinical outcomes are uniquely tied to the surgeon's technical performance—such as surgical wound infection, others are attributed to the anesthesiologist's technical performance (failed intubation, TEE-related esophageal complications, and awareness during general anesthesia or recall). With their intraoperative interventions, anesthesiologists can impact and change the ultimate clinical outcome. Some distinct examples are blood conservation efforts, multimodal analgesia protocols, and preoperative anemia clinics. More recently, *shared outcome measures* have been endorsed by the anesthesiology quality organizations, in which anesthesiologists and surgeons have shared accountability. Examples of such shared clinical outcomes are mortality rate, acute renal failure, stroke, and prolonged mechanical ventilation, among others.

4. **Cardiac anesthesiology database:** The use of large databases to collect, analyze, and share outcomes is critical for the improvement of anesthesia quality of care, as they enable physicians to identify variations in anesthesiology practices and their impact on patients' outcomes. A collaboration between the STS and the Society of Cardiovascular Anesthesiologists culminated with the creation of an *Adult Cardiac Anesthesiology Section of the STS database* in 2014. The goal is to report metrics related to cardiac anesthesia management, identify practice patterns among different institutions, and demonstrate the value of cardiac anesthesiology in the perioperative care of cardiac surgery patients.[6] This database includes an extensive list of measures that are in compliance with the requirements set by the regulatory and quality organizations. These include process measures such as adherence to blood conservation strategies, pain assessment scores, temperature management, as well as clinical outcomes, which may be affected by the cardiac anesthesia management—operative mortality, stroke, renal failure, and prolonged postoperative intubation.

CLINICAL PEARL

The Adult Cardiac Anesthesiology Section of the STS database collaboration emerged as a model of joint accountability and aimed to measure the performance of the "cardiac perioperative team," in addition to demonstrate the value of cardiothoracic anesthesiologists in the perioperative outcomes of cardiac surgery.

5. **ASPIRE:** One of the largest national anesthesiology quality databases is the *ASPIRE (Anesthesiology Performance Improvement and Reporting Exchange) initiative*, which uses data from the Multicenter Perioperative Outcomes Group. The ASPIRE database uses voluntary reporting of electronic perioperative data from private or academic anesthesiology practices to generate institution-specific or provider-specific performance reports, across various domains of anesthesia care, comparing them to their own department, or to other member centers of the ASPIRE registry. The act of measurement and feedback is itself what drives performance improvement, not necessarily a specific intervention, and it is very applicable to modern healthcare (the Hawthorne effect).

CLINICAL PEARL

With their perioperative interventions, anesthesiologists can impact the clinical course and influence patients' outcomes. For this reason, anesthesiologists' performance should be measured and feedback provided either individually or as a group.

E. **Value-Based Healthcare**

1. **Fee-for-service payment:** Healthcare is undergoing a major transformation transitioning from *fee-for-service* (eg, volume of cardiac operations) to *fee-for-value* (improved outcomes ultimately leading to reduced complications and lower costs). The *value-based care delivery model* was proposed to align the goal to improve clinical care and patient outcomes, while optimizing the costs incurred in this process. The change is mandated by the ever-growing healthcare costs in the United States, which do not necessarily lead to improved clinical outcomes. Studies have shown similar survival rates for certain medical conditions, despite higher diagnostic and therapeutic procedures in U.S. centers compared to other countries.[7]

2. **Quality payment system:** The Merit-Based Incentive Payment System (MIPS) ties reimbursement to quality and costs. Through MIPS, the CMS requires physician practices to report the accepted quality metrics and outcomes. The *bundled payment program* as introduced by the CMS stipulates that the total expenditure of a procedure or episode of care is predetermined. By reducing the complications and cost of care, medical centers retain a higher proportion of the payment. On the flip side, those centers caring for patients with higher acuity may be penalized under this model.[8] Acute myocardial infarction and CABG are examples of mandatory bundled payments.

3. **Anesthesiologists' role in improving outcomes:** Anesthesiologists have a unique opportunity to enhance outcomes in the value-based era by development of *preoperative care clinics*, designed to address modifiable risk factors, showing the enormous value of preventative care. Many quaternary centers have already established preoperative care clinics led by anesthesiologists to optimize patients for upcoming cardiac surgery in regard to preoperative anemia, malnutrition, prehabilitation, smoking cessation, pain, and frailty.

CLINICAL PEARL

The CMS aim to reimburse all healthcare organizations according to the value-based care model by 2025. This model projects that anesthesiology services will be reimbursed not by the hours of care provided, but will incorporate quality of care, as defined by accepted team-based outcome metrics.

F. **Metric-Driven Strategy**

1. **Six Sigma:** Six Sigma is a metrics-driven strategy initially applied in the manufacturing industry, whose main goal is quality improvement through standardization and elimination of variation, resulting in decreased defects or errors. The term *Six Sigma* originates from measuring six standard deviations between the average and the acceptable limit of performance. The *Lean methodology* focuses on creating value by reducing waste. The combination of the two methodologies is "Lean Six Sigma," which proposes increased efficiency and maximized outcomes. Applied to healthcare, reduction of defects translates into reduction in medical errors. Lean Six Sigma is a valuable strategy toward value-based healthcare. Lean Six Sigma has the following elements: *define* (focus on patient values), *measure* (create database), *analyze* (scientific approach), *improve* (communicate and implement the change), and *control* (sustain the gains realized). Many healthcare organizations have used the Lean Six Sigma methodology to reduce surgery cancellation, medication errors, and patient visit waiting time and to increase OR efficiency.

2. **Lean Six Sigma for the operating room:** More specifically in the cardiac ORs, the Lean Six Sigma principles have been used to analyze and improve upon:

   a. **Reduce idle time:** Reduce OR turnover time, shorten time for chest closure, decrease patient's waiting time at the preoperative clinic

   b. **Minimize inventory waste:** Equipment maintenance, surplus of medical supplies, which result in expired items and medication waste

   c. **Eradicate defects (medical errors):** Effective handoffs, universal protocol and procedural checklists, standardized clinical pathways for high-risk patients

d. **Transportation:** Optimize patient and caregiver movement, such as locating the cardiothoracic ORs and intensive care unit (ICU) in the same geographic area

e. **Overprocessing:** When time, efforts, and recourses do not improve quality of care and may even cause harm, such as needless blood tests, which may lead to unnecessary transfusions, or daily chest x-ray, which increases the patient's radiation dose[9]

G. **Quality Improvement Program Development**

1. **Implementation:** The implementation of quality improvement initiatives starts with hospital leadership and requires a rigorous structure that extends to the frontline caregivers. The most effective model of quality program is the one that ensures the local quality initiatives align with the organizational objectives. Examples of successful implementation of quality initiatives in cardiac surgery are physician-led introduction of procedural checklists, implementation of evidence-based care protocols (central line placement bundle, basic and advanced life support algorithms), "huddles," and debriefings. High-impact quality initiatives require complex strategic plans involving clinician, financial, informational technology, and statistical participation. The structure includes defining the aim, data collection and analysis, pre- and postintervention measurement, education, and practice improvement changes.

2. **High reliability:** The concept of high reliability assumes that accidents can be prevented at a system level, through good organizational design and management. Characteristics of high-reliability organizations include a commitment of the organization to promote safety, high levels of redundancy in safety measures, and a strong culture for speaking up. They also strive for improving teamwork and relationship building, group performance, and communication, which are often the source of medical errors.

3. **Disproportionate higher acuity:** Large subspecialized academic centers disproportionately serve the sickest and most complicated of all cardiac surgery patients, who may not be acceptable surgical candidates at smaller, lower volume medical centers. At the same time, in the era of value-based healthcare, they must nevertheless meet the state and professional organizations' quality targets and may be penalized for serving patients with higher acuity, despite the fact that patients may still have survival benefit from the surgery.

4. **Institutional quality improvement:** The strategy of implementing a quality improvement program at the institutional level is aimed toward reducing the variations in clinical care based upon individual physician preferences and is commonly described as "the institution's way."[10] It is a cultural transition from individual physician-preferred practice to a multidisciplinary and standardized approach. Protocols are developed to address the most impactful aspects of clinical management of high-risk patients, through the implementation of clinical pathways, preoperative risk assessment, rigorous outcomes measurement and analysis, multispecialty involvement to ensure continuum of care, role clarity, and exemplary teamwork and communication. Variation in clinical management of common cardiac conditions is only acceptable with respect to the patients' unique medical conditions and not with respect to differences due to a provider's subjective preference.

5. **Just culture:** The "traditional culture" of medicine creates an expectation of perfection and attribute errors to carelessness or incompetence. Liability concerns discourage reporting of errors and working on solutions. Among the four types of behavior that lead to patient harm (human error, negligence, rule violation, and reckless conduct), *human errors* comprise the majority of adverse events. A "human error"–centered workplace assumes that the individual inadvertently causes an undesirable outcome. In contrast, a "just culture" workplace provides a psychologically safe environment for health professionals that, in turn, leads to a safer environment for patients.

CLINICAL PEARL

The main principles of the "just culture" movement are to develop a local culture of safety in which speaking up is enabled, to create a blameless reporting system to capture and analyze errors, and to communicate back the lessons learned. This process leads to transparency and accountability, as well as to commitment of the entire team to contribute to the culture of safety.

6. **Reporting systems:** The majority of *reporting systems* within healthcare organizations are voluntary and rely on providers to report patient safety concerns; these should be afforded guaranteed legal protection from data discoverability. Such systems aim to identify vulnerabilities in work systems and patterns of errors, based on the organization's own data. The voluntary nature of reporting systems results in the collection of only a small percentage of the actual events. These data are not an epidemiologic data set, therefore, and do not represent the true frequency of events or trends in events over time. Higher reporting rates of adverse events have been consistently linked to better clinical outcomes because they are used to remedy the weaknesses and prevent future identical events. It should be a priority of the organization's leadership to create a culture in which providers feel safe and supported to report their own safety events and those of other providers.

H. **The "Swiss Cheese" Model of System Failure**

1. **Medical errors:** Most people view medical errors as a "performer issue" rather than a failure in the process of delivering care in a complex delivery system. On the contrary, preventing errors and improving patient safety require systems solutions in order to modify the conditions that contribute to errors. There are two types of medical errors, both well represented in the cardiac ORs.[11] *Active errors* occur at the level of the caregiver—a surgeon, a nurse, or an anesthesiologist. Their effect is obvious and discovered immediately. For example, an anesthesiologist sets up a wrong medication in an infusion pump, which causes an undesirable hemodynamic effect in the patient during surgery. *Latent errors* tend to be out of the direct control of the caregiver and include things such as poor design, incorrect installation, faulty equipment, lack of backup strategies, and poorly structured workspaces. More often than not, root cause analysis focuses on the more obvious active errors (comes down to individual performance) and fails to identify the latent errors, which remain hidden in the system design. Correction of the latent errors is slow and resource intensive. An example of a latent error is the similarity between two medications, which creates the opportunity for an error. It requires creating infusion medication labels, which sharply distinguish the two medications, rearranging the pharmacy station to allow for physical separation and incorporating technology to improve the safety of medication administration, such as barcode scanners.

2. **Swiss cheese model:** *The Swiss cheese model* suggests that multiple layers of hidden (latent) failure, represented by the holes in the cheese slices, have to occur before serious harm reaches the patient (active error). It is an effective model for investigating the cause of serious safety events and identifying important system weaknesses. Safety depends on increasing the number of safety layers and preventing the holes from aligning. An example of analysis of an error occurring using the "Swiss cheese" sequence of events is presented in Figure 32.1.

CLINICAL PEARL

One of the most successful examples of the effectiveness of the Swiss cheese model in the eradication of latent errors is the decrease in patient harm from medication errors (Figure 32.2).

I. **Categorization of Safety Events and Process Improvement**

1. **Sentinel events:** *Sentinel events* are defined as an unanticipated death or permanent loss of function, not related to the natural course of the patient's illness. A comprehensive list of the most frequently reviewed sentinel events within the 2022 Report of The Joint Commission is presented in Table 32.4. Sentinel events from this list that could occur in a cardiothoracic OR setting include wrong procedure (type, patient, site, and side), unintended retained foreign body, medication errors, and delay in treatment. The common factors contributing to The Joint Commission's most frequently reviewed events were inadequate staff-to-staff communication during transfer of care and sign out, policies not followed, and inadequate patient education.[12] *Precursor events* are those adverse events that result in temporary mild or moderate harm. *Near-miss events* are defined as errors that do not reach the patient; however, they represent serious potential safety risks and should be viewed critically as a potential patient threat.

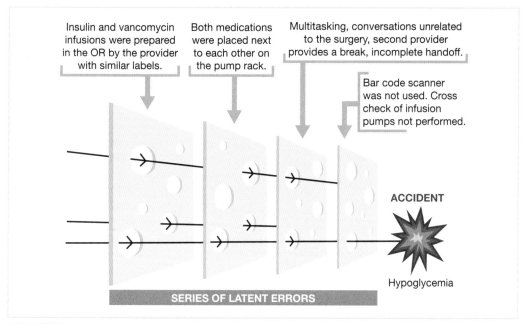

FIGURE 32.1 The Swiss cheese model of systemic failure leading to an adverse event. Event summary: A 54-year-old male patient is undergoing coronary artery bypass grafting and requires vancomycin infusion over 60 minutes as a perioperative antibiotic prophylaxis. The resident had three infusion medications that the patient will eventually need during surgery on the pump rack—insulin, vancomycin, and epinephrine, all of which have been mixed and labeled. After induction of anesthesia, the resident intended to start vancomycin, however, inadvertently infused insulin 100 U over 60 minutes. After central line placement, a break was provided by another resident. When the infusion was complete, the second resident noticed that insulin was infused, instead of vancomycin. Immediate blood glucose check showed blood glucose of 28 mg/dL. OR, operating room. Created at the Cleveland Clinic as per Dr Geube.

2. **Root cause analysis:** *Root cause analysis* was adopted in healthcare in the 1990s from other high-risk industries, during the early movement for improvement of patient safety in hospitals. It is a systematic analytical process that aims to establish the course of the adverse event (*what* happened), the factors leading to the event (*why* it happened), and the circumstances around it, in an attempt to identify a strategy (*how*) to prevent future events. The goal is to implement changes that address how the *system* broke down in order

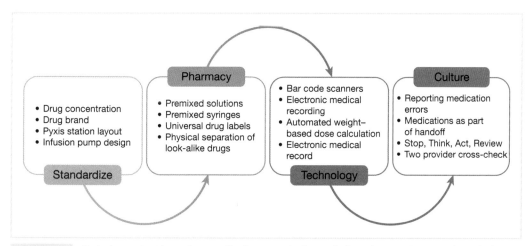

FIGURE 32.2 Reducing patient harm from medication errors in the cardiothoracic operating room through elimination of latent errors in the work system.

TABLE 32.4 The Joint Commission's Top 10 Most Frequently Reviewed Sentinel Events (January 2021-June 2022)

Sentinel Event Type	CY 2021	Q1 & Q2 CY 2022
Fall	480	199
Wrong surgery[a]	116	19
Delay in treatment	105	25
Unintended retention of a foreign object	94	30
Suicide	70	26
Assault/rape/sexual assault	59	16
Self-harm	47	11
Fire	42	10
Medication management	31	12
Clinical alarm response	24	7

[a]Wrong surgery includes wrong site, wrong procedure, wrong patient, and wrong implant.
© The Joint Commission. Sentinel Event Data: General Information & 2022 Q1, Q2 Update. Joint Commission Resources; 2022:11. Reprinted with permission.

to prevent future failure and not simply to provide education, which has not been found to be an effective and sustainable solution for the prevention of future events. State-regulatory agencies mandate root cause analysis for all sentinel events and when significant patient harm occurs.

3. **Morbidity and mortality review:** *Mortality and morbidity conferences* are regularly scheduled department/specialty-specific or multidisciplinary confidential group discussions of patient complications or deaths. It is part of the departmental quality and patient safety program and should include all members of the team. The goal is to review the incident, identify the cause of the incident and potential areas for change of existing systems, and finally to provide education to caregivers in an attempt to prevent a repeat incident.

4. **Peer review:** *Clinical peer review* is a process whereby physicians review the performance and decision-making of other physicians, within their own specialty or another specialty in order to ensure that the standards of care are being met. There are three indications for initiating a peer review in current hospital practice. Hospitals are required by The Joint Commission to perform peer review for accreditation purposes when privileges are requested for new physicians. Second, peer review can be requested for a physician in the case of an adverse event. The review aims to determine if the physician deviated from the accepted standard of practice, if there was a noncompliance with accepted policies, or if negligence was the cause for the event. Finally, some practices use the peer-review process for quality improvement as peers review each other's performance, for example, review of the completeness and accuracy of intraoperative TEE images and reports.

J. **Mitigating Risk: Crisis Management and Teamwork Training**
1. **Complex system:** The cardiac OR is an example of a complex system composed of multiple independently structured units—surgeons, anesthesia, perfusion, nursing, physician assistants, engineers, techs, and, last but not least, equipment and technology. It is a work environment of high risk, high pace, and high complexity, which, therefore, has a unique set of safety risks and hazards.

2. **Human error:** The likelihood of human error increases with the number of monitors and tasks that OR personnel have to manage at any given time. The *cognitive workload* of anesthesia clinicians in cardiac ORs is higher than in other anesthesia locations due to the multiple monitoring systems, alarm alerts, multiple infusions, and the need for frequent interventions. Observational studies have shown that there may be >100 disruptions per cardiac case.[13]

3. **Operating room distractions:** *OR noise* is one of the biggest factors for distraction in this setting. Noise as high as 80 dB (the level of noise produced by a lawn mower) has been

recorded in the OR, which can negatively affect the team's performance by reducing their concentration and affecting communication. *Alarms,* while designed to warn providers of an imminent threat to the patient's condition, are a common source of noise and distraction in cardiac ORs. Studies have found that 90% of alarms are false positives and may lead to alarm fatigue and distraction. Adopting the "sterile cockpit" *concept* from aviation helps to minimize noise and interruptions during critical stages of the surgery, such as anesthesia induction and emergence, as well as during institution of or separation from cardiopulmonary bypass.

CLINICAL PEARL

Reducing the noise and distractions in the OR is fundamental to avoid errors. Adopting the "sterile cockpit" model ensures that all team members pay attention during the critical stages of surgery when the cognitive workload is the highest, such as induction and emergence from anesthesia, as well as during transition to or from cardiopulmonary bypass.

4. **Communication:** *Communication failures* in U.S. hospitals are responsible for up to 87% of untoward events in the perioperative period. The highest potential for communication breakdown occurs during transitions of care between locations or providers, within the team, or between different teams. An effective tool to prevent communication breakdown is *closed-loop communication*, which involves active listening, followed by confirmation that the message was received and understood. Repeating the information using *numeric and phonetic* clarification ensures accuracy and safety, especially when critically important values are reported. One example is sharing the results of the activated clotting time immediately before commencing cardiopulmonary bypass by spelling out "4-9-0" rather than stating "four hundred and ninety," which may be confused with four hundred and nineteen.

CLINICAL PEARL

Use closed-loop communication techniques to ensure proper transfer of critical information. Use phonetic and numeric clarifiers to ensure clarity and safety. Facilitate briefings, huddles, plan-of-care rounds, and debriefings to improve the effective communication within and between the teams.

5. **Handoff risks:** The Joint Commission defines the *handoff* as a process of transferring patient-specific information within or between teams in a variety of settings, to ensure continuity and safety of care. The handoff is not only giving and receiving a report, rather it is the active process of transferring responsibility. Higher complexity and longer procedure times predispose cardiac surgery patients to handoff failures due to the involvement of multiple providers in the patient care. A recent observational study found that intraoperative anesthesia handoffs were associated with higher mortality in cardiac surgery patients[14;] however, it is possible that longer and more complex cases have a higher number of handoffs and thus higher mortality. The risk of losing information during handoff should be carefully weighed against the fatigue and burnout associated with having one provider complete the case, by working excessively long hours. Interventions proven effective in reducing medical errors by improving communication are the standardized *transfer-of-care handoffs.*[15] They improve the content and structure of the sign-out process and provide standardization, so critical information is not omitted. Knowing that handoffs are associated with worse outcomes should focus attention on improved quality and also minimize the number of handoffs.

CLINICAL PEARL

Intraoperative assignments should minimize handoffs and interruptions during cardiac surgery. Rare and high-complexity cases should be completed by one anesthesiology team. Handoffs should be standardized in order to avoid omitting important information. Handoffs should not occur during critical periods of the surgery—induction of anesthesia, transition to and from cardiopulmonary bypass, and before transport out of the OR.

6. **Patient huddle:** *Multidisciplinary briefings (huddles)* should involve the entire OR team and aim to reduce omission of pertinent information. Information such as allergies, blood availability, arterial and venous access, necessary equipment (type of valves, or size of endovascular grafts), and cannulation strategy are typically discussed.

7. **Plan-of-care approach:** Holding plan-of-care rounds in the ICU is an approach that occurs at the bedside and requires the participation of intensivists, bedside nurses, and respiratory specialists to ensure that the treatment plan is communicated to all involved caregivers, as well as to the patient and their family.

8. **Checklists:** A *procedural checklist* is a standardized tool for verification of all critically important steps common for all procedures (type, site, and laterality of the procedure; antibiotic requirements; fire risk; and necessary equipment). Checklists and *memory aids* can also provide an effective step-by-step management of a crisis situation, such as a fire—code red (RACE—Rescue, Alarm, Contain, Extinguish/Evacuate and PASS—Pull, Aim, Squeeze, Sweep). Adopting checklists for crisis management is meant to decrease errors from omission (forgetting an important step) or error of commission (improper implementation of a procedure). In order for the checklist to effectively improve outcomes, they have to be simple, evidence based, and practical (easy to implement). One of the most effective checklists implemented to date is the central line placement bundle, resulting in significant reduction of central line–associated infectious and noninfectious complications.

9. **Simulation:** *Simulation-based training* has emerged as a valuable tool for teaching and assessing procedural skills and teamwork in medicine. Simulators have become an integral part of cardiac anesthesia training of technical skills (lung isolation techniques, TEE, vascular access) or team management skills (cardiac arrest, malignant arrhythmias, extracorporeal life support) by providing a learning environment with realistic physiologic data and real equipment without the potential for patient injury. A summary of the work system factors that have a significant impact on improving patient safety and quality of care in cardiac surgery patients is provided in Table 32.5.

K. **Barriers to Quality Improvement and Future Directions**

1. **Value-based payment:** The CMS is transitioning physicians' compensation to value-based compensation, adjusted for performance measures. Part of the reported measures must be outcome measures. Creating risk-adjusted outcome metrics for performance assessment of individual anesthesiologists is challenging. A recent study using a population-based reporting registry for cardiac surgery in New York State found that the relative contribution of cardiothoracic anesthesiologists to the clinical outcomes was proportionally one-fourth of that of cardiac surgeons and that the variation among the cardiothoracic anesthesiologists' metrics was minimal.[16] The study failed to identify high- or low-performing individuals, and the authors raised concerns regarding the feasibility of the pay-for-performance model. These findings do not rule out the possibility of performance variation among cardiothoracic anesthesiologists and the need for *individual scorecards*; however, the metrics must be meaningful for patients and must contain actionable feedback for providers.

2. **Clinical care standardization:** The pressures associated with value-based care payments based on clinical outcomes present a major challenge for high-volume academic centers that perform *high-risk, complex cardiac surgery*. This can be successfully managed by

TABLE 32.5 Summary of Work System Factors That Improve Patient Safety and Quality of Care in Cardiac Surgery Patients

Factor	Intervention
Physical environment	Standardized OR layout (fluid bags, IV tubing, airway equipment)
	Standardized medication stations (similar layout in all ORs, induction agents are placed together, as well as emergency vasoactive medications)
	Decrease OR clutter
	Minimize distractions and disruptions
	"Sterile cockpit" during critical portions of surgery
Teamwork and communication	Preoperative briefings and huddles
	Plan-of-care rounds
	Postoperative debriefings
	Closed-loop communication
	Standardized handoffs
Tasks and cognitive workload	Universal protocol and procedural checklists
	Incorporate breaks to reduce fatigue
	Incorporate technology to reduce errors—(bar code scanning of medications, blood product scanning for verification)
Organizational processes	"Just culture"
	Facilitate debriefings and multidisciplinary conferences
	Create safety events reporting systems

IV, intravenous; OR, operating room.

implementing standardized clinical care using protocols and pathways; multidisciplinary training that emphasizes teamwork, effective communication, and escalation; and the use of rigorous measures and data to analyze and act upon quality metrics and outcomes. This is an opportunity for the cardiothoracic anesthesiologist to provide leadership in organizing the elements of perioperative care and promote safety and efficiency in their high-performing teams.

3. **Safety event reporting:** Despite significantly improved clinical outcomes in patients undergoing cardiac surgery (current mortality rate 1%-3%), cardiothoracic surgical and anesthesia teams must continue to work on *eliminating preventable harm*. The key to minimizing patient safety events is to establish a rigorous, transparent, and nonpunitive safety event reporting system. Incorporating automated trigger tools such as *notification alerts* through the electronic anesthesia record (administration of naloxone or flumazenil, coding dose of epinephrine) will significantly improve the capture of intraoperative events.

4. **Culture of safety:** The key to success of patient safety programs is the leadership focus on the culture of safety to replace punitive actions. The organizations find a quick solution by analyzing the performer and recommend mitigating measures, such as additional training. Instead, the focus is on the efforts to *eliminate the latent errors* at an organizational level, which are incorporated in the system design and precede the human errors. Without eliminating latent errors, the system will continue to malfunction and will result in repeated incidents.

5. **High reliability:** Training *high-reliability teams* with a focus on communication, teamwork, effective leadership, and a culture of safety are the pillars of patient safety. Our medical community has recognized that humans will continue to make mistakes. Healthcare organizations should develop mechanisms through high team performance systems that will create an environment in which a potential trap is identified before it becomes a patient injury. Efforts should not be focused on *zero human error*, but rather on *zero patient harm*.

IV. **Ethical and Legal Issues**

A. **Introduction**

1. As cardiothoracic and vascular anesthesia evolves in the 21st century, developing an expertise in clinical ethics has emerged as a basic competency for anesthesiologists managing a myriad of ethical issues, while using effective communication skills and critical reflection. Ethical concerns range from evaluating patient capacity for informed consent, conveying the limitations of do-not-resuscitate (DNR) orders in the OR, and resolving intractable conflicts in end-of-life (EOL) care between patients, surrogates, and clinicians. A basic ethical analysis should consider at least four topics during the perioperative evaluation: the surgical or medical indications, quality of life before and after an intervention, specific patient preferences, and any contextual features affecting the intervention, such as financial, religious, or social matters.[17] This section briefly describes some common ethical and legal topics that anesthesiologists may encounter in the daily practice of cardiothoracic and vascular anesthesiology.

B. **Informed Consent**

1. **Moral obligation:** Obtaining *informed consent* is a moral obligation predicated on one of the dominant principles of Western medical ethics: respect for personal autonomy.[18] This fundamental ethical principle supports the privileged right of patients to decide what will and will not be done to their bodies.

2. **Ethical obligation:** Informed consent for anesthesia and surgery involves two distinct processes: (1) an ethical obligation to *disclose* the *relevant risks, benefits, and alternatives* associated with a cardiothoracic procedure to the patient and (2) a compliance requirement that satisfies the legal and administrative obligations of informed consent as documented in the (electronic) medical record. These processes necessitate an assessment of the patient's ability to comprehend the proposed intervention or the patient's medical capacity for decision-making. This ability to evaluate a patient's "decision-making capacity" is an essential element of the informed consent process and, in rare circumstances, may require psychiatric, ethical, and even legal consultations.[19]

3. **Informed consent:** Informed consent processes are specifically pertinent to cardiothoracic and vascular surgery since the procedures themselves often involve major risks for complications and morbidity. Legal challenges for informed consent usually focus on whether the clinician provided the necessary or material information needed for appropriate decision-making by a legally competent patient. In the past, courts have required any one of three standards for determining the type of information to disclose to patients for appropriate informed consent. However, the *reasonable patient standard* has been adopted by most courts in the country because it is based on what information a *reasonable patient* needs to know to make *reasonable decisions* about medical interventions.

4. **Exceptions:** Exceptions for informed consent include emergency procedures where delaying a surgical treatment for consent jeopardizes the patient's health. In this instance, consent is implied because a reasonable person would consent to such a surgical intervention in emergency circumstances.

5. **Surrogate decision-making:** Surrogate decision-making describes the process of physicians relying on family or proxies appointed by patients to make healthcare decisions on their behalf. The typical hierarchy of surrogates starts with court-appointed guardians, followed by surrogates selected by patients, most often family members or close friends. When patients lack medical capacity for decision-making, surrogates and clinicians typically rely on two standards for decision-making: substituted judgment and best interests.

6. **Substituted judgment:** Substituted judgment advises surrogates to construct decisions based on what the patient would make under the circumstances through a process of thoughtful consideration of that patient's specific healthcare values, goals, and preferences. Disagreements with the substituted judgment transpire when inconsistencies in the patient's expressed preferences and values are exposed, when there is a lack of knowledge of the patient's preferences, and in situations where substituted judgment seemingly conflicts with the patient's best interests.

7. **Best interests standard:** The best interests standard is typically used for legally incompetent patients who lack both decision-making capacity and advance directives, indicating that the specific values and preferences of the patient are unknown. This standard, predicated on the ethical principles of beneficence and nonmaleficence, obligates anesthesiologists and surgeons to weigh the benefits and burdens of surgical interventions viz-à-viz the patient's best interests at the time of consent. Limitations associated with the best interests standard include difficulties in making judgments about the presumed quality of life after a procedure as well as any inherent paternalistic bias. Paternalism arises when a physician overrides a patient's expressed wishes based on a clinical presumption that a physician feels is in the patient's best interests at a particular moment in time.

8. **Advance directives:** Traditionally, these standards are viewed as a hierarchy. For example, substituted judgment takes precedence over best interests when patients have made their preferences known in the recent past, even though they are now unable to provide consent or refusal. This is the rationale for patients completing advance directives: These are documents that empower competent patients to formally express their preferences regarding their goals of care in advance and, more significantly, allow patients to appoint surrogates with the requisite authority to make healthcare decisions should the patient lose medical capacity for decision-making. An advance directive process reaffirms personal autonomy and encourages patients to engage in a thoughtful and ongoing consideration of their values, goals, and preferences, specifically for EOL care. Advance directives also assume hierarchal precedence over the substituted judgments and best interests standards in most circumstances.

CLINICAL PEARL

Standards for decision-making when patients lack medical capacity or legal competence include advance directives, substituted judgments, and best interests of the patient with justifiable exceptions, such as unintended negative consequences.

C. **Confidentiality (Patient Privacy)**
   1. **Respecting confidentiality:** The duty to respect a patient's privacy and maintain confidentiality harkens back to the Hippocratic Oath. This ancient duty for the physician rested on loyalty and usefulness of confidential information for the therapeutic relationship. However, modern medical ethics predicates this duty on respect for patient autonomy and the recognition that every individual has a unique worth and dignity.[20]
   2. **Challenge of confidentiality:** Despite the tradition of the Hippocratic Oath, maintaining confidentiality is increasingly difficult with computerized access to medical records, which invites serious breaches of protected health information (PHI). Beginning in 1996, the federal government implemented a series of health privacy regulations known as the *Health Insurance Portability and Accountability Act* (HIPAA) that mandates physicians and healthcare institutions adopt procedures that safeguard PHI predicated on the principle that patients have the right to control their own health information. The risk of ignoring HIPAA, even for seemingly innocuous actions, can lead to dire personal and professional consequences.[21]
   3. **Duty of confidentiality:** Privacy and confidentiality are understood as prima facie duties, meaning clinicians are obligated to honor these principles unless a stronger moral duty takes precedence. Justifiable exceptions for privacy and confidentiality include the public reporting of infectious diseases, child abuse, elder abuse, and domestic violence to public health officials.

CLINICAL PEARL

The duty to protect patient confidentiality is grounded in the principle of respect for autonomy and further encoded in federal law by what is commonly referred to as HIPAA regulations.

6

D. Conflict of Interest

1. **Definition:** The term "conflict of interest" (COI) has been variously defined as conditions or considerations that direct professional judgment of clinicians away from their primary interest, which is care of the patient in the OR. These considerations are secondary to the welfare of the patient and range from personal financial interests to clinical affiliations with research or industry funding. Secondary interests can also be imposed by institutions, such as financial decisions meant to benefit the institution or leadership at the expense of professional ethics or the institutional mission.[22]

2. **Inclusions:** COIs can occur when physicians are consciously or unconsciously influenced by financial or academic links to industry that may not serve a patient's best interests. COIs also include personal or professional rewards in the form of paid speakerships, professional advancement, and prestige. Other COIs with patient care may include submitting to production pressure, concealing errors to protect professional reputations, or discouraging patient safety and quality initiatives because of their impact on efficiency and time management.

3. **Challenges:** Not every COI should be interpreted as unethical, illegal, or unprofessional, nor can every COI be avoided. The challenge is recognizing and resolving identified COIs, usually by acting in the best interest of the patient. In addition, hospitals and institutions must embrace responsibilities for implementing policies and procedures defining financial relationships for staff clinicians, publishing disclosures of COIs, promoting and modeling appropriate professional behavior, prohibiting specified actions and situations, and affirming the primacy of patient interests over clinician and institutional self-interests.[22]

E. End-of-Life Care and Ethical Conflicts

1. **End-of-life care:** EOL care is a frequent source of conflict among cardiothoracic and vascular surgery patients. Anesthesiologists and surgeons often receive requests to either withhold or withdraw life-sustaining therapy, such as mechanical ventilation or ventricular assist devices. Similarly, clinicians may receive demands from surrogates to escalate therapies in clinically dire circumstances, such as implementing mechanical circulatory support (MCS) when a patient is dying from multisystem organ failure. With advancements in cardiopulmonary life-sustaining therapies, particularly ECMO and MCS, it is essential for cardiac anesthesiologists and surgeons to be skilled in both the art of communication for EOL conversations and management of ethical conflicts between patients, surrogates, and even clinicians.

2. **Legal protection of rights:** Two seminal legal cases, Quinlan and Cruzan, affirmed the right of every patient with decision-making capacity to refuse as well as consent to life-sustaining treatment.[23] Because cardiopulmonary resuscitation (CPR) is traditionally initiated without a physician order, a DNR order is required in advance for withholding CPR. However, the use of the DNR order in the OR was perceived as conflicting with the safe practice of anesthesia care. Change came about in the early 1990s when the *ASA* and the *American College of Surgeons* recommended a mandatory reevaluation of preoperative DNR orders before proceeding with surgery. Through consideration and clarification of the goals for surgery and EOL care, a goal-directed perioperative DNR can preserve the goals of anesthetic and surgical care in the OR with agreed limitations to the DNR.[24] A *review and revise* process of a preexisting DNR integrates a process for assessing the patient's goals of care, reviewing any advance directives, and securing authorization to manage anesthetic or surgical events considered temporary and reversible by clinicians.

CLINICAL PEARL

Anesthesiologists evaluating a patient presenting for surgery with an intact DNR order should review the indications for the order and seek to either suspend, revise, or retain the order based on the patient's goals of care.

3. **Extracorporeal membrane oxygenation:** The use of ECMO for preoperative bridging, intraoperative cardiopulmonary support, and postoperative care has become a valuable tool in the care of patients with refractory cardiac and pulmonary failure. However, the rapid expansion of ECMO raises ethical questions about the use of this technology in patients, given its clinical uncertainty regarding long-term outcomes. Consequently, a lack of clarity in elucidating the goals of patient care as well as clinical ambiguity can lead to unique challenges involving conflict with the ethical principles of patient autonomy, beneficence, maleficence, and justice.[25] For example, does ECMO serve as a bridge to recovery, or is it a bridge to mechanical circulatory device and/or transplantation? Or, is ECMO a bridge to decision for EOL care and terminal discontinuation? The concept of "bridge to nowhere" defines a patient with minimal chance for recovery or transplantation and who would die almost immediately if ECMO was discontinued. This circumstance can lead to intractable disagreements among surrogates and clinicians about its ongoing use, especially when there is negligible hope for patient recovery.

4. **Other ethical dilemmas:** Other sources of ethical conflicts include patient selection, informed consent, patient or surrogate confusion about the goals of ECMO, emergency implementation of ECMO, limited quality of life data, and the quality and costs of ECMO programs. The Extracorporeal Life Support Organization offers certification of ECMO programs that emphasize the following: institutional multidisciplinary clinical training, formal guidelines and procedures for patient selection, allocation protocols when access to ECMO support is limited, a formal consent process, family engagement and education, continuing quality improvement assessments, use of time-limited trials for ECMO, and consultation with palliative care, hospice, and clinical ethics for institutional ECMO programs.[26]

5. **Mechanical circulatory support:** MCS is increasingly used in the management of end-stage heart failure. MCS includes left ventricular assist devices (LVADs), biventricular assist devices, and total artificial hearts. However, MCS complicates the dying process with its requirement for device deactivation. Ethical conflicts and disagreements between clinicians and surrogates occur because of low use of advance directives, high rates of surrogate decision-making in situations of patient incapacity, and increased incidence of complications and deaths in both the hospital and the ICU. Moreover, it is not rare for some clinicians to argue against deactivating an LVAD because they perceive equivalence to physician-assisted suicide or euthanasia. However, the principle of autonomy supports the right of competent patients to refuse unwanted medical treatment, including termination of MCS when used in the natural progression of end-stage heart failure. Other principles that support a patient's justification for deactivation of MCS include patient consent to LVAD deactivation and a detailed determination of the burdens outweighing the benefits of the device, especially with impending death.[27]

CLINICAL PEARL

Recent studies suggest a lack of insight among some clinicians who regard LVAD deactivation as equivalent to physician-assisted suicide and/or euthanasia despite the intention of deactivation being to avoid prolonged suffering and dying from the disease process.

6. **Best practices:** Best practice for EOL care of patients on MCS requires multidisciplinary consensus and collaboration on all these issues. Programmatic use of device-specific deactivation protocols, prior advance directives confirmed by multidisciplinary discussions with patient and family, and palliative care, hospice support, and clinical ethics services have the potential for minimizing ethical dilemmas in patients with MCS and improving EOL care.[27]

7. **Potentially inappropriate treatments:** Patients or surrogates sometimes insist on cardiothoracic surgical interventions that are either harmful or nonbeneficial for patients. The term *futility* is often loosely employed to describe a medical intervention offering little therapeutic value, negligible change in quality of life, or minimal impact on the goals of care for a patient. Use of this term increases the risk of intractable ethical dilemmas, given that clinician judgments regarding *futility* are often in error when employed to estimate prognosis and quality of life. Moreover, when clinicians unilaterally make decisions to withhold or withdraw treatment interventions based on their perception of futile care, they risk accusations of abusing their power by acting unilaterally and further alienating patients and surrogates. In a stricter sense, the concept of *futility* is said to describe an intervention that has no pathophysiologic rationale. Given the controversy over the meaning of *futility*, a recent consensus statement recommends using the term "potentially inappropriate treatments" to describe medical or surgical interventions with marginal benefit for patient care while competing ethical considerations argue against these interventions.[28] The same consensus statement further recommends hospitals and healthcare institutions establish guidelines and processes for adjudicating intractable ethical conflicts caused by futile care or potentially inappropriate treatments that include fair processes of conflict resolution, intensive communication, negotiation, and procedural oversight by ethics consultants or legal counsel.[28]

F. **Transplant Ethics**

1. **Fundamental bioethical principles:** Patients with end-stage heart and lung disease who receive heart and lung transplantation have an opportunity to improve both length and quality of life. However, heart and lung transplantation raises difficult questions of informed consent, acceptable risk in donation, fair and just allocation of organs, and the hastening of donor death. For these reasons, the procedure relies on the four foundational principles of bioethics to support the medical and surgical enterprises involved in transplantation. Given that the number of patients needing heart and lung transplantations far exceeds the supply of donated organs, ethical principles are necessary to maintain the public trust and ensure a fair and just allocation of donated organs. Hence, the transplant process must be transparent, legally regulated, and open to both national and international scrutiny.[29]

7

CLINICAL PEARL

Adherence to the four foundational bioethics for both organ donation and transplant recipient selection is essential for the preservation of transparency, accountability, and trust in the heart and lung transplantation process.

2. **Autonomy:** The principle of autonomy applies to the organ donor by considering the interventions needed before organ procurement to secure the best graft condition for recipient survival. This means that organ donation becomes an important part of EOL care. Informed consent for organ donation must be free of coercion for both living donors and families of deceased donors. The principle of beneficence supports allocating scarce organs to those patients who will receive the greatest medical benefit as measured by survival and quality of life. The principle of justice not only guides the fair and equitable distribution of donated organs but also considers waiting list times, medical needs, geographic locale, and anticipated benefits of the transplantation.

3. **Transplant tourism:** Transplant tourism is defined as the movement of organs, donors, and recipients across borders, contradicting the ethical principles of transplant medicine as defined by the *International Society for Heart and Lung Transplantation.*[30] The sale of organs from both live and deceased donors violates the *Universal Declaration of Human Rights.* Harvesting organs for transplantation from the bodies of executed prisoners also breaches the principle of voluntary donation as does the selling of organs for transplantation. Many families struggle to comprehend the definition of death, especially brain criteria for death, leading to lower permission rates for organ donation. The practice of donation after circulatory death, known as DCD, has several ethical concerns, such as ambiguity related to the precise amount of time required before establishing a diagnosis of death and whether the process of harvesting organs contributes to the death of the donor.[31] One proposal to increase the donations of cadaveric organs is to presume consent for organ donation on the part of the patient or family unless they object otherwise.

G. **Professionalism**
   1. **Patients first:** To state that the primary concern of an anesthesiologist is the patient's best interests, not their personal convenience or well-being seems cliché. Nevertheless, respecting the physician-patient relationship takes on greater significance for the anesthesiologist working with surgeons in the cardiothoracic and vascular ORs and the postoperative ICUs. In these settings, patients are at their most vulnerable and solely dependent on the care team day and night for extended periods of time. This intensity of experience and unique patient vulnerability distinguishes the duty of professionalism in cardiothoracic anesthesiology and surgery.[32]
   2. **Ethical principles:** The ethical principles supporting professionalism in anesthesiology are based on the same ethical and moral framework in much of this discussion: respect for patient autonomy, acting in the patient's best interests, weighing the surgical intervention for a balance between benefit and harm, and an equitable distribution of resources and benefits. In addition, there are other rules that apply to the professional-patient relationship: privacy, confidentiality, as well as veracity and fidelity.[20]
   3. **Commitment to excellence:** These moral rules extend the anesthesiologist's fiduciary duty to include commitment to excellence in patient care. This commitment obligates a maintenance of competency in the practice of CTA and continuing certification, development of effective communications skills for patient advocacy and conflict resolution, and a disciplined work ethic. One eminent cardiac anesthesiologist challenged the profession at the end of the 20th century by famously stating that an anesthesiologist "who ignores patient values and ethical issues is not a complete physician and does not live up to the profession of an oath to put the welfare of patients above self-interests."[33] The reality is that the culture of both cardiothoracic and vascular anesthesia and surgery observe an uncompromising "moral imperative to do the right thing," meaning that its practitioners must be able to ignore their personal commitments, extreme stress, and profound fatigue while working together to provide the best outcome for their patient.[34]

V. **Summary**
Practicing excellence in cardiothoracic and vascular anesthesia requires that anesthesiologists maintain fluency in the ethical issues associated with their specialty. This includes not only the customary issues of informed consent, decisional capacity, surrogate decision-making, confidentiality, and EOL care; it also embraces the ethical concerns associated with transplantation, ECMO, MCS, research design, recognition of COIs related to business and organizational demands, as well as professional advocacy for greater access to healthcare.[19] The practice of cardiothoracic and vascular anesthesiology calls for constant mindfulness of the ethical obligations embedded in every clinical encounter between patient and anesthesiologist in the 21st century.

REFERENCES

1. Gawande A, Thomas E, Zinner M, Brennan T. The incidence and nature of surgical adverse events in Colorado and Utah in 1992. *Surgery*. 1999;126:66-75.
2. Kohn LT, Corrigan J, Donaldson MS. *To Err Is Human: Building a Safer Health System*. National Academy Press; 2000.
3. American Society of Anesthesiologists. Relative value guide* 2022 book. https://www.asahq.org/shop-asa/mk2022rvg
4. American Society of Anesthesiologists. Statement on transesophageal echocardiography. Accessed January 20, 2024. https://www.asahq.org/standards-and-practice-parameters/statement-on-transesophageal-echocardiography
5. Fleisher L. Quality anesthesia. Medicine measures, patients decide. *Anesthesiology*. 2018;129:1063-1069.
6. Del Rio M, Abernathy J, Taylor M, et al. The adult cardiac anesthesiology section of STS adult cardiac surgery database: 2020 update on quality and outcomes. *J Cardiothorac Vascul Anesth*. 2021;35:22-34.
7. Ryan A. Will value-based purchasing increase disparities in health care? *N Engl J Med*. 2013;369:2472-2474.
8. Mahajan A, Esper S, Cole D, et al. Anesthesiologists's role in value-based perioperative care and healthcare transformation. *Anesthesiology*. 2021;134:526-540.
9. Lawal A, Rotter T, Kinsman L, Sari N, Harrison L, Jeffery C, Kutz M, Khan M, Flynn R. Lean Management in healthcare: definition, concepts, methodology and effects reported (systematic review protocol). *Systematic Reviews*. 2014;3:103.
10. Ibrhim M, Szeto W, Gutsche J, et al. Transparency, public reporting and a culture of change to quality and safety in cardiac surgery. *Ann Thorac Surg*. 2022;114:626-635.
11. Merry A, Weller J, Mitchell S. Improving the quality and safety of patient care in cardiac anesthesia. *J Cardiothorac Vascul Anesth*. 2014;28(5):1341-1351.
12. 2022 Joint Commission. Sentinel event data summary. Accessed January 20, 2024. https://www.jointcommission.org/resources/sentinel-event/sentinel-event-data-summary/
13. Wahr J, Abernathy J. Improving patient safety in the cardiac operating room: doing the right thing the right way, every time. *Curr Anesthesiol Rep*. 2014;4:113-123.
14. Sun L, Jones P, Wijeysundera D, et al. Association between handover of anesthesiology care and 1-year mortality among adults undergoing cardiac surgery. *JAMA Netw Open*. 2022;5(2):e2148161.
15. Gleicher Y, Mosko J, McGhee I. Improving cardiac operating room to intensive care unit handover using a standardized handover process. *BMJ Open Qual*. 2017;6:e000076.
16. Glance L, Hannan E, Fleisher L, et al. Feasibility of report cards for measuring anesthesiologist quality for cardiac Surgery. *Anesth Analg*. 2016;122:1603-1613.
17. Jonsen AR, Siegler M, Winslade WJ. *Clinical Ethics: A Practical Approach to Ethical Decisions in Clinical Medicine*. 8th ed. McGraw-Hill Education; 2015.
18. Berg JW, Lidz CW, Appelbaum PS. *Informed Consent: Legal Theory and Clinical Practice*. 2nd ed. Oxford University Press; 2001.
19. Appelbaum PS. Assessment of patients' competence to consent to treatment. *N Engl J Med*. 2007;357:1834-1840.
20. Beauchamp T, Childress J. *Principles of Biomedical Ethics*. 7th ed. Oxford University Press; 2013:302-349.
21. Lo B, Dornbrand L, Dubler NN. HIPAA and patient care: the role of professional judgment. *JAMA*. 2005;293(14):1766-1771.
22. Lo B, Field MJ, eds. *Conflict of Interests in Medical Research, Education, and Practice*. Institute of Medicine of the National Academies; 2009:45-87.
23. Waisel DB, Truog RD. The end-of-life sequence. *Anesthesiology*. 1997;87:676-686.
24. Truog RD, Waisel DB, Burns JP. DNR in the OR: a goal-directed approach. *Anesthesiology*. 1999;90:289-295.
25. Enumah ZO, Carrese J, Choi CW. The ethics of extracorporeal membrane oxygenation: revisiting the principles of clinical bioethics. *Ann Thorac Surg*. 2021;112:e61-e67.
26. Wirpsa MJ, Carabini LM, Neely KJ, et al. Mitigating ethical conflict and moral distress in the care of patients on ECMO: impact of an automatic ethics consultation protocol. *J Med Ethics*. 2021;47:e63.
27. Pak ES, Jones CA, Mather PJ. Ethical challenges in care of patients on mechanical circulatory support at end-of-life. *Curr Heart Fail Rep*. 2020;17:153-160.
28. Bernat JL. Medical futility: definition, determination, and disputes in critical care. *Neurocrit Care*. 2005;2:198-205.
29. DeVita MA, Caplan AL. Caring for organs or for patients? Ethical concerns about the Uniform Anatomical Give Act. *Ann Intern Med*. 2007;147:876-879.
30. Holm AM, Fedson S, Courtwright A, et al. International society for heart and lung transplantation statement on transplant ethics. *J Heart Lung Transplant*. 2022;41(10):1307-1308.
31. Jericho BG. Organ donation after circulatory death: ethical issues and international practices. *Anesth Analg*. 2019;128:280-285.
32. Lowenstein E. Cardiac anesthesiology, professionalism and ethics: a microcosm of anesthesiology and medicine. *Anesth Analg*. 2004;98:927-934.
33. Hug CC. Rovenstine lecture: patient values, hippocrates, science, and technology: what we (physicians) can do versus what we should do for the patient. *Anesthesiology*. 2000;93(2):557.
34. Berian JR, Ko CY, Angelos P. Surgical professionalism: the inspiring surgeon of the modern era. *Ann Surg*. 2016;263(3):428-429.

Index

Note: Page number followed by *f* and *t* indicates figure and table only.